SIXTH EDITION

BROWSE'S INTRODUCTION TO THE SYMPTOMS & SIGNS OF SURGICAL DISEASE

SIXTH EDITION

BROWSE'S INTRODUCTION TO THE SYMPTOMS & SIGNS OF SURGICAL DISEASE

Edited by

James A. Gossage BSc MS FRCS
Consultant General Upper GI Surgeon
Guy's and St Thomas' NHS Foundation Trust, London, UK

Matthew F. Bultitude MBBS MRCS MSc FRCS(Urol)
Consultant Urological Surgeon and Clinical Director for Transplant, Renal and Urology,
Guy's and St Thomas' NHS Foundation Trust, London, UK

Steven A. Corbett BSc PhD FRCS FRCS(Tr&Orth)
Consultant Orthopaedic Surgeon
Guy's and St Thomas' NHS Foundation Trust, London, UK
Fortius Clinic, London, UK

Associate Editors

Katherine M. Burnand FRCS(Paed Surg)
Consultant Paediatric Surgeon, St George's Hospital, London, UK

Rajiv Lahiri BSc MD(res) FRCS
Senior Fellow in HPB Surgery, Royal Surrey County Hospital, Guildford, UK

Emeritus Editor

Kevin Burnand MBBS FRCS MS
Emeritus Professor of Surgery, Kings College, London, UK

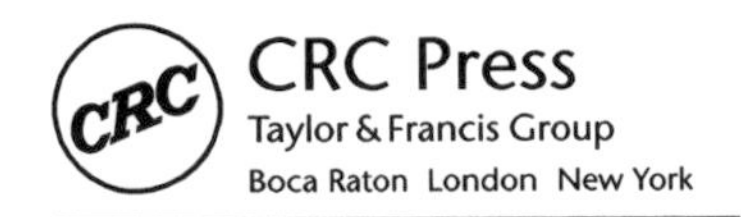

CRC Press is an imprint of the
Taylor & Francis Group, an **informa** business

CRC Press
Taylor & Francis Group
6000 Broken Sound Parkway NW, Suite 300
Boca Raton, FL 33487-2742

Printed on acid-free paper

International Standard Book Number-13: 978-1-138-33040-5 (Hardback)
978-1-138-33008-5 (Paperback)

Visit the Taylor & Francis Web site
at http://www.taylorandfrancis.com

and the CRC Press Web site
at http://www.crcpress.com

Contents

Companion website – visit www.routledge.com/cw/gossage for digital resources to supplement this textbook including self-assessment material, video animations and an image library.

Professor Sir Norman Browse

Norman was born in 1931 within the sound of "Bow Bells" which he said entitled him to be called a "Cockney"! He was educated in East London and won a scholarship to East Ham Grammar School.

From here, he was accepted for medical training at St Bartholomew's Hospital Medical School in the city of London. He did his national service in the RAMC on Cyprus after qualification before he began his surgical training with Professor Robert Milnes-Walker in Bristol.

He then went to the USA as a Harkness fellow at the Mayo clinic where he was supervised by John Sheppard. He wrote his thesis and a book on "the Physiology and Pathology of bed rest" based on his research carried out at the Mayo.

He returned to the post of lecturer at the academic department of surgery at the Westminster Hospital under the chairmanship of Professor Harold Ellis (where Sir Roy Calne was the senior lecturer and Sir Barry Jackson was the SHO!)

He was appointed to the senior lectureship in the academic department of surgery at St Thomas' Hospital in 1966 under the chairmanship of Professor John Kinmonth while still in his early 30's. Over the next 30 years, he developed his skills in vascular surgery, research and teaching. He was promoted reader and then given a personal chair in vascular surgery before taking over the chairmanship of the academic department of surgery at St Thomas' when Professor Kinmonth retired in 1981.

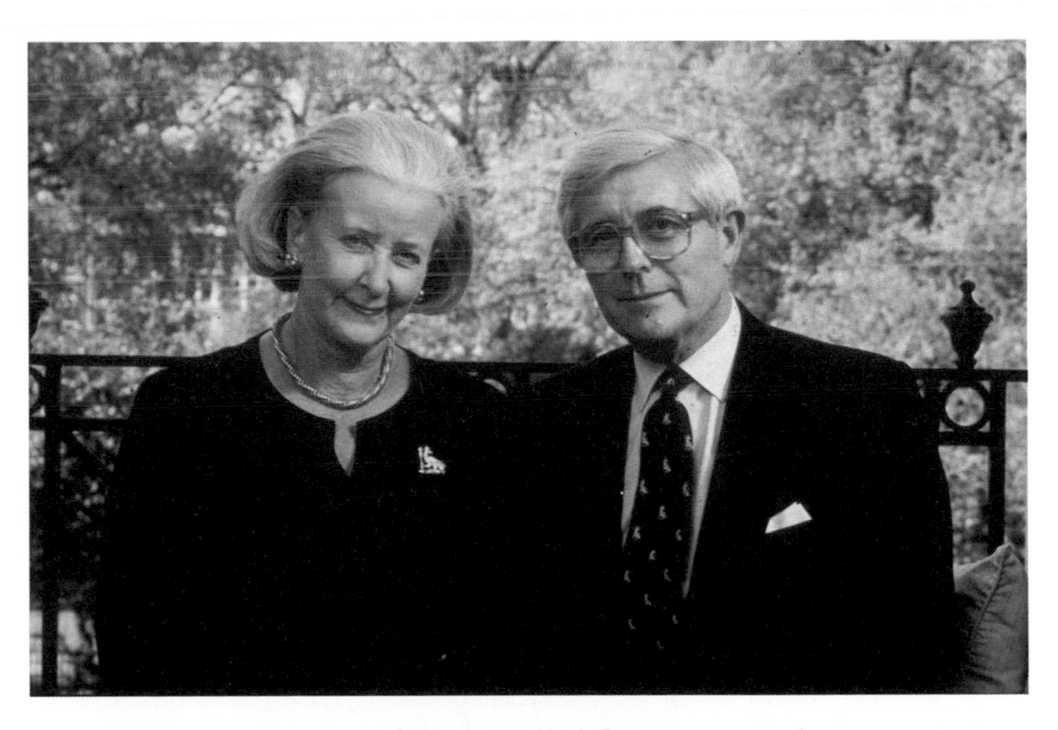

Sir Norman and Lady Browse

During this time, he wrote many seminal papers on venous thrombosis, venous ulceration, atheroma and aneurysm formation, congenital vascular malformations and lymphoedema. He also wrote books on venous and lymphatic disease and contributed chapters to many other surgical books. He gave many prestigious lectures and was a visiting professor at famous universities all over the world.

He was on the court of examiners of the Royal College of Surgeons of England, the Specialist Advisory Committee in Surgery and was then elected to the council of the RCS England before becoming its President in 1992. During his time in office, he made many far reaching changes including the development of the "Exit Examination" and the Research Fellowship scheme which has provided £40 million pounds to date for young surgeons to carry out a period of research in their training.

He wrote the first edition of this book in 1978 and it became an immediate best seller because of its clear and well-structured approach, combined with excellent illustrations and clinical pictures. The first edition was dedicated to his wife Jeanne who he met at medical school who was from the island of Alderney. The Browses retired to this island and Norman was elected as its President for nine years.

Jeanne died just over a year before Norman who died on September 12th, 2019 at the age of 87.

Foreword

Since the last edition of this book, both Sir Norman and Lady Browse have died on their beloved Island of Alderney. Norman was my boss, my mentor and then my colleague and friend. I was honoured when he asked me to help him with the preparation of the fourth edition and I suggested that we ask my friends John Black and Bill Thomas to join us in bringing the book up to date. Norman and the three of us had an interest in all the sub- specialities that make up "general surgery" and we were all recognised as enthusiastic undergraduate and post- graduate teachers.

Norman had an agile and organised mind, and he recognised the importance of a clear structure and the use of repetition in teaching trainees of all levels about conditions requiring surgical treatment. He was always professional and courteous to the patients in his care and meticulous in his questioning and clinical examination. His clinical notes were legible, accurate and comprehensive. He was recognised throughout the United Kingdom as an excellent 'second opinion' for patients with complex problems and was referred patients from all over the world with specialist vascular disorders for assessment and treatment where possible. He was a neat and precise surgeon who achieved and published excellent results in challenging operations.

His practice was based on an accurate clinical diagnosis and he always championed the importance of a careful history and a meticulous clinical examination before any special investigations were ordered or obtained. Not for him, the blanket diagnostic test of a 'CT or ultrasound scan' of the abdomen in a patient presenting with abdominal pain before a differential diagnosis had been developed!

He strongly disapproved of 'surgical pathways' and 'clinical protocols' which he felt removed the need for brain usage and encouraged a false sense of security. He disliked the widespread use of protocols which he thought risked missing aberrant and rare conditions in patients who fell outside the norm and he felt could be extremely dangerous if rigidly applied.

He believed in constructing a differential diagnosis that could be whittled down until the correct diagnosis became apparent, rather than a problem-orientated approach or the development of a working diagnosis which, he also held, reduced the need for lateral thought.

It is ironic that when he himself developed marked dyspnoea on Alderney several years before his death he was referred to specialist cardiac services on the 'mainland' where he underwent two unnecessary coronary interventions without improvement before the correct diagnosis of 'pulmonary fibrosis' was eventually reached! So much for modern clinical acumen!

This book has stood the test of time because it has been written in straightforward English, clearly structured and filled with excellent clinical pictures and diagrams. This ethos has been maintained. It is more comprehensive than the first edition with some of the more idiosyncratic and rare conditions having been downsized or removed. The fifth edition was longer (which Norman did not like), as a consequence of the more comprehensive coverage of the sub-specialities, but this edition has been rigorously pruned and unhelpful illustrations removed.

All the present editors and subeditors are well known to me and were selected because they have excellent track records in teaching and writing about surgery. As a consequence, the book retains its close association with Guy's and St Thomas' hospitals although many of the chapters have been revised by clinicians from other institutions.

Most of the original 'Browse Book' remains as new surgical diseases are rare, but fresh eyes and minds have ensured that outdated material has been removed and unhelpful illustrations culled. Self-assessment feedback has been added and hopefully future editions will make use of more multimedia platforms.

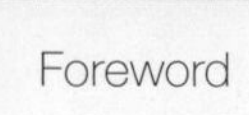

I like to think that Norman would be pleased with the new 6th edition and I would like to thank all the editors and contributors for all their hard work in producing such a tangible memorial to an outstanding surgical clinician.

Kevin Burnand

Contributors

Adil Ajuied BSc(Hons) MSc FRCS(Tr&Orth)
Consultant Orthopaedic Surgeon
Guy's and St Thomas' NHS Foundation Trust
Honorary Senior Clinical Lecturer
King's College London
London, UK

Peter Bullock FRCS MRCP
Consultant Neurosurgeon
King's College Hospital
Honorary Neurosurgeon
Guy's and St Thomas' NHS Foundation Trust and The Maudsley Hospital
London, UK

Matthew F Bultitude MBBS MRCS MSc FRCS(Urol)
Consultant Urological Surgeon and Clinical Director for Transplant, Renal and Urology
Guy's and St Thomas' NHS Foundation Trust
London, UK

Katherine M Burnand FRCS(Paed Surg)
Consultant Paediatric Surgeon
St George's Hospital
London, UK

Ben Challacombe MS FRCS (Urol)
Consultant Urological Surgeon and Honorary Senior Lecturer
Guy's and St Thomas' NHS Foundation Trust and King's College
London, UK

Steven A Corbett BSc PhD FRCS FRCS(Tr&Orth)
Consultant Orthopaedic Surgeon
Guy's and St Thomas' NHS Foundation Trust and Fortius Clinic
London, UK

Mark George BSc MS FRCS
Consultant Colorectal Surgeon
Guy's and St Thomas' NHS Foundation Trust
London, UK

James A Gossage BSc MS FRCS
Consultant General Upper GI Surgeon
Guy's and St Thomas' NHS Foundation Trust
Honorary Senior Lecturer
King's College
London, UK
Honorary Senior Lecturer
Karolinska Institute
Sweden

Jason R Harvey MBBS FRCSEd FRCS(Tr&Orth)
Consultant Spinal Surgeon
Wessex Spinal Unit
Southampton University Hospital
Southampton, UK
Fortius Clinic
London, UK

Ian P Holloway MBBS FRCS(Tr&Orth)
Consultant Orthopaedic Surgeon and Clinical Director for Orthopaedics
London North West University Healthcare NHS Trust
London, UK

David Houlihan-Burne MBBS(Hons) BSc(Hons) MRCS FRCS(Tr&Orth)
Consultant Knee Surgeon
Fortius Clinic
London, UK
Three Rivers Knee & Sports Injury Clinic
Middlesex, UK

Johnathan G Hubbard MD FRCS(Gen) FEBS(Endocrine)
Consultant Endocrine Surgeon
Guy's and St Thomas' NHS Foundation Trust
Kings College Hospital
London, UK

Kavan S Johal BMedSci(Hons) BMBS(Hons) MPhil FRCS(Plast)
Specialist Registrar in Plastic Surgery
Guy's and St Thomas' NHS Foundation Trust
London, UK

Richard Keen BSc PhD FRCP
Consultant in Metabolic Bone Disease
Royal National Orthopaedic Hospital
Stanmore, UK

Rajiv Lahiri BSc MD(res) FRCS
Senior Fellow in HPB Surgery
Royal Surrey County Hospital
Guildford, UK

Richard Leach MD FRCP
Consultant Physician and Honorary Reader in Medicine
Clinical Director Pulmonary and Critical Care Medicine
Guy's and St Thomas' NHS Foundation Trust
London, UK

Mark McGurk MD FRCS DLO FDSRCS
Professor of Oral & Maxillofacial Surgery
Director of Head & Neck Centre
UCL Division of Surgical Interventional Sciences
King Edward VII's Hospital
London Bridge Hospital
UCL Hospital
London, UK

Bijan Modarai FRCS
Professor and King's Chair
Vascular and Endovascular Surgery
Guy's and St Thomas' NHS Foundation Trust
London, UK

Pari-Naz Mohanna MBBS BSc MD FRCS(Plast)
Consultant Plastic and Reconstructive Surgeon
Guy's and St Thomas' NHS Foundation Trust
London, UK

Jenna Morgan MBChB MRCS(Ed) DipMedEd PhD
NIHR Clinical Lecturer in Surgery
Department of Oncology and Metabolism
University of Sheffield
Sheffield, UK
Higher Surgical Trainee
Doncaster and Bassetlaw Teaching Hospitals NHS Foundation Trust
Doncaster, UK

Ashish Patel FRCS
Clinical Senior Lecturer
Vascular Surgery
King's College Hospital
Guy's and St Thomas' NHS Foundation Trust
London, UK

Jonathan Rees FRCP FFSEM MD
Consultant Rheumatologist and Sports Physician
Fortius Clinic
Honorary Senior Lecturer
Queen Mary College
London, UK

Andrew Roche MBChB MSc FRCS(Tr&Orth)
Consultant Foot and Ankle Surgeon
Chelsea & Westminster Hospital
Fortius Clinic
London, UK

Arun Sahai PhD FRCS(Urol)
Consultant Urologist and Honorary Senior Lecturer
Department of Urology
Guy's and St Thomas' NHS Foundation Trust
London, UK

Donald Sammut FRCS FRCS(Plast)
Consultant Hand Surgeon
OneWelbeck Clinic
Marylebone, London
Circle Bath Hospital
Bath, UK

Samer Saour MB BCH BAO MSc FRCS(Plast)
Consultant Plastic Surgeon
St George's Hospital
London, UK

Glyn Towlerton MBBS(Hons) BSc MRCP FRCA FFPMRCA FIPP
Consultant in Pain Medicine
Chelsea & Westminster Hospital NHS Foundation Trust
London, UK

Navin Vig MBBS BDS FRCS(OMFS) PhD
Specialty Registrar, Oral & Maxillofacial Surgery and Clinical Research Fellow
UCL Hospital
London, UK

W James White MBBS BSc(Hons) FRCS(Tr&Orth)
Consultant Trauma and Orthopaedic Surgeon
Guy's and St Thomas' NHS Foundation Trust
London, UK

Lynda Wyld BMedSci MBChB(Hons) PhD FRCS(GenSurg) FEBS
Professor of Surgical Oncology
Department of Oncology and Metabolism
University of Sheffield
Sheffield, UK
Honorary Consultant Oncoplastic Breast Surgeon
Doncaster and Bassetlaw Teaching Hospitals NHS Foundation Trust
Doncaster, UK

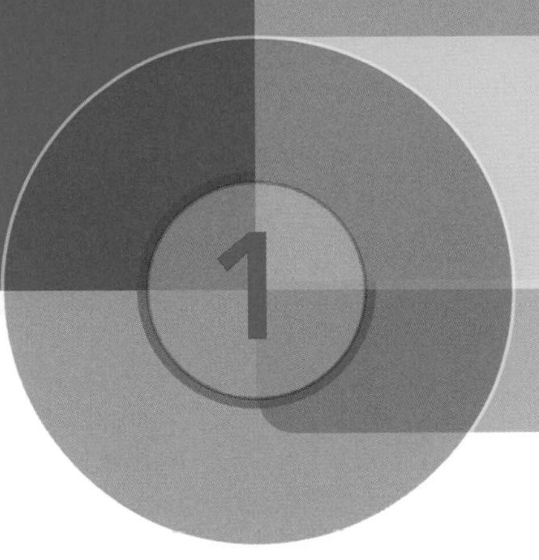

History-taking and clinical examination

JAMES A GOSSAGE AND RAJIV LAHIRI

You must be alert from the moment you first see the patient. Use your eyes, ears, nose and hands in a systematic fashion to collect information from which you can deduce the diagnosis. The ability to appreciate an unusual comment or minor abnormality can lead you to the correct diagnosis. This skill only develops from the diligent and frequent practice of the routines outlined in this chapter. *Always give the patient your whole attention and never take short cuts.*

In the outpatient clinic, have patients walk into the consulting room to meet you, rather than finding them lying undressed on a couch in a cubicle. General malaise and debility, breathlessness, cyanosis and difficulty with particular movements or an abnormal gait are much more obvious during exercise. Patients like to know to whom they are talking. They are probably expecting to see a specific doctor. *You should tell patients your name, and explain why you are seeing them.*

A parent, spouse or friend who is accompanying the patient can often provide valuable information about changes in health and behaviour not noticed by the patient. Remember, that many patients are inhibited from discussing their problems in front of a third person. It can also be difficult if the relative or friend, with the best of intentions, constantly replies on behalf of the patient. When the time comes for the examination, the friend or relative can be asked to leave and further questions can then be asked in private. It is also often helpful if a chaperone is present.

Talk with patients or, better still, let them talk to you. At first, guide the conversation, but do not dictate it. Treat patients as rational, intelligent human beings. They know what worries them better than you do, but they are visiting a doctor to obtain a diagnosis and if necessary receive treatment. *At all stages, explain what you are doing, and why you are doing it.*

All questions should be put in simple plain language, *avoiding medical terms and jargon*, and using lay expressions as much as possible. When a patient is not fluent in English, an interpreter is required. When conducting an interview through an interpreter, keep your questions short and simple, and have them translated and answered one at a time.

You should not use leading questions. Allow patients to choose their own answers. Do not say, 'Did the pain move to the right-hand side?' This is a leading question because it implies that it should have moved in that direction, and an obliging patient will sometimes answer yes just to please you. The patient should be asked whether the pain ever moves. When the answer is yes, the supplementary question is 'Where does it go to?' If, however, patients fail to understand the question, a number of possible answers may have to be proposed, which can then be confirmed or rejected.

Remember that a question that you do not think is leading the patient may be interpreted incorrectly if they do not realize that there is more than one answer. For example, 'Has the pain changed?' can be a bad question, as there are a variety of ways in which the pain can change. It can alter in severity, nature, site, etc., but the patient may be so disturbed by the intensity of the pain that they think only of its severity and forget the other features that have altered. In such situations, it often helps to include possible answers to the question, for example, 'Has the pain moved to the top, bottom, or side of your abdomen or anywhere else?', 'Has the pain got worse, better or stayed the same?' or 'Can you walk as far, less far or the same distance that you could a year ago?'

The patient should provide the correct answer providing you ask the question correctly. Do not be overconcerned about the questions – worry about the answers, and accept that it will sometimes take a long time and a great deal of patience and perseverance to get a good history.

At some stage, you will read the referral letter, which may suggest a diagnosis. It is often better to read this after you have taken your own history as it can bias your independent opinion.

How to take the history

The history should be taken in the order described below and in Revision panel 1.1. *Try not to write and talk to the patient at the same time.* It is, however, important to document dates and times and drug history and dosage accurately, which you may not recall after you have finished the examination and left the room. Brief notes as you talk to the patient are therefore essential.

Always make sure you know, and record, the patient's name, age, sex and occupation. Whenever you write a note about a patient, whether it is a short progress report or a full history, make sure that you write down the date and time that the patient was seen.

THE PRESENT COMPLAINT/ PROBLEM

Start by asking the patient what is their main complaint and record the answer. Ask the patient to use their own words to describe exactly what it is that they have found to be wrong with themselves, and not what they have been told is wrong, perhaps by another doctor. It is also worth asking 'What is the problem that you want me (e.g. the surgeon) to sort out?' If you ask 'What is the matter?', the patient will often tell you what they think is their diagnosis, or what they have been told by others. *It is better not to know what the patient thinks is the diagnosis, or the diagnoses given by other doctors* (see the point about referral letters above), because neither may be correct. Try to tease out the patient's complaints and problems and come to your own conclusions!

Complaints should be listed in order of severity, with a record of precisely when and how they started. Whenever possible, it should be noted why the patient is more concerned with one complaint than another.

HISTORY OF THE PRESENT COMPLAINT

The full history of the main complaint or complaints must be recorded in detail, with precise dates. It is important to get right back to the beginning of the problem. For example, a patient may complain of a recent sudden attack of indigestion. When further questioning reveals that similar symptoms occurred some years previously, their description should be included in this section.

REMAINING QUESTIONS ABOUT THE AFFECTED SYSTEM

When a patient complains of indigestion, for example, it is sensible, after recording the history of the indigestion, to move on at this point to other questions about the alimentary system.

SYSTEMATIC DIRECT QUESTIONS

These are direct questions that every patient should be asked, because the answers may amplify your knowledge about the main complaint and will often reveal the presence of other disorders of which the patient was unaware, or thought irrelevant. An absence of associated symptoms is often just as important as positive answers. The standard set of direct and important supplementary questions is described in detail below because they are so important. *It is essential to know them by heart because it is very easy to forget to ask some of them.*

Revision panel 1.1

SYNOPSIS OF A HISTORY

Names. Age and date of birth. Sex.

Marital status. Occupation. Ethnic group.

Hospital or practice record number

Present complaints or problems

Preferably in the patient's own words

History of the present complaint

Include the answers to the direct questions concerning the system of the presenting complaint

Systematic direct questions

a. ***Alimentary system and abdomen***

Appetite. Diet. Weight. Nausea. Dysphagia. Regurgitation. Flatulence. Heartburn. Vomiting. Haematemesis. Indigestion pain. Abdominal pain. Jaundice. Abdominal distension. Bowel habit. Nature of stool. Rectal bleeding. Mucus. Slime. Prolapse. Incontinence. Tenesmus

b. ***Respiratory system***

Cough. Sputum. Haemoptysis. Dyspnoea. Hoarseness. Wheezing. Chest pain. Exercise tolerance

c. ***Cardiovascular system***

Dyspnoea. Paroxysmal nocturnal dyspnoea. Orthopnoea. Chest pain. Palpitations. Ankle swelling. Dizziness. Limb pain. Walking distance. Colour changes in hands and feet

d. ***Urogenital system***

Loin pain. Frequency of micturition including nocturnal frequency. Poor stream. Dribbling. Hesitancy. Dysuria. Urgency. Precipitancy. Painful micturition. Polyuria. Thirst. Haematuria. Incontinence

In males: Problems with sexual intercourse and impotence

In females: Date of menarche or menopause. Frequency. Quantity and duration of menstruation. Vaginal discharge. Dysmenorrhoea. Dyspareunia. Previous pregnancies and their complications. Prolapse. Urinary incontinence. Breast pain. Nipple discharge. Lumps. Skin changes

e. ***Nervous system***

Changes of behaviour or psyche. Depression. Memory loss. Delusions. Anxiety. Tremor. Syncopal attacks. Loss of consciousness. Fits. Muscle weakness. Paralysis. Sensory disturbances. Paraesthesias. Dizziness. Changes of smell, vision or hearing. Tinnitus. Headaches

f. ***Musculoskeletal system***

Aches or pains in muscles, bones or joints. Swelling joints. Limitation of joint movements. Locking. Weakness. Disturbances of gait

Past medical history

Previous illnesses. Operations or accidents. Diabetes. Rheumatic fever. Diphtheria. Bleeding tendencies. Asthma. Hay fever. Allergies. Tuberculosis. Sexually transmitted diseases. Tropical diseases

Drug history

Include all prescription and over the counter medications. Always check for allergies

Immunizations

BCG. Diphtheria. Tetanus. Typhoid. Whooping cough. Measles

Family history

Causes of death of close relatives. Familial illnesses in siblings and offspring

Social history

Marital status. Sexual habits. Living accommodation. Occupation. Exposure to industrial hazards. Travel abroad. Leisure activities. Smoking. Number of cigarettes smoked per day. Drinking. Units of alcohol drunk per week

The only way to memorize this list is by practice, which means taking as many histories as possible and writing them out in full. The answers to every question must be recorded.

Revision panel 1.2

CLASSIFICATION OF THE AETIOLOGY OF DISEASE

Congenital

- Genetic
- Sporadic

Acquired

- Traumatic
- Inflammatory:
  - Physical
  - Chemical
- Infection:
  - Viral
  - Bacterial
  - Rickettsial
  - Spirochaetal
  - Protozoal
  - Fungal
  - Helminthic
  - Mycoplasm
  - Prions
- Neoplastic:
  - Benign
  - Malignant
  - Primary:
    - Carcinoma
    - Sarcoma
    - Others
- Secondary
- Degenerative
- Autoimmune
- Proliferative
- Metabolic
- Hormonal
- Mechanical
- Vascular
- Self-induced
- Psychosomatic
- Iatrogenic

The alimentary system (see Chapters 15 and 16)

Appetite Has the appetite increased, decreased or remained the same? If it has decreased, is this caused by a loss of appetite, or is it because of apprehension as eating always causes pain?

Diet What type of food and when does the patient eat? Are they vegetarian, or do they avoid any particular foods?

Weight Has the patient's weight changed, and if so, by how much and over how long a time? Many patients never weigh themselves, but they usually notice if their clothes have got tighter or looser, and friends may have told them of a change in physical appearance.

Teeth and taste Can they chew their food? Do they have their own teeth? Do they get odd tastes and sensations in their mouth? Are there any symptoms of water brash or acid brash? (This is the sudden filling of the mouth with watery or acid-tasting fluid – saliva and gastric acid, respectively.)

Swallowing Do they have any difficulty (dysphagia) or pain (odynophagia) in swallowing? If so, ask about the type of food that causes difficulty, for example solids, liquids or both, and the level at which they feel the food sticking. Also ask about the duration and progression of these symptoms, and whether swallowing is painful.

Regurgitation Do they regurgitate? This means the effortless return of food into the mouth. It is different from vomiting, which is associated with a powerful involuntary contraction of the abdominal wall. If they do regurgitate, what comes up? Is it fluid or solid? Regurgitated food is either digested, or recognizable and undigested? How often does regurgitation occur and does anything, such as bending over, stooping or straining, precipitate it?

Flatulence Does the patient belch frequently? Does this relate to any other symptoms?

Heartburn This is a burning sensation experienced behind the sternum, caused by the reflux of acid into the oesophagus. Patients may not realize that this symptom comes from the alimentary tract, which is why it must be specifically asked about. If patients do experience heartburn, how often does it happen and does anything precipitate it, such as lying flat or bending over?

Vomiting This is the forcible ejection of gastric or intestinal contents through the mouth as the result of involuntary spasms of the oesophagus, stomach and abdominal wall. If patients do vomit, how often do they do so? Is the vomiting preceded by nausea? What is the nature, colour and volume of the vomit? Is it recognizable food from previous meals, digested food, clear acidic (burning) fluid or bile-stained fluid (bitter-tasting)?

Is the vomiting preceded by another symptom such as indigestion pain, headache or giddiness? Does it follow eating, and what is its relationship to food? Is it effortless?

Haematemesis This is defined as the vomiting of blood. Always ask if patients have ever vomited blood because it is such an important symptom. Old, altered blood looks like coffee grounds.

Some patients have difficulty in differentiating between vomited or regurgitated blood and coughed-up blood – *haemoptysis* (see Chapter 2). Haemoptysis is usually pale pink and frothy.

When patients have had a haematemesis, always ask whether they have had a recent nose bleed. They may be vomiting swallowed blood.

Patients are rarely able to make useful guesses at the amount of blood vomited up, and the addition of gastric juice makes questions on the volume of blood vomited of little value. Associated collapse and/or faintness suggests major blood loss has occurred.

Indigestion or abdominal pain (dyspepsia) This is correctly defined as difficulty in digesting food and is usually accompanied by discomfort or abdominal pain and often by heartburn and belching (see above). Some patients call all abdominal pains indigestion; the difference between a discomfort after eating and a pain after eating may be very small.

It is therefore better to concentrate on elucidating the important features of the pain or discomfort, its site, time of onset, severity, nature, progression, duration, radiation, course and precipitating, exacerbating and relieving factors.

Jaundice This is a yellow colouration of the tissues as a consequence of excessive quantities of bile pigments accumulating in the blood (see Chapter 15).

Have the patient's skin or eyes ever turned yellow? When did this happen, and how long did it last? Were there any accompanying symptoms such as fever, abdominal pain, loss of appetite or weight loss? Did the skin itch?

Did the faeces or urine change colour?

Have they had any recent injections, drugs or blood transfusions?

Have they been abroad, and what immunizations have they had?

Abdominal distension Have they noticed that their abdomen has become swollen (distended)? What brought this to their attention? When did it begin, and how has it progressed? Is it constant or variable?

What factors are associated with the distension?

Is it painful? Does it affect their breathing?

Is it relieved by belching, vomiting, passing flatus or defaecation?

Have they lost weight or had any urinary problems?

If female, could they be pregnant, and when was their last period?

Defaecation This is the act of discharging bowel contents though the anus (see Chapter 16). How often does the patient defaecate per day? Are the actions regular or irregular?

What are the physical characteristics of the stool?:

- *Colour:* Brown, black, pale yellow, white, silver, bloody?
- *Consistency:* Hard, soft, frothy or watery?
- *Size:* Bulky, pellets, string- or tape-like?
- *Specific gravity:* Does it float or sink?
- *Smell:* Is it particularly foul?

Beware of the terms 'diarrhoea' (a frequent and copious discharge of liquid faeces) and 'constipation' (an infrequent or difficult bowel evacuation of hard faeces). These terms are often misinterpreted by the patient, and should not be written in the notes without also recording the frequency of bowel action and the consistency of the faeces (see Chapter 16).

Rectal bleeding Has the patient ever passed any blood in the stool?

Was it bright or dark? Were the amounts large or small, and on how many occasions did it occur?

Was it mixed in with or on the surface of the stool, or did it appear only after the stool had been passed? Was the blood only present on the toilet paper?

Flatus or mucus passage per rectum Is the patient passing more gas (flatus) than usual, or has it

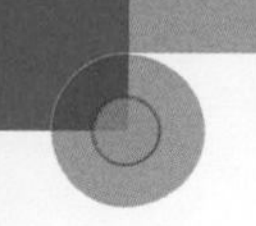

ceased? Has the patient ever passed mucus (slime) or pus (yellow/green opaque liquid)?

Pain on defaecation Does this occur? If so, when does the pain begin – before, during, after or at times unrelated to defecation? Are there any other aggravating or relieving factors?

Prolapse and incontinence Does anything come out of the anus on straining? Does it return spontaneously or have to be pushed back?

Is the patient continent of faeces and flatus? If not, does anything cause incontinence, such as standing or coughing? Are they aware that they are being incontinent, and is it associated with a severe urge to pass stool?

Have they had any injuries or anal operations in the past?

If they are female, what is their obstetric history?

Tenesmus Do they experience a constant and urgent desire to pass stool (see Chapter 16)?

The respiratory system (see Chapter 2)

Cough This is the abrupt/explosive expulsion of air from the lungs through partially closed vocal cords, causing a characteristic noise and often producing mucus (sputum).

How long have they had a cough, and how often do they cough? Does the coughing come in bouts?

Does anything, such as a change of posture, precipitate or relieve the coughing?

Is it a dry or a productive cough (with sputum)?

Sputum This is the mucus/pus that is coughed up. What is the quantity (teaspoon, dessertspoon, etc.) and the colour (white, clear or yellow) of the sputum?

Some patients only produce sputum in the morning or when they are in a particular position.

Haemoptysis This is coughed-up blood (see Chapter 2).

Has the patient noticed it? Was it frothy and pink, which is suggestive of heart failure? Were there red streaks in the mucus, or clots of blood?

What quantity was produced? How often does the haemoptysis occur?

Shortness of breath/dyspnoea (see Chapter 2) Do they become breathless? Is dyspnoea present at rest? Do they wheeze (make a rasping or whistling sound, which suggests asthma)?

How many stairs can they climb? How far can they walk on a level surface before the dyspnoea interferes with this or stops them? Can they walk and talk at the same time?

Is it present when sitting, or made worse by lying down? Dyspnoea on lying flat is called *orthopnoea*. How many pillows do they need at night?

Does the breathlessness wake them up at night – this is called *paroxysmal nocturnal dyspnoea* – or get worse if they slip off their pillows?

The severity of the dyspnoea can be graded numerically (see Chapter 2).

Is the dyspnoea induced or exacerbated by external factors such as allergy to animals, pollen or dust? Does the difficulty with breathing occur on breathing out or in?

Pain in the chest (see Chapter 2) Ascertain the site, severity and nature of the pain. Chest pains can be continuous, pleuritic (made worse by inspiration), constricting (see below) or stabbing.

The cardiovascular system (see Chapter 2)

Cardiac symptoms

Breathlessness/dyspnoea These are defined by the same questions as those described above.

Orthopnoea and paroxysmal nocturnal dyspnoea These symptoms are particularly associated with heart failure (see Chapter 2).

Pain Cardiac pain typically begins in the midline behind the sternum (retrosternal), but may occasionally be experienced in the epigastrium. It is often described as constricting or band-like. The patient should be asked if the pain radiates to the neck or to the left arm, and whether it is exacerbated by exercise or excitement and relieved by rest (all suggestive of cardiac pain).

Palpitations These are episodes when the patient becomes aware of a sudden fluttering or thumping of the heart in the chest. These symptoms are indicative of an arrhythmia but can be caused by extrasystoles.

Ankle swelling/oedema Do either the ankles or legs swell? When do they swell? What is the effect on the swelling of bed rest and/or elevation of the leg?

It is important to consider cardiac failure in patients with ankle oedema, although there are a number of other causes of ankle swelling (see Chapters 2 and 10).

Dizziness, headache and blurred vision These are some of the symptoms associated with hypertension and postural hypotension. They can also be caused by neurological, vestibular or ocular disorders (see Chapter 3).

Peripheral vascular symptoms (see Chapter 10)

Does the patient get pain in the leg muscles on exercise, which interferes with walking (*intermittent claudication*)? Does it occur in the thigh, buttocks, calf or foot? How far can the patient walk before the pain begins? Is the pain so bad that they have to stop walking? How long does the pain take to wear off? Can the same distance be walked again?

In a man, a recent loss of penile erections in association with buttock claudication suggests occlusion of the abdominal aorta or internal iliac artery (*Leriche's syndrome*).

Is there any pain in the limb at rest? Which part of the limb is painful (typically the foot)? Does the pain interfere with sleep? What positions relieve the pain (typically, hanging the foot over the side of the bed or getting up and walking around). Do analgesic drugs provide any relief?

Are the extremities of the limbs cold? Are there colour changes in the hands, particularly in response to cold, classically from white, to blue, before turning red? Raynaud's phenomenon (see Chapter 10) is rarely associated with all the typical changes in colour.

Does the patient experience any paraesthesias in the limb (tingling or numbness), which indicates critical ischaemia and a limb at risk?

Has the patient experienced any transient weakness of the limbs (transient *ischaemic attack*), loss of vision (*amaurosis fugax*, or fleeting blindness) or difficulty with speech? These symptoms may presage a full-blown stroke (see Chapter 10).

The urogenital system (see Chapters 17 and 18)

Urinary tract symptoms

Pain Has there been any pain in the loin (kidney), groin (ureter) or suprapubic region (bladder)? What is its nature and severity? Does it radiate to the groin or scrotum, suggesting a ureteric calculus?

Micturition How frequently does the patient pass urine, and how many times by day and by night?

Is the volume and frequency excessive (*polyuria*)? Is the patient thirsty? Do they drink excessive volumes of water, suggesting diabetes?

Is micturition painful (*dysuria*)? What is the nature and site of the pain?

Is there any difficulty with micturition, such as a need to strain or to wait to get started? How is the stream? Can it be stopped at will? Is there any dribbling at the end of micturition? These symptoms suggest prostatic pathology.

Does the bladder feel empty at the end of micturition, or do they have to pass urine a second time (*double micturition*; see Chapter 17)?

Haematuria (blood in the urine) Has the patient ever experienced this? Where in the stream and how often did it occur? Was there any associated pain?

Pneumaturia The patient may notice bubbles in the urine, suggesting a fistula between bladder and bowel.

Incontinence of urine Does this occur with urgency or on coughing and straining (*stress incontinence*)? Does it occur continuously without awareness (true), or is it associated with discomfort and a full bladder (overflow)? In females, is there any history of prolapse with stress incontinence? It is also important to take a complete obstetric history.

Genital tract symptoms – male

Scrotum, penis and urethra Has the patient any pain in the penis or urethra during micturition or on intercourse? Is there any difficulty with retraction of the foreskin, or has there been any purulent urethral discharge now or in the past (sexually transmitted infections)?

Has the patient noticed any pain or swelling of the scrotum, and can he achieve an erection and satisfactory ejaculation? Is the patient fertile?

Genital tract symptoms – female

Menstruation When did menstruation begin (the *menarche*)? When did it end (the *menopause*)? What is the duration and quantity of the menses? Is

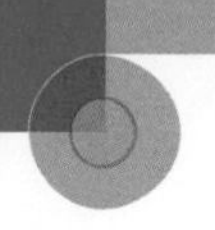

menstruation associated with pain (*dysmenorrhoea*)? What is the nature and severity of the pain? Is there any abdominal pain midway between the periods (mittelschmerz)? Has the patient noticed any pain on intercourse (*dyspareunia*)?

Has the patient had any *vaginal discharge*? What is its character and amount?

Has she noticed any *prolapse of the vaginal wall* or cervix or any *urinary incontinence*, especially when straining or coughing (stress incontinence)?

Pregnancies Record details of the patient's pregnancies – number, dates and complications.

Breasts (see Chapter 13) Do the breasts change during the menstrual cycle? Are they ever painful or tender, and does this occur premenstrually (cyclical breast pain)?

Has the patient noticed any swellings or lumps in the breasts? Did she breast-feed her children? Has there been any nipple discharge or bleeding? Has she noticed any skin changes over the breasts, or any change in contour?

The nervous system (see Chapter 3)

Mental state Is the patient placid or nervous? Has the patient noticed any changes in their behaviour or reactions to others? Patients will often not appreciate such changes themselves, and these questions may have to be asked of close relatives.

Does the patient get depressed and withdrawn, or are they excitable and extroverted?

Brain and cranial nerves Does the patient ever have seizures (epilepsy)? What happens during a seizure? It is often necessary to ask a relative or a bystander to describe the seizure. Did the patient lie still or jerk about, bite their tongue or pass urine? Was the patient sleepy after the seizure? Was there any sense (an *aura*) that the seizure was about to develop? Has there been any subsequent change in the senses of smell, vision and hearing?

Is there a history of *headache*? Where is it experienced? How long has it been occurring, and when does it occur? Are the headaches associated with any visual symptoms (migraine, hypertension, tension and raised intracranial pressure)?

Has the face ever become weak or paralysed? Have any of the limbs been paralysed (strokes or demyelinating disease), or has the patient ever experienced pins and needles in a limb (paraesthesias)?

Has there ever been any buzzing in the ears (tinnitus), or *dizziness* (vestibular symptoms)?

Has there ever been any loss of speech (*aphasia*)? Can the patient speak clearly and use words properly? Do they know what they want to say but cannot express it (*expressive dysphasia*)?

Peripheral nerves Are any limbs or part of a limb weak or paralysed? Is there ever any loss of skin sensation? Does the patient experience any tingling or pins and needles in the limbs (paraesthesias), suggestive of peripheral neuropathy or nerve compression?

The musculoskeletal system

Ask if the patient suffers from pain, swelling or limitation of the movement of any joint. What precipitates or relieves these symptoms? What time of day does this occur? Are any limbs or groups of muscles weak or painful?

Can the patient walk normally?

Are there any known congenital musculoskeletal deformities?

PREVIOUS HISTORY OF OTHER ILLNESSES, ACCIDENTS OR OPERATIONS

Record, with dates, the history of any conditions that are not directly related to the present complaint.

Ask specifically about a previous diagnosis of ischaemic heart disease, asthma, hypertension, diabetes, rheumatic fever, tropical diseases and bleeding tendencies. The likelihood of intimate contact with carriers of the human immunodeficiency virus (HIV) and of other sexually transmitted infections should be explored, especially if the patient's lifestyle is considered to be high risk.

DRUG HISTORY

Ask whether the patient is taking any drugs. Specifically, enquire about insulin, steroids, antidepressants, diuretics, antihypertensives, hormone replacement therapy and the contraceptive pill.

Patients usually remember about drugs they are taking that have been prescribed by a doctor, but often forget about self-prescribed drugs.

HISTORY OF ALLERGIES

Patients should be specifically questioned on their known allergies to drugs, especially penicillin and other antibiotics, and also to adhesive plaster. A history of hay fever, asthma and eczema is worth noting as is any previous episodes of anaphylaxis.

Write all the patient's known allergies in large letters on the front of their notes.

IMMUNIZATIONS

Check the vaccination history in accordance with the UK childhood schedule. Check for any reactions. Many individuals, especially medical staff, will also have been immunized against viral hepatitis, and this is worth recording.

FAMILY HISTORY

Enquire about the health and age, or cause of death, of the patient's first-degree relatives who have died or have familial diseases.

Also ask about any children who may have died or developed specific diseases. Draw a family tree if there is an obvious familial disorder (e.g. neurofibromatosis).

You will need information about the mother's pregnancy if the patient is a child. Did she take any drugs during pregnancy? What was the birth weight? Were there any difficulties during delivery? Was the physical and mental development normal in early life?

SOCIAL HISTORY

Record the patient's marital status, and the type and place of their dwelling (e.g. lives in a hostel or of no fixed abode).

Ask about the patient's sexual orientation and their occupation, with special regard to contact with hazards such as dust, asbestos and chemicals.

What are the patient's leisure activities?

Has the patient travelled extensively or lived abroad? List the countries and the dates if these appear to be relevant. Does the patient smoke? If so, what do they smoke? Record the frequency, quantity and duration of their smoking habit.

Does the patient drink alcohol? Record the type and quantity consumed (in units/week) and the duration of the habit. 1 unit = a very small glass of whisky, half a small glass of wine or a half/third of a pint of beer.

A detailed history of pain

Pain is an unpleasant sensation of varying intensity. We have all experienced pain. It can come from any of the body's systems, but there are certain features common to all pains that should always be recorded.

Tenderness is pain induced by a stimulus, such as pressure from the doctor's hand, or forced movement. Remember that *the patient feels pain – the doctor elicits tenderness*. It is possible for a patient to be lying still without pain and yet have an area of tenderness. Patients may complain of tenderness if they happen to have pressed their fingers on a painful area or have discovered a tender spot by accident. Thus, tenderness can be both a symptom and a physical sign.

A careful history of 'a pain' frequently provides the diagnosis, so you must question the patient closely about each of the following features (Revision panel 1.3).

SITE

Many factors may indicate the source of the pain, but the most valuable indicator is its site.

It is of little value to describe a pain as 'abdominal pain'; you must try to be more specific. Although patients do not describe the site of their pain in anatomical terms, they can normally point to the site of maximum intensity, which you should convert into an exact anatomical description.

When the pain is indistinct in nature and spreads diffusely over a large area, you must illustrate the area in which the pain is felt and the point (as indicated by the patient) of maximum discomfort.

It is also worthwhile asking about the depth of the pain. Patients can often tell you whether the pain is near to the skin or deep inside. *Splanchnic pain* from an organ, which is experienced through the autonomic system, is poorly localized to the midline, while *somatic pain* from the body's surface layers is well localized.

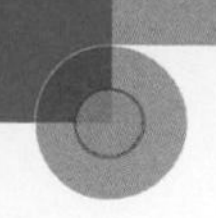

Revision panel 1.3

FEATURES OF A PAIN THAT MUST BE ELICITED AND RECORDED

Site

Time and mode of onset

Record the time and date of onset, and the way the pain began – suddenly or gradually

Severity

Assess the severity of the pain by its effect on the patient

Nature/character

Aching, burning, stabbing, constricting, throbbing, distending, colicky

Progression

Describe the progression of the pain. Did it change or alter?

The end of the pain

Describe how the pain ended. Was the end spontaneous, or brought about by some action by the patient or doctor?

Duration

Record the duration of the pain

Relieving and exacerbating factors

Radiation

Record the time and direction of any radiation of the pain; remember to ask if the nature of the pain changed at the time it moved

Referral

Was the pain experienced anywhere else?

Cause

Note the patient's opinion of the cause of the pain

TIME AND MODE OF ONSET

It may be possible to pinpoint the onset of the pain very precisely, but if this cannot be done, the part of the day or night when the pain began should be recorded. Ask if the pain began gradually or suddenly.

When pain has a truly acute/sudden onset, patients often remember the time precisely, or exactly what they were doing at the time. This occurs when a viscus perforates or a blood vessel splits (dissects) or ruptures.

Inflammation, infarction or obstruction of a hollow viscus all produce a pain of more insidious onset.

You should record the calendar dates on which the pain occurred, but it is also very useful to add in brackets the time interval between each episode and the current examination, because it is these intervals, rather than the actual dates, that are more relevant to the problems of diagnosis.

For example, write, 'Sudden onset of severe epigastric pain on 16th September, 2013, at 11.00 a.m. (3 days ago)'; remember that such comments are useless if you forget to record the date and time of the examination.

SEVERITY

Individuals react differently to pain. What is a 'severe pain' to one person might be described as a 'dull ache' by another. Avoid adjectives used by a patient to describe the severity of their pain. A far better indication of severity is the effect of the pain on the patient's life:

- Did it stop the patient going to work?
- Did it make the patient go to bed?
- Did they use any analgesia?
- Did they have to call their doctor?
- Did it wake the patient up at night, or stop them going to sleep?
- Was the pain better lying still, or did it make them roll around?

The answers to these questions provide a better indication of the severity of a pain than words such as mild, severe, agonizing or terrible. Your assessment of the way the patient responds to their pain, formed while you are taking the history, may influence your diagnosis.

NATURE OR CHARACTER OF THE PAIN

Patients often find it difficult to describe the nature of their pain, but some of the adjectives that are commonly used, such as aching, stabbing, burning, throbbing, constricting, distending, gripping or colicky, are clearly recognized by most people.

'Burning and throbbing' sensations are within everyone's experience. Almost everyone has experienced a burning sensation in the skin, so when a patient spontaneously states that their pain is 'burning' in nature, it is likely to be so. Most have experienced a throbbing sensation at some time in their life from an inflammatory process such as toothache, so this description is also usually accurate.

A 'stabbing pain' is sudden, severe, sharp and short-lived.

The adjective 'constricting' suggests a pain that encircles the relevant part (chest, abdomen, head or limb) and compresses it from all directions. A pain that feels like an iron band tightening around the chest is typical of angina pectoris, and is almost diagnostic of this.

When patients speak of 'tightness' in their chest or limb, do not immediately assume that they have a constricting pain. They may be describing a tightness caused by distension, which may occur in any structure that has an encircling and restricting wall, such as the bowel, bladder, an encapsulated tumour or a fascial compartment. Tension in the containing wall may cause a pain that the patient may describe as 'distension', 'tightness' or a 'bursting feeling'.

A 'colicky pain' comes and goes like a sine wave. It feels like a migrating constriction in the wall of a hollow tube that is attempting to force the contents of the tube forwards. It is not a word that many patients use, and it is dangerous to ask them if their pain is 'colicky' without giving an example such as intestinal colic during an episode of diarrhoea, and many females have suffered colicky pains with their periods or in labour. Remember that not all recurring, intermittent pain is necessarily colic; it should also have a gripping nature.

'Just a pain, doctor.' Many pains have none of the features mentioned above and defy description! They may vary in severity from a mild discomfort or ache, to an agonizing pain that makes the patient think they are about to die. When a patient cannot describe the nature of their pain, do not press the point. You will only make them try to fit their description to your suggestions, which may be misleading.

PROGRESSION OF THE PAIN

Once it has started, a pain may progress in a variety of ways:

- It may begin at its maximum intensity and remain at this level until it disappears.
- It may increase steadily until it reaches a peak or a plateau, or conversely it may begin at its peak and decline slowly.
- The severity may fluctuate. The intensity of the pain at the peaks and troughs of the fluctuations, and the rate of development and regression of each peak, may vary.
- The pain may disappear completely between each exacerbation.
- The time between the peaks of an abdominal colic indicates the likely site of a bowel obstruction. In upper small bowel obstruction, the frequency of the colic is approximately every 1–2 minutes, whereas in the ileum it is every 20 minutes, and in the large bowel every 30–60 minutes.
- It is essential to find out how the pain has progressed and ascertain the timing of any fluctuations before its nature can be determined.

END OF THE PAIN

A pain may end spontaneously, or as a result of some action taken by the patient or doctor. The end of a pain is either sudden or gradual. The way in which a pain ends may give a clue to the diagnosis, or indicate the development of a new problem.

Patients always think that an improvement in their pain means that they are getting better. They are usually right, but sometimes their condition may have become worse, for example, an intestinal perforation relieving the colic but causing peritonitis and septicaemia.

DURATION OF THE PAIN

The duration of a pain will be apparent from the time of its onset and end, but it is nevertheless worthwhile stating the duration of the pain in your notes. The length of any periods of exacerbation or remission should also be recorded.

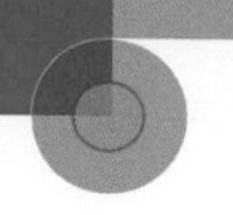

FACTORS THAT RELIEVE THE PAIN

Position, movement, a hot-water bottle, aspirins and other analgesics, food or antacids may all relieve the pain. The natural response to a pain is to search for relief. Sometimes patients try the most bizarre remedies, and many convince themselves that these help, so accept some of their replies to this question with caution.

FACTORS THAT EXACERBATE THE PAIN

Anything that makes the pain worse, such as movement, eating or opening the bowels, should be recorded.

The type of stimulus that exacerbates a pain will depend on the organ from which it emanates and on its cause. For example, intestinal pains may be made worse by eating particular types of food, while musculoskeletal pains are affected by joint movements, muscle exercise and posture. If the initial description has indicated the source of the pain, you can ask direct questions about these potential triggers.

RADIATION AND REFERRAL

You should always ask if the pain is experienced anywhere else or has moved from its initial site.

Radiation This is the extension of the pain to another site while the initial pain persists. For example, patients with a posterior penetrating duodenal ulcer usually have a persistent pain in the epigastrium, but the pain may also radiate to the back. The extended pain usually has the same character as the initial pain.

A pain that occurs in one site and then disappears before reappearing in another site is not radiation: it is a new pain in another place.

Referred pain This is pain that is felt at a distance from its source. For example, inflammation of the diaphragm causes a pain experienced only at the tip of the shoulder (Figure 1.1). Referred pain is caused by the inability of the central nervous system to distinguish between visceral and somatic sensory impulses.

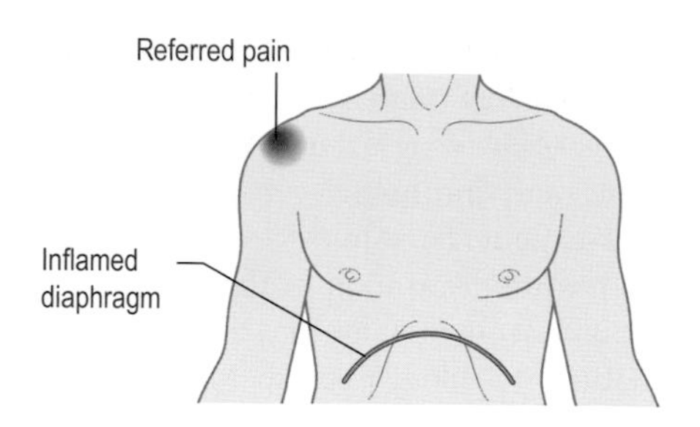

Figure 1.1 Pain referral.

CAUSE

It is important to ask patients what they think is the cause of their pain. Even if they are hopelessly wrong, you may get some important insight into their worries.

PSYCHOGENIC CAUSE

A patient's pain may appear disproportionate or exaggerated. The patient whose symptoms do not fit any known pattern, or who, while complaining of severe pain, appears quite unconcerned ('la belle indifference') may well be neurotic, hysterical or fabricating their symptoms and even physical signs.

A diagnosis of Munchausen's syndrome (see Chapter 15) or psychogenic cause should only be made when all possible organic causes for the patient's symptoms have been excluded. In this situation, your clinical experience is your greatest help.

Clinical examination

The following chapters of this book each deal with a specific region of the body and its surgical diseases. The methods of examination peculiar to each region are described in detail in the relevant chapter.

The emphasis to date in this introductory chapter has been on the importance of taking a precise and full history, but it now moves on to a description of the basic plan of a physical examination.

Your ability to perform a thorough clinical examination can only be improved by frequent bedside practice. Examine as many patients as you can, as this experience increases fluency. Repetition is the secret of learning. This axiom applies as much to the doctor as it does to the sportsman or the concert pianist. Your visual, tactile and aural appreciation of the patient's physical signs will improve by repeatedly exercising these senses.

Experienced clinicians usually begin the routine physical examination with a *provisional or differential diagnosis* in mind that has been gleaned from the history. The full impartial systematized examination is then often modified to look for specific signs that confirm or refute the working diagnosis. When, however, a sign is elicited that refutes this, the astute clinician returns to the textbook routine.

Students and trainees must not follow this method. Although it is understandable and practical when used by an experienced consultant surgeon in a busy clinic, it is inherently dangerous! Students must discipline themselves to use the standard textbook routine for every physical examination if mistakes are to be avoided. When this is abandoned, some parts of the examination will be omitted, which can have serious consequences.

The easiest way to ensure that your examination is complete is to learn the routine by heart and repeat it to yourself during the examination. While looking at a lump, say to yourself 'site, size, shape, ...'. If you do not do this, you will find, when you come to present the case or write the notes, that you have forgotten to elicit some of the lump's physical features, necessitating a re-examination of the patient.

Always maintain the basic pattern of looking, feeling, tapping and listening:

- Inspection.
- Palpation.
- Percussion.
- Auscultation.

In the musculoskeletal system, percussion and auscultation are replaced by moving the joint (look, feel, move).

NOTE: It is often best to examine initially the part of body that is the source of the patient's complaint, before completing the full examination of all other systems.

GENERAL ASSESSMENT/ APPEARANCE

The first part of the physical examination is performed when taking the history. While you are talking to the patient, you can observe the patient's general demeanor and their attitudes to their disease. These observations will inevitably affect the manner in which you conduct the examination. Your instructions will need to be extremely simple if the patient appears slow, or coaxing and gentle if the patient is shy or embarrassed.

The patient's general mental state, their memory and their use of words should be noted. A number of terms are used to describe various speech and communication disorders (see Chapter 3). When a patient has been admitted as an emergency, especially if they have been injured, it is important to record their level of consciousness using the Glasgow Coma Scale (see Chapters 3 and 5).

You can also observe a number of physical characteristics when taking the history, such as posture, mobility, weight, colour of the skin, facial appearance and general body build. These should be looked at in detail and recorded at the start of the examination.

Colour

One of the first things to observe is the colour of the patient's skin. Although minor colour variations are easier to appreciate in fair-skinned people, they are also visible on careful inspection in dark-skinned people.

Pallor/anaemia

Normal skin colour varies depending upon the thickness of the skin, the state of the skin circulation and the degree and type of pigmentation. Pallor of the skin usually indicates anaemia providing the skin thickness and circulation appear to be normal (Figure 1.2a, b).

Anaemia is best detected by looking at the colour of the mucous membranes:

- Look at the colour of the conjunctiva on the inner side of the lower eyelid.
- Look at the colour of the buccal mucous membrane.

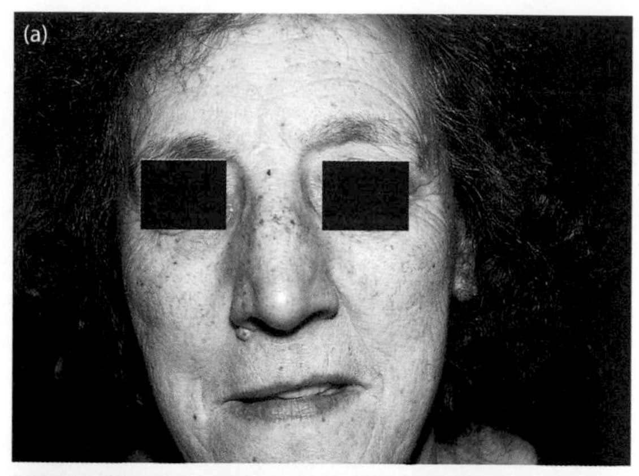

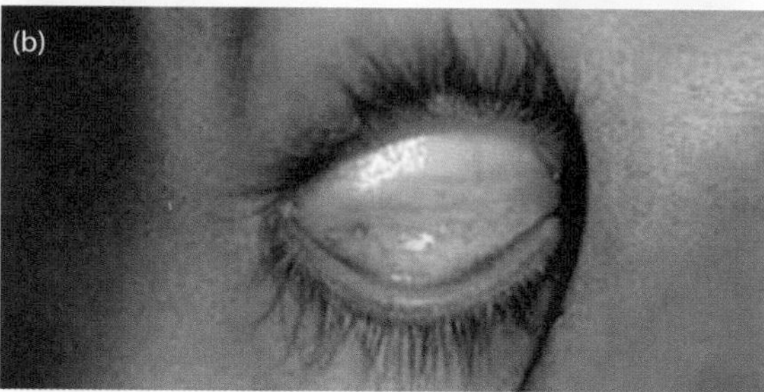

Figure 1.2 ANAEMIA. (a) The patient is very pale. (b) Pale conjunctiva.

- Stretch the skin of the palm and look at the colour of the palmar creases; then compare the colour of the patient's palm against your own palm.

Cyanosis

Cyanosis is the purple–blue colour imparted to the skin and mucus membranes by deoxygenated blood within them. It is most apparent in areas with thin skin and a rich blood supply, such as the lips, tongue, fingernails and ear lobes. Cyanosis is difficult to see in black skin and also hard to detect when the patient is anaemic.

There are two categories of cyanosis:

- *Central cyanosis*, when the defect lies in the cardiopulmonary circulation (Figure 1.3) (see Chapter 2).
- *Peripheral cyanosis*, when poor tissue perfusion causes excessive deoxygenation in the peripheral tissues (see Chapter 10).

The cyanosis is central if it is caused by cardiopulmonary disease, and the patient's extremities

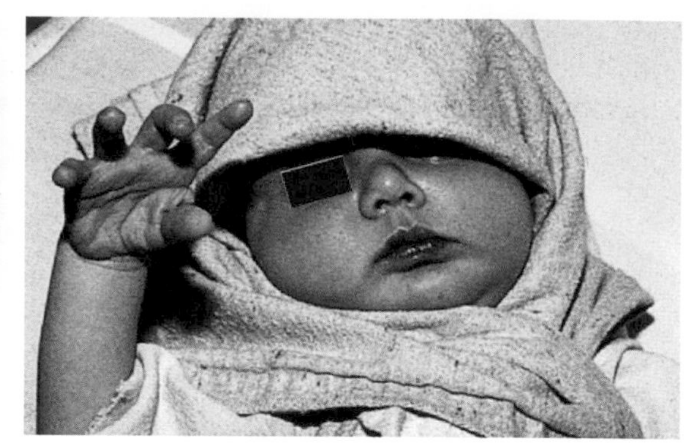

Figure 1.3 A child with central cyanosis and blue lips.

are usually warm. It is best appreciated by inspecting the inner aspect of the lips (Figure 1.3). When the cyanosis is caused by a peripheral abnormality, the extremities such as the fingers, toes and nose are blue and cold, but the central organs such as the lips and tongue remain pink.

Polycythaemia

An excess of circulating red blood cells gives the patient a purple–red, florid appearance (Figure 1.4).

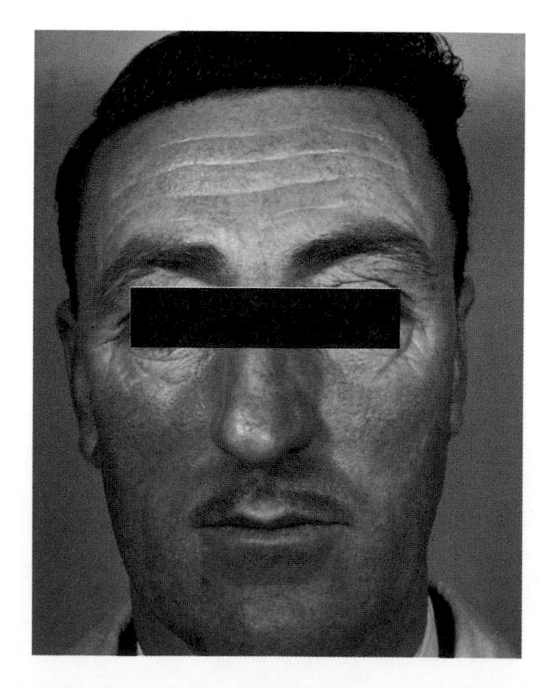

Figure 1.4 A patient with polycythaemia. Note: florid purple–red appearance.

Polycythaemia may be mistaken for cyanosis, from which it differs, in that *the colour of all the skin is heightened*, especially the colour of the cheeks, the neck and the backs of the hands and feet. The discolouration of peripheral cyanosis is usually limited to the tips of the hands, feet and nose.

Jaundice

Jaundice is a yellow discolouration of the skin caused by an excess of bilirubin (bile pigment), a breakdown product of haemoglobin, in the plasma.

The yellow colour is first visible in the white background of the sclerae (Figure 1.5), but as the jaundice increases, the skin turns yellow.

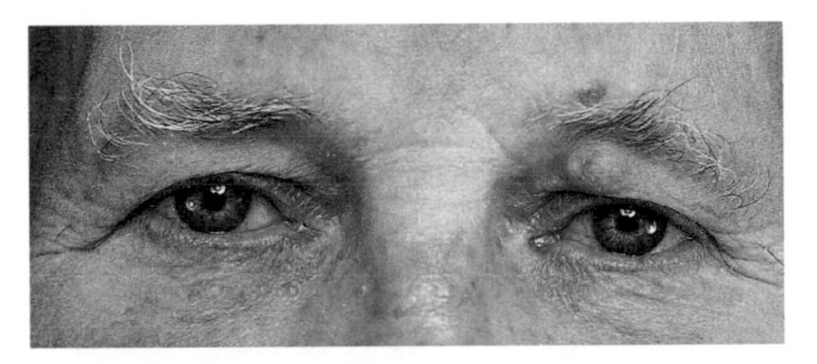

Figure 1.5 Jaundice. The sclerae have yellow discolouration.

With the onset of jaundice, white skin first turns a pale lemon yellow. As the bilirubin level increases, the skin becomes yellow–orange and sometimes almost brown. The skin eventually turns a yellow–grey–green colour in patients with primary biliary cirrhosis, when severe jaundice has existed for many years.

Jaundice can be caused by:

- excessive haemolysis – prehepatic jaundice.
- by liver malfunction – hepatic jaundice.
- by obstruction of the bile ducts – posthepatic jaundice.

The symptoms, signs and cause of jaundice are discussed in more detail in Chapter 15.

Brown pigmentation

An increase in the natural brown pigmentation of the skin (melanin) can be generalized or localized. The causes of this are discussed in more detail in Chapter 4.

The patient's size, shape and physical characteristics

When you look at a patient, you will subconsciously put them into one of four categories: their body will look normal, wasted or overweight, or have some skeletal or sexual characteristics that look out of proportion.

The principal conditions that cause these changes in body build are now briefly discussed.

Wasting/cachexia

There are many causes of wasting. Almost all serious diseases cause some loss of appetite and weight, so only the common conditions are listed in Revision panel 1.4.

The degree of wasting is apparent from the way in which the skeleton, particularly around the shoulder girdle, becomes visible. Folds of loose skin may be present on the arms, trunk and buttocks.

Revision panel 1.4

COMMON CAUSES OF WASTING

In children

Severe gastroenteritis
Malabsorption syndromes

In young adults

Tuberculosis
Haematological disorders
Anorexia nervosa

In middle age

Diabetes
Thyrotoxicosis
Carcinoma

In old age

Carcinoma
Gross cardiorespiratory disease
Sarcopenia

All age groups

Starvation

Overweight/obesity

Patients with normal skeletal and sexual proportions whose bodies are bigger than they should be are most likely to be obese from overeating (Figure 1.6)! Three important medical disorders are known to cause an increase in weight that can easily be mistaken for obesity (Revision panel 1.5).

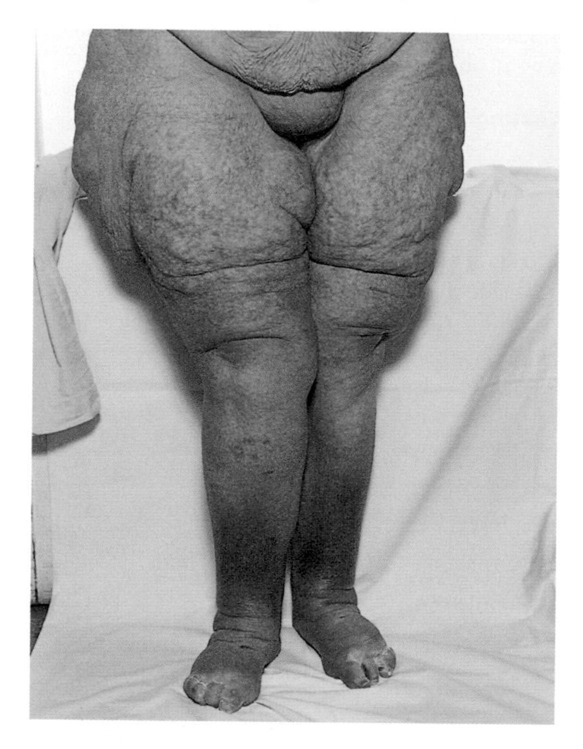

Figure 1.6 Morbid obesity usually affects the whole body, but may, as in this patient, be predominantly confined to the buttocks and thighs.

Revision panel 1.5

COMMON CAUSES OF AN INCREASE IN WEIGHT

- Obesity
- Pregnancy
- Interstitial fluid retention (renal, cardiac or hepatic failure)
- Localized fluid retention (massive ovarian cysts, ascites)
- Myxoedema
- Cushing's syndrome

Water retention

Chronic glomerular nephritis, hypoproteinaemia, hepatic failure and cardiac failure all cause an increase in body weight as a consequence of 'fluid retention'. The whole body swells, but the swelling is most noticeable in the dependent parts.

These patients have oedema of the ankles and legs, or the sacral region if they have been confined to bed, and also in the loose tissues of the face, especially in the skin below the eyes. The swelling around the eyes is often the first symptom and is present when the patient wakes up.

Ankle oedema and sacral oedema 'pit', which is an indentation in the subcutaneous tissue produced by prolonged digital pressure.

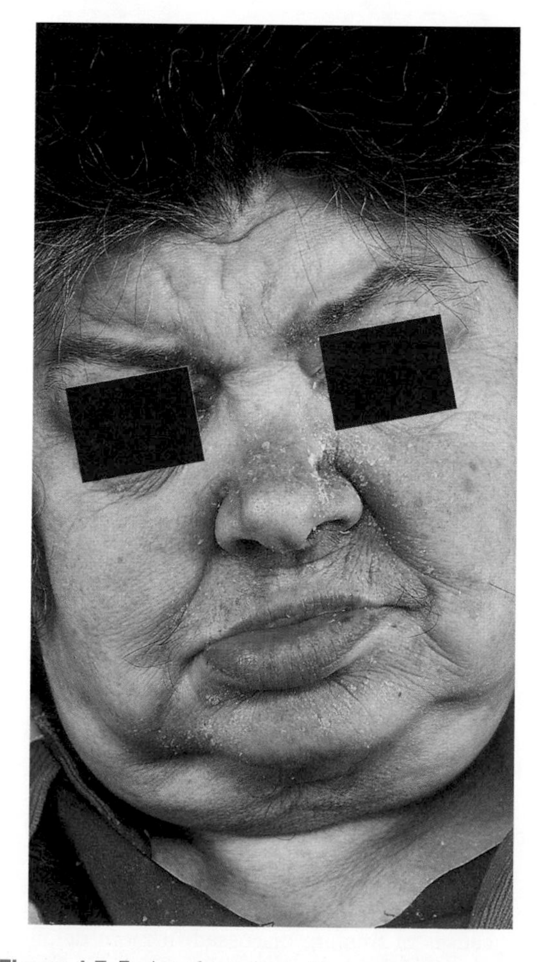

Figure 1.7 Facies of a patient with myxoedema.

Myxoedema/severe hypothyroidism

This is caused by a deficiency of thyroid hormone, usually as a result of autoimmune destruction of the thyroid gland (see Chapter 12). Patients with the condition develop a puffy face with a 'peaches and cream' complexion (Figure 1.7), a generalized, non-pitting increase in the subcutaneous tissues of the trunk and limbs and a dulling of thought, speech and action.

Cushing's syndrome

Cushing's syndrome is caused by an excess of adrenal glucocorticoids. The iatrogenic prescription of corticosteroids as a medical treatment is the most common cause. The majority of patients with endogenous Cushing's syndrome have a pituitary adenoma that secretes adrenocorticotrophic hormone, and the rest have adrenal adenomas, adrenal hyperplasia, neurofibromas or a paraneoplastic syndrome with exogenous adrenocorticotrophic hormone production, from, for instance, a carcinoma of bronchus.

The patient puts on weight, particularly on the face, neck and trunk (centropedal obesity), while the arms and legs stay thin. The face becomes 'moonshaped' (Figure 1.8b), and the rounded, thickened shoulders are often described as a 'buffalo hump'.

There is excess of lanugo hair, and an increase in skin pigmentation with thinning, leading to red–purple striae in the skin that has been stretched, particularly in the skin of the abdomen (Figure 1.8a). Back pain from osteoporosis, hypertension and oedema are common.

Bodily disproportion

A variety of skeletal abnormalities and a few rare disorders of general body development are usually associated with chromosomal abnormalities that will be apparent from your initial general inspection (Figures 1.9, 1.10 and 1.11). The common conditions are shown in Revision panel 1.6 and some are discussed in more detail in other chapters in the book.

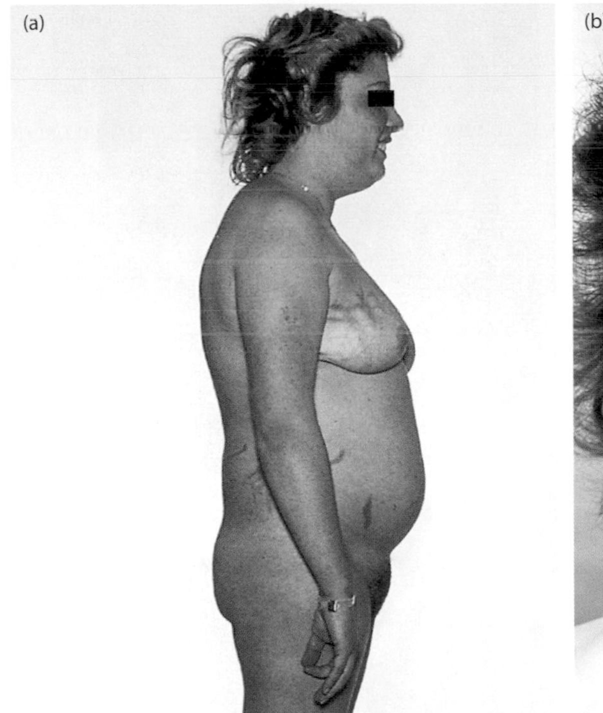

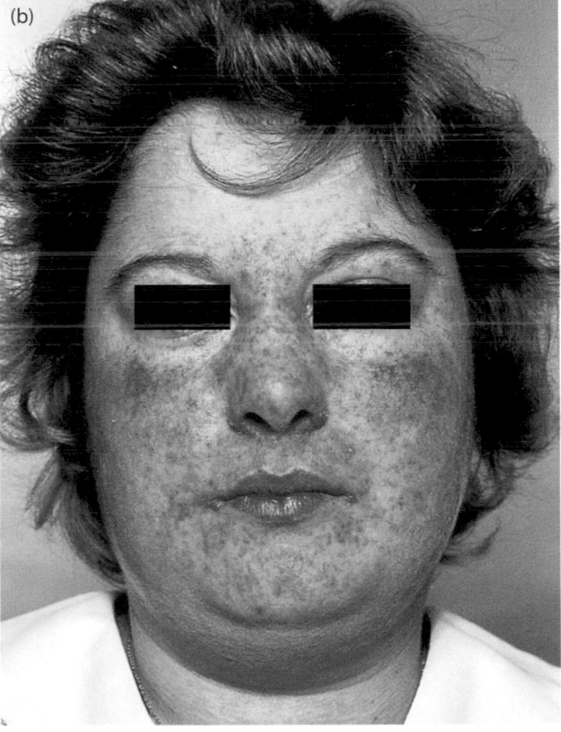

Figure 1.8 CUSHING'S SYNDROME. (a) Centropedal obesity with thin arms and legs. Red striae can be seen on the abdomen and breasts. (b) A round 'moon' face, some early hypertrichosis and an unusually florid acneiform rash.

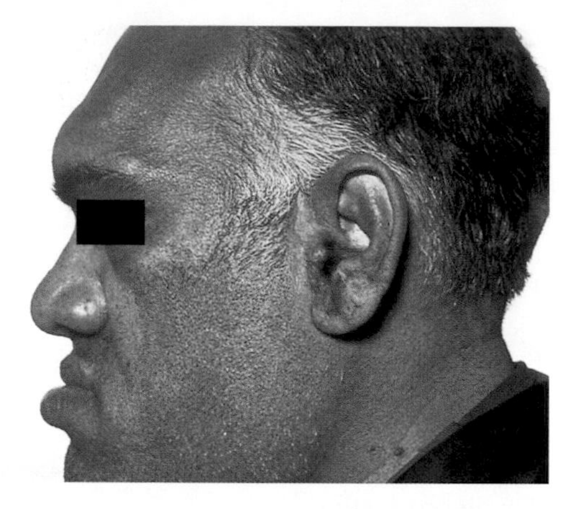

Figure 1.9 Acromegaly. A heavy head with a prominent nose, chin and lips. These patients also have long arms and large hands and feet.

Bell's palsy

Bell's palsy is an idiopathic lower motor paralysis of the facial nerve affecting the muscles of facial expression (Figure 1.12). The absence of tone in the facial muscles makes the affected side of the face look smooth and droopy. The corner of the mouth droops, the nasolabial creases become asymmetrical and less noticeable, and the lower eyelid droops. The asymmetry of the mouth can be increased by asking the patient to bare their teeth. The lids fail to close on the affected side when they attempt to shut their eyes.

Scleroderma

This is an autoimmune collagen disease that causes progressive thickening of the skin of the face. This reduces the patient's ability to use their muscles

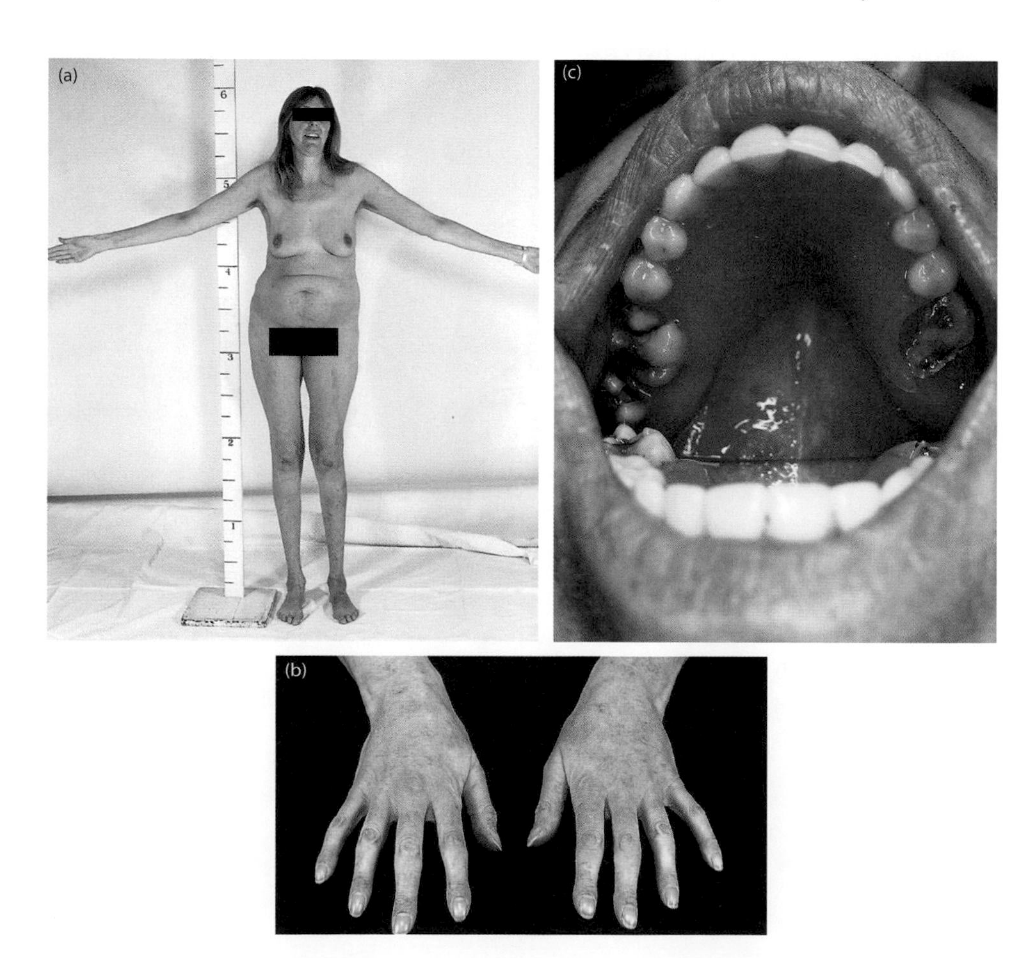

Figure 1.10 MARFAN'S SYNDROME. (a) The patient is tall and slim with long arms. (b) The long spindly fingers of a person with Marfan's syndrome. (c) The high-arched palate of Marfan's syndrome.

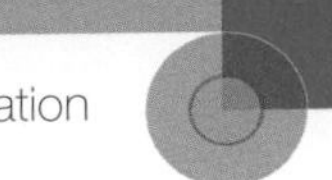

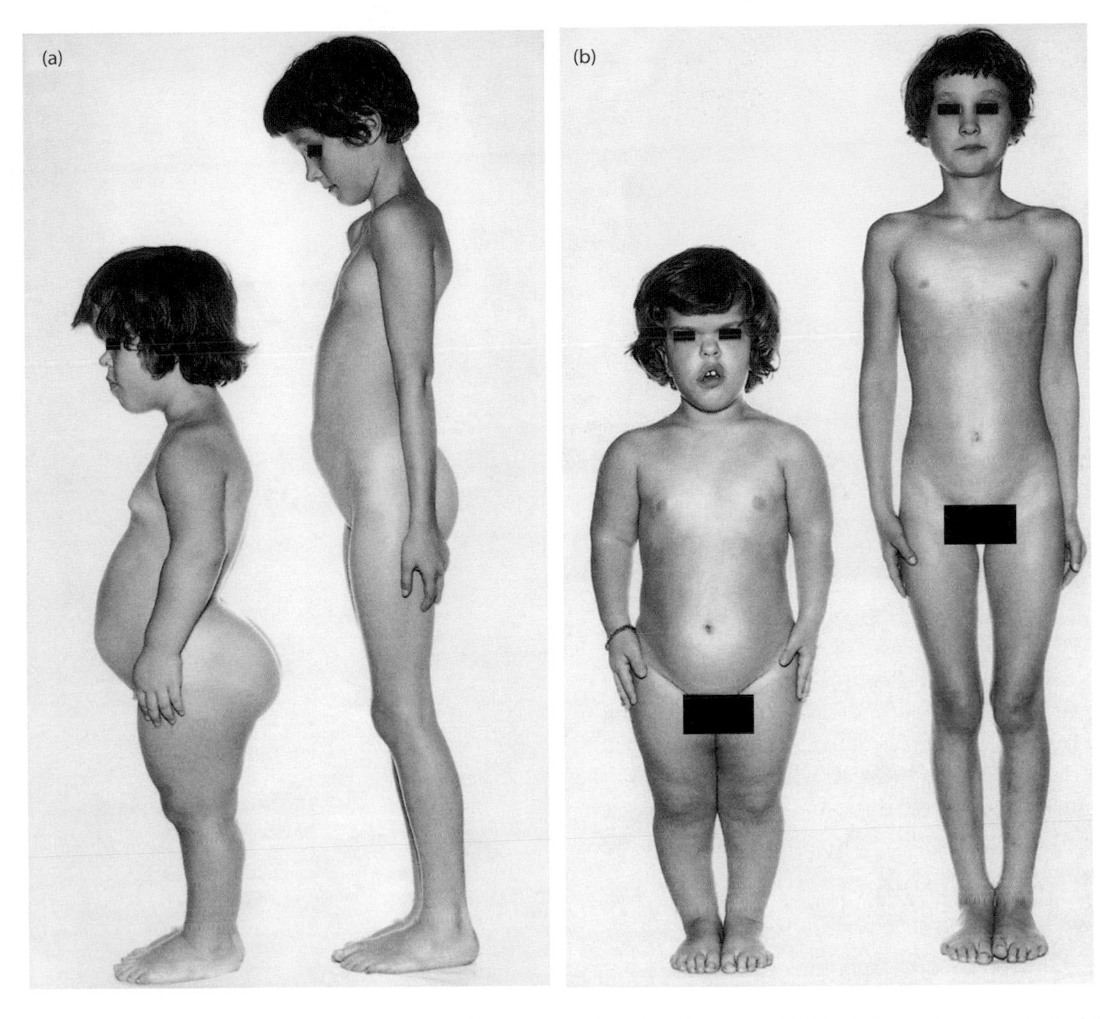

Figure 1.11 DWARFISM. (a, b) An achondroplastic child standing beside a normal child of the same age. The facial and skeletal abnormalities are obvious. Note that the umbilicus of the achondroplastic child is below the mid-point of the vertical height.

Revision panel 1.6

DIAGNOSES MADE ON INITIAL GENERAL INSPECTION

- Paget's disease (osteitis deformans) (see Chapter 6)
- Acromegaly (Figure 1.9)
- Marfan's syndrome (Figure 1.10)
- Kleinfelter's syndrome (see Chapter 18)
- Turner's syndrome
- Dwarfism (Figure 1.11):
  - Achondroplasia
  - Renal dwarfism
  - Congenital hypothyroidism/pituitary insufficiency

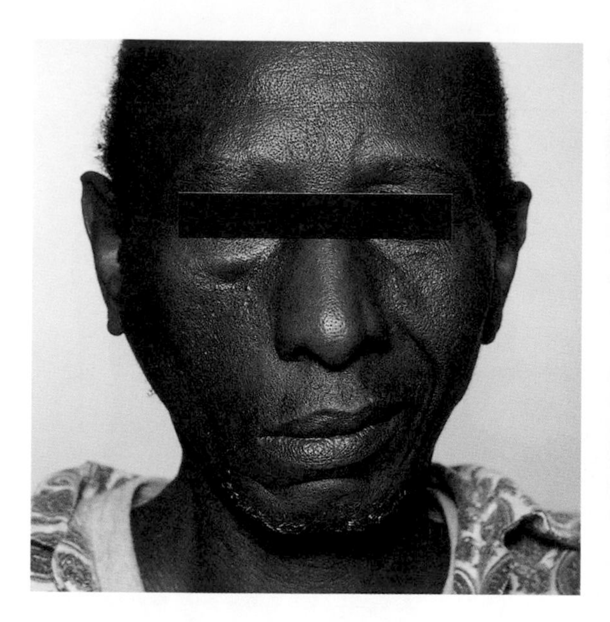

Figure 1.12 Right-sided Bell's palsy.

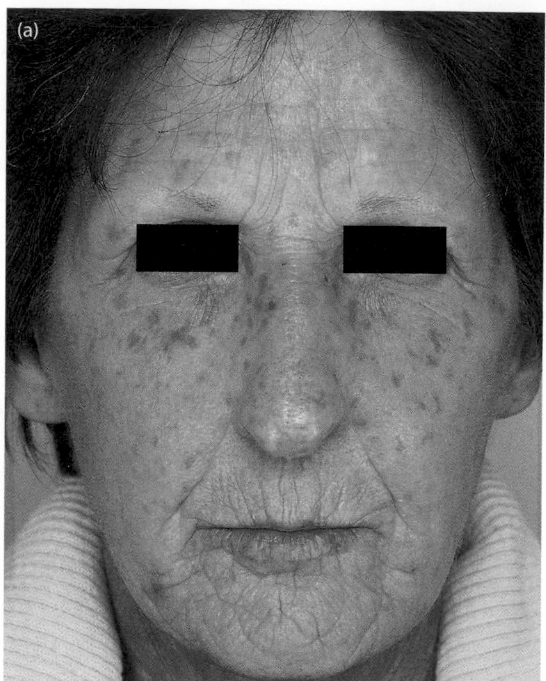

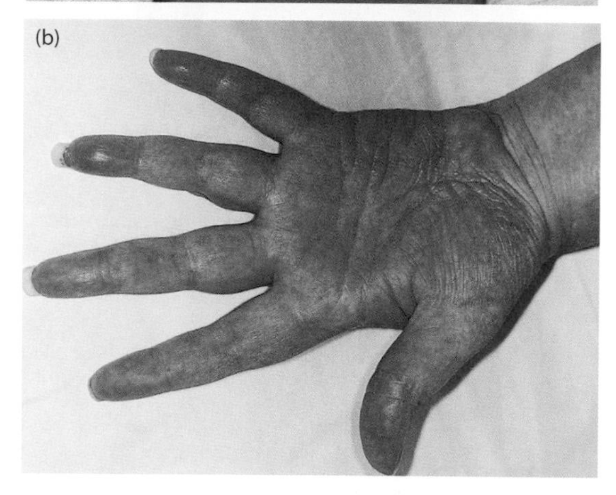

Figure 1.13 SCLERODERMA. (a) Note the tight skin, small mouth, fine wrinkles around the eyes and small telangiectases. (b) The spindle-shaped fingers of scleroderma.

of facial expression. The thick skin has a pale, waxy appearance. The mouth is constricted (microstomia), and jaw movements become restricted (Figure 1.13).

Telangiectases appear on the cheeks, around the mouth and across the nose, and fine, white, horizontal scars appear on the neck. Difficulty with swallowing may be experienced.

Down's syndrome

Down's syndrome is a congenital abnormality usually associated with an extra chromosome 21 (trisomy 21). It affects approximately 1 infant in 700. Males and females of all races are equally affected.

The dominant facial characteristic is that the outer ends of the palpebral fissures slant upwards and there are prominent epicanthic folds (mongoloid appearance) (Figure 1.14). The face and nasal bridge are flattened, and the tongue protrudes. Affected children often have a squint and one-third have congenital heart disease. Mental retardation, floppiness and a short stature are the dominant features.

Abnormal skull shape including hydrocephalus

Abnormalities of the shape of the skull are described in Chapter 3.

The baby may be born with a large head (hydrocephalus, Figure 1.15), often now detected by prenatal ultrasound, or the head may become enlarged after delivery if adequate drainage is not provided. There may be an associated meningomyelocele (Figure 1.16).

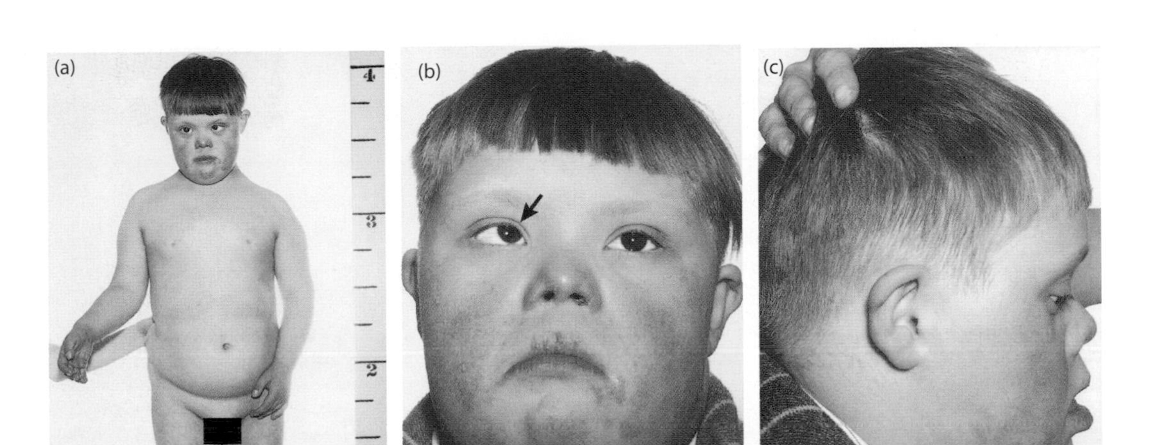

Figure 1.14 DOWN'S SYNDROME. (a) The short stature, floppiness and typical facial features of Down's syndrome. (b) Prominent epicanthic folds (arrow). (c) Face and nasal bridge flattened.

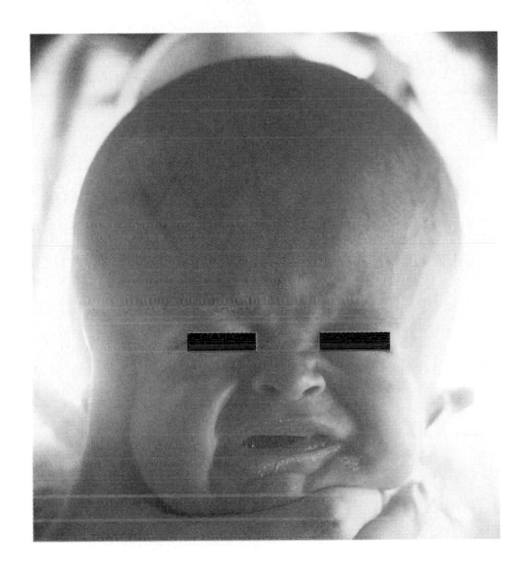

Figure 1.15 Congenital hydrocephalus. The bright light behind the baby's head reveals the thinness of the bones of the skull.

EXAMINATION OF THE HANDS

Make early physical contact with the patient in the examination by holding their hand and counting the pulse. The physical contact that is essential for the clinical examination forges a bond between you and the patient.

The features that can be observed by examining the hands are as follows:

Pulse See Chapters 2 and 10.

Nails Look at the colour and shape of the nails:

- Spoon-shaped nails (*koilonychia*) are associated with anaemia (Figure 1.17).
- Clubbing of the nails occurs in pulmonary and cardiopulmonary disease and various gastrointestinal disorders (Figure 1.18).

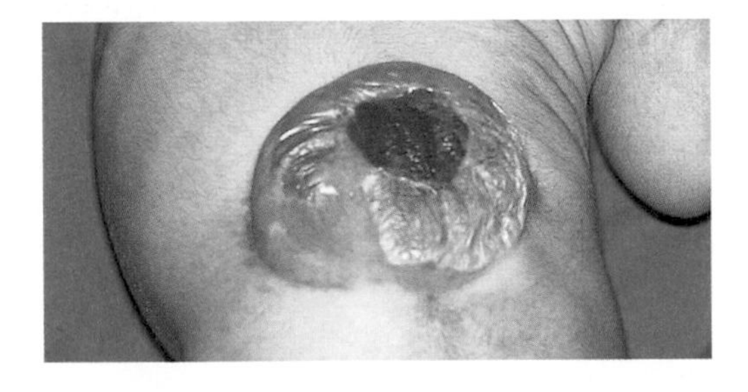

Figure 1.16 A meningomyelocele of the spine.

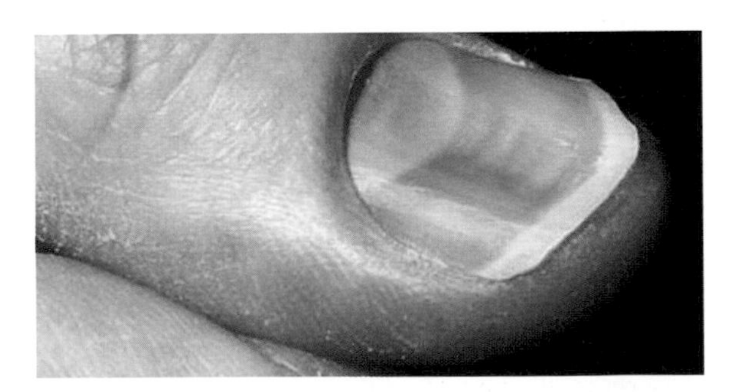

Figure 1.17 Koilonychia.

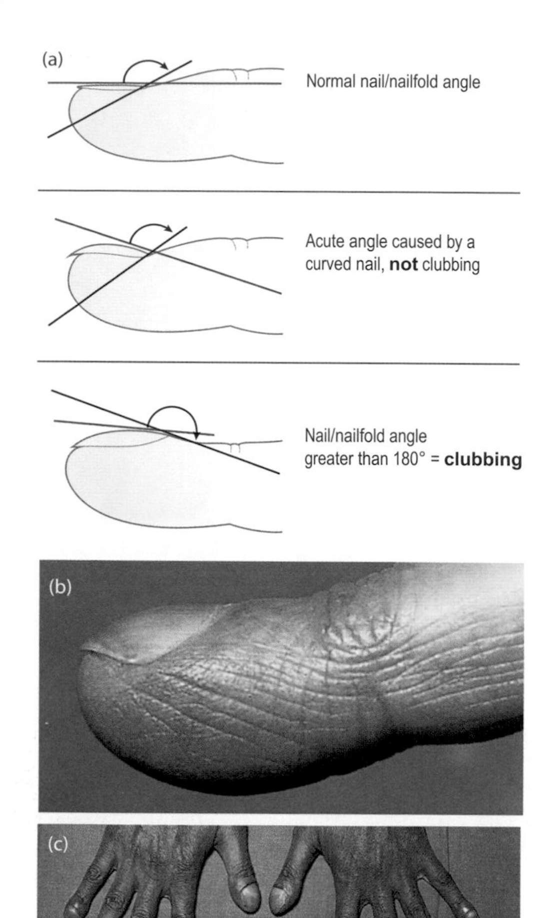

Figure 1.18 CLUBBING. (a) Normal and abnormal nail/nailfold angles. (b) Finger clubbing at more than 180°. (c) Clubbing of all the fingers. Note the swelling of the terminal phalanges.

- Splinter haemorrhages under the nails are caused by small arterial emboli (Figure 1.19).
- Pits and furrows are associated with skin diseases such as psoriasis.

Temperature Observe the temperature of the hands – but remember that it will be affected by the air and room temperatures.

Moisture Are the patient's palms sweating excessively?

Colour Pallor of the skin of the hands, especially in the skin creases of the palm and in the nail beds, suggests anaemia. Reddish-blue hands occur in polycythaemia.

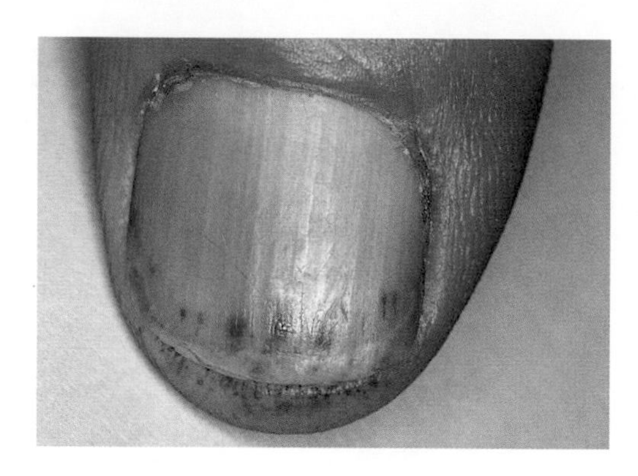

Figure 1.19 Splinter haemorrhages caused by small arterial emboli.

The fingers may be stained with nicotine.

Callosities The position of any callosities may reflect the patient's occupation.

EXAMINATION OF THE EYES

Look for any asymmetry of the position, size or colour of the eyes, and especially for any abnormality in the width of the palpebral fissures. This can be caused by *ptosis* (droopy eyelids) or *proptosis* (exophthalmos) when the eyeball is pushed forwards, pushing the lids apart.

The *size* and equality of the two pupils should be recorded (dilated, constricted or unequal).

The *reaction* of the pupil to light is checked by shining a bright light off and on the pupil.

The pupil's reaction to accommodation is assessed by asking the patient to look into the distance and then to refocus on a finger held close to their eye.

The *eye movements* are examined by fixing the patient's head with one hand while asking them to watch your finger as it travels upwards and downwards and inwards and outwards to the full extremes of movement. Patients should be asked if they experience any *double vision (diplopia)* in any particular position. While the eye movements are being tested, the presence of any *strabismus (squint)* can usually be easily seen, which may be *concomitant (divergent or convergent)* or *paralytic*.

Look for the presence of *nystagmus* (oscillations of the eye characterized by a slow drift and a rapid jerk back) at the inward and outward extremes of movement.

Inspect the lids, conjunctiva, cornea and lens. *Styes, Meibomian cysts* and *blepharitis* may inflame the lids or cause a swelling. The edges of the eyelids may be everted or inverted (*ectropion* or *entropion*) and the eye may water (*epiphora*) if the tear duct or lacrimal sac is blocked.

A painful red eye may be caused by *acute conjunctivitis* (when there is usually an associated discharge), *acute iritis* (when the anterior chamber of the eye is inflamed), *acute glaucoma* (which is associated with severe pain and a misty cornea), *acute keratitis* (from a corneal ulcer, seen as a cloudy opacity) or an inflamed sclera in *episcleritis*.

When an elderly patient has a gradual loss of eyesight, they are likely to have a *cataract* (which can be confirmed by finding a loss of part or the whole of the 'red-reflex' when a powerful light is shone on the pupil).

Other possible causes of gradual loss of vision including *optic nerve or retinal damage*, can only be detected by inspecting the retina through an ophthalmoscope. This requires practice, and you should take every opportunity to use the ophthalmoscope by inspecting the retinas of all the patients you examine.

Ophthalmoscopy is best carried out in a darkened room to ensure that the pupils are dilated. The ophthalmoscope is an illuminated lens system that can be focused on the retina. Patients are asked to stare fixedly at a point on the wall behind the examiner. The instrument is switched on and held by its handle in the right hand. The examiner then places his right eye against the lens opening and his left hand on the patient's forehead above their right eye. He then looks through the aperture of the ophthalmoscope, and brings the instrument very close to the patient's right pupil by placing his forehead against his left hand on the patient's forehead.

The light can be watched illuminating the fundus through the pupil, as the instrument and the patient's eye are brought close together. The approach should be slightly from the temporal side, at an angle of 10–15° to the direct line, to avoid noses colliding! When the pupils are level, this approach usually ensures that the optic nerve disc is the first part of the fundus to come into view. If the disc is not seen, a retinal artery should be followed back until the edge of the pale-yellow disc is seen.

The optic disc is 'cupped' by chronic glaucoma and swollen by papilloedema (Figure 1.20).

Other abnormalities that can be detected by careful fundoscopy of the rest of the retina include haemorrhages and exudates (in diabetes and hypertension), retinal emboli and infarcts and occasionally retinal detachment. At the end of the examination, the patient should be asked to look directly at the light of the ophthalmoscope in order to inspect the macula.

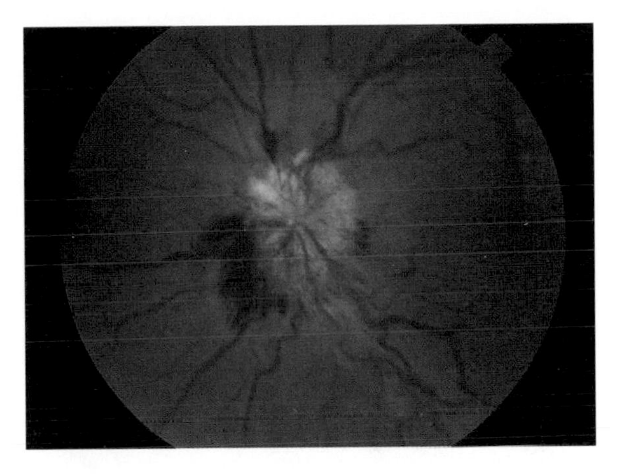

Figure 1.20 Papilloedema, a diagnostic sign of a chronically raised intracranial pressure, most often caused by a space-occupying intracranial tumour or a chronic subdural haematoma. (Courtesy of Dr E. Graham.)

A few common disorders of the eyes

Arcus senilis

This is a white rim around the outer edge of the iris caused by sclerosis and cholesterol deposition in the edge of the cornea (Figure 1.21). It is common in the elderly. It may be associated with hyperlipoproteinaemia and often coexists with generalized atherosclerosis (see Chapter 10).

Xanthelasma

These are painless opaque yellow 'fatty' plaques in the skin of the eyelids (Figure 1.22). One or two on the eyelids do not necessarily indicate any underlying disease, but they are known to be associated with hyperlipidaemia and arterial disease.

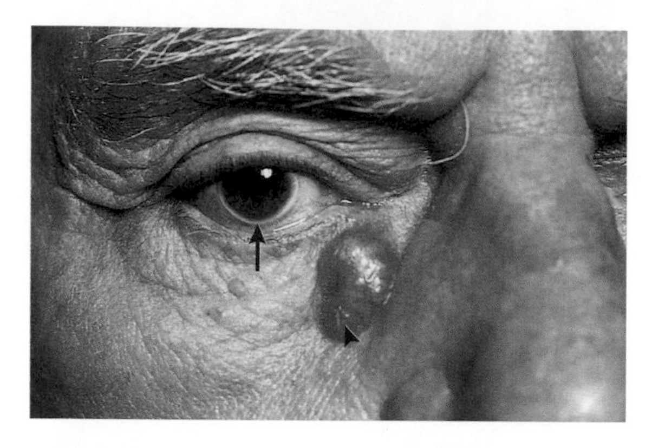

Figure 1.21 Arcus senilis: a thin white rim around the iris (arrow). It is a common abnormality and does not indicate advanced arterial disease. Note that the patient also has a basal cell carcinoma (arrowhead).

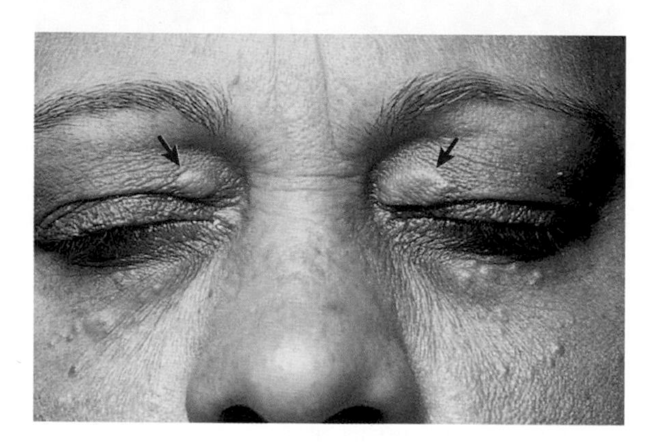

Figure 1.22 Xanthelasma of the upper eyelid (arrows).

Exophthalmos (Proptosis)

This is the forward protrusion of the eye from its normal position in the orbit. In the normal eye, the lower eyelid just touches the lower edge of the iris (the inferior limbus), provided the lower lid is normal, while the upper lid crosses the eye midway between the pupil and the superior limbus. The first sign of exophthalmos is the appearance of sclera below the inferior limbus. The proptosis has to be considerable before sclera is visible above the superior limbus (Figure 1.23).

The position of the upper eyelid is also altered by the tone of the levator palpebrae superioris muscle. Retraction of the upper eyelid reveals sclera above the superior limbus. You will not mistake this for exophthalmos if you remember to check the position of the lower eyelid.

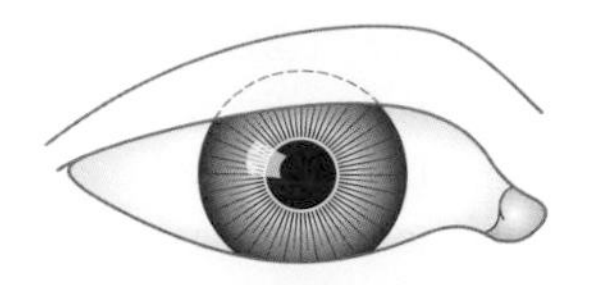

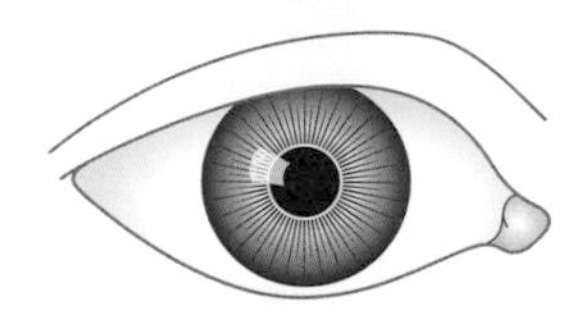

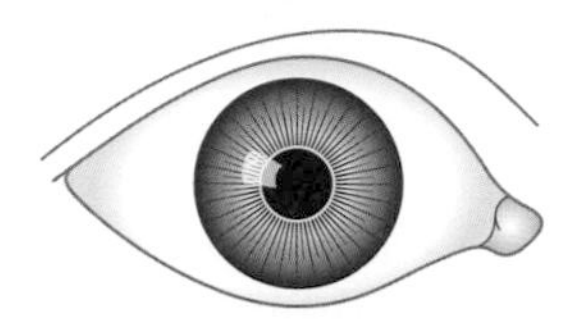

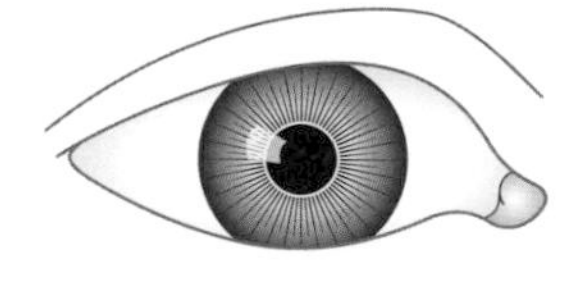

Figure 1.23 Exophthalmos/proptosis: the relations of the eyelids to the iris.

When the eye is pushed forwards, four secondary physical signs appear:

1. The patient can look up without wrinkling the forehead.
2. Convergence is restricted.
3. The patient blinks less often than normal.
4. The patient may not be able to close their eyes, and corneal ulceration may develop.

The conjunctiva becomes oedematous if the protrusion interferes with the venous and lymphatic drainage of the conjunctiva. This is called *chemosis*.

The causes of exophthalmos and pulsating exophthalmos are summarized in Revision panels 1.7 and 1.8.

Ectropion

In this deformity, the eyelids are everted (Figure 1.24) because of atonia or weakness of the obicularis oculi muscles, or scarring and contracture of the lids. When the eyelid becomes everted, the tear duct is separated from the conjunctiva, which causes *epiphora* (weeping), conjunctival inflammation and exposure keratitis.

Revision panel 1.7

CAUSES OF EXOPHTHALMOS

Endocrine

Thyrotoxicosis (before, during and after its onset)
Cushing's syndrome (rare)

Non-endocrine

Congenital deformities of the skull (craniostenosis, oxycephaly, hypertelorism)

Orbital or periorbital tumours

Periorbital meningioma
Optic nerve glioma
Orbital haemangioma
Lymphoma
Osteoma
Pseudotumour (granuloma)
Carcinoma of the antrum
Neuroblastoma

Inflammation

Orbital cellulitis
Ethmoid or frontal sinusitis

Vascular causes

Cavernous sinus arteriovenous fistula

Eye disease

Severe myopia
Severe glaucoma (buphthalmos)

Revision panel 1.8

CAUSES OF PULSATING EXOPHTHALMOS

Carotid artery–cavernous sinus arteriovenous fistula
Aneurysm of the ophthalmic artery
Vascular neoplasm in the orbit
Cavernous sinus thrombosis

Entropion

This is present when the eyelid inverts. It is usually caused by traumatic scarring or trachoma. It causes pain, irritation and epiphora.

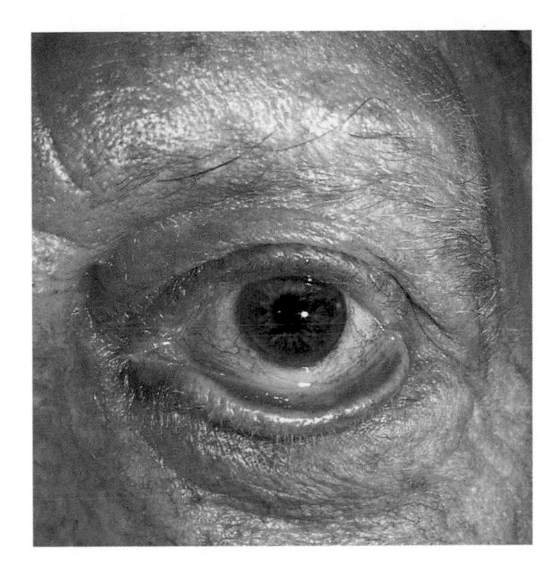

Figure 1.24 Ectropion: eversion of the lower eyelid.

Subconjunctival haemorrhage

This is a bleed occurring between the conjunctiva and the sclera (see Figure 5.6). It is usually spontaneous and harmless, but can be associated with a fractured base of skull, hypertension, blood dyscrasia, anticoagulation, choking (asphyxia) or scurvy.

Horner's syndrome

This is the set of physical signs that follow interruption of the sympathetic nerve supply to the head and neck arising from the first and second thoracic segments of the spinal cord.

The sympathetic nerves pass to the three cervical ganglia, before synapsing with postganglionic nerves to the structures of the head and neck. These nerves can be interrupted by trauma or disease anywhere along this pathway.

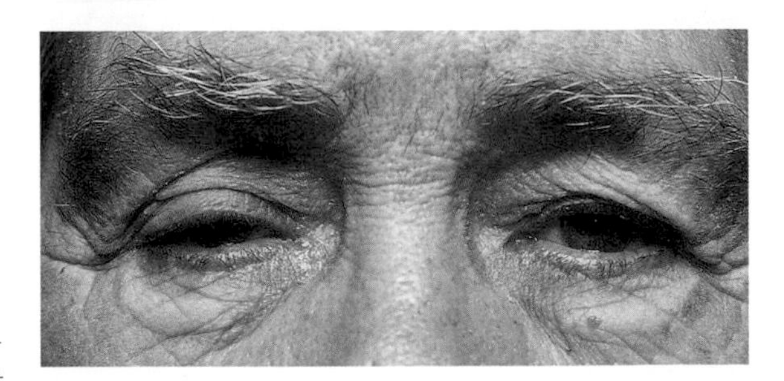

Figure 1.25 Horner's syndrome.

Absence of sympathetic tone causes *miosis* (narrowing of the pupil), *ptosis* (drooping of the eyelid), *vasodilatation* and *anhidrosis* (absence of sweating) over the cheek and eye (Figure 1.25). The condition is considered further in Chapter 2.

The causes of Horner's syndrome, with the common cause in bold, are:

- Tumours; including in the apex of the lung (*Pancoast tumour*) and the neck.
- Brain lesions – posterior inferior cerebellar artery thrombosis.
- Spinal cord lesions – syringomyelia, tumours.
- Injuries to the lower roots of the brachial plexus.
- Surgical excision of the inferior cervical ganglion (cervical sympathectomy).
- Aneurysm and dissection of the carotid artery.

Revision panel 1.9

HORNER'S SYNDROME

A small pupil (*myosis*)
Drooping of the upper eyelid (*ptosis*)
A warm, pink cheek (*vasodilatation*)
Absence of sweating (*anhidrosis*)
Nasal congestion (*nasal vasodilatation*)
Apparent enophthalmos

Ptosis

Horner's syndrome, myasthenia gravis (Figure 1.26) and any cause of paralysis of the IIIrd cranial nerve can cause ptosis (see Chapter 3). Some cases are congenital and many are idiopathic (see Revision panel 1.10).

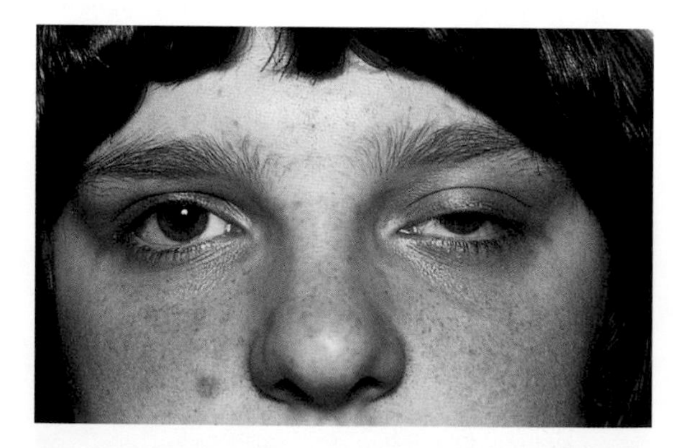

Figure 1.26 Left-sided ptosis in myasthenia gravis. The eye signs of generalized diseases are often asymmetrical and sometimes even unilateral.

Revision panel 1.10

CAUSES OF PTOSIS

Inflammation
Tumours
Excess eyelid skin
Muscle weakness (myopathies, myasthenia) (Figure 1.26)
IIIrd cranial nerve palsy

EXAMINATION OF THE EARS AND NOSE

These must be examined after the eyes. This is often forgotten during routine examination. Examination of these structures is especially important if there is any possibility of disease in the head and neck.

Clinical examination of the ear requires an *auroscope*. This instrument directs a beam of light down a conical metal speculum; the ear is then viewed through a lens. The speculum should be gently inserted into the external auditory meatus, while the ear is retracted upwards and backwards to straighten the external auditory canal. Wax may be present and must be removed before the tympanic membrane can be seen. The whole of the tympanic membrane can only be seen if the angle of the speculum is altered.

Normal tympanic membranes vary in *colour, translucency and shape* – so you should look at as many normal tympanic membranes as possible. The tympanic membrane may be normal, torn by *injury*, bulging and inflamed (*acute otitis media*), or perforated (*chronic otitis media*).

The external auditory canal may contain wax or foreign bodies. You may see otitis externa (dermatitis), blood or pus.

A few common disorders of the ear and nose

Bat ears

These are ears that jut out from the side of the head rather than lying flat against it (Figure 1.27).

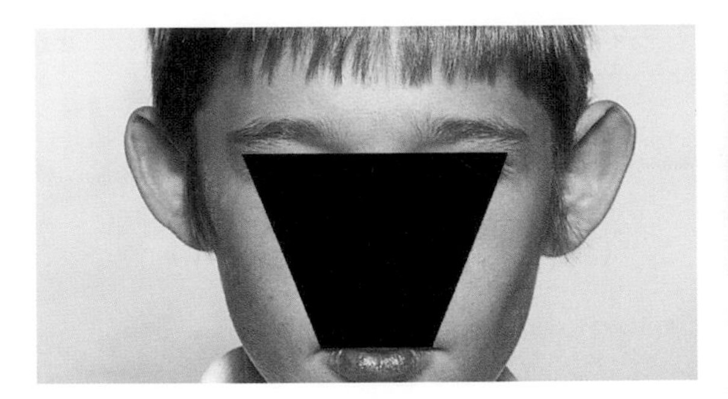

Figure 1.27 Bat ears.

Cup-shaped ears that protrude from the side of the skull are a feature of Down's syndrome.

Cauliflower ears

Cauliflower ears are ears distorted by multiple subperichondral haematomas caused by repeated trauma (Figure 1.28). They occur in boxers, wrestlers and rugby players.

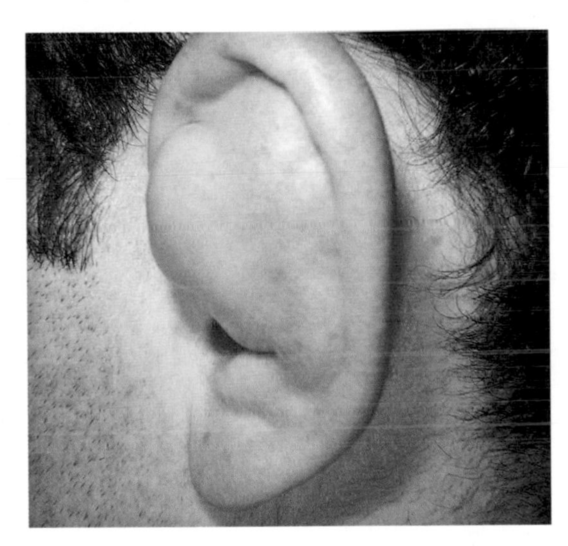

Figure 1.28 A 'cauliflower ear'. The swelling is a subperichondral haematoma and is almost blocking the external auditory meatus.

Keloid nodules

Many females and males have their ears pierced. The scar tissue may overgrow and produce a large nodule inside the lobe of the ear, especially if the hole becomes infected or the patient has any 'keloid' tendency. The nodule is firm and spherical, and may become pedunculated (Figure 1.29).

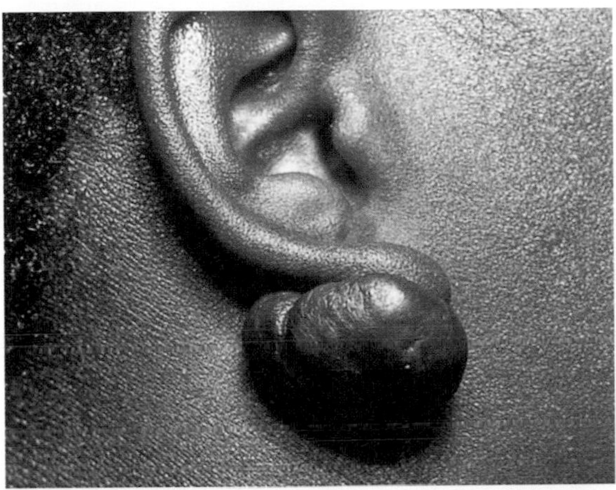

Figure 1.29 Keloid scars at the site of ear piercing. The mass of scar tissue usually protrudes from the posterior aspect of the ear lobe. Keloid scars are more common in black patients.

Accessory auricles

These are small pieces of skin-covered cartilage separate from the pinna. They are found on the side of the face just in front of the tragus (Figure 1.30). They are present from birth and cause no symptoms.

Saddle nose

The bridge of the nose is depressed and widened due to congenital abnormalities such as achondroplasia, hypertelorism (wide-set eyes) or destruction of the nasal cartilages caused by leprosy, cutaneous leishmaniasis or congenital syphilis.

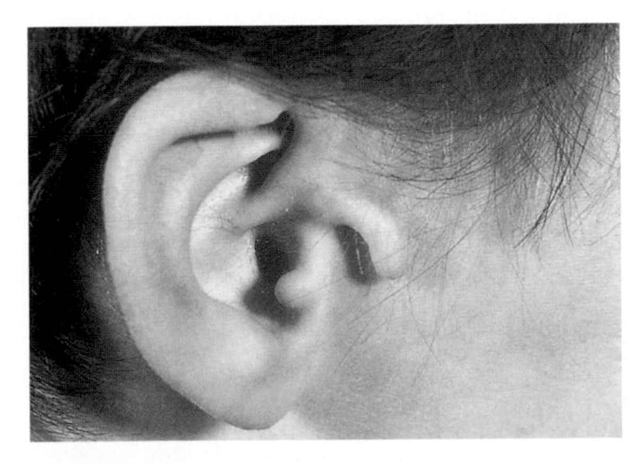

Figure 1.30 An accessory auricle.

Rhinophyma

This is a thickening of the skin over the tip of the nose caused by hypertrophy and adenomatous changes in its sebaceous glands (Figure 1.31). It is not caused by an excessive intake of alcohol, but can be exacerbated by it.

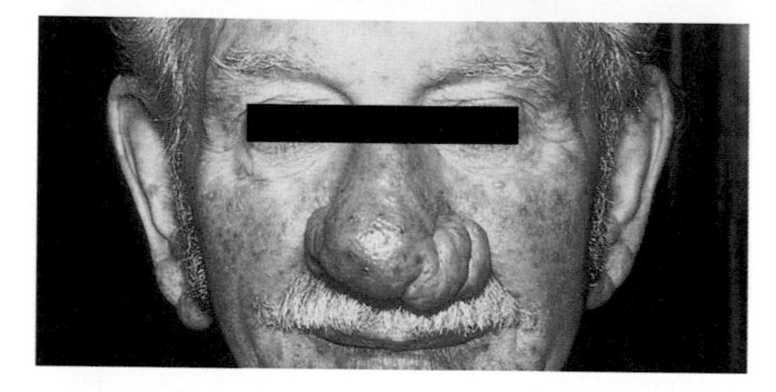

Figure 1.31 Rhinophyma.

EXAMINATION OF THE HEART, LUNGS AND PLEURA

The pulse and blood pressure must be measured and inspection palpation, percussion and auscultation carried out on the chest wall as described in Chapter 2.

EXAMINATION OF THE MOUTH

Note the colour and state of the lips. Ask to see the patient's tongue; observe its movement, symmetry and surface. Look at the teeth and gums. Use a spatula to inspect the soft palate, tonsils and posterior wall of the oropharynx (see Chapter 11).

EXAMINATION OF THE NECK

The important features to examine in the neck are the jugular veins, the trachea, the thyroid and the lymph glands (see Chapter 12).

EXAMINATION OF THE ABDOMEN

Examination of the abdomen is described in detail in Chapter 15. A large number of patients with surgical disease have intra-abdominal pathology, so a good technique for abdominal examination is essential.

Examination of the abdomen follows the standard pattern:

- Inspection for asymmetry, distension, masses, visible peristalsis and skin discolouration.
- Palpation for superficial and deep tenderness, the normal viscera (liver, spleen and kidneys) and any abnormal masses.
- Percussion of the liver and splenic areas and any other masses.
- Auscultation for bowel sounds and vascular bruits.
- Examination of hernia orifices.
- Rectal examination and vaginal examination.

There are three things that should always be remembered:

1. Palpate the supraclavicular lymph glands.
2. Feel the femoral pulses.
3. Examine the genitalia.

NOTE: Always remember to listen to the abdomen, and always carry out a rectal examination.

EXAMINATION OF THE LIMBS

There are four main tissues to be examined in a limb:

- Bones and joints (see Chapters 6, 7 and 8).
- Muscles and soft tissues (see Chapters 6, 7 and 8).
- Arteries and veins (see Chapter 10).
- Central nervous system and peripheral nerves (see Chapter 3).

The examination of these structures is covered elsewhere in the book.

TEST THE URINE, FAECES AND SPUTUM

It is important to note the colour and smell of the urine before using the dipstick for testing it for sugar, blood, ketones and protein.

Look at the faeces if the patient complains that they are abnormal. This can be inspected on the glove used for rectal examination (see Chapter 16).

Look at the sputum if the patient is producing any.

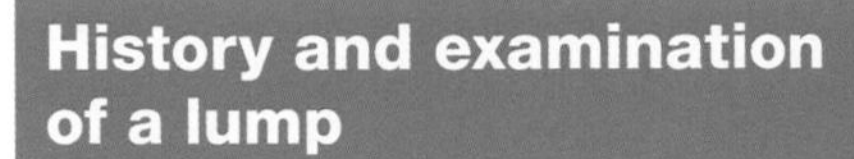

History and examination of a lump

History

Most patients with a lump feel it frequently and should be able to answer the following (Revision panel 1.11):

1. **When was the lump first noticed?**
   It is important to be precise with dates and terminology. Do not write 'the lump first appeared 6 months ago', when you mean 'the lump was first noticed 6 months ago'. Many lumps may exist for months, even years, before the patient notices them.
2. **What made the patient notice the lump?**
   There are four common answers to this question:
   - 'I felt or saw it when washing.'
   - 'I had a pain and found the lump when I felt the painful area.'
   - 'Someone else noticed it and told me about it.'
   - 'I found it on self examination', for example a breast lump in a female.

Revision panel 1.11

HISTORY OF A LUMP OR ULCER

Duration

When was it first noticed?

First symptom

What brought it to the patient's notice?

Other symptoms

What symptoms does it cause?

Progression

How has it changed since it was first noticed?

Persistence

Has it ever disappeared or healed?

Multiplicity

Has (or had) the patient any other lumps or ulcers?

Cause

What does the patient think caused it?

3. **What are the symptoms of the lump?**
   The lump may be painful, and if it is, you must take a careful history of the pain, as described earlier in this chapter (see page 9). Pain is usually associated with inflammation, not neoplastic change. Many patients expect cancer to be painful and therefore often ignore a malignant lump just because it does not hurt.
   The characteristic feature of pain associated with acute infection is its throbbing nature. A lump may be disfiguring or interfere with movement, respiration or swallowing. Describe the history of each symptom carefully.
4. **Has the lump changed since it was first noticed?**
   The patient should be able to tell you if the lump has got bigger or smaller, or has fluctuated in size and when they noticed a change in size.
5. **Does the lump ever disappear?**
   A lump may disappear on lying down, or during exercise, and yet be irreducible at the time of your examination.
   The patient should always be asked if the lump ever disappears completely, because this physical characteristic is peculiar to only a few types of lump.
6. **Has the patient ever had any other lumps?**
   You must ask this question because it might not have occurred to the patient that there could be any connection between their present lump and a previous lump, or even a coexisting one (e.g. neurofibromas or lipomas).
7. **What does the patient think caused the lump?**
   Lumps occasionally follow injuries or systemic illnesses known only to the patient.

Examination

Site/position The location of a lump must be described in exact anatomical terms, using distances measured from bony points. Do not guess distances; use a tape measure (Revision Panel 1.12).

Colour and texture of the overlying skin The skin over a lump may be discoloured, may be inflamed or may have become smooth and shiny, or thick and rough.

Shape Remember that lumps have three dimensions. You cannot have a circular lump because a

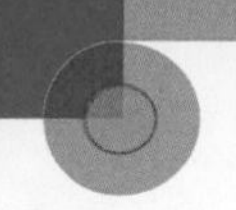

Revision panel 1.12

EXAMINATION OF A LUMP

Local examination

- Site
- Size
- Shape
- Surface
- Depth
- Colour
- Temperature
- Tenderness
- Edge
- Composition:
  - Consistency
  - Fluctuation
  - Fluid thrill
  - Translucency
  - Resonance
  - Pulsatility
  - Compressibility
  - Bruit
- Reducibility
- Relations to surrounding structures – mobility/fixity
- Regional lymph nodes
- State of local tissues:
  - Arteries
  - Nerves
  - Bones and joints

circle is a plane figure. Many lumps are not spherical, elliptical or hemispherical, but have an asymmetrical outline. In these circumstances, it is permissible to use descriptive terms such as *dumb-bell shaped, pear shaped* or *kidney shaped*.

Size Once the shape has been established, it is possible to measure its dimensions. Remember that all solid objects have at least three dimensions: *width, length and height or depth*, although the latter may be impossible to measure clinically. Asymmetrical lumps will need more measurements to describe them accurately, and sometimes a diagram will clarify your written description.

Surface The first feature of the lump that you will feel will be its surface. It may be *smooth or irregular*. An irregular surface may be covered with smooth bumps, rather like cobblestones, which can be called *bosselated*, or may be irregular or rough. There may be a mixture of surfaces if the lump is large.

Temperature Is the lump hot or of normal temperature? Assess the skin temperature with the dorsal surfaces of your fingers, because they are usually dry (free of sweat) and cool.

Tenderness Is the lump tender? If so, is the whole lump tender? Always try to feel the non-tender part before feeling the tender area, and watch the patient's face to ensure that you are not causing discomfort as you palpate.

Edge The edge of a lump may be *clearly defined or indistinct*. It may have a definite pattern.

Composition Any lump must be composed of one or more of the following:

- Calcified tissues such as bone, which make it *bony-hard*.
- Tightly packed cells, which make it *solid or firm or rubbery* depending on the tissue of origin and the individual's stromal response.
- Extravascular fluid, such as urine, serum, cerebrospinal fluid, synovial fluid or extravascular blood, which make the lump *soft and cystic*.
- *Gas*, which makes it soft and compressible.
- *Intravascular blood*, which makes it pulsatile.

The physical signs that help you decide the composition of a lump are: consistency, fluctuation, a fluid thrill, translucency, resonance, pulsatility, compressibility and bruits.

Consistency The consistency of a lump may vary from very soft to very hard. As it is difficult to describe hardness, it is common practice to compare the consistency of a lump to well-known objects. A simple scale for consistency is as follows:

- *Stony hard:* Not indentable – usually bone or calcification.
- *Firm:* Hard but not as hard as bone – similar to an unripe apple or pear.
- *Rubbery but slightly squashable:* similar to a rubber ball.

- *Spongy:* Soft and very squashable, but still with some resilience, like a sponge.
- *Soft:* Squashable and with no resilience, like a balloon.

The consistency of a lump is dependent not only upon its structure, but also on the tension within the lump. *Some fluid-filled lumps feel hard, some solid lumps are soft;* therefore, the final decision about composition of a lump (i.e. whether it is fluid or solid) rarely depends solely upon an assessment of the consistency.

Fluctuation Pressure on one side of a fluid-filled cavity makes all the other surfaces protrude (Figure 1.32). This is because an increase of pressure within a cavity is transmitted equally and at right angles to all parts of its wall. When you press on one aspect of a solid lump, it may or may not bulge out in another direction, but it will not bulge outwards in every other direction.

Fluctuation is elicited by feeling at least two other areas of the lump between the thumb and index finger of the left hand while pressing on a third central point with the index finger of the right hand (Figure 1.32). The lump fluctuates and contains fluid if two areas on opposite aspects of the lump bulge out when a third area is pressed in. This examination should be carried out in two planes, the second at right angles to the first.

Fluid thrill A percussion wave is easily conducted across a large fluid collection or cyst but not across a solid mass. The presence of a fluid thrill is detected by tapping one side of the lump, by flicking the middle finger of the right hand against the thumb, and feeling the transmitted vibration when it reaches the other side, where the second detecting left hand is placed (Figure 1.33). When it is present, a fluid thrill is a diagnostic and extremely valuable physical sign.

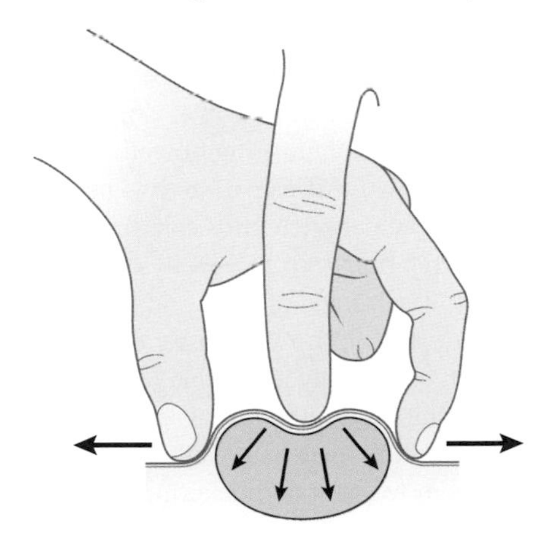

Figure 1.32 Fluctuation.

> **NOTE:** Beware – a percussion wave can be transmitted along the wall of a large swelling.

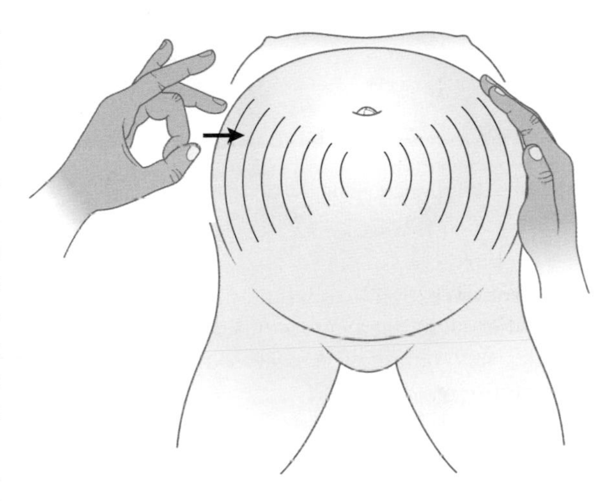

Figure 1.33 Fluid thrill.

This is prevented by placing the edge of the patient's or an assistant's hand on the lump midway between the percussing and palpating hands. Percussion waves cannot be felt across small fluid-filled lumps because the wave moves so quickly that the time gap cannot be appreciated or distinguished from the mechanical shaking of the tissue caused by the percussion.

Translucency *(transillumination)* Light passes easily through clear fluids but does not pass through solid tissues. A lump that transilluminates must contain water, serum, lymph or plasma. Highly refractile light can also appear to transilluminate through a large lipoma (see page 145), while blood and other opaque fluids do not transmit light.

Transillumination requires a bright pinpoint light source and a darkened room. The light should be placed on one side of the lump, not directly on top of it. Transillumination is present when the whole lump glows at a distance from the light source (Figure 1.34).

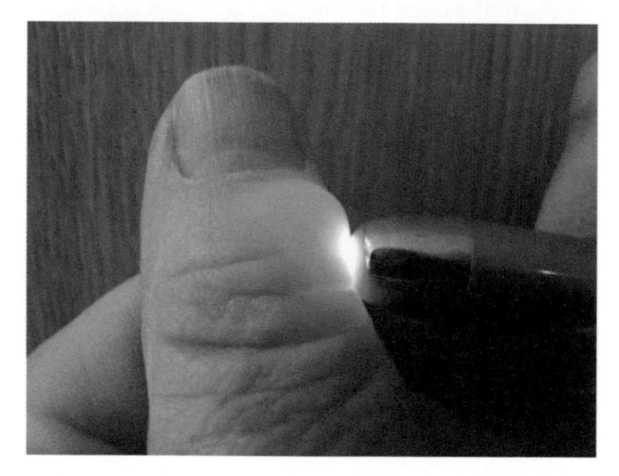

Figure 1.34 Transillumination of a ganglion of the thumb. Note: Light is visible beyond the site of application.

Resonance Solid and fluid-filled lumps sound dull when percussed. A gas-filled lump, such as a hernial sac containing bowel, sounds hollow and resonant.

Pulsatility Lumps may pulsate because they are near to an artery and are moved by its pulsations (*transmitted pulsation*) or because they are connected with the heart or arterial system (*expansile pulsation*). The most common cause of expansile pulsation is an aneurysm, with, rarely, very vascular tumours.

Always let your hand rest still for a few seconds on every lump to discover if it is pulsating. When a lump pulsates, you must find out whether the pulsations are transmitted or are expansile. Place a finger (or fingers if the lump is large) of each hand on opposite sides of the lump and feel if they are pushed *outwards and upwards*. When they are, the lump has an expansile pulsation. When they are pushed only *upwards*, the lump has a transmitted pulsation (Figure 1.35).

Compressibility Some fluid-filled lumps can be compressed until they disappear. When the compressing hand is removed, the lump re-forms. This finding is a common feature of *vascular malformations and fluid collections* that can be pushed back into a cavity, a joint or a cistern (see Chapter 10). *Compressibility should not be confused with reducibility* (see below). A lump that is reducible – such as a hernia – can be pushed away into another place but will often not reappear spontaneously without the stimulus of coughing or gravity.

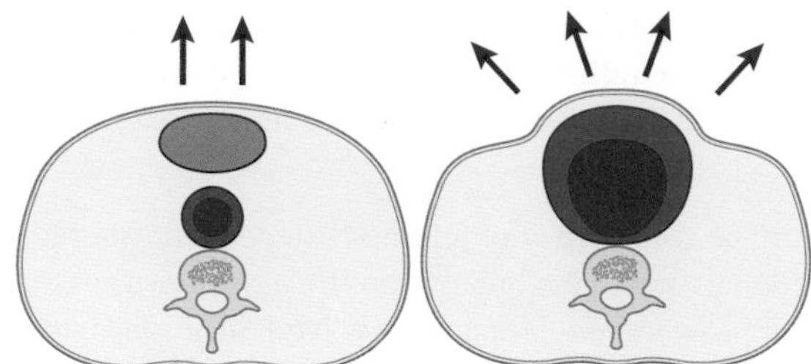

Figure 1.35 Transmitted versus expansile pulsation.

Reducibility You should always see if a lump is reducible (disappears) by gently compressing it. A reducible lump becomes smaller and then moves to another place as it is compressed. It may disappear quite suddenly after appropriate pressure has been applied. The lump may return, when you ask the patient to cough, expanding as it does so. This is called a *cough impulse* and is a feature of *hernias*. The reduction can be maintained by pressing over the point at which the lump finally disappeared.

In some ways, the differences between compressibility (see above) and reducibility are semantic.

Bruits Always listen over a lump with your stethoscope. A systolic bruit or a machinery murmur (throughout both systole and diastole) may be audible over vascular lumps that contain an arteriovenous fistula. Audible bowel sounds can be heard over a hernia containing bowel.

Relations By careful palpation, it is usually possible to decide which structure contains the lump, and what its relation is to the overlying and deeper tissues. The attachment of skin and other superficial structures to a lump can easily be determined because both are readily accessible to the examiner and any limitation of their movement easily felt. The lump should be gently moved while the skin is inspected for movement or 'puckering'.

Attachment to deeper structures is more difficult to determine. *The underlying muscles must be tensed* to see if this reduces the mobility of an overlying lump or makes it easier or more difficult to feel

(Figure 1.36). The former indicates that the lump is attached to the fascia covering the superficial surface of the muscle or to the muscle itself; the latter that the lump is within or deep to the muscles.

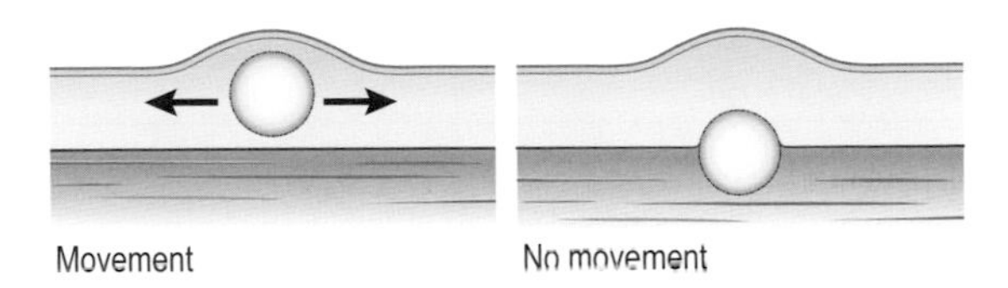

Figure 1.36 Attachment of lumps to the skin and deep tissue.

Lumps that are attached to bone do not move.

Lumps that are attached to or arising from vessels or nerves may be moved from side to side across the length of the vessel or nerve, but not up and down along their length.

Lumps in the abdomen that are freely mobile usually arise from the intestine, its mesentery or the omentum (see Chapter 15).

Lymph glands Never forget to palpate the lymph glands that would normally drain lymph from the region occupied by the lump:

- The skin, muscles and bones of the limbs and trunk drain to the axillary and inguinal glands.
- The head and neck to the cervical glands.
- The intra-abdominal structures to the preaortic and para-aortic glands.

Local tissues It is important to examine the overlying and nearby skin, subcutaneous tissues, muscles and bones, and the local circulation and nerve supply of adjacent tissues. This is most relevant when examining an ulcer, but some lumps are associated with a local vascular or neurological abnormality, so this part of the examination must not be forgotten as, for example, skin ulceration can occur over a locally advanced breast cancer.

General examination It is often tempting to examine only the lump about which the patient is complaining. This will lead to misdiagnosis.

NOTE: You must always examine the whole patient.

History and examination of an ulcer

An ulcer is *a dissolution of the continuity of an epithelium* (i.e. an epithelial defect, not a wound). Unless their ulcers are painless or in an inaccessible part of the body, patients notice ulcers from the moment they begin, and can describe most of their clinical features.

History

The questions to be asked concerning an ulcer follow a pattern similar to those asked about a lump.

1. **When was the ulcer first noticed?**
   Ask the patient when the ulcer began and whether it could have been present for some time before it was noticed. The latter often occurs with neurotrophic ulcers on the sole of the foot.
2. **What drew the patient's attention to the ulcer?**
   The most common reason is pain, but the 'sore' or defect may be visible. Occasionally, the presenting feature is bleeding, or a purulent discharge, which may be foul smelling.
3. **What are the symptoms of the ulcer?**
   The ulcer may be painful. It may interfere with daily activities such as walking, eating or defaecation. Record the history of each symptom.
4. **How has the ulcer changed since it first appeared?**
   The patient's observations about changes in size, shape, discharge and pain are likely to be accurate. If the ulcer has healed and broken down, record the features of each episode.
5. **Has the patient ever had a similar ulcer on the same site, or elsewhere?**
   Obtain a complete history of any previous ulcer.
6. **What does the patient think caused the ulcer?**
   Many patients believe they know the cause of their ulcer, and they are often right. In many cases, it is trauma. When possible, the severity and type of injury should be assessed. A large ulcer following a minor injury suggests that the skin was abnormal before the injury.

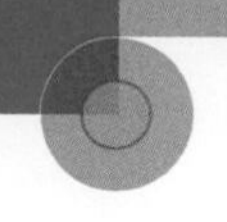

Examination

The examination of an ulcer follows the same pattern as the examination of a lump. When an ulcer has an irregular shape that is difficult to describe, draw it in your notes and add the dimensions. When an exact record of size and shape is needed, place a thin sheet of sterile transparent plastic sheet over the ulcer and trace around its edge with a felt-tipped pen.

After recording the site, size and shape of the ulcer, you must examine the base (surface), edge, depth, discharge and surrounding tissues, the state of the local tissues and local lymph glands and complete the general examination.

Base The base, or floor, of an ulcer usually consists of slough or granulation tissue (capillaries, collagen, fibroblasts, bacteria and inflammatory cells), but recognizable structures such as tendon or bone may be visible. The nature of the floor occasionally gives some indication of the cause of the ulcer:

- Solid brown or grey dead tissue indicates full thickness skin death.
- Syphilitic ulcers (nowadays rare) have a slough that looks like a yellow–grey wash-leather.
- Tuberculous ulcers have a base of bluish unhealthy granulation tissue.
- Ischaemic ulcers often contain poor granulation tissue, and tendons and other structures may lie bare in their base.

The redness of the granulation tissue reflects its underlying vascularity and indicates the ability of the ulcer to heal. Healing epidermis is seen as a pale layer extending in over the granulation tissue from the edge of the ulcer.

Edge There are five types of edge (Figure 1.37).

A flat, gently sloping edge This indicates that the ulcer is shallow, and this type of ulcer is usually relatively superficial. *Venous ulcers* usually have this type of edge, but so do many other types of ulcer. The new skin growing in around the edge of a healing ulcer is pale pink and almost transparent.

A square-cut or punched-out edge This follows the rapid death and loss of the whole thickness of the skin without much attempt at repair of the defect. This form of ulcer is most often seen in the foot where pressure has occurred on an insensitive piece of skin, i.e. a *trophic ulcer* secondary to a neurological defect.

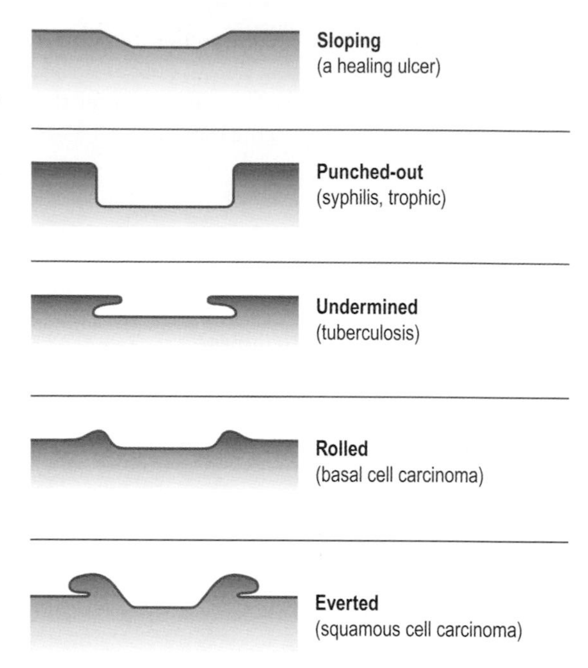

Figure 1.37 The varieties of ulcer edge.

The classic textbook example of a punched-out ulcer is the ulcer of *tertiary syphilis*, but these lesions are rare today in Europe. Most of the punched-out ulcers that are now seen are caused by the neuropathy of *diabetes and peripheral arterial ischaemia* or, outside Europe and North America, *leprosy*.

An undermined edge When an infection in an ulcer affects the subcutaneous tissues more than the skin, the edge becomes undermined. This type of ulcer is commonly seen in the buttock as a result of *pressure necrosis*, because the subcutaneous fat is more susceptible to pressure than the skin; however, the classic textbook example is the *tuberculous ulcer* – which is now uncommon in Europe and North America.

A rolled edge This develops when there is slow growth of tissue in the edge of the ulcer. A rolled edge is typical, and almost diagnostic, of a *basal cell carcinoma* (*rodent ulcer*). The edge is usually pale pink or white, with clumps and clusters of cells visible through the paper-thin superficial covering of squamous cells. Telangiectases are commonly seen in the pearly edge.

An everted edge This develops when the tissue in the edge of the ulcer is growing so rapidly that it spills out of the ulcer to overlap the normal skin. An everted edge is typical of a *squamous cell carcinoma* and is seen in the skin, in the bowel, in the bladder and in the respiratory tract.

Depth Record the depth of the ulcer in millimetres, and anatomically by describing the structures it has penetrated or reached.

Discharge The discharge from an ulcer may be serous, sanguineous, serosanguinous or purulent. There may be a considerable quantity of discharge, which is easily visible, or it may only be apparent from inspection of the patient's dressings.

Revision panel 1.13

FOUR BASIC EXAMINATION TECHNIQUES

Inspection
Palpation
Percussion
Auscultation

And with a joint

Look
Feel
Move

You may be unable to see the features of the ulcer if it is covered with coagulated discharge (a scab). This may have to be removed to examine the ulcer properly. Students should not do this without the permission of the doctor in charge of the patient.

Relations Describe the relations of the ulcer to its surrounding tissues, particularly those deep to it. It is important to know if the ulcer is adherent or invading deep structures such as tendons, periosteum and bone – which may indicate the presence of osteomyelitis.

The local lymph glands must be carefully examined. They may be enlarged because of secondary infection or secondary tumour deposits, and they may be tender.

Local tissues Pay particular attention to the local blood supply and innervation of the adjacent skin. Many ulcers in the lower limbs are secondary to vascular and neurological disease. There may also be evidence of previous ulcers that have healed.

General examination This is very important because many systemic diseases as well as many skin diseases present with ulcers. Examine the whole patient with care, looking especially at their hands and facies, which can supply important clues to the diagnosis.

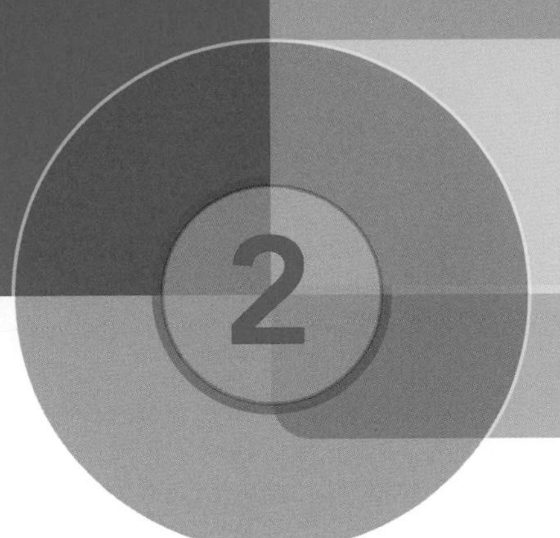

The heart, lungs and pleura

RICHARD LEACH

Introduction

The chest is an airtight cage. Its movements and pressure changes enable ventilation of the lungs, whilst the bony chest wall protects the lungs, trachea, heart, great vessels, thymus and oesophagus.

The main symptoms of chest disease – *chest pain, cough and shortness of breath* – are common to a number of disorders affecting the heart, lungs, pleura, chest wall and mediastinum. There is considerable overlap in the clinical signs of heart and lung disorders.

Some diseases of the chest are symptomless and may be without clinical signs. For example, the first presentation of ischaemic heart disease can be a fatal episode of ventricular fibrillation, whilst lung cancer may be detected incidentally when a chest X-ray is performed for a completely different reason.

EXAMINATION OF THE CHEST WALL AND LUNGS

Inspection

Cyanosis caused by cardiopulmonary disease is most easily appreciated by inspecting the inner aspect of the lips (see pages 13, 14).

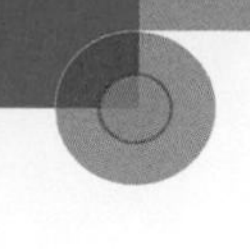

Count the rate of respiration and notice the rhythm. A slow respiratory rate occurs in patients with cerebral compression or damage, while rapid respiration is often seen in patients with ventilation–perfusion mismatch.

A fluctuating respiratory rate and volume, interspersed with periods of *apnoea* (cessation of breathing) and episodes of *tachypnoea* (rapid breathing), is called *Cheyne–Stokes* or periodic respiration. It is caused by variations in the sensitivity of the respiratory centre to normal stimuli, and occurs commonly in patients with heart failure and severe cerebrovascular accidents.

Compare the duration of inspiration and expiration and note whether respiration seems to require extra voluntary effort. Watch the chest during inspiration to see if there is any inward (paradoxical) movement of the intercostal spaces. This is usually caused by obstruction to the inflow of air into the lungs, but in an injured patient may indicate instability of a segment of the chest wall (e.g. flail segment) (see Chapter 5, Figure 5.4).

Record any abnormality in the shape of the chest. The two common deformities are funnel chest (*pectus excavatum*) and pigeon chest (*pectus carinatum*) (see Figures 2.29 and 2.30).

Palpation

Trachea Check that the trachea is in a central position at the suprasternal notch (Figure 2.1). The trachea is deviated *away from* a 'tension' pneumothorax and *towards* a collapsed lung.

Chest expansion Spread your hands around the patient's chest so that your thumbs just meet in the midline. Ask the patient to take a deep breath. Your thumbs should be dragged apart to a distance roughly equivalent to half the chest expansion. When the expansion is asymmetrical, it will be felt and seen.

Chest expansion is the difference between the circumference of the chest at full inspiration and full expiration, measured at the level of the nipples (T4). Unilateral changes in expansion are associated with lung collapse, consolidation and interstitial lung disease.

Apex beat The apex beat is the lowest and most lateral point of the cardiac impulse. It is situated in the fifth intercostal space in the mid-clavicular line (Figure 2.2). It is shifted laterally if the heart enlarges, and moves medially or laterally when the mediastinum changes position. The mediastinum moves to one side if it is pulled over by a collapsed, contracted lung, or pushed over by air or fluid in the

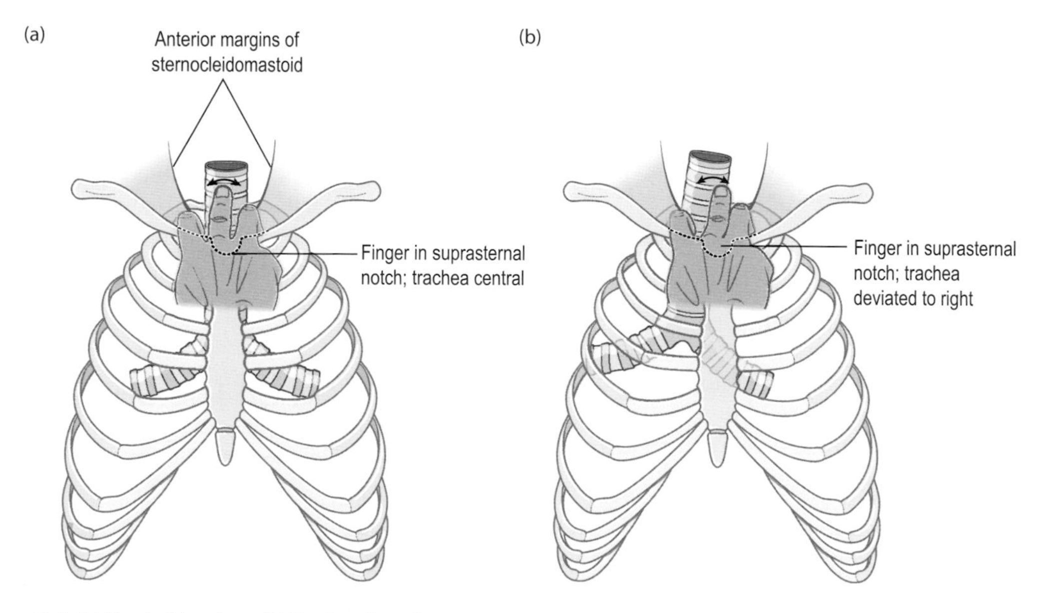

Figure 2.1 (a) Central trachea. (b) Deviated trachea.

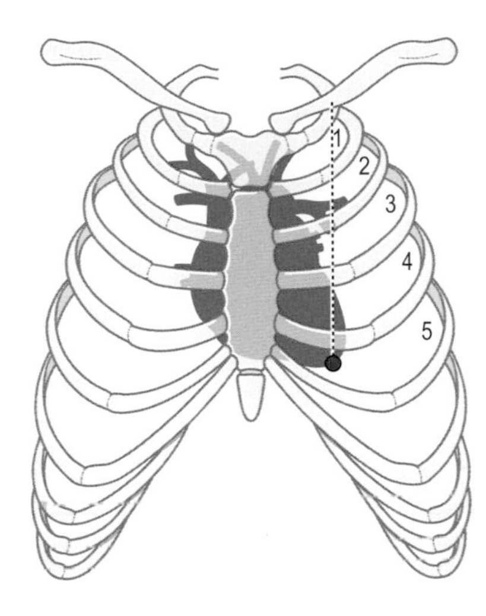

Figure 2.2 The apex beat is normally felt in the fifth intercostal space in the mid-clavicular line.

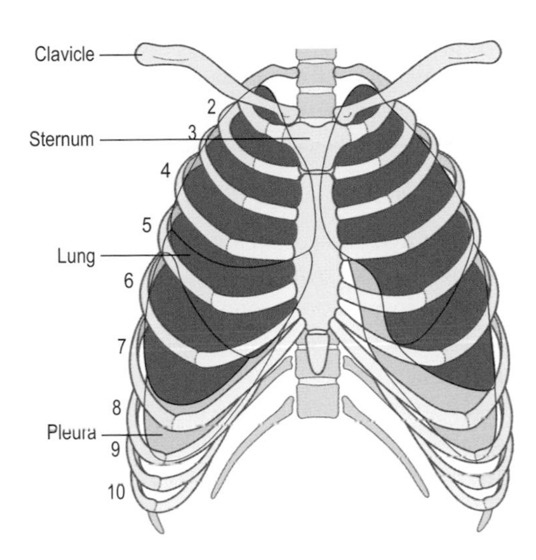

Figure 2.3 The surface markings of the lungs.

opposite pleural cavity (tension pneumothorax or pleural effusion).

Tactile vocal fremitus To detect this, place your whole hand firmly on the chest and ask the patient to say '99'. The vibrations that you can feel with your hand are called the *vocal fremitus*. Compare the strength of these vibrations on either side of the chest, front and back, and over the apical, middle and basal zones of the lung.

A blocked bronchus leading to lung collapse or a layer of fluid or air between the visceral and parietal layers of the pleura (pleural effusion) suppresses the conduction of sound waves and reduces the intensity of the palpable fremitus.

Regional lymph nodes The axillary and supraclavicular lymph nodes may be enlarged by infection (e.g. tuberculosis or malignant lung/gastric tumours [metastases]).

Percussion

The whole of the surface of both lungs must be percussed. The surface markings of the lungs are shown in Figure 2.3.

Place the left hand flat on the chest wall, keeping the middle finger, which you intend to strike, straight and firmly applied to the underlying skin. Tap the centre of the middle phalanx of this middle finger with the tip of the middle finger of the right hand by forcibly flexing the right wrist (Figure 2.4). Listen carefully to the sound and compare it with the sound produced by percussing the same area on the other side of the chest.

Percuss over the whole of the front and back of both lung fields. The two areas most often forgotten are the lateral zones high in the axillae and the anterior aspect of the lung apices behind the clavicles. Percuss the latter area by striking the clavicle directly with the percussing finger.

The normal chest gives a resonant sound when percussed, a sound that is, to some extent, felt by the percussing finger as well as being heard. Anything solid in the pleural space or in the substance of the lungs decreases the resonance and makes the sound dull. Any extra air, whether in the pleural space (a

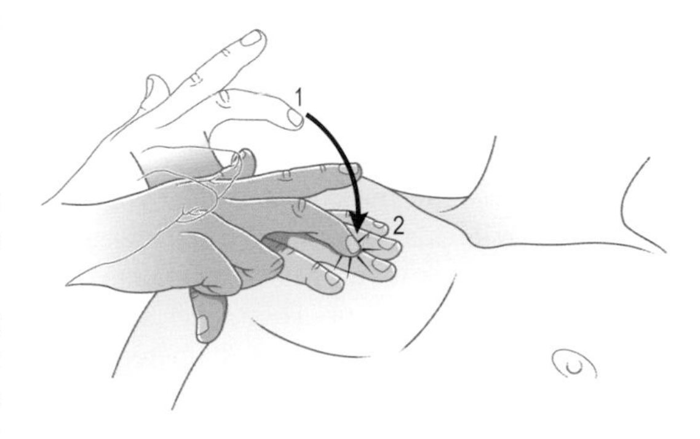

Figure 2.4 Percussion (see text above).

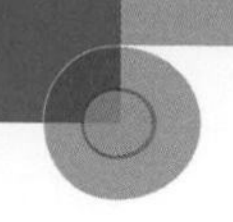

pneumothorax) or in the lung substance (an emphysematous bulla or multiple bullae), makes the sound more resonant (hyper-resonance).

Auscultation

The normal sounds of breathing can be heard all over the chest except over the heart and spine. A longer 'rustling' inspiratory sound is followed immediately by a shorter, softer, expiratory sound. There is no gap between the two phases. This noise is known as *vesicular breathing* and is caused by the movement of air in and out of the smaller bronchioles and alveoli. It produces a rustling noise.

The sound of air moving in the larger bronchioles and main bronchi is heard over the lung fields when the periphery of the lung has been solidified by pneumonia or collapse (*atelectasis*). This sound is harsher and louder than the low rustle of vesicular breathing. The inspiratory and expiratory phases are of equal length and separated by a short, silent gap. This is called *bronchial breathing.* The quality of the sound and the presence of the gap are the two distinguishing features.

When the lung alveoli are full of fluid, exudate or pus (*consolidation*) but the air passages remain patent, the thickened lung transmits the sound from the larger bronchi, and bronchial breathing indicates an area of consolidated lung.

Absent breath sounds

Breath sounds are abolished or diminished by any process that reduces the normal conduction of sound through the lung substance and chest wall. The common causes are bronchial obstruction (producing collapse of the distal part of the lung), pleural effusion and a large pneumothorax.

Added sounds

Wheezes These are the unmistakable whistling sounds made by air passing through narrowed air passages. They are commonly heard in patients with asthma or chronic bronchitis. Their pitch depends upon the velocity of airflow and the diameter of the bronchioles from which they originate.

Crackles These are caused by air passing through bronchioles containing water, mucus or pus. They may be coarse or fine.

Pleural rub The visceral and parietal layers of the pleura normally slide easily over one another without causing any sound. If the pleura is inflamed, the roughened pleural surfaces rubbing together during inspiration and expiration can produce a noise that is similar to walking in fresh snow. It is a mixture of grating and squeaking sounds. The patient often complains of pleuritic pain over the area where the rub can be heard.

EXAMINATION OF THE HEART AND CIRCULATION

It is common practice to feel the pulse when you take the patient's hand at the beginning of the examination (see above). Any abnormalities detected at this stage require reassessment by further careful palpation of the radial pulse. (see Chapter 10)

The pulse

The following features should be observed and recorded.

The rate Count for 15 seconds or longer, especially if the pulse feels irregular, and express the rate in beats/minute.

The rhythm The pulse beat may be regular or irregular. When the pulse is irregular, it may have a regular recurring pattern or be totally irregular. The latter is called an *irregularly irregular* pulse and indicates *atrial fibrillation* (Figure 2.5).

The volume The examining fingers can appreciate the expansion of the artery with each beat, and consequently get an impression of the amount of blood passing through the artery. Patients with a high cardiac output have a strong pulse. Patients in haemorrhagic (hypovolaemic) shock have a weak, thin, 'thready' pulse.

The nature of the pressure wave Every pressure wave has definable characteristics such as the rate of increase and decrease of pressure, and the height of the pressure. The shape of the pulse wave can be

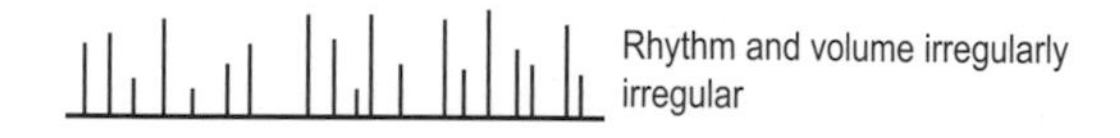

Figure 2.5 Atrial fibrillation.

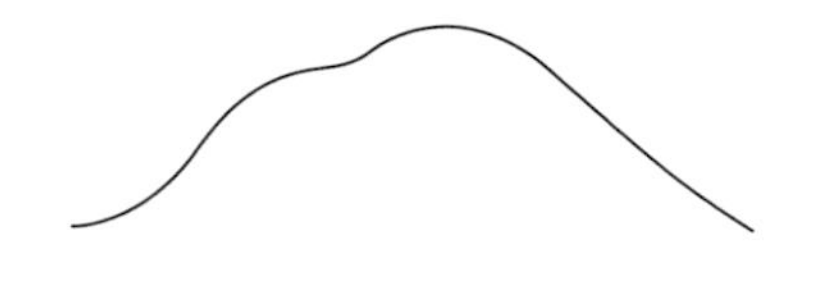

Figure 2.6 An anacrotic pulse.

appreciated more easily over the carotid than the radial artery.

A steep rise followed by a rapid fall, with a large pulse pressure (high peak), is called a *collapsing* or *water-hammer pulse* and is typical of *aortic regurgitation*. Conversely, a *tight aortic stenosis* causes a flattened pulse with a slow rise and fall, called an *anacrotic pulse* (Figure 2.6).

Compare the pulses of both wrists This should always be done because a stenosis or occlusion of the subclavian artery, or an aortic dissection, can produce asymmetrical pulses.

Measure the blood pressure

The blood pressure is usually measured in the brachial artery with a sphygmomanometer. The cuff, which must fit snugly and be at least 10 cm wide (as a narrow cuff gives false readings), should be firmly wrapped around the middle of the upper arm and inflated above the systolic pressure. It should then be slowly deflated until the start of blood flow is detected by listening over the brachial artery at the elbow with a stethoscope or by palpating the pulse at the wrist. This pressure is the *systolic blood pressure*.

The sounds that indicate the commencement of flow in the brachial artery below the cuff are caused by turbulent blood flow. They were first described by Korotkoff and are known as *Korotkoff sounds*.

The cuff is further deflated until the Korotkoff sounds suddenly diminish or, more often, disappear. This is the *diastolic pressure*.

It is worth repeating both measurements on several occasions with the patient sitting and lying down and again at the end of the examination when the patient is more relaxed. Remember that the readings from a very fat arm will be falsely high by as much as 10 mmHg.

NOTE: Whenever there is the possibility of disease of the aorta and its branches, the blood pressure should be measured in both arms.

Inspect the head and neck

The signs particularly indicative of cardiovascular disease are cyanosis, plethora, xanthomata, arcus senilis and dyspnoea.

Jugular venous pressure

The pressure in the great veins is slightly greater than the pressure in the right atrium. The pressure in the right atrium is one of the most important indicators and influences of cardiac activity. An increase in the right atrial pressure increases cardiac output by stimulating an increase of cardiac contractility and rate.

The pressure in the right atrium can be estimated clinically from the pressure in the internal jugular veins. In a normal person reclining at 45°, the great veins in the neck are collapsed, and there should be no visible venous pulsations above the level of the manubrio-sternal joint. When the patient is reclining at 45°, this is at the same level as the mid-point of the clavicles (Figure 2.7). The venous pulse is seen as a double pulse wave followed by a pause, and may be elevated or visualized by compressing over the liver to increase the venous return.

The right atrial pressure is raised if there are visible pulsations in the internal jugular veins when the patient is reclining at 45°. The vertical distance between the upper limit of the venous distension and the level of the clavicle should be estimated by eye and expressed and recorded in centimetres.

Obstruction of the great veins in the superior mediastinum will also cause distension of the neck veins, but there is no visible venous pulse wave within the distended veins.

Neck arteries

The carotid, subclavian and superficial temporal pulses should be palpated in the head and neck. The whole length of the subclavian and carotid arteries should be auscultated for bruits, especially over the sternoclavicular joints, in the supraclavicular fossae

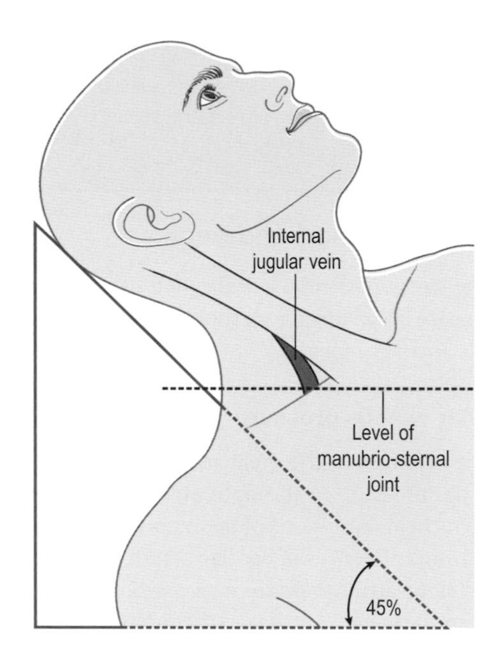

Figure 2.7 Measurement of jugular venous pressure.

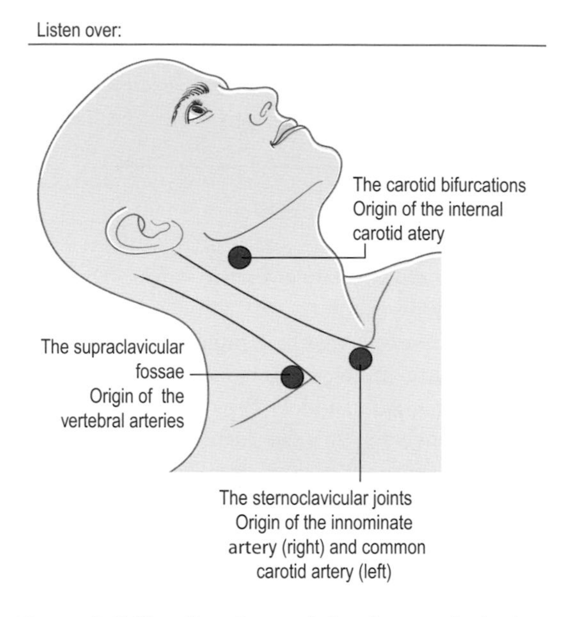

Figure 2.8 The sites of auscultation for vascular bruits on the neck.

and at the level of the hyoid bone just below the angle of the jaw. These sites correspond to the origins of the subclavian, vertebral and internal carotid arteries, respectively (Figure 2.8).

Examination of the heart

Inspection The heart may be seen to be beating rapidly or to be heaving up the chest wall with each beat.

Palpation Place your whole hand firmly on the chest wall, just below the left nipple, and ascertain the strength of the cardiac impulse. It may be weak, normal or heaving in nature.

The *apex beat* is the lowest and most lateral point at which the cardiac impulse can be felt. It should be in the fifth intercostal space, in the mid-clavicular line (an imaginary vertical line that passes through the middle of the clavicle). The apex beat moves laterally and may be felt in the mid-axillary line if the heart is enlarged.

It may also be possible to feel vibrations, called *thrills*, which correspond to audible heart murmurs. Thrills may be felt during systole, during diastole or throughout the whole cardiac cycle.

Remember to palpate the back of the chest. Thrills from abnormalities of the aorta, such as a *patent ductus arteriosus or a coarctation of the aorta*, are conducted posteriorly as well as anteriorly.

Percussion The area of cardiac dullness should be delineated by percussion.

Auscultation The whole of the anterior aspect of the heart must be examined with the stethoscope, but the areas where the sounds from the four valves are best heard are shown in Figure 2.9.

Begin by listening at the apex of the heart (the mitral area) before listening over the aortic, pulmonary and tricuspid areas. Identify the *first and second heart sounds.*

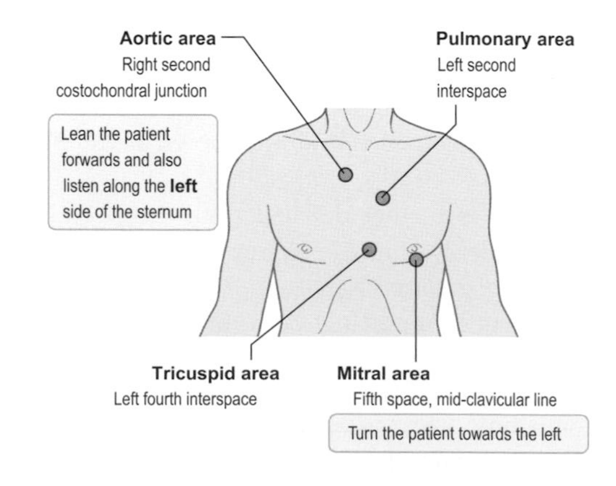

Figure 2.9 Areas of cardiac auscultation.

The heart sounds are traditionally described as sounding like the words *lub-dub*; that is to say, the first sound is slightly longer and softer than the second sound. As this is not always the case, it is wise to confirm that the sound you believe to be the first sound corresponds to the beginning of the cardiac impulse or coincides with the subclavian or carotid pulse.

Having decided which sound is which, listen carefully to the *second sound*. It may be sharper and shorter than usual – almost a *click* – or it may be *split*. A double, or split, second sound occurs when the aortic and pulmonary valves close asynchronously. A double sound can be heard when the sounds are 0.2 or more seconds apart and indicates *pulmonary hypertension*.

Next, listen carefully to the intervals between the two main sounds, and between diastole and systole, for any *additional heart sounds or murmurs*.

Murmurs are caused by turbulent flow and the vibration of parts of the heart. They may vary in nature from a low-pitched rumble to a high-toned swish. Try to decide whether the murmur occupies the whole or part of diastole or systole and whether its intensity changes.

Think of the way you are going to record your findings (Figure 2.10), two blocks for the main heart sounds (M and T, and A and P) and a zig-zag line for the murmur. Imagine your drawing as you listen to the sound and you will find it easier to define the timing of the murmur.

The sounds at the apex, from the mitral valve, can be made louder by asking the patient to turn over onto their left side; the aortic valve sounds can be amplified by asking the patient to lean forwards.

Always listen to the heart sounds at the back of the chest. The murmur of a patent ductus or coarctation can often be heard over the aorta, posteriorly, just to the left of the midline.

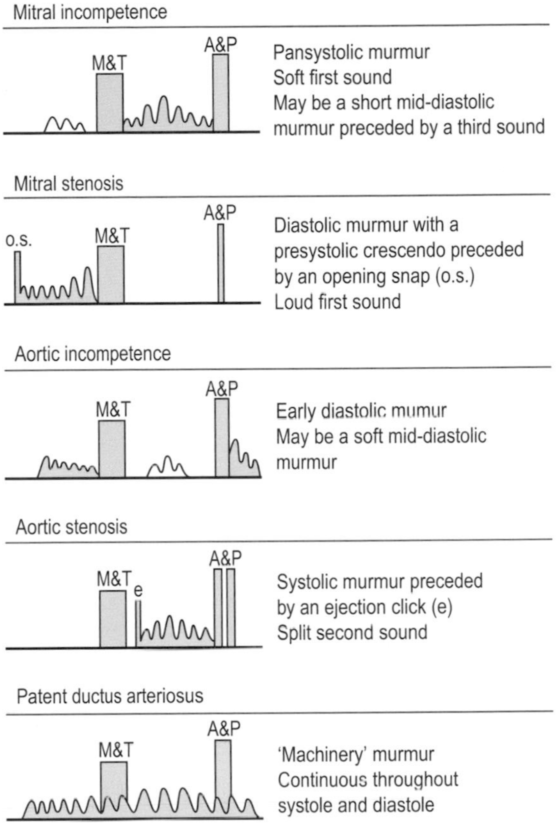

Figure 2.10 The sounds of some common cardiac abnormalities. M & T, first heart sound; A & P, second heart sound.

Test for oedema

Oedema commonly appears first in the feet and ankles, but may be more apparent in the sacral and buttock regions if the patient has been bedridden for some time. Cardiac oedema is very soft and 'pits' easily. The common causes of ankle oedema are listed in Revision panel 2.1.

Revision panel 2.1

COMMON CAUSES OF ANKLE SWELLING

- Dependency/immobility
- Pregnancy
- Heart failure
- Low plasma proteins
- Chronic venous insufficiency
- Deep vein thrombosis
- Lymphatic insufficiency
- Chronic renal failure (nephrotic syndrome)

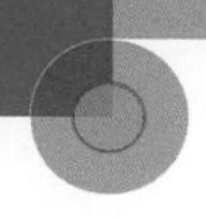

Revision panel 2.2

CAUSES OF BREATHLESSNESS

Airways

- Asthma
- Chronic obstructive pulmonary disease
- Airways obstruction (e.g. tumour of the trachea or major bronchi, inhaled foreign body, sputum retention)/tracheomalacia

Lung parenchyma

- Pneumonia
- Pulmonary oedema
- Interstitial lung disease (pulmonary fibrosis)
- Chronic obstructive pulmonary disease/ emphysema/bullous lung disease
- Primary and metastatic lung cancer
- Bronchiectasis
- Pulmonary haemorrhage/pulmonary contusion

Pleural space

- Pleural effusion
- Pneumothorax
- Pleural tumour (e.g. mesothelioma)
- Haemothorax
- Empyema

Heart and pulmonary vasculature

- Valvular heart disease
- Ischaemic heart disease
- Pulmonary embolus/pulmonary hypertension
- Cardiomyopathies
- Arrhythmias
- Pericardial effusion
- Cyanotic congenital heart disease

Chest wall and diaphragm

- Trauma (fractured ribs) with associated pain
- Flail chest
- Diaphragmatic hernia
- Diaphragmatic paralysis

Mediastinum

- Mediastinal lymphadenopathy
- Large mediastinal mass

Other

- Anaemia
- Hyperthyroidism

BREATHLESSNESS

Breathlessness is usually the result of lung or heart disease, although it can be caused by severe anaemia (see Chapter 1). The causes are summarized in Revision panel 2.2.

Dyspnoea is the sensation of breathlessness experienced by patients. It is usually first felt during exercise, such as climbing hills and stairs. As symptoms become more severe, patients may be breathless on minimal exertion (e.g. dressing or brushing their teeth) or even at rest.

CHARACTERISTICS OF BREATHLESSNESS

Onset and duration

Dyspnoea of *acute onset* is usually noticed at rest. Development over a few minutes suggests an inhaled foreign body, a pneumothorax, severe acute asthma, a pulmonary embolism or pulmonary oedema (often from an acute myocardial infarction or decompensation of pre-existing heart failure).

Development over a slightly longer period – typically hours to days – is more characteristic of pneumonia, acute asthma, chronic obstructive pulmonary disease exacerbations, retained secretions, a haemothorax, an empyema or pulmonary haemorrhage.

Chronic breathlessness is often first noticed on exercise and increases with time. In airway obstruction secondary to an endobronchial tumour, a pleural effusion, a pericardial effusion or anaemia, symptoms develop over weeks or months.

The onset of breathlessness can be much more insidious, perhaps over several years, with many patients attributing their symptoms to 'old age'. Conditions that present like this include interstitial lung disease and chronic obstructive pulmonary disease. Mediastinal masses, hyperthyroidism and cardiac disorders (including ischaemic heart disease with heart failure, valvular heart disease and the cardiomyopathies) also develop slowly.

Severity

The severity of chronic breathlessness from lung disease is graded according to the Medical Research

Revision panel 2.3

MRC DYSPNOEA SCALE

1. Not troubled by breathlessness except on strenuous exercise
2. Short of breath when hurrying or walking up a slight hill
3. Walks slower than contemporaries on level ground because of breathlessness, or has to stop for breath when walking at own pace
4. Stops for breath after walking about 100 m or after a few minutes on level ground
5. Too breathless to leave the house, or breathless when dressing or undressing

Revision panel 2.4

NEW YORK HEART ASSOCIATION FUNCTIONAL CLASSIFICATION

1. Cardiac disease present, but no symptoms and no limitation in ordinary physical activity, such as walking and climbing stairs
2. Mild symptoms (mild shortness of breath and/or angina) and slight limitation during ordinary activity
3. Marked limitation in activity caused by symptoms, even during less-than-ordinary activity such as walking short distances (20–100 m). Comfortable only at rest
4. Severe limitations, with symptoms even at rest. Mostly bedbound

Council Dyspnoea Scale, a useful measure of disability (Revision panel 2.3).

The equivalent scale for heart disease is the New York Heart Association Functional Classification (Revision panel 2.4). A higher New York Heart Association class is associated with a worse prognosis.

Effect of posture

Orthopnoea is the sensation or worsening of breathlessness when lying flat caused by redistribution of blood volume from the lower extremities to the lungs, with resulting pulmonary oedema secondary to heart failure. Patients often sleep with several pillows or in an upright position.

Trepopnoea is breathlessness experienced while lying on one side, but not on the other. It is a symptom of unilateral chest disease (such as a collapsed lung secondary to endobronchial obstruction). The patient tends to lie with the diseased side upwards, as this eases symptoms by increasing perfusion to the good lung (reducing ventilation/perfusion mismatch through the diseased lung).

Nocturnal breathlessness

Paroxysmal nocturnal dyspnoea occurs in patients with heart failure. The mechanism is similar to orthopnoea. After several hours' sleep, the patient wakes with a frightening sensation of suffocation. Pulmonary congestion decreases when the patient sits upright and symptoms usually subside after half an hour.

Associated symptoms

Fatigue and lethargy are commonly associated with chronic dyspnoea. Patients report a progressive reduction in exercise tolerance. Anorexia and weight loss may also occur.

Pneumothorax

A pneumothorax is a collection of air within the pleural space resulting in lung collapse. It can cause respiratory and eventually haemodynamic distress, depending on the size and type of pneumothorax (Figure 2.11).

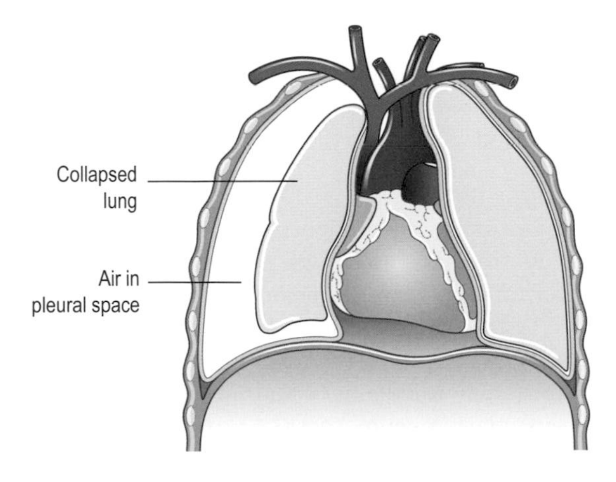

Figure 2.11 Pneumothorax.

Revision panel 2.5

CAUSES OF PNEUMOTHORAX

Primary

Apical bleb or bulla

Secondary

Chronic obstructive pulmonary disease and emphysema
Cystic fibrosis
Cavitating infections and tumours (e.g. tuberculosis)
Pneumocystis jiroveci (carinii) pneumonia in AIDS patients
Alpha-1 antitrypsin deficiency
Connective tissue disorders
Catamenial pneumothorax (associated with menstruation)
Trauma (blunt or penetrating)

Primary spontaneous pneumothoraces are caused by a ruptured apical subpleural 'bleb' (a 1–2 mm thin walled, probably congenital, cyst) or bulla. Secondary spontaneous pneumothoraces are the result of underlying lung disease. The most common cause is a ruptured bulla on a background of emphysema. Other causes are listed in Revision panel 2.5.

History

Age Primary spontaneous pneumothoraces occur in young adults (peak age 16–30 years). Secondary pneumothoraces tend to occur in late middle and old age.

Symptoms The two main symptoms are shortness of breath and pleuritic chest pain localized to the side of the pneumothorax. The onset is usually sudden. There may have been similar episodes before, but the first episode is often very frightening for the patient.

Previous history

In primary spontaneous pneumothorax, there are no predisposing factors. Smoking is only a risk factor for recurrence. A history of chronic lung disease, particularly chronic obstructive pulmonary disease as a result of smoking, will almost certainly be present in middle-aged and elderly patients with a secondary pneumothorax. Marfan's syndrome (see Chapter 1) is associated with an increased incidence of pneumothorax in younger people.

Examination

General appearance Patients who present with a primary pneumothorax are typically tall (>190 cm), thin and usually male (M:F ratio 6:1).

The stigmata of the underlying chest disease may be present in patients with a secondary pneumothorax. Patients with chronic obstructive pulmonary disease may have a barrel-shaped chest and pursed-lip breathing.

Inspection Tachypnoea (a respiratory rate of more than 20 breaths per minute) is often present. Respiratory rates may be significantly higher with a large pneumothorax or when there is severe underlying chest disease. Tachycardia is common, but evidence of shock indicates a tension pneumothorax (see below). In severe cases, there may be central cyanosis but surgical emphysema is uncommon (Figure 2.12).

Palpation The trachea is usually central in the case of a simple pneumothorax. Deviation to the contralateral side occurs in tension pneumothorax. Surgical emphysema is sometimes palpable just beneath the skin covering the anterior chest wall and neck.

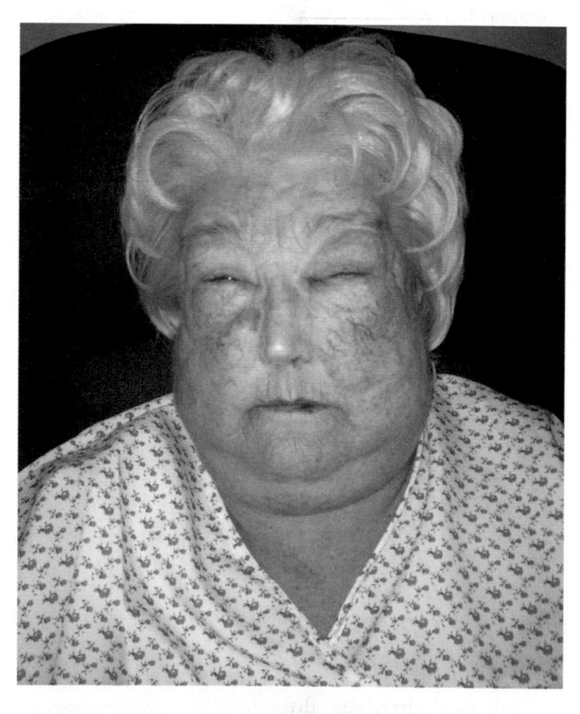

Figure 2.12 Gross surgical emphysema in a patient with a drained pneumothorax and ongoing air leak. Pressure applied by fingers gives a 'dent' and feels like egg shells cracking.

Percussion Classically, a hyper-resonant, or *tympanic*, percussion note is detected on the ipsilateral side.

Auscultation Air entry on the ipsilateral side is quiet or absent, while breath sounds and air entry on the contralateral side should be normal. A crackling sound will be heard as the stethoscope compresses the skin if surgical emphysema is present.

TENSION PNEUMOTHORAX

This uncommon but dangerous condition occurs if a breach in the visceral pleura covering the lung acts as a one-way valve between the lung and the pleural space. The volume and pressure of air in the pleural space increase with every breath, causing movement of the mediastinum away from the pneumothorax, reduced venous return to the heart and eventually shock (Figure 2.13).

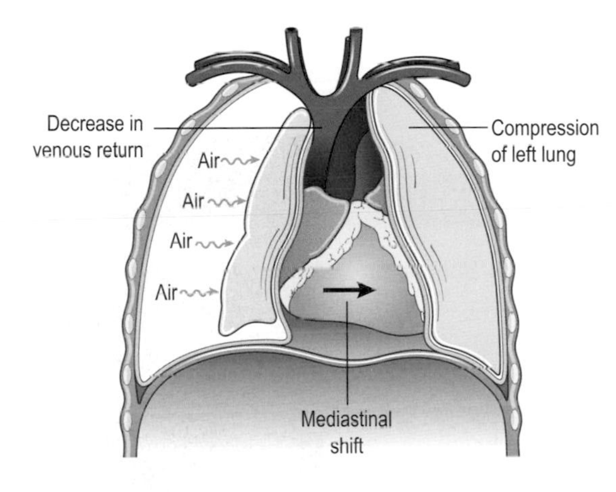

Figure 2.13 Tension pneumothorax.

Examination

On examination, there will be distended neck veins, deviation of the trachea to the contralateral side and signs of shock if left untreated. Urgent measures are needed to avoid death.

Pleural effusion

This is defined as fluid in the pleural space, formed when the rate of pleural fluid production is greater than the rate of resorption (Figure 2.14). Increased production of fluid occurs in diseases

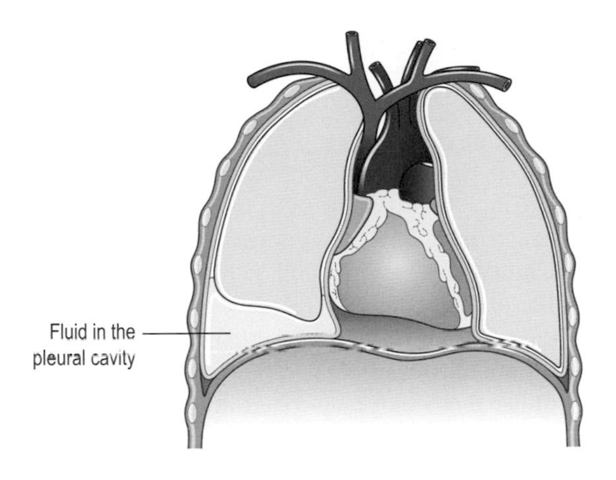

Figure 2.14 Pleural effusion.

Revision panel 2.6

CAUSES OF A PLEURAL EXUDATE

Chest

- Pneumonia (may lead to empyema)
- Other infections (e.g. tuberculosis)
- Malignancy (e.g. mesothelioma, lung cancer, metastatic disease)
- Pulmonary embolus
- Trapped lung, where the lung cannot expand because of a constricting coat caused by infection or tumour

Gastrointestinal tract, abdomen and pelvis

- Acute pancreatitis
- Subphrenic abscess
- Meig's syndrome (associated ovarian tumour)

Iatrogenic

- Radiation therapy
- Postsurgery (e.g. coronary artery bypass, liver transplant)
- Collagen vascular disease
- Rheumatoid arthritis
- Systemic lupus erythematosus
- Granulomatosis with polyangiitis

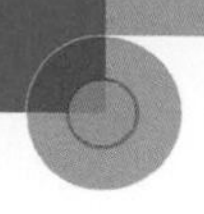

causing pleural inflammation or in heart failure, while reduced fluid resorption can be caused by tumour deposits.

Bilateral effusions tend to be transudates, characterized by a protein content of less than 30 g/L, occurring in heart failure, hypoalbuminaemia, liver failure, renal failure or hypothyroidism.

Unilateral effusions tend to be exudates with a higher protein content. The many causes are shown in Revision panel 2.6. Pleural infection and malignancy are most common.

Other fluids that may collect in the pleural space include blood (haemothorax), chyle (chylothorax) and gastric contents (e.g. following oesophageal perforation).

History

Age Patients with pleural effusions are usually elderly because the underlying diseases are more common in this age group.

Symptoms Shortness of breath and chest discomfort are the two main symptoms. There is usually a progressive increase in the severity of symptoms over several months. In patients with pneumonia, this may be days or weeks, and after an oesophageal rupture the effusion is immediate (see Chapter 15).

Occasionally, chest pain is severe, especially with pleural malignancy. The pain is usually pleuritic in nature. Invasion of the chest wall can cause deep-seated pain. Weight loss and general malaise may also occur.

Previous history

Occupational exposure to asbestos makes mesothelioma more likely (see below). A history of previously treated malignancy, particularly cancers of the lung or breast or a cancer of gynaecological origin, may indicate a metastatic relapse.

Examination

Effusions of more than 300 mL are usually detectable clinically at the lung bases.

General appearance There may be stigmata of the underlying cause, such as rheumatoid arthritis, systemic lupus erythematosus or heart failure. Wasting and cachexia are present in advanced metastatic malignancy.

Inspection A high respiratory rate indicates a large effusion, bilateral effusions or a patient with little respiratory reserve.

Reduced chest wall movement is sometimes seen on the side of the effusion.

Palpation The trachea is usually central, except with massive effusions, when it may be deviated away from the affected side.

Tactile vocal fremitus is reduced over the effusion.

Percussion The percussion note over the fluid is described as *stony dull.*

Auscultation Air entry is reduced or absent under the fluid. Sometimes bronchial breathing can be heard in the collapsed lung just above the fluid level. Vocal resonance is reduced, differentiating the effusion from consolidation.

Chylothorax produces physical signs identical to those of a pleural effusion. Half of the cases are caused by trauma, most commonly iatrogenic damage to the thoracic duct during chest surgery. Malignancy (lymphoma or metastatic disease) accounts for the bulk of the remaining cases.

Mesothelioma

Mesotheliomas are rare malignant tumours arising from the mesothelial layer of the pleura. In almost all cases, the cause is asbestos exposure, typically 30–40 years earlier. The incidence in the UK has peaked at around 2600 new cases per year, and is projected to fall by ~50% by 2035.

History

Dyspnoea results from either the presence of a pleural effusion or the mass effect of the pleural tumour. The underlying lung may not able to re-expand after drainage of an effusion if it is encased by tumour on the visceral pleural surface (*trapped lung*).

Chest pain is either pleuritic, or more deep-seated and 'gnawing' in nature as a consequence of chest wall and intercostal nerve invasion.

Examination

On examination, the physical signs are those of a pleural effusion.

Empyema

An empyema is a collection of pus in the pleural space (Figure 2.15).

An empyema develops from a parapneumonic effusion complicating a pneumonia. Only a small proportion of these effusions go on to become empyemas.

An iatrogenic empyema can complicate chest surgery or chest drain insertion.

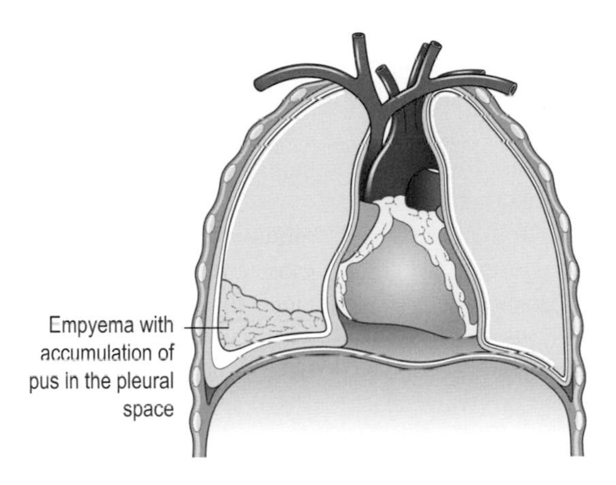

Figure 2.15 Empyema.

There are three stages in the development of an empyema:

1. **Exudative**. A simple pleural effusion becomes complicated by infection.
2. **Fibrinopurulent**. A macroscopically purulent effusion develops with fibrin deposition, which may cause the effusion to become loculated.
3. **Organizing/chronic**. The pus is viscous and both the visceral and parietal pleurae become thickened, encasing the lung.

History

Age An empyema complicating a pneumonia can occur at any age.

Symptoms There is often a history of a respiratory tract infection, or symptoms of general malaise, over the previous few weeks or months.

Patients may be *breathless* caused by lung compression by the pleural pus, restriction of normal chest wall and lung excursion by scar tissue over the parietal and visceral pleura, or lung consolidation.

Vague ipsilateral chest discomfort or pleuritic chest pain is sometimes a dominant feature.

Fever is common, and the patient may experience sweats and rigors.

A *cough with purulent sputum* may still persist from the original pneumonia.

Examination

General appearance Although some patients look relatively well, others show signs of systemic sepsis (hypotension, tachycardia and respiratory distress).

A swinging fever, typical of a collection of pus, is often seen, and the patient may appear flushed and sweaty.

Inspection Chest movement may be reduced on the affected side. The trachea is only deviated if there is associated lung collapse (deviated to the ipsilateral side) or a massive effusion (deviated to the contralateral side).

Palpation Vocal resonance is reduced over an empyema, and there may be reduced chest wall excursion.

Percussion A dull or stony dull percussion note is characteristic of an effusion or empyema.

Auscultation Air entry is usually reduced or absent over the empyema.

Untreated, serious complications can develop (Revision panel 2.7).

Revision panel 2.7

COMPLICATIONS OF AN EMPYEMA

Bronchopleural fistula (invasion into the bronchial tree)
Empyema necessitatis (invasion through the chest wall with spontaneous external drainage)
Hemithorax contraction secondary to chronic pleural fibrosis
Osteomyelitis (Figure 2.16)
Death

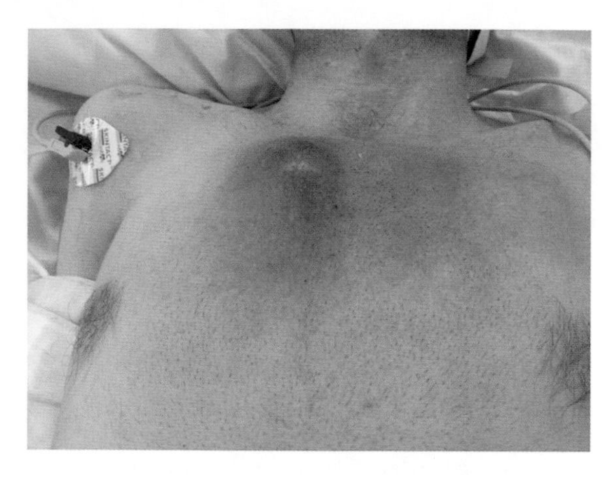

Figure 2.16 Sternal osteomyelitis in an intravenous drug user following a traumatic sternal fracture.

Pulmonary embolism

Pulmonary embolism is usually a complication of venous thromboembolic disease (see Chapter 10) (Revision panel 2.8). Less frequently, air, fat and amniotic fluid embolize to the lungs. Reduced pulmonary blood flow, local inflammation and right heart strain are responsible for the ensuing signs and symptoms.

History

Age Although the incidence increases with age, pulmonary emboli can occur at any age.

Symptoms Many pulmonary emboli are symptomless, while some present as sudden death.

Revision panel 2.8

RISK FACTORS FOR DEEP VEIN THROMBOSIS/PULMONARY EMBOLUS

- Immobility
- Surgery
- Pregnancy
- Obesity
- Cancer
- Increasing age
- Genetic thrombophilias (e.g. protein C deficiency, protein S deficiency, antithrombin III deficiency, antiphospholipid syndrome)
- Acquired prothrombotic disorders (e.g. nephrotic syndrome)

The most common clinical presentation is with a sudden onset of breathlessness, often accompanied by pleuritic chest pain. The pain may heighten the sensation of breathlessness by preventing deep inspiration. Haemoptysis occasionally occurs.

Some patients present with a *swollen painful leg* secondary to an underlying *deep venous thrombosis* (see Chapter 10, page 364).

Examination

Inspection Patients who have had a massive pulmonary embolism may be centrally and peripherally cyanosed (see Chapter 1), with tachypnoea and signs of cardiovascular collapse (tachycardia, hypotension, cool peripheries).

A raised jugular venous pressure is indicative of right heart strain.

Even in severe cases, examination of the chest is often normal except for the presence of tachypnoea.

Auscultation A pleural rub may appear later in the disease process. Right ventricular strain can produce a loud second heart sound as a result of loud pulmonary valve closure. Fixed splitting of the second heart sound may develop.

Lung cancer

Lung cancer is the most common cause of cancer death in the world. Smoking is the main risk factor, and around one in 10 smokers develop lung cancer. Around 40,000 new patients are diagnosed each year in the UK, of whom less than 10% survive 5 years.

There are two main histological types: small cell, and non-small cell.

- *Non-small cell* tumours comprise 80–85% of all lung cancers and include adenocarcinomas (~35–40%), squamous cell carcinomas (~20–30%) and large cell carcinomas (~10%).
- *Small cell* tumours are less common (10–15%) and are part of a spectrum of neuroendocrine lung malignancies that includes carcinoid tumours and large cell neuroendocrine carcinomas.

Common sites of distant spread include the mediastinal lymph nodes, the liver, the adrenal glands, the bones and the brain. Metastases are more common in small cell carcinoma than in other types.

History

Age The incidence of lung cancer increases with age and is uncommon before the age of 50 years.

Symptoms Around one-fifth of patients are symptomless when diagnosed, their lung cancer being picked up incidentally on a routine chest X-ray. These patients are likely to have operable disease, but those with symptoms tend to have more advanced disease.

Patients may also present acutely with chest sepsis, thromboembolic disease, hypercalcaemia or other symptoms of metastatic disease.

Shortness of breath may be caused by:

- Pneumonia, lobar collapse or lung collapse distal to an obstructing bronchial tumour.
- Partial obstruction of the major airways (trachea or main bronchi) by endobronchial tumour, causing impaired airflow.
- Extrinsic compression of the major airways by mediastinal invasion or mediastinal lymphadenopathy.
- Invasion and occlusion of a pulmonary artery.
- Pulmonary emboli.
- Pleural or pericardial effusions secondary to metastatic spread of disease or direct pleural or pericardial invasion.
- Diaphragmatic palsy caused by invasion of the phrenic nerve.
- Underlying chronic obstructive pulmonary disease or emphysema.
- Anaemia.

Cough is a common symptom. It may have an insidious onset and is often persistent and non-productive in nature. Coughs are caused by local irritation of the airways or recurrent chest infections secondary to bronchial obstruction.

Haemoptysis may occur but is usually of small volume.

Chest pain can occur in more peripheral tumours. Pleuritic pain may be a consequence of repeated chest infections and pleural inflammation. Invasion of the chest wall produces a localized deep, gnawing pain. Subsequent involvement of the intercostal nerve causes pain referred anteriorly to the affected dermatome.

Non-specific symptoms such as loss of appetite, weight loss, malaise, fatigue and low-grade fevers are common. Significant weight loss is a poor prognostic sign.

Other symptoms caused by local spread include:

- Stridor from involvement of the major airways by either endobronchial tumour or extrinsic compression.
- Facial swelling as a result of superior vena cava obstruction secondary to mediastinal lymphadenopathy or invasive right hilar tumours.
- Dysphagia from direct invasion or extrinsic compression of the oesophagus.
- Hoarseness from invasion of the recurrent laryngeal nerve (usually the left nerve because of its origin in the aortopulmonary window and long course in the chest).
- Arm pain (brachial plexus invasion in a Pancoast tumour, see below).
- Palpitations from pericardial involvement.

Symptoms from distant spread are present in 30–40% of patients at diagnosis. These include:

- Bone metastases, causing bone pain and pathological fractures.
- Brain metastases, resulting in space-occupying symptoms such as headache and nausea, and central nervous system signs.
- Liver metastases with abdominal pain and jaundice (see Chapter 15).
- Paraneoplastic syndromes (Revision panel 2.9).

Risk factors Ninety per cent of patients with lung cancer will be current or ex-smokers. A smoking history should be expressed in pack years – one packet of 20 cigarettes a day for 1 year equates to a pack year (7300 cigarettes!).

A previously cured lung cancer and exposure to asbestos or radon gas (e.g. from soil/bedrock) are other risk factors for lung cancer.

Examination

General appearance Cachexia may be the result of metastatic lung cancer or pre-existing emphysema.

Jaundice suggests liver metastases, while anaemia may be the result of significant or prolonged haemoptysis or the consequence of chronic disease.

Finger clubbing is a paraneoplastic syndrome (see page 77).

Examination of the neck may reveal metastatic cervical lymphadenopathy (see Chapter 12, page 404).

Revision panel 2.9

PARANEOPLASTIC SYNDROMES ASSOCIATED WITH LUNG CANCER

Endocrine/metabolic

Water retention with hyponatraemia (syndrome of inappropriate antidiuretic hormone secretion)
Hypercalcaemia (parathormone-like hormone)
Cushing's syndrome (adrenocorticotrophic hormone)
Gynaecomastia

Neurological

Peripheral neuropathy
Polymyositis
Eaton–Lambert syndrome

Skeletal

Finger clubbing
Hypertrophic pulmonary osteoarthropathy

Cutaneous

Hyperkeratosis
Hyperpigmentation
Dermatomyositis
Acanthosis nigricans

Distended neck veins are seen in both superior vena cava obstruction and pericardial effusion. The face and chest wall may also be engorged, swollen and plethoric in superior vena cava obstruction (Figure 2.17).

Horner's syndrome is the result of invasion of the stellate sympathetic ganglion, normally by a *Pancoast tumour* (see Chapter 1, page 26). Direct spread into the pericardium can produce arrhythmias or signs of cardiac tamponade (see below).

Examination of the respiratory system is often normal, but there may be signs of pneumonia, pleural effusion, lobar collapse, lung collapse or airway compression.

Inspection Stridor (see below) may be audible from the end of the bed, and is the result of critical airway narrowing. It is often associated with an increased respiratory effort.

Unilateral reduced chest movement can be caused by the collapse of a lobe or a lung secondary to bronchial obstruction.

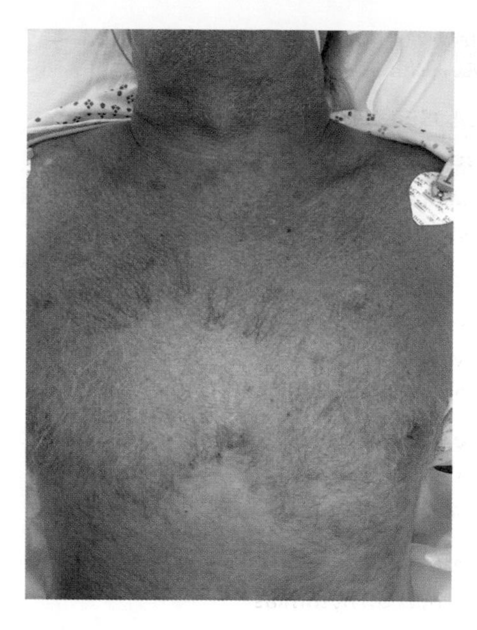

Figure 2.17 Acute superior vena cava obstruction secondary to locally advanced non-small cell lung cancer. The upper half of the torso is erythematous with engorged veins and venous flaring.

Palpation The trachea is deviated to the side of any lobar or lung collapse. By contrast, reduced chest movement with tracheal deviation to the contralateral side is seen with massive pleural effusions.

Percussion This is dull over a collapsed lung or a pleural effusion.

Auscultation Stridor or a wheeze may be heard over an area of major airway compression or partial obstruction.

Air entry is reduced over the affected lobe or throughout the whole lung in lobar or lung collapse respectively.

Coarse upper airways noises may be heard throughout if there are problems clearing secretions past an obstruction.

A localized area of bronchial breathing may be present over the collapsed lung.

Heart failure

Heart failure is the end result of all diseases of the heart. Over the age of 65 years, around 1 in 10 people will have heart failure. The causes are shown in Revision panel 2.10.

> **Revision panel 2.10**
>
> **CAUSES OF HEART FAILURE**
>
> **Ischaemic heart disease**
>
> Myocardial infarction
> Ongoing myocardial ischaemia
>
> **Hypertension**
>
> **Valvular heart disease**
>
> Mitral valve disease
> Aortic valve disease
>
> **Congenital heart disease**
>
> Atrial septal defect
> Ventricular septal defect
>
> **Cardiomyopathy**
>
> **Cardiac arrhythmias**
>
> **Alcohol and drugs**
>
> Alcohol
> Beta-blockers, calcium antagonists
>
> **Pericardial disease**
>
> Constrictive pericarditis
> Pericardial effusion
>
> **Primary right heart failure**
>
> Cor pulmonale
> Pulmonary embolism
> Primary pulmonary hypertension
> Tricuspid valve regurgitation

History

Shortness of breath/dyspnoea is the most common symptom and is the result of pulmonary oedema or reduced cardiac output. It is not a symptom specific for heart failure, but when accompanied by orthopnoea or paroxysmal nocturnal dyspnoea, heart failure is the likely diagnosis. Its severity is graded according to the New York Heart Association Functional Classification (see Revision panel 2.4).

Nocturnal cough or wheeze can also occur with pulmonary oedema.

Reduced exercise tolerance, with lethargy, fatigue and exertional dyspnoea, is due to reduced cardiac output, muscle wasting and loss of sleep from paroxysmal nocturnal dyspneoa.

Ankle swelling and tender hepatic enlargement are other common but non-specific symptoms of right heart failure (itself usually a consequence of left heart failure).

Previous history

Previous ischaemic heart disease, hypertension and valvular heart disease are common.

Examination

Inspection Cachexia and muscle wasting occur in severe heart failure, but in less severe forms there may be few physical signs.

Examination of the pulse may reveal tachycardia (as a result of sympathetic overdrive) or *pulsus alternans* (the poor prognostic sign of alternating weak and strong beats sometimes seen in left ventricular failure). Arrhythmias are also common, especially atrial fibrillation.

Distended neck veins (elevated jugular venous pressure) result from elevated right heart pressures (Figure 2.18).

Oedema of the ankles and feet is a common but non-specific sign – immobility is a more common cause of ankle swelling. In gross heart failure, tender hepatomegaly and ascites may be present.

Palpation A displaced apex beat indicates an enlarged heart, while right ventricular heave is a sign of right heart failure.

Auscultation Fine, usually bilateral inspiratory crepitations (crackles) heard at the lung bases indicate the presence of pulmonary oedema.

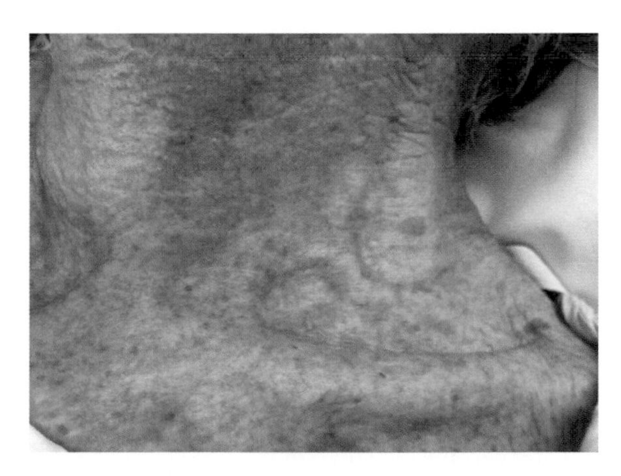

Figure 2.18 Distended neck veins in a patient with heart failure.

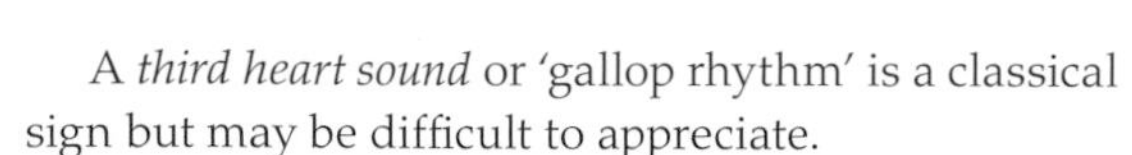

A *third heart sound* or 'gallop rhythm' is a classical sign but may be difficult to appreciate.

A *murmur* should be heard if the heart failure is secondary to valvular heart disease.

Valvular disease

MITRAL REGURGITATION

Mitral regurgitation is the most common heart valve disorder. It is often the result of 'floppy' valve prolapse or myxomatous degeneration. In the past, rheumatic heart disease was a common cause, usually associated with a degree of mitral stenosis.

Functional mitral regurgitation occurs as a result of left ventricular enlargement often caused by ischaemic heart disease. It can also occur with papillary muscle dysfunction or infarction following a myocardial infarction, or from valvular destruction in infective endocarditis.

Mitral regurgitation leads to volume overload (and increased preload) of the left heart because a significant proportion of the potential cardiac output is ejected back into the left atrium during systole, increasing pulmonary vascular pressure and the risk of pulmonary oedema.

History

Initially, mitral regurgitation is symptomless as the heart compensates by left atrial enlargement and left ventricular hypertrophy. As the regurgitation becomes more severe, the heart decompensates, with breathlessness on exertion, fatigue and other symptoms of heart failure/pulmonary oedema.

Palpitations are very common, and usually the result of atrial fibrillation.

Examination

General features The *irregularly irregular pulse* of atrial fibrillation is common, and a tachycardia may be present in those patients with decompensated heart failure. With more severe regurgitation, other signs of heart failure such as ankle oedema and a raised jugular venous pressure are likely.

Palpation The apex beat may be displaced to the left and become hyperdynamic.

Auscultation A pansystolic murmur loudest at the apex indicates mitral regurgitation. The murmur can radiate to the axilla or lower left back. Its loudness is not necessarily related to the severity of the regurgitation. *There may be a third heart sound* and subsequent heart failure is associated with the bilateral inspiratory crepitations of pulmonary oedema.

MITRAL STENOSIS

Beta-haemolytic *Streptococcus* throat infections cause rheumatic fever, associated heart disease and most cases of mitral stenosis. Bacterial antigens cross-react with various tissues including the heart valves, joints and basal ganglia (Sydenham's chorea). The valve commissures become fused, the leaflets thickened and the chordae shortened.

In countries where rheumatic fever is endemic (those with overcrowding and poor living conditions), mitral stenosis is the most common heart valve abnormality.

Narrowing of the mitral valve orifice leads to an increased pressure gradient across the valve during diastole. As the stenosis becomes more severe with time, the obstruction to the forward flow of blood becomes greater, resulting in increased left atrial pressures, atrial dilatation complicated by thrombosis, atrial fibrillation and pulmonary oedema from increased pulmonary vascular pressures. Right heart failure will also develop.

History

Initial symptoms are experienced 15–20 years after the first episode of rheumatic fever.

Breathlessness is the most common symptom, and is often worse on lying flat.

Fatigue and other symptoms of heart failure develop as the stenosis becomes more severe with reduced cardiac output. Associated heart failure can cause haemoptysis.

Palpitations are commonly the result of atrial fibrillation, the risk increasing with the degree of stenosis.

Thromboembolic disease presents most commonly as a *stroke* secondary to cerebral emboli due to thrombosis associated with atrial fibrillation in a dilated left atrium. Other sites for emboli are the legs and mesenteric vessels.

Examination

Inspection The term *'mitral facies'* refers to the red cheeks but otherwise pallid complexion of those with severe mitral stenosis. It is not a specific sign and is seen in some normal individuals.

Cachexia is not uncommon (see Chapter 1) and progresses with the severity of the stenosis, as do the other signs of heart failure.

Atrial fibrillation is common, particularly in the later stages of the disease.

Palpation The increased shock of closure of the mitral valve may be appreciated as a 'tapping' apex beat. Sometimes the murmur of mitral stenosis can be felt as a thrill, which may be described as feeling like the back of a purring cat. A left parasternal or right ventricular heave indicates pulmonary hypertension and right heart failure.

Auscultation An opening snap is heard immediately after the second heart sound, followed by a low-pitched mid-diastolic murmur. These added sounds are heard best with the patient turned towards their left side.

AORTIC REGURGITATION

Aortic regurgitation often coexists with aortic stenosis, as any pathological process that restricts valve opening can also impair valve closure. Causes of regurgitation include rheumatic fever, a congenital bicuspid aortic valve, infective endocarditis, aortic dissection and syphilis. Dilatation of the aortic root and ascending aorta as a result of Marfan's syndrome or annuloaortic ectasia is another cause (see Chapter 1).

The result is volume overload and increased preload of the left heart. A proportion of the cardiac output flows back into the left ventricle from the aorta during diastole. This leads to left ventricular hypertrophy and dilatation, and eventually to heart failure if left untreated.

History

Patients with acute aortic regurgitation secondary to infective endocarditis or aortic dissection can present with acute heart failure and cardiovascular collapse. Those with chronic aortic regurgitation may, however, be symptomless for a considerable period of time because the left ventricle adapts to the volume overload. As the heart begins to decompensate, symptoms of heart failure appear.

Examination

Inspection In the later stages of the disease, signs of heart failure may be obvious. A number of specific signs can be attributed to the low diastolic blood pressure and wide pulse pressure found in aortic regurgitation:

- *Water hammer pulse*: accentuation of the radial pulse when lifting the arm.
- *Quincke's sign*: capillary pulsation in the nail beds.
- *De Musset's sign*: head nodding in time with the heart beat.
- *Pulsatile liver*: more often associated with tricuspid incompetence.

Palpation The apex beat is hyperdynamic and may be displaced laterally in later stages of the disease.

Auscultation An early diastolic murmur is almost always heard, loudest at the lower left sternal edge. It is sometimes easier to hear when the patient leans forward and pauses at the end of expiration. As the left ventricle decompensates with time, a third heart sound or gallop rhythm develops.

A regurgitant jet of blood can interfere with the opening of the mitral valve and produce an apical mid-diastolic murmur similar to that of mitral stenosis. This is called an *Austin Flint murmur*.

AORTIC STENOSIS

The most common cause of aortic stenosis is senile aortic calcification, followed by secondary calcification of a congenitally bicuspid aortic valve.

Rheumatic heart disease accounts for most of the remaining cases.

Narrowing of the aortic valve orifice leads to an increased pressure gradient across the valve during systole. Obstruction to the forward flow of blood from the left ventricle through the aortic valve and into the aorta leads to pressure overload (and increased afterload) that is compensated for by left ventricular hypertrophy. As the aortic stenosis becomes increasingly severe, left ventricular pressure increases, causing ventricular dilatation, and subsequent heart failure.

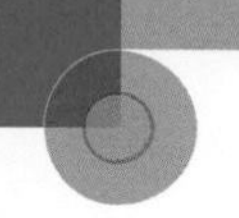

History

Age Senile calcification is uncommon before the age of 65 years. With a bicuspid aortic valve, calcification and stenosis occurs in middle age.

The triad of symptoms Most patients with mild to moderate aortic stenosis, and many with severe stenosis are symptomless. As the stenosis becomes more severe, symptoms of angina, breathlessness and syncope (Stokes-Adams attacks) may follow.

The stage at which the symptoms appear is a good prognostic indicator. The onset of angina is associated with a median survival of 5 years, syncope with 3 years and breathlessness and other symptoms of heart failure with only 2 years.

Examination

Pulse The pulse is typically slow-rising or low in volume.

Palpation In severe stenosis with preserved ventricular function, a thrill may be felt in the second right intercostal space, at the sternal notch or over the carotid arteries.

Auscultation The murmur of aortic stenosis is an ejection systolic murmur heard loudest in the second right intercostal space. It radiates to the neck and can be confused with a carotid bruit. As the heart begins to fail, the murmur becomes softer.

TRICUSPID REGURGITATION

This rarely develops in isolation, and the valve usually becomes incompetent as a consequence of high right-sided pressures with subsequent right ventricular dilatation. The most common cause is left heart failure. Another cause of such functional regurgitation is cor pulmonale. Infective endocarditis in intravenous drug users can result in destruction of the valve, causing regurgitation.

Examination

Inspection The jugular venous pressure is raised, with large visible V waves occurring in systole. Peripheral oedema is often present.

Palpation A large pulsatile liver may be palpable in the right hypochondrium. Ascites may also be present.

Auscultation A pansystolic murmur is usually heard, loudest at the lower left sternal edge on inspiration.

PULMONARY VALVE DISEASE

This is rare. Pulmonary stenosis is congenital and can occur at the level of the pulmonary valve, below the valve (right ventricular outflow tract) or above the valve (pulmonary artery). It most commonly occurs in isolation, but is associated with other conditions such as tetralogy of Fallot (see page 59).

In severe pulmonary stenosis, the right atrial pressures rises and can force open the foramen ovale, causing a right to left shunt of deoxygenated blood and central cyanosis. In less severe cases, right heart failure can develop over time, producing the signs of elevated jugular venous pressure, peripheral oedema and hepatomegaly.

Pulmonary regurgitation is usually acquired and may be the result of pulmonary hypertension (e.g. cor pulmonale), infective endocarditis, rheumatic fever, carcinoid syndrome or trauma (usually iatrogenic following surgery for pulmonary stenosis or tetralogy of Fallot). The symptoms that predominate are those of the underlying cause. Right ventricular hypertrophy produces a right ventricular heave on examination. The subsequent development of right heart failure produces the signs described above.

Infective endocarditis

This is an infection of the endocardium that results in 'vegetations' on the heart valves from a repeated cycle of bacterial infection and platelet and thrombus deposition.

In intravenous drug abusers, the tricuspid valve is most commonly affected, as this is the first valve the infected material meets. In other cases, there is often pre-existing congenital or acquired valve pathology, and the left-sided valves (aortic and mitral) are usually affected.

Any bacteraemic episode can potentially cause endocarditis, Gram-positive cocci predominating. Causes include dental surgery or poor dental hygiene, any other surgery and long-term central venous lines.

History

Age The elderly are most at risk.

Symptoms *Fever* is the principal symptom, with night sweats, rigors, lethargy, muscle aches and general malaise, easily confused with influenza. Once a heart valve becomes regurgitant as a consequence of local tissue destruction, the symptoms of heart failure become apparent.

Neurological symptoms can result from septic emboli to the brain.

Risk factors include previous heart valve disease, a history of rheumatic fever, the insertion of prosthetic valves, congenital heart disease and intravenous drug abuse.

Pyrexia of unknown origin Endocarditis should be suspected in any immunocompromised patient with a persistent fever.

Examination

General examination A fever is invariably present, usually with anaemia and a raised erythrocyte sedimentation rate. Nowadays, the classic vascular phenomena secondary to septic emboli or an immune complex-mediated vasculitis are only occasionally seen. These include splinter haemorrhages (see Figure 1.19, page 22), Janeway lesions (erythmatous non-tender lesions on the soles or palms), Osler's nodes (painful nodules on the finger pulps or digits) and Roth's spots (retinal haemorrhages with pale centres).

Septic emboli to the brain are not uncommon, and neurological signs will be present in 15% of patients.

Chest A *new or changing murmur*, most commonly of aortic regurgitation, is heard in one-third of patients. Signs of heart failure such as a gallop rhythm or the bi-basal inspiratory crackles of pulmonary oedema occur in those with valve incompetence.

Congenital heart disease

There are many congenital cardiac anomalies. They can be divided into septal defects, obstructive defects and cyanotic defects. The most common are:

- Septal defect:
  - Atrial septal defect.
  - Ventricular septal defect.
- Obstructive defects:
  - Aortic stenosis (see above).
  - Pulmonary stenosis (see above).
  - Coarctation of the aorta.
- Cyanotic defects:
  - Tetralogy of Fallot.
  - Transposition of the great vessels.

Other conditions affect the great vessels but are commonly classified with the congenital heart defects, including patent ductus arteriosus.

PATENT DUCTUS ARTERIOSUS

This common congenital cardiac defect (5–10% of all cases) results from failure of the ductus arteriosus to close at birth (Figure 2.19). When the shunt is large, oxygenated blood flows from the systemic circulation into the pulmonary circulation, raising the pulmonary arterial and right heart pressures, and causing pulmonary vascular engorgement and hypertension. The left ventricle is subject to volume overload, and will fail with time if left untreated.

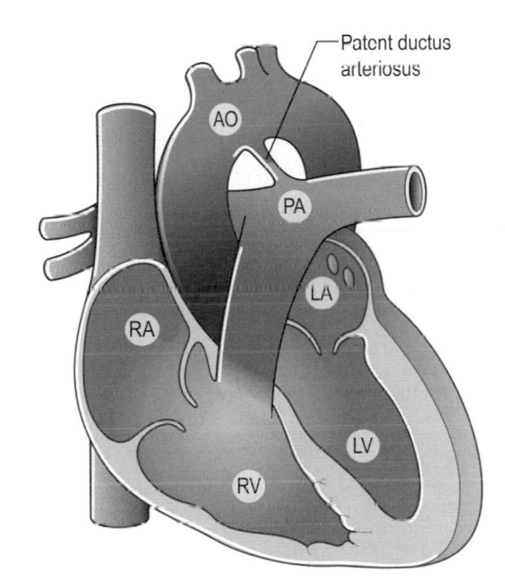

Figure 2.19 Patent ductus arteriosus. AO aorta; LA left atrium; LV left ventricle; PA pulmonary artery; RA right atrium; RV right ventricle.

Many patients with small shunts have few symptoms and signs throughout life. Symptoms include dyspnoea and fatigue on exertion with failure to grow.

On examination, the pulses are bounding with cyanosis of the lower body when shunt reversal occurs from pulmonary hypertension. A continuous 'machinery' murmur is heard best in the left second intercostal space. Signs of heart failure eventually develop, occurring more quickly with larger shunts.

ATRIAL SEPTAL DEFECT

The atria are connected through the foramen ovale before birth to allow oxygenated blood arriving in the right atrium from the placenta to bypass the non-functional fetal lungs and enter the systemic left heart circulation. When the lungs expand at birth, pulmonary vascular resistance drops, and the right atrial pressure falls below that of the left atrium. The flap valve (septum primum) in the foramen ovale closes and seals to the septum secundum (Figure 2.20). Failure of this process results in a patent foramen ovale. An ostium secundum atrial septal defect forms if this is associated with abnormal development of the septum secundum.

Three patterns of atrial septal defect are recognized: ostium secundum (as above, accounting for 80% of atrial septal defects), and two less common but more complex defects (ostium primum and sinus venosus defects).

The compliant right ventricle allows a large left to right shunt, eventually causing the right heart size to increase and the pulmonary pressure to rise. In some cases, the pulmonary arterial pressure may rise sufficiently to reverse the shunt. This rare occurrence is known as *Eisenmenger's syndrome*.

Symptoms are often absent for many years, but some children may suffer from recurrent chest infections, fatigue and shortness of breath on exertion.

Decompensation usually occurs between 30 and 50 years of age, and is indicated by decreased exercise tolerance, fatigue, dyspnoea, palpitations secondary to atrial arrhythmias and syncopal attacks.

Some patients present in adulthood with *paradoxical emboli*. Thrombi from the lower limb veins pass through the defect into the systemic circulation and may cause strokes.

On examination atrial fibrillation or flutter is present.

Right ventricular dilatation and hypertrophy may be detected as a right heart 'heave'.

There is a fixed wide split of the second heart sound, which does not alter with respiration. An ejection systolic murmur is produced by increased flow across the pulmonary valve. Flow across the atrial septal defect cannot be heard.

Cyanosis and finger clubbing indicate the onset of Eisenmenger's syndrome.

VENTRICULAR SEPTAL DEFECT

Many congenital ventricular septal defects close spontaneously in early life. In children with persistent and large defects, blood flows into the right ventricle from the higher pressure left ventricle, causing pulmonary hypertension (Figure 2.21). There is an increased incidence in children with Down's syndrome and other congenital conditions.

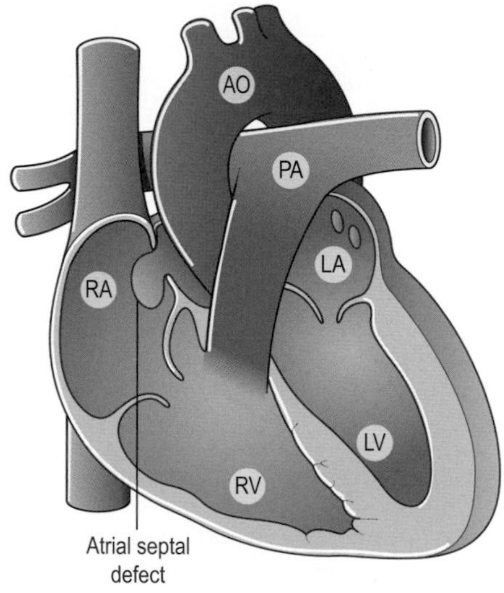

Figure 2.20 Atrial septal defect.

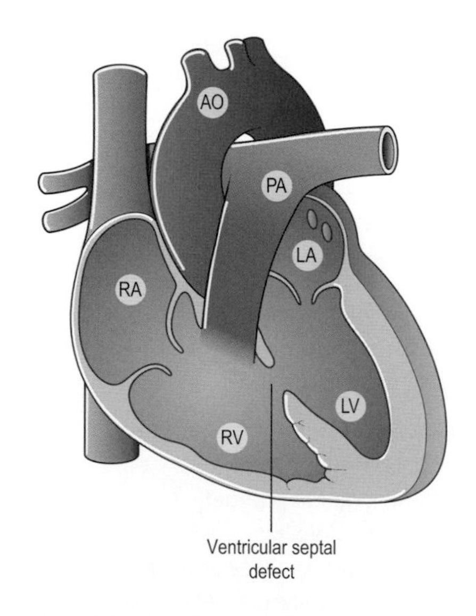

Figure 2.21 Ventricular septal defect.

A ventricular septal defect may also be acquired in adulthood as a complication of myocardial infarction (see below).

Symptoms are usually minimal at first, but dyspnoea, recurrent chest infections, poor feeding and failure to thrive develop in children with large defects causing cardiac failure.

On examination there is often evidence of an enlarged and displaced apex beat with a right heart heave and a thrill.

There is fixed splitting of the second heart sound, and a loud pansystolic murmur heard best at the left sternal edge.

Cyanosis indicates Eisenmenger's syndrome (see above).

COARCTATION OF THE AORTA

Coarctation means 'narrowing' and refers to obstruction of blood flow in the aorta, usually just distal to the origin of the left subclavian artery around the level of the ductus arteriosus. The defect varies in severity and length from a long-narrow-segment stenosis to a discrete shelf. To supply blood to the lower body, large collaterals form between the branches of the subclavian arteries and the intercostals (causing rib *notching*), and *upper limb hypertension* develops.

Males are affected twice as commonly as females. Associations include Turner's syndrome and left-sided congenital cardiac defects.

Symptoms may be absent in mild cases, and only present in later life with hypertension and its complications. Neonates with severe coarctations may present with cardiovascular collapse as the ductus closes. Between these two extremes, symptoms include dyspnoea, poor feeding and failure to thrive.

Increasing dyspnoea, faintness, chest pain and fatigue indicate the onset of heart failure. Headaches and nosebleeds may be caused by the associated hypertension, and impaired circulation to the lower limbs may cause *intermittent claudication* (see Chapter 10, page 336).

On examination there are weak femoral and feet pulses that contrast with bounding 'hypertensive' pulses in the upper limbs. An associated discrepancy in the blood pressure of 20 mmHg or more (the pressure being higher in the brachial vessels) is diagnostic. Palpation of the peripheral pulses will reveal a radial-femoral delay.

An abnormal pulsation or thrill may be felt in the suprasternal notch. An ejection systolic murmur situated over the coarctation in the left infraclavicular area and/or under the left scapula, is often heard.

TETRALOGY OF FALLOT

The four components are:

- Ventricular septal defect.
- The aorta over-riding the defect (straddling the ventricular septal defect), causing it to receive deoxygenated blood from the right ventricle.
- Obstruction of the right ventricular outflow tract/pulmonary valve.
- An abnormally thick right ventricular wall (Figure 2.22).

A proportion of the deoxygenated blood in the right ventricle passes through the ventricular septal defect into the left ventricle and aorta, producing varying degrees of cyanosis. When the child becomes upset, the right ventricular outflow tract muscle can contract, exacerbating the obstruction and causing

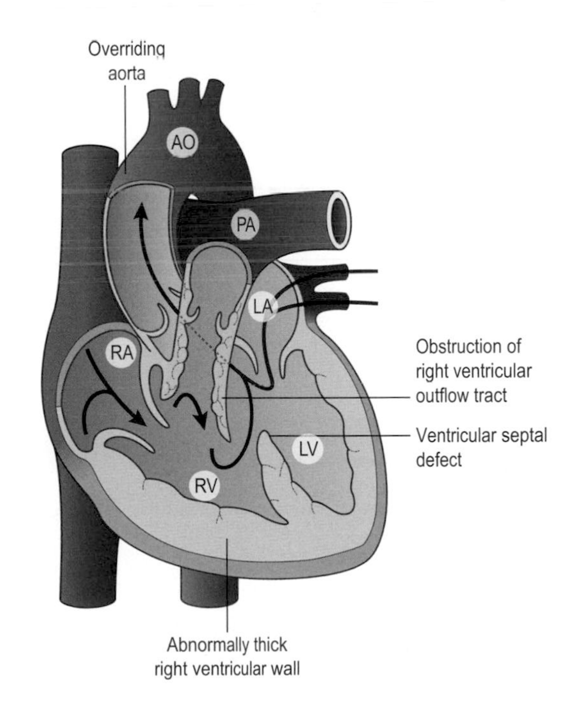

Figure 2.22 Tetralogy of Fallot.

more right to left shunting of deoxygenated blood. The resulting cyanotic episodes are known as *blue spells* or *tet spells* and may be associated with breathlessness, limpness and occasionally syncope.

History

Symptoms The child may be 'blue' or *cyanotic* at birth, or become blue when active, feeding or upset. In older children, a characteristic squatting posture may relieve the hypoxaemia caused by these spells by kinking the femoral arteries, raising the systemic resistance, reducing the right to left shunt by forcing more blood through the lungs.

Examination

Central cyanosis suggests the diagnosis. Finger clubbing develops early. A right ventricular heave is often present.

Cardiac murmurs range from almost imperceptible to very loud; the systolic murmur from the pulmonary stenosis is heard best at the left sternal edge and is associated with a palpable thrill. It may disappear during a cyanotic spell.

TRANSPOSITION OF THE GREAT VESSELS

In this rare condition, the aorta arises from the right ventricle, and the pulmonary artery from the left ventricle. Survival after birth is dependent on arterial and venous blood mixing through various septal defects and a patent ductus arteriosus. The condition is incompatible with life without surgical intervention.

Cyanosis is usually present at birth, and a number of murmurs indicate the existence of the shunts described above.

Left atrial myxoma

This rare benign tumour can present in three distinct ways:

- As the tumour enlarges, it can obstruct blood flow, mimicking mitral stenosis, causing dyspnoea, orthopnoea and paroxysmal nocturnal dyspnoea. There may be a mid-diastolic murmur and a 'tumour plop' (a sound related to movement of the tumour) that varies with posture.
- A distal embolus or stroke may occur. All recovered embolic material should always be sent for histological examination.
- There may be non-specific symptoms of fever and malaise, with raised inflammatory markers.

COUGH

A cough is a forced expulsion of air from the lungs, initially against a closed glottis, accompanied by a characteristic sound. It may be a voluntary manoeuvre or an involuntary reflex. Its purpose is protective, and it serves to clear secretions, foreign bodies or other irritants from the airways. An occasional cough is a normal and necessary part of everyday life, but a persistent or troublesome cough may be the first symptom of underlying disease.

By far the most common cause of an acute cough is a viral upper respiratory tract infection. A chronic cough is most commonly caused by postnasal drip, asthma, eosinophilic bronchitis or gastro-oesophageal reflux disease. Other causes are listed in Revision panel 2.11.

CHARACTERISTICS OF A COUGH

History

Duration A cough lasting less than 3 weeks is termed acute, while one lasting more than 8 weeks is termed chronic. An acute cough will, in all likelihood, be benign in nature, and is usually caused by a viral upper respiratory tract infection. Sudden onset cough may be the result of an inhaled foreign body.

A chronic cough is also likely to be benign, but a careful history and examination may reveal a more sinister underlying disease process.

Sputum production Most coughs are dry or non-productive. The production of significant amounts of sputum suggests pathology of pulmonary origin.

Sputum is mucus from the lower airways. Its colour or consistency may provide clues to the underlying disease:

- Mucoid sputum is clear or white and seen commonly in smokers with chronic bronchitis.

- Purulent sputum is usually the result of underlying infection and has a thick yellow or green appearance. It may be present acutely (upper respiratory tract infection, pneumonia, lung abscess) or in a chronic infection (chronic bronchitis, bronchiectasis).
- Rust-coloured sputum is typical of pneumococcal and *Klebsiella* pneumonia.
- Blood-streaked sputum, or haemoptysis, occurs in acute infection or lung cancer.
- Large-volume haemoptysis is much less common, and tends to occur in chronic inflammatory conditions (bronchiectasis, aspergillosis, tuberculosis).
- White or pink and frothy sputum is seen in acute pulmonary oedema. The pink colour is caused by red blood cells in the alveoli. Chronic and copious amounts of frothy sputum (*bronchorrhoea*) may be seen with adenocarcinoma of the lung.

Diurnal variation

Most patients cough less at night as the cough reflex is, to some degree, suppressed. The cough in chest infection does not lessen overnight and may wake the patient and the characteristic 'early morning (4 a.m.) cough' of asthma is caused by physiological night-time airways narrowing. Some conditions become worse on lying flat (e.g. pulmonary oedema, gastro-oesophageal reflux) and may manifest themselves as a nocturnal cough.

Association with eating, drinking or talking

A cough associated with eating, or one that occurs in the immediate postprandial period, may be the result of gastro-oesophageal dysmotility (see Chapter 15).

Associated symptoms

Although an acute cough is usually benign and self-limiting, certain additional symptoms suggest more serious pathology:

- Haemoptysis of small volume may be a symptom of lung cancer or an inflammatory or infective process.

Revision panel 2.11

CAUSES OF COUGH

Infective

Viral upper respiratory tract infections
Bacterial infection (acute bronchitis)
Pneumonia
Tuberculosis
Aspergillosis
Bronchiectasis
Lung abscess

Airways

Asthma
Eosinophilic bronchitis
Chronic obstructive pulmonary disease
Inhaled foreign body
Allergy
Endobronchial tumours (e.g. lung cancer, carcinoid tumour, metastatic disease)

Other lung disease

Lung cancer
Interstitial lung disease
Sarcoidosis
Cystic fibrosis

Heart

Pulmonary oedema

Drugs

Angiotensin-converting enzyme inhibitors

Environment

Smoking (chronic bronchitis)
Pollution

Other

Postnasal drip (secondary to rhinitis or sinusitis)
Gastro-oesophageal reflux
Oesophageal dysmotility
Mediastinal masses
Psychogenic

- Shortness of breath occurring acutely with a cough is often caused by acute bronchitis, but asthma, an inhaled foreign body or anaphylaxis must be excluded.
- Fever and cough of acute onset may indicate pneumonia.
- Acute-onset pleuritic chest pain with a cough may result from underlying pneumonia. A more gradual onset of symptoms may also represent an infective process, but lung cancer must be considered in the differential diagnosis. Mediastinal masses may also cause these symptoms but are much less common.
- Weight loss can be dramatic, and is most commonly seen with lung cancers and chest sepsis.

Specific sounding coughs

- A barking cough is characteristic of *croup*.
- Pertussis, or *whooping cough*, is so-named because of the high-pitched 'whoop' sound made by an affected child when inhaling air immediately after coughing.
- A *bovine cough*, weak and non-expulsive, is associated with hoarseness from recurrent laryngeal nerve palsy, often from a lung cancer.

COMPLICATIONS OF ACUTE AND CHRONIC COUGH

Vomiting and syncope may be seen following bouts of severe coughing.

In parous females, a cough can induce stress incontinence.

Rib fractures are uncommon but can occur following episodes of severe coughing.

Chronic cough may result in development of an abdominal hernia.

Inhaled foreign body

The inhalation of objects is more common in young children. Because of the small size of the airways, there is a greater chance of complete obstruction. Adults also inhale foreign bodies, commonly teeth and crowns (often while undergoing a dental examination), food (especially peas and peanuts), coins, pins and tacks.

Because of the shape of the bronchial tree, most inhaled objects *lodge in the right main bronchus*, bronchus intermedius or right lower lobe segmental bronchi. Occasionally, life-threatening complete obstruction or partial obstruction of the larynx or trachea may occur.

History

In adults, the most common symptoms of lower respiratory tract inhalations are cough, wheeze or stridor and breathlessness of acute onset, but many cases are symptomless. There is usually a clear history of an inhalation event. The symptoms and signs of pneumonia predominate when a patient presents late. They may be unaware or have forgotten that they had inhaled anything. Complete or partial obstruction of the larynx or trachea presents acutely and may be fatal. It is most commonly the result of food aspiration.

Examination

Physical examination is often unremarkable, but tachypnoea may be evident. Proximal obstruction of a lung will cause collapse of the lung with tracheal deviation to that side, with possible reduced air entry and a localized wheeze. Complete obstruction of the larynx or trachea causes rapid onset cyanosis, a silent chest, marked respiratory distress (with paradoxical movements of the chest and diaphragm), loss of consciousness and death.

Depending on degree of obstruction, partial obstruction is associated with varying degrees of stridor, respiratory distress and paroxysmal coughing.

Pneumonia

Pneumonia is inflammation and consolidation of the lung, normally caused by infection. Most cases are bacterial or viral, but fungi and parasites may be responsible, particularly in immunocompromised patients. Non-infectious causes including the idiopathic interstitial lung diseases (e.g. usual interstitial pneumonia), organizing pneumonia, drug reactions and lipoid pneumonia are usually classified independently.

Infective pneumonia, is classified as community-acquired or hospital-acquired pneumonia. Community-acquired pneumonia refers to pneumonia contracted by a person with little contact with healthcare systems. Most cases (>50%) of community-acquired pneumonia are caused by *Streptococcus pneumoniae* (the pneumococcus) but ~10% of cases are from atypical organisms like *Legionella* or *Mycoplasma*. Hospital-acquired pneumonia refers to pneumonia that develops >48 hours after hospital admission.

This classification is important because hospital-acquired pneumonia is caused by different bacterial organisms to community-acquired pneumonia and has a higher mortality. About 80% of hospital-acquired pneumonia is caused by gram-negative organisms (e.g. *Pseudomonas, E. coli*) with 20% from to staphylococci. These organisms are frequently more resistant to antibiotic therapy.

Pneumonia is a significant cause of death in the very young and the very old, in patients with chronic illness and in patients admitted to hospital. It is also a significant cause of postoperative death.

History

Age All ages are affected, but those older than 65 years are most at risk.

Symptoms The onset may be rapid, with significant symptoms developing in less than 24 hours.

Cough is common and may produce purulent sputum. In pneumococcal infection, this classically has a rusty colour.

Haemoptysis is occasionally seen.

Non-specific symptoms *Malaise* and *fatigue* are present in most cases. *Fever* may be associated with sweats and rigors. Joint and muscle aches are frequent.

Shortness of breath is reported by two-thirds of patients, often exacerbated by severe, sharp, inspiratory *pleuritic chest pain* that can prevent adequate ventilation and lead to respiratory failure.

Hiccough is an occasional symptom.

Previous history

Smoking is the biggest risk factor in those who were previously fit and well.

Specific conditions that increase the risk of pneumonia include a history of chronic obstructive pulmonary disease, other chronic illness, alcohol dependency, immunocompromise and gastro-oesophageal reflux disease. Malnutrition and immobility are other factors.

In some patients, an episode of pneumonia may be the first presentation of lung cancer but is often accompanied by non-specific symptoms such as weight loss and fatigue.

Examination

General appearance Some individuals look relatively well. Others are very ill, with cardiovascular compromise (tachycardia, hypotension) and signs of respiratory distress (tachypnoea, central cyanosis). Confusion is common in the elderly.

Inspection *Tachypnoea* is common in unwell patients. Reduced chest movement on the affected side is sometimes seen.

Palpation The trachea is normally central, but collapse of a lobe or lung results in deviation towards the affected side.

Increased tactile vocal fremitus results from a better conduction of sound through consolidated lung. This will be absent if there is an associated pleural effusion.

Percussion The percussion note will be dull over the affected area.

Auscultation Air entry may be reduced or *bronchial breathing heard over the area of consolidated lung,* particularly at the bases. Coarse inspiratory crackles are common.

Increased vocal resonance (i.e. the patient's voice [or whisper in whispering *pectoriloquy*] can be heard more clearly over consolidated lung) with reduced air entry differentiates lung consolidation from a pleural effusion.

A *pleural rub* is occasionally heard and occurs as inflamed pleural surfaces move against each other during both inspiration and expiration.

Lung abscess

This is a localized collection of pus contained within a cavity formed by the disintegration of the surrounding lung parenchyma. Multiple abscesses may be present in the immunocompromised patient.

A primary lung abscess is either caused by aspiration or as a complication of pneumonia.

Secondary lung abscesses occur as a result of another pathology such as metastatic septic emboli, an obstructing bronchial carcinoma or an infected bulla.

Anaerobic organisms (particularly *Bacteroides*) are commonly isolated from the pus, having gained access from aspiration or periodontal disease. Aerobic, gram-positive bacteria such as *Streptococcus pneumoniae* and *Staphylococcus aureus* are increasingly common.

History

Age Lung abscesses are more common in the elderly as they are more likely to develop pneumonia or suffer from dysphagia and aspiration and to have poor oral health.

Symptoms *Cough* and *fever* are the most common symptoms. Later in the disease process, as the abscess drains spontaneously into the bronchial tree, the cough produces pus, which tastes and smells foul in anaerobic infections.

Haemoptysis occurs in one-third of patients.

Night sweats and rigors may accompany the fever.

General symptoms include malaise, fatigue and weight loss.

Shortness of breath is sometimes a feature and may be exacerbated by pleuritic chest pain.

Previous history

Aspiration is a cause of primary lung abscess, and risk factors such as alcohol abuse, recent dental work and bulbar palsy may be present.

A lung abscess should be considered in any patient who has failed to respond to the treatment of pneumonia (although an empyema is more likely).

Examination

General appearance *Cachexia* and *fever* are usually present. The fever is often swinging and associated with a tachycardia.

Finger clubbing is seen in one-third of patients.

Some patients, particularly those with aerobic infections, can be very unwell with high fever, signs of respiratory failure, and cardiovascular compromise, with tachycardia and hypotension.

Chest signs may be absent but are often the same as in pneumonia and lung consolidation. A dull percussion note with reduced air entry and reduced vocal resonance will be present when a pleural effusion or empyema has complicated the lung abscess.

Bronchiectasis

Bronchiectasis is a chronic condition characterized by abnormal and permanent dilatation of the subsegmental bronchi. Its pathogenesis involves previous infection related to impairment of bronchial drainage, airway obstruction or impaired immunity (Figure 2.23).

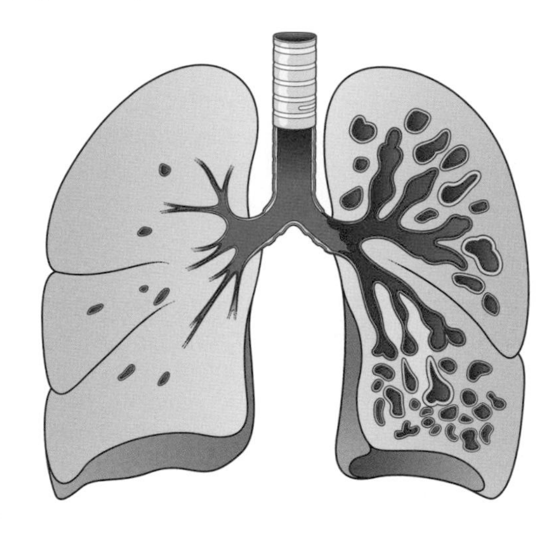

Figure 2.23 Bronchiectasis (dilated bronchi).

History

Age Bronchiectasis is most common in young people with cystic fibrosis and in those over the age of 60 years.

Symptoms *Cough* is the dominant symptom. While this may be unproductive, the majority of patients produce large volumes of purulent, often foul-smelling sputum, which may cause embarrassment.

Repeated respiratory tract infections cause shortness of breath, wheezing and pleuritic chest pain.

Halitosis is noticed by patients or those around them, and may indicate an exacerbation.

Haemoptysis is common and, on occasion, massive.

Previous history

Congenital causes of bronchiectasis include:

- Cystic fibrosis.
- Hypogammaglobulinaemia.
- Alpha-1 antitrypsin deficiency.
- Kartagener's syndrome (failure of ciliary motility).

While previous or recurrent bacterial infection is the most common cause of acquired bronchiectasis, other associations include childhood whooping cough (pertussis), aspergillosis, AIDS, tuberculosis, ulcerative colitis, rheumatoid arthritis and male infertility.

Examination

General appearance Cachexia and evidence of weight loss may be present. Finger clubbing is seen only in patients with severe disease, but nasal polyps and chronic sinusitis are common.

Auscultation All manner of added sounds, including crackles, wheezes and squeaks can be heard throughout all lung fields. These sounds are more pronounced during exacerbations.

CHEST PAIN

Pain in the chest is a common presenting symptom. It may arise from almost any structure within the thorax, including the heart, pericardium, lungs, pleura, chest wall, oesophagus, mediastinum or thoracic spine. Some causes are benign and self-limiting, while others are immediately life threatening. The causes are listed in Revision panel 2.12.

Revision panel 2.12

CAUSES OF CHEST PAIN

Heart

Chronic stable angina
Acute coronary syndromes
Aortic dissection
Aortic stenosis

Pericardium

Pericarditis
Pericardial cyst

Mediastinum

Mediastinitis
Oesophagitis
Oesophageal tumour
Oesophageal motility disorders
Ruptured oesophagus
Other mediastinal masses (e.g. thymoma, lymphadenopathy, germ-cell tumour, neurogenic tumour, foregut cysts)
Spontaneous pneumomediastinum (Hamman's syndrome)

Pleura

Pneumonia
Pulmonary embolus
Pneumothorax
Pleural effusion/empyema
Tumour (e.g. invasive lung cancer, mesothelioma, metastatic disease)

Chest wall and spine

Trauma (e.g. rib fractures)
Tumour (e.g. invasive lung cancer, secondary bony deposits, mesothelioma, primary chest wall sarcomas)
Vertebral collapse (e.g tumour, osteoporosis) with intercostal nerve compression
Costochondritis
Tietze's syndrome (see Chapter 13)

CHARACTERISTICS OF CHEST PAIN

Site

Central, retrosternal or midline chest pain normally arises from structures in the midline such as the heart, pericardium and oesophagus. Similarly, mediastinal masses are likely to cause central chest pain or discomfort.

It is unusual for lateral structures such as the lung, pleura or lateral chest wall to cause midline pain and, in these, pain tends to be localized to the site and side of origin.

Radiation

Pain felt distant to the site of the cause may either be *referred*, or from an *extension* of the underlying disease. Occasionally, referred pain is the only feature (e.g. left arm pain from cardiac ischaemia), making the diagnosis difficult.

History of referred pain

Myocardial ischaemia classically causes central chest pain. Common sites of radiation include the arms (especially the left), neck, jaw, epigastrium and back.

Aortic pathology such as a dissection may present with symptoms identical to myocardial ischaemia, or with back pain between the shoulder blades.

Oesophageal pain, such as in reflux disease or oesophageal spasm, may also be very similar to cardiac pain in terms of site and radiation.

Lung cancers invading the chest wall, chest wall tumours, neurogenic tumours arising in the paravertebral region and pleural disease may produce pain localized to the site of origin. Often, however, intercostal nerve involvement causes neurogenic pain felt in the dermatome of the affected nerve. If this is only felt anteriorly, it mimics conditions causing midline chest or abdominal pain.

Extension of the underlying disease process

As an aortic dissection extends from the ascending aorta to the descending aorta, pain may migrate from the retrosternal area to the back. Mediastinal tumours are often symptomless, but may cause central chest pain. Spread into the pleural cavity may produce more lateral symptoms. Pneumothorax is often associated with sharp pleuritic chest pain on the affected side. Extension of air into the mediastinum can result in central chest pain.

Character

The central aspect of cardiac pain is often described as 'crushing', 'heavy', 'tight', 'like a band around my chest' or 'like a weight on my chest'. Interestingly, referred cardiac pain often has a different quality (e.g. 'severe ache').

Oesophageal pain can mimic cardiac pain in character as well as site, as can pain from other mediastinal pathology.

Aortic dissection may produce a 'tearing' sensation, often felt between the shoulder blades.

Pleural pain is sharp or stabbing in nature, and any pleural or chest wall pathology can cause it. It results from inflammation of the pleural surfaces, and the pain is felt as they move against one another, typically on deep breathing, coughing, laughing or sneezing. Chest wall invasion by tumour does not always produce pleuritic pain. It tends to be dull, gnawing or aching.

Severity

Severity of pain is subjective, depending on personal tolerance and on the situation. For example, a chest injury sustained on the rugby pitch will be tolerated better than a similar injury in the home.

Myocardial infarction, aortic dissection, oesophageal rupture and multiple rib fractures typically cause severe pain but bizarrely, some patients experience little or no pain. This is more likely in the elderly, and in those with autonomic neuropathy from diabetes.

Onset and duration

Pain of a few seconds duration is unlikely to be significant (e.g. precordial catch syndrome).

The pain of chronic stable angina usually lasts minutes, whereas pain from a myocardial infarction may last for hours.

Acute diseases causing pleural pain, such as pneumothorax, usually produce pain with an acute onset, which may be persistent.

Tumours of the mediastinum and chest wall are often symptomless, but there may be pain with an insidious onset that persists.

Frequency and periodicity

There is no chest equivalent to the colicky pain of intestinal origin. The pain tends to be constant, the exception being pleuritic chest pain related to breathing.

Precipitating and aggravating factors

The symptoms of chronic stable angina are usually brought on by exercise. As the coronary artery disease progresses and blood flow to the heart reduces, symptoms appear with progressively less exertion, even on brushing the teeth. Other precipitating factors include emotional stress, cold weather and eating.

Pleuritic pain is classically worse on inspiration. Sometimes it may only be felt on deep inspiration, while at others times pain may be experienced even during shallow respiration. Other aggravating factors include any chest movement, including coughing, laughing and sneezing.

Pericarditis causes a sharp central pain, typically aggravated by lying flat and relieved by sitting up or leaning forward. Like pleuritic pain, it is worse on inspiration.

Oesophageal pain is often identical to cardiac pain, and telling the two apart can be difficult. Precipitation by eating or aggravation by posture is more likely with oesophageal pain, while exercise is associated with cardiac pain.

Musculoskeletal chest wall pain, in common with pleuritic pain, is aggravated by any form of chest movement, including inspiration. Local pressure may precipitate or exacerbate the pain. Tenderness over the costal cartilages suggests costochondritis and pressing on the sternum causes pain over the sites of rib fractures.

Relieving factors

Sometimes an action or event coincides with the spontaneous resolution of pain, and the patient wrongly attributes this as a relieving factor. There are, however, true relieving factors classically associated with different causes of chest pain.

The central chest pain of stable chronic angina typically passes off after a few minutes of rest or use of sublingual nitrates. Failure to resolve with rest or nitrates suggests a different diagnosis, such as acute coronary syndrome or non-cardiac pain.

Oesophageal pain is often similar to cardiac pain, and confusingly may also be relieved by nitrates. *Relief of symptoms with antacids suggests an oesophageal cause.*

Partial relief of musculoskeletal and pleuritic pains may be achieved by keeping as still or as rigid as possible.

ASSOCIATED SYMPTOMS AND SIGNS

Pain is often associated with features that are the result of sympathetic over-stimulation, such as tachycardia and hypertension. Nausea and sweating are frequently associated with the severe pain of acute coronary syndrome.

Regurgitation of gastric acid in association with central chest pain is not seen with cardiac ischaemia and is typical of gastro-oesophageal reflux disease. Breathlessness, however, is commonly seen with cardiac ischaemia but not with oesophageal disease.

Chronic stable angina

Angina, or angina pectoris, is the symptom of chest pain or discomfort experienced during transient cardiac ischaemia. The most common cause is atherosclerosis of the coronary arteries. As a consequence, coronary artery blood flow is reduced, and pain develops when the heart is asked to work harder during exercise. Other conditions that reduce coronary artery blood flow include coronary artery spasm (known as *variant or Prinzmetal's angina*) and neointimal hyperplasia within a coronary stent or in areas of previous coronary angioplasty. Angina is also a late and worrying symptom in aortic valve stenosis (see above).

History

Age and sex The likelihood of angina increases with age. In the UK, it is rare before the age of 45 years and unusual before 55 years. The incidence of angina then increases steeply with each decade of life, and is higher in males than females. Over the age of 75 years, 14% of males and 8% of females experience angina as a symptom of ischaemic heart disease.

Symptoms The main symptom is *central retrosternal chest pain or discomfort brought on by effort or exercise.* Other precipitating factors include stress, cold weather and large meals. The pain is variously described as 'tight', 'band-like', 'constrictive' or 'heavy'. Radiation to the jaw or neck may produce a 'choking' sensation. Other sites of radiation include the arms (principally the left arm) and the back. The pain abates after a few minutes of rest or the use of sublingual nitrates.

The severity of angina pain is not necessarily related to the degree of ischaemia. Indeed, myocardial ischaemia may be silent, particularly in patients with autonomic neuropathy (such as diabetics).

The thresholds for the precipitation of angina symptoms are summarized by the Canadian Cardiovascular Society angina classification (Revision panel 2.13). Patients in classes 3 and 4 have a worse prognosis than those in classes 1 and 2.

Angina can be aggravated by anaemia, hyperthyroidism and obesity.

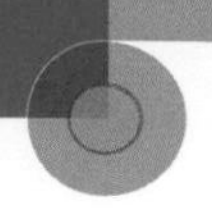

Revision panel 2.13

CANADIAN CARDIOVASCULAR SOCIETY ANGINA CLASSIFICATION (2016)

Class 0: Symptomless angina: Mild myocardial ischemia with no symptoms.
Class 1: Angina only with strenuous exertion and rapid or prolonged ordinary activity.
Class 2: Angina with moderate exertion causing slight limitation of ordinary activities. Occurs when walking uphill or climbing stairs at a normal pace or with meals, emotional stress and in the cold or wind.
Class 3: Angina with mild exertion: Having difficulties walking one or two blocks or climbing one flight of stairs at normal pace.
Class 4: Angina at rest: No exertion needed to trigger angina.
(Class 0 is not part of the official classification)

Patients with ischaemic heart disease and angina often experience breathlessness and autonomic symptoms such as nausea with their pain.

Pain caused by oesophageal pathologies such as oesophageal motility disorders and reflux disease is the most important differential diagnosis (see above).

Risk factors include smoking, a family history of ischaemic heart disease, obesity, advancing age and a sedentary lifestyle. Their presence makes myocardial ischaemia a more likely diagnosis.

Previous history

Hypertension, diabetes and hypercholesterolaemia are additional risk factors. Patients with renal failure are also at significant risk. A history of peripheral vascular or cerebrovascular disease is more likely in patients with ischaemic heart disease.

Examination

General appearance There are frequently no abnormal physical signs in patients with chronic stable angina. Nicotine staining of the fingers may be seen in smokers.

Xanthelasmata, or cholesterol deposits in the skin of the eyelids, are a sign of hypercholesterolaemia (see Chapter 1).

Similarly, a *corneal arcus* may also indicate hypercholesterolaemia in young patients, but in older people is a relatively non-specific sign.

Blood pressure should be checked, as hypertension is a major risk factor.

The pulse will normally be regular, but cardiac ischaemia is a known cause of atrial fibrillation, in which case, the pulse will be irregularly irregular. Signs of heart failure, such as raised jugular venous pressure and ankle oedema should also be sought.

Chest examination This is usually normal. If there is an element of heart failure, fine inspiratory crackles may be heard at both lung bases. Mitral regurgitation as a result of cardiac ischaemia may result in a pansystolic heart murmur.

Acute coronary syndromes

The acute coronary syndromes occur following occlusion of a coronary artery, usually by thrombus formation over the site of a ruptured atherosclerotic plaque within the wall of the coronary artery. They are almost always accompanied by central chest pain. There are three patterns:

1. ST elevation myocardial infarction (STEMI).
2. Non-ST elevation myocardial infarction (NSTEMI).
3. Unstable angina.

A *STEMI* is characterized by electrocardiogram (ECG) changes typical of myocardial ischaemia (ST elevation or new left bundle branch block) with evidence of myocardial damage (raised serum cardiac markers such as troponin I or T).

An *NSTEMI* does not produce typical ECG changes, but there is biochemical evidence of myocardial damage.

Unstable angina typically has neither ST elevation on ECG nor positive serum cardiac markers.

Symptoms are often identical for all three syndromes.

History

The age, risk factors and previous history are the same for the acute coronary syndromes as for chronic stable angina. It is the onset, severity and resolution of symptoms that differentiate the two. While many patients presenting with an acute coronary syndrome have a history of chronic stable angina, it is often the first presentation of ischaemic heart disease.

Symptoms The predominant symptom is *central, retrosternal chest pain*, often with *radiation to the neck, jaw, arms or back*.

In those with a previous history of chronic stable angina, the pain is often described as being more severe or oppressive in nature. Whereas stable angina is brought on by effort and is relieved after a few minutes by rest or sublingual nitrates, the acute coronary syndromes have an *unpredictable onset or occur at rest*. Furthermore, pain is not relieved by rest or nitrates and may persist for many minutes or indeed hours.

Patients often have a sense of impending doom or death. Sympathetic symptoms such as nausea, vomiting and sweating are more prominent than in stable angina, particularly for inferior STEMIs.

Acute left ventricular failure is a potential complication of acute coronary syndromes, and sudden onset breathlessness and orthopnoea are presenting features. Rhythm disturbances such as atrial fibrillation, atrial flutter, ventricular ectopics, heart block and ventricular tachycardia are also common, causing palpitations, light-headedness or syncope. Ventricular fibrillation leading to sudden death is not uncommonly the first presentation of ischaemic heart disease.

Examination

General appearance As with stable angina, the stigmata of smoking or hypercholesterolaemia may be evident.

The patient often looks unwell, with autonomic signs such as *sweating, pallor and vomiting* as a consequence of the pain.

Tachycardia A *weak and rapid pulse* indicates cardiogenic shock that can complicate some acute coronary syndromes, particularly STEMIs. *Arrhythmias* may also be detected. The blood pressure may be elevated as a result of either long-standing hypertension or the acute pain. Low blood pressure with cool peripheries, peripheral cyanosis, sweating and pallor indicates cardiogenic shock, and there may be other signs of heart failure such as a raised jugular venous pressure.

Chest In the presence of heart failure, fine inspiratory crackles are heard at the lung bases.

Auscultation of the heart is usually normal unless there is concomitant valvular heart disease.

Complications of myocardial ischaemia may produce additional signs:

- A gallop rhythm indicates left ventricular failure.
- Ischaemic rupture of the chordae tendineae will result in acute mitral regurgitation and a pansystolic murmur.
- Postinfarct VSD causes a harsh systolic murmur, loudest at the lower left sternal edge.
- Some patients who survive a large full-thickness infarct may develop a left ventricular aneurysm. This may lead to heart failure, and arrhythmias.

Aortic dissection

A dissection forms when a tear at a weak spot in the intimal lining of the aorta allows blood to enter and separates the muscular layers of the vessel forming a false lumen.

Two-thirds of cases originate in the ascending aorta, with the remainder in the arch or proximal descending aorta. Whilst the false lumen may remain localized, the pressure of the blood can force it to extend (*dissect*) proximally towards the heart or distally towards the aortic iliac bifurcation. The process can then occlude branches of the aorta (the coronary, carotid or coeliac arteries), or the thinned outer layer of the aorta can rupture, usually fatally (Figure 2.24).

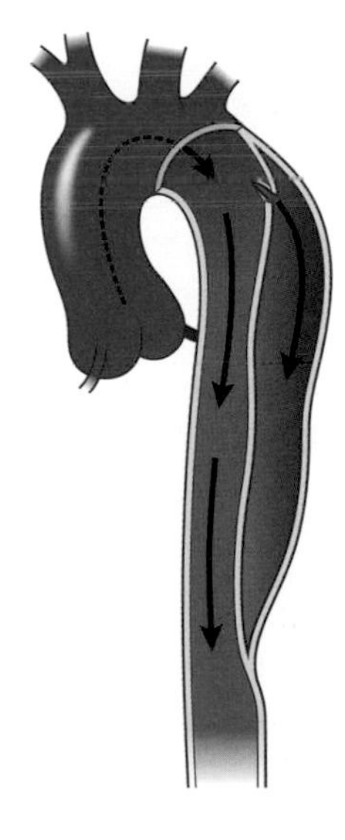

Figure 2.24 Aortic dissection.

The Stanford classification divides aortic dissections into two groups:

- Type A dissections involve the ascending aorta and require immediate surgery.
- Type B dissections do not involve the ascending aorta and can be managed conservatively without initial surgery, although endovascular stenting or surgery may be required later to treat complications.

History

Age Most patients are over 60 years old, and dissection is twice as likely in males. Many patients die before reaching hospital.

Symptoms *Pain* is the principal symptom and is related to the site of the dissection. Central chest pain, not dissimilar to angina, is experienced in dissections involving the ascending aorta. The onset is usually sudden, and it is sometimes described as *tearing in nature.*

Back, or intrascapular, pain is a feature of dissections involving the descending aorta. Pain that began centrally radiating to the back is ominous, indicating possible extension of the dissection.

Sharp, central, pleuritic-type pain may indicate involvement of the pericardial sac and the impending development of cardiac tamponade.

Involvement of the arteries to the heart or aortic branches can result in end-organ damage and further symptoms.

One-third of type A dissections involve the aortic valve, causing aortic regurgitation and symptoms of heart failure.

Involvement of the coronary arteries may produce additional *symptoms of myocardial ischaemia,* although these are difficult to separate from the symptoms of the dissection itself.

Neurological symptoms and *stroke* occur with occlusion of the aortic arch branches.

Extension distally may produce *abdominal pain* (coeliac and mesenteric vessels) or symptoms of lower limb ischaemia.

Risk factors Hypertension is the most common risk factor.

Other predisposing conditions include connective tissue disorders such as Ehlers–Danlos syndrome (Figure 2.25) and Marfan's syndrome (see Chapter 1) and bicuspid aortic valve.

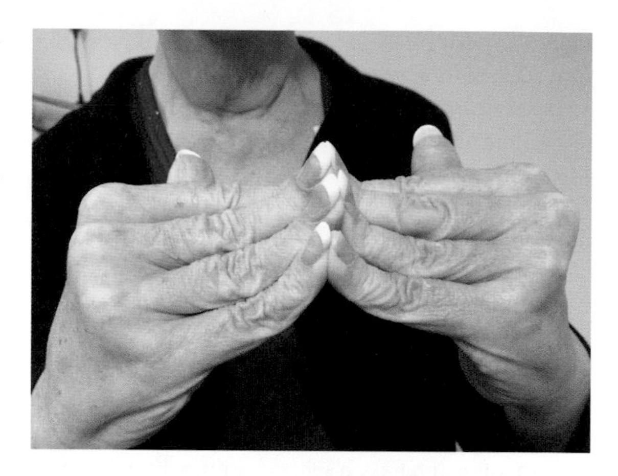

Figure 2.25 Hyperflexibility of the fingers in Ehlers–Danlos syndrome. This condition is a risk factor for aortic dissection.

Hypervolaemic states such as pregnancy in conjunction with connective tissue abnormalities may initiate dissection.

Previous history

Recent cardiac surgery, particularly on the aortic valve, can predispose to dissection.

Examination

General appearance The surviving patients may have obvious stigmata of underlying connective tissue disorders, or signs of stroke or limb ischaemia. Paraplegia, if present, is a result of spinal artery occlusion.

Blood pressure is variable. Pain or long-standing hypertension may result in high blood pressure, but loss of blood, cardiac failure or cardiac tamponade is associated with hypotension.

Hypotension is more common in type A dissections and is a poor prognostic sign. Aortic regurgitation results in a low diastolic pressure with a wide pulse pressure.

If the blood pressure is measured in an ischaemic upper limb, there will be apparent hypotension. Check the peripheral pulses first. The pulses in he left arm may be impalpable.

Auscultation Auscultation of the heart reveals an early diastolic murmur if the dissection has caused aortic regurgitation. Muffled heart sounds suggest cardiac tamponade.

Pleural fluid collections can develop from either rupture of the aorta or an inflammatory reaction to the dissection process. The left chest is usually involved, with signs of a pleural effusion (see above). If severe aortic regurgitation has complicated the dissection, there will be signs of pulmonary oedema (fine bi-basal crackles).

Mediastinal masses and tumours

Masses arising in the mediastinum are inaccessible to clinical examination. Modes of presentation are:

- No symptoms, with an incidental finding on imaging studies such as a chest X-ray or CT scan.
- Chest pain, normally central; paravertebral masses may produce pain in the affected dermatome.
- Shortness of breath as a result of airway compression or invasion by large mediastinal masses or lymphadenopathy; or diaphragmatic paralysis from phrenic nerve damage.
- Cough
- Dysphagia from compression of the oesophagus.
- Fever or night sweats in mediastinal lymphadenopathy caused by lymphoma, sarcoidosis or tuberculosis.
- General malaise.
- Muscle weakness secondary to myasthenia gravis associated with a thymoma.

One-half of all mediastinal masses are symptomless. The presence of symptoms or signs is more likely to represent a sinister pathology.

Anatomically, the mediastinum is divided into the superior, anterior, middle and posterior compartments. A more useful surgical description of the mediastinum divides it into three compartments: anterior (containing the thymus gland, fat and lymph nodes), visceral (containing the trachea and main stem bronchi, lymph nodes, heart, pericardium, great vessels, oesophagus and thoracic duct) and paravertebral (containing the sympathetic chain and thoracic spinal ganglia).

The cause and sites of mediastinal masses are listed in Revision panel 2.14.

Revision panel 2.14

SITES AND CAUSES OF MEDIASTINAL MASSES

Anterior compartment

Thymoma or thymic hyperplasia
Thyroid (retrosternal goitre)
Germ cell tumours
Lymphadenopathy

Visceral compartment

Tracheal and bronchial tumours (e.g. lung cancer, benign tracheobronchial tumours)
Lymphadenopathy
Foregut cysts (bronchogenic, oesophageal)
Pericardial cysts
Cardiac tumours
Aortic aneurysm
Oesophageal tumours
Hiatus hernia

Paravertebral compartment

Neurogenic tumours (e.g. neurofibroma, schwannoma, ganglioneuroma, phaeochromocytoma)
Lymphadenopathy

OTHER SYMPTOMS/SIGNS

Stridor

Stridor is the harsh, high-pitched or wheezing sound of breathing associated with a partially obstructed airway. Turbulent and restricted airflow occurs secondary to either intrinsic obstruction or extrinsic compression of the airway, anywhere between the larynx and the main bronchi. The onset of stridor is always an emergency and must be investigated promptly.

Revision panel 2.15

CAUSES OF STRIDOR

Laryngeal disease

Infection (croup, epiglottitis, retropharyngeal abscess)
Tumour (laryngeal papillomatosis, laryngeal cancer)
Oedema (instrumentation of airway, anaphylaxis)

Endobronchial disease

Lung cancer
Primary tracheal tumours
Metastatic cancer (e.g. renal cell)
Locally invasive cancer (e.g. lung, oesophagus, thyroid)
Inhaled foreign body
Benign stenosis (e.g. secondary to prolonged intubation or tracheostomy)

Extrinsic compression

Mediastinal lymphadenopathy (e.g. metastatic lung cancer, lymphoma)
Mediastinal tumours (thymoma, germ cell tumour)
Thyroid swelling
Thoracic aortic aneurysm
Vascular anomalies (e.g. vascular ring secondary to a double aortic arch)

Other

Tracheomalacia

Stridor is loudest in inspiration and is accentuated by coughing. It is often, although not always, associated with shortness of breath.

A sudden onset is typical of an inhaled foreign body, while a gradual onset may be from endobronchial malignancy or extrinsic compression by tumour masses (Revision panel 2.15).

Haemoptysis

Haemoptysis is the clearing of blood or blood-stained sputum from the lungs by coughing. It is sometimes difficult to differentiate from bleeding from the nasopharynx, or the oesophagus and stomach.

Revision panel 2.16

CAUSES OF HAEMOPTYSIS

Inflammation and infection (including tuberculosis and *Aspergillus*)
Bronchiectasis
Lung cancer and other tumours of the tracheobronchial tree
Trauma (e.g. pulmonary artery catheter, penetrating trauma)
Pulmonary embolus
Pulmonary arteriovenous malformations
Mitral stenosis

Massive haemoptysis describes potentially life-threatening bleeding into the bronchial tree. There are no accepted criteria for the volume (but usually >0.5 L over 24 h) or rate (>100 mL/h) of bleeding constitutes massive haemoptysis but the principal threat is asphyxiation (drowning) rather than exsanguination.

The causes of simple haemoptysis are the same as those for massive haemoptysis (Revision panel 2.16). While small-volume haemoptysis in a smoker may be a symptom of lung cancer, massive haemoptysis is more commonly caused by an inflammatory process.

Distended neck veins

Distention of the neck veins is most commonly the result of a raised jugular venous pressure secondary to heart failure. Consequently, there are normally other signs of right heart failure including ankle swelling.

Any pathology that interferes with drainage of the blood from the head and neck into the heart via the brachiocephalic veins and superior vena cava can cause distension of the neck veins (Revision panel 2.17).

PERICARDIAL EFFUSION

A pericardial effusion is a collection of fluid in the non-distensible pericardial sac that encloses the heart. Cardiac tamponade (literally 'packing') ensues if the pressure is sufficient to impair cardiac function. The cause may be benign (usually inflammatory) or malignant (invariably metastatic) (Revision panel 2.18).

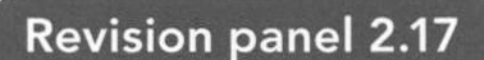
Revision panel 2.17

CAUSES OF DISTENDED NECK VEINS

Cardiac disease

Left and right heart failure
Cor pulmonale
Pulmonary embolism
Primary pulmonary hypertension
Tricuspid valve regurgitation

Pleural disease

Tension pneumothorax
Massive pleural effusion
Massive haemothorax

Pericardial disease

Constrictive pericarditis
Pericardial effusion
Cardiac tamponade

Superior vena cava obstruction

Locally invasive tumours
Thrombosis

Revision panel 2.18

CAUSES OF A PERICARDIAL EFFUSION

Pericarditis

Idiopathic
Viral
Bacterial (including tuberculosis)
Post-myocardial infarction (Dressler's syndrome)
Collagen disease (e.g. systemic lupus erythematosus)
Uraemia of renal failure

Malignant

Metastatic spread (lung cancer and other cancers such as breast)
Direct spread (lung cancer)

Trauma

Postcardiac surgery

Other

Hypothyroidism

History

Symptoms Small pericardial effusions are usually symptomless. As the effusion becomes larger, there may be central chest discomfort. Breathlessness, light-headedness and syncope are symptoms of impending cardiac tamponade.

When pericarditis is the cause, this usually causes pleuritic central chest pain, worse on inspiration and lying flat, but eased by sitting up and leaning forwards.

Previous history

A myocardial infarction within the previous 2–6 weeks suggests *Dressler's syndrome* (pericardial effusion, fever and pleuritic pain).

Postcardiotomy syndrome after cardiac surgery is similar, and probably has the same autoimmune cause.

Examination

General examination In the presence of a pericardial effusion, the stroke volume of the heart cannot increase. Tachycardia is the only way to increase the cardiac output. Tamponade with hypotension and shock will eventually follow (see below).

The jugular venous pressure is usually raised, and there may be a paradoxical rise on inspiration, known as *Kussmaul's sign* (not to be confused with Kussmaul's breathing in acidosis).

Other signs of right heart failure, such as ankle swelling, may also be present.

Auscultation of the heart in acute pericarditis may reveal a *pericardial friction rub*, best heard at the lower left sternal edge with the patient leaning forwards. The heart sounds are muffled or distant with significant effusions.

CARDIAC TAMPONADE

Cardiac tamponade is caused by fluid accumulation within the limited pericardial space which increases the right heart pressure. Diastolic ventricular filling is impaired, decreasing preload and stroke volume, which reduces normal cardiac function. Tachycardia develops to maintain cardiac output. Eventually, the heart can no longer compensate, and shock ensues.

As little as 100 mL of fluid in the pericardial sac is enough to cause tamponade. It is seen most commonly after trauma and cardiac surgery.

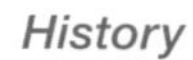

History

Patients feel generally unwell and complain of breathlessness, fatigue, light-headedness and fainting.

Examination

The classical triad of signs in cardiac tamponade is known as *Beck's triad*. This consists of:

- *Hypotension* (reduced stroke volume and cardiac output).
- *Distended neck veins* (impaired diastolic filling of the heart).
- *Muffled heart sounds* (the presence of pericardial fluid).

Other signs include tachypnoea, tachycardia, *pulsus paradoxus* (an exaggerated drop in blood pressure during inspiration) and a reduced level of consciousness.

SUPERIOR VENA CAVA OBSTRUCTION

The superior vena cava is a short segment of the venous system connecting the junction of the left and right brachiocephalic veins with the right atrium. It drains blood from the arms, head, neck and upper thorax. It is a thin-walled, low-pressure conduit and is susceptible to external compression and obstruction by mediastinal pathology.

The most common cause of superior vena cava obstruction is lung cancer from either invasive right-sided tumours or metastatic mediastinal lymph nodes. Other causes are shown in Revision panel 2.19.

History

Age Except for mediastinal tumours, the other causes occur in older age groups.

Symptoms The most common symptom is breathlessness, usually of gradual onset. At the same time, the *neck and face swell*, most pronounced in the morning. This improves during the day because standing aids venous drainage of the head.

Examination

There is *obvious swelling and venous congestion, with flaring* of the arms, neck, face and anterior chest wall.

Revision panel 2.19

CAUSES OF SUPERIOR VENA CAVA OBSTRUCTION

Benign

Fibrosing mediastinitis
Great vessel arterial aneurysm
Retrosternal goitre
Thrombosis (e.g. trauma, antiphospholipid syndrome)

Malignant

Lung cancer
Mediastinal lymphadenopathy (e.g. lymphoma, metastatic disease)
Mediastinal masses (e.g. thymoma, germ cell tumours)

Iatrogenic thrombosis

Internal jugular and subclavian central venous lines
Transvenous pacing systems

Veins over the anterior chest wall may become very prominent, as venous blood finds alternative routes to the right atrium if the condition becomes chronic (Figure 2.26).

Chest and cardiac trauma

Chest trauma will be covered fully in Chapter 5.

AORTIC RUPTURE

This serious injury occurs in severe high-speed deceleration accidents such as car crashes. The site of rupture is just beyond the left subclavian artery at the level of the ligamentum arteriosum.

In patients who survive the initial incident, the adventitia remains intact, temporarily containing the bleeding. The diagnosis is suspected from finding weak femoral pulses or unequal blood pressures in the two arms.

Investigation usually reveals a wide mediastinum.

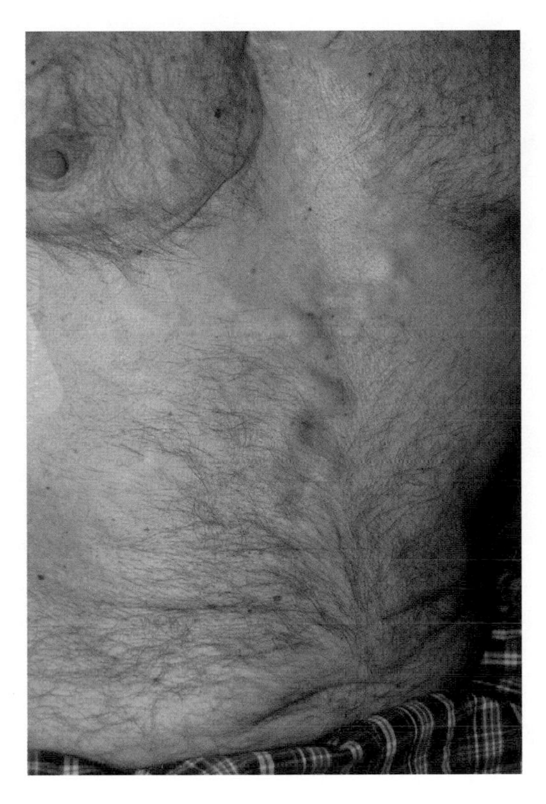

Figure 2.26 Chronic superior vena cava obstruction secondary to trauma. There are enlarged and tortuous superficial veins over the anterior chest wall.

BLUNT CARDIAC INJURY

The heart is compressed between the sternum and the vertebral column.

The patient dies immediately if the heart ruptures but myocardial contusions can occur. These behave like myocardial infarcts (see above).

Very occasionally, heart valves rupture. Presentation is with symptoms of acute regurgitation.

PENETRATING CARDIAC INJURY

An appropriately sited entry wound (normally medial to the nipple) and evidence of tamponade or hypovolaemia suggest the diagnosis (see Chapter 5).

Chest wall abnormalities

The chest wall may be an abnormal shape, which is either congenital or acquired later in life (Revision panel 2.20).

Pectus deformities are common, and occur in more than 1 in every 1000 children. Trauma (including iatrogenic) is probably the most common cause of acquired chest wall deformity.

Primary chest wall tumours (chondromas and sarcomas) are rare (Figure 2.27).

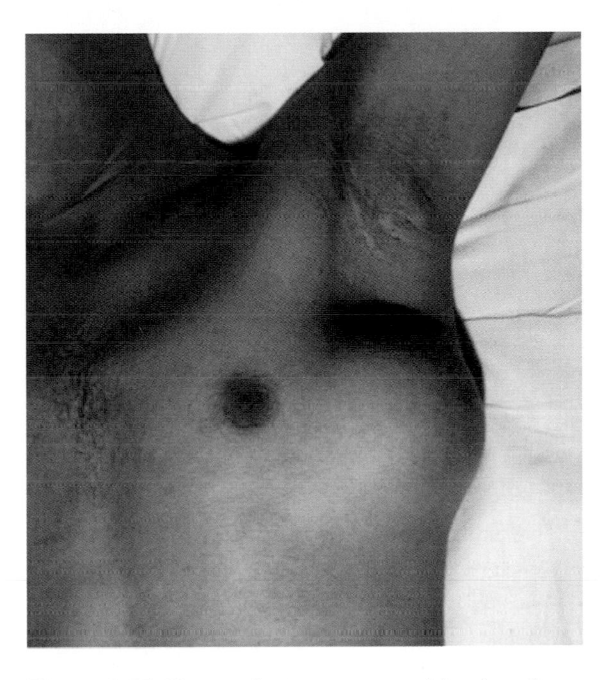

Figure 2.27 Chest wall osteosarcoma arising from the left fourth rib laterally just below the axilla.

Revision panel 2.20

CAUSES OF CHEST WALL DEFORMITY

Congenital

- Pectus excavatum
- Pectus carinatum
- Poland syndrome

Acquired

- Trauma (e.g. rib fractures, sternal fracture)
- Iatrogenic (e.g. thoracoplasty)
- Lung hernia
- Thoracic aortic aneurysm
- Benign tumours (e.g. chondroma)
- Malignant tumour (e.g. metastasis, primary sarcoma)

Lung hernias usually occur following a thoracic or cardiac operation (Figure 2.28), but can occur spontaneously following a bout of severe coughing.

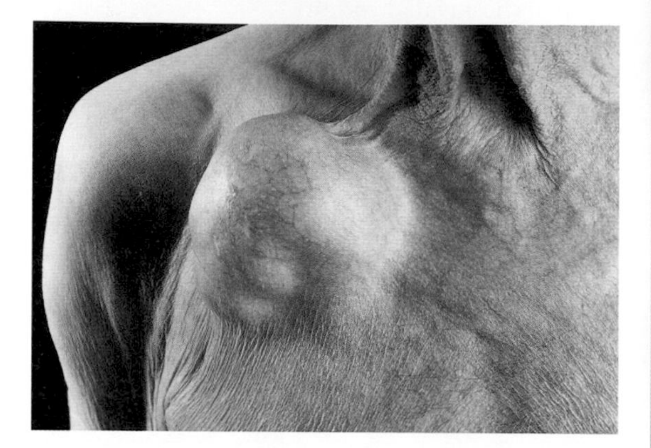

Figure 2.28 Lung hernia. This occurred following placement of a chest drain in a patient with bullous emphysema.

Syphilitic ascending thoracic aortic aneurysms eroding the anterior chest wall are now exceptionally rare.

PECTUS DEFORMITIES

Pectus excavatum is a depression of the anterior chest wall, and is sometimes known as funnel chest (Figure 2.29).

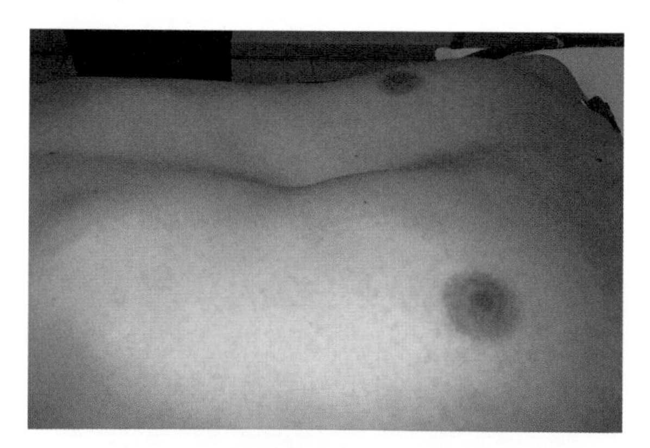

Figure 2.29 Symmetrical pectus excavatum deformity.

Pectus carinatum is the opposite, with protrusion of the anterior chest wall (Figure 2.30). It is sometimes called pigeon chest. The cause is thought to be abnormal growth patterns of the costal cartilages. Excavatum and carinatum deformities can coexist.

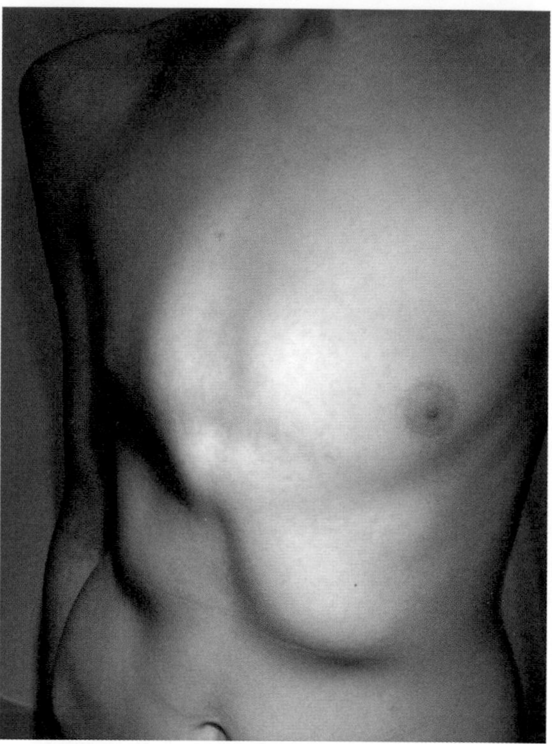

Figure 2.30 Pectus carinatum deformity, more marked on the right.

History

Age Pectus deformities often become apparent during adolescent growth spurts.

Symptoms The major symptom, and the reason why surgical correction is offered, is sensitivity about the shape of the chest causing lack of confidence, depression and an inability to interact with peers.

Vague chest pains, fatigue and shortness of breath on exertion are sometimes reported.

Previous history

Scoliosis (see Chapter 9) is associated with both deformities. Pectus excavatum is often present in Marfan's syndrome (see Chapter 1).

Examination

General appearance In addition to an assessment of the pectus deformity, look for costal flaring and scoliosis.

Auscultation of the heart in Marfan's syndrome may reveal a murmur of either mitral or aortic regurgitation.

Finger clubbing

The pathological process leading to finger clubbing is not established but growth factor secretion (e.g. in lung cancers) and disorders of prostaglandin metabolism (e.g. in idiopathic clubbing) are the most likely causes. It is a common sign in chest disease and is most frequently seen as a paraneoplastic syndrome, in chronic chest sepsis or in chronic cyanotic conditions. Lung cancer is the most common pulmonary cause, and congenital cyanotic heart disease – in which a right-to-left shunt exists – is the most common cardiac cause. Other causes are listed in Revision panel 2.21.

Revision panel 2.21

CAUSES OF FINGER CLUBBING

Non-suppurative lung disease

Lung cancer (usually non-small cell)
Interstitial lung disease
Tuberculosis

Suppurative lung disease

Lung abscess
Bronchiectasis
Cystic fibrosis

Pleural disease

Empyema
Mesothelioma
Solitary fibrous tumour

Heart disease

Congenital cyanotic heart disease
Infective endocarditis
Atrial myxoma

Abdominal disease

Malabsorption syndromes
Inflammatory bowel disease
Cirrhosis

Others

Hyperthyroidism
Familial/idiopathic

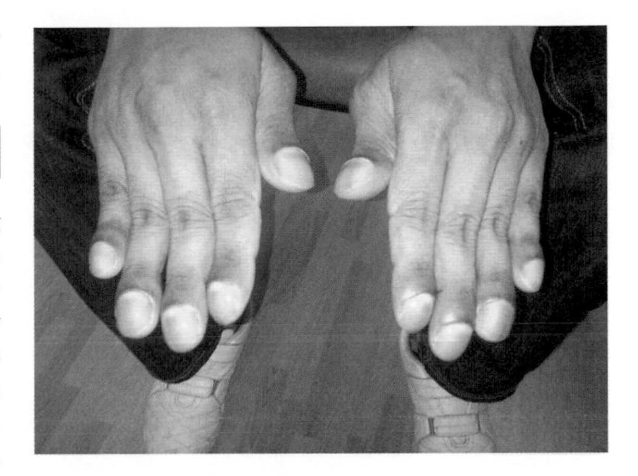

Figure 2.31 Idiopathic clubbing that developed over 4 years in a healthy 22-year-old man.

Finger clubbing (Figure 2.31) is characterized by:

- A fluctuant nail bed.
- Loss of the nail bed angle.
- Increased curvature of the nail.
- Swelling and thickening of entire finger pulp, producing the classic drumstick appearance.

Ankle swelling

Ankle swelling as a result of right heart dysfunction and peripheral oedema is a classical sign of heart failure. It is more commonly associated with immobility, and is most marked in low-protein states (for example, in postoperative patients who are recovering from complications or nephrotic syndrome).

Peripheral oedema is characterized by ankle swelling that pits on sustained pressure with an examining thumb, 'pitting oedema' (Figure 2.32). The causes are listed in Revision panel 2.22.

Cyanosis

Cyanosis is the blue discolouration of the skin or mucous membranes seen when there are high levels of deoxygenated haemoglobin (1.5–5 g/dL) in the blood.

Central cyanosis is a sign of arterial hypoxia, and is noticed when the arterial oxygen saturation falls below 85%. The lips or tongue take on a bluish tinge, and it can be present in any condition causing severe hypoxaemia (see Figure 1.3).

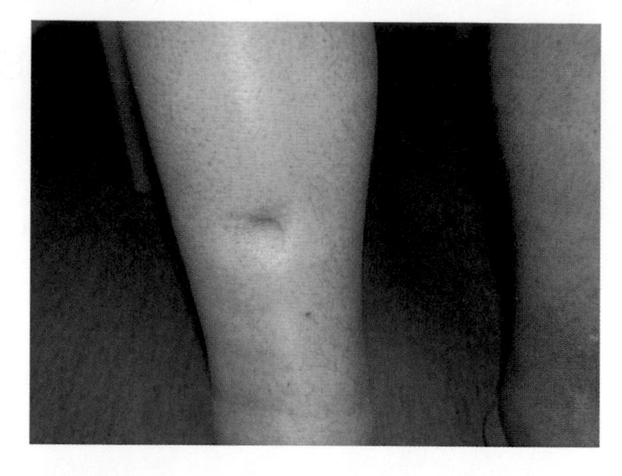

Figure 2.32 Gross pitting ankle oedema in a patient with heart failure. There is a thumb indentation on the right shin.

Revision panel 2.22

CAUSES OF PERIPHERAL OEDEMA

Immobility
Right heart failure (often from left heart failure)
Hypoalbuminaemia
Deep vein thrombosis
Venous stasis and insufficiency
Pregnancy
Calcium antagonists

Peripheral cyanosis refers to a blue discolouration of the fingers and toes. It is also seen in hypoxia, but is additionally observed as a result of poor tissue perfusion. Examples include low cardiac output states such as shock or severe heart failure, and local vasoconstrictive states such as Raynaud's phenomenon (see Figure 10.22a).

Horner's syndrome

The most common thoracic cause of Horner's syndrome is lung cancer. Tumours at the apex of the upper lobes can invade the surrounding structures, including the brachial plexus, subclavian vessels, chest wall and vertebral bodies. These so-called *Pancoast tumours* may also invade the stellate ganglion of the sympathetic chain, causing an ipsilateral Horner's syndrome (Figure 2.33).

Interruption of the sympathetic nervous supply to the face produces:

- Ptosis (a droopy eyelid).
- Miosis (a constricted pupil).
- Anhidrosis (a dry cheek due to a lack of sweating).
- Enophthalmos (a sunken eyeball).

Other causes within the chest include high paravertebral mediastinal tumours (normally neurogenic in origin), trauma and intercostal chest tube drains.

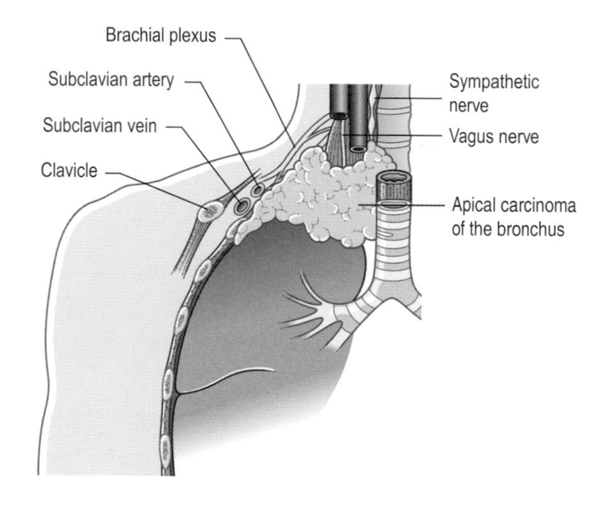

Figure 2.33 Pancoast tumour.

Acknowledgements

The contribution of Timothy Batchelor to this chapter in the 5th edition is gratefully acknowledged.

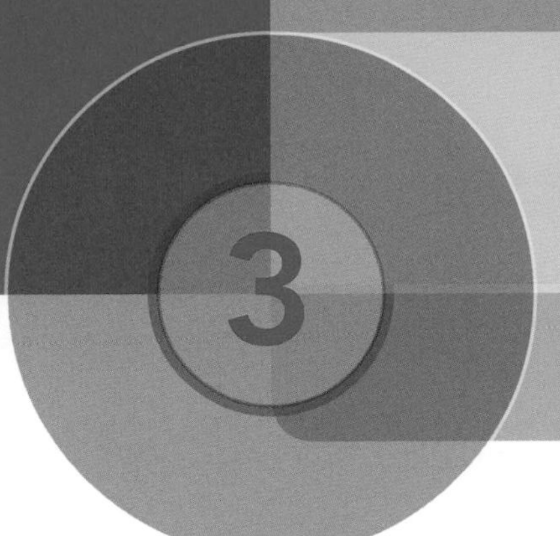

The brain, central nervous system and peripheral nerves

PETER BULLOCK

In the nervous system, it is usually possible to localize the likely pathology by clinical assessment alone, because the different functions are located in different sites connected by well-defined anatomical pathways. Advances in neurological imaging have not reduced the importance of taking a full history and carrying out a thorough examination.

HISTORY

A full neurological examination requires the co-operation of a patient who has the capacity to make decisions about their own care. Neurological illness frequently results in impairment of this capacity, but a modified history and examination can still be undertaken. Broadly, this will follow the same strategy as a full neurological examination starting with assessment of higher mental functions then proceeding through cortical function, cranial nerve examination and the long tracts before moving onto the peripheral nervous system and taking into account indices affected by autonomic function, for example blood pressure on standing up from lying down.

In the UK, the Mental Capacity Act is designed to protect people who may lack mental capacity to make decisions about their care and treatment. It applies to people aged 16 years and over. Formal independent assessment of capacity may need to be undertaken in cases where there is uncertainty or disagreement.

First, establish the patient's age, whether they are right- or left-handed and their occupation. Then try to assess their mental status. The ability to give a history may be impaired by neurological disease, and help will be needed from family members, paramedics or other witnesses to the event (see Chapter 5).

For a child, include details of the birth, early milestones and school progress.

The nervous system is bilaterally symmetrical, and establishing the correct side is vital, *so write out 'right' or 'left' in full*. It is also important to understand the impact of the condition on the patient's day-to-day activities.

Start with open questions, but then supplement the information with direct questions such as 'What do you mean by weakness?'

At the end of the history, it is worth going through a summary with the patient because they will often remember further details of their condition.

Neurological symptoms arising from cranial conditions

Common neurological symptoms include:

- Headache.
- Fits.
- Visual disturbance.
- Weakness.
- Deafness.
- Loss of balance.

INTRACRANIAL CONDITIONS PRESENTING WITH SEVERE HEADACHE

Headache is a common complaint at all ages, but severe headaches in a sick patient must not be ignored (Revision panel 3.1).

Subarachnoid haemorrhage usually presents as the *worst headache the patient has ever experienced*, as if they have been struck over the head with a hammer. This pattern of headache must not be missed as there is major risk of further bleeds. Misdiagnosis as 'sinusitis' or 'atypical migraine' is common even although the patient has described the headache as:

- 'Like no other, worst at the beginning'.
- 'As though I have been hit over the head'.
- 'Definitely the worst headache of my life'.

Pituitary apoplexy also presents with *sudden onset of severe headache and may involve loss of vision and disturbed eye movements*. It may be caused by a spontaneous bleed into an existing pituitary macroadenoma and the patient may also be taking anticoagulants.

Acute hydrocephalus can arise as a result of a blocked ventriculoperitoneal shunt or rarely from a colloid cyst of the third ventricle blocking the foramina of Monro, causing acute obstruction. Early diagnosis is vital to avoid rapid deterioration and death.

Revision panel 3.1

CAUSES OF ACUTE HEADACHE

Infection

Meningitis
Encephalitis
Ventriculoperitoneal shunt infection and blockage
Subdural empyema
Brain abscess

Vascular

Arteriovenous malformation
Subarachnoid haemorrhage
Intracerebral haemorrhage
Vascular dissection
Pituitary apoplexy
Venous thrombosis

Increased intracranial pressure

Hydrocephalus
Tumours

Local causes

Temporal arteritis
From the eye (acute angle-closure glaucoma)
Sinusitis

Headaches associated with nausea and giddiness are common after a head injury and may not settle for days or weeks. Increasing headache after a head injury in the elderly or a patient on anticoagulants suggests a chronic subdural collection.

Raised intracranial pressure from any cause (tumour, haematoma, abscess or hydrocephalus) typically causes *severe, progressive headaches that are worse in the morning and are often accompanied by vomiting*. When a person is asleep in the recumbent position, there is a relative rise in pCO_2 and a degree of vasodilatation. This relative expansion of the vascular space, with the loss of compliance as a result of the space-occupying lesion, leads to an exponential rise in pressure, manifesting as an intense headache that can wake the patient. Vomiting and hyperventilation follow the onset of the headache, which can in turn ease the headache, only for it to return the next day. Such headaches always require *urgent referral*.

Headache with a fever, photophobia and neck stiffness is characteristic of *meningitis*, and can progress to a subdural empyema.

A *cough headache* experienced 'intensely at the back of the head' is a presenting feature of a *type 1 Chiari malformation*, which is associated with herniation of the cerebellar tonsils through the foramen magnum.

There are therefore several important questions to be explored with any patient with a headache:

- Severity.
- Character.
- Duration.
- Speed of onset.
- Distribution – hemicranial or symmetrical?
- Are you unwell?
- What provokes the headache?
- What makes it better?
- Is it different from previous headaches?
- Is there any aura or accompanying visual symptoms or nausea?
- Is there conjunctival injection or hyperaemia or tearing?
- Are there associated focal neurological deficits or cranial neuropathy?

NOTE: Never forget that the headache may be the result of a brain haemorrhage, although most headaches are the result of migraines or tension.

INTRACRANIAL CONDITIONS PRESENTING WITH 'FITS'

A 'fit' will always provoke major concerns for the patient and their family.

The diagnosis of 'epilepsy' is usually straightforward, but exclude:

- Blackout from a cardiac event.
- Simple faint (vasovagal attack).

It is important to establish whether the fit was *focal* and stayed focal, or whether it became *generalized*. Did the 'twitching' start in the face or arm?

Was there any weakness after the attack (postictal weakness, *Todd's paresis*)?

Family and friends may describe:

- A brief blank look and 'lip-smacking' in a *petit mal attack*.
- Major body movements in a generalized tonic/clonic *grand mal attack*.

Many patients bite their tongue and are incontinent during a generalized fit.

In an acutely unwell patient, the following conditions must be considered:

- Infection.
- Stroke.
- Head injury.
- Cerebral haemorrhage.
- Supratentorial brain tumour.
- Metabolic disorder.

Continuous seizure activity without interruption is a medical emergency and may quickly result in brain injury. It is termed *status epilepticus* and may be convulsive or non-convulsive. It is diagnosed after 5 minutes of continuous seizure activity and treatment must be initiated to prevent neuronal death within 30 minutes.

Partial or generalized epilepsy is a frequent symptom of frontal and temporal lobe tumours.

Seizures beginning after adolescence should always raise the suspicion of an underlying brain tumour.

When recording the history of a 'fit', ask what the patient experienced, as well as what was observed by family or friends. Ask about the onset of the fit:

- Were there any warning symptoms?
- Were there any abnormal tastes or smells?
- Were there any 'butterflies' in the stomach?

These may indicate an origin in the temporal lobe.

Subsequent attacks often follow a particular pattern, and can be triggered by lack of sleep, alcohol and stress.

NOTE: A brain abscess carries the highest risk of long-term fits.

INTRACRANIAL CONDITIONS PRESENTING WITH DISTURBANCE OF VISION (VISUAL LOSS AND DOUBLE VISION)

Failing vision

The cause is ocular (cataract, macular degeneration and glaucoma) more often than neurological.

Is the visual loss *monocular* or *binocular*? Monocular visual loss arises in one eye or optic nerve. Binocular visual loss, such as a *homonymous hemianopia*, is related to the visual pathways posterior to the optic chiasm.

A vascular cause such as *amaurosis fugax* (fleeting blindness) should be suspected from the history (see Chapter 10). Smoking, diabetes and hypertension are associated factors.

Coexisting headache or retro-orbital pain raises the possibility of *retro-orbital neuritis*, a *carotid dissection* or an *expanding aneurysm*.

Other important elements in the history are the speed and degree of visual loss, whether it is painful and the exact pattern of the defect.

Neurosurgical causes for visual loss

Tumours in the suprasellar region compressing the optic nerves and chiasm. *Meningiomas and pituitary tumours* present with gradual painless visual loss. Compression of the optic nerves and chiasm leads to a reduction in the peripheral visual fields, sometimes unnoticed for years. The patient will eventually present with visual failure when the tumour is much larger and the central visual fields are lost, limiting reading and writing.

Pituitary apoplexy with headache is associated with rapid loss of vision in one or both eyes, often with temporal visual field loss, and is caused by haemorrhage in a pre-existing pituitary tumour.

Raised intracranial pressure can lead to transient loss of vision with postural change (obscuration). It is often described as a brief blackout, like a curtain coming down, and lasting only seconds.

Look for *papilloedema* (see Figure 3.4, page 86).

In the elderly, transient visual loss can be caused by *temporal arteritis*, which, without treatment, can lead to irreversible blindness. There may be tenderness and prominence of the temporal artery and 'claudication' on chewing.

Double vision (diplopia)

To identify which group of muscles are involved ask whether the double vision is:

- Worse looking up or down.
- Worse looking left or right.
- Better with the head tilted.

If the double vision is worst in one particular direction, *horizontal, vertical or diagonal*, this will indicate which muscle and hence which nerve is involved. For example, if the left lateral rectus is weak, double vision will be maximal looking to the left.

> **NOTE:** A painful IIIrd nerve palsy with ptosis, a dilated pupil and an inability to move the eye in any direction but outwards is a classical presentation of an expanding aneurysm behind the eye (Figure 3.1).

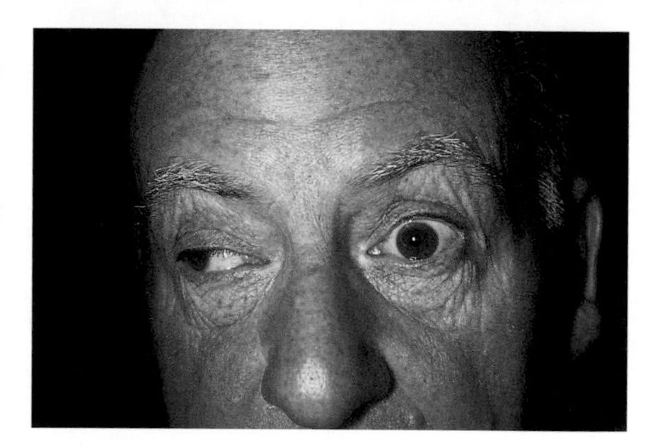

Figure 3.1 IIIrd cranial nerve palsy.

A pupil-sparing IIIrd nerve palsy is often attributed to diabetes and an ischaemic neuropathy.

When a tumour or aneurysm involves the cavernous sinus there is a characteristic combination of IIIrd, IVth and VIth cranial nerve palsies, often with proptosis. If the branches of the trigeminal nerve are also involved, there is altered sensation over the cheek or the forehead.

Painless diplopia secondary to an isolated IVth or VIth cranial nerve palsy is often unexplained.

When the eyes obviously point in different directions and there is no complaint of double vision, there must be a long-standing squint, or an accompanying loss of vision in one eye with the squint (*amblyopia*).

INTRACRANIAL CONDITIONS PRESENTING WITH WEAKNESS (FOCAL NEUROLOGICAL DEFICIT)

Focal neurological deficits such as weakness of the arm or leg allow the site of the pathology to be localized whatever its cause (Table 3.1).

The motor homunculus is a cortical representation of control of movements (Figure 3.2). It is important to *distinguish cortical from spinal motor paresis.* A parasagittal meningioma compressing the medial aspect of the motor strip in the posterior frontal region can give rise to a stiff spastic leg.

INTRACRANIAL CONDITIONS PRESENTING WITH DEAFNESS AND LOSS OF BALANCE

Deafness is common and has many causes. Ask directly about:

- Speed of onset.
- Degree of hearing loss.
- Unsteadiness.
- Facial numbness.
- Change of voice.
- Difficulty swallowing.

Table 3.1 Localization of pathology within the brain

Site of focal lesion	Symptom
Frontal lobe	Dementia and personality change with hemiparesis
Temporal lobe	Auditory or olfactory hallucinations, memory impairment, visual field defect and with dominant lobe, dysphasia
Parietal lobe	Hemiparesis with sensory neglect and visual field defect
Occipital lobe	Contralateral visual field defect
Posterior fossa	Cranial nerve palsies and ipsilateral ataxia

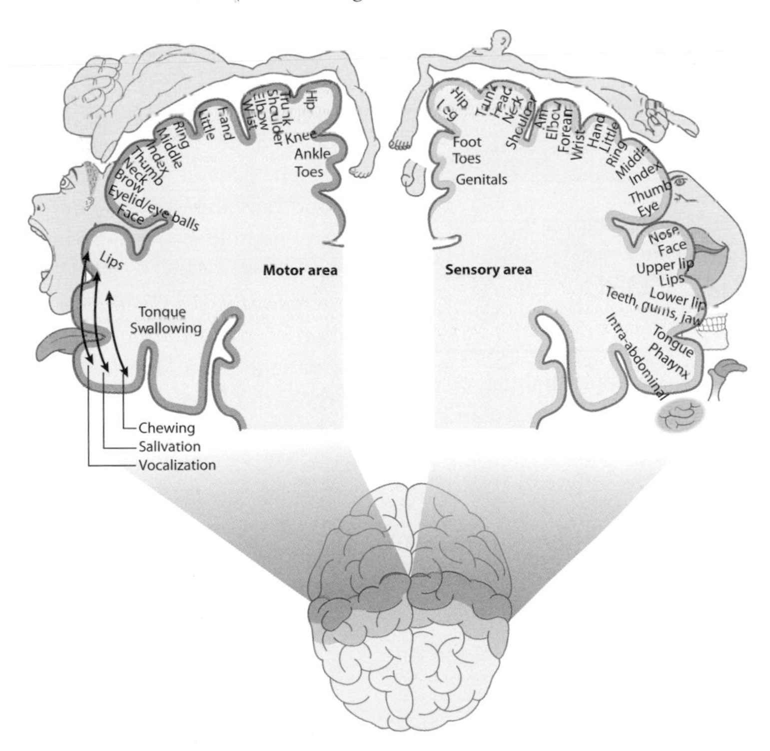

Figure 3.2 Motor and sensory homunculus.

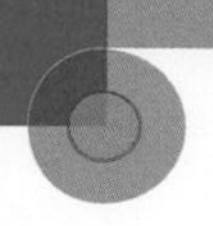

Unilateral progressive deafness may indicate the early stages of an infratentorial tumour such as a vestibular schwannoma or a meningioma.

As these tumours enlarge, they distort the brainstem, which produces multiple cranial nerve palsies, seen with any space-occupying lesion in the cerebellopontine angle.

Early symptoms with small tumours include:

- Unilateral hearing loss.
- High-pitched tinnitus.
- Unsteadiness.

Examination reveals a sensorineural hearing loss. In contrast, a conductive deafness may be caused by chronic otitis media.

Symptoms of a vestibular schwannoma correlate closely with tumour size. Large tumours can cause facial pain or numbness from trigeminal nerve compression, as well as unsteadiness from brainstem distortion.

Bilateral symptoms are rare and suggest type 2 neurofibromatosis.

Very large tumours cause brainstem signs with ataxia, double vision and eventually hydrocephalus. Lower cranial nerve involvement produces hoarseness and difficulty in swallowing.

Neurological symptoms arising from spinal conditions

These are also discussed in Chapter 9.

CHRONIC SPINAL CORD COMPRESSION

Cervical myelopathy causes abnormalities of gait and weakness or stiffness of the legs. It can also present with a loss of manual dexterity, difficulty in writing and abnormal sensations, which patients describe as numb, clumsy hands.

Signs of spasticity are often present, but loss of sphincter control and urinary incontinence are unusual.

ACUTE SPINAL CORD COMPRESSION

The clinical features of acute cord compression are:

- Progressive paraparesis.
- A 'sensory level' (the sensory segmental level of the spinal cord below which sensation to a pin or light touch is impaired).
- Often disturbance of sphincter control.
- Back pain, usually intense.

Speed of onset

An *acute onset* is typically associated with *transverse myelitis or a bleed* from a *spinal arteriovenous malformation*.

Infection and malignant tumours present with a steady *deterioration over some weeks*.

A *slow painless progression* over months suggests a *benign intradural tumour* such as a *meningioma or schwannoma*.

Evidence of cutaneous neurofibromatosis (see Chapter 4) increases the likelihood of a spinal tumour. Long-standing plexiform neurofibromas are known to undergo late malignant transformation.

NEUROLOGICAL EXAMINATION

You need to become confident with the ophthalmoscope, red pin and reflex hammer.

Observe the patient as they enter the room, noting their general appearance, mood and mobility, and how they sit and stand, undress and dress. Several neurological conditions can be diagnosed at this point.

Acromegaly (see Chapter 1) is caused by the stimulation of growth after normal growth has ceased. The patient has a large face and large hands, with overgrowth of the soft tissues of the face, nose, lips and tongue, and of the frontal sinuses and jaw (see Figure 1.9).

The *neurocutaneous syndromes* (see Chapter 4) are readily diagnosed on sight:

- *Type 1 neurofibromatosis*: café-au-lait patches, subcutaneous nodules, plexiform neuromas with a risk of sarcomatous change.
- *Sturge–Weber syndrome*: epilepsy and a port wine stain on the forehead.
- *Tuberous sclerosis*: adenoma sebaceum on the cheeks and nose, subungual fibromas.

Head and spine

Measure the circumference of a large or abnormally shaped head with a tape measure. Over 60 cm is abnormal. Larger heads can indicate:

- Chronic hydrocephalus (see Chapter 1).
- Acromegaly (see Chapter 1).
- Paget's disease in the elderly (Figure 3.3).

Often standard headwear, caps and hats will not fit (see Chapter 6).

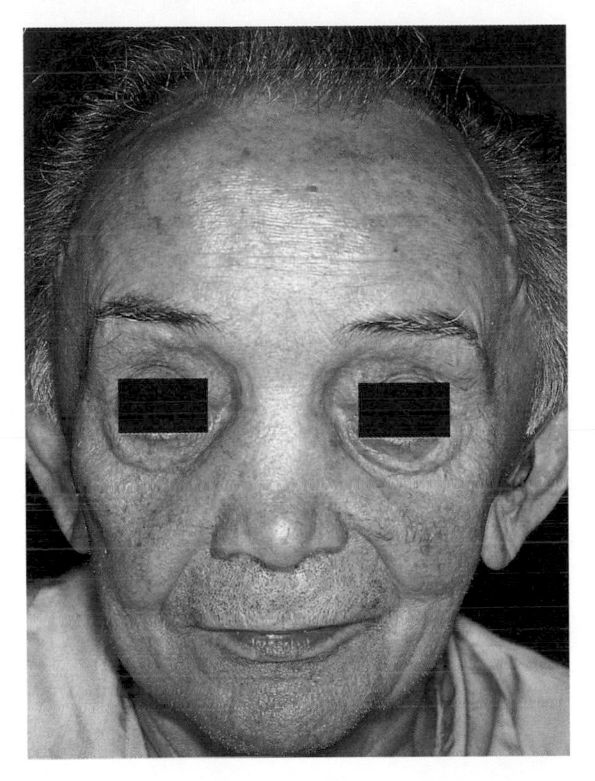

Figure 3.3 Paget's disease. Large head circumference.

Scalp swellings are inspected and palpated. Determine whether they are mobile in relation to the skull, such as a dermoid of the scalp (see Chapter 4), or are fixed to the skull and hard, such as an osteoma of the skull (see Chapter 6). Very rarely, a hard, bony lump indicates an underlying meningioma.

In the elderly, feel the temporal arteries looking for tenderness and thickening. In a patient with the headache of temporal arteritis, the abnormal arteries stand out.

Listen with your stethoscope over the closed eye, the cheek and the mastoid area if there is a proptosis. There will be bruit – a whooshing noise if there is a caroticocavernus fistula or a cerebral arteriovenous malformation.

Inspect the spine for any midline cutaneous abnormalities such as an *angioma, dimple or hairy patch* (see Chapter 9) that may be a cutaneous manifestation of underlying spinal dysraphism (see Chapter 9).

Examine the spine with the patient standing. Note any deformity or swelling. Look for kyphosis and scoliosis. Assess the full range of movement, with the patient bending forwards and backwards, with lateral flexion and with rotation to either side. Note any fatty swelling such as a lipoma over the lower spine, also in keeping with dysraphism. Palpate for tenderness and paravertebral spasm.

The neurological examination starts with the higher functions and then works systematically down from the head to the arms and legs.

Explain what you are doing and why.

> **NOTE:** The examination finishes as you watch the patient leave the consulting room.

Practical neurological examination

TESTING OF HIGHER CORTICAL FUNCTION

Assess the patient's orientation in time and place. Ask their views of current events, perhaps sport results or newspaper headlines. Routine tests of memory and intellectual function are undertaken if there are doubts about short-term memory.

A useful test is to ask the patient to memorize three objects immediately and recall them immediately after 5 minutes. An alternative is to ask them to carry out a serial subtraction of seven from 100.

Any speech or language disorder should become evident during the history-taking.

Do not use the term 'confused'. It is better to state whether the patient is fully orientated or disorientated, and whether they can express themselves or not, that is, they are *dysphasic*.

Dysphasia can make patients appear muddled because of difficulty in expressing themselves.

Other tests of language include reading and the ability to execute spoken commands and name objects.

Visual spatial difficulties can be assessed by asking the patient to copy a figure or draw a clock face with hands.

Further assessment can be undertaken using tools that specifically assess and document higher function, for example, the Mini Mental State examination.

EXAMINATION OF THE CRANIAL NERVES

Examine the cranial nerves systematically to ensure that all 12 nerves are tested on every occasion.

I Olfactory nerve

The sense of smell can be tested formally with bottles containing cloves or cinnamon. You can use orange peel or soap if these are not available. The nose is supplied by the Ist (smell only) and Vth cranial nerves.

An *anosmic patient* can still sense noxious agents such as ammonia through the trigeminal nerve, but can taste only salt, sweet, sour and bitter, not enough to savour food or wine. They cannot smell smoke if there is a fire.

Neurological loss of smell results from *head injury or a large anterior skull base tumour* such as a bifrontal meningioma presenting with dementia and anosmia.

Nasal causes of anosmia such as *sinusitis and polyps* are more common.

II Optic nerve

Fundoscopic examination is key.

Look for swelling of the optic disc (*papilloedema*) in any patient with suspected raised intracranial pressure (Figure 3.4). The optic disc is normally pale pink or yellow with crisp margins. An early sign of papilloedema is the loss of venous pulsation. Standing the patient up increases the pulsation if there is any doubt. Blurring of the optic disc is characteristic, particularly on the temporal side, and retinal haemorrhages are common.

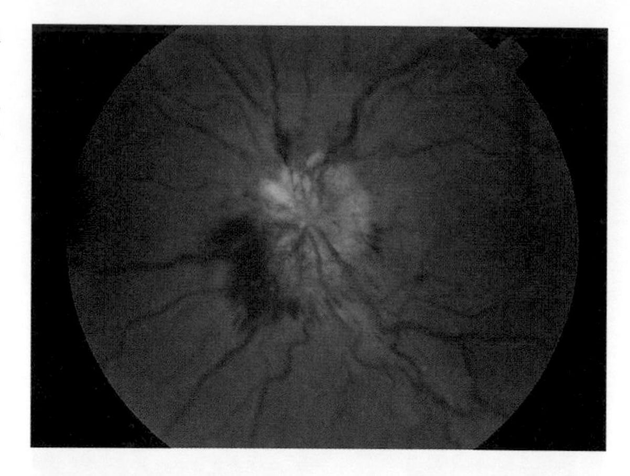

Figure 3.4 Papilloedema.

The visual acuity is often normal, with a concentric restriction of the visual fields and enlargement of the blind spot (see below). Note that papilloedema may not occur in elderly patients who have raised intracranial pressure.

Optic atrophy (pallor of the optic disc) secondary to chronic compression is found in patients with expanding lesions in the suprasellar region, pituitary tumours, meningioma and aneurysms (Figure 3.5).

Confidence using the ophthalmoscope requires practice at every opportunity. The pupil gets smaller with age, so learn to use the instrument on younger patients or colleagues. A darkened room helps.

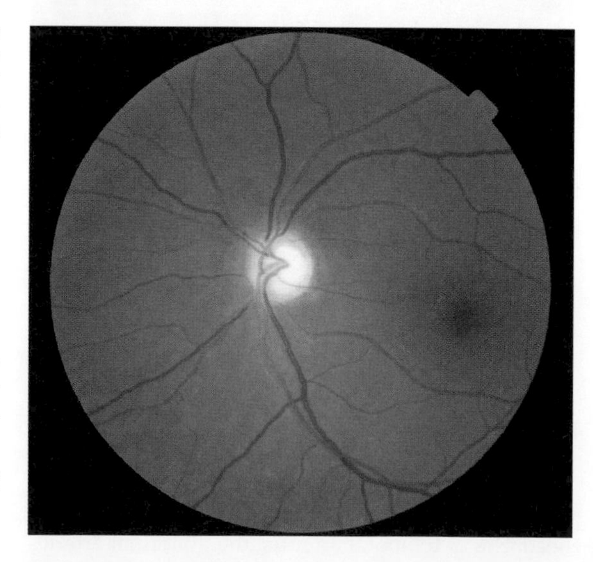

Figure 3.5 Optic atrophy.

Visual acuity is a test of how well patients see using their central visual field.

Distant vision is tested with a well-illuminated Snellen chart, at a distance of 6 m. Details can be found in ophthalmology texts.

Asking the patient to read newspaper headlines is a crude alternative.

Impaired vision can be graded as the ability to count fingers, detect hand movements and tell light from dark.

Near vision is tested with reading cards with varying sizes of print.

Visual fields can be tested rapidly and reliably at the bedside.

Sit directly in front of the patient. Ask them to close one eye and look straight at you with the other. Keeping your hand midway between you and the patient, move your hand holding a red pin beyond your own visual field. Then gradually move the pin towards the midline until you can see it.

The visual field is normal if you and the patient see the red colour at the same time. Any abnormality can be investigated further by testing each quadrant.

Visual pathways (Figure 3.6)

The visual pathways are important in localizing cerebral lesions because they travel from the temporal lobe through the parietal lobe to the occipital cortex. The pattern of visual field loss enables the lesion to be localized.

A lesion of the optic radiation leads to a *homonymous hemianopia or quadrantanopia.*

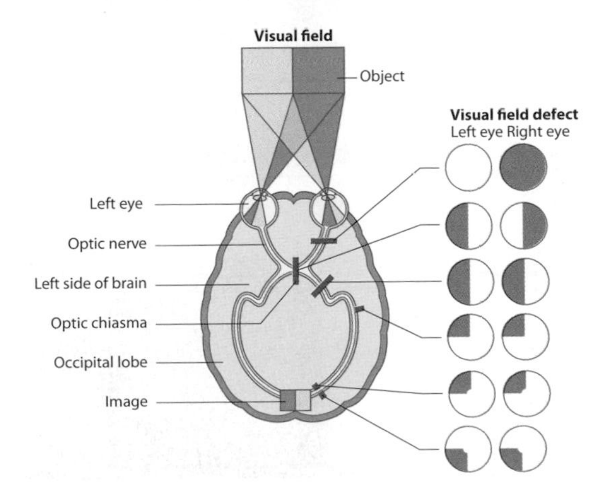

Figure 3.6 Visual pathways.

Lesions of the optic nerve lead to *monocular visual loss,* and those of the optic chiasm to *bitemporal hemianopia.*

Lesions of the optic tract, optic radiation or geniculostriate tract cause varying degrees of *homonymous hemianopia.*

Lesions of the striate cortex, particularly if vascular, can be associated with sparing of macular vision. Some fibres course inferiorly around the occipital horn of the lateral ventricle (Meyer's loop), and lesions here cause a *homonymous upper quadrantanopia.*

Lesions affecting the upper, more direct fibres of the tract cause a *homonymous lower quadrantanopia.*

The *pupils* are inspected for size, shape and reaction to light. Horner's syndrome (see Chapter 1) and Holmes Adie syndrome will be obvious.

Eye movements

There are six muscles attached to each eye. To test the eye movements, ask the patient to keep their head still and follow your finger, and to tell you if they see double at any stage.

Draw a large H to test lateral and vertical movements.

The medial and lateral rectus are involved in horizontal movement.

The inferior and superior rectus are involved in vertical movements.

Torsional movements are controlled by the inferior and superior obliques.

III Oculomotor nerve

This supplies four of the six extrinsic eye muscles, as well as the levator palpebrae superioris and the muscle of accommodation. When it fails to function, the eye turns downwards and outwards, the upper lid droops (ptosis) and the pupil becomes fixed (not responding to light or accommodation) (Figure 3.7).

Sometimes individual muscles supplied by the IIIrd nerve can be paralysed.

To test the *superior rectus muscle,* ask the patient to 'look up'.

To test the *inferior rectus,* ask the patient to 'look down'.

Oculomotor function is examined by looking for ptosis, the size of the pupils, and their reactivity to light and accommodation.

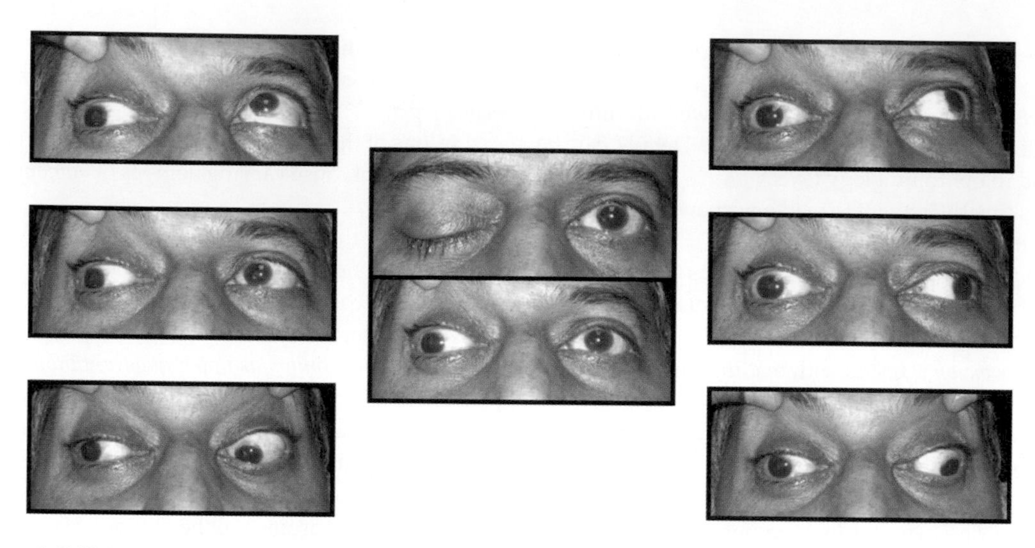

Figure 3.7 IIIrd nerve palsy. Ptosis and difficulty looking up and down.

Remember that the IVth and VIth cranial nerves also have a role in eye movements. Attention should be paid to the direction in which maximal diplopia is noted by the patient, because this indicates the most likely weak muscle and responsible cranial nerve.

IV Trochlear nerve

This supplies the superior oblique muscle, which turns the eye downwards and outwards. If the nerve is damaged, the eye will look inwards (Figure 3.8) and the patient will experience diplopia below the horizontal plane, for example when walking downstairs.

V Trigeminal nerve

This has three main divisions and is sensory to the face and up to the crown of the head (vertex). Test sensation close to the midline and compare the two sides. Note that the angle of the jaw is supplied by the great auricular nerve from the C2 and C3 roots. The

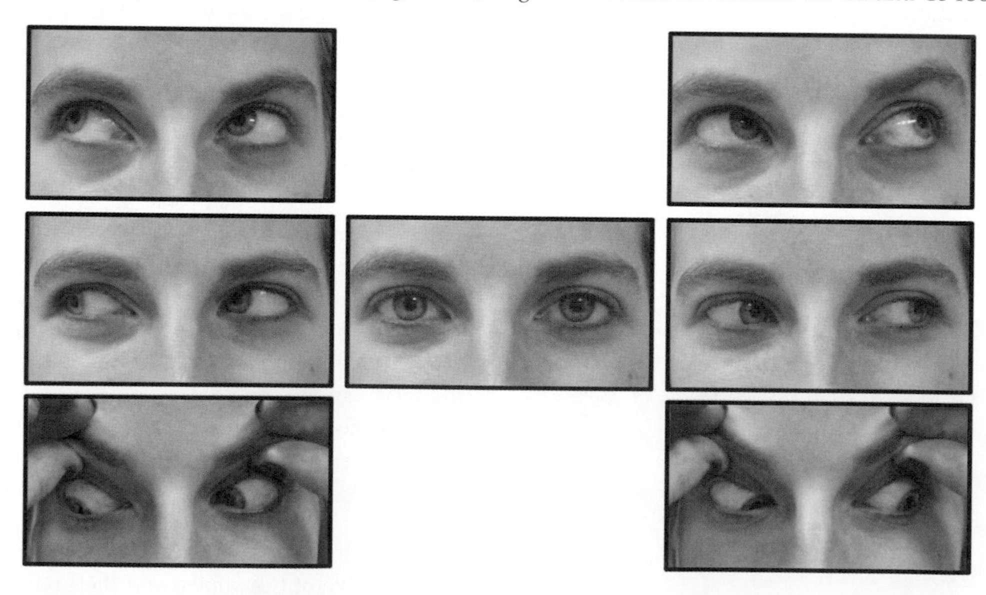

Figure 3.8 Damage of the right IVth cranial nerve.

cutaneous distribution of the ophthalmic, maxillary and mandibular divisions are shown in Figure 3.9.

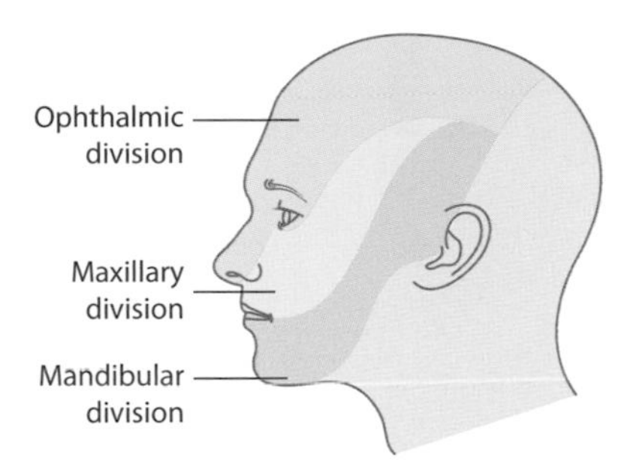

Figure 3.9 Trigeminal nerve sensory distribution.

The *corneal reflex* has the Vth nerve as its afferent pathway and the VIIth nerve as its efferent. It therefore assesses the facial nerve as well as the trigeminal nerve. It is tested by touching the cornea of the eye with a twisted pointed roll of tissue paper or cotton wool. This normally elicits a blink. The reflex/blink is lost if the ophthalmic division is damaged.

The *trigeminal nerve also supplies the muscles of mastication*. Motor fibres of the trigeminal nerve run in its mandibular division to the masseter, temporalis and medial and lateral pterygoid muscles.

Ask the patient to clench the teeth and feel the contraction of the temporalis and masseter.

Do not test power by trying to close an open jaw. This may cause dislocation. If there is Vth nerve damage, the jaw deviates towards the side of the lesion, pushed across by the unopposed pterygoid muscles.

VI Abducens nerve

This nerve supplies the lateral rectus muscle, which turns the eye outwards. If it is damaged, the eye does not move when the patient tries to look sideways and there is diplopia, maximal when looking towards the side of the lesion (Figure 3.10).

A VIth nerve palsy can occur with any rise in intracranial pressure, so it is not a useful localizing sign.

VII Facial nerve

This is the motor nerve to the muscles of facial expression.

To test the facial nerve:

- Ask the patient to look up – the forehead should wrinkle (Figure 3.11a).

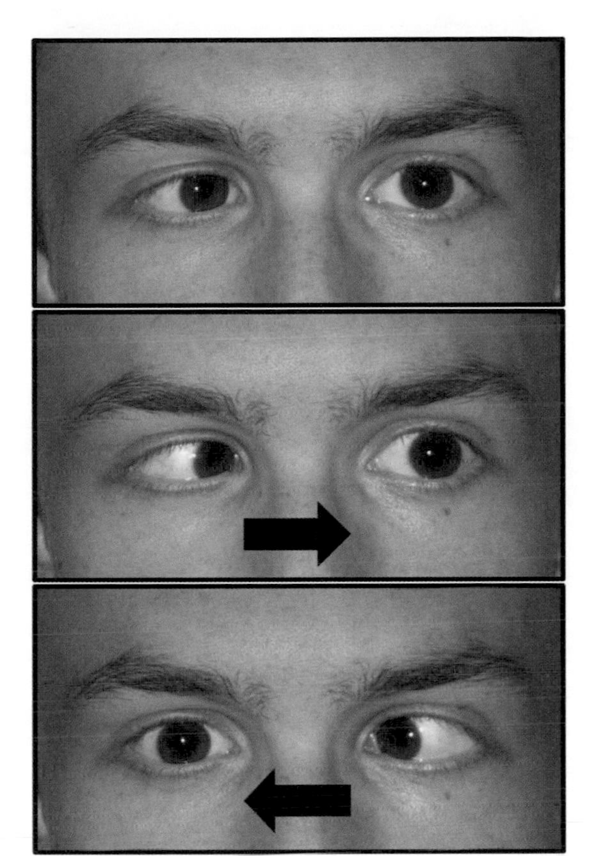

Figure 3.10 Bilateral VIth cranial nerve palsies.

- Ask them to close their eyes tightly. Any weakness is obvious (Figure 3.11b).

With a facial nerve lesion, the *ability to blink is lost* and the eyelids do not cover the eye fully.

When the patient is asked to show you their teeth, the mouth becomes asymmetrical.

The patient cannot whistle.

Any damage to the tract of the nerve distal to the nucleus (lower motor neuron, LMN) causes paralysis of the whole of one side of the face (see Figure 1.12).

There is bilateral representation and function of the forehead is persevered if there is an upper motor neuron lesion.

Facial movements should also be observed with the patient talking and smiling, as a mild UMN weakness may be missed at rest.

The most important sensory function of the facial nerve is taste to the anterior two-thirds of the tongue via the chorda tympani. Taste may be tested using sweet, sour, salt and bitter substances.

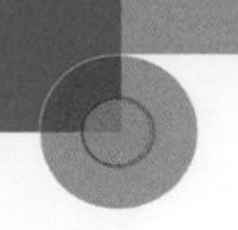

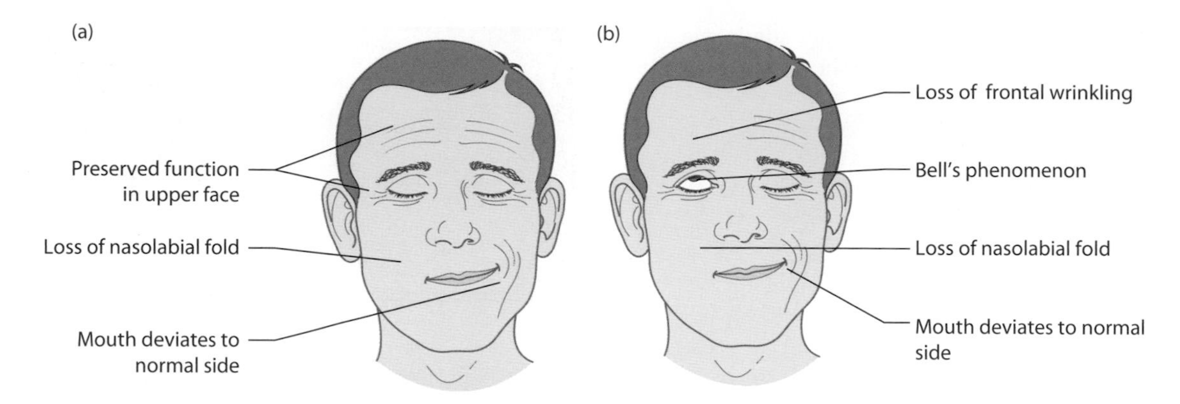

Figure 3.11 FACIAL NERVE PALSY. (a) Wrinkling of the forehead, UMN. (b) Weakness of eye closing, LMN.

VIII Auditory nerve

This nerve has two distinct components, both passing through the internal auditory meatus:

- The *cochlear* (auditory) division is responsible for hearing and transmits sound from hair cells in the organ of Corti within the inner ear.
- The *vestibular* division is responsible for balance and transmits information from the semicircular canals.

This nerve may be damaged by fractures of the base of the skull or compressed by acoustic neuromas.

Hearing can be tested simply by whispering in one ear while the opposite ear is closed by pressure on the tragus. The patient is asked to repeat what they can hear.

Hearing loss is either *conductive*, when the sound does not reach the cochlea, or *sensorineural*, where there is dysfunction of the cochlea, the auditory nerve or the brain itself. First look with an auroscope to ensure there is no obstruction in the outer or middle ear causing conductive deafness.

Rinne's and Weber's tests distinguish sensorineural hearing loss from conductive hearing loss.

- **Rinne's test.** Hold a vibrating tuning fork next to the external auditory meatus until the patient indicates that the sound can no longer be heard. The base of the tuning fork is then placed on the mastoid process. If the sound can still be heard, the patient has a conductive deafness (*negative* Rinne's test).
- **Weber's test.** Place the tuning fork on the centre of the forehead. Normally, both ears hear the sound equally. If there is sensorineural deafness, the sound will be loudest in the normal ear. If there is conductive deafness, the sound will be loudest in the abnormal ear.

Nystagmus, a rapid, brief to and fro movement of the eyes, suggests impairment of the vestibular division of the auditory nerve. The patient may complain of giddiness, and the abnormal eye movements may be seen on extremes of gaze.

The Romberg and stepping tests are also useful in evaluating vestibular function (see below).

IX Glossopharyngeal nerve

This nerve is the sensory nerve of the posterior third of the tongue. It also supplies the taste receptors and sensory endings of the mucous membrane of the pharynx.

It can be assessed by testing the *gag reflex*.

X Vagus nerve

The vagus nerve carries motor function to the soft palate.

When patients are asked to open the mouth widely and say 'Aarrh', the soft palate should move upwards symmetrically. If one side of the palate is paralysed, the uvula will be pulled towards the functioning side.

Lesions of the glossopharyngeal nerve usually also involve the vagus nerve as they travel together through the jugular foramen, where they can be compressed by, for example, a glomus jugular tumour.

The IXth and Xth nerves control the pharynx and larynx and are tested together. The voice and the ability to cough and swallow are functions of the two nerves. Loss of function should be suspected if the patient is hoarse or has a bovine cough. They are then at risk of aspiration and chest infection.

XI Spinal accessory nerve

This nerve arises from the medulla and upper spinal cord. It is a pure motor nerve and supplies the trapezius and sternomastoid muscles.

The function of these muscles is tested by asking the patient to shrug the shoulders and to turn the head against resistance.

It is very rare to have a spontaneous XIth nerve palsy. The usual cause is damage during surgical dissection of the posterior triangle of the neck (Figure 3.12).

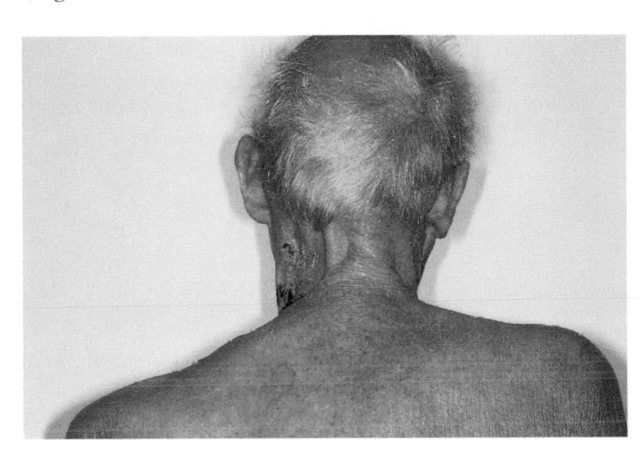

Figure 3.12 Spinal accessory nerve. Damaged by block dissection of neck on the left side.

XII Hypoglossal nerve

This is also a purely motor nerve and supplies the muscles of the tongue. When one hypoglossal nerve is paralysed, the tongue is wasted on that side and the tongue deviates towards the weak side (Figure 3.13).

EXAMINING MOTOR FUNCTION

Start by inspecting and testing the tone of the resting muscles (Revision panel 3.2). *Wasting and reduced tone indicate an LMN lesion.* Muscle bulk can be assessed by comparing the maximum circumference of the calves or thighs (Figure 3.14).

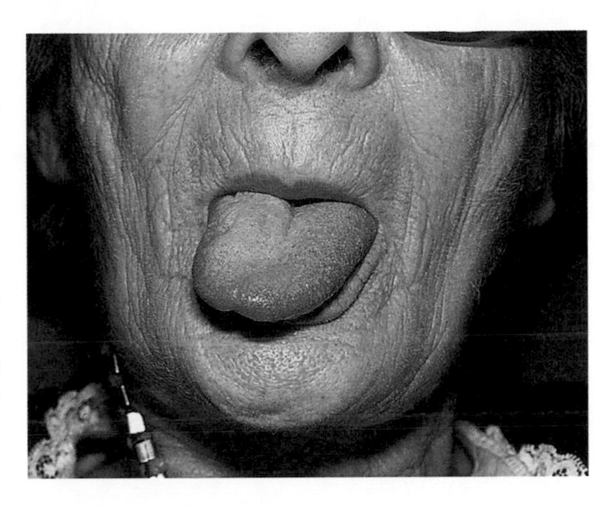

Figure 3.13 Hypoglossal nerve. Damaged by right carotid endarterectomy.

Revision panel 3.2

TYPES OF WEAKNESS AND REGION AFFECTED

Monoplegia: Single limb
Hemiplegia: One side of the body, arm and leg
Paraplegia: Both lower limbs
Quadriplegia: All four limbs

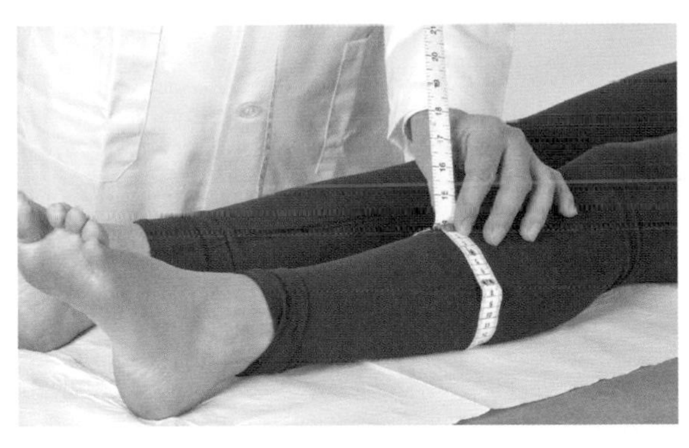

Figure 3.14 Measuring to assess muscle bulk.

There should be no more than 1 cm difference. *With a UMN lesion, there is no wasting*; increased spinal activity maintains the muscle bulk.

- Examine the upper limbs with the patient sitting (Figure 3.15).
- Examine the lower limbs with the patient supine.

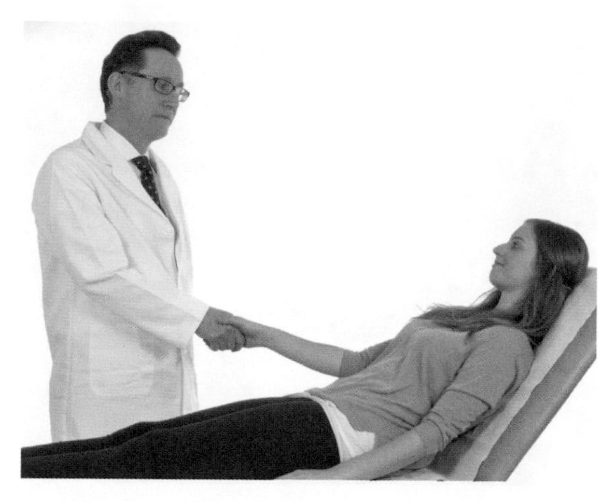

Figure 3.15 Examining the upper limbs with the patient seated.

- Examine the range of spinal movements with the patient standing.

Ask the patient to stand on their toes, testing S1, and then on their heels, testing L4/5. Then ask them to stand on each leg, and then hop on each leg, thus checking power and coordination.

Watch the patient walking.

Look out for proximal weakness, which may be indicated by difficulty with getting out of a chair.

Upper limb

Power is graded from 0 to 5.

Fine finger movement is tested by asking the patient to pretend to play the piano.

The fingers are spread wide, testing the intrinsic muscles of the hand supplied by T1 (Figure 3.16).

The fingers are brought together and held straight, which tests the long extensors (C8) (Figure 3.17) and curled to test the flexors (Figure 3.18).

The fist is clenched and locked at the wrist. Resistance to movement assesses muscle power.

Test elbow flexion (C6) and extension (C7) (Figure 3.19).

Finally, test the power of shoulder abduction (C5) (Figure 3.20).

Upper limb reflexes

These are supinator (C6) (Figure 3.21) biceps (C6) (Figure 3.22), triceps (C7) (Figure 3.23) and deltoid (C5).

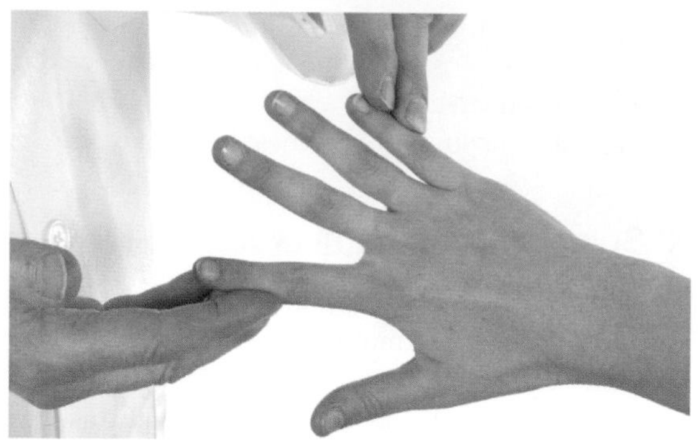

Figure 3.16 Testing the power of the intrinsic muscles of the hand (T1).

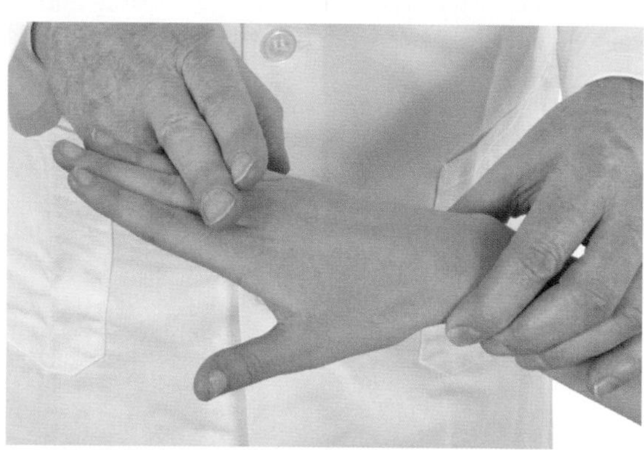

Figure 3.17 Testing the power of the long extensors of the hand (C7/8).

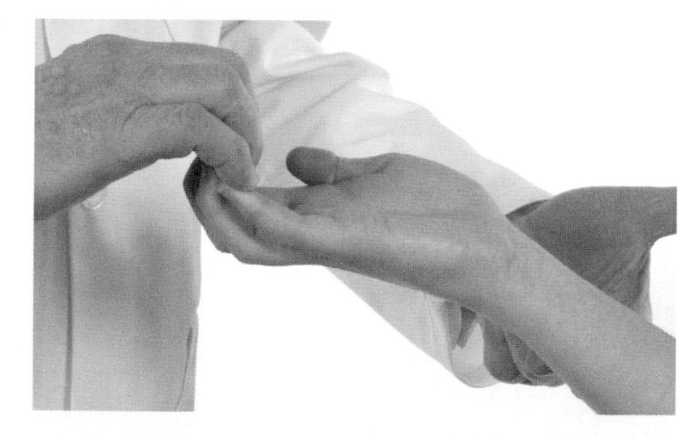

Figure 3.18 Testing the long flexors (C8).

The tendon hammer is held lightly at the far end and swung smoothly onto the tendon covered by your finger or thumb. This allows you to see and feel the reflex, or its absence.

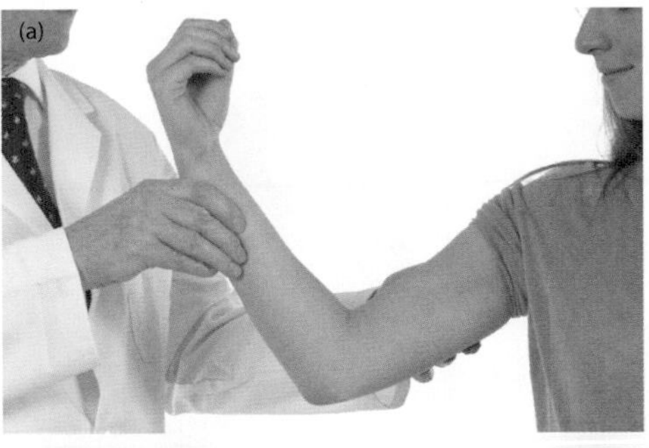

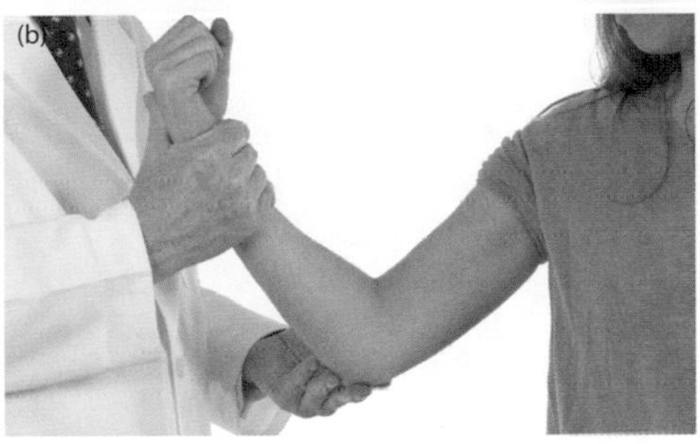

Figure 3.19 ELBOW FLEXION AND EXTENSION. (a) Testing the power of extension of the elbow (C7). (b) Testing the power of flexion of the elbow (C5/6).

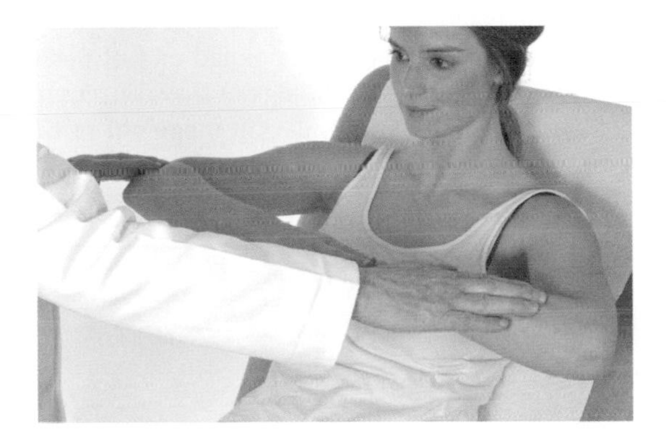

Figure 3.20 Testing the power of shoulder abduction (C5).

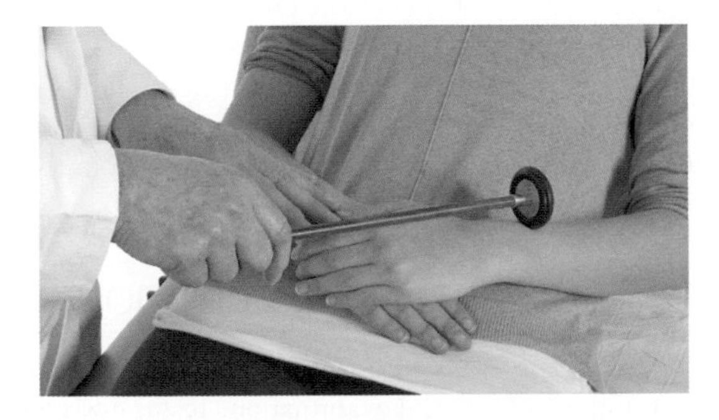

Figure 3.21 Supinator (C6) reflex.

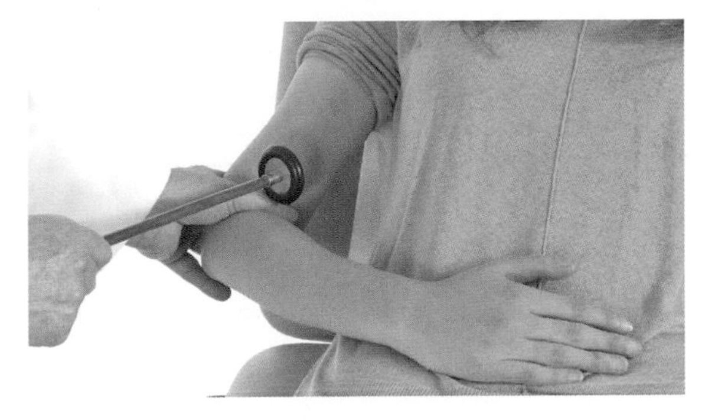

Figure 3.22 Biceps (C5/6) reflex.

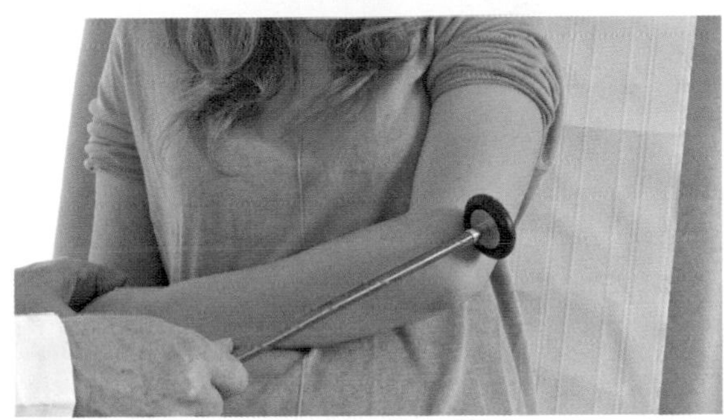

Figure 3.23 Triceps (C7) reflex.

An 'inverted' or paradoxical reflex is a useful localizing sign, particularly in patients with multilevel cervical myelopathy. On testing, the biceps reflex (C6) is absent, but there is brisk finger flexion (C8) (Figure 3.18). This indicates an LMN lesion at C6 level (absent reflex) and a UMN lesion at C8 (finger flexion brisk).

Rapid screening tests

Ask the patient to hold their arms out straight. If one arm drifts down or the wrist pronates, there may be pyramidal weakness. A rising arm is a sign of a cortical sensory loss in the parietal region with loss of spatial awareness.

Oscillation of the arms indicates a cerebellar problem with lack of coordination.

Simple tests of coordination

Ask the patient to alternately touch their nose and the examiner's finger and run a heel down their contralateral shin.

These should always be part of your examination.

Lower limb

With the patient supine, begin with straight leg raising, which should be to 80–90°. Look for muscle wasting, and then test power, tone and reflexes (Figure 3.24).

Start distally at the ankles, with dorsiflexion (L4/5) and plantar flexion (S1/2) (Figure 3.25).

Place the patient's heels together and test inversion (L4) (Figure 3.26a) and eversion (L5) (Figure 3.26b).

Movements at the knee and hip are then examined (Figure 3.27).

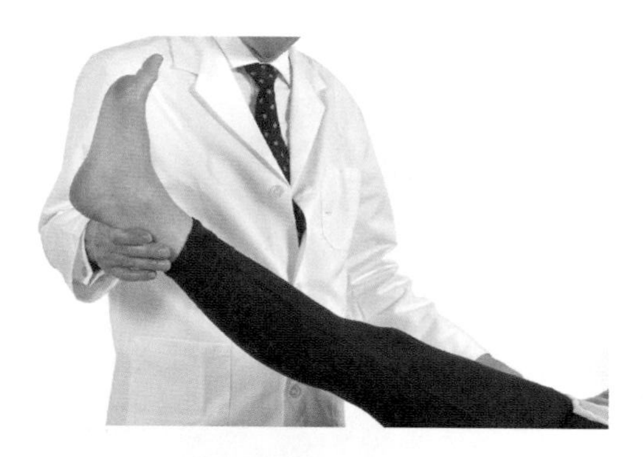

Figure 3.24 Straight leg raising.

(a)

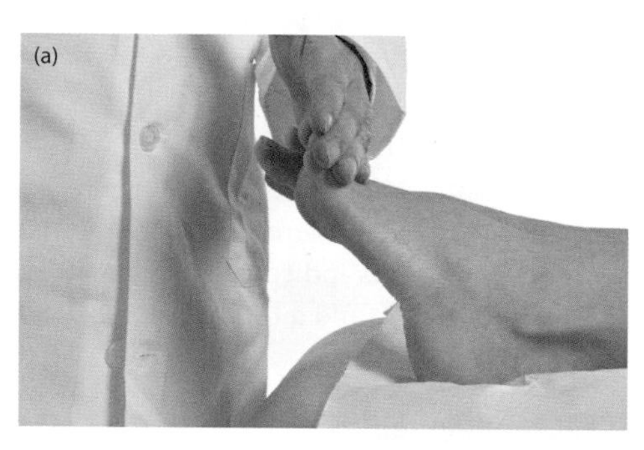

(b)

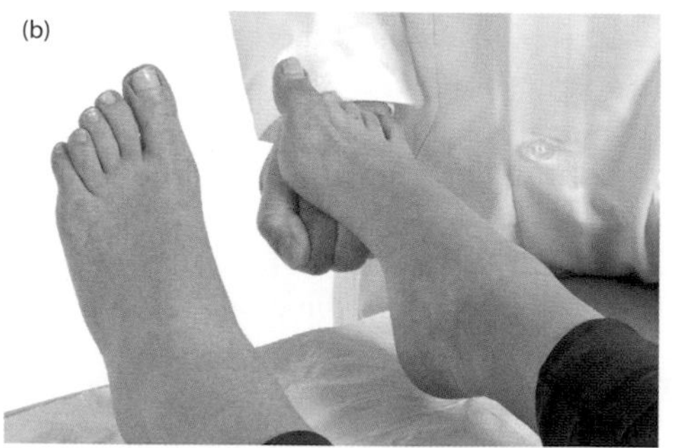

Figure 3.25 DORSIFLEXION AND PLANTAR FLEXION. (a) Testing dorsiflexion of the ankle (L4/5). (b) Testing plantar flexion of the ankle (S1/2).

(a)

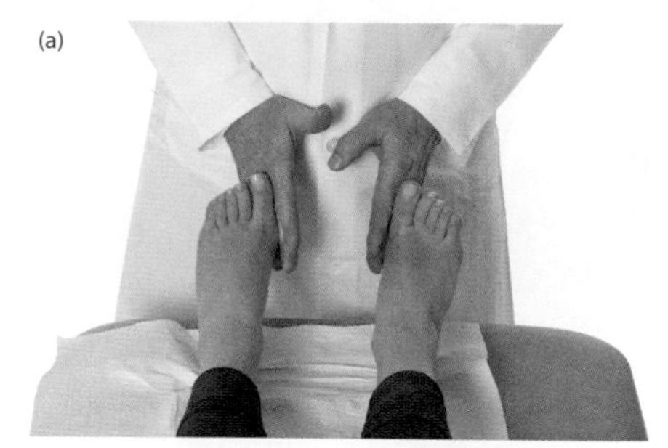

(b)

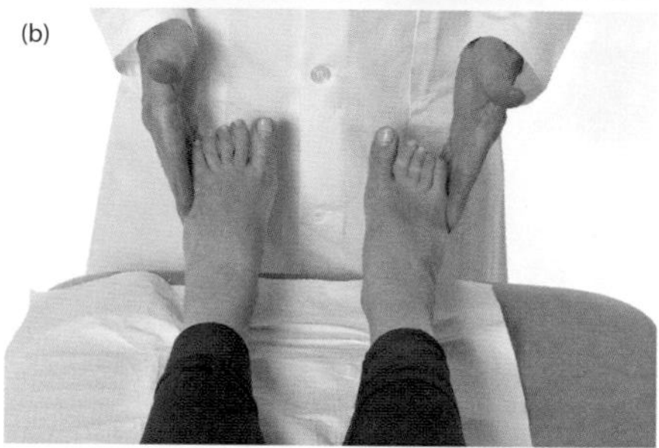

Figure 3.26 INVERSION AND EVERSION OF THE ANKLE. (a) Testing inversion of the ankle (L4). (b) Testing eversion of the ankle (L5).

Test the patellar and ankle reflexes (Figure 3.28). Gently draw a thumbnail or pointed end of patellar hammer along the outer edge of the sole (Figure 3.28). If there is tonic dorsiflexion (upgoing) of the big toe accompanied by fanning of the other toes, this is a positive plantar reflex, called Babinski's sign.

> **NOTE:** *Always check the peripheral pulses.* Claudication may be vascular or neurological, and the presence or absence of pulses can be indicative (see Chapter 10).

Finally, ask the patient to lie prone so the back can be inspected, and test perineal sensation.

The patient may sometimes be unable to stand, as for example in acute lumbar disc prolapse with sciatica. It is possible to gain diagnostic information from the reflexes and restricted straight leg raising.

EXAMINING SENSORY FUNCTION

This is the most time-consuming and difficult part of the neurological examination. Test the whole body, with different methods.

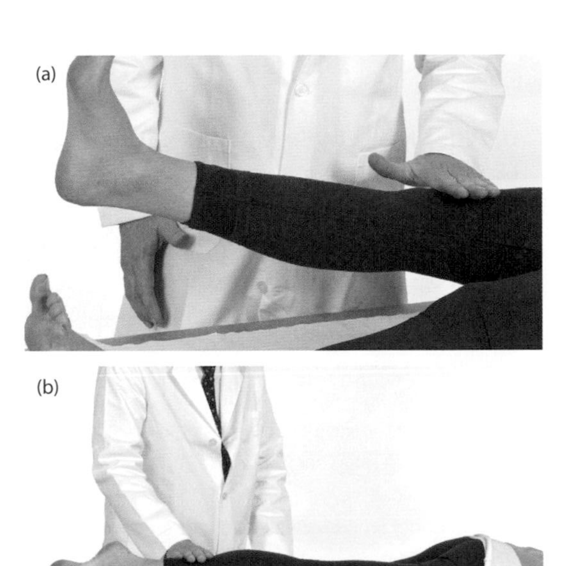

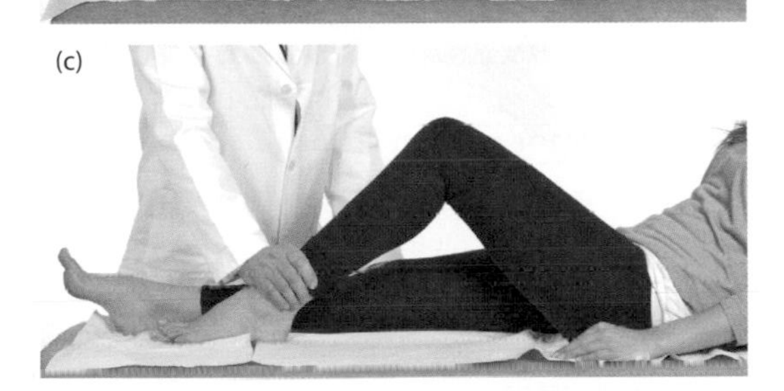

Figure 3.27 TESTING POWER OF MOVEMENTS OF THE KNEE AND HIP. (a) Hip flexion (L1, L2, L3). (b) Hip extension (L5, S1). (c) Knee extension (L3, L4).

Some variations in sensation are actually normal. For example, the outer aspect of the thigh is less sensitive than the inner.

Start with a general survey of sensation to light touch and pinprick. Any obvious abnormality can then be looked at in more detail.

When mapping numbness, test the region with reduced sensation before the area with normal sensation. This makes it easier for the patient to recognize the difference.

The examination should include a testing of sensations subserved by:

- The *lateral spinothalamic pathway* – pain, temperature.
- The *anterior spinothalamic tract* – touch/deep pressure.

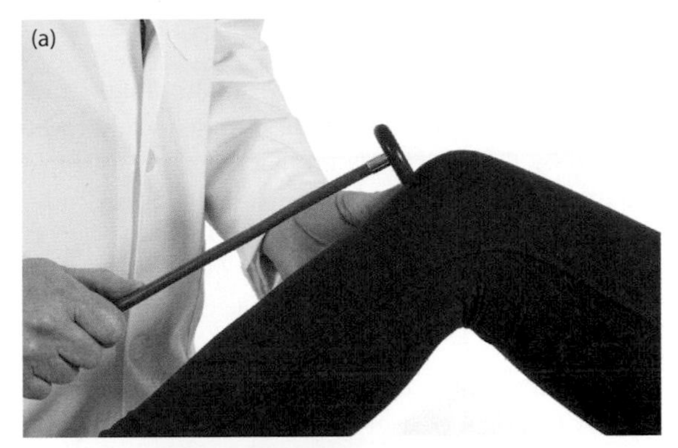

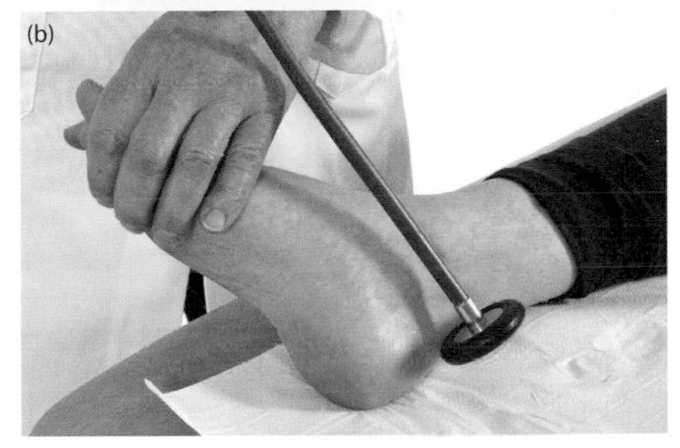

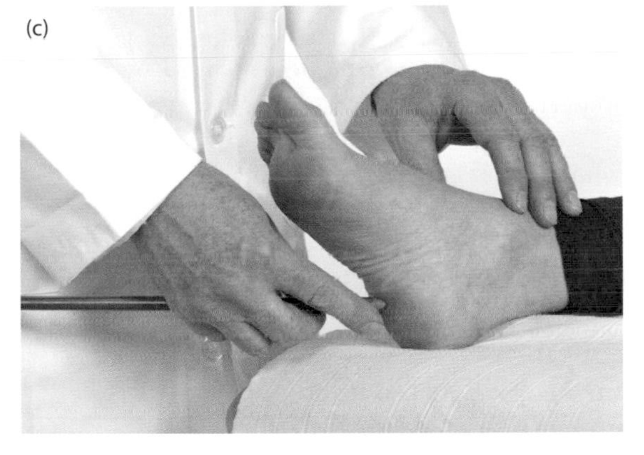

Figure 3.28 TESTING LOWER LIMB REFLEXES. (a) The knee reflex L3/L4. (b) The ankle reflex S1. (c) Testing the plantar response.

- The *posterior column/medial lemniscal system* – light touch, proprioception, vibration and position sense.

> **NOTE:** The sensory level is vital to establish in patients presenting with cord compression.

Perception of passive motion

Proprioception is first tested in the fingers and toes, as any abnormality here is more likely to be noticed by the patient. Then move proximally. Hold the digit laterally and ask the patient if you are moving it up or down.

Vibration sense

Vibration sense is tested by placing a low frequency tuning fork over a bony prominence. Explain that you want to see if the patient detects vibration and not just pressure. Vibration and position sense are usually lost together, vibration sense usually more obviously. With increasing age, vibration sense is commonly reduced in the feet.

REFLEXES

These can be both seen and felt, as described above.

Increased reflexes may indicate UMN disease but remember that reflexes are often brisk in the young or anxious patient.

Decreased or absent reflexes are a sign of a LMN lesion and will often be accompanied by reduced tone and loss of muscle bulk (Revision panel 3.3).

At the start of the examination explain (as always) what you are going to do, and make sure the patient is warm and relaxed.

Test the biceps, triceps, supinator, patellar, Achilles and plantar reflexes.

Revision panel 3.3

UPPER AND LOWER MOTOR NEURON LESIONS

Upper motor neuron lesions

There is damage above the level of the anterior horn cell, anywhere from the spinal cord to the primary motor cortex. There is:

- No muscle wasting
- Increased tone – spasticity like a clasp knife due to hypersensitivity of the stretch reflex
- Weakness in a typical pattern, termed 'pyramidal'
- In the upper limbs – weak abductors and extensors
- In the lower limbs – weak abductors and flexors
- Increased reflexes causing slow involuntary contractions (clonus)
- Up-going plantar response (extensor)

Lower motor neuron lesions

Damage below the level of the anterior horn cell resulting in:

- Muscle wasting
- Fasciculations – rapid twitches
- Decreased tone
- Flaccid weakness
- Decreased tendon reflexes
- Plantar response that is down-going or absent (flexor)

GAIT AND STANCE

This usually concludes the examination of the neurological system.

An abnormality of gait and stance may be the only neurological abnormality if there is a midline cerebellar lesion.

Asking the patient to walk heel to toe may unmask subtle problems with balance not seen with their normal gait.

A *spastic gait* is a stiff scraping walk often tripping over kerbs.

An *ataxic gait* can be the result of cerebellar disease or to loss of the dorsal column pathways caused by vitamin B12 deficiency or syphilis (sensory ataxia). The patient will describe being unsteady in the dark and having difficulty walking across rough ground. They often have a loud slapping step and rely on visual clues.

A *Parkinson's gait* is short shuffling steps with difficulty starting and stopping. There may be resting tremor and a lack of facial expression.

Perform the *Romberg test*. Ask the patient to stand still with their heels together and eyes closed. The test is positive if the patient loses balance. The usual cause is a sensory problem in the posterior columns.

SPECIFIC INTRACRANIAL CONDITIONS

Head injury

When taking a history and examining a patient with a head injury who is conscious and alert, it is important to decide whether the patient has suffered a superficial head injury or a brain injury.

Try to establish a clear history of the forces involved and the speed of the accident. Question any available witness, police or attending paramedics for further information.

Record the Glasgow Coma Scale score in all patients. This is an essential tool in the assessment and management of patients with a head injury. Establish the best score in eye opening, verbal response and motor examination (Table 3.2) (Revision panel 3.4).

Table 3.2 The Glasgow Coma Scale

	Patient response	Score
Eye opening	Spontaneous	4
	To speech	3
	To pain	2
	None	1
Best verbal response	Orientated	5
	Confused	4
	Inappropriate words	3
	Incomprehensible sounds	2
	None	1
Best motor response	Obeys commands	6
	Localizes to pain	5
	Normal flexion	4
	Abnormal flexion	3
	Extends to pain	2
	None	1

Assess the *post-traumatic amnesic period,* which is a good guide to the severity of the injury. This is the time from the accident to the recovery of full orientation. Amnesia for a significant length of time indicates diffuse head injury. Post-traumatic amnesic of less than 1 hour is graded mild, 1–24 hours moderate and more than 24 hours severe.

Revision panel 3.4

SEVERITY OF HEAD INJURY

Severe head injury

Glasgow Coma Scale score 3–8

Moderate injury

Glasgow Coma Scale score 9–14

Minor head injury

Glasgow Coma Scale score 15

Examine the head looking for lacerations and bruising, shaving the hair if necessary. An apparently innocent laceration may be a sign of penetrating injury.

Look for blood or cerebrospinal fluid leaking from the ear or nose. This indicates a skull base fracture, with a risk of meningitis (see below).

Look for bruising behind the ear over the mastoid process (*Battle's sign*). This reflects a fracture of the middle cranial fossa (see Figure 5.9).

Bruising around the eyes (*panda sign*) indicates a fracture of the anterior skull base (see Figure 5.7).

Decide whether this is a *closed* or an *open head injury*. Patients with compound depressed fractures may not have been knocked out and may be fully alert and orientated by the time they arrive at hospital. Examine the wound for foreign bodies. Feel around the laceration as a depressed fracture may not be directly under the wound.

CONCUSSION

This means temporary loss of consciousness occurring from the time of impact.

It can be *moderate,* with complete recovery in less than 5 minutes, or *severe* if the patient is unconscious for more than 5 minutes.

The majority of patients do not deteriorate but still require neurological monitoring until the symptoms have resolved. They may also be under the influence of drugs or alcohol and have no reliable companion at home.

Postconcussive syndrome includes headache, mild impairment of memory, giddiness and alteration of mood. These symptoms usually regress spontaneously but can persist for weeks or months.

HEAD INJURY AND REDUCED CONSCIOUS LEVEL

You must decide if there are *focal signs or* whether it is a *diffuse head injury.*

A patient with focal neurological signs, such as a unilateral dilated pupil who is flexing to pain on one side and extending on the other with a deteriorating conscious level, is very likely to have an expanding intracranial haematoma such as an *acute subdural haematoma.*

In contrast, a patient who is involved in a high-speed accident who is deeply unconscious from the time of the accident with symmetrical pupils and no lateralizing signs is more likely to have suffered a diffuse head injury (diffuse axonal injury) without any intracerebral haematoma.

This is the most severe form of diffuse brain injury and is the most common cause of prolonged post-traumatic coma that is not the result of a mass lesion or ischaemia. It is characterized by small haemorrhages from microscopic shearing injuries between the grey and white matter tracts, involving the corpus callosum, rostral mid brain and superior cerebellar peduncles.

Patients frequently show abnormal posturing and autonomic dysfunction in addition to their prolonged coma. The intracranial pressure is often normal.

The prognosis is generally poor, with half dying.

Cerebral contusion is focal brain injury caused by the impact of the brain surface against the internal ridges of the skull. Cerebral contusions are common in the frontal and temporal poles, as a result of impact against the corrugations in the floor of the skull.

A characteristic pattern of cerebral contusion is the *coup and contrecoup* injury. The coup occurs at the point of impact and the contrecoup at the point diametrically opposite (Figure 3.29).

A contusion can cause fits or may lead to an expanding haematoma producing late deterioration.

> **NOTE:** The neurological condition of patients with severe brain injury is notoriously fluctuant. Any deterioration in a patient's condition may require urgent intervention, so such patients must be monitored carefully, and any change acted upon.

Many patients with head injuries are found unconscious at the scene of a high-speed accident, with focal neurological signs. Associated extracranial injuries are common, so that the primary brain injury is compounded by secondary damage from ischaemia and hypoxia. Swelling and bleeding from the surface of the hemisphere at the site of impact is also common. The blood clot can cover the whole hemisphere and cause major brain shift (see below) with elevated intracranial pressure (Figure 3.30).

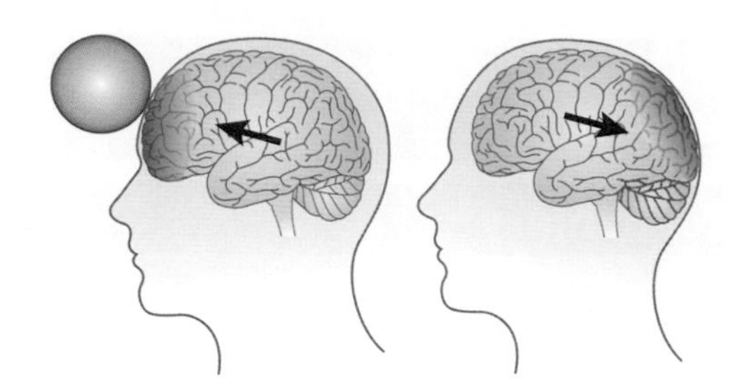

Figure 3.29 Coup and contrecoup in cerebral contusion.

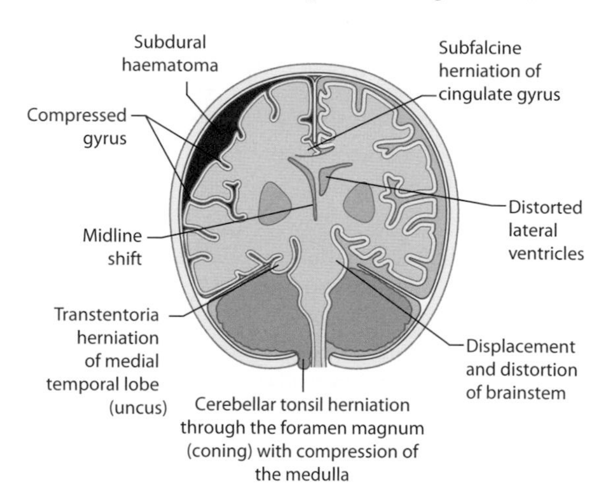

Figure 3.30 Lateral and vertical brain shift caused by expanding space-occupying lesion (e.g. a haematoma).

BRAIN SHIFT AND HERNIATION

In brain herniation, a rise in intracranial pressure displaces the brain either downwards or across a fixed intracranial structure, leading to deepening coma.

Major herniations are common in severe head injuries. As the brain shifts, the brainstem is compressed against the contralateral tentorial edge. This results in an *ipsilateral dilated pupil* and a *contralateral hemiplegia*. Initial midbrain dysfunction progresses to involve the brainstem.

Brainstem signs are associated with deepening coma and imminent death. They include profound bradycardia, raised blood pressure and an irregular respiratory pattern.

Coning is an example of brain herniation. There is vertical displacement of the hindbrain. The cerebellar tonsils and lower brainstem become impacted in the foramen magnum, often producing irreversible brainstem ischaemia (see Figure 3.30).

EXTRADURAL HAEMATOMA

A fracture, commonly of the temporal bone, tears an adjacent meningeal vessel, and a haematoma develops in the extradural space (Figure 3.31). This increases the intracranial pressure (which is normally less than 20 mmHg). The brain itself is often initially undamaged. The rapidly expanding haematoma in the middle cranial fossa displaces the brain medially, causing the inner aspect of the temporal lobe (uncus) to be stretched over the free edge of the tentorium. This compresses the ipsilateral IIIrd cranial nerve and posterior cerebral artery, resulting in a dilated pupil on the side of the injury (Figure 3.32), and then posterior cerebral ischaemia, which produces paralysis on the opposite side because of the crossed nerve tracts.

Symptoms Typically, a young person is struck forcibly on the side of the head, and there may be no loss of consciousness. There is headache from local bruising and the underlying fracture. There follows a progressive deterioration in the clinical condition, with increasing headache, vomiting and drowsiness progressing to coma. There is often no lucid interval but rather progression of signs and symptoms of raised pressure.

Signs There is bruising and swelling over the temporal area of the skull where the impact occurred. Deterioration to a contralateral hemiplegia and an ipsilateral dilated pupil can occur within hours and requires urgent surgery.

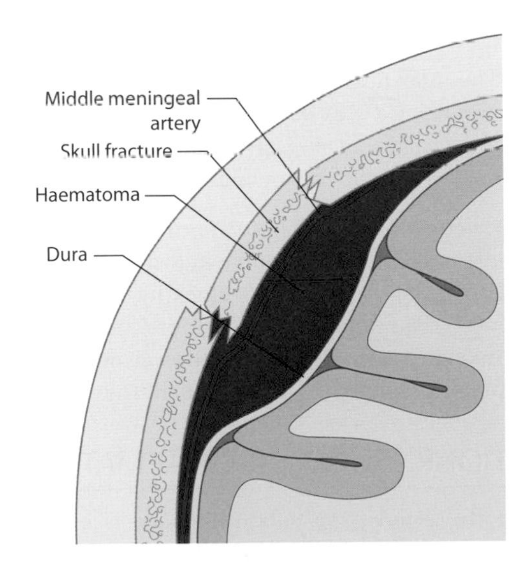

Figure 3.31 Extradural haematoma formation after a skull fracture and torn middle meningeal artery.

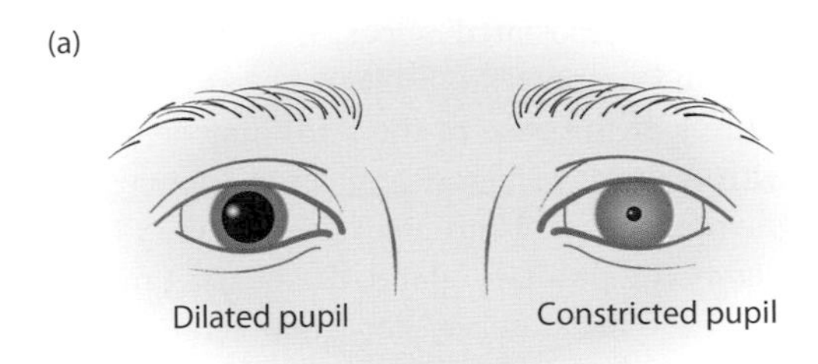

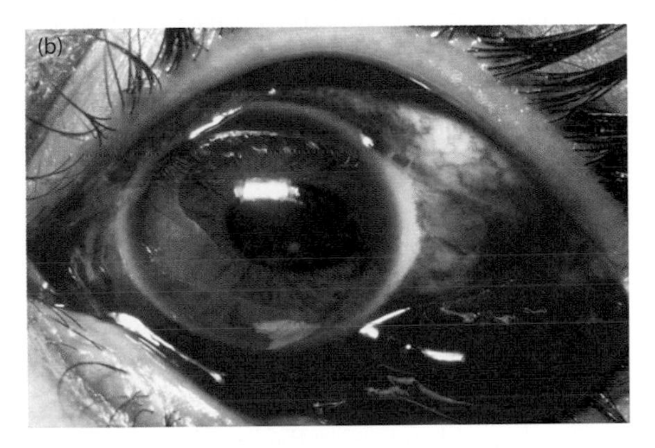

Figure 3.32 FIXED DILATED PUPIL. (a) Fixed dilated pupil with decreased conscious level due to expanding space-occupying lesion. (b) Traumatic fixed dilated pupil.

PENETRATING BRAIN INJURIES

Low-velocity injuries, such as those produced by a knife blade, cause local injury to the brain along the track but may not cause loss of consciousness or leave a permanent neurological deficit. The prognosis is good if no vital structures are torn.

High-velocity injuries, by a bullet, produce widespread damage to the brain, from the missile itself and from the associated shock wave. Patients in coma have a very poor prognosis.

Fractures of the base of the skull may be associated with leakage of blood and cerebrospinal fluid from the nose or ear. There may also be injury to the optic nerve, the pituitary gland, the hearing mechanisms and the facial nerve. Persistent cerebrospinal fluid rhinorrhoea carries the risk of meningitis and tension pneumocephalus.

INJURIES OF THE BRACHIAL PLEXUS

It is important to remember the possibility of a brachial plexus injury in any unconscious patient, especially when there are fractures of the shoulder girdle, proximal humerus or first rib. Complete plexus lesions can be caused by trauma to the cervical spine, gunshot wounds, stabbings, fractures of the clavicle, dislocations of the humerus and motorcycle accidents (in which the shoulder and neck are forcibly pulled apart, causing complete or partial disruption of the plexus).

The prognosis relates to the level of the damage. There are three main types of injury:

- **Root avulsion.** The nerve roots are avulsed from the spinal cord within the vertebral column. Spontaneous improvement is unlikely, and the injury is not amenable to surgical repair.
- **Rupture outside the vertebral column.** Spontaneous improvement is unlikely, but the injury may benefit from surgical repair.
- **Nerve damage without rupture.** A neuropraxia or axonotmesis (see later in the chapter) with preservation of the nerve sheaths is likely to improve spontaneously.

In road traffic accidents, a low-velocity injury points to neuropraxia and axonotmesis, while a high-velocity impact is more likely to produce a complete disruption of the plexus.

The clinical picture depends on the level of injury (Figure 3.33):

- In *root damage*, there will be paralysis of the scapular muscles and the diaphragm, and a Horner's syndrome.
- In *upper plexus damage*, sensation is lost over the C5 and C6 dermatomes. There is paralysis of the deltoid, the external rotators of the shoulder and the biceps, resulting in loss of shoulder abduction and inability to externally rotate the arm. Elbow flexion and forearm supination are weak. The internally rotated arm hangs against the trunk in the 'waiter's tip' position.
- *Isolated lower plexus damage* is rare. Sensation is lost over the inner ulnar aspect of the arm. The small muscles of the hand are paralysed, producing a claw hand.
- In *total plexus damage*, there is a numb flail upper limb with severe muscle wasting.

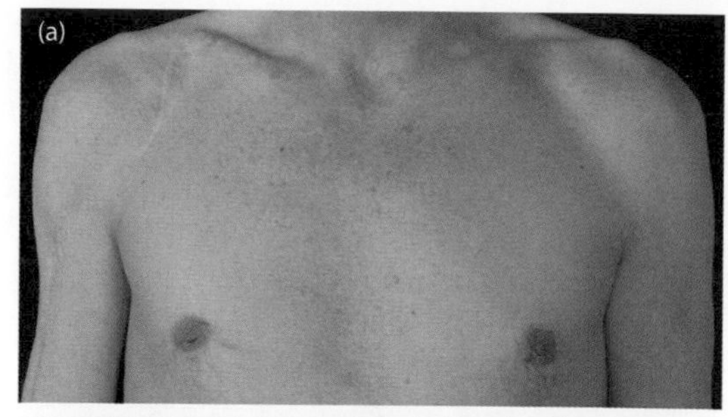

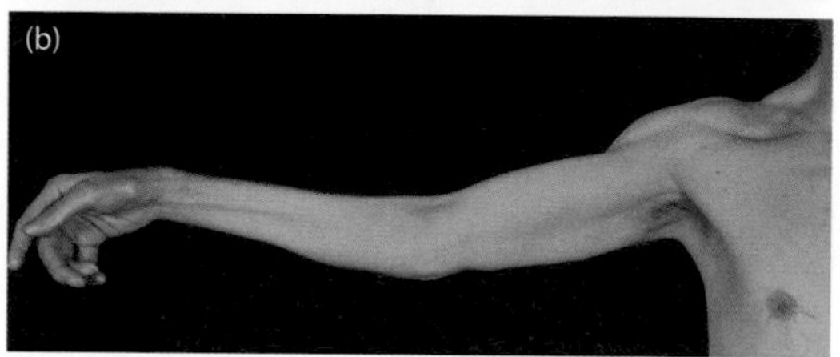

Figure 3.33 BRACHIAL PLEXUS INJURY FROM MOTORCYCLE ACCIDENT, RUPTURE OCCURRED OUTSIDE VERTEBRAL COLUMN. (a) Preservation of the deltoid (C5). (b) All other muscles are wasted, and the hand is clawed.

In a conscious patient, a careful examination of sensation and motor function will distinguish a brachial plexus injury from a radiculopathy (see Revision panel 9.1). Pain and sensory changes are generally dominant in a plexus injury, and the sensory changes do not follow typical dermatomal patterns.

CHRONIC SUBDURAL HAEMATOMA

In the elderly, the subdural space is enlarged because of brain atrophy. Relatively minor head injuries such as striking the head against a door can tear a cortical bridging vein. The subsequent chronic

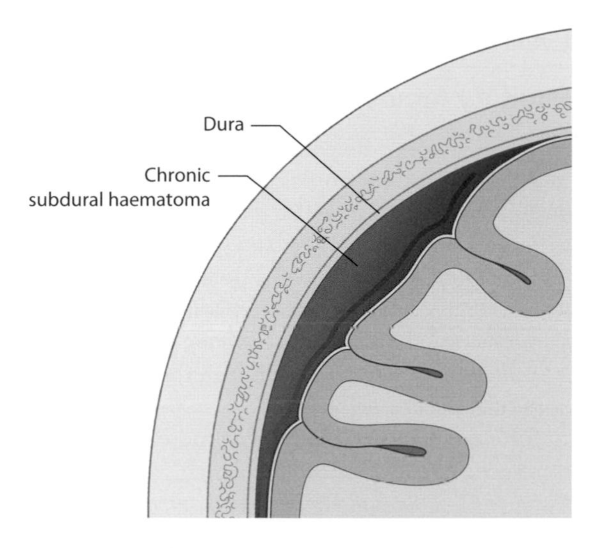

Figure 3.34 Chronic subdural haematoma.

subdural venous haematoma enlarges slowly, with episodes of rebleeding (Figure 3.34).

Time of onset Clinical presentation is typically 6–8 weeks after a minor head injury.

Risk factors The risk factors are advanced age and cerebral atrophy, coagulopathy, anticoagulants and alcohol abuse.

Symptoms These are of raised intracranial pressure, namely headache and drowsiness.

Signs The haematoma causes a mass effect, leading to hemiparesis, dysphasia and tremors.

Differential diagnosis The clinical picture can easily be mistaken for a stroke, but the prognosis can be good, because there is no primary brain injury.

Brain tumours

Presentation This depends on the location and speed of growth of the tumour. In general, a brain tumour can present with the signs of raised intracranial pressure, focal signs and/or fits. Progressively severe headaches and vomiting are typical symptoms. Drowsiness is an early sign of raised intracranial pressure. Hemiparesis and ataxia are examples of focal signs.

Family history The vast majority of primary brain tumours are sporadic. Of the small number that are familial, there is usually a hereditary disease known to be associated, such as tuberous sclerosis, neurofibromatosis, familial polyposis or Li–Fraumeni syndrome.

Symptoms The most common presentation is a progressive, usually motor neurological deficit, followed by headaches and then fits.

> **NOTE:** Brain tumours are classified by tumour location as supratentorial or infratentorial, and by tumour type.

Frontal brain tumours characteristically present with *mental apathy* and *personality change* and dementia. Anosmia in such a patient would suggest a meningioma arising from the floor of the anterior cranial fossa.

Temporal tumours will often present with *fits* and *speech disturbance* if the dominant hemisphere is involved. On examination, there may be a contralateral hemiparesis and a visual field defect.

Parietal tumours classically present with a *contralateral weakness* depending on which region of the motor strip is involved.

Patients with *occipital tumours* are often found to have a *visual field defect.*

Infratentorial tumours (cerebellum/brainstem) often present with *loss of balance (ataxia)* and *disturbance of vision. Headache,* when present, is often severe due to obstructive hydrocephalus.

The location of the headache is not normally related to the site of the tumour, although rarely downward displacement of the cerebellar tonsils can cause severe neck pain.

Brain tumours may be intrinsic, namely arising from the brain itself, or they may be extrinsic and arise from the surrounding structures (Revision panel 3.5).

Revision panel 3.5

INTRINSIC AND EXTRINSIC BRAIN TUMOURS

Intrinsic tumours

Cerebral metastases
Astrocytoma
Oligodendroglioma
Ependymoma

Extrinsic tumours

Meningioma
Pituitary adenoma
Schwannoma

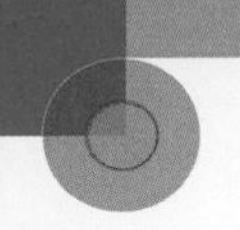

INTRINSIC TUMOURS

Gliomas, the most common type, are classified by cell type and histological grade. The incidence of high-grade glioma is increasing as the population grows older.

Grade 1 gliomas, such as the well-circumscribed pilocytic astrocytoma, occur in children and young adults and can involve both the cerebellum and the cerebral hemispheres. They generally carry a good prognosis.

Grades 2, 3 and *4* are infiltrating astrocytomas and usually involve the cerebral hemispheres and spare the cerebellum. The prognosis deteriorates with increasing grade.

Grades 3 and *4* are clearly malignant tumours with a poor prognosis.

Older patients tend to have more aggressive higher-grade tumours.

The mean ages for these tumours are:

- Grade 2 astrocytoma in adults – 34 years.
- Anaplastic grade 3 astrocytoma – 41 years.
- Grade 4 malignant glioblastoma multiforme – 63 years.

It is very unusual for a primary tumour of the central nervous system to spread outside the brain and spinal cord. Rarely, an aggressive primary tumour of the central nervous system such as a high-grade glioma will metastasize within the craniospinal axis (Revision panel 3.6).

Revision panel 3.6

CEREBRAL METASTASES

These are the most common intracranial tumours
Their incidence is increasing as more patients survive the primary treatment of carcinomas
Common primary tumours for blood-borne metastases are:
- Lung carcinoma
- Breast carcinoma
- Kidney carcinoma
- Gastrointestinal carcinoma
- Melanoma

EXTRINSIC TUMOURS

Pituitary tumours

These present with endocrine dysfunction caused by either overproduction of hormones or underproduction because of pressure from a tumour leading to failure of the rest of the gland (hypopituitarism).

Prolactinomas (lactotroph) secrete excessive prolactin, and a microprolactinoma is typically responsible for *amenorrhoea* and *galactorrhoea* in young females.

Somatotroph adenomas produce excessive growth hormone, causing acromegaly.

Pituitary tumours may also produce *adrenocorticotrophic hormone* causing Cushing's disease (see Chapter 1), or *thyroid-stimulating hormone* leading to thyrotoxicosis (see Chapter 12).

Functioning tumours are seen more often in younger age groups and are generally small benign adenomas.

Non-functioning tumours typically occur in the elderly. Symptoms do not appear until the tumour has reached a considerable size (macroadenoma). The tumour fills the pituitary fossa and grows upwards to compress the optic chiasm and optic nerves. The central crossing fibres are compressed, resulting in a *bitemporal hemianopia* (see Figure 3.6).

There may be associated hypopituitarism, but the visual loss is usually the presenting feature.

Craniopharyngiomas

These arise in the suprasellar region, often from the pituitary stalk, so the endocrine dysfunction produced is diabetes insipidus, because of a loss of antidiuretic hormone. This causes polyuria and polydipsia.

Craniopharyngiomas occur more frequently in the young, causing short stature from a lack of growth hormone. The local mass effect causes headaches and visual loss is usually asymmetrical.

Meningiomas

These arise from meningothelial cells of the arachnoid layer, a membranous layer surrounding the brain and spinal cord. They occur primarily at the base of the skull, in the parasellar regions and over the cerebral convexities. They are usually solitary, except in neurofibromatosis type 2.

Ninety per cent of meningiomas are benign, but a few are atypical or frankly malignant. There are many histological varieties of benign meningioma, including syncytial, fibrous and transitional, but the distinction is usually of little clinical significance.

Meningiomas typically grow very slowly and can reach a considerable size without producing symptoms.

Symptoms and signs often present in the middle-aged and elderly include *progressive motor weakness*, *visual disturbance* and *infrequent headaches*.

Symptomless meningiomas are often uncovered in the elderly after a stroke or head injury and can usually simply be kept under periodic review.

Vestibular schwannomas (acoustic neuromas)

These are benign tumours of myelin-forming cells of the VIIIth cranial nerve. They cause unilateral deafness that may be preceded or accompanied by tinnitus.

In the early stages, there is nothing to find apart from deafness, but as the tumour gradually enlarges, there is displacement and distortion of the brainstem. The diagnosis should be considered in any patient with unilateral deafness.

Brain haemorrhage

Twenty per cent of strokes are caused by a cerebral haemorrhage, the rest being caused by a thrombosis or embolism.

SPONTANEOUS INTRACRANIAL HAEMORRHAGE

Causes of spontaneous intracranial haemorrhage vary with age (Revision panel 3.7). In the elderly, vascular disease associated with hypertension is common, but in younger patients, coagulopathy is more likely.

Clues to the cause of an intracranial bleed may be gleaned from the site. For example, hypertensive haemorrhage tends to damage the basal ganglia, and a lobar haematoma is seen with amyloid angiopathy.

Revision panel 3.7

RISK FACTORS FOR INTRACRANIAL HAEMORRHAGE

General

- Increasing age
- Male gender
- Hypertension
- Smoking
- Diabetes
- Alcohol abuse

Underlying vascular conditions

- Arteriovenous malformation
- Aneurysm
- Cavernoma
- Amyloid angiopathy
- Cerebral venous thrombosis

Abnormal haemostasis

- Anticoagulant drugs
- Antiplatelet drugs
- Coagulation disorders
- Thrombolytic drugs

Other causes

- Drug abuse (cocaine)
- Moyamoya syndrome
- Haemorrhage into a primary or secondary brain tumour

SUBARACHNOID HAEMORRHAGE FROM BERRY ANEURYSMS

Cerebral aneurysms occur at the branching points of the cerebral arteries around the circle of Willis, in the subarachnoid space (Figure 3.35). They are commonly known as *berry aneurysms* because of their size and shape.

Incidence As many as 1% of adults in the UK are affected.

Age They are increasingly common with age.

Sex Berry aneurysms are twice as common in females.

Risk factors Hypertension and smoking.

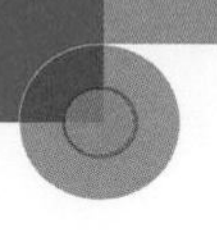

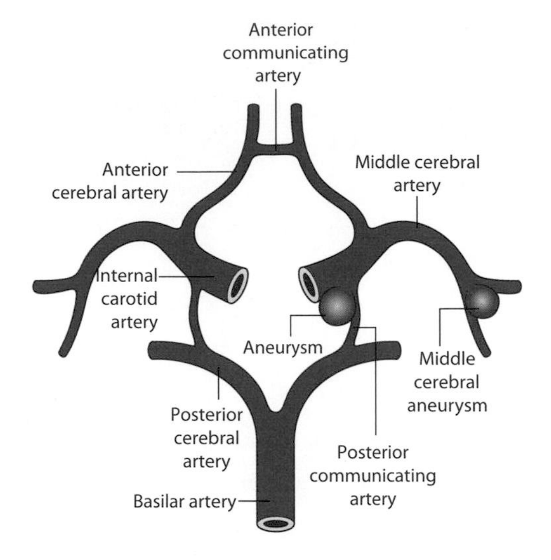

Figure 3.35 Circle of Willis with sites of aneurysm formation. These may rupture and cause subarachnoid haemorrhage.

Symptoms There are usually no symptoms from an unruptured aneurysm, although large lesions can compress surrounding brainstem structures and can, for example, interfere with vision. Patients may experience a less severe, sentinel headache a few days before a major rupture.

The major bleed causes a severe headache and may cause the patient to lose consciousness or develop localizing signs.

Where there is no neurological deficit, the decision to investigate this group of patients is then based on the history alone.

Signs The patient with a typical subarachnoid is *drowsy* and *disorientated with neck stiffness*. The site of the ruptured aneurysm will dictate the presence of any focal signs. Vasospasm can occur in the weeks after the initial bleed, leading to cerebral ischaemia with further neurological deficit.

CEREBRAL ARTERIOVENOUS MALFORMATION

Incidence They are only one-tenth as common as cerebral aneurysms.

Pathology The malformations develop in early life and are usually solitary lesions. Most exhibit somatic mutations of the recurrent aphthous stomatitis/MAPK signalling pathway resulting in abnormal angiogenesis. There is shunting of blood from arteries to veins.

Symptoms and signs Some patients describe a pulsatile noise in the head, but the usual presentation is with an intracerebral haemorrhage that may be intraparenchymal, intraventricular or subarachnoid. This haemorrhage may produce severe headache, fits and/or a stroke.

CAVERNOMA

This lesion is a cavernous haemangioma of the brain, spinal cord or cauda equina, and consists of vascular channels under low pressure. It is often small and looks like a blackberry. One-quarter are multiple.

Aetiology Cavernomas are often familial. Multiple sporadic lesions may result from radiation.

Symptoms The cavernoma may enlarge and present as a space-occupying lesion. Once a lesion bleeds there is a small risk of further local small bleeds. Fits may also be a symptom of repeated haemorrhage.

Signs When the cavernoma is in the posterior fossa or the spinal cord, there may be a progressive neurological deficit resulting from repeated local bleeds.

Infections of the brain

CEREBRAL ABSCESS

A brain abscess may be the result of a local spread of infection from the frontal sinuses, mastoids or teeth, or less commonly via the bloodstream from the heart or lungs.

Presentation The classical triad is *fever, headache* and *focal neurological signs*.

Fever is often absent or low grade.

Headache is often accompanied by drowsiness because there is raised ICP.

The focal signs depend on the site of the abscess:

- Fits suggest a frontal or temporal lobe abscess.
- A temporal lobe abscess arising from a chronic middle ear infection can present with a contralateral hemiparesis and a visual field defect.
- Nystagmus and ataxia suggest a cerebellar abscess arising from the middle ear.

SUBDURAL EMPYEMA

Infection from the sinuses or skull bones may be confined to the subdural space. It may cause thrombosis of the cortical veins leading to infarction and swelling of the brain.

Symptoms Because of the confined space, the headache is severe and rapidly progressive.

Signs The patient is unwell with a high fever and neck stiffness from meningeal irritation.

There is often tenderness over the infected sinus.

Eventually, the patient, who is often young, develops fits, a decreasing conscious level and hemiparesis.

TRAUMATIC CEREBROSPINAL FLUID LEAK AND MENINGITIS

A skull base fracture involving the anterior or middle fossa may lead to a cerebrospinal fluid leak. The fluid may initially be bloodstained but becomes clear. This is a compound fracture, and meningitis can follow.

The bacteria responsible depend on the site: *Pneumococcus* from the nose, and multiple organisms such as *Staphylococcus, Pseudomonas* and coliforms from the ears.

Air may pass into the cranium under pressure if a patient with cerebrospinal fluid rhinorrhoea blows their nose, causing a *tension pneumocephalus* and collapse.

Hydrocephalus

This is *excessive accumulation of cerebrospinal fluid* caused by a disturbance of its formation, flow or absorption.

The volume of cerebrospinal fluid in an adult is 120–150 mL, and the normal production of cerebrospinal fluid is 450 mL/24 hours. Therefore, the cerebrospinal fluid is recycled three times every day.

Types of hydrocephalus:

- *Communicating hydrocephalus* occurs when there is impaired cerebrospinal fluid reabsorption by the arachnoid granulations and leads to increased cerebrospinal fluid pressure and ventricular enlargement. It is generally safe to undertake lumbar puncture in this group of patients, but not in patients with an obstructive hydrocephalus.
- *Non-communicating* or *obstructive hydrocephalus* occurs when the cerebrospinal fluid outflow tracts are obstructed, such as at the exit foramina (Magendie and Luschka) of the fourth ventricle (see Figure 1.15).
- *Hydrocephalus ex vacuo* occurs when compensatory ventricular enlargement develops secondary to brain atrophy.
- *Arrested hydrocephalus* usually occurs as a result of an incomplete obstruction in a communicating hydrocephalus where cerebrospinal fluid production is balanced by absorption. The intracranial pressure is normal, despite the ventricles remaining dilated. The head circumference may be increased if the hydrocephalus is congenital and presenting in infancy. These patients can decompensate after a head injury later in life.
- *Normal-pressure hydrocephalus* is a condition in which the ventricles remain enlarged after a previous period of raised pressure.

ACUTE HYDROCEPHALUS

The causes of acute hydrocephalus are shown in Revision panel 3.8.

Revision panel 3.8

CAUSES OF HYDROCEPHALUS

Acute

Posterior fossa tumours
Cerebellar haemorrhage or infarction
Colloid cyst of the third ventricle
Ependymoma of the fourth ventricle
Subarachnoid haemorrhage
Trauma
Acute meningitis

Chronic

Slow-growing posterior fossa tumours
Subarachnoid haemorrhage
Chronic meningitis

NOTE: No demonstrable cause (30% of cases).

History

There is headache and vomiting because of the raised intracranial pressure. There may be diplopia caused by a VIth nerve palsy.

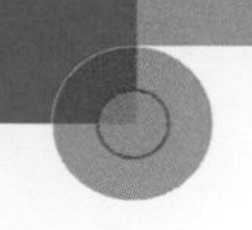

Occasionally, there is rapid loss of consciousness and death. For example, acute hydrocephalus with a colloid cyst blocking the foramina of Monro.

Examination

On examination, there may be an impaired conscious level and an inability to look upwards (*Parinaud's syndrome*, a result of compression of the upper brainstem). Papilloedema may be present.

CHRONIC HYDROCEPHALUS

Presentation is usually in the elderly with a decline in intellect and memory, an ataxic gait and urinary incontinence.

Peripheral nerve injury

There are three grades of peripheral nerve injury.

NEURAPRAXIA

Axonal continuity is maintained, and nerve conduction is preserved both proximal and distally but not across the injured segment. This type of injury is usually reversible, and a full recovery may occur within days to weeks.

It results from:

- Direct mechanical compression.
- Ischaemia secondary to vascular compromise.
- Metabolic derangements.
- Diseases or toxins causing demyelination.

In the last two categories, conduction is restored once either the metabolic derangement has been corrected or remyelination occurs.

AXONOTMESIS

This is a more severe grade of nerve injury in which there is interruption of the axons with preservation of the surrounding myelin and connective tissue sheath. It is followed by degeneration of the axon and myelin distal to the site of injury, occurs over several days and is called *Wallerian degeneration*.

Electrical stimulation of the disconnected distal nerve stump does not produce nerve conduction or muscle contraction. Recovery can occur from axonal regeneration through the preserved Schwann cells and their basal lamina. The Schwann cells proliferate and form longitudinal conduits through which the axons regenerate.

This type of injury usually recovers, but over a period of months. The timing and degree of recovery depend on the extent of the retrograde axonal loss. Peripheral nerve fibres usually regenerate at approximately 1 mm per day (1 per month). More proximal injuries take longer to recover.

NEUROTMESIS

In the most severe grade of peripheral nerve injury, there is disruption of the axon, myelin and connective tissue components of the nerve. Therefore, recovery through regeneration is impossible.

Division may be obvious, but sometimes the continuity of the nerve appears intact although intraneural fibrosis has blocked axonal regeneration. Continuity of the nerve can only be re-established by surgery to remove scar tissue and restore alignment.

It is often difficult to diagnose the grade of nerve injury by clinical examination at the time of injury. In general, movement recovers before sensation.

Examination

First, grade the strength of the individual muscles or muscle groups. Then perform a sensory examination, testing for light touch, pinprick, two-point discrimination, vibration and proprioception. Look carefully at the autonomous zones of a nerve where there is minimal overlap from adjacent nerves.

Map out the distribution of the sensory loss to determine whether it corresponds to a dermatome or a single nerve (Figure 3.36).

Tinel's sign is paraesthesia distal to the injury, described by the patient as tingling, that is elicited by tapping over the nerve. It indicates a partial lesion or the beginning of regeneration of the nerve and can be used to map nerve regeneration. The presence of this sign does not, however, guarantee motor recovery.

A *return of sweating* signifies sympathetic nerve fibre regeneration.

Reflex changes are sensitive indicators of nerve damage.

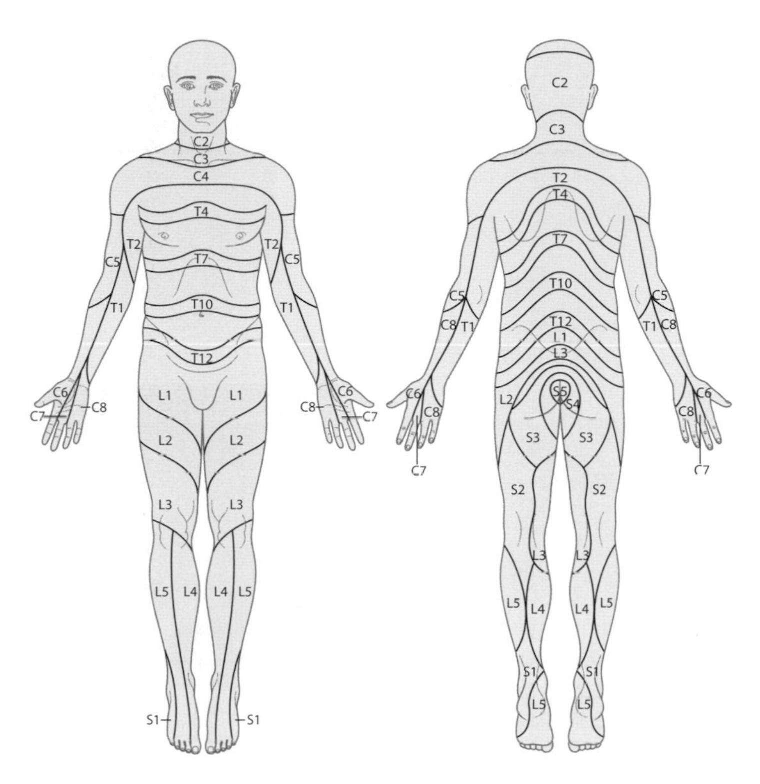

Figure 3.36 Upper and lower limb dermatomes.

NERVES OF THE UPPER LIMB

Median nerve

The nerve can be damaged by:

- Penetrating injuries of the arm and forearm.
- Lacerations at the wrist.
- Wrist dislocation.
- Carpal tunnel compression.

Sensory loss The median nerve is sensory to the palmar aspect of the thumb, index and middle fingers, and the dorsal aspect of the distal phalanx and half of the middle phalanx of the same fingers. It also supplies sensation to the radial side of the palm.

Motor malfunction If the injury is at wrist level, there is:

- Wasting of the muscles of the thenar eminence.
- Loss of abduction and opposition of the thumb (Figure 3.37).

If the injury is above the antecubital fossa (elbow level), there is:

- Wasting of the muscles of the forearm and thenar eminence.
- Loss of flexion of the thumb and index finger.
- Holding of the hand in the 'benediction' position, with the ulnar fingers flexed and the index finger straight.

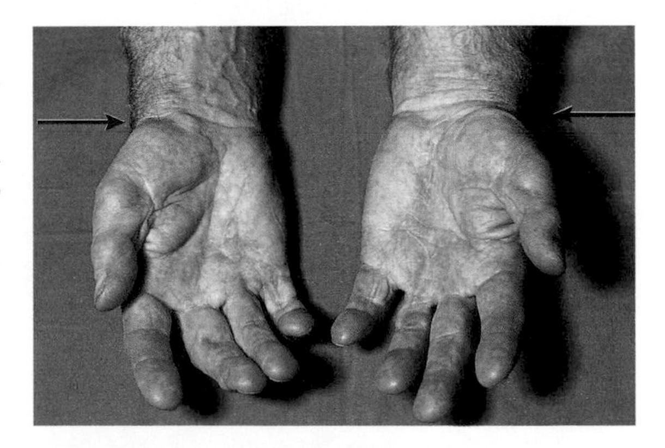

Figure 3.37 Bilateral median nerve compression with wasting of the thenar eminences.

Ulnar nerve

This nerve can be damaged by:

- Compression or injury at the elbow.
- Penetrating injuries of the arm or forearm.
- Fractures of the medial epicondyle.
- Lacerations at the wrist.
- Long-standing marked cubitus valgus.

Sensory loss The ulnar nerve is sensory to the anterior and posterior surfaces of the little finger, and the ulnar side of the ring finger. It also provides sensation to the skin over the front and back of the hypothenar eminence.

Motor malfunction If the injury is at wrist level, there is:

- Wasting of the hypothenar eminence and between the metacarpals.
- Loss of flexion of the little and ring fingers.
- A 'claw' hand, in which the ring and little fingers are hyperextended at the metacarpophalangeal joints and flexed at the interphalangeal joints (Figure 3.38).
- An absence of both abduction and adduction of the fingers, with a positive Froment's sign (inability to hold a sheet of paper between thumb and index finger) (Figure 3.39).

If the injury is at elbow level, there is:

- Wasting of the intrinsic muscles of the hand and hypothenar eminence.
- A claw hand without the flexion of the terminal interphalangeal joints because of paralysis of half the deep flexors of the fingers.
- A positive Froment's sign.

If the injury is well above the elbow, there is:

- Wasting of the intrinsic muscles of the hand and hypothenar eminence.
- Loss of flexion of the little and ring fingers.
- A 'claw' hand in which the ring and little fingers are hyperextended at the metacarpophalangeal joints without flexion of the interphalangeal joints.
- Absence of both abduction and adduction of the fingers, with a positive Froment's sign.
- A paralysed flexor carpi ulnaris.

(a)
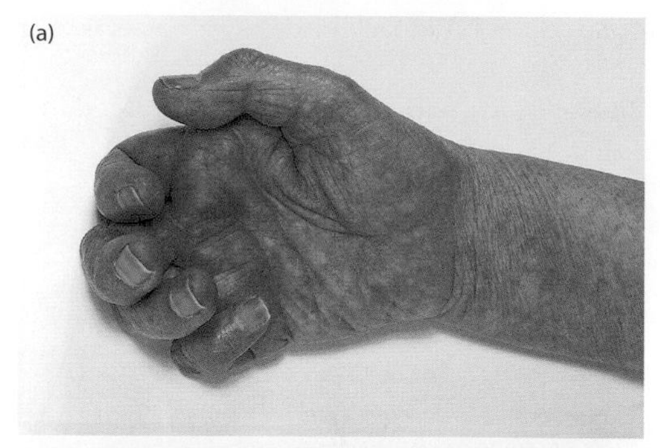

(b)
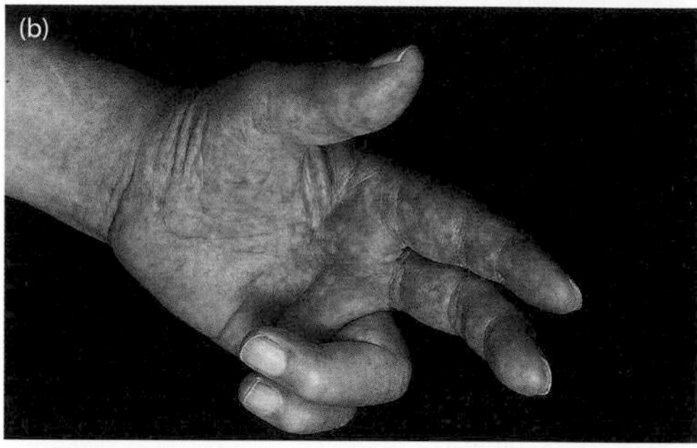

Figure 3.38 (a) Claw hand in syringomyelia. (b) Ulnar nerve lesion.

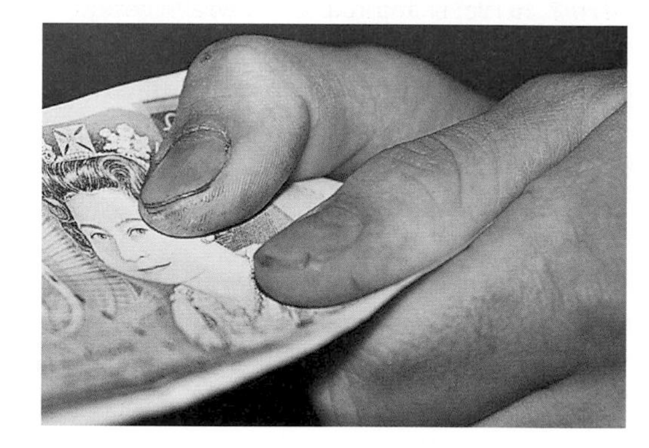

Figure 3.39 Froment's sign.

Radial nerve

This nerve can be damaged by:

- Fractures of the humeral shaft.
- Prolonged pressure from a crutch in the axilla.
- Penetrating injuries of the back of the arm or forearm.

Sensory loss The radial nerve supplies sensation to a small area on the lateral aspect of the first metacarpal and the back of the first web space and thumb.

Motor malfunction If the nerve is injured in the axilla:

- There will be dropping of the wrist with inability to extend (Figure 3.40).
- The triceps will be paralysed, so the elbow will not extend.

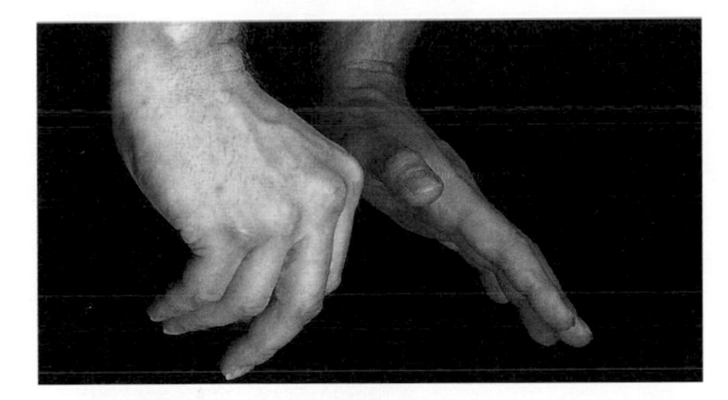

Figure 3.40 Wrist drop of right hand, caused by radial/posterior intraosseous nerve damage.

If the nerve is injured as it wraps round the humerus in its middle third:

- The brachioradialis, an elbow flexor, is spared.
- There is still a wrist drop and loss of triceps action.

If the injury is to the posterior interosseous nerve:

- The hand deviates radially during wrist extension.
- There is an inability to maintain opposed finger extension.

Quick screen of the motor function of the nerves of the upper limb

Three simple tests will give you an idea of which nerve is injured:

- Median nerve: Abduction of thumb (Figure 3.41a).
- Ulnar nerve: Abduction of little finger (Figure 3.41b).
- Radial nerve: Extension of the wrist (Figure 3.41c).

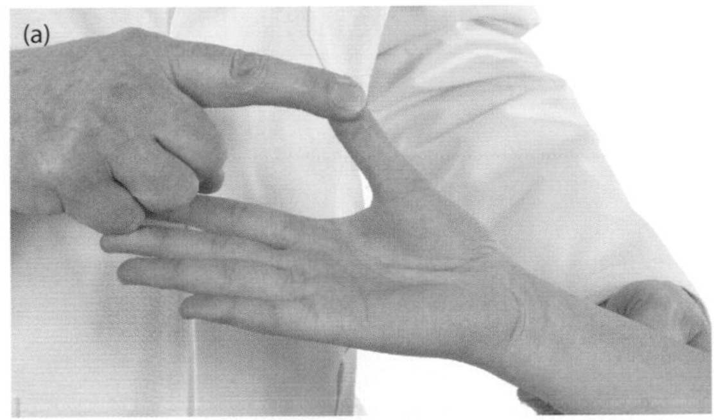

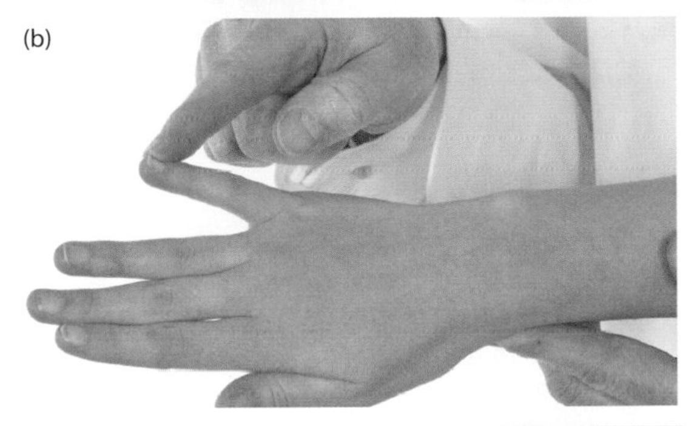

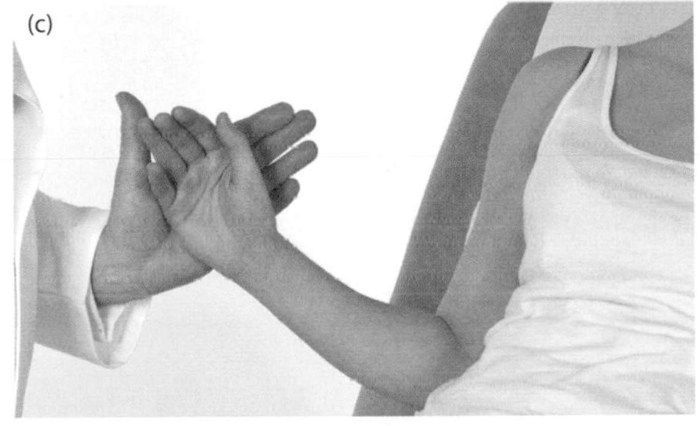

Figure 3.41 QUICK SCREEN OF MOTOR FUNCTION IN THE UPPER LIMB. (a) Median nerve – abduction of the thumb. (b) Ulnar nerve – abduction of the little finger. (c) Radial nerve – extension of the wrist.

Axillary nerve

This nerve can be damaged by:

- Shoulder dislocation or fracture.
- Penetrating axillary injuries.

Sensory loss The loss covers a small area over the deltoid equivalent to the C5 dermatome.

Motor malfunction The deltoid muscle is paralysed, so shoulder abduction is lost.

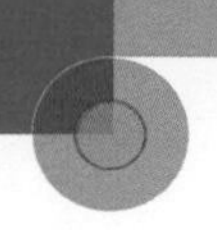

NERVES OF THE LOWER LIMB

Femoral nerve

This nerve can be damaged by:

- Knife or bullet injuries to the femoral triangle.
- Iatrogenic injuries also occur.

Sensory loss is over the anterior and medial surfaces of the thigh.

Motor malfunction The quadriceps muscles are paralysed, causing weakness of knee extension.

The patellar tendon reflex is lost.

Sciatic nerve

This nerve can be damaged by:

- Usually knife and gunshot wounds (e.g. knee-capping).
- Gluteal injections, hip replacement surgery and repair of acetabular fractures.
- Compound fracture dislocation of the hip.

Sensory loss is variable, depending on the level of nerve damage.

Motor malfunction The muscles of the lower leg are paralysed and later become wasted. The limb is 'flail'.

The ankle jerk is lost.

Common peroneal nerve

This nerve is easily damaged as it winds around the neck of the fibula.

This nerve can be damaged by:

- Local trauma.
- External pressure from a splint or plaster.
- Iatrogenic damage during surgery on the limb, usually caused by poor positioning.

Sensory loss Sensation is lost over the outer side of the leg foot and sole.

Motor malfunction There is foot drop with weakness of eversion and dorsiflexion of the ankle.

Quick screen of the motor function of the nerves of the lower limb

Test plantar flexion (Figure 3.42a) and dorsiflexion (Figure 3.42b).

[Insert the following - see p183 for example heading style]'

(a)

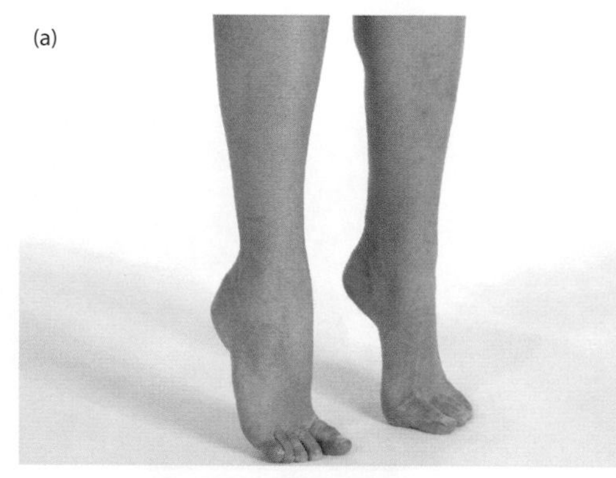

(b)

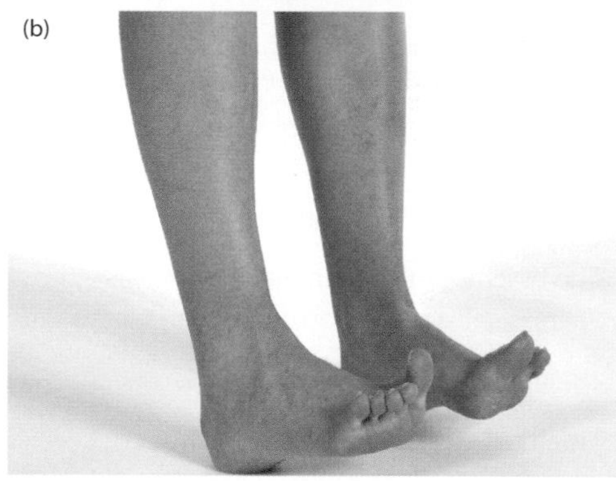

Figure 3.42 QUICK SCREEN OF MOTOR FUNCTION IN THE LOWER LIMB. (a) The patient standing on their toes to test plantar flexion S1, S2. (b) The patient standing on their heels to test dorsiflexion L4/5 and exclude any foot drop.

Acknowledgements

The contribution of Mr Aabir Chakraborty, BSc, MBBS, PhD, FRCS (Neurosurg), Consultant Neurosurgeon, University Hospital Southampton NHS, UK in the updating of this chapter is gratefully acknowledged.

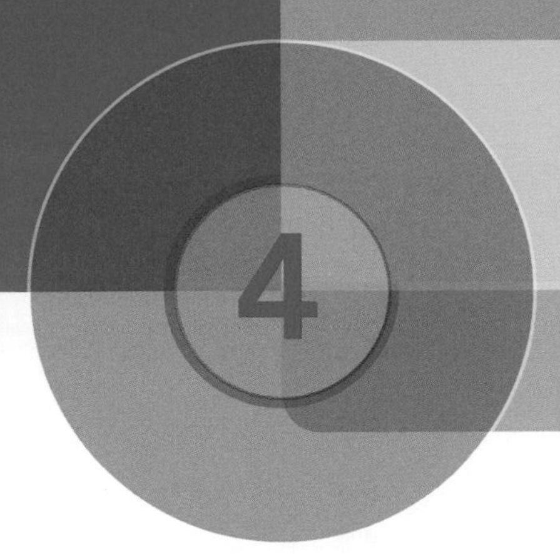

The skin and subcutaneous tissues

KAVAN S JOHAL, SAMER SAOUR AND PARI-NAZ MOHANNA

Anatomy and function

The skin is a complex organ that provides protection from ultraviolet light and microbiological invasion. It has an *important sensory role,* containing mechanoreceptors, thermoreceptors and nociceptors (for pain sensation). It also *controls body temperature,* is important in *maintaining fluid balance* and provides *immunological surveillance.*

The skin consists of two layers: *the epidermis,* derived from *the ectoderm,* and *the dermis,* derived from *the mesoderm.*

THE EPIDERMIS

The epidermis is a stratified squamous epithelium composed of five layers:

- Stratum germinativum – containing basal cells.
- Stratum spinosum – containing prickle cells.
- Stratum granulosum – containing granular cells.
- Stratum lucidum – a clear layer present only in the palms of the hands and soles of the feet.
- Stratum corneum – containing keratinized cells.

The thick cells of the stratum corneum protect against trauma and bacterial invasion, and also insulate against fluid loss.

Melanoblasts, derived from the neural ectoderm of the anterior horn cells, migrate into the basal layers of the epidermis. They produce the pigment melanin in response to a number of stimuli, and transfer this to the nearby keratinocytes through their dendritic processes.

Langerhans cells are also present in the epidermis, and are part of the monocyte–macrophage system, which processes antigens.

Merkel cells are mechanoreceptors present in the epidermis.

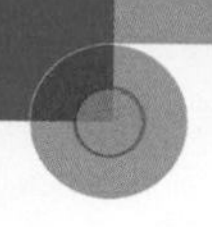

The hair and nails are derived from modified keratin by invagination of the epidermis.

THE DERMIS

The dermis is made up of collagen bundles and various proteoglycans that form a supporting framework for the blood vessels, lymphatics, nerves, sebaceous glands, sweat glands and hair follicles. The dermis also contains histiocytes and mast cells, which can act as antigen-presenting cells and are part of the reticuloendothelial system.

The dermis is subdivided into the papillary dermis and the deeper reticular dermis, which sits on the deep fascia.

Diagnosis of skin conditions

This chapter concentrates on the common skin problems that are likely to be seen in a surgical clinic. The important features that should be elicited in the history and examination are summarized in Revision panel 4.1.

It is difficult to draw up a set of simple diagnostic pathways suitable for all skin lesions because they have such varied features. For example, a basal cell carcinoma can be a raised nodule, a flat plaque or an ulcer, and can be skin coloured, pearly white, brown or pink. It is therefore better to learn the physical features of each skin lesion, and the best way to do this is by examining as many patients with 'skin conditions' as you can. *The diagnosis relies heavily on careful inspection and pattern recognition.* Tactile and auditory skills are less important.

GENERAL EXAMINATION

Always examine every skin blemish carefully before making a diagnosis, however familiar the condition.

Skin lesions have two basic distinguishing features: *their colour and their relationship to, and effect on, the overlying epidermis.* The overlying epidermis is likely to be raised and look abnormal if abnormal tissue is present in the superficial part of the dermis. An ulcer will develop if a localized area of the epidermis is destroyed. Alternatively, the overlying epidermis

Revision panel 4.1

FEATURES OF THE HISTORY AND EXAMINATION OF A LUMP OR SKIN LESION THAT MUST BE ELICITED

History

- Age
- Sex, ethnic group, occupation
- First local symptom
- Other symptoms
- Duration of symptoms
- Development of symptoms
- Persistence of symptoms
- Multiple or single lesions
- Systemic symptoms (direct questions)
- Possible cause
- Family history
- Social history

Local examination

- Site
- Shape
- Size
- Colour
- Temperature
- Tenderness
- Surface
- Edge
- Ulcer (edge, base, depth, discharge, surrounding tissues)
- Composition/contents:
  - Consistency
  - Fluctuation
  - Resonance
  - Fluid thrill
  - Translucency
  - Pulsatility
  - Compressibility
  - Bruit
- Reducibility
- Relations to surrounding structures
- Lymph drainage
- State of local tissues (arteries, nerves, bones and joints)

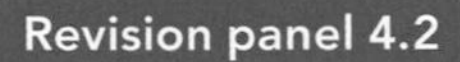

TERMS USED TO DESCRIBE SKIN PATHOLOGY

Macule – a localized change in colour of the skin that is not elevated (or palpable) or freckled

Papule – a small, solid elevation, flat-topped, conical, round, polyhedral, follicular (hairy), smooth or scaly

Vesicle – a small collection of fluid between the dermis and epidermis (a blister)

Bulla – a collection of fluid larger than a vesicle, under the epidermis

Wheal – a transient elevation of the skin caused by oedema

Cyst – a tumour that contains fluid

Naevus – a lesion present from birth, composed of mature structures normally found in the skin but present in excess, or in an abnormal disposition. The term 'naevus' is also used to describe lesions composed of naevus cells, as in melanocytic or pigmented naevi

Papilloma – a benign overgrowth of epithelial tissue (raised from the surface)

Tumour – literally, a swelling; commonly but inaccurately used to mean a malignant swelling

Hamartoma – an overgrowth of one or more cell types that are normal constituents of the organ in which they arise; the most common examples are haemangiomas, lymphangiomas and neurofibromas

Ulcer – an area of 'dissolution' of an epithelial surface

may be stretched but remains normal if there is an abnormality deep in the dermis. The terms used to describe the clinical appearances of different skin conditions are summarized in Revision panel 4.2.

It is possible, therefore, to subdivide all skin lesions into three categories:

- Those with an intact but abnormal epidermis.
- Those in which an area of the overlying epidermis is destroyed (ulcers).
- Those covered with a normal epidermis.

In the last of these, the bulk of the pathology is likely to be in the subcutaneous tissues, and even though it may be derived from a skin structure (e.g. a sebaceous gland), it is usually classified as a subcutaneous lesion.

The colour of a skin lesion may be helpful in making a diagnosis. Skin lesions may be black, brown, yellow, red or normal skin colour.

The following classification, based on the condition of the overlying epidermis and its colour, gives some idea of the multitude of lesions that you must learn to recognize.

EPIDERMIS INTACT BUT ABNORMAL (FIGURE 4.1)

- Black:
  - Gangrenous skin.
  - Early pyoderma gangrenosum.
  - Early anthrax pustule.
- Brown:
  - Freckles.
  - Seborrhoeic keratosis.
  - Moles of all varieties.
  - Malignant melanoma.
  - Pigmented basal or squamous cell carcinoma.
  - Café au lait patch.
  - Pigmentation following a bruise, thrombophlebitis or venous hypertension (the epidermis may be normal in these conditions).
- Greyish-brown:
  - Wart.
  - Seborrhoeic keratosis.
  - Keratoacanthoma.
- Yellow–white:
  - Xanthoma.
  - Lymphangioma.
  - Pustules of furunculosis and hidradenitis, subcutaneous calcinosis.

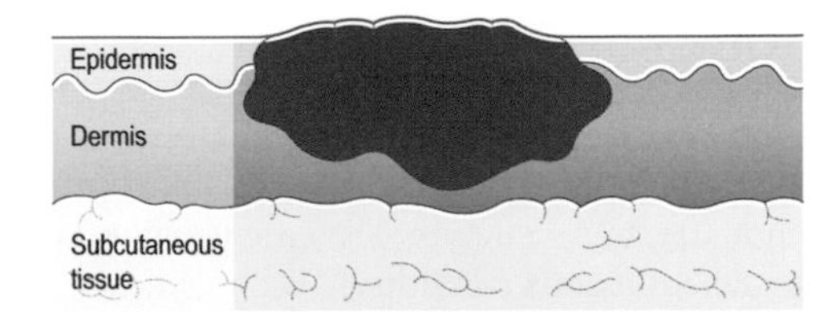

Figure 4.1 Epidermis intact but abnormal.

- Red–blue:
  - Strawberry naevus.
  - Port wine stain.
  - Spider naevus.
  - Campbell de Morgan spot.
  - Telangiectases.
  - Pyogenic granuloma.
- Skin colour:
  - Papilloma.
  - Early basal and squamous cell carcinoma.
  - Keloid scar.
  - Keratoacanthoma.

DESTRUCTION OF THE OVERLYING EPIDERMIS: ULCERATION (FIGURE 4.2)

- Sloping edge: A venous, ischaemic, trophic or neuropathic ulcer.
- Punched-out edge: An ischaemic, trophic or syphilitic ulcer.
- Undermined edge: Chronic infection (tuberculosis, carbuncle), pressure sore.
- Rolled or everted edge: Malignant ulceration.

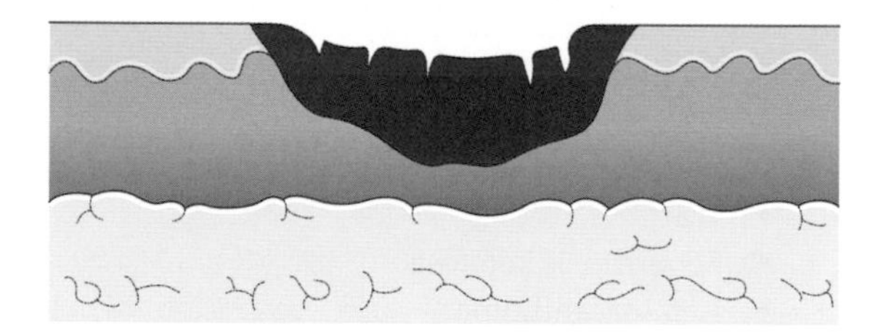

Figure 4.2 Destruction of the overlying epidermis – ulceration.

OVERLYING EPIDERMIS NORMAL (FIGURE 4.3)

Although these lesions may have arisen from a skin structure, their mass is beneath the skin and does not affect its structure. They are usually classified as subcutaneous conditions.

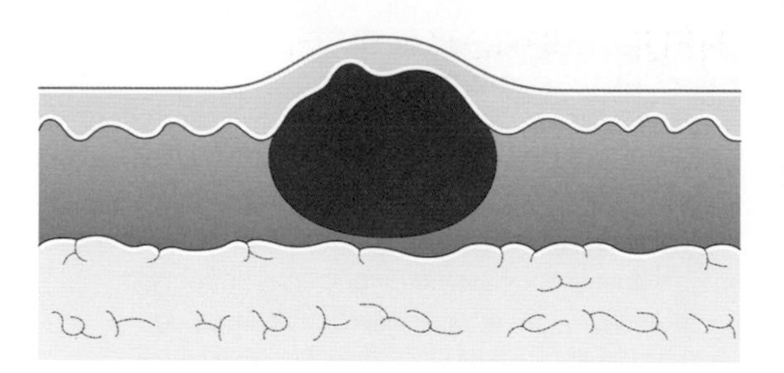

Figure 4.3 Overlying epidermis normal.

CONGENITAL SKIN DISORDERS

These may be genetic or non-genetic. *The latter are more common and mostly hamartomas,* i.e. tumour-like malformations in which there is an overgrowth of normal tissues arranged in an irregular fashion. The common congenital skin disorders are summarized in Revision panel 4.3.

Genetic skin disorders

Rare genetic skin disorders such as ichthyosis (a disorder of keratin formation that looks like lizard scales) or epidermolysis bullosa (in which the skin develops massive blisters after friction or minor trauma) are only likely to be encountered in a specialist dermatology clinic, whereas inherited neurofibromatosis is much more commonly seen in a surgical clinic.

Revision panel 4.3

CONGENITAL SKIN DISORDERS

Genetic

Alopecia
Ichthyosis vulgaris
Epidermolysis bullosa
Neurofibromatosis
Plantar keratosis

Non-genetic

Hamartomas (e.g. capillary haemangiomas, lymphangiomas, venous angiomas)
Dermoid cysts

NEUROFIBROMATOSIS

This is an autosomal dominant condition in which *multiple neurofibromas are present at birth and increase in number.* The condition is associated with a number of related abnormalities, such as:

- Fibroepithelial skin tags (Figure 4.4).
- Patches of light brown discolouration of the skin (café-au-lait patches) (Figure 4.5).
- Neuromas on major nerves, especially the acoustic nerve (acoustic neuroma) and the sensory roots of the spinal nerves (dumb-bell neuroma).
- *Malignant change to a neurofibrosarcoma* (seen in 5% of neuromas).
- *Phaeochromocytoma* of the adrenal gland, which commonly coexists.

Several types are recognized, the commonest of which are:

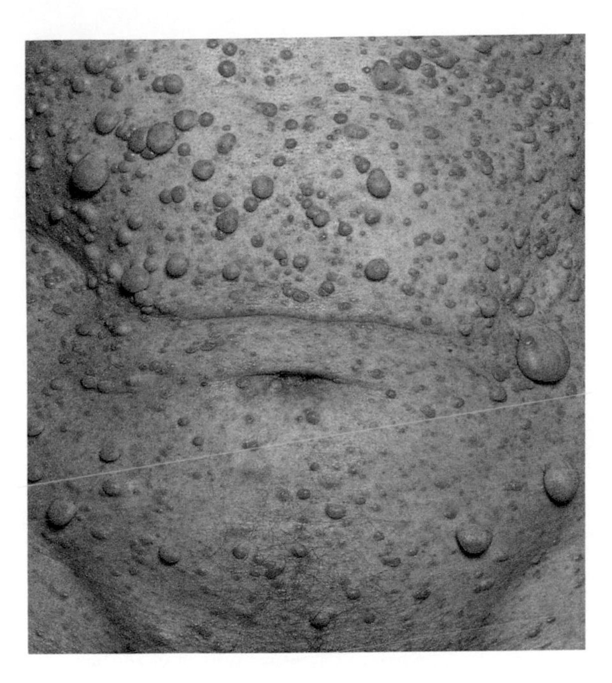

Figure 4.4 Multiple neurofibromatosis.

Neurofibromatosis type 1 (von Recklinghausen's disease)

- Cafe-au-lait spots (macules), axillary/inguinal freckling, optic gliomas, Lisch nodules of the iris, optic gliomas.
- This is the commonest type, affecting around 90% of all cases.

Neurofibromatosis type 2

- Rarer, central neurofibromatosis. Vestibular schwannomas, intracranial meningiomas and peripheral nerve schwannomas are recognized.

History

Most neurofibromas are present at birth, but they increase in size and number during life. As the disease is inherited through a dominant gene, one of the patient's parents and half of their brothers and sisters will be affected.

Examination

The patient is covered with *nodules of all sizes* (see Figure 4.4). Some are in the skin, some are tethered to it, and some become pedunculated. The nodules vary in consistency from soft to firm and may be a darker pink than the surrounding skin. Careful inspection of the skin nearly always reveals irregular patches of pale brown pigmentation. The pigment is melanin, and the patches are known as *café-au-lait patches* (see Figure 4.5). These are a diagnostic feature of von Recklinghausen's disease.

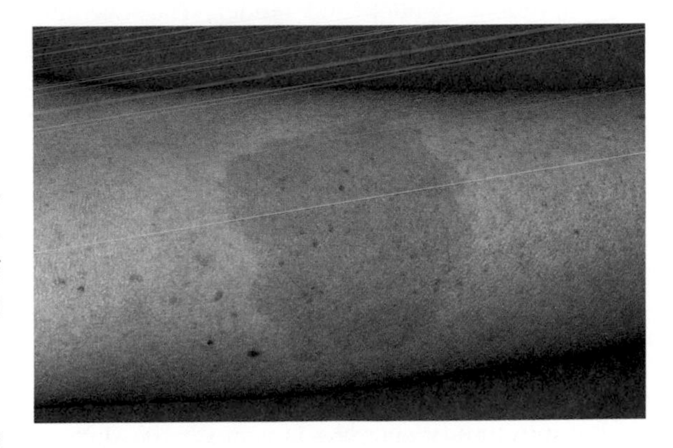

Figure 4.5 A café-au-lait patch on the forearm.

The blood pressure should be measured, as a coexisting *phaeochromocytoma* may cause hypertension. Neurological abnormalities are also common. It is important to test hearing and to examine the spinal nerves, to exclude the presence of major nerve malfunction caused by neuromas on the acoustic and spinal nerves (see Chapter 3).

Non-genetic congenital skin disorders

Almost all of the following conditions are hamartomas.

BENIGN PAPILLOMA

A benign papilloma of the skin is a simple overgrowth of all layers of the skin, with a vascular core (Figure 4.6). This is a hamartoma, and should be called a 'skin tag'.

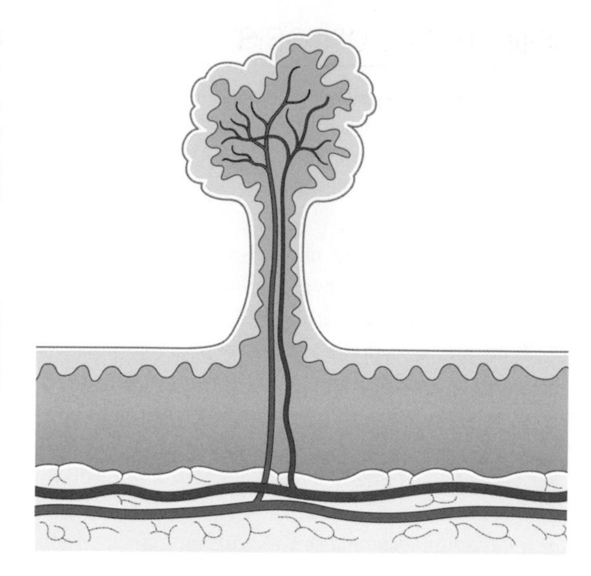

Figure 4.6 A papilloma is an overgrowth of all layers of the skin with a central vascular core.

History

Age They can appear at any age, and a few are congenital.

Symptoms May catch on clothing or rub (as pedunculated), may become red and swollen and ulcerate, or even infarct if it is injured.

The skin that forms a papilloma contains sweat glands, hair follicles and sebaceous glands. All of these structures can become infected and make the papilloma swollen and tender. The swelling can look like a carcinoma if the granulation tissue that forms in response to the infection becomes exuberant.

Examination

Site Papillomas occur anywhere on the skin.

Shape and size They vary from a smooth, raised plaque to a papilliferous, pedunculated polyp (Figure 4.7). Their size is equally variable.

Colour Normal skin.

Composition Soft and incompressible.

Lymph glands Normal.

Local tissues Normal.

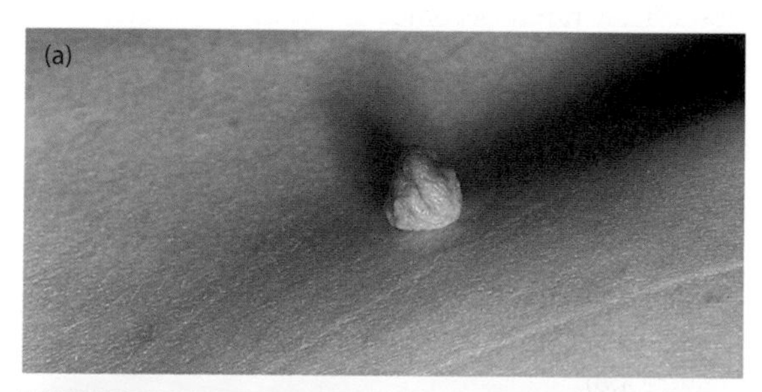

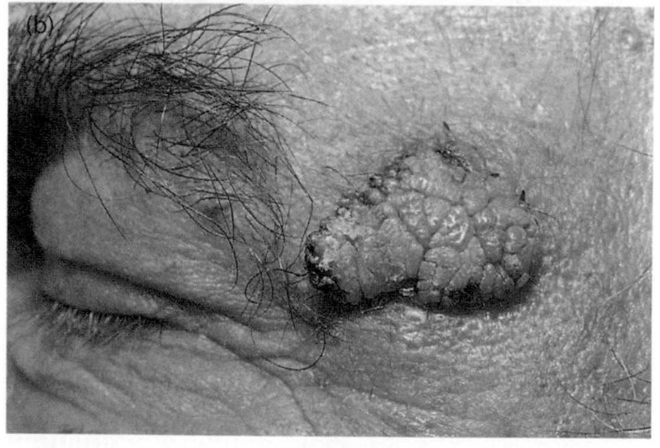

Figure 4.7 PAPILLOMAS. (a) A smooth papilloma with a narrow pedicle. (b) A sessile polyp with excess epithelium covering the clefts and corrugations.

CONGENITAL DERMOID CYST

This cyst lies beneath the skin and is lined by 'skin'. The two ways in which a piece of skin can become trapped deep to the normal skin are:

- As an accident during antenatal development.
- Following an injury, which implants some skin into the subcutaneous tissue.

Dermoid cysts are therefore either congenital or acquired. When considering congenital dermoid cysts, the potential for intracranial communication means that the majority should be imaged with ultrasound/MRI, especially if midline.

History

Duration May be present at birth, but usually become obvious a few years later when they begin to distend. Rarely multiple.

Symptoms Most congenital dermoid *cysts occur in the head and neck,* and parents are therefore concerned about their 'unsightliness' as well as the diagnosis. They rarely become very large or infected.

Examination

Site Congenital dermoid cysts develop where the skin dermatomes fuse. They therefore occur in the midline of the trunk, and are particularly common in the neck and face, along the lines of fusion of the ophthalmic and maxillary facial processes, especially at the inner and outer ends of the upper eyebrow (Figure 4.8).

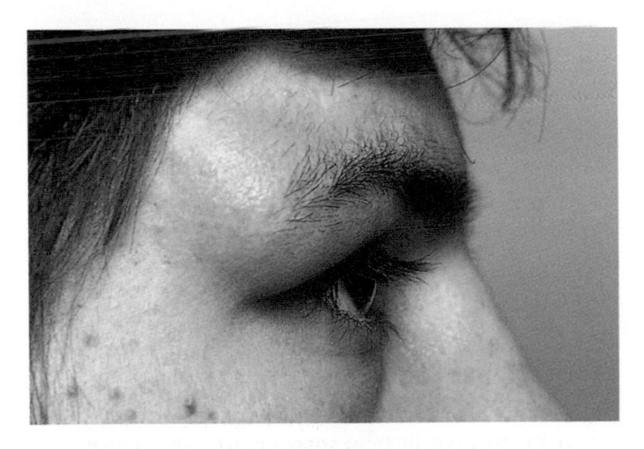

Figure 4.8 A right external angular dermoid cyst, so called because it lies beneath the outer end of the eyebrow over the external angular protuberance of the skull. This is a congenital dermoid cyst.

Shape and size They are usually ovoid or spherical and 1–2 cm in diameter.

Surface Their surface is smooth.

Composition Cysts on the face often feel soft, not tense and hard. *They fluctuate,* but only transilluminate if they contain clear fluid, instead of the usual thick, opaque mixture of sebum, sweat and desquamated epithelial cells. They are not pulsatile, compressible or reducible.

Relations Dermoid cysts lie deep to the skin, in the subcutaneous tissue. Unlike sebaceous cysts, they are not attached to the skin.

Haemangiomas/lymphangiomas

These are vascular hamartomas in which the blood and lymphatic vessels are irregularly arranged. They have many forms, such as *strawberry naevus, port wine stain, spider naevus, vin rosé patch and Campbell de Morgan spot.* Virtually all are various shades of pink or red, but each one has distinctive features. The majority blanch on pressure.

STRAWBERRY NAEVUS

The name is an accurate description because this bright red 'tumour', which sticks out from the surface of the skin, looks just like a strawberry. The term 'naevus' is correct because strawberry naevi are present at birth. They are congenital intradermal haemangiomas (Figure 4.9).

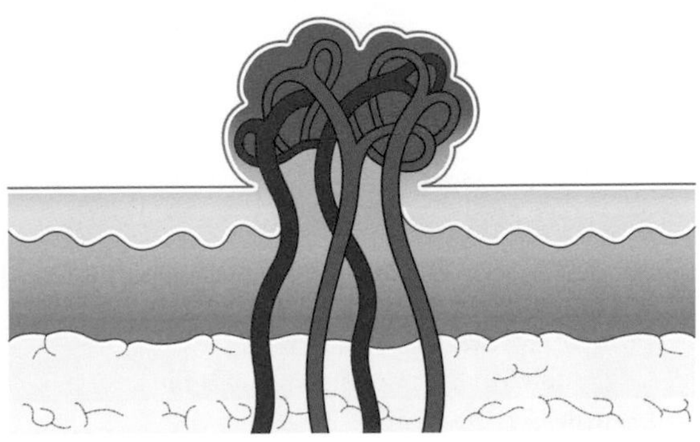

Figure 4.9 Diagram showing that a strawberry naevus is an intradermal and subdermal collection of dilated blood vessels.

History

Age Strawberry naevi *are present at birth.*

Sex They are equally distributed.

Duration *They often regress spontaneously,* months to years after birth.

Symptoms The child is almost always brought to the clinic because the red lump is disfiguring or a nuisance. Naevi that are rubbed or knocked may ulcerate and bleed. When they are on the buttocks, they can get wet and infected. More than one strawberry naevus may be present.

Examination

Site They can occur on any part of the body, but are most common on the *head and neck.*

Shape and size They protrude from the skin surface. Small naevi are sessile hemispheres, but as they grow, they can become pedunculated.

They are *usually 1–2 cm in diameter,* but they can become quite large (5–10 cm).

Surface Their surface is irregular, but covered with a smooth, pitted epithelium. There may be small areas of ulceration covered with scabs.

Colour They are either bright or dark red (Figure 4.10).

Consistency A strawberry naevus is soft and compressible, but not pulsatile. *Gentle sustained pressure squeezes most of the blood out of the 'tumour', leaving it collapsed, crinkled and colourless.*

Relations Strawberry naevi are confined to the skin, and are freely mobile over the deep tissues.

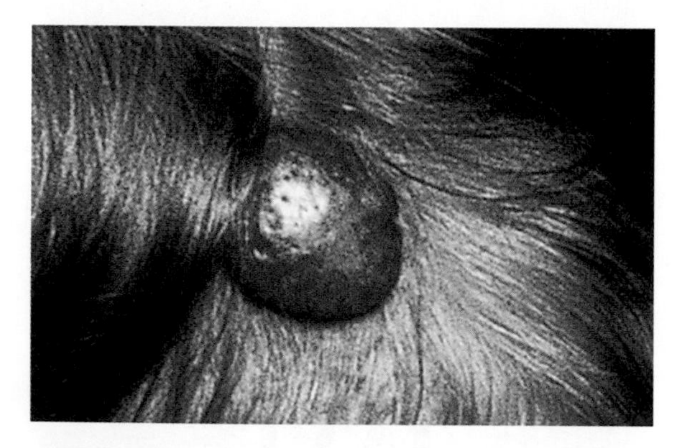

Figure 4.10 A close-up view of a strawberry naevus on the scalp, showing the smooth epithelial covering and little pits, which, with the red colour, make the lesion look like a strawberry.

Lymph nodes Unaffected.

Local tissues Unchanged.

PORT WINE STAIN

This is an extensive intradermal haemangioma, which is mostly made up of small venules and capillaries (Figure 4.11). It gives the skin a deep purple–red colour; hence its name.

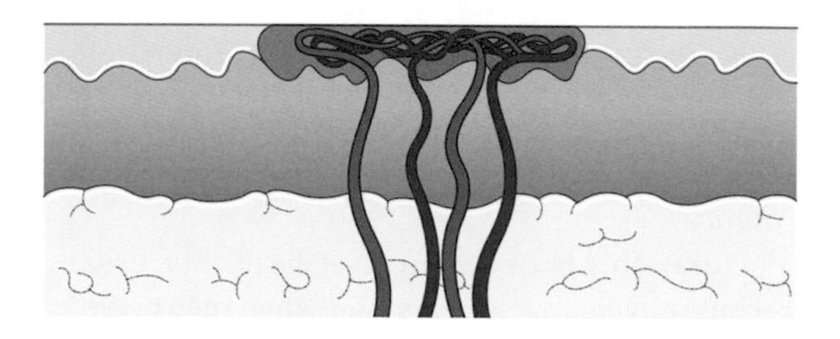

Figure 4.11 A port wine stain is a collection of dilated venules and capillaries just below the epidermis.

History

Age *Present at birth,* do not change in size relative to the size of the rest of the body, although colour may.

Symptoms Patient and parental distress is common because of the visibility of lesions, especially those on the face. Occasionally, small vessels within the stain become prominent and bleed.

The port wine stain may be part of a more extensive vascular deformity.

Examination

Site Port wine stains are common on the *face,* and at the *junctions between the limbs and the trunk,* i.e. the shoulders, neck and buttocks. They may appear localized to a dermatome and can be associated with glaucoma or other syndromes such as *Sturge–Weber.*

Shape and size Both are very variable.

Surface Usually smooth, but the vessels can be prominent and may bleed.

Colour Their *distinctive feature is their deep purple–red colour* (Figure 4.12). There may be paler areas at the edge of the patch. The colour can be diminished by local pressure, but pressure rarely returns the skin to its normal colour because all the blood vessels within the patch are abnormal.

Local tissues There may be some dilated subcutaneous veins beneath and around the lesion.

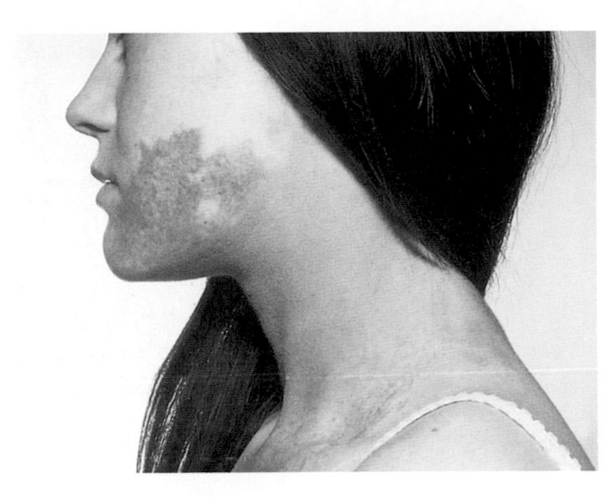

Figure 4.12 An extensive port wine stain of the lower face and neck.

VENOUS ANGIOMA

Venous angiomas are usually situated in the deeper levels of the subcutaneous tissues and can extend into the muscles or joints (see Chapter 10). There are often some irregularly arranged distended blue veins in the skin over the surface of the subcutaneous soft mass that empty with pressure.

> **NOTE:** It is always wise to listen over the swelling for a bruit (see below).

SPIDER NAEVUS

This consists of a solitary dilated skin arteriole feeding a number of small branches that leave it in a radial manner (Figure 4.13).

> **NOTE:** It is an acquired condition, and may be associated with a generalized disease such as cirrhosis.

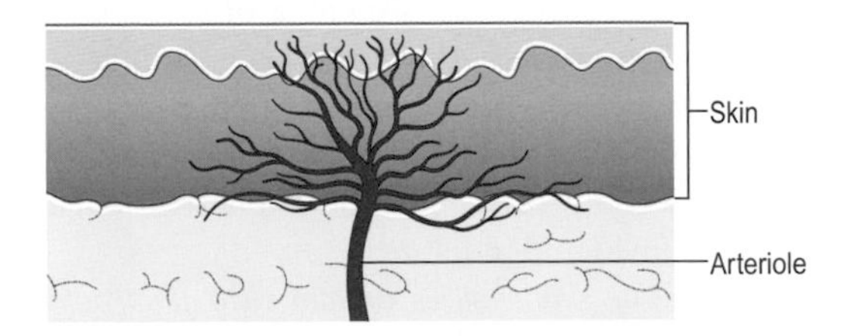

Figure 4.13 A spider naevus is a solitary dilated arteriole with visible radiating branches.

History

Spider naevi are rarely noticed by the patient unless they are in a prominent position on the face. They cause no symptoms. They are usually multiple, and tend to increase in number over the years. *It is important to enquire about the patient's consumption of alcohol* because they are known to be associated with chronic liver disease.

Examination

Site Spider naevi appear on the *upper half of the trunk, the face and the arms*. This is the area of drainage of the superior vena cava, but it is not clear how this could affect their distribution.

Shape and size They look like little red spiders (Figure 4.14). The central arteriole is 0.5–1.0 mm in diameter, and the radiating vessels usually spread for a varying distance of 1–2 mm.

Colour The central arteriole is bright red, and the vessels radiating from it are of a similar colour.

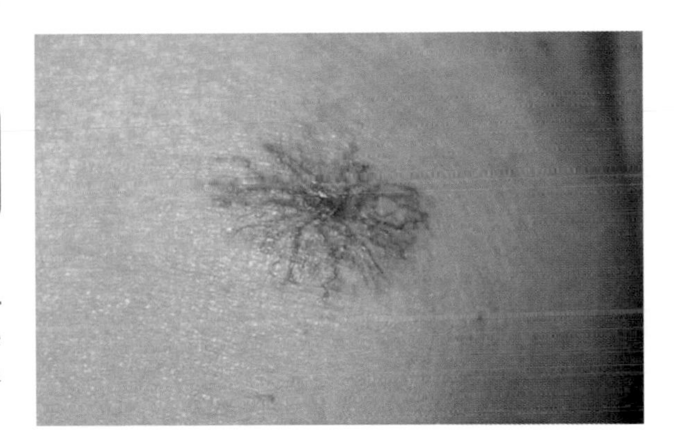

Figure 4.14 A spider naevus.

Compressibility Spider naevi are not tender, and fade completely when compressed. *Compression of the central arteriole with the head of a pin makes the radiating 'legs' fade.* They refill as soon as the pressure is released.

Local tissues Normal.

General examination *They are known to be associated with liver cirrhosis* (other stigmata of liver disease may be present, see Chapter 15) and also liver tumours/oestrogen-producing tumours.

VIN ROSÉ PATCH

This is a congenital intradermal vascular abnormality in which mild dilatation of the vessels in the subpapillary dermal plexus gives the skin a pale pink colour. It is often associated with other vascular abnormalities such as extensive haemangiomas, giant limbs caused by arteriovenous fistulas and lymphoedema (see Chapter 10).

A vin rosé patch can occur anywhere, is rarely causes symptoms and usually does not require any treatment.

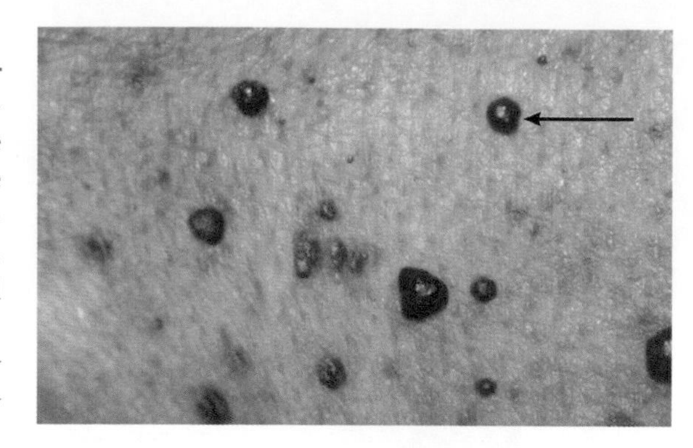

Figure 4.15 A Campbell de Morgan spot.

CAMPBELL DE MORGAN SPOT

This is *a bright red,* clearly-defined spot caused by a collection of dilated capillaries fed by a single or small cluster of arterioles. The cause of these spots is unknown, and they are not associated with any other disease.

History

Age Increase with age, rarer <45 years old.

Duration Appear spontaneously, alone or occasionally as a cluster.

Symptoms Non-painful/tender, rarely disfiguring.

Examination

Site Usually develop on the trunk, occasionally on the limbs and rarely on the face.

Shape and size Circular and have a sharp edge, which is sometimes slightly raised. They are usually 1–3 mm in diameter.

Colour They have a *uniform deep red or purple colour* that makes them look like drops of dark red paint or sealing wax just under the epidermis (Figure 4.15).

Compressibility Although they comprise a collection of dilated capillaries, they do not always empty when compressed, although they always fade slightly.

LYMPHANGIOMA CIRCUMSCRIPTUM

This is a circumscribed cluster of many small dilated lymph sacs in the skin and subcutaneous tissues that *do not connect* with the normal lymph system. These blind sacs may be clusters of lymph sacs that failed to join into the lymph system during its development. Large, translucent lymph cysts confined to the subcutaneous tissues are called *lymphatic malformations* (see Chapter 12).

History

Sex *They are present at birth,* but may not be noticed until the skin vesicles appear a few years later. They are equally common in males and females.

Symptoms They are usually noticed by the child's parents, who consult the doctor because they are concerned about the disfigurement. The vesicles *sometimes leak clear fluid,* and when very prominent, the vesicles can be rubbed by clothes and may get infected and painful.

Development As the years pass, the subcutaneous cysts enlarge and become prominent, and the number and extent of the skin vesicles increases.

Examination

Site *They are found at the junction of the limbs with the trunk,* i.e. around the shoulder, axilla, buttock and groin.

Shape and size They may present as a single or multiple lumps. A large area of skin may be involved – the whole of the buttock or shoulder may be abnormal – and most lymphangiomas cover an area 5–20 cm across by the time that they present.

Surface Their surface is smooth, but their edge is often ill defined and indistinct.

Colour *The skin vesicles contain clear fluid, which looks watery or yellow. Blood in the vesicles turns them red–brown or even black* (Figure 4.16).

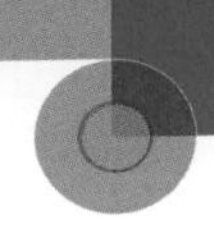

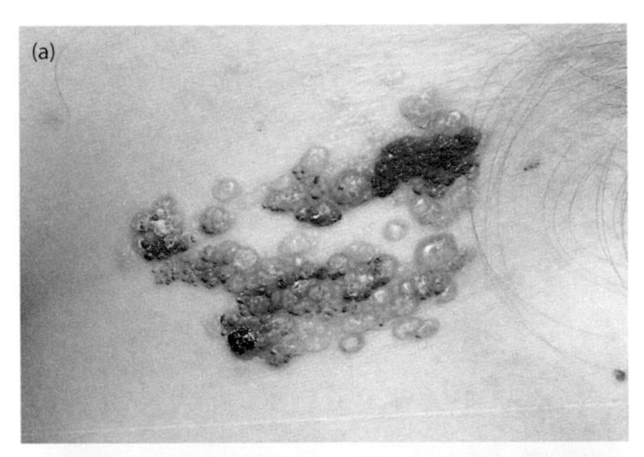

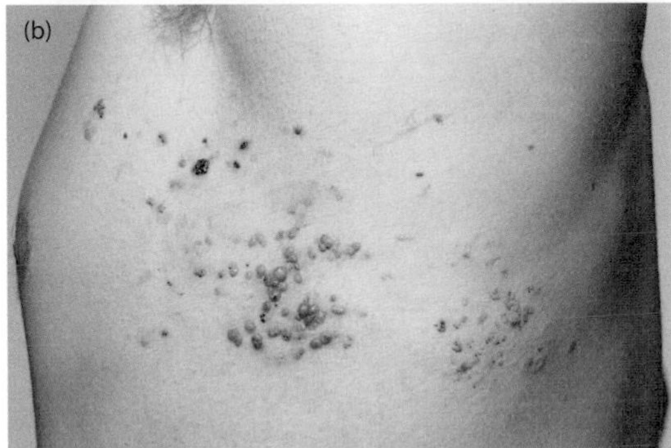

Figure 4.16 LYMPHANGIOMATA CIRCUMSCRIPTUM. (a) Many of the vesicles are red, black or brown because they contain old blood. (b) This malformation involves the whole of the side of the chest just below the axilla.

Overlying skin The subcutaneous cysts make the abnormal area bulge slightly, but the edges of this swelling are indistinct. The skin contains vesicles of varying sizes and colour, ranging from 0.5 to 3 or 4 mm in diameter (Figure 4.16).

Composition *The whole swelling is soft and spongy*, although as it is usually composed of multiple cysts, it does not fluctuate. Occasionally, it may contain one or two large cysts, which may fluctuate. The mass is not compressible. The dark red or brown vesicles do not fade with pressure.

Lymph glands The local lymph glands are not enlarged unless the lymphangioma has become infected.

ARTERIOVENOUS FISTULAS

These may cause a swelling in the skin or subcutaneous tissues, which may have a vascular appearance. The veins are also often distended, but *careful inspection may reveal pulsation, which is confirmed by palpation.* Arteriovenous fistulas are not compressible, but *should have a loud machinery murmur situated over them* providing that they have a high flow (see Chapter 10).

ACQUIRED DERMATOLOGICAL CONDITIONS

Conditions of the skin caused by trauma including burns

KELOID AND HYPERTROPHIC SCARS

An incised wound heals in four phases:

- *Haemostasis*, in which the gap in the tissue is filled by blood and fibrin.
- This is then followed by the *inflammation phase*, where there is an influx of mononuclear cells (monocytes and macrophages) into the wound.
- *The proliferation phase* involves the production of fibrous tissue/collagen in the wound.
- Reorganization then follows in the *remodelling phase* to give the wound its maximum strength.

This process, which is called *healing by primary intention*, is remarkably well controlled. Most surgical scars in the skin are thin lines containing the minimum amount of scar tissue.

Hypertrophic scar

Sometimes, however, the fibrous tissue response is excessive, and the result is a hypertrophic or keloid scar.

In a *hypertrophic scar*, excessive amounts of fibrous tissue form (organized bundles of type III collagen), *but this is confined to the scar; i.e. it is between the incised skin edges* (Figures 4.17 and 4.18). Hypertrophic scars are quite common, particularly if there has been some additional stimulus to fibrous tissue formation during healing, such as infection or excessive tension, both of which are common complications of scars crossing skin creases.

Hypertrophic scars only enlarge for *2–3 months*.

Normal scar

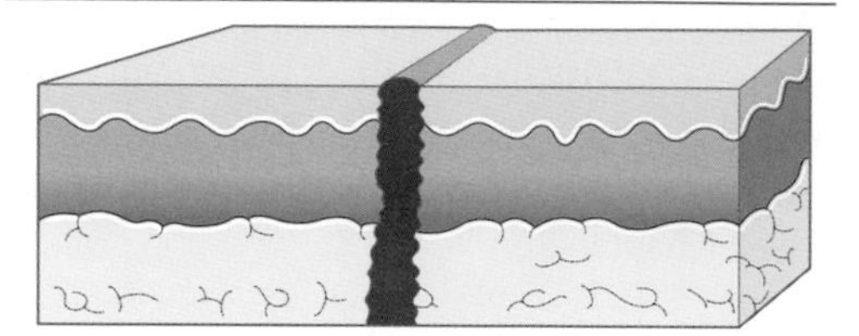

Hypertrophic scar

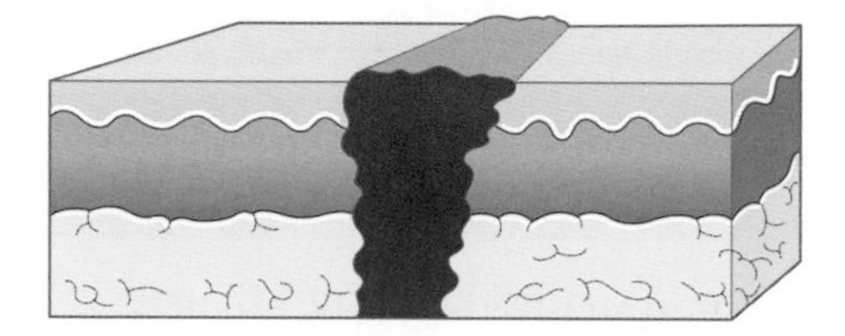

Keloid scar

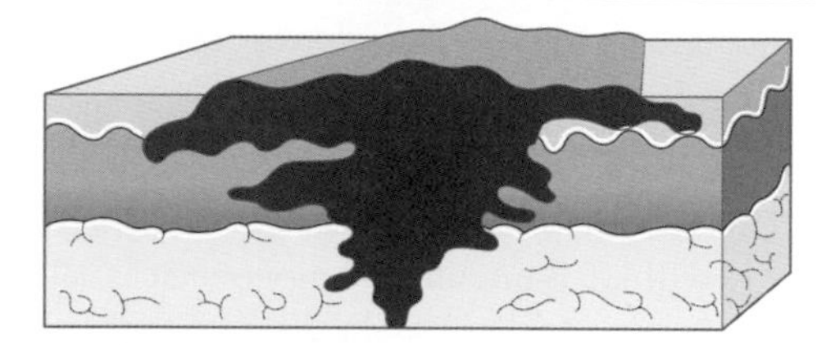

Figure 4.17 Normal, hypertrophic and keloid scars.

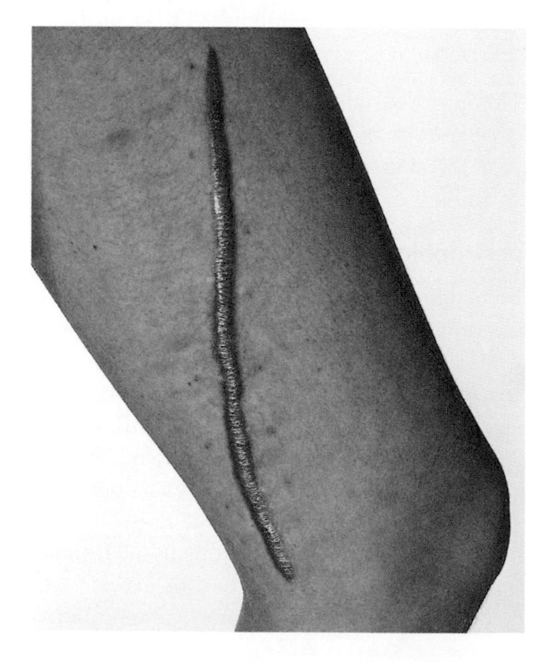

Figure 4.18 A hypertrophic scar on the medial side of the thigh.

Keloid scar

This occurs when the hypertrophy and overgrowth of the fibrous tissue extend beyond the original wound into normal tissues (Figure 4.19). This means that the scar has some of the characteristics of a locally invasive malignant neoplasm.

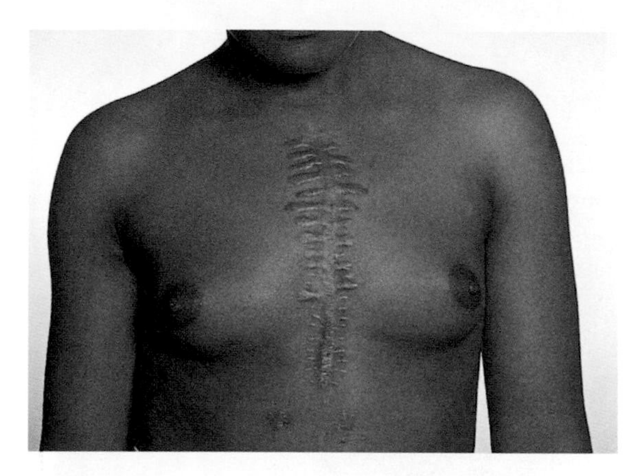

Figure 4.19 A keloid scar after a median sternotomy.

The tendency to produce keloid scars is a congenital trait, *common in Afro-Caribbean individuals*. Some tribes exploit the trait for the production of decorative scars on the face and trunk.

Keloid scars continue to enlarge for *6–12 months* after the initial injury. They are almost certainly the result of a local release of fibroblast growth factors, which are unsuppressed.

Poorly organized type I and type III collagen are seen microscopically.

As a keloid scar grows, it can become very unsightly, it is often tender to the touch, and it may itch. Although the disfigurement produced by a hypertrophic scar may be as great as that of a keloid scar, it is important to try to distinguish the two abnormalities because *hypertrophic scars do not recur* after they have been excised if the causative factors are eliminated, whereas *keloid scars will recur unless special measures are taken.*

ACQUIRED IMPLANTATION DERMOID CYSTS

History

These cysts develop when a piece of skin survives after being forcibly implanted into the subcutaneous tissues by an injury – often a small, deep cut or stab. The patient may not remember the initial injury.

Symptoms Implantation dermoid cysts are usually small and tense. They may be painful and tender because they usually occur in areas subject to repeated trauma. Cysts on the fingers may interfere with grip and touch.

Examination

Site Implantation dermoid cysts are *commonly found where injuries are likely to occur, such as the fingers*. Surprisingly, surgical incisions rarely cause these cysts.

Shape and size The cysts are spherical, smooth and small, about 0.5–1.0 cm in diameter (Figure 4.20).

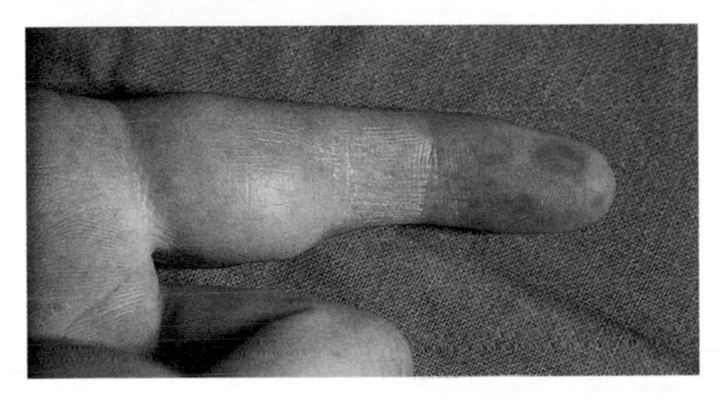

Figure 4.20 An implantation dermoid cyst that appeared following a small stab wound.

Composition Implantation dermoid cysts feel *hard and tense, sometimes stony hard*. Their small size makes the detection of their cystic nature – *fluctuation – difficult*. The deduction that they are cystic usually depends solely on their shape. They may *transilluminate*.

Relations A scar is usually present in the overlying skin. The cyst may be tethered to the deep aspect of the scar or even lie within it. The deeper structures should be normal, and the cyst is freely mobile over them unless they were involved in the initial injury.

Lymph glands The regional lymph glands should be normal.

Differential diagnosis A *sebaceous cyst* (see below) is often confused with an implantation dermoid. The history of an old injury and the presence of a scar are the most significant diagnostic features.

PYOGENIC GRANULOMA

Small capillary loops develop in a healing wound to knit it together and provide sustenance and support for the covering epithelium. In the base of a healing ulcer, these capillary loops form a layer of bright red tissue known as *granulation tissue*.

When the capillary loops grow too vigorously, they may form a protruding mass of tissue that becomes covered with epithelium and is called a *pyogenic granuloma*. (It is probably neither pyogenic nor granulomatous.) Its surface is often ulcerated and infected. The infection is a secondary event and probably not the initiating stimulus.

History

Age Any age.

Symptoms There may be a history of a minor injury, usually a cut or scratch, but the patient often cannot remember the initial injury. They sometimes occur in response to a chronic infection such as a paronychia.

The patient complains of a skin lump that *bleeds easily and discharges serous or purulent fluid. The lump usually grows rapidly* (it may double in size in a few days), and as a consequence many patients think it is a tumour. The bleeding, weeping and pain stop when it is completely covered with epithelium.

Examination

Site Pyogenic granulomas are commonly found where injuries are most likely to occur, such as the hands and face.

Shape and size They begin as a hemispherical nodule that grows upwards and outwards (Figure 4.21).

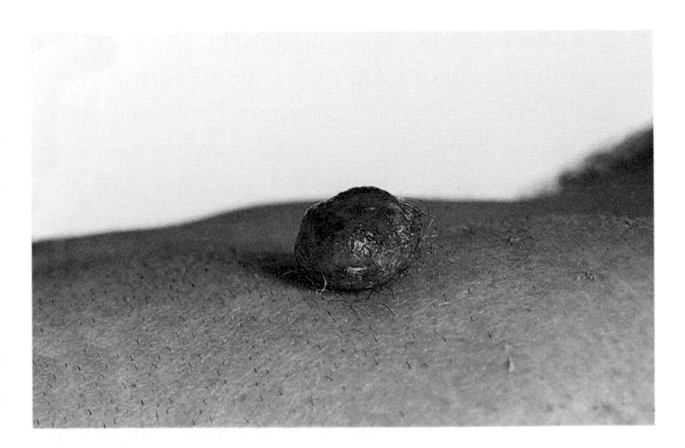

Figure 4.21 A pyogenic granuloma on the skin of the chest.

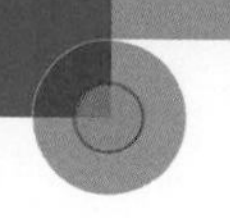

The lump is rarely more than 1 cm across because its blood supply becomes inadequate. Growth from a few millimetres to full size can occur in a few days.

Surface Before the surface is epithelialized, it has a covering of dried blood or plasma and *bleeds easily*.

Colour At first, they are the *bright red colour* of healthy granulation tissue (Figure 4.21), but as they get bigger and less vascular, they *fade to a pale pink*. When they become covered with epithelium, they *turn pink or white*.

Tenderness and composition Sometimes slightly tender, soft.

Relations Confined to the skin.

Complications They bleed easily when knocked, and can break off at their base. The granuloma may reform in the next few days, or the base can re-epithelialize.

Natural history Once the granulations have become completely covered with epithelium, the nodule begins to shrink, but it rarely disappears completely.

Differential diagnosis The important conditions to exclude are:

- Squamous cell carcinoma.
- Non-pigmented melanoma.
- Kaposi's sarcoma.

A history of trauma and the very rapid growth are the particular features of a pyogenic granuloma, but an excisional biopsy is often needed to confirm the diagnosis.

FAT NECROSIS

Dead fat becomes hard and fibrous. The skin then becomes tethered or fixed to it, and indrawn.

In the breast, which is an organ that is frequently knocked and bruised, fat necrosis may be mistaken for a carcinoma (see Chapter 13). The buttock is also a common site of fat necrosis, particularly in patients who have frequent subcutaneous injections, such as those with diabetes (Figure 4.22).

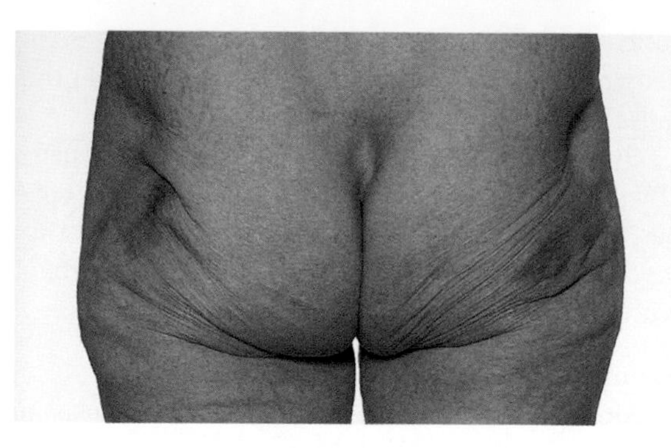

Figure 4.22 Fat necrosis of the buttock fat caused by repeated injections of insulin. Note the tethering, indrawing and pigmentation of the skin. Beneath these areas were hard lumps of necrotic fat.

COMMON ULCERS OF THE SKIN

An ulcer is a *dissolution* of the continuity of an epithelial surface. Ulcers follow traumatic removal, or death and desquamation by disease, of the whole or part of an epithelium, and most occur in the lower limb (see Chapter 1).

Ulcers are discussed here because trauma is often the final cause of the skin breakdown, although there are many underlying causes that make the skin susceptible to injury and impede subsequent healing. The common causes are listed in Revision panel 4.4.

Revision panel 4.4

CAUSES OF ULCERATION OF THE SKIN OF THE LOWER LIMB

Venous: 60% (one-half varicose and one-half post-thrombotic)
Ischaemic: 20% (one-quarter have an associated venous cause)
Collagen disease: 5% (rheumatoid and systemic lupus erythematosus)
Neuropathic: 2%
Traumatic: 1%
Neoplastic: 1%
Many rare causes: 5%
Unknown: 6%

Venous ulcers

Venous ulcers are characteristically found in the *lower medial third of the lower limb*. They are described in detail in Chapter 10.

Ischaemic ulcers

Arterial insufficiency usually manifests terminally in limbs. It is rare to see ulcers caused by arterial disease at the base of the limbs or on the trunk. Ischaemic ulcers are described in detail in Chapter 10.

Trophic ulcers

A trophic ulcer is an ulcer that has developed as the result of *the patient's insensitivity to repeated trauma*. These ulcers are commonly associated with those forms of neurological disease that cause loss of the appreciation of pain and light touch in weight-bearing areas (see Chapters 3 and 10).

Neoplastic ulcers

Ulcers due to basal and squamous cell carcinomas are described in detail later in this chapter (see page 151).

Metastases from distant or underlying cancers can appear in the skin, and may ulcerate and have features similar to those of a primary carcinomatous ulcer – *an everted edge and a proliferating base.*

BURNS

The skin can be burnt by heat, irradiation, electrical or chemical noxious stimuli.

A *heat burn* is usually caused by direct flames, an explosion, contact with a hot object, steam or hot fluid. Burns caused by steam or hot water are called *scalds*. All burns cause local inflammation, and *systemic effects occur if more than 20% of the total body surface area is burnt.*

Assessment and resuscitation As in a major injury (see Chapter 5), these two must proceed simultaneously. *Intravenous access and fluid replacement are essential* in any patient who has a sizeable burn, and cannulae should be placed in large veins in an area of unburnt skin.

The size and depth of the burn must be carefully assessed. The burn size is measured as a percentage of total body area using the *Rule of nines* (Figure 4.23). For a child, this must be modified – the head and neck being scored as 18% and the lower limbs downgraded from 18% to 14%.

The burn depth can be subdivided into superficial, superficial dermal, mid-dermal, deep dermal and full thickness (Figure 4.24).

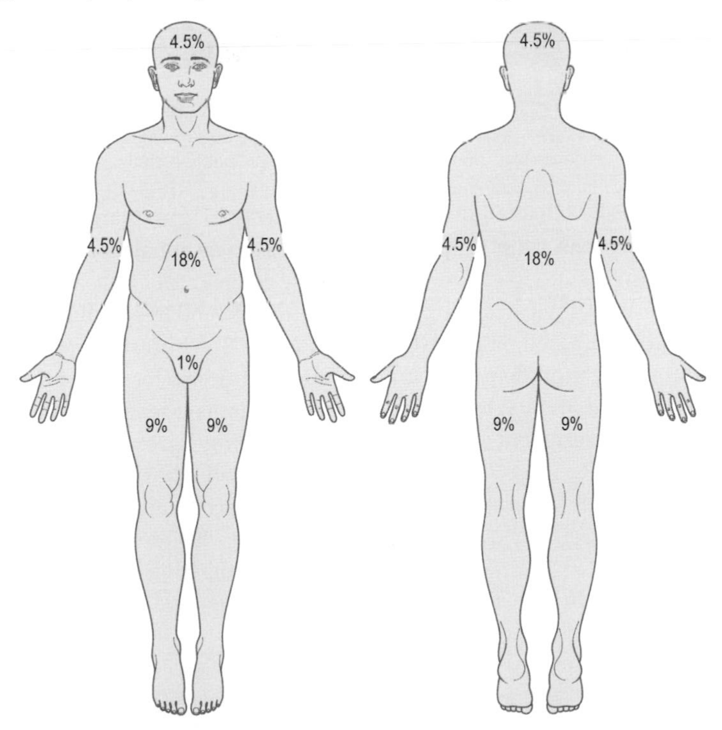

Figure 4.23 The 'Rule of nines' method for calculating the proportion of the body surface that has been burnt.

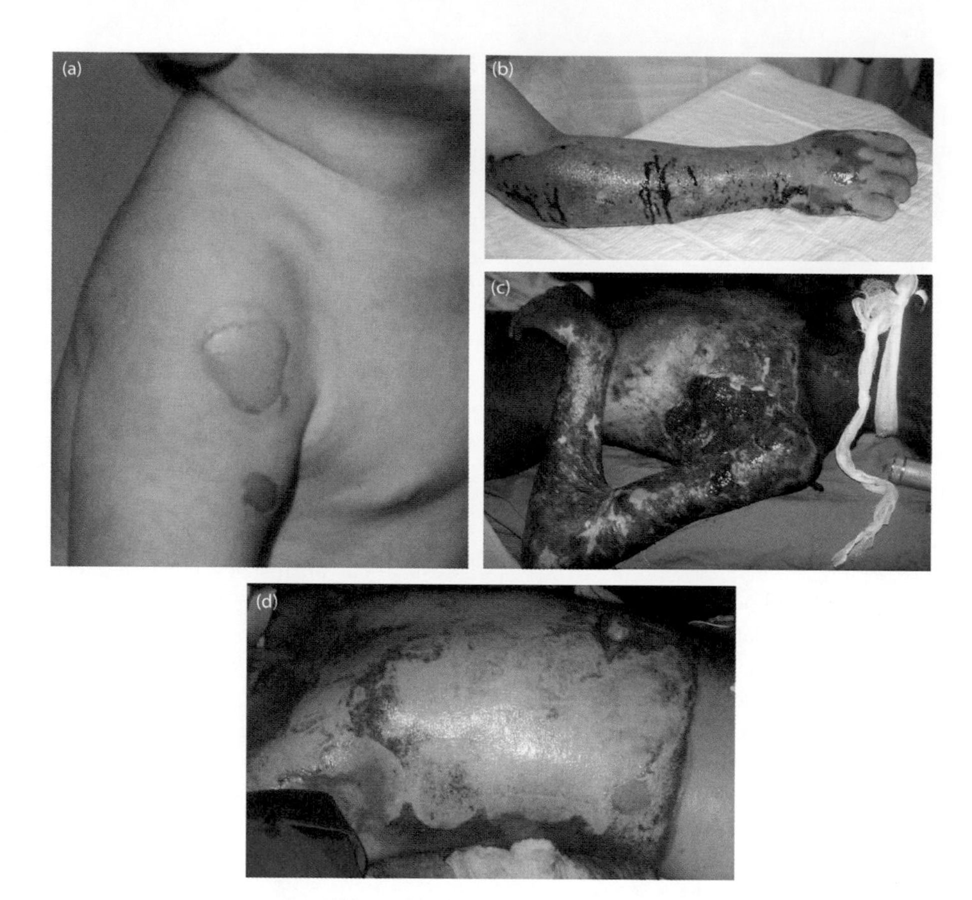

Figure 4.24 BURNS. (a) A superficial burn: hyperaemia, blistering and pain. (b) A mixture of partial-thickness and full-thickness burns. (c) A partial-thickness burn: loss of epithelium, some superficial capillary bleeding and a few pale patches that may turn out to be deeper burns. (d) An extensive scald, probably mostly a partial-thickness burn.

Superficial burns are usually blistered and very painful, while full-thickness burns are often pale or white, with absent sensation.

A number of formulae exist for calculating the patient's early fluid requirement based on the extent and depth of the burn, the weight of the patient and the time the burn was sustained. It must be stressed that early and adequate fluid replacement is the most important initial treatment.

Clinical features

Pain *This is the main symptom,* especially in patients with superficial burns.

Skin sensation Sensation must be carefully tested whenever a full-thickness burn is suspected, *and retested 24 hours later,* when the lack of sensation may be easier to determine.

Airway It is important to assess the face, mouth and airways, as an inhalation injury of their lining commonly complicates extensive burns. Burns around the mouth, nose and lips are highly indicative of *an inhalation injury.* The buccal mucous membrane and tongue must be inspected for mucosal burns. An urgent anaesthetic review is essential if airway burns are suspected.

Breathing Special attention must be paid to any circumferential burns of the neck or chest, as these may constrict breathing. The occurrence of stridor or a difficulty with breathing is an indication for endotracheal intubation and ventilation, especially if the patient is unconscious.

> **NOTE:** The airway and breathing must be carefully monitored.

Circulation The state of the circulation must be repeatedly assessed, as burns are associated with *massive losses of fluids, electrolytes and protein from their surface, and red cell damage or destruction occurs,* especially in full-thickness burns.

The pulse, blood pressure, central venous pressure, urine output and haematocrit must be carefully monitored in all patients with major burns. Failure to maintain an adequate circulation may be followed by renal failure and eventually multiorgan failure. The latter may proceed septicaemia from secondary infection in and around the burns.

Circumferential burns of the limbs or digits may cause peripheral ischaemia, and need urgent release.

Depigmentation This is a rare problem that can occur in Afro-Caribbean races after extensive scarring and burns.

Electrical burns

Most electrical burns come from faulty home appliances or the careless touching of electrodes. In high-voltage burns, such as lightening strikes, survival is uncommon because the depolarization usually causes severe cardiac arrhythmias and arrest.

A severe local burn develops at the point of entry, and adjacent nerves and muscles are often damaged. Deep tissue damage can lead to metabolic derangements, compartment syndromes, arterial and venous thrombosis and even visceral damage if the entry point is over the torso.

Radiation injury

The initial skin injury caused by radiation often resembles a standard thermal burn. The clinical evidence of the commonly associated lung/bowel damage and bone marrow depression appears later.

Many patients exposed to high doses of radiation die from pulmonary complications or aplastic anaemia, and those who survive the early systemic effects may die later from radiation-induced malignant change in organs such as the thyroid gland.

Chemical burns

Most chemical burns are caused by contact with acids or alkalis; a few are caused by phosphorus and phenols. Chemical burns of the skin can be avoided by wearing protective clothing and washing off the contaminant as quickly as possible. *They have the same clinical appearance as full/partial-thickness thermal burns.*

The oral ingestion of corrosive chemicals may destroy the lining of the oesophagus and cause life-threatening complications and serious long-term morbidity.

Infections of the skin

Skin and subcutaneous infections are common, especially when the skin is breached. *The cardinal signs of rubor, calor, dolor and tumour* are usually present in all infections, and patients are invariably pyrexial.

BACTERIAL INFECTIONS

Impetigo

This a relatively rare *staphylococcal infection* that causes blistering of the hands and face. Vesicles form and rupture, and are covered with a honey coloured crust. They may form circinate or gyriform patterns. Fresh blisters form daily, and many develop inflammatory halos. A microbiological swab should be sent for culture. Patients are usually referred to dermatology clinics.

Furunculosis (boils)

Furuncles and boils are caused by infection entering a hair follicle. This first produces pus and then a central core of necrotic tissue. *When only pus is present, it is called a furuncle; when it contains a solid core, it is called a boil.*

Boils are often multiple and associated with general debility, or underlying disease such as diabetes. They can occur on any part of the body, but are *common in the skin of the head and neck, axillae and groins.* They begin as a hard, red, tender area, which gradually enlarges and causes a throbbing pain. The tissue in the centre of the infected area eventually dies and forms a thick yellow slough. The lump then becomes fluctuant, the centre of the covering skin sloughs, and the pus and necrotic core are discharged.

Subcutaneous abscess

Abscesses in the subcutaneous tissue are common and usually follow the implantation of bacteria by a penetrating injury, or infection in a haematoma.

The common infecting organism is *Staphylococcus aureus*, but almost any organism can cause an abscess if the local conditions are favourable to its growth. An abscess is a pocket of pus (dead cells, exudate and bacteria) surrounded by granulation tissue.

History

Age All ages and both sexes.

Hygiene Poor social conditions/bodily hygiene increase the chances of an infection following a minor injury such as a pinprick.

Symptoms The principal complaint is of *a throbbing pain* that gets steadily worse and keeps the patient awake at night.

The patient notices an area of *thickening and tenderness* at the site of the pain, which slowly turns into a hard mass. The mass may discharge spontaneously, with relief of the symptoms, before the patient attends the doctor.

Previous history Patients who are debilitated, diabetic or drug addicts may have had previous abscesses as a result of their underlying disease and frequent injections.

Habits Enquire about the drug-taking habits of the patient if you have cause to think that the abscess might have followed a self-administered injection.

Examination

The four classical signs of an abscess (the *signs of Celsus*) are tumour, rubor, calor and dolor (*swelling, redness, heat and pain*).

Site Areas subjected to trauma are more susceptible. The hands are common sites for subcutaneous infection (see Chapter 7).

Injections are usually given into the buttock or thigh, so these are also common sites for abscesses.

Self-administered injections by intravenous drug users are usually given into the veins in the cubital fossa and groin.

Shape and size Initially induration is seen. As the pus forms, this patch turns into a definite mass that is usually spherical. The mass may become large, and lose its spherical shape if the pus begins to spread through the subcutaneous tissues.

Surface The inner surface of an abscess is a layer of granulation tissue that is inseparable from the indurated inflamed tissues around it. Thus, an abscess does not have a definable outer surface, even though its contents may be easy to feel.

Colour *The overlying skin is red.*

Temperature The skin over an abscess is *hot*.

Tenderness Abscesses become increasingly tender as the tension in the pocket of pus increases.

Edge The edge is not palpable, as the induration and oedema gradually merge into the normal tissues.

Composition In the early stages, an abscess feels hard and solid. As the pus forms, the centre of the area becomes soft and, if it is not too tender to press, *fluctuant*.

Relations The skin over a subcutaneous abscess is invariably involved in the inflammatory process, so it is red, oedematous and fixed to the underlying mass.

The skin becomes white and then black as it dies and sloughs away if the pus points towards the skin. When the dead skin separates, the pus can escape from the abscess. Deep fixation depends upon the size and direction of spread of the abscess.

Lymph glands Draining glands may be enlarged, tender and may even suppurate.

Local tissues The local tissues should be normal, apart from those close to the abscess that are involved in the inflammation. There may be scars from previous abscesses.

General examination A large abscess can cause considerable systemic disturbance. The patient looks pale and ill, but *may be sweating and having rigors* and episodes of flushing. The temperature and pulse are elevated.

Carbuncle

A carbuncle is a spreading necrotizing infection in the subcutaneous tissues, with pus and slough formation, similar to the changes that occur in a boil, but with *many points of discharge* through holes in the skin that appear when patches of necrotic skin slough. The subcutaneous tissue necrosis is much more extensive than the reddened area of overlying skin (Figure 4.25).

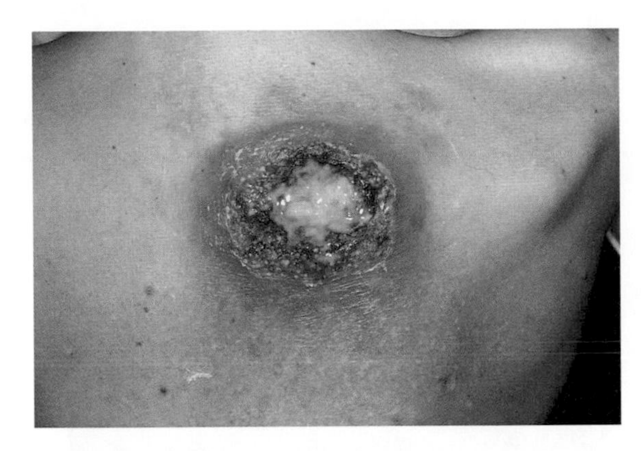

Figure 4.25 A carbuncle.

Sinuses and fistulas

Sinus

A sinus is a tract lined by granulation tissue that connects a cavity (usually an old abscess) with an epithelial surface, for example the skin (Figure 4.26).

A sinus produces a serous or purulent discharge and fails to close if it has one of the reasons outlined in Revision panel 4.5:

- The cavity is inadequately drained.
- It is caused by a specific chronic infection (e.g. actinomycosis, tuberculosis, syphilis).
- A foreign body (e.g. stitch material) is present at the bottom of the sinus.
- The cavity has epithelialized.
- The cavity has undergone malignant change.
- The surrounding tissues have poor vascularity or have been *irradiated*.

Sinuses commonly follow surgical wound infections and necrosis of tumours (Revision panel 4.5)

Revision panel 4.5

CAUSES OF A CHRONIC ABSCESS OR PERSISTENT SINUS

Inadequate drainage
Specific chronic infection, e.g. tuberculosis
Foreign body, or base e.g. a stitch
Epithelialization of the cavity
Malignant change in the wall of the cavity
Arises in irradiated or ischaemic tissues

Fistula

A fistula is a pathological connection between two epithelial surfaces (Figure 4.27), for example bowel and the skin, the bowel and another loop of bowel, or the bowel and the bladder.

Fistulas are usually lined with granulation tissue, but the tract can become epithelialized.

They form when a chronic abscess bursts in two directions, connecting two epithelial surfaces. They persist if they have to transmit the contents of one of

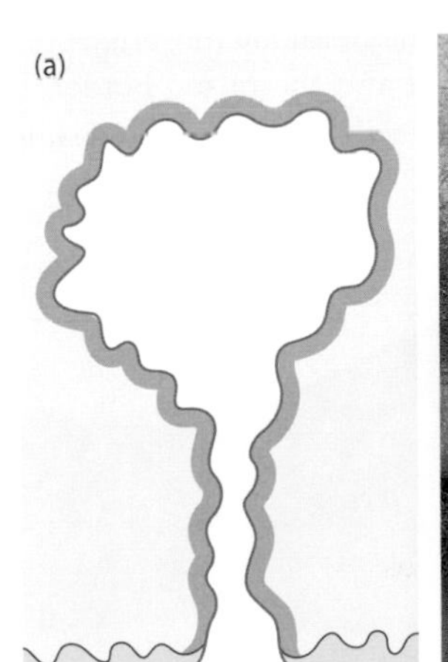

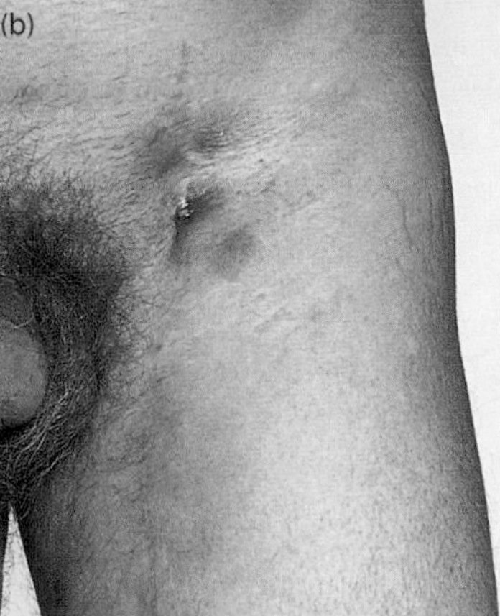

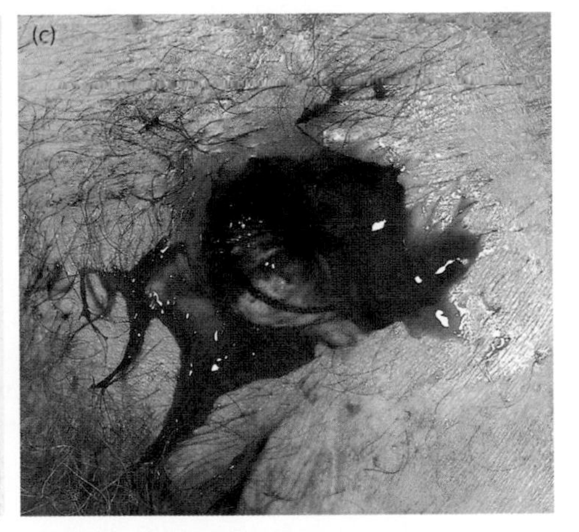

Figure 4.26 SINUS. (a) A sinus is a connection between a cavity lined with granulation tissue and an epithelial surface. (b) A discharging sinus from the centre of a groin wound. (c) The same wound 3 weeks later. The sinus has opened widely to reveal its cause – an infected Dacron arterial graft.

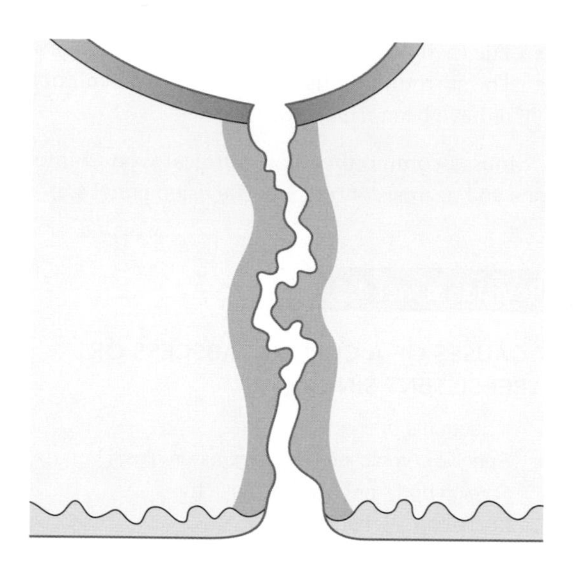

Figure 4.27 A fistula is a connection between two epithelium-lined surfaces.

the epithelium-lined cavities to the other if the former's normal outflow is obstructed.

They do not resolve until the cause of the abscess has been eradicated (see above for the factors that delay abscess closure) or the obstruction to the emptying of the viscus has been removed.

The common fistulas seen in surgical practice are between the anal canal and the perianal skin and the bowel (see Chapter 16).

Hidradenitis suppurativa

Whereas boils are infections in the hair follicles, *hidradenitis is an infection of the apocrine sweat glands.* It is most often seen in the axillae and groins. White individuals living in tropical countries are especially prone.

Patients present with multiple tender swellings in the axillae or groins (Figure 4.28), which enlarge and then discharge pus. The condition is made worse if there is an underlying systemic disease, such as diabetes. The site and the chronic recurring nature of this condition make it unpleasant and disabling.

Erysipelas and cellulitis

Erysipelas is an infection in the skin and subcutaneous tissues caused by a pathogenic *Streptococcus.*

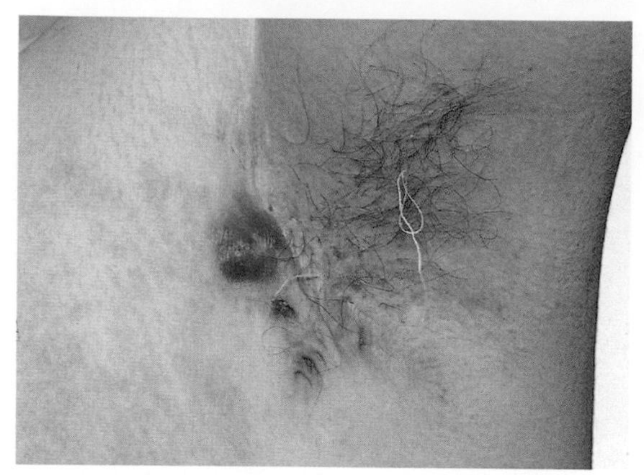

Figure 4.28 Hidradenitis suppurativa. Infected and inflamed apocrine glands.

Whereas *Staphylococcus* commonly causes a localized infection and pus formation, *Streptococcus* spreads easily through the skin and *produces a diffuse cellulitis.* The erythrotoxins produced by *Streptococcus* make the infected area red, hot, tender and oedematous (Figure 4.29). *Oedema of the reddened skin gives the involved area a raised border – a diagnostic clinical appearance.* The patient has a high temperature, tachycardia and general debility. Streptococcal infections rarely form thick pus.

Careful examination may reveal a source of entry for the organism, such as a small cut or a scratch. Erysipelas is especially common when there is pre-existing oedema caused by venous or lymphatic insufficiency.

Infection of the skin and subcutaneous tissues caused by other organisms, without the bright red discolouration of the skin and the raised border, is called *cellulitis.* A patch of cellulitis may necrose and suppurate.

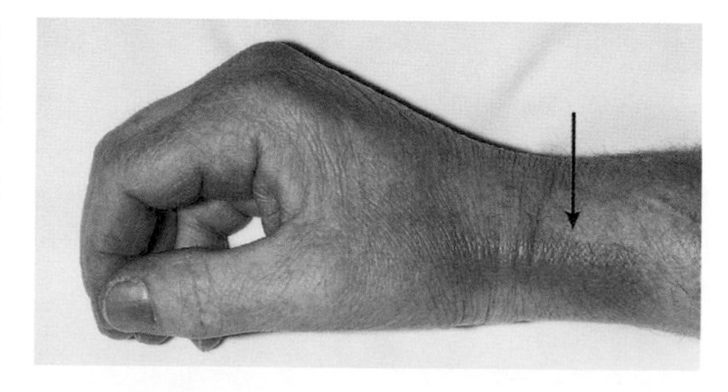

Figure 4.29 Erysipelas.

Erysipeloid

This is a gram-positive coccal infection that is present in *shellfish, meat and poultry*. It commonly affects fishermen, fishmongers and butchers. It occurs in the hands, usually as a purple–red papule with a well-defined edge, and may spread to other fingers.

Anthrax

This is a spore-forming, highly resistant bacterium that is found in animal carriers and is present in wood, hide and bones. It causes *a black, malignant-looking sore on the skin* (Figure 4.30), and patients may die rapidly from pulmonary complications.

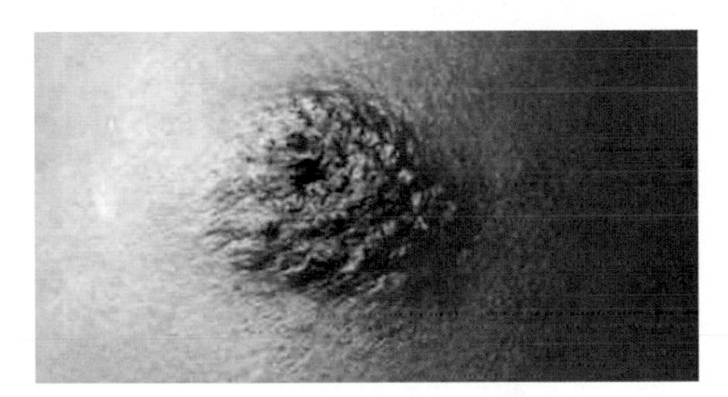

Figure 4.30 An anthrax pustule.

Tuberculosis

Tuberculosis of the skin is a rarity. Primary tuberculosis of the skin produces a persistent ulcer with undermined edges. This is more commonly seen now in an unhealed BCG vaccination site. The associated lymph glands are enlarged and may suppurate.

Lupus vulgaris

This is the well-recognized cutaneous form of tuberculosis that often affects the head and neck of children. The skin is red, telangiectatic and scaly. When it is compressed with a glass slide, it appears to be composed of pale yellow-brownish nodules (apple jelly) (Figure 4.31). It is slowly progressive and causes massive scarring.

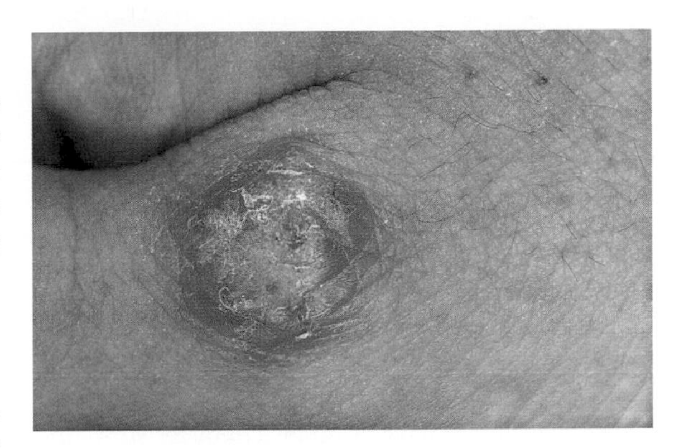

Figure 4.31 Lupus vulgaris: an apple jelly appearance.

Syphilis

Syphilis is rare in the UK, although its incidence has increased slightly in recent years.

The primary sore (chancre) This is acquired by sexual intercourse, biting or kissing, and develops between 3 and 6 weeks after inoculation. *The common sites for chancres are the penis and the vulva,* but they can occur on the *cervix, lips, fingers, nipple or anus*. A chancre is usually a 1 cm or less solid papular ulcer, with an indurated base that can be lifted up like a button in the skin (Figure 4.32). Approximately 1 week after its appearance, one or more of the regional lymph glands become enlarged. Affected glands are not painful and feel rubbery. They are called bubos.

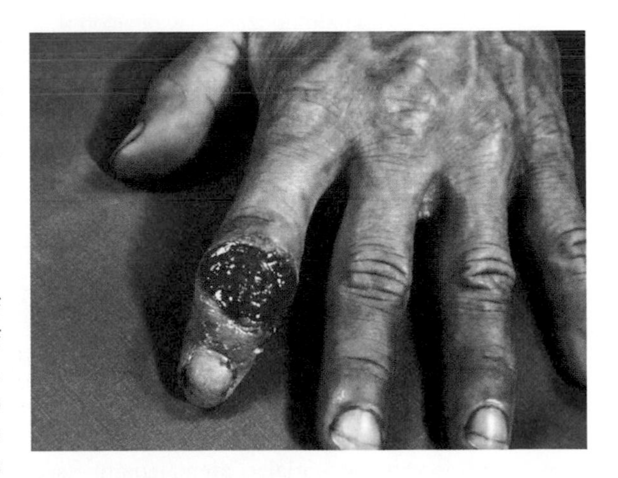

Figure 4.32 A syphilitic chancre.

The secondary stage This develops 5–6 weeks later if the primary condition is not treated. This is the result of organisms disseminating through the bloodstream. *A widespread polymorphic rash develops* that is not itchy and consists of macules, papules and scaly lesions. Patients often complain of associated malaise, headaches and limb pains.

At first, *the macules are pink or copper coloured and oval in shape, with an ill-defined edge. They are widely distributed on the trunk, limbs, palms of the hands and soles of the feet.*

The papules have similar characteristics and become florid and scaly, appearing in groups, often with an annular pattern, which makes them look almost like psoriasis. This is associated with a *generalized lymphadenopathy.*

Enlargement of the epitrochlear lymph glands is said to be characteristic.

Superficial erosions may then develop in the buccal mucosa, appearing as tender, red patches. When these are covered by adherent mucus, they are likened to snail tracks. It is, therefore, always important to *look in the mouth, and fold back the lips.*

Flat, moist plaques that are purple in colour may appear in the perianal and vulval skin, at the angle of the mouth, and in any of the skin flexures (e.g. armpits and groins). These are called condylomata lata.

A patchy loss of hair often occurs that gives patients a 'moth-eaten' appearance.

Tertiary syphilis This begins 2–10 years after the initial infection.

Serpiginous or arcuate nodules may develop that are either scaly or ulcerated. These leave central scars that may be mistaken for lupus vulgaris (see above), although the latter is usually much more chronic in its development.

Gummas can also develop at this stage. They start as a small nodule in the subcutis, but then enlarge and become red before ulcerating. *The ulcer associated with a gumma is discrete, punched out (see above) and characteristically has a wash-leather slough in its base* (Figure 4.33).

Leukoplakia of the mouth and tongue This is another manifestation of the tertiary stage of syphilis. The epithelium appears thickened and white. This condition is potentially premalignant (see Chapter 11).

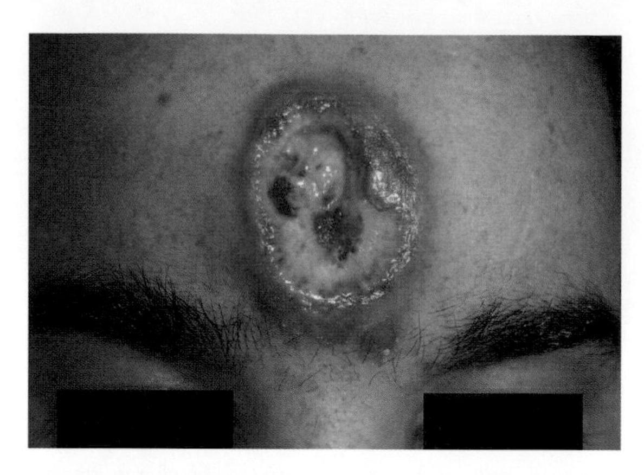

Figure 4.33 A gumma.

Aortic aneurysms (see Chapter 10) and tabes dorsalis are other important complications of the tertiary stage. Tabes is the result of damage to the posterior spinal columns causing loss of deep pain and proprioception, resulting in a 'stamping gait' (see Chapter 3).

The quaternary or final stage Untreated, syphilis can progress to involve the cardiovascular (aortitis, aneurysms, narrowing of the aorta) and neurological systems (neurosyphilis with general paresis, meningovascular syphilis and/or tabes dorsalis). Fortunately, this is now rare today with antibiotic therapy.

Congenital syphilis

This is almost extinct in the home-born population of the UK because of routine serological screening in pregnancy. Affected children develop a bullous eruption on their palms and soles a few days after birth. The liver enlarges, and the affected neonate develops 'snuffles' from severe nasal discharge that obstructs the breathing. The bridge of the nose eventually 'caves in'. The long bones develop osteochondritis and periostitis, causing deformity.

Diagnosis

The diagnosis of primary syphilis is usually made by scarifying the chancre, transferring the resultant discharge onto a microscope slide and examining it with dark-ground illumination for the *presence of spirochaetes.* A number of serological tests are useful for detecting active or prior infection.

Leprosy (Hansen's disease)

This may appear in any part of the world because of the ease of air travel and shifts of large populations to seek asylum. It must always be considered in a patient from a tropical country presenting with an *unusual rash*. It is spread by prolonged contact.

The 'tuberculoid' form is most commonly seen in the UK. *The skin usually contains sharply defined asymmetrical areas of hypopigmentation with dry, scaly surfaces.* Alternatively, there may be infiltrated, raised, hyperpigmented plaques with sharply demarcated erythematous edges. These may resemble vitiligo, but differ in that some pigment remains. These plaques or patches are insensate.

The ulnar, peroneal and greater auricular nerves are commonly thickened and easily palpable. *Foot drop and ulnar palsy are common.* Eventually, the insensate fingers are damaged by repeated trauma/infection and may result in shortening via auto-amputation (Figure 4.34).

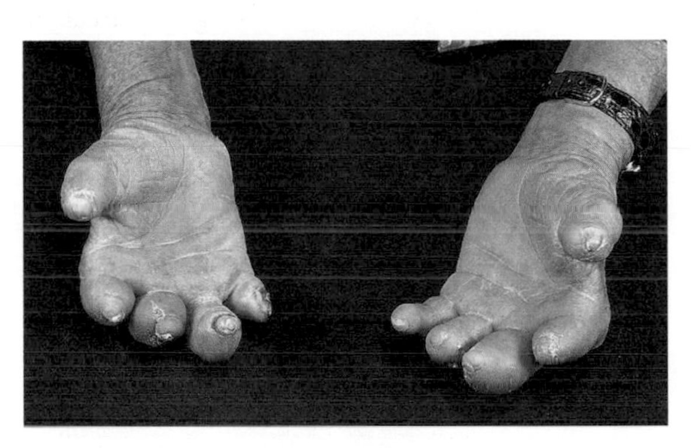

Figure 4.34 Leprosy of the hands.

Patients with lepromatous leprosy have no resistance to the spread of organisms. The early skin lesions are small, ill defined, erythematous macules that have a smooth and shiny surface. These become infiltrated to form plaques and nodules, especially in the face and pinnae. The polyneuritis described above is a late manifestation of this form of disease.

Diagnosis

The diagnosis is made by biopsy and nasal scrapings, when the microbacteria may be seen within the granulomas, consisting of epithelioid cells surrounding histiocytes and lymphocytes. Serological tests are also available.

VIRAL INFECTIONS

Viral warts

Papilliferous patches of overgrown hyperkeratotic skin whose growth has been stimulated by the *human papilloma virus*.

History

Age Any age, but are most common in children, adolescents and young adults.

Duration They grow to their full size in a few weeks, but may be present for months or years before a patient complains about them. Patients may be unconcerned.

Symptoms Warts are disfiguring. Multiple warts on the fingers can interfere with fine movements. They are painful only if they are rubbed or become infected.

Progression Once present, they may persist unchanged for many years, or regress and disappear spontaneously. 'Kiss lesions' may appear on adjacent areas of skin that make frequent contact. Warts occur in crops and may come and go spontaneously.

Family history They may occur in other members of the family.

Examination

Site *Commonly found on the hands*, but may appear on other exposed areas that are frequently touched by the hands, such as the face, arms and knees.

Shape and size They arise *as flat-topped, angular, smooth or hemispherical macules that are less than 1 cm in diameter* (Figure 4.35).

Surface Their surface is rough and hyperkeratotic, and often covered with fine filiform excrescences.

Colour Warts are *greyish-brown*.

Composition Firm and non-compressible.

Lymph glands The regional lymph glands are not enlarged.

Differential diagnosis Squamous papilloma, molluscum contagiosum and condylomata lata are other conditions that may be considered in the differential diagnosis.

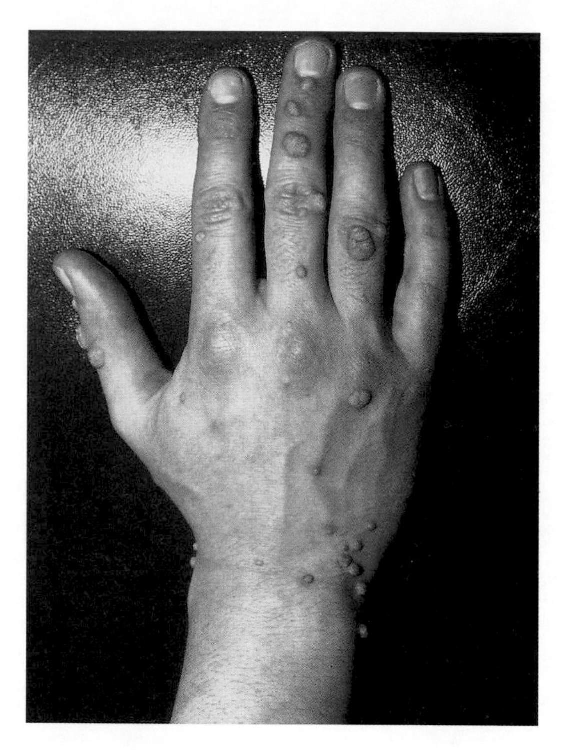

Figure 4.35 Viral warts.

Plantar warts

Warts on the soles of the feet (verrucas) appear as flat tender plaques that are fundamentally the same as any other wart, but they have a different appearance because they are pushed into the skin (Figure 4.36). They must be differentiated from *callosities and corns* (see Chapter 8).

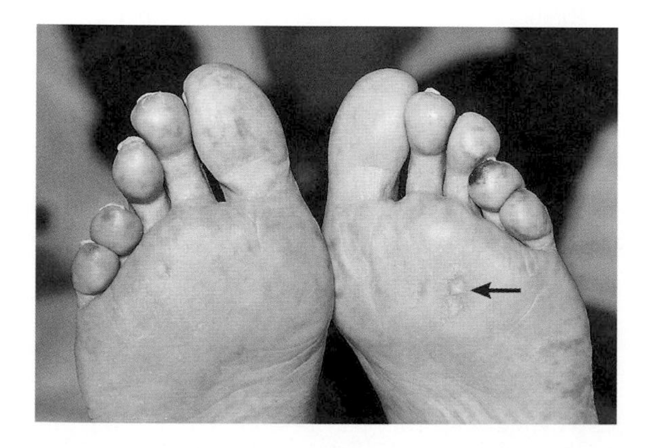

Figure 4.36 A plantar wart (verruca) (arrow).

Molluscum contagiosum

These are discrete, pearly, rounded nodules with umbilicated centres; when squeezed, they release a white exudate that contains virus. They are usually grouped in one area of the trunk.

Herpes simplex

This is the most common skin virus, with more than 60% of the population infected and remaining carriers throughout their lives. The primary infection often passes unnoticed, but it may cause a *severe gingivo-stomatitis with fever and local lymphadenopathy*. The mouth often contains a crop of 'aphthous' ulcers (see Chapter 11). Vesicles may be present over the face, the neck and even the eyes. The attack subsides in 10–14 days, but the virus remains latent in the epithelial cells of the buccal and nasal mucosa. The micro-organisms may proliferate again in response to a noxious stimulus such as a fever, sunlight, pneumonia or immune suppression.

History

Patients usually complain of a painful localized sore on their lip, which develops blisters that discharge and then crust over.

Examination

Site *Most lesions occur at the mucocutaneous junctions, particularly on the lips and angle of the mouth*, but they may appear on the nail clefts, trunk, genitalia, cheeks and natal cleft.

Shape and size A burning, uncomfortable papule develops that is usually oval or elliptical. It is slightly raised and very tender.

Surface The papular surface is smooth at first, but becomes covered in a crop of small vesicles (Figure 4.37) that break to leave a crust. This heals in 7–10 days, and the skin returns to normal.

Lymph glands The lymph nodes are rarely enlarged.

Herpes zoster

This skin rash is thought to be caused by *reactivation of the chickenpox virus*, which can lie dormant for many years in the anterior horn cells of the spinal cord.

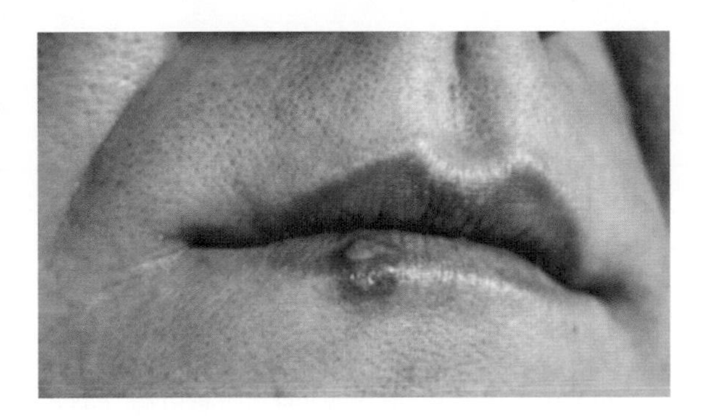

Figure 4.37 Herpes simplex.

History

Age It usually occurs after the age of 45 years.

Onset It can develop within a week of re-exposure to the varicella virus. Reactivation can be the result of tuberculosis or tumour.

Symptoms Pain occurs over the distribution of the nerve roots involved *before the rash develops*.

Examination

Site The rash can occur in any cutaneous dermatome(s). It appears in a continuous line, or as patches throughout these segments (Figure 4.38). The trigeminal nerve may be involved, and if the virus enters the ophthalmic branch, the eye will be affected.

Rash Initially, there is a *raised patch of erythema*, which rapidly becomes covered with a cluster of umbilicated vesicles. These quickly become infected and haemorrhagic before necrotic crusts form. There may be severe photophobia, with a red, watering eye if the ophthalmic division of the trigeminal nerve is involved.

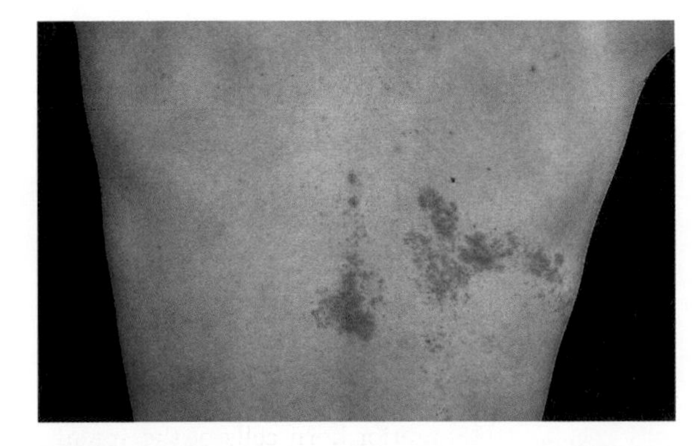

Figure 4.38 Herpes zoster in the T12 dermatome.

Resolution The pain improves as the rash clears (usually after 10 days). Sometimes severe cutaneous necrosis can leave disfiguring scars and there may be persisting pain.

NOTE: Do not forget that herpes zoster may be the cause of severe abdominal pain before the rash develops and the diagnosis is clear (see Chapter 15).

FUNGAL INFECTIONS

Candida (moniliasis)

This is a normal component of the body's flora and is present in the skin, mouth, vagina and gut of us all. *Clinical problems only develop when there is a reduction in the normal defence mechanism that leads to infection*. It may present in a number of different ways.

Oral candida

The buccal mucosa and tongue of infants or adults on prolonged courses of antibiotics may become covered in white spots or plaques (see Chapter 11).

Flexural intertrigo

Scattered soft macules may appear in the skin flexures, especially in the submammary areas and axillae of obese females. Patients with these problems should be checked for coexisting diabetes.

Balanitis

Monilial balanitis can be a problem in uncircumcised males (see Chapter 18).

Chronic paronychia

Prolonged water immersion (as seen in some professions such as nursing, bar staff) causes the nail fold to separate from the nail plate, which allows the fungus to gain access.

Established infection causes a painful red swelling at the base of the nail, which may become thickened, opaque and soft.

The differential diagnosis of a chronic fungal paronychia includes herpetic or bacterial paronychia, collagen diseases and Buerger's disease (see Chapter 10).

Tinea pedis (athlete's foot)

This is a common condition caused by one of three fungi. Damage to the protective barrier function of the skin caused by athlete's foot may predispose to the entry of bacteria that can cause cellulitis, especially in patients with chronic lymphoedema (see Chapter 10).

History

Age and sex *It is common in fit, young male athletes and swimmers,* who pick it up in showers and communal baths.

Symptoms *Patients usually complain of itching, maceration and fissure formation in the interdigital spaces of the toes, most often in the space between the fourth and fifth toes.* It often improves in winter and worsens in summer. The sole of the foot may itch and develop vesicles, and a rash may arise on the palms. Lymphangitis and cellulitis may complicate the condition (see page 130).

Examination

Site *Always* inspect between the toes.

Rash Maceration, odour and fissure formation with desquamation may be present (Figure 4.39). These may spread onto the dorsum of the foot. Asymmetry is characteristic. A vesicular eruption with bullae may be present on the soles of the feet and the palms of the hands. The nails may become distorted, white and soft.

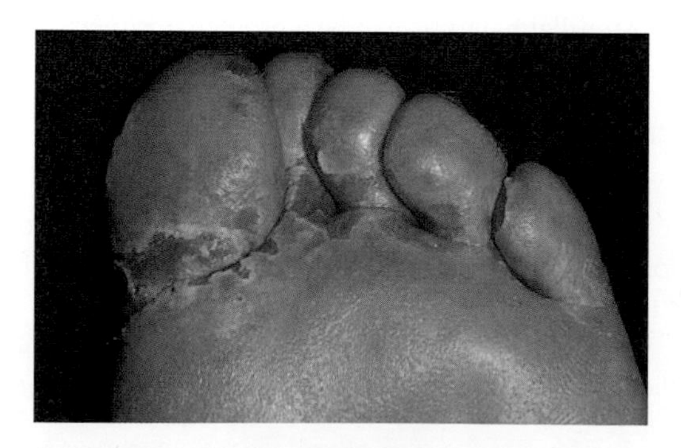

Figure 4.39 Tinea pedis.

The fungus may spread to the limbs and trunk, especially the groins, where annular lesions may develop.

INFESTATIONS

Scabies

This is the result of invasion of the epidermis by the *Acarus scabies* mite. The adult female is about 0.5 mm in length, and is only just visible to the naked eye. The male is half this size.

The fertilized female moves over the body until it finds a place to burrow through the horny layer (stratum corneum) of the skin. The female remains here for the rest of her life, laying two or three eggs per day for several weeks. These hatch in 3–4 days, and the larvae leave the burrow and enter the hair follicles to mature. The adult mites then escape onto the skin, where mating occurs. This cycle then begins again, roughly every fortnight.

History

An *erythematous rash develops around the burrows* 1 month after infestation. This is usually followed by a generalized urticarial reaction. The skin then begins to itch, especially at night. Other family members are often affected.

Examination

An *urticarial rash* is usually present, which in adults consists of wheals developing mostly on the trunk and limbs. *Vesiculation* may be present on the hands and limbs, which may become ecze matous or infected.

NOTE: Sixty per cent of burrows are on the hands and wrists, the remainder being on the soles of the feet, the genitalia, the axillae, the elbows and the buttocks.

Confirmation of diagnosis *The diagnosis is confirmed by finding burrows* (Figure 4.40). A magnifying lens, a good light and a sterile needle are required. The mite is visible at the anterior end of

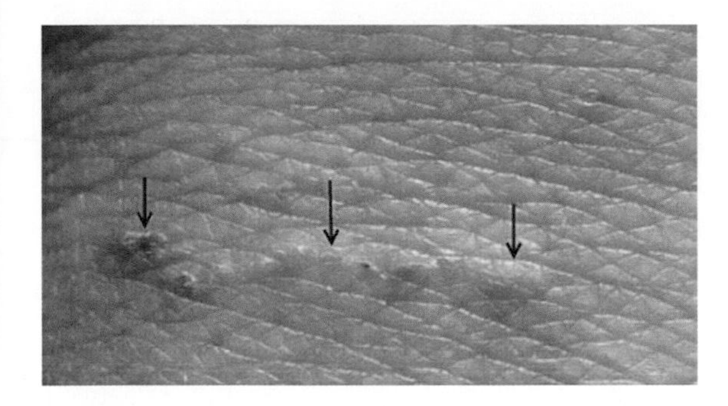

Figure 4.40 A scabies burrow.

the burrow as a white oval with a black dot at its front. The needle is inserted into the burrow, which is opened up, and the mite adheres to the tip of the needle. The mite is then put on a microscope slide and inked around, (Figure 4.41) and the diagnosis is confirmed.

The differential diagnosis includes other causes of generalized itching (see below).

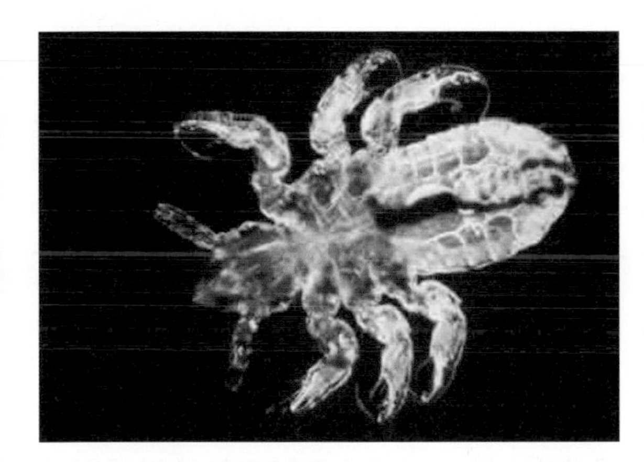

Figure 4.41 A scabies mite.

Pediculosis capitis

Infestation with head lice is common in schoolchildren. Severe infestation causes intolerable itching, and there is often secondary infection and enlarged cervical lymph glands.

Nits are present on the shafts of the hairs.

Pruritus

This is itching of the skin caused by a local or general abnormality. The presence of multiple skin scratches (excoriation) is usually obvious. The causes include:

- Skin diseases:
  - Urticaria.
  - Eczema.
- Local irritation:
  - Local allergy, e.g. washing powder.
  - Parasites (see above).
  - Discharge, e.g. rectal or vaginal.
- General disease:
  - Jaundice from accumulation of bile salts.
  - Hodgkin's disease.
  - Uraemia.
  - Thyrotoxicosis.
  - Iron deficiency or polycythaemia.
  - Diabetes.
  - HIV infection.
- Psychogenic causes.

Benign skin lumps

SEBORRHOEIC KERATOSIS (SENILE WART, SEBORRHOEIC WART, VERRUCA SENILIS, BASAL CELL PAPILLOMA)

This is a benign overgrowth of the basal layer of the epidermis containing excess small, dark-staining basal cells, which raise it above the level of the normal epidermis (Figure 4.42) and give it a semi-transparent, oily appearance.

History

Age Senile warts occur in both sexes but, as the name implies, they become more common with advancing years. *Most people over the age of 70 years have one.*

Duration They are slow growing, beginning as a minute patch that gradually increases in area. Patients have invariably had the lesion for months or years before complaining about it.

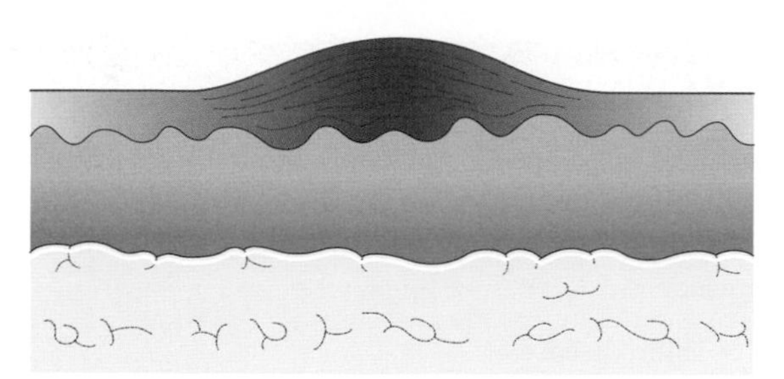

Figure 4.42 A seborrhoeic keratosis. The plaque consists of an excess number of basal cells and will peel off.

Symptoms As it gets bigger, it becomes disfiguring, and may start to catch on clothes. It seldom bleeds, but may get infected and it may itch. It sometimes contains sufficient melanin in the lesion to make the patient think it is a mole.

Progression Senile warts gradually increase in area, but not in thickness. They can suddenly fall off, uncovering a pale pink patch of skin.

Examination

Site They occur on any part of the skin except those areas subjected to regular abrasion, such as the palms of the hands and the soles of the feet. *The majority are found on the back of the trunk.*

Shape and size They form a raised plaque of hypertrophic, slightly greasy skin, with a square-cut and distinct edge. *They appear 'stuck on' and vary in size from a few millimetres to 2–3 cm in diameter* (Figure 4.43).

Surface They have a rough, sometimes papilliferous, surface.

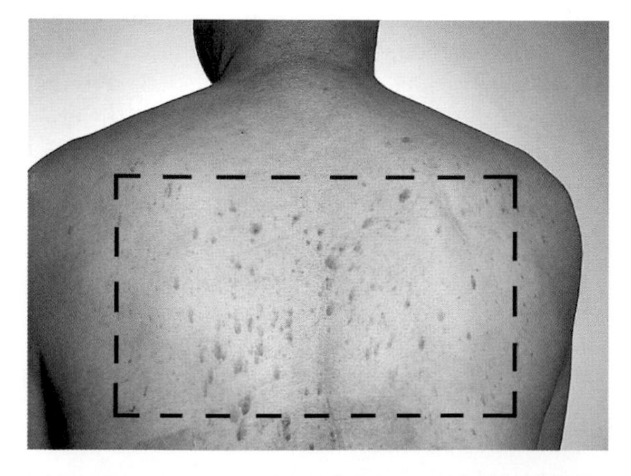

Figure 4.43 A patient whose back was covered with seborrhoeic keratoses.

Colour Their colour varies from pale yellow to dark brown, depending on the thickness of the epithelium and the quantity of melanin in the underlying skin (Figure 4.44).

Bleeding into a plaque after trauma makes the lesion swell and turn brown – changes that may be confused with malignant change in a melanoma.

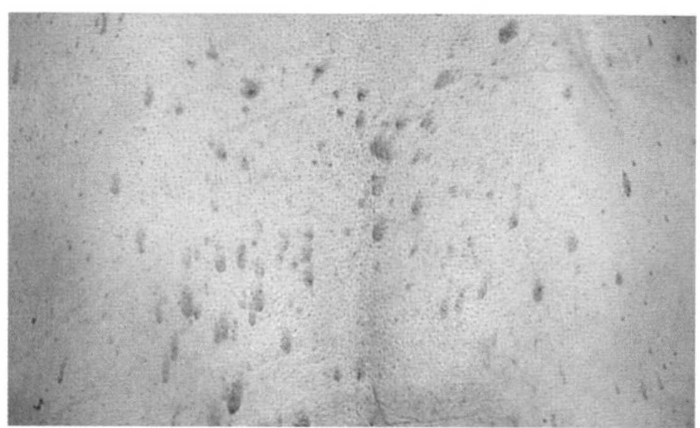

Figure 4.44 The area outlined in the Figure 4.43 is enlarged here.

An infected keratosis may become swollen and tender and be confused with a pyogenic granuloma or squamous cell carcinoma.

Consistency Seborrhoeic warts are a little harder and stiffer than normal skin. The surrounding tissues are healthy, but there are often other seborrhoeic warts nearby. They have a greasy, soapy feel.

Special diagnostic feature Because seborrhoeic keratoses are patches of thick squamous epithelium, they can be picked off. They feel *stuck on.* When a wart is peeled off, it leaves a patch of pale pink skin, and one or two fine surface capillaries that bleed slightly. No other skin lesion behaves like this.

> **NOTE:** Never pick hard at the edge of any skin lesion for fear of damaging it. Interfering in this way with a malignant tumour may hasten its local spread.

KERATOACANTHOMA (ADENOMA SEBACEUM, MOLLUSCUM PSEUDOCARCINOMATOSUM)

This is a self-limiting overgrowth of hair follicle cells, which spontaneously regresses. *It is often mistaken for a squamous cell carcinoma because it grows so rapidly.*

History

Rapidly growing lesions in adults, are often unsightly but not painful. *The lump takes 2–4 weeks to grow, and 2–3 months to regress. The cause is unknown.* It may be a self-limiting benign neoplasm or an unusual response to a viral infection.

Examination

Site Keratoacanthomas are often found as solitary lumps on the face (Figure 4.45), but can occur anywhere where there are sebaceous glands.

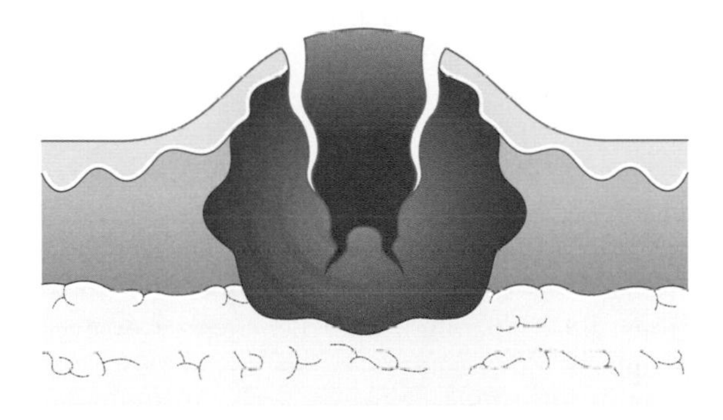

Figure 4.45 A keratoacanthoma is an overgrowth of hair follicle cells that produce a central plug of keratin. When the plug separates, the lesion usually undergoes spontaneous regression.

Shape and size The lump is hemispherical or conical, and looks like a volcano when the central slough appears and the surrounding skin retracts (Figure 4.46). *The nodule is usually 1–2 cm in diameter by the time the centre of the lump begins to necrose.*

Consistency The bulk of the lesion is firm and rubbery, but the central core is hard.

Colour The lump has a normal skin colour, but the necrotic centre is brown or black (Figure 4.47).

Relations The lump is confined to the skin, and is freely mobile over the subcutaneous tissues.

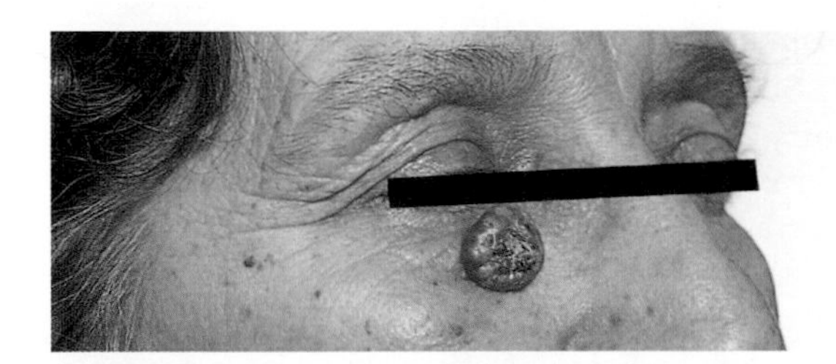

Figure 4.46 A large keratoacanthoma on the face.

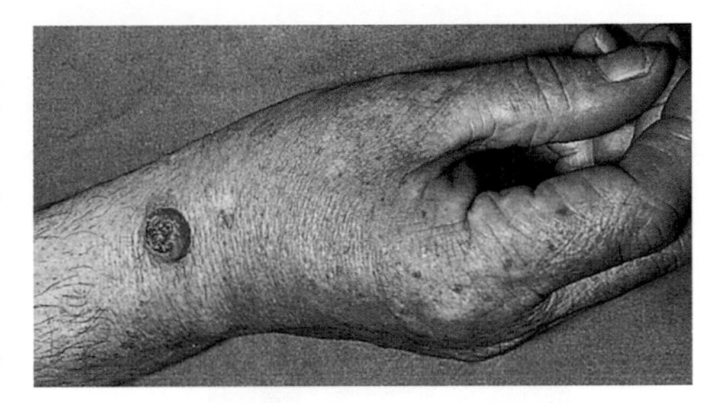

Figure 4.47 A keratoacanthoma on the wrist. The slough is just beginning to separate.

Lymph glands The local lymph glands should not be enlarged.

Natural history The central core eventually separates and the lump collapses, leaving a deep indrawn scar.

Differential diagnosis *A keratoacanthoma must be differentiated from a squamous cell carcinoma.* The latter grows more slowly, and eventually becomes an ulcer. Due to diagnostic uncertainty Keratocanthomas are often excised for pathological examination because of diagnostic uncertainty.

HISTIOCYTOMA (DERMATOFIBROMA, SCLEROSING ANGIOMA)

This is a benign neoplasm of the fibroblasts of the dermis. Its name is derived from the many histiocytes that are present between the fibroblasts. The overlying epidermis is normal. It has also been suggested that it may be a haemangioma with a marked desmoplastic response.

History

Age Lesions appear on the skin of young and middle-aged adults.

Sex Both sexes are equally affected.

Symptoms The patient complains of a slow-growing lump on the skin.

Examination

Site They can occur anywhere, but are slightly more common on the skin of the limbs.

Shape As they grow, they form a hemispherical lump, which then flattens into a thick disc (Figure 4.48). The edges of the disc may overhang its base.

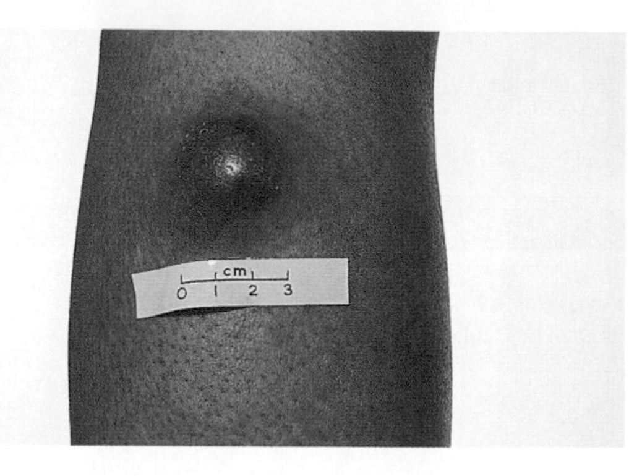

Figure 4.48 A large histiocytoma on the calf.

Size Most patients complain of these tumours when they are 1–2 cm across, but they can grow to a considerable size if they are neglected.

Surface and colour The overlying skin is inseparable from the lump. The epidermis is usually a normal colour but may contain haemosiderin, which gives it a brown appearance like a mole.

Tenderness Non-tender.

Composition These tumours usually have a rubbery or spongy consistency.

Relations They are in the skin.

Lymph drainage The local lymph glands should not be enlarged.

Local tissues Normal.

SEBACEOUS CYST

The skin is kept soft and oily by the sebum secreted by sebaceous glands. *When an opening of one of these glands becomes blocked, it distends with its own secretion, and ultimately becomes a sebaceous cyst.* These are more correctly called *pilar* or *trichilemmal cysts* when they develop in the scalp, as they arise from infundibular parts of hair follicles and have no function.

History

Age Any age particularly 20–40 years old, but rarely before adolescence.

Duration Sebaceous cysts are slow growing and have usually been present for some years before the patients may request removal.

Symptoms Sebaceous cysts *most frequently arise on the scalp,* and the most common complaint is of a lump that gets scratched when the patient is combing their hair. Such scratches may get infected, and when infection develops in a cyst, it enlarges rapidly and becomes acutely painful.

A slow discharge of sebum from a wide punctum sometimes hardens to form a *sebaceous horn.*

Infection of the cyst wall and the surrounding tissues produces a boggy, painful, discharging swelling known as *Cock's peculiar tumour.* This only happens if an infected cyst is neglected.

Development Sebaceous cysts usually enlarge with time, but the increase in size is accelerated if the cyst becomes infected. A cyst will sometimes discharge its contents through its *punctum* (sebaceous gland opening), and then regress or even disappear.

Multiplicity Sebaceous cysts are often multiple (Figure 4.49).

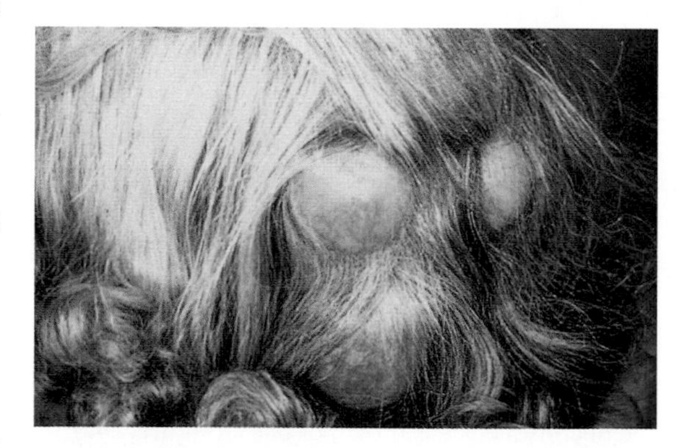

Figure 4.49 Three sebaceous cysts on the scalp. Note that you cannot see a punctum, a common finding.

Examination

Site Most sebaceous cysts are found in the hairy parts of the body. *The scalp, scrotum, neck, shoulders and back are the common sites,* but they can occur wherever there are sebaceous glands. There are no sebaceous glands on the palms of the hands and soles of the feet.

Shape and size Most sebaceous cysts are tense and spherical. Even on the scalp, where there is the unyielding skull beneath them, they remain spherical by bulging outwards and stretching the overlying skin (Figure 4.50). They can vary from a few millimetres to 4–5 cm in diameter, but most patients seek advice before they become very large.

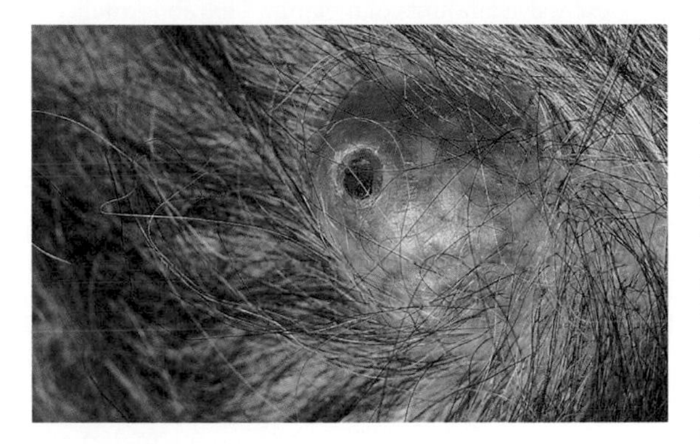

Figure 4.50 A punctum of a sebaceous cyst.

Surface The surface of a sebaceous cyst is smooth.

Edge Well defined and easy to feel, as it is usually lying in subcutaneous fat.

Colour The skin over the cyst is usually normal, although a *'punctum' or pit may be visible as a dark spot* (Figure 4.50).

Tenderness Uncomplicated sebaceous cysts are not tender. Pain and tenderness indicate infection.

Temperature Normal unless infection present.

Composition Most sebaceous cysts feel hard and solid. They are occasionally so tense that it is *not possible to elicit fluctuation,* especially if there is no firm underlying tissue to press them against. On the scalp, the resistance of the underlying skull aids detection of fluctuation.

They do not transilluminate because they are full of sebum.

Relations They arise from a skin structure but lie in the subcutaneous tissues, although they are attached to skin. Their point of discharge is usually along a hair follicle and, as the cyst grows, this point of fixation is often pulled inwards to become a *small punctum* (Figure 4.50). *Only one-half of the cysts that you will see have a visible punctum,* but when one is present it is a useful diagnostic sign. All sebaceous cysts are attached to the skin even if there is no punctum. The area of attachment may be quite small, but it prevents the cyst moving independently of the skin. Sebaceous cysts are not attached deeply.

Lymph glands The local lymph glands should not be enlarged.

A sebaceous horn

This arises from a sebaceous cyst when the contained sebum slowly exudes from a large central punctum before drying and hardening into a conical spike (Figure 4.51). The friction from clothes and washing normally removes the secretions of the gland as soon as they appear. *A sebaceous horn can therefore only grow if the patient fails to wash!*

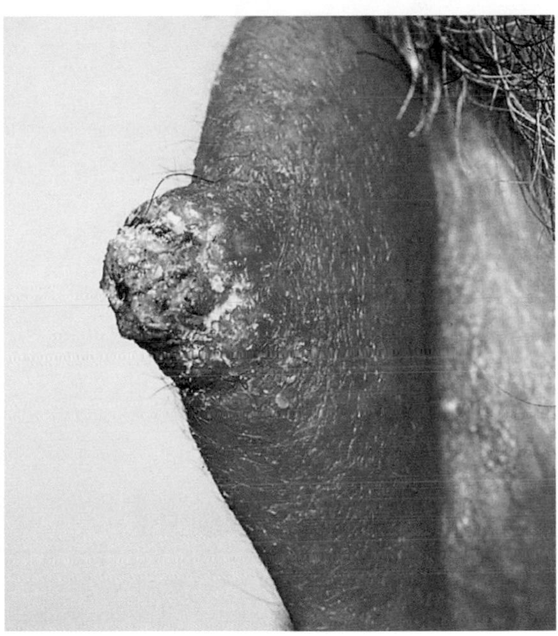

Figure 4.51 A sebaceous horn on the ear. The 'horn' is simply the hardened sebaceous material (epithelial cells and sebum) extruding from the cyst.

Cock's peculiar tumour

Cock's peculiar tumour is an *infected, open, granulating, oedematous sebaceous cyst.* It looks angry, sore and malignant, *and is often mistaken for a squamous cell carcinoma of the scalp.* Granulation tissue arising from the lining of the cyst heaps up and bursts onto the skin, giving the lesion an everted edge (Figure 4.52).

The infection in the cyst wall and surrounding tissues makes the whole area oedematous, red and tender. The regional lymph glands may be enlarged.

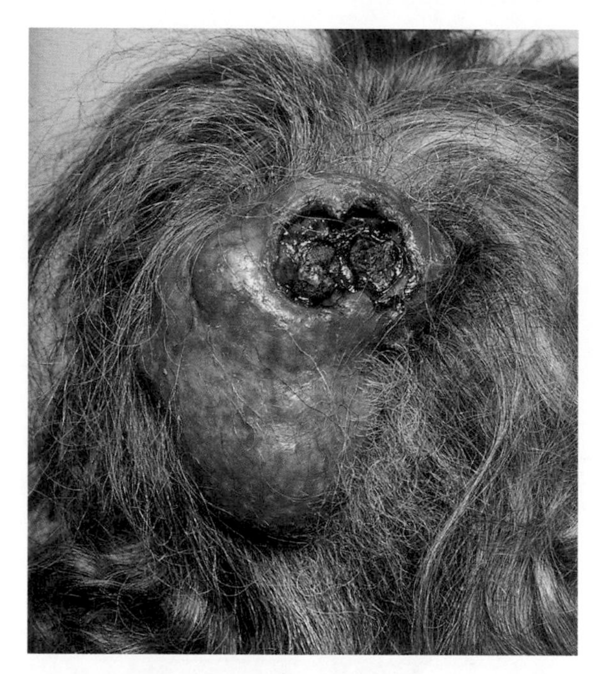

Figure 4.52 Cock's peculiar tumour. This is a mass of granulation tissue protruding from the base of a previously infected and ruptured sebaceous cyst.

PIGMENTED NAEVI (MOLES)

The word 'mole' is a lay term used to describe a brown spot or blemish on the skin. The brown pigment is melanin. There are three ways in which an excess of melanin may be produced to colour the skin brown (Figure 4.53):

- There may be a normal number of melanocytes, in their normal position, each producing excess melanin. This abnormality is called a *freckle* or *ephelis*. It is not called a mole because it does not contain an increased number of melanocytes.
- There may be an increased number of melanocytes, in their normal position, each producing normal amounts of melanin. This abnormality is called a lentigo.
- There may be an increased number of melanocytes, in abnormal clusters at the dermo-epidermal junction, producing normal or excessive amounts of melanin. This abnormality is called a *mole* or *pigmented naevus*.

A mole becomes a *malignant melanoma if the melanocytes invade adjacent tissues or show signs of abnormal and excessive multiplication.* It is called a *dysplastic naevus* if there are some nuclear abnormalities but no evidence of invasion.

The three benign pathological entities described above often have similar macroscopic features, and it is therefore safest to call all benign melanin-producing lesions moles or pigmented naevi, and to call all malignant melanin-producing tumours malignant melanomas.

Pathology

Whereas the clinical appearance of pigmented naevi is infinitely variable and almost unclassifiable, moles can be defined according to their microscopic appearance (Figure 4.53). Melanocytes are normally found in small numbers among the cells of the basal layer of the epidermis. They first cluster in this layer, and then migrate into the dermis if they proliferate.

The mature adult mole consists of clusters of melanocytes in the dermis, and is therefore called an *intradermal naevus. This can be flat or raised, smooth or warty, and hairy or non-hairy.* Most of the moles on the arms, face and trunk are of this variety, and they hardly ever turn malignant.

There will be clusters of cells at various stages of maturity in the epidermis and the dermis if the growth and movement of the melanocytes stop before they have all migrated into the dermis. This lesion is called a *compound cellular naevus.*

The naevus is called a *junctional naevus if the melanocytes remain close to the junction between the epidermis and dermis.* These naevi are immature and unstable, and can turn malignant. The majority of malignant melanomas begin in junctional moles. Many of the moles on the palms of the hands, the

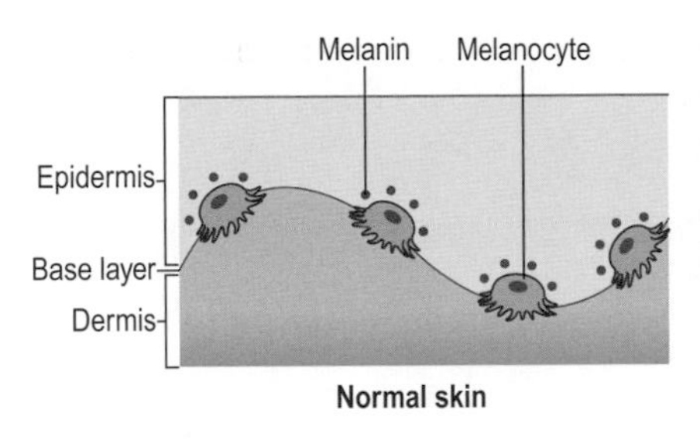

Normal skin

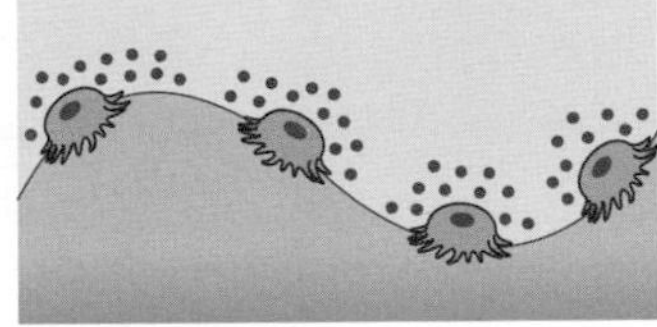

Freckle (ephelis)
Normal number of melanocytes, in normal position, producing excess melanin

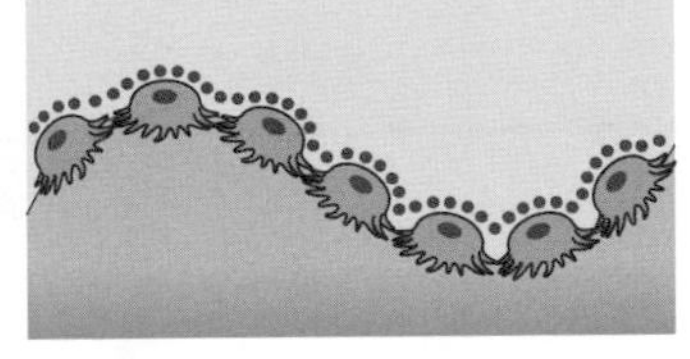

Lentigo
Excess melanocytes, each in normal position, producing normal amounts of melanin

Pigmented naevus/mole
Excess melanocytes, in clusters, variable but usually excess melanin production

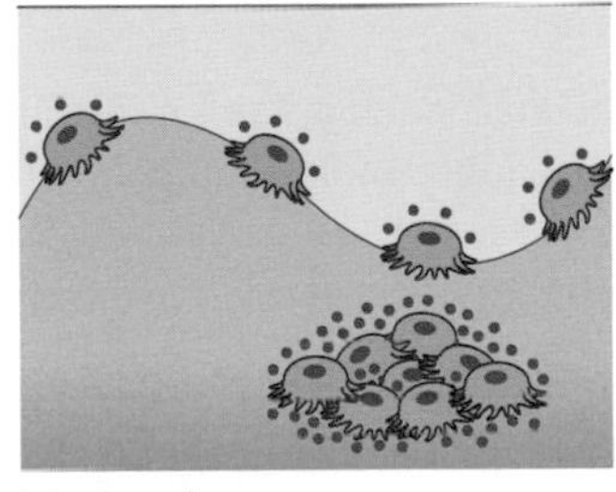

Intradermal naevus

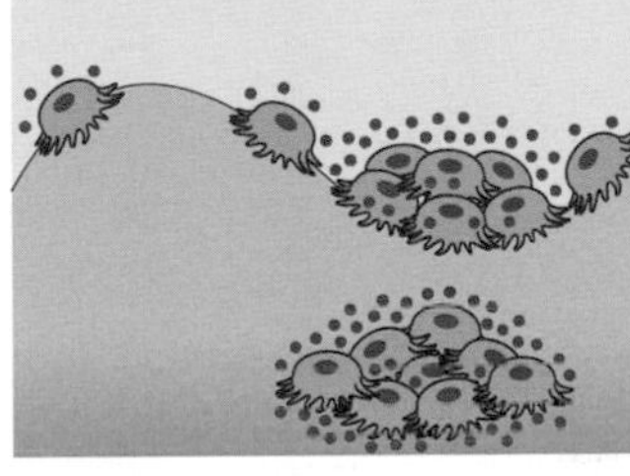

Compound naevus

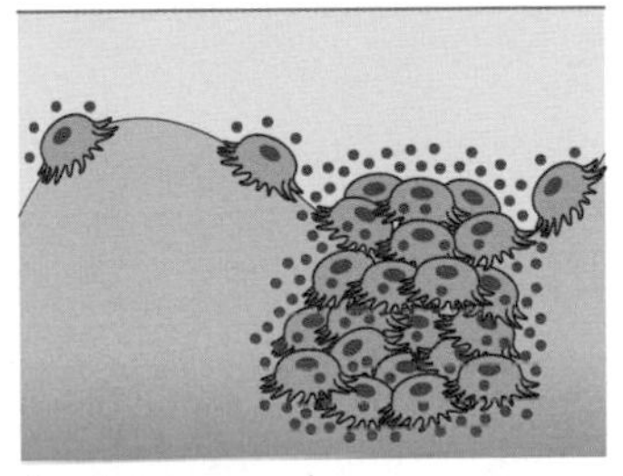

Junctional naevus

Figure 4.53 The histological varieties of pigmented spots and blemishes.

soles of the feet and the external genitalia are of the junctional variety.

Melanocytes that have never reached the epidermis, and therefore lie in the deep dermis or subcutaneous tissues, may still proliferate and produce excess melanin. The resulting lesion has a *blue appearance and is called a blue naevus.*

History

Age Everyone, except for albinos, has a few moles at birth, but the number increases during life. It has been estimated that most Caucasian individuals have *15–20 moles.* During childhood and adolescence, these may become more pigmented or completely regress. A mole on a child may be clinically and histologically difficult to distinguish from a malignant melanoma if it enlarges and becomes darker, but true malignant change is uncommon before puberty.

Ethnic group They are more common in Causcasians living in hot countries, such as Australia, because the skin is exposed to more ultraviolet light. Moles do occur in Afro-Caribbean individuals, particularly in the less pigmented areas such as the soles of feet and palms of the hands, but are rare.

Symptoms They rarely cause any serious symptoms, but may be disfiguring, protrude above the skin surface and catch on clothes. *Itching or bleeding suggests the possibility that malignant change has occurred* (see below).

Examination

Site Moles can occur on any part of the skin, but are most common on the limbs, face, neck and trunk.

Size Most are 1–3 mm in diameter.

Colour Their colour varies from light brown to black and does not fade with pressure. Amelanotic naevi do occur, but without their pigment they are unlikely to be recognized. Pigmented naevi may regress. A mole surrounded by a white halo of regression is known as a *halo naevus* (Figure 4.54).

Composition Moles usually have a soft consistency and are indistinguishable, by palpation, from the surrounding tissues.

Lymph glands The local lymph glands should not be enlarged.

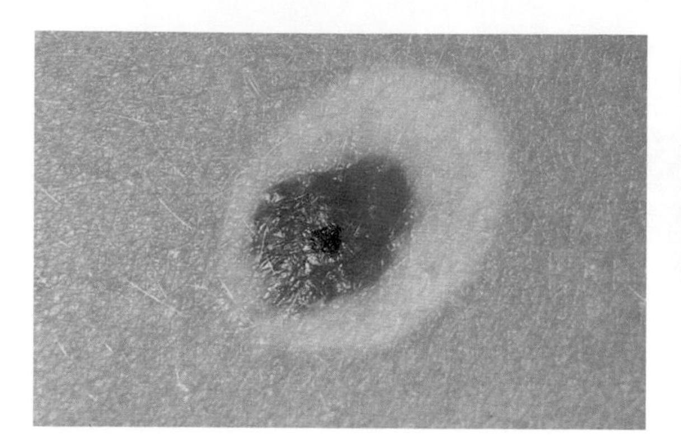

Figure 4.54 A 'halo' naevus. This mole is regressing. It has faded and the skin around it has become depigmented.

Shape and surface There are four clinical varieties of mole:

- *Hairy mole* is a common variety. It is flat, or very slightly raised above the level of the surrounding skin, with a smooth or slightly warty epidermal covering, and has hairs growing from its surface (Figure 4.55). The presence of hairs means that the mole also contains sebaceous glands that can become infected and cause changes such as swelling and tenderness, which may be indistinguishable from malignant change. Hairy moles are always intradermal naevi.
- *Non-hairy or smooth mole* is also a common variety. The epithelium is smooth and not elevated. The brown pigment looks as if it is deep in the skin (Figure 4.56) – deeper than that of the hairy mole – but this is just an optical illusion. Non-hairy moles may be intradermal, junctional or compound naevi.
- *Blue naevus* is a mole deep in the dermis. The thick overlying layers of dermis and epidermis mask the brown colour of the melanin and make it look blue (Figure 4.57). The overlying skin is often smooth and shiny. This is an uncommon type of mole, more often seen in children. It usually occurs on the face, the dorsum of the hands and feet, and the buttocks.
- *Lentigo* is an area of pigmentation that appears in late adult life and is prone to undergoing malignant change (Figure 4.58) (see below).

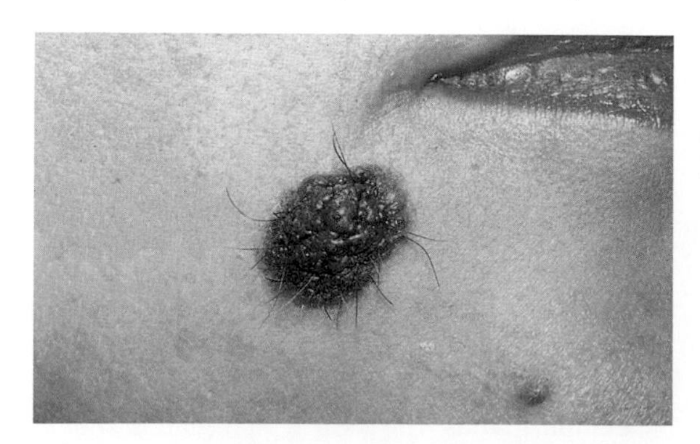

Figure 4.55 A hairy mole.

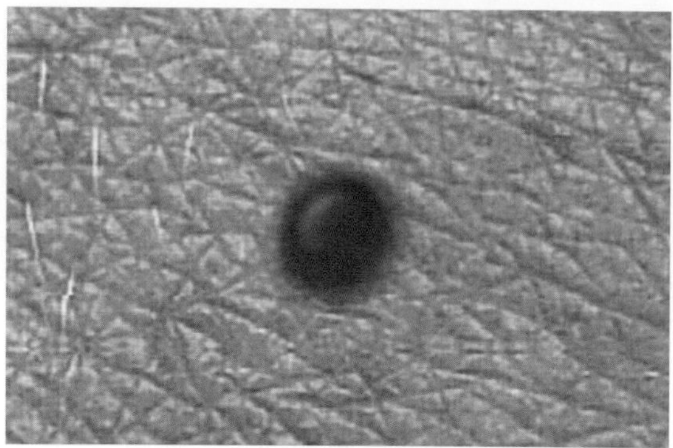

Figure 4.56 A smooth mole.

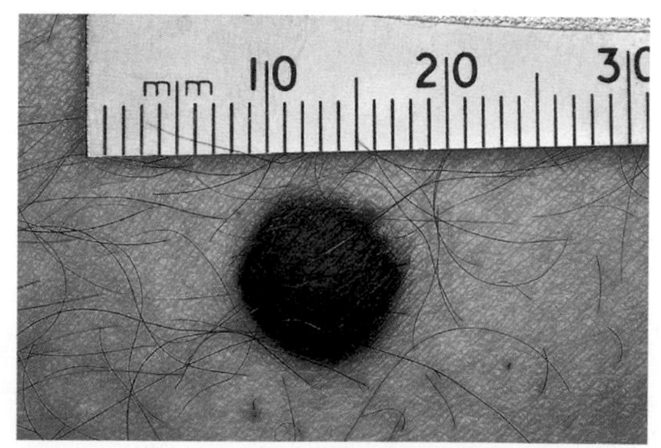

Figure 4.57 A blue mole.

There are two other varieties of melanotic skin pigmentation: the café-au-lait patch (see page 115) and the circumoral moles of the *Peutz–Jegher syndrome* (see Chapter 11).

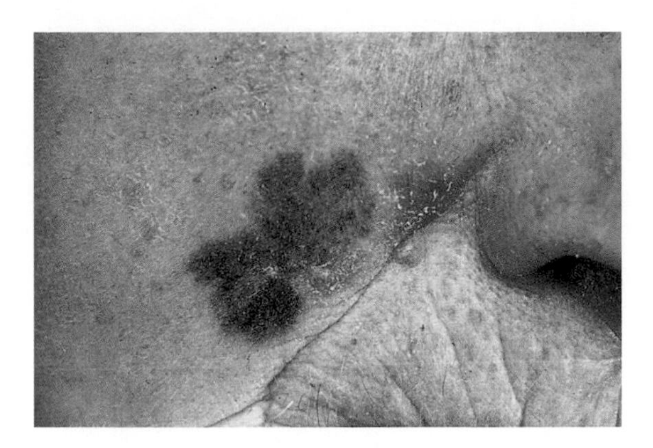

Figure 4.58 A Hutchinson's lentigo on the face.

Benign subcutaneous swellings

LIPOMA

This is a cluster of fat cells that have become overactive and so enlarged that they have become palpable lumps. *They are never malignant.*

Liposarcomas, which often develop in the retroperitoneal tissues (see Chapter 15), arise *de novo.*

History

Age All ages, but uncommon in children.

Duration They usually grow slowly for months or years before being noticed. They rarely regress.

Symptoms Most patients present because they have noticed a lump and want to know what it is. *The lump may be unsightly* or interfere with movement, especially if it becomes pedunculated or very large (Figure 4.59).

Multiplicity Patients often have many lipomas, or have had others excised in the past. Multiple contiguous lipomas cause enlargement and distortion of the subcutaneous tissues. This condition is called *lipomatosis*. It usually occurs in the buttocks and sometimes in the neck.

Multiple lipomatosis (Dercum's disease) is a condition in which the limbs and sometimes the trunk are covered with lipomas of all shapes and sizes. These can be painful and may contain angiomatous elements (angiolipomas).

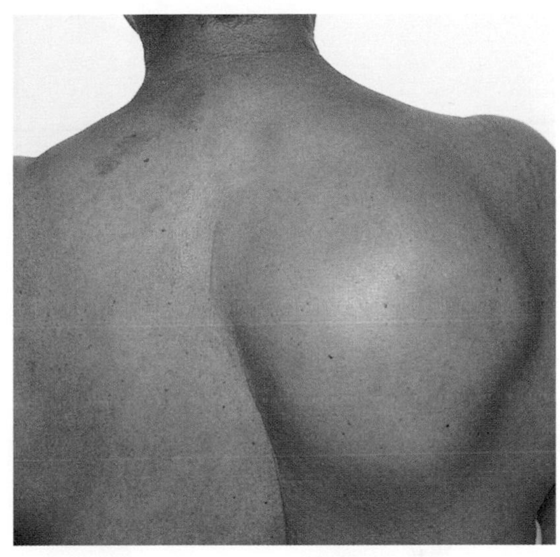

Figure 4.59 A large lipoma overlying the scapula.

Examination

Site They are most common in the subcutaneous tissues of the upper limbs, chest, neck and shoulders, but they can occur anywhere.

Colour The overlying skin is normal. Veins over the lipoma may be more visible.

Tenderness Lipomas are not usually tender, but angiolipomas are.

Temperature The temperature of the overlying skin is normal.

Shape and size They are usually spherical, but subcutaneous lipomas that develop between the skin and the deep fascia are usually discoid or hemispherical.

Most lipomas are lobulated, as fat in the body is in the form of lobules. The lobules can be seen and felt on the surface and at the edge of the lump (Figure 4.60). Lipomas come in all sizes.

Surface The surface feels smooth, but firm pressure reveals the depressions between the lobules, which become more prominent with firm palpation or gentle squeezing. This increases the pressure within the lipoma and makes each lobule bulge out between the fine strands of fibrous tissue that surround it (Figure 4.61).

Edge The edge is not circular but a series of irregular curves corresponding to each lobule. Because the edge is soft, compressible and sometimes quite

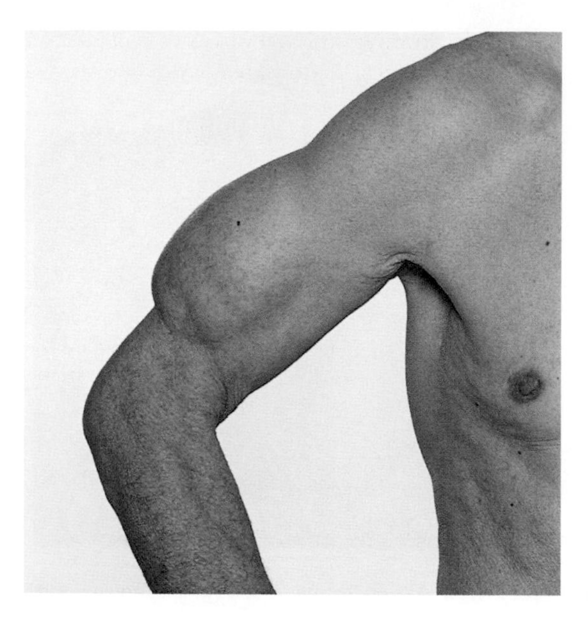

Figure 4.60 A lipoma in the subcutaneous tissues of the upper arm. Note the lobulation.

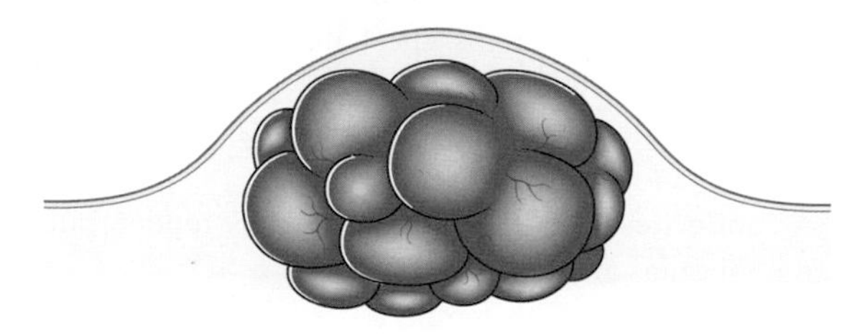

Figure 4.61 Lobulation.

thin, it slips away from the examining finger. This has been described as the 'slip sign'. It is not a very useful or diagnostic feature.

Evidence of lobulation on the surface and at the edge is the most significant physical sign.

Composition Most lipomas contain a soft but solid jelly-like fat when they are cut open immediately after removal.

Lipomas often give the impression of fluctuating, but careful examination reveals that they are just yielding to pressure, spreading out in all directions because they are soft. They do not become more tense and prominent in the plane at right angles to the palpating finger. The larger the lipoma, the more it appears to fluctuate, but fat at body temperature is solid, not liquid.

Lipomas do not transilluminate in that they do not pick up and transmit light from a torch shone beside them, but they may light up if light is shone directly across them. They do not have a fluid thrill, and they do not reduce or pulsate.

The physical signs of pseudo-fluctuation and transillumination make them appear cystic, a false impression that emphasizes the diagnostic importance of finding lobulation.

Relations Lipomas may arise within deep structures, such as muscles. These lipomas are fixed deeply, and may become more prominent if they are pushed out of the muscle (Figure 4.62), or disappear if they are drawn into the muscle when it contracts.

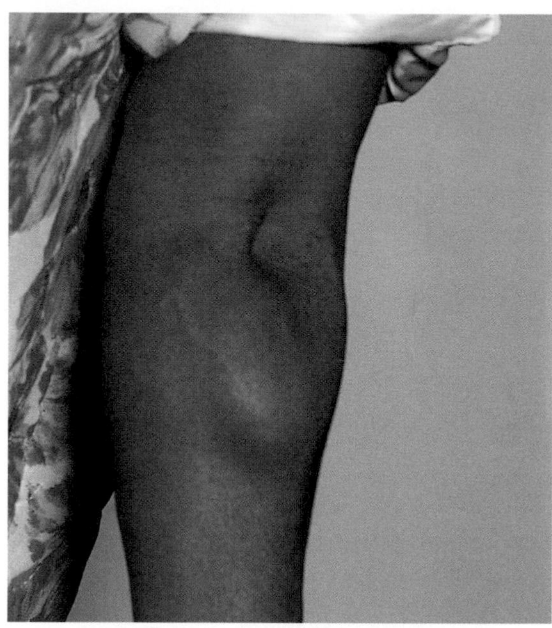

Figure 4.62 A lipoma in the forearm. This swelling became more prominent and fixed when the forearm muscles were contracted, showing that it was superficial to the muscle, but attached to its fascia.

Subcutaneous lipomas are not attached superficially or deeply, and can be moved in all directions.

Lymph glands The regional lymph glands are not enlarged.

Local tissues The surrounding tissues are normal, but other lipomas may be present.

GANGLION

A ganglion is a *myxomatous degeneration of fibrous tissue.* Ganglia can occur anywhere in the body, but they are common where there is a lot of fibrous tissue, i.e. around the joints.

History

Age The majority present between the ages of 20 and 70 years, and they are rare in children.

Duration They grow slowly over months or years.

Symptoms *They are not painful.* Most patients seek advice because they wish to know the diagnosis or because the lump is disfiguring. Some ganglia slip away between neighbouring bones, giving the false impression that they are reducing into the joint, but a true ganglion should not connect with or empty into a joint. Ganglia may rupture into the subcutaneous tissues and disappear.

Examination

Site Most ganglia are found near joint capsules and tendon sheaths, but they can occur anywhere. *Ninety per cent arise on the dorsal and ventral surfaces of the wrist joint and hand* (Figure 4.63).

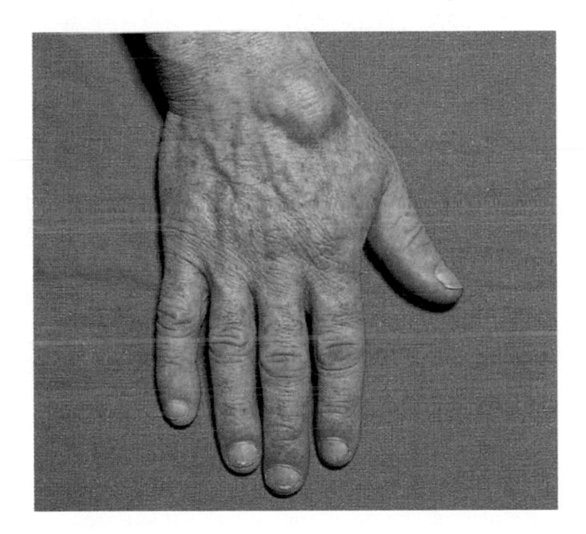

Figure 4.63 A soft multilocular ganglion on the back of the wrist.

Shape and size Ganglia are spherical. Some are multilocular and feel like a collection of cysts. They come in all sizes. Small ganglia (0.5–1.0 cm) tend to be *tense and spherical*. Large ones, which can be up to 5–6 cm across, are flattened and soft.

Surface They have a smooth surface.

Composition Ganglia feel solid, but their consistency varies from soft to hard. The gelatinous material within them is very viscous, *but most ganglia fluctuate*, provided they are not very small or very tense.

They usually transilluminate brilliantly (Figure 4.64).

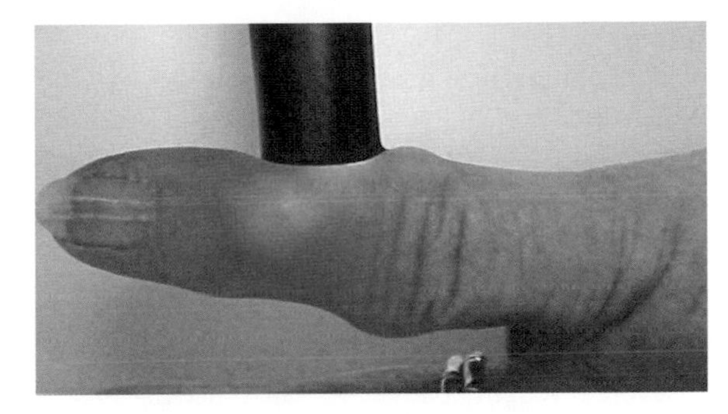

Figure 4.64 A ganglion transilluminating.

Reducibility A ganglion may slip away between deeper structures when pressed, giving the false impression that its contents have reduced into the joint.

Relations Ganglia are usually attached to the fibrous tissue from which they originate. They are not attached to the overlying skin, which should be freely mobile over them. The mobility of a ganglion depends on the extent and nature of its deep attachment. When the tissue of origin is part of a joint capsule, tendon sheath or intramuscular septum, the ganglion becomes less mobile when these structures are made tense. Therefore, remember to palpate ganglia in all positions of the underlying joint, and with the surrounding muscles relaxed and tense.

Differential diagnosis The three common swellings found close to joints are:

- Bursae.
- Cystic protrusions of the synovial cavity of arthritic joints.
- Ganglia.

The first two are usually soft; the ganglion is tense. The joint is normal bursae or ganglia.

SUBCUTANEOUS BURSAE

Bursae are fluid-filled cavities, lined with a flattened endothelium similar to synovium, that develop between tendons, bones and skin to allow tissues

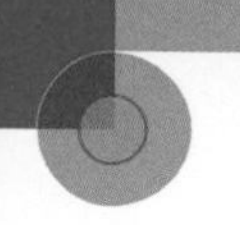

to slide easily. A considerable number of bursae are always present. Others called *adventitious bursae* develop wherever there is friction between two layers of tissue.

History

Age Bursae are uncommon in the young, and they usually appear in middle and later life as a result of prolonged friction between skin and bone, associated with the patient's occupation or with a deformity produced by injury or arthritis.

Symptoms *Pain and an enlarging swelling* at the site of repeated trauma are the common presenting symptoms, and may stop the patient working. A severe throbbing pain and a rapid increase in size indicates the presence of infection.

Development The swelling usually appears to develop rapidly, even though the bursa has probably been present for many years. The increase in fluid within the bursa is usually secondary to minor infection or trauma.

Multiplicity Bursae are often symmetrical, for example on both knees or elbows.

Cause The patient often knows the cause of the swelling (prolonged friction or a skeletal deformity), and may have had a similar complaint before.

Examination

Site Subcutaneous bursae occur where there is friction between skin and bone. The common sites are (Figure 4.65):

- Between the skin and olecranon: *student's elbow.*
- Between the skin and patella: *carpet-layer's knee.*
- Between the skin and patellar ligament: *clergyman's knee.*
- Between the skin and the head of the first metatarsal: *bunion.*

Shape and size *Bursae are usually circular in outline with an indistinct edge,* but their depth, or thickness, can vary from a few millimetres to 3–4 cm.

Surface The surface feels smooth providing it is not attached to the skin.

Colour The overlying skin is usually thickened, and often appears shiny, white and cracked.

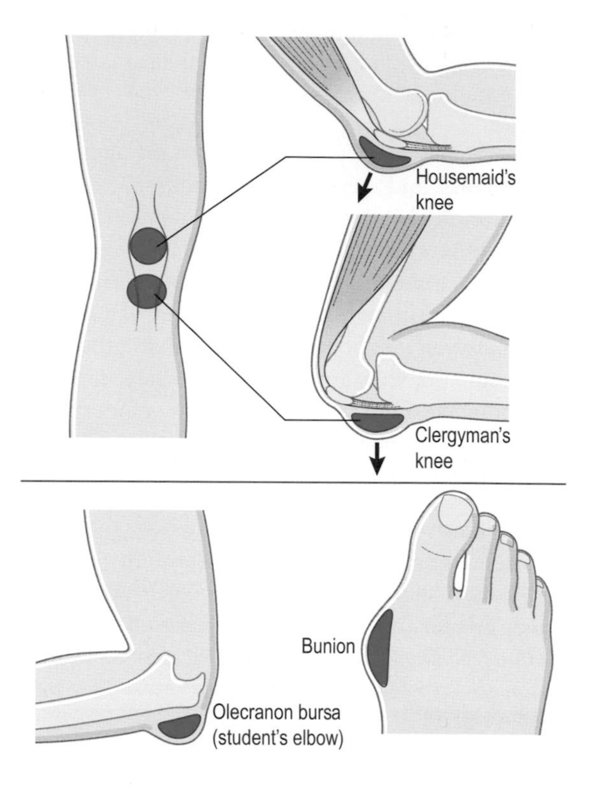

Figure 4.65 The common adventitious bursae.

Tenderness They are only tender if they become very tense or inflamed. The overlying skin then turns red and hot.

Composition They contain a clear viscous fluid, similar to synovial fluid, which gives them a soft or spongy consistency.

They fluctuate, transilluminate and may have a fluid thrill. These signs may be difficult to elicit if the wall of the bursa is thick, or the quantity of contained fluid small.

Relations The deep and superficial surfaces of a bursa are usually firmly attached to the two tissues it separates, so that the friction occurs between the lubricated inside surfaces of the bursa. *This makes the bursa immobile and the walls impalpable.*

Local tissues The bones and joints beneath the bursa must be carefully examined because a bursa may have developed to ease the movement of the skin over a skeletal abnormality such as an exostosis or deformed joint. The overlying skin is often thickened and cracked.

Complications Bursae can become inflamed by repeated trauma and by conditions that cause inflammation of the synovial surfaces, such as rheumatoid arthritis and gout. They also commonly become infected.

General examination Even though the patient complains of one lump, examine the same area on the other limb because *symmetrical bursae are common.* Also look for other skeletal abnormalities and joint diseases.

SPORADIC NEUROFIBROMA

Multiple familial neurofibromatosis (von Recklinghausen's disease) has already been discussed on page 115.

Sporadic neurofibromas are *benign tumours* that contain a mixture of neural (ectodermal) and fibrous (mesodermal) elements. They are often multiple. Tumours that are derived from nerve sheaths (the neurilemmoma, also known as the schwannoma), are very rare.

History

Age Neurofibromas can appear at any age, but usually present in adult life.

Symptoms Most cause no discomfort, and they rarely grow to be disfiguring. When they are related to a nerve trunk, they may be tender, and the patient may get tingling sensations in the distribution of the affected nerve.

Multiplicity They are often multiple.

Examination

Site They can occur anywhere in the skin and subcutaneous tissues. *The forearms seem to be most often affected,* perhaps because they are the part of the body most frequently palpated by the patient.

Shape and size Neurofibromas are *usually fusiform,* with their long axes lying along the length of the limb. They are rarely more than a few centimetres in length (Figure 4.66).

Composition They have the consistency of *firm rubber.*

Relations The surrounding structures are normal. Subcutaneous neurofibromas are mobile within the subcutaneous tissues but move most freely in a direction at right angles to the course of the nerve to which they are connected.

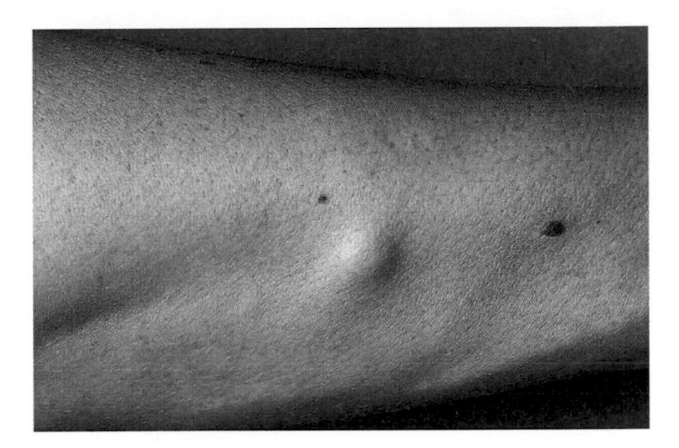

Figure 4.66 A neurofibroma on the leg of a patient with five other similar lesions.

PLEXIFORM NEUROFIBROMA

Although this is a very rare condition, it is mentioned because it is one of those conditions that can cause considerable diagnostic confusion if the doctor has never heard of it.

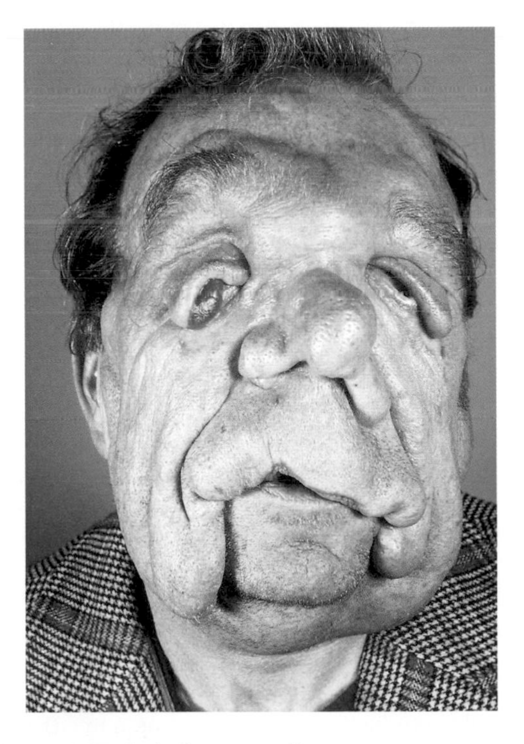

Figure 4.67 A plexiform neurofibroma.

It is an excessive overgrowth of neural tissue in the subcutaneous layers, which gives the tissues a swollen and oedematous appearance. It is sometimes called elephantiasis neurofibromatosis (Figure 4.67) 'The Elephant Man'.

It is often misdiagnosed as lymphoedema (see Chapter 10), so remember the condition when presented with a child with an apparent overgrowth of the soft tissues of the hand or foot. The diagnosis can only be made by the pathologist.

Tumours of the skin appendages

These arise from the sebaceous glands, sweat glands, eccrine and apocrine glands and hair gland cells. Most are benign and have exotic names. The majority are relatively benign, such as basal cell carcinomas (see page 151), but 5–10% are malignant and liable to local recurrence. All arise as subcutaneous pink, brown or red/white nodules on different parts of the body, but mainly in the head and neck.

SEBACEOUS GLAND TUMOURS

These include the *naevus sebaceous of Jadassohn, sebaceous adenoma* and *sebaceous carcinoma,* which is rare. They are all solitary subcutaneous tumours that are either soft and warty, or firm.

ECCRINE (SWEAT) GLAND TUMOURS

These include the *eccrine poroma*, the *spiradenoma* and the *acrospiroma*. These all present as solitary subcutaneous lumps, which can be reddish-pink or red–blue coloured.

Syringomas also arise from the sweat glands, and present as multiple flesh-coloured or yellow papules on the faces of females.

Cylindromas (turban tumours) are rare tumours that arise from the sweat glands of the head and scalp. They present as solitary or multiple, pink, spherical or slightly flattened nodules, which may coalesce to look like a turban, hence the common name (Figure 4.68). They are soft with an ill-defined edge.

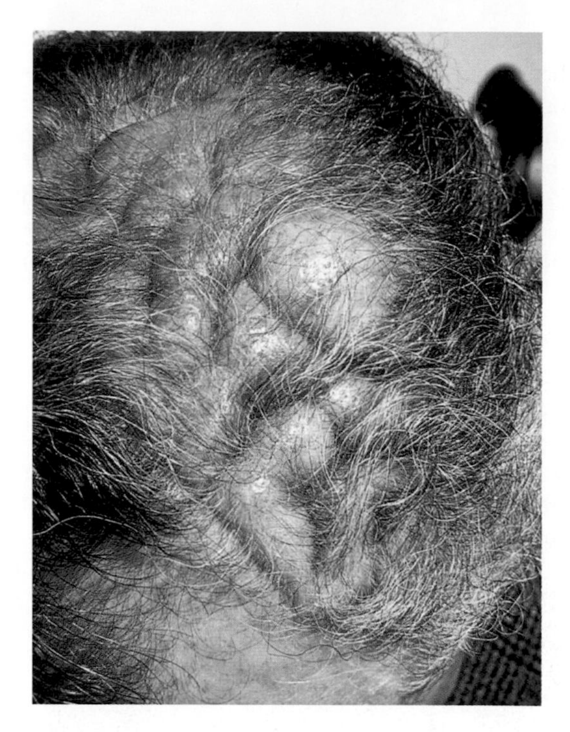

Figure 4.68 A 'turban' tumour.

APOCRINE GLAND TUMOURS

These include *apocrine hidrocystomas* and the *syringocystadenoma papilliferum*.

HAIR GLAND TUMOURS

These include *trichofolliculomas, trichoepitheliomas, trichilemmomas* and *pilomatrixomas,* many of which are hamartomas.

Premalignant skin lesions

SOLAR KERATOSIS

Prolonged exposure of the skin to sunlight can cause areas of hyperkeratosis of the skin, which may undergo malignant change.

History

The patient notices the gradual appearance of thickened patches of skin, which are not painful but can become unsightly.

Natural history Solar keratoses grow slowly, and the patients, usually elderly males who have worked out of doors for many years, ignore them. Any change in size or appearance should arouse suspicion.

Examination

Site They are commonly found on the *backs of the fingers and hands, on the face and on the rim of the ears.*

Shape and size Beneath their horny surface layer, there is a raised plaque of skin that may vary in diameter from a few millimetres to 1 cm and protrude above the skin surface (Figure 4.69). The whole of the strip of skin along the rim of the pinna may be affected.

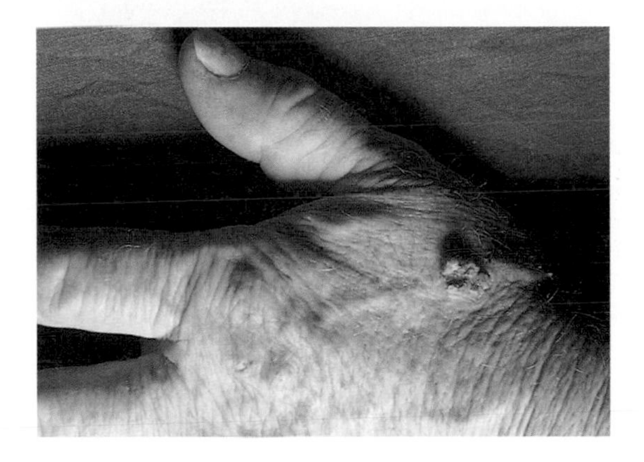

Figure 4.69 A solar keratosis on the back of the hand.

Colour The thickened patches of skin have a yellow–grey or red–brown colour.

Composition The keratinous layer is very hard, and clearly part of the underlying skin.

Relations They are confined to the skin, and if a nodule or patch is tethered to the underlying structures, it has already turned into a squamous carcinoma.

Lymph glands The local lymph glands should not be enlarged unless one of the keratoses has become a squamous cell carcinoma.

BOWEN'S DISEASE

This also is a precancerous lesion. It presents as a *cluster of flat, pink, papular patches that are covered with crusts.* The patches and the adjacent skin have a pale brown, thickened appearance. (Figure 4.70). Patients usually believe they have a patch of eczema.

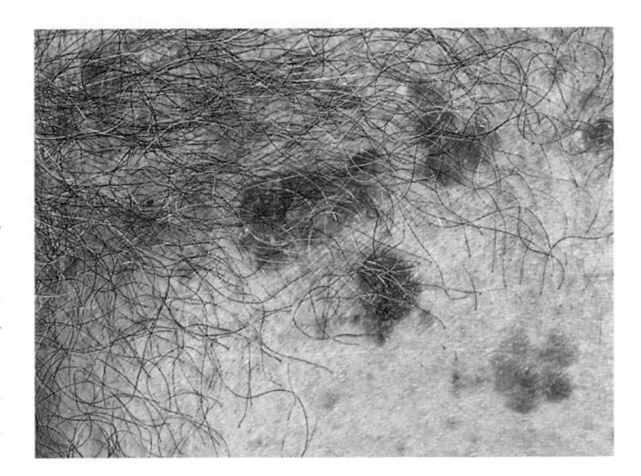

Figure 4.70 Bowen's disease on the skin of the chest.

When the crusts are removed, the papules can be seen to have a wet, oozy, slightly bloody, papilliferous surface.

HUTCHINSON'S LENTIGO

This is a large area of pigmentation that commonly appears and slowly enlarges on the face and neck in late adult life (after the age of 60 years). The surface is smooth, but there may be raised, rough nodules (see Figure 4.58, page 145), which correspond to areas of junctional activity and become the sites of malignant change, alongside pale areas of regression. Areas of malignant change cause an increase in pigmentation that may pass unnoticed because the background pigmentation is so dark.

This mole is different from other moles because of two special features: *its late development and its high incidence of malignant change.* It may be 'premalignant' or 'frankly malignant' from the start: an example of malignant change 'in situ'.

Malignant diseases of the skin

BASAL CELL CARCINOMA (RODENT ULCER)

This is a locally invasive carcinoma of the *basal layer of the epidermis.* Metastasis is extremely rare, but infiltration into adjacent tissues is recognized. It is common in exposed skin, especially in countries where there is a high incidence of ultraviolet irradiation, i.e. bright sunlight.

History

Age The incidence increases with age because it is related to the duration of exposure of the skin to ultraviolet light.

Geography It is the most common cancer in Europe, Australia and the USA, and is showing a worldwide increase in incidence.

Ethnic group It is rare in dark-skinned races.

Sex Males are affected more often than females.

Duration The lesions grow very slowly and have often been present for months or years before the patient seeks advice.

Symptoms The principal complaint is of a *persistent nodule* or *an ulcer with a central scab* that repeatedly falls off and then re-forms. The tumour eventually becomes disfiguring. It may itch or be painful, and if it is neglected, it eventually becomes a deep infected ulcer. A large, neglected ulcer destroying one side of the face is now rare.

Development These tumours grow very slowly and may have been present for months or years before the patient presents. The long history gives a false impression that the lesion is 'benign and unimportant'.

Persistence Some spread rapidly through the skin, leaving a central scar.

Multiplicity They are often multiple.

Predisposing factors The most significant aetiological factors appear to be a genetic predisposition and an exposure to ultraviolet radiation.

Examination (Revision panel 4.6)

Site They are commonly found on the face above a line drawn from the *angle of the mouth to the lobe of the ear* (Figure 4.71). This does not mean that they do not occur in other sites; all exposed skin is susceptible, particularly on the scalp, neck, arms and hands.

Size Most patients complain of the *nodule* or *ulcer* (Figure 4.72) when it is quite small, but they can grow to a considerable size if they are neglected (Figure 4.73). A few grow outwards from the skin to become a fungating mass on the skin surface (Figure 4.74), but the majority erode deeply, destroying the underlying tissues and forming a deep cavity (see Figure 4.73) – hence the name 'rodent'.

Revision panel 4.6

VARIOUS CLINICAL APPEARANCES OF BASAL CELL CARCINOMAS

- Nodule
- 'Cystic' (a large, seemingly transparent nodule)
- Ulcer
- Deeply eroding ulcer: the 'rodent' ulcer
- Pigmented nodule
- Geographical (advancing edge, healing centre)

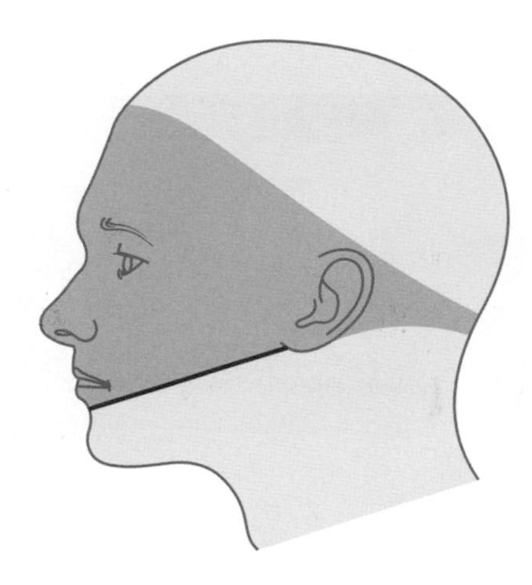

Figure 4.71 Basal cell carcinomas commonly appear in the shaded area.

Shape Some of the many macroscopic appearances are shown in Figures 4.72–4.74. The tumour always starts as a nodule. *When the central epithelium dies, the resulting ulcer develops a rolled edge* (see Chapter 1). This means that the edge is raised up and rounded, but not everted. The nodule can become quite large and look like a cyst if the centre of the tumour does not necrose and ulcerate (see Figure 4.72a). It is however not cystic, because it is solid and non-fluctuant, although the term 'cystic rodent ulcer' is unfortunately sometimes used to describe this appearance.

Colour The raised portion of the tumour – its edge if it is annular, or its centre if it is a nodule – is smooth, glistening and slightly transparent. This gives the impression that there are *pearl-white nodules* of tissue just below the epidermis (see Figure 4.72b). These

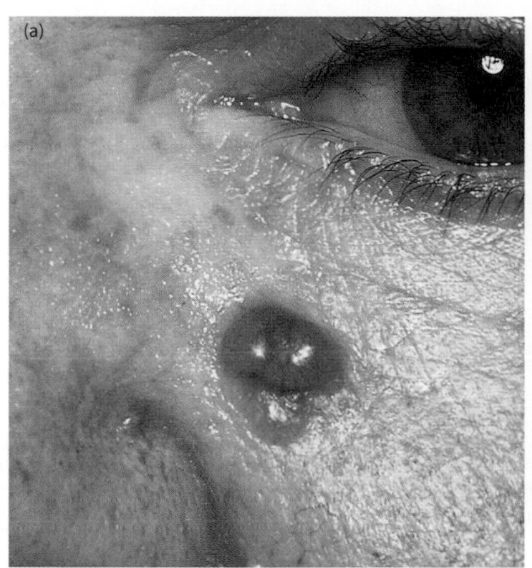

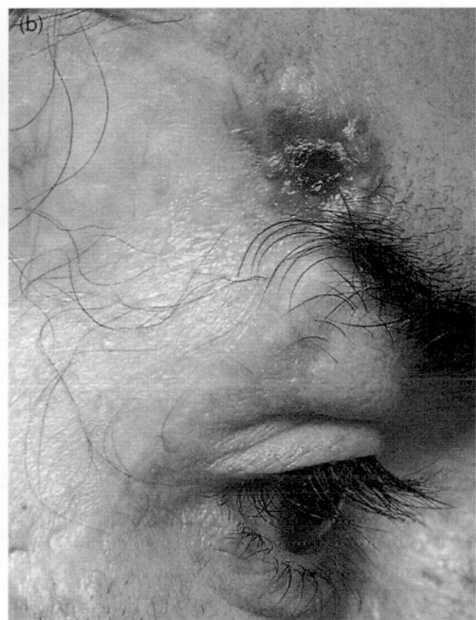

Figure 4.72 BASAL CELL CARCINOMAS. (a) An early nodule just below the eye. These nodules are sometimes mistakenly thought to be cystic. (b) A recurrent basal cell carcinoma at the edge of a skin graft placed to cover the skin defect from a previous excision 7 years earlier.

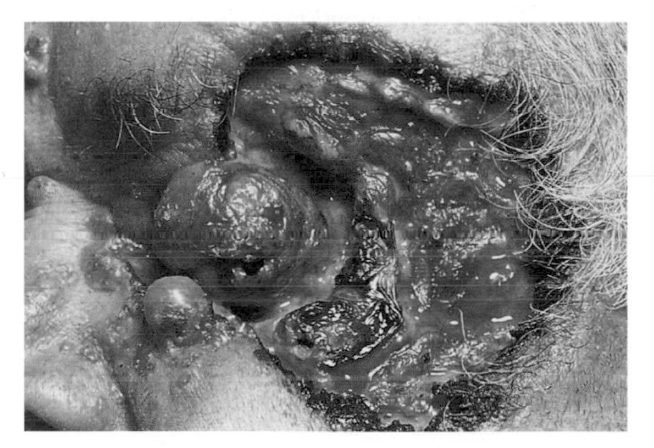

Figure 4.73 A true 'rodent ulcer'. The basal cell carcinoma has destroyed the orbit and the eye.

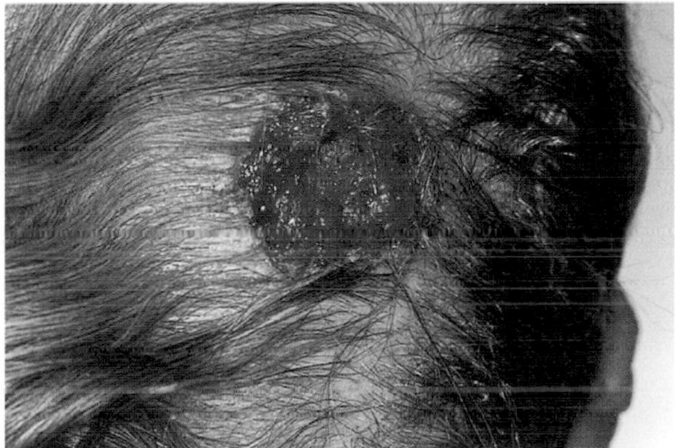

Figure 4.74 A raised, wet, weeping basal cell carcinoma that was thought by the patient to be a patch of eczema.

nodules also give the ulcerating variety its typical 'rolled edge'.

The whole lesion may be coloured brown by excess melanin (a pigmented basal cell carcinoma) (Figure 4.75).

Surface The surface of the nodular variety is covered by fine, distinct blood vessels, which may give it a pink hue (see Figure 4.72a).

Edge When the nodule first ulcerates, the rolled edge is circular, but as the malignant cells spread, its shape becomes irregular. The raised edge may be the only clue to the diagnosis if the ulcer heals. An irregular raised edge around a flat white scar is sometimes called a 'geographical' or 'forest fire' basal cell carcinoma (see Figure 4.72b). When the ulcer erodes into deeper structures, the edge becomes more prominent and florid, but not everted (see Figure 4.72b).

Base The base of a small rodent ulcer is covered with a coat of dried serum and epithelial cells, and will bleed slightly if this layer is picked off. The bases of deeply eroding ulcers consist of fat, bone, muscle or other structures covered by poor-quality granulation tissue (see Figure 4.73).

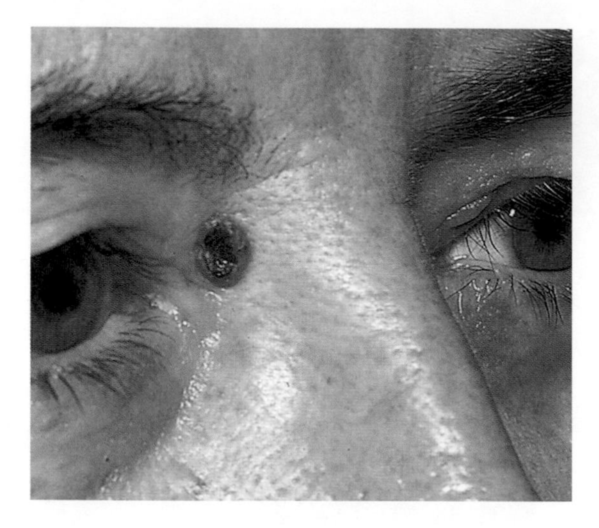

Figure 4.75 A pigmented basal cell carcinoma.

Depth Long-standing ulcers may erode deep into the face, destroying skin and bone, and exposing the nasal cavity, air sinuses and even the eye (see Figure 4.73). Such extensive lesions are now uncommon.

> **NOTE:** Hence the name 'rodent' because the tissues look as if they have been gnawed by a rat.

Lymph glands The local lymph glands should not be enlarged.

Relations A small tumour is confined to the skin, and is freely movable over the deep structures. Fixation of the ulcer indicates that it has invaded deeply.

Differential diagnosis (Table 4.1) *A rodent ulcer can resemble a squamous cell carcinoma.* The long history and the rolled edge are the clinical features that indicate its basal cell origin.

A *keratoacanthoma* (see above) that is just beginning to slough at its centre can also look like an early rodent ulcer, but the short history and the deep slough should suggest the correct diagnosis.

Sweat gland tumours and *malignant melanomas* are other differential diagnoses that should be considered.

SQUAMOUS CELL CARCINOMA (EPITHELIOMA)

This is a carcinoma of the cells of the epidermis that normally migrate out towards the surface to form the superficial keratinous squamous layer. The tumour cells infiltrate the epidermis, the dermis and adjacent tissues.

Microscopic examination reveals tongues of tumour cells spreading in all directions, and clusters of cells with concentric rings of flattened squamous cells at their centre. These onion-like clumps of cells are often called 'epithelial pearls', but are only seen under the microscope.

History

Age The incidence of squamous cell carcinoma of the skin increases with age.

Causes The following are all associated with an increased incidence of these tumours:

- Prolonged exposure to sunlight.
- Solar keratoses.
- Bowen's disease.

Table 4.1 The diagnostic features of the four common surgical skin lesions

	Duration of growth	Physical features
Squamous cell carcinoma	Few months	Occasional bleeding Nodule or ulcer with everted edge
Basal cell carcinoma	Many months or years	Nodule or ulcer with rolled edge and permanent scab
Keratoacanthoma	Few weeks	Nodule with central hard necrotic core No bleeding Spontaneous regression
Pyogenic granuloma	Few days	Soft red nodule that becomes covered with epithelium Bleeds easily

- Certain chemicals and irradiation.
- The presence of old scarring.
- Following burns, or chronic ulcers.

Cancer of the scrotal skin was once common in chimney sweeps (see Chapter 18).

Duration The ulcerating tumour has usually been present for 1 or 2 months before the patient presents. It may grow quite large before being noticed if it is in an inaccessible part, such as in the middle of the back.

Symptoms The patient complains of a lump, or of bleeding and discharge from an ulcer. *Bleeding is more common with squamous than basal cell carcinomas.*

The tumour may become *painful* if it invades deep structures.

Patients occasionally notice *enlarged lymph glands,* and are unaware of the primary tumour. *Dissemination of tumour cells throughout the body is a late event.*

Development The ulcer or nodule enlarges steadily and inexorably. The edges become more prominent and florid (see Chapter 1).

Multiplicity There may be multiple tumours in skin affected by exposure to ultraviolet light or chemicals.

Examination

Site They can occur on any part of the skin, *but are more common on the exposed skin of the head and neck, hands, forearms and upper trunk.* They also develop in skin subjected to repeated chemical or mechanical irritation.

Colour The everted edge of a carcinomatous ulcer is usually a dark red–brown colour because it is very vascular (Figure 4.76). The whole ulcer may be covered with old coagulated blood or serum.

Tenderness The ulcer is not usually tender.

Shape and size They begin as small nodules on the skin. As they enlarge, the centre becomes necrotic and sloughs, and the nodule turns into an ulcer. This is initially circular with prominent everted edges (Figure 4.77), but can become any shape as it enlarges.

Edge Squamous cell carcinomas have an *everted edges* because the excessive tissue growth raises them above and over the normal skin surface (see Figures 4.76 and 4.77).

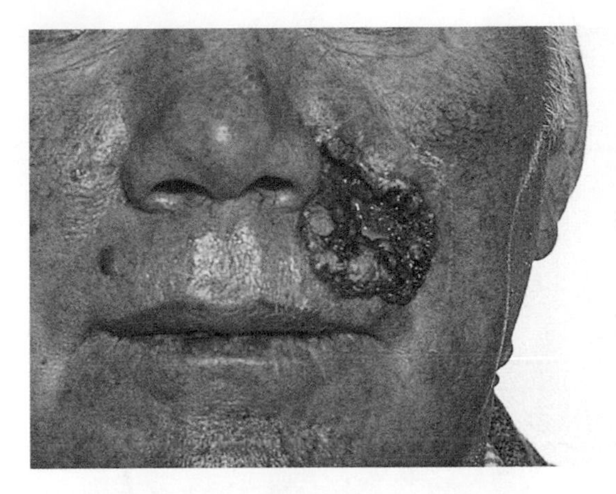

Figure 4.76 A squamous cell carcinomatous ulcer on the face, with an everted edge and a necrotic base.

Base The base of the ulcer consists of necrotic tumour covered with serum and blood (Figure 4.78). There is usually some granulation tissue, but this tends to be pale and unhealthy. Deep tissues may be exposed.

Depth The depth of the ulcer is affected by the nature of the underlying tissues and the virulence of the tumour. Soft tissues are easily invaded, and when they slough they leave a deep ulcer (Figure 4.78).

Discharge The discharge can be copious, bloody, purulent and foul-smelling. This is often the patient's most depressing and debilitating symptom.

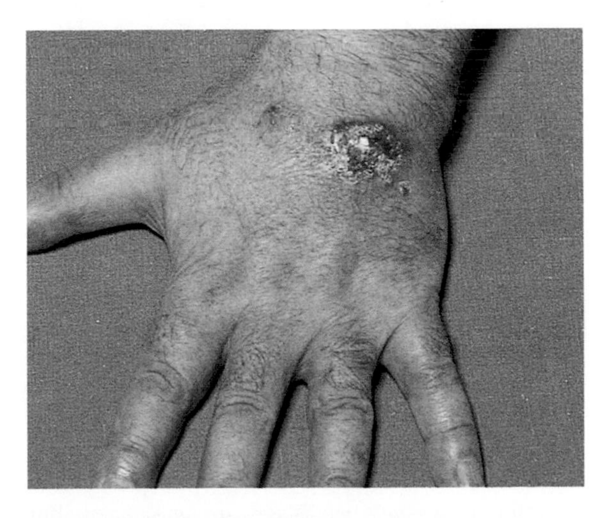

Figure 4.77 A squamous cell carcinomatous ulcer on the hand, whose edge is not yet everted but is raised and almost everted on the proximal side.

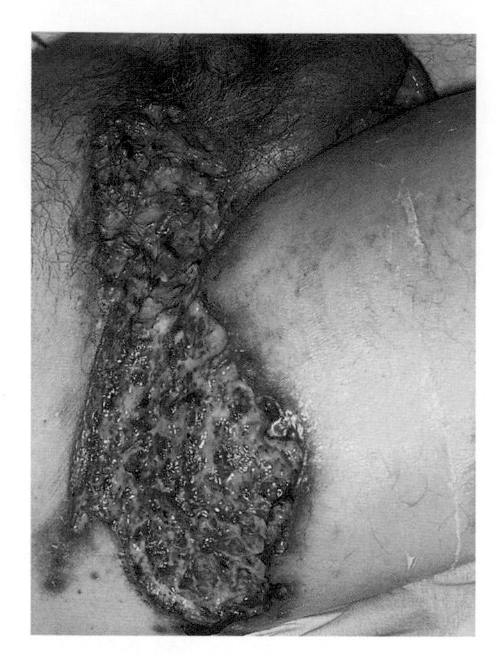

Figure 4.78 An extensive squamous cell carcinoma of the skin of the groin and scrotum.

Relations These vary according to the extent of the malignant infiltration. The tumour has spread beyond the skin and subcutaneous tissues into tendon, bone and muscle if the ulcer is immobile.

Lymph glands The local lymph glands are *often enlarged,* but this does not always mean that they contain tumour. In about one-third of patients, the lymphadenopathy is caused by infection, which subsides after excision of the ulcer. Nevertheless, it should be assumed that palpable lymph glands contain metastases.

Local tissues The surrounding tissues may be oedematous and thickened, and there may be subcutaneous spread into nearby nerves. Invasion of local blood vessels can cause thrombosis and tissue ischaemia. These are features of the late stages of the disease.

Complications Infection and bleeding are the common complications. *Bleeding can sometimes be massive and fatal.*

General examination All the lymph glands that might contain metastases should be palpated (see Chapter 1). *Distant metastases are uncommon,* but hepatomegaly or a pleural effusion is indicative of systemic spread.

Differential diagnosis The differential diagnosis is summarized in Revision panel 4.7.

Revision panel 4.7

DIFFERENTIAL DIAGNOSIS OF A SQUAMOUS CELL CARCINOMA

- Tumours of the skin appendages
- Cutaneous secondary deposits
- Basal cell carcinomas
- Keratoacanthomas
- Malignant melanomas
- Solar keratoses
- Pyogenic granulomas
- Infected seborrhoeic warts

MARJOLIN'S ULCER

This is an eponym for a squamous cell carcinoma that arises in a long-standing ulcer or benign burn scar. The most common ulcer to become malignant is a *long-standing venous ulcer* (see Chapter 10, page 363).

These carcinomas are very similar to the idiopathic variety, except that they may not be so florid. Their edge is not always raised and everted, and there may be pre-existing chronic ulceration or scarring (Figure 4.79). Unusual nodules or changes in a chronic ulcer or a scar should be viewed with suspicion, especially if they increase in size and develop an offensive discharge.

MALIGNANT MELANOMA

Because of the confusion that has arisen from using the word 'melanoma' to describe a benign lesion and 'malignant melanoma' to describe a malignant one, *use the terms 'mole' or 'pigmented naevus' for benign lesions, and 'malignant melanoma' for malignant lesions.*

As the melanocyte originates from the neural crest and so is neuroectodermal in origin, it could be argued that malignant change in melanocytes should be called a carcinoma. Terms such as 'melanocarcinoma' and even 'melanosarcoma' only add to the confusion. It is therefore best to use the well-established descriptive term 'malignant melanoma'.

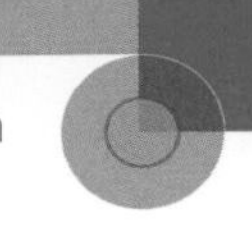

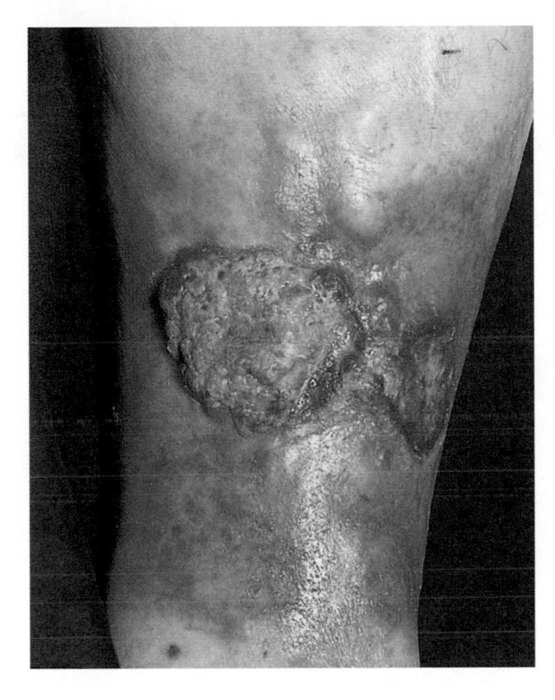

Figure 4.79 A Marjolin's ulcer. The lipodermatosclerosis, pigmentation and scarring caused by long-standing venous hypertension and ulceration can be seen around the central neoplastic ulcer.

Cardinal symptoms of malignant change in a mole

- **Change in the surface.** One of the earliest signs associated with malignant change is a loss of the normal skin markings (creases) over the mole. The skin may also become rough and scaly (Figure 4.80).
- **Itching.** This is an early and significant symptom, often associated with a pale pink halo around the mole (Figure 4.81).
- **Increase in size, shape or thickness.** The patient usually complains that a long-standing mole, or a recently developed brown spot, has grown steadily over a period of a few weeks or months. The mole or part of the mole may become wider and thicker, often changing from a flat plaque to a *nodule* (Figure 4.81). Alternatively, the mole may simply change in outline (Figure 4.82).
- **Change in colour.** Malignant melanocytes usually produce more melanin, so the mole gets *darker*. The colour change is often patchy, with some areas becoming almost *black*, others turning *blue–purple* with the increased vascularity, and some areas not changing at all. Very occasionally, the malignant melanocytes do not produce melanin, so that the new growth is pink (Figure 4.83).

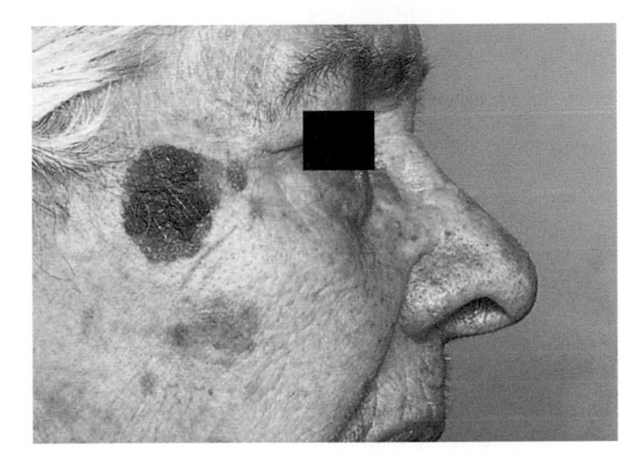

Figure 4.80 Rough and scaly skin over a malignant melanoma arising in a Hutchinson's lentigo.

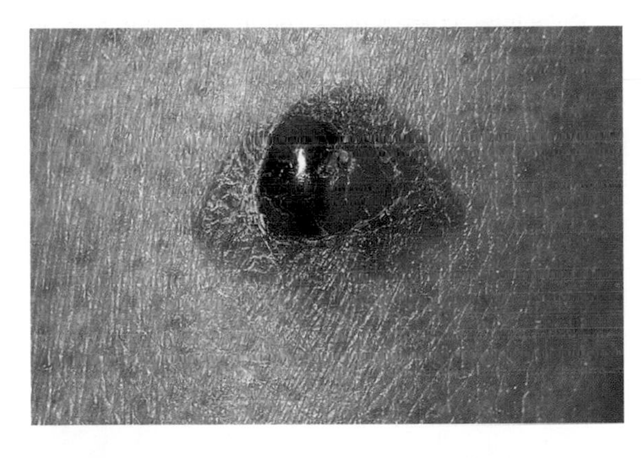

Figure 4.81 A halo of pigment around a nodular melanoma.

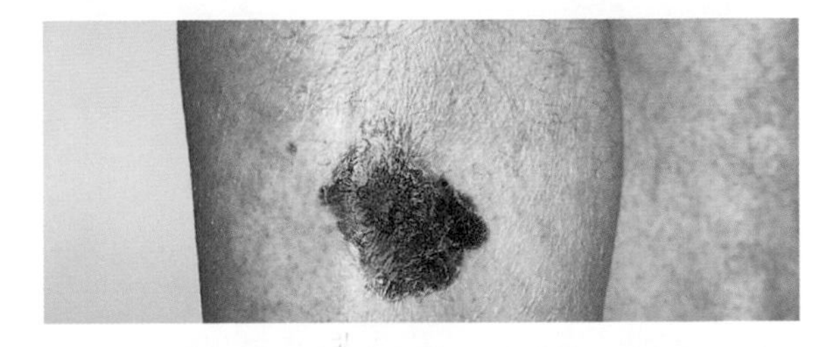

Figure 4.82 A change in outline of pre-existing mole.

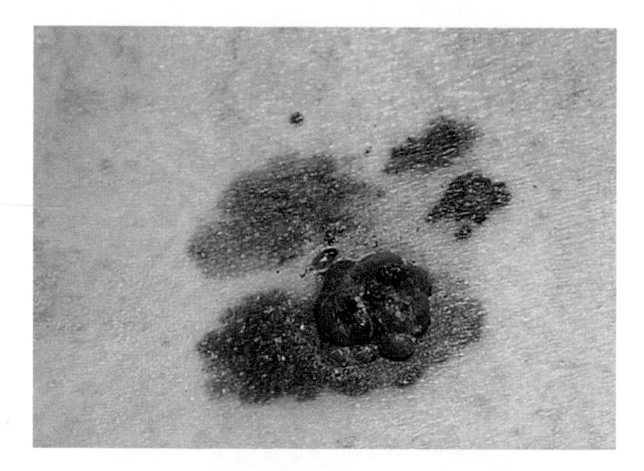

Figure 4.83 A superficial spreading melanoma with a 'pink' amelanotic area.

- **Bleeding.** As the tumour cells multiply, the overlying epithelium becomes anoxic, and either ulcerates spontaneously or breaks down after a very minor injury. Bleeding is usually slight and a late sign.
- **Evidence of local or distant spread.** The pigment produced by the malignant melanocytes may spread diffusely into the surrounding skin to produce a *brown halo* around the primary lesion (see Figures 4.81–4.84). The malignant cells may also spread through the skin in the intradermal lymphatics. When they stop migrating and multiply, they become small intradermal nodules. Small nodules around the primary lesion are called *satellite nodules* (Figure 4.84).

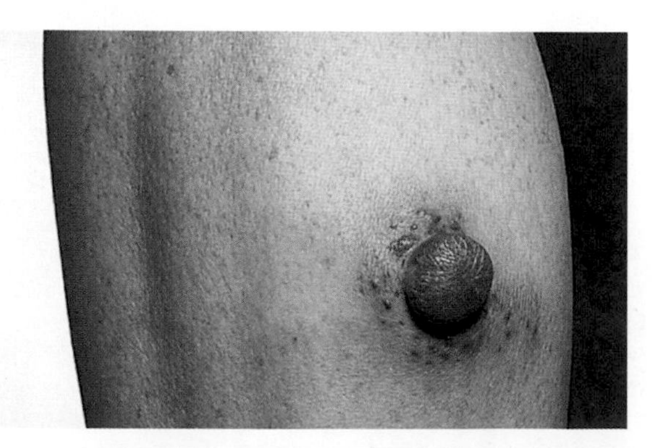

Figure 4.84 Satellite nodules around a nodular melanoma.

Patients occasionally notice enlarged lymph glands in the groin or axilla.

NOTE: Not all malignant melanomas arise in pre-existing pigmented naevi.

All the changes listed above can develop in a few weeks or months (Revision panel 4.8).

Revision panel 4.8

CHANGES THAT SUGGEST THAT A MOLE HAS TURNED MALIGNANT

- Loss of normal surface markings (e.g. skin creases)
- Change in size, shape or thickness
- Change in colour
- Itching
- Bleeding/ulceration
- Halo:
  - Pink (inflammatory reaction) – early
  - Brown (pigment) – late
- Satellite nodules

History

Age Malignant melanoma is very rare before puberty, although it has been reported in children. Most cases occur in patients aged 20–30 years or more.

Sex Malignant melanoma occurs equally in both sexes, but is found more often in the lower limbs in females and on the trunk in males. At younger ages more females are affected and *vice versa* in elderly groups.

Ethnic group Malignant melanoma is common in white individuals and rare in black ones.

NOTE: People with fair complexions, red hair and a tendency to freckle are more susceptible.

Cause Melanocytes are stimulated by ultraviolet light. White-skinned people living in those parts of the world that enjoy abundant sunlight, such as

Australia and *the west coast of the USA*, have a high incidence of malignant melanoma. Those who work out of doors in these regions, especially those with a history of repeated episodes of sunburn, are particularly susceptible.

Symptoms The cardinal features have already been described. The common reasons for seeking medical advice are a change of size or colour, bleeding and the appearance of a brown halo or satellite nodules. It is usually the cosmetic disfigurement caused by an enlarging mole that brings the patient to the doctor, but more than 25% of lesions arise *de novo*, i.e. in normal skin rather than in a pre-existing lesion.

> **NOTE:** Malignant melanomas often itch, but are not painful.

The patient has sometimes observed the changes described above, but if the mole is on the sole of the foot or the back of the trunk where it cannot be seen, the patient may present with lymph gland enlargement or symptoms caused by distant metastases, such as *weight loss, dyspnoea* or *jaundice*.

Multiplicity Multiple malignant melanomas are very rare, but there are often multiple secondary nodules around a primary lesion. Two concurrent primary lesions are very uncommon.

Examination

Site The majority of malignant melanomas are found on the *limbs, head, neck and trunk*. They are uncommon on the palms of the hands and the soles of the feet (except in black Africans). They may arise in the subungual tissues, at the mucocutaneous junction and in the mouth and the anal margin.

Shape and size When first noticed, the area of malignant change is usually quite small (0.5–2 cm in diameter), but the mole in which the change has begun may be of any size. When a malignant melanoma is neglected, it becomes a large, florid tumour, protruding from and overlapping the surrounding skin (Figure 4.85).

Surface When the tumour is small, it is covered by smooth epithelium. When the epithelium dies, from ischaemic necrosis, the resulting ulcer is covered with a crust of blood and serum. Bleeding and subacute infection may make the surface of the tumour wet, soft and boggy.

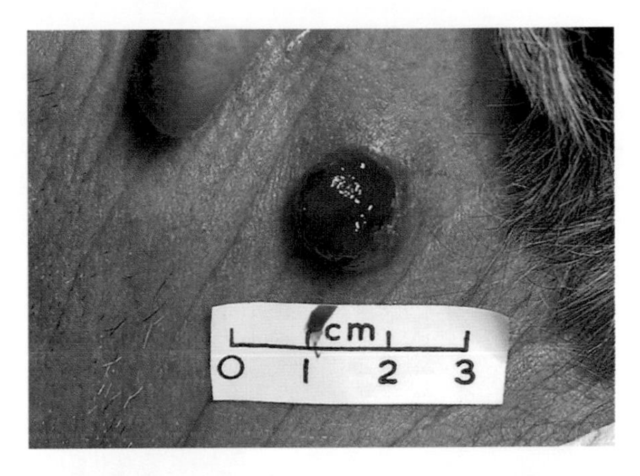

Figure 4.85 A large nodular melanoma.

Colour Malignant melanomas may be any colour from a *pale pinkish-brown to black*. If they have a rich blood supply, they develop a purple hue. Variations in the colour are common, some areas being very black and others pale. *Amelanotic melanomas are rare* but do occur (Figure 4.86).

Temperature and tenderness A malignant melanoma is no warmer than the surrounding skin, and is not tender.

Composition The primary tumour has a firm consistency. Small satellite nodules feel hard.

Relations The malignant tissue is within the skin and moves with it.

Lymph glands The local lymph glands may be enlarged.

Surrounding tissues There may be a halo of brown pigment in the skin around the tumour (see Figures 4.81–4.83), and satellite nodules in the skin

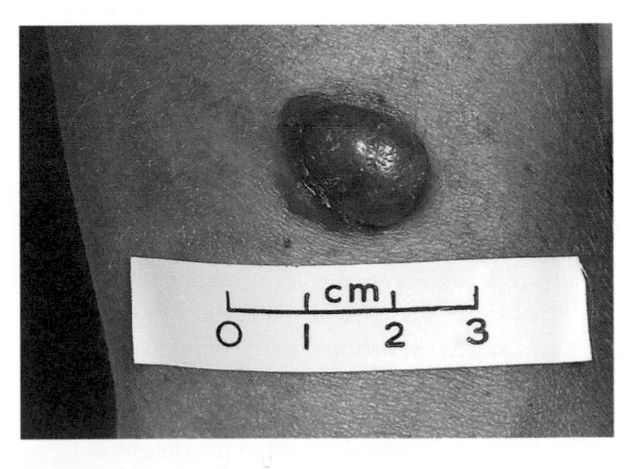

Figure 4.86 An amelanotic melanoma.

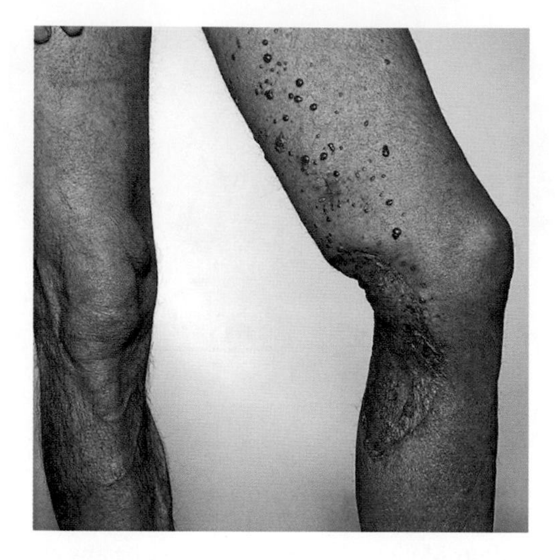

Figure 4.87 Multiple metastatic nodules of melanoma previously excised.

and subcutaneous tissue between the primary tumour and the nearest lymph glands (Figures 4.84 and 4.87). It is important to feel all the subcutaneous tissues along the course of the lymphatics that drain the melanoma, as nodules of metastatic melanoma may be palpable.

Clinical types

Although the above description indicates that a malignant melanoma may have many forms, there are *four common clinical types:*

- *Superficial spreading melanoma* is the most common variety (see Figures 4.82 and 4.83). It may occur on any part of the body, and is usually palpable but thin, with an irregular edge and a *variegated colour.*
- *Nodular melanoma* is thick and protrudes above the skin (see Figure 4.85). It has a smooth surface and a regular outline, and may arise *de novo*. It may become ulcerated, and then often bleeds.
- *Lentigo maligna melanoma* is a malignant melanoma arising in a patch of Hutchinson's lentigo (see Figure 4.80). The malignant areas are thicker than the surrounding pigmented skin and usually darker in colour, but seldom ulcerate.
- *Acral lentiginous melanoma* is a rare type of malignant melanoma, but important to remember because it is often misdiagnosed as a chronic paronychia or a subungual haematoma. It presents as an irregular, expanding area of brown or black pigmentation on the palm or sole, or beneath a nail (see Figure 4.94).
- *Amelanotic melanomas* occasionally occur (see Figure 4.86).

General examination Malignant melanoma spreads via the lymphatics to the regional lymph glands. It may then spread in the bloodstream to the lungs, liver and brain. Pleural effusions, hepatomegaly, jaundice and neurological abnormalities are indications of distant metastases. Blood-borne secondary deposits in the skin and subcutaneous tissues are not uncommon.

OTHER RARER BUT IMPORTANT LESIONS

Merkel cell carcinoma

Rare tumours; initially thought to arise from Merkel cells (mechanoreceptors of neural crest origin), they may more likely have B-lymphocyte origins. Up to 80% may be associated with the Merkel cell polyomavirus which causes gene mutations, possibly in immune-depleted individuals. The tumour may be very locally aggressive and also has the propensity to metastasize.

History

Usually present as rapidly growing *solitary red/purple nodules,* usually in sun-exposed sites on the head and neck. More common in men and after the age of 50.

Examination

The initial lesion is often solitary and may be irregular. The colour is *classically pink/red* (Figure 4.88). Sometimes there may be confusion with basal cell carcinoma. Examination of the lymph node basins is key, 10–20% of patients may have metastases at presentation and a significantly higher proportion may develop them.

Sebaceous carcinoma

Rare tumors of sebaceous glands present as yellow nodules/plaques often around the eye (Figure 4.89) (75%) and usually in elderly patients. They may exhibit aggressive local/distant spread. Some can be part of syndromes, such as Muir–Torre.

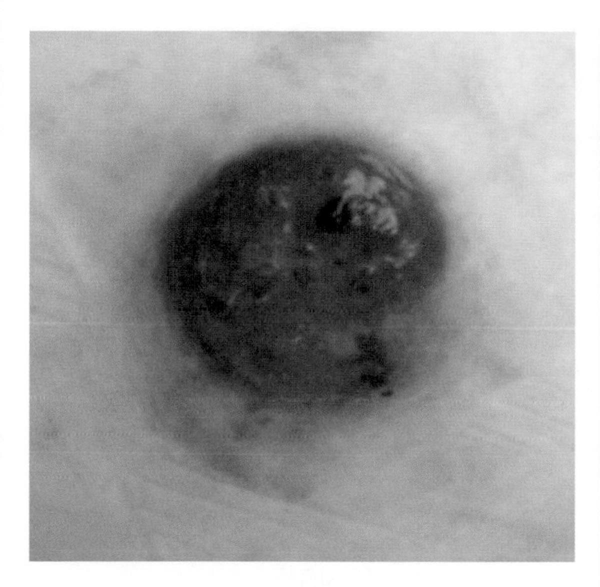

Figure 4.88 Merkel cell carcinoma.

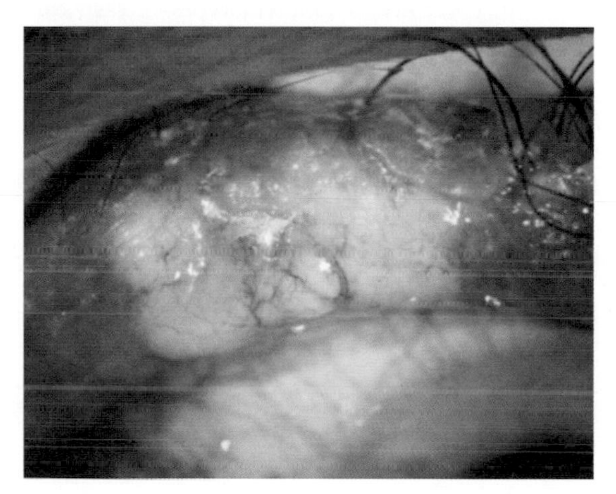

Figure 4.89 Upper eyelid sebaceous carcinoma.

Dermatofibrosarcoma protuberans

These tumours tend to be slow-growing, usually presenting as a plaque or nodule that may be red-brown in colour (Figure 4.90). They are commonly found on the trunk in those between 20 and 50 years of age. These tumours tend to be locally aggressive but rarely metastasize.

MYCOSIS FUNGOIDES

This is a rare skin lymphoma that occasionally presents in a surgical clinic. It begins as a patch of thickening and reddening of the skin, which enlarges into a plaque that may ulcerate. The tumours may be multiple. It is often associated with a generalized lymphoma.

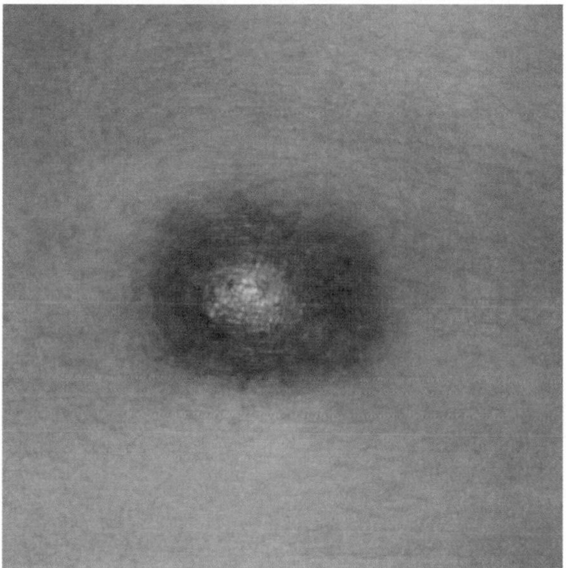

Figure 4.90 Dermatofibrosarcoma protuberans

KAPOSI'S SARCOMA

Kaposi's sarcoma is a cutaneous sarcoma that, before the appearance of human immunodeficiency virus (HIV) infection, was a rare sporadic condition in Europe, but not uncommon and endemic in sub-Saharan Africa.

The variety not associated with HIV infection runs a slow, indolent course, and is only very rarely associated with spread to the intestine or generalized malignant lymphoma.

The variety associated with HIV infection and acquired immunodeficiency syndrome (AIDS) runs an aggressive course, and is usually associated with systemic tumour infiltration of the lymph glands, intestine, mucous membranes, lungs and other organs.

History

Patients complain of the presence of *painless nodules or plaques in and beneath the skin, which often appear first in the legs*. There are likely to be a multitude of systemic symptoms if the patient has AIDS.

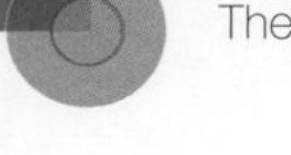

Examination

The nodules are *red, hemispherical* and *painless* (Figure 4.91). They lie in the subcutaneous tissues, but the overlying skin is often red, adherent to and involved in the disease process. The overlying skin may break down into an ulcer.

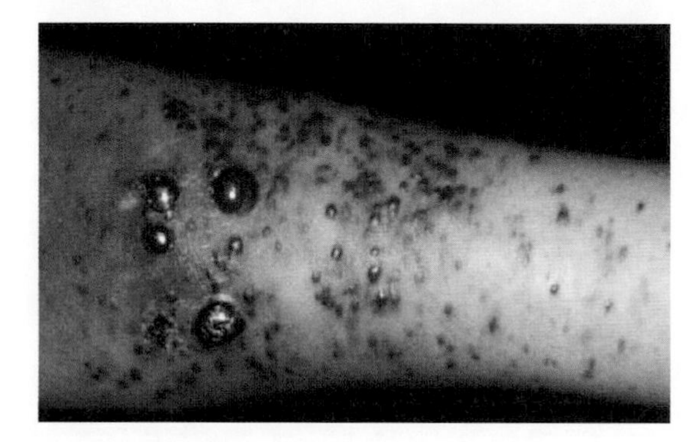

Figure 4.91 Kaposi's sarcoma.

Other common skin conditions sometimes seen in surgical patients

HYPERHIDROSIS

This is an excessive quantity of sweat released without an appropriate heat stimulus. It most commonly affects the *axilla, hands, feet and groins.* It is closely associated with vasospastic disorders and is more common in females.

The skin becomes soggy, white, moist and macerated. Clothes may become saturated with sweat and offensive. It can cause social embarrassment when shaking hands, and interfere with writing.

Generalized hyperhidrosis can be associated with thyrotoxicosis, which must be excluded by careful examination and special tests (see Chapter 12).

ECZEMA/DERMATITIS

This is a red, weepy, vesicular rash that usually has an immune cause (Figure 4.92). There are constitutional 'endogenous' factors in all patients with eczema, but 'exogenous' sensitizing factors are also very important. The condition may be inherited, when it is often associated with hay fever and asthma. It can also be initiated by an allergy, drugs or infection, or physical problems such as an injury, scratching or varicose veins.

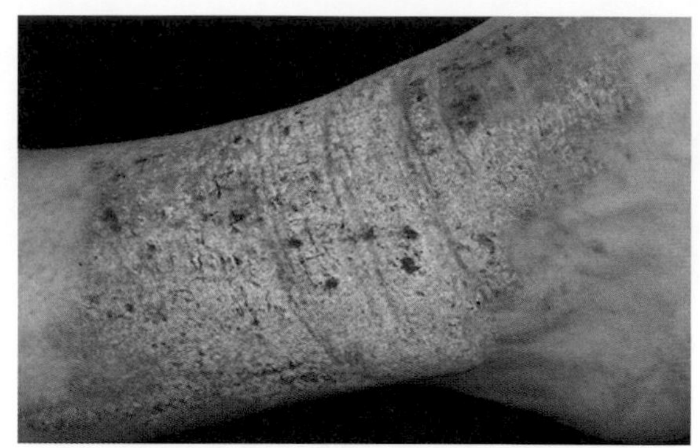

Figure 4.92 Eczema.

DRUG ERUPTIONS

A whole variety of different types of rash can occur in response to drugs, including *maculopapular rashes, eczema, purpura, urticaria and generalized desquamation.*

Patients occasionally develop severe malaise, pyrexia and generalized lymphadenopathy. A drug eruption must be considered in any patient who develops a rash (Revision panel 4.9).

Revision panel 4.9

COMMON CAUSES OF DRUG ERUPTION

- Antibiotics
- Barbiturates
- Non-steroidal anti-inflammatory drugs
- Diuretics
- Chlorpromazine

URTICARIA

This used to be called 'hives', and is the development of allergic wheals in the skin in response to a noxious stimulus. *The condition is caused by the degranulation of mast cells, which release histamine.* In some patients, the cause proves impossible to identify, and these cases are called idiopathic. Nettle stings, jelly-fish stings and insect bites are recognized causes, as are morphine and atropine.

The term *angioneurotic oedema* is used to describe a form of 'urticarial' swelling of the tongue, eyelids, lips and larynx that comes on intermittently and for which there is no known cause. A family history is occasionally present, indicating a genetic factor.

ACNE AND SYCOSIS BARBAE

These are conditions in which the ducts of the sebaceous glands become blocked by overactivity. They may then become inflamed and secondarily infected. The condition causes comedos (blackheads) and blind cysts, which may turn into sebaceous cysts. Severe scarring may result. The condition declines after the age of 20 years.

PSORIASIS

This condition occurs in *1–2% of the white population*, usually beginning between the ages of 5 and 25 years. About one-third of those affected have a family history of the condition, which may have an autoimmune cause.

It presents as *sharply demarcated, red, raised, oval plaques mainly situated over the elbows, knees and scalp* (Figure 4.93). The plaques have a silver, scaly surface, and the pattern of distribution varies widely. Psoriasis is often associated with an *arthritis of the hands*, which has to be distinguished from rheumatoid arthritis. One-quarter of those affected develop *pits in the nails*, which are often thick, opaque and discoloured, and break easily.

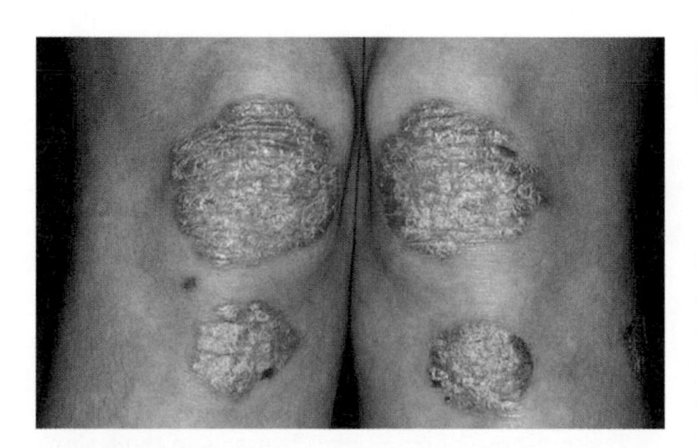

Figure 4.93 Psoriasis.

PITYRIASIS ROSACEA

This is the most common cause of a *slightly itchy skin rash in a young person.*

It usually starts with a single red, oval, scaly macule, which often develops over the lower abdomen or shoulder. Three or 4 days later, a characteristic rash appears over the trunk, consisting of both macules and papules. The rash does not involve the skin below the upper thighs and arms, and has a 'vest and pants' distribution.

The long axes of the macules are arranged along the line of skin cleavage (Langer's lines). They typically have a fawn centre with a pink surround. Scaling is often present at the junction with normal skin. The rash usually clears completely in 6–12 weeks.

The differential diagnosis includes *drug sensitivity, tinea pedis, guttate psoriasis* and *secondary syphilis.*

LICHEN PLANUS

An itchy rash develops on the wrists and forearms of adults before usually spreading to the trunk and legs. The face and scalp are almost never affected. *The characteristic papules are flat-topped, shiny, purple and commonly polygonal in shape.* They are often umbilicated and appear in scratch marks (the *Koebner phenomenon*). They may become warty and form larger plaques, which can coalesce.

Delicate, white striae, annular lesions or white dots may be present on the buccal mucosa, tongue or inside of the lips. Painless oral ulceration may also develop. Its course is very variable, but it usually lasts 3–6 months.

The fingernails

Inspection of the nails often yields useful information about the patient's general health (see Chapter 1). *The nails are usually pale pink while the most common cause of nail pallor is anaemia.* Another sign of anaemia in the hands of white-skinned races is a loss of skin crease colour. When the hand is relaxed, the palmar skin creases are slightly darker than the rest of the skin, but if the skin of the palm is stretched, the creases turn a deep red. This deep red colour is not visible if the patient is anaemic.

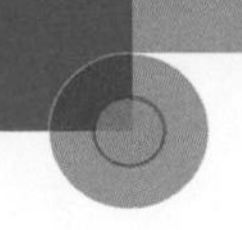

SPLINTER HAEMORRHAGES

Splinter haemorrhages are small extravasations of blood from the vessels of the nail bed caused by *minute arterial emboli.* They are long, thin, red–brown streaks, their long axis running towards the end of the finger. Their colour and shape make them look like splinters of wood beneath the nail (see Figure 1.19).

The presence of splinter haemorrhages is an important physical sign because they are usually caused by emboli from a *bacterial endocarditis or a fulminating septicaemia*. They may also occur in rheumatoid arthritis, mitral stenosis and severe hypertension.

CLUBBING

Clubbing of the nails is a term used to describe the *loss of the normal angle between the surface of the nail and the skin covering the nail bed* (see Figure 1.18). Some causes of clubbing are listed in Revision panel 4.10.

Revision panel 4.10

SOME CAUSES OF CLUBBING

- Congenital
- Carcinoma of the bronchus
- Chronic lung disease:
  - Alveolitis
  - Bronchiectasis
  - Cystic fibrosis
  - Congenital cyanotic heart disease
- Ulcerative colitis/Crohn's disease

If you look at your finger from the side, you will see that the plane of the nail and the plane of the skin covering the base of the nail bed form an angle of 130–170° (see Chapter 1). In clubbed nails, there is hypertrophy of the tissue beneath the nail bed, which makes the base of the nail bulge upwards, and distorts nail growth so that the nail becomes curved. The planes of the nail and the skin covering the nail bed then meet at an angle greater than 180°.

It is possible to have a very curved nail but still have a normal nail–nailfold angle, so do not look only at the shape of the nail when assessing clubbing – *look at the whole finger.* The terminal phalanx may enlarge to make the end of the finger bulbous (Revision panel 4.11).

Revision panel 4.11

SIGNS OF CLUBBING

- Increased nail–nailfold angle
- Increased longitudinal and transverse nail curvature
- Bulbous terminal phalanges
- Spongy nail bed

SPOON-SHAPED NAILS (KOILONYCHIA)

A normal nail is convex transversely and longitudinally, the degree of curvature varying considerably from person to person. Loss of both these curves produces a hollowed-out spoon-shaped nail (koilonychia) (see Figure 1.17).

When a patient complains that their nails have changed from a normal to a spoon shape, it is very likely that they have developed anaemia following chronic loss of blood, usually from menorrhagia or haemorrhoids.

SUBUNGUAL HAEMATOMA AND MELANOMA

A blow on a nail can cause bleeding beneath it. A collection of blood beneath the nail is called a subungual haematoma. If it appears at the time of the injury, the patient usually makes their own diagnosis, and only comes for treatment if it is painful.

Sometimes the patient does not notice the injury, and comes complaining of a brown spot beneath the nail. It is then important to decide whether the brown spot is haemosiderin or melanin – *a haematoma or a mole.* A haematoma is usually reddish-brown, with sharp edges. A melanoma is brown with a greyish tinge, and has indistinct edges (Figure 4.94).

The presence of small blood vessels in the lesion, seen using a hand lens, indicates that it is cellular.

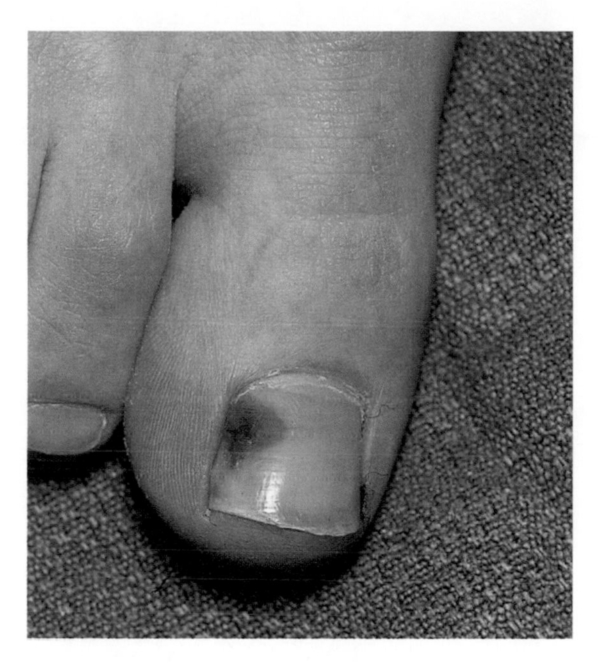

Figure 4.94 A subungual melanoma.

The patient may be able to tell you that it has moved down the nail with nail growth, or stayed still. *Haematomus move down the nail; melanomas do not move.*

If it is not possible to make a definite clinical diagnosis, the patient should be managed as if they have a melanoma until you prove otherwise.

GLOMUS TUMOUR

This is a very rare tumour, but is mentioned because it can cause a great deal of pain, and often occurs beneath the nail. It is an *angioneuromyoma*.

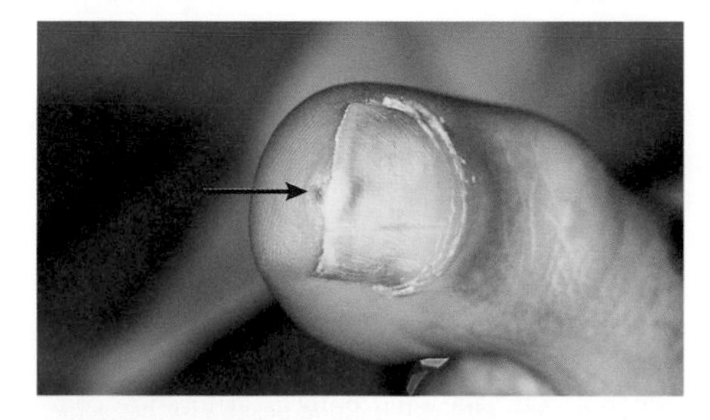

Figure 4.95 A glomus tumour.

The patient complains of severe pain every time the nail is touched. Examination usually reveals a small, purple–red spot beneath the nail (Figure 4.95). The colour is caused by the angiomatous nature of the tumour; the pain comes from its abnormally rich nerve supply.

Glomus tumours can occur in any part of the skin but are most often found in the hands.

CHANGES IN THE NAILS ASSOCIATED WITH GENERALIZED DISEASES (REVISION PANEL 4.12)

- Psoriasis: Pitting, ridges, poor growth.
- Myxoedema: Brittle nails.
- Cirrhosis of the liver: White nails.
- General debilitating illnesses: Transverse furrows (Beau's lines).
- Anaemia: Koilonychia.
- Telangiectasia: Rendu–Osler–Weber syndrome.
- Gout (and pseudogout).

Revision panel 4.12

COMMON NAIL ABNORMALITIES

Loosening
Fungal infections
Pitting
Clubbing (see Revision panel 4.11)
Longitudinal ridges
Local damage (paronychia)
Transverse ridges
Thickening and twisting (onychogryphosis)
Systemic illness (including psoriasis, thyroid myxoedema)

The toenails

The toenails may show the same changes in response to local or generalized disease that have been described for the fingernails. Paronychia and other forms of infection are far less common, but fungal infection (athlete's foot) between the toes and near the nails is very common (see above).

ONYCHOGRYPHOSIS

The normal nail is a thin plate that slides along the nail bed (Figure 4.96). When the sliding mechanism fails, the nail begins to thicken and heap up until it appears to be growing vertically out of the nail bed. It then curves over the end of the toe and looks like a 'ram's horn' – an onychogryphosis (Figures 4.96 and 4.97).

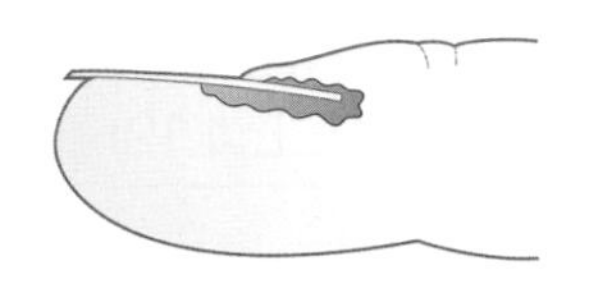

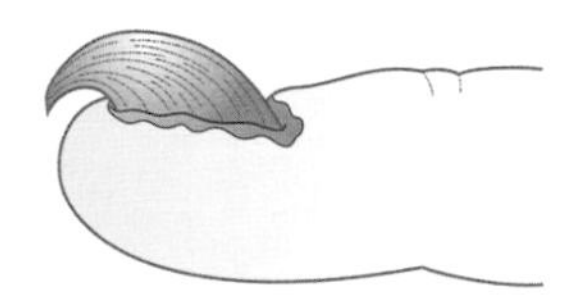

Figure 4.96 Onychogryphosis.

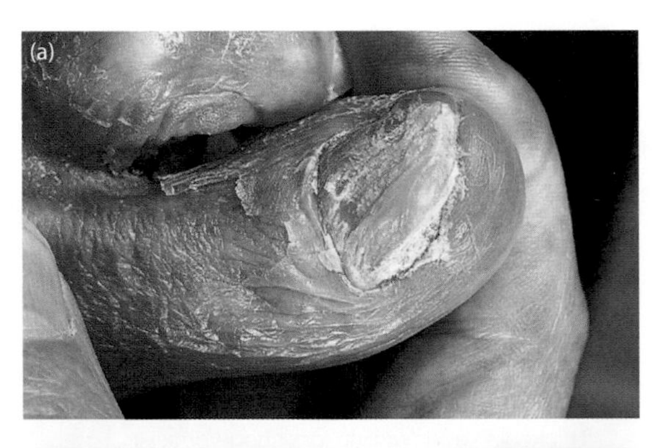

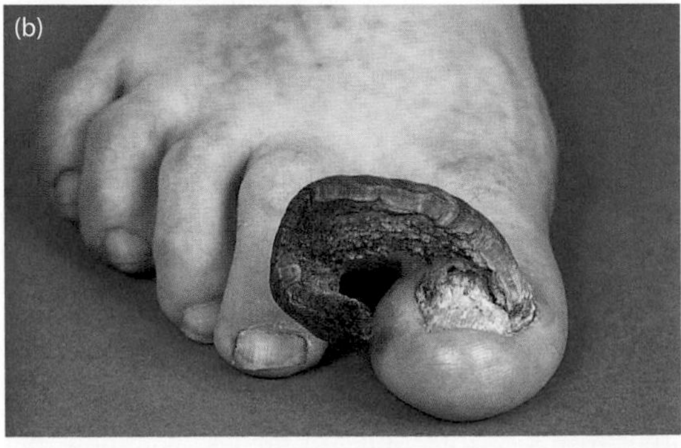

Figure 4.97 ONYCHOGRYPHOSIS. (a) Mild onychogryphosis. (b) Severe onychogryphosis.

It can occur in young people after an injury to the nail bed, but is most common in elderly people, when the sliding mechanism presumably fails in old age.

INGROWING TOENAIL

This is a common condition in which the great toenail appears to be growing or digging into the soft tissues at the side of the toe. An ingrowing toenail usually has an irregular jagged edge, which digs into the skin of the lateral fold. The damage is exacerbated when the skin at the side of the toe is forced upwards during walking. The precipitating factor is often an attempt by the patient to cut off the corner of the nail, which then gets torn off, leaving a jagged spike at the edge (Figure 4.98).

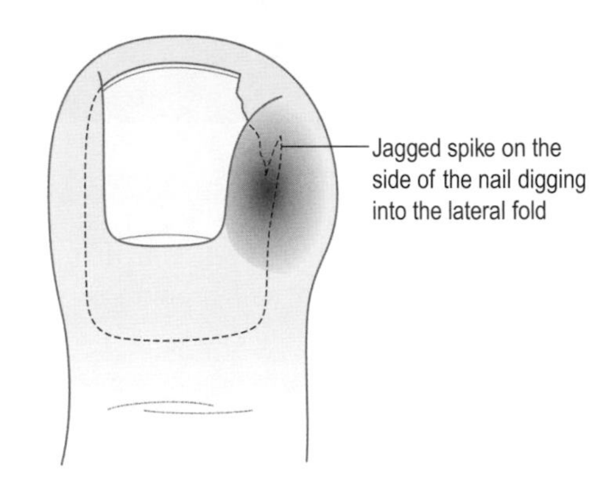

Figure 4.98 Ingrowing toenail.

History

Age and sex Ingrowing toenails are commonly found in adolescent and young adult males. Games such as football, and less stringent hygiene in young boys and males, may contribute to the sex difference.

Symptoms The principal symptom is pain. The toe is sore and painful when walking. It throbs at night if it gets badly infected. There may be a purulent or serous discharge from beneath the lateral nailfold. The skin at the lateral nailfold becomes prominent, oedematous and soggy.

Examination

Site The lateral side of the nail (between the great and second toe) is affected more than the medial side, but both sides and both great toes are commonly affected.

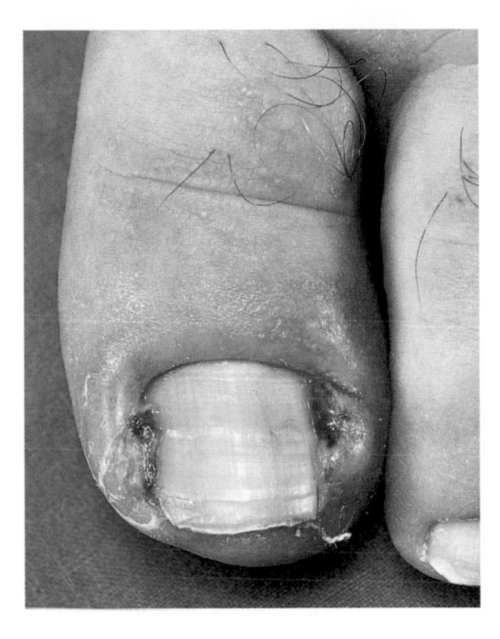

Figure 4.99 Ingrowing toenail.

Colour The skin of the lateral nailfold is reddish-blue, and red granulation tissue may be visible between the skin fold and the nail (Figure 4.99).

Tenderness The swollen skin and the nail are tender. When there is extensive infection, the whole toe is tender, and movement of the interphalangeal joint is painful.

Shape The increase in the bulk of the lateral nailfold makes the great toe appear wide, but the nail itself does not look abnormal. It may be possible to see the extent to which the nail is digging into the tissues if the nailfold can be pulled away from the nail without causing too much pain.

Lymph glands The inguinal lymph glands may be enlarged if there has been long-standing infection, but this is uncommon.

Complications Inadequate excision of the nail bed may result in the regrowth of spikes of nail.

Major injuries

RAJIV LAHIRI

This is the only chapter in this book where basic 'management' (first aid and resuscitation) is discussed with the symptoms and signs of major injuries.

NOTE: This is a deliberate decision as resuscitation and assessment are carried out simultaneously in patients with major injuries.

The physical signs produced by injury are usually more evident and immediately significant than a detailed history, especially if the patient is unconscious. Obtaining a history of the type of injury and the possible forces involved, from the patient, family members, friends, onlookers or first-aiders who witnessed the event, is always helpful, but must not interfere with the initial rapid clinical assessment and resuscitation of the patient. Information on the injured person's habits, such as drug or alcohol addictions, may also be very helpful.

The Advanced Trauma Life Support course (ATLS) has established the value of a standardized approach to trauma assessment and management, especially for the lone practitioner faced with one or more patients who have sustained severe injuries. This chapter follows the ATLS approach using an 'ABCDE' mnemonic that is easy to remember in stressful circumstances.

When an initial assessment has been made at the site of the injury, it must be repeated in the hospital. Patients presumed to have sustained major injuries should be taken straight to the resuscitation area for their primary hospital survey. Increasingly worldwide, major trauma is managed in dedicated trauma centres and critically injured patients are diverted to these centres.

Patients thought to have minor injuries should still be carefully assessed by an experienced doctor as soon as possible, as apparently stable patients may have sustained serious injuries, which may have passed undetected during the initial assessment, especially when an influx of many injured patients overwhelms local resources.

First aid

First-aiders should ensure that there is no immediate danger to themselves before approaching a casualty. Many injured patients are best served by leaving them where they are until experienced help arrives, provided the environment is not continuing to damage or threaten them. Provided the injured patient has a strong pulse, is breathing normally and is not overtly bleeding, this is invariably the correct course of action.

It is, of course, important to obtain help as soon as possible so that there is always someone available to stay with the patient to monitor their pulse and breathing, and provide moral support.

The widespread availability of smartphone technology has improved the first-aider's ability to summon help.

NOTE: Under no circumstances should an injured patient be given anything to eat or drink.

The primary survey and management at the site of the event

This is carried out under the five easily remembered headings of 'ABCDE':

- **A**irway & cervical spine control.
- **B**reathing & ventilation.
- **C**irculation & haemorrhage control.
- **D**isability (neurological evaluation).
- **E**xposure and environmental control.

This approach is particularly important when assessing patients with multiple injuries.

AIRWAY AND CERVICAL SPINE CONTROL

The signs of an obstructed airway are stridor (noisy breathing), increased respiratory effort, cyanosis (a blue colour) and apnoea (not breathing) (see Chapter 2).

It is essential to protect and secure an adequate airway. The lungs cannot oxygenate the blood if *the airway is obstructed by the jaw and tongue falling back, swollen soft tissues, vomit, blood or direct damage to the upper airway.*

The airway of unconscious patients lying on their back often becomes obstructed by their own intraoral soft tissues, but before they are rolled into the supine or semi-prone position, or the neck is extended, always consider an *associated cervical spinal injury* (see Chapter 9). All patients found to be unconscious

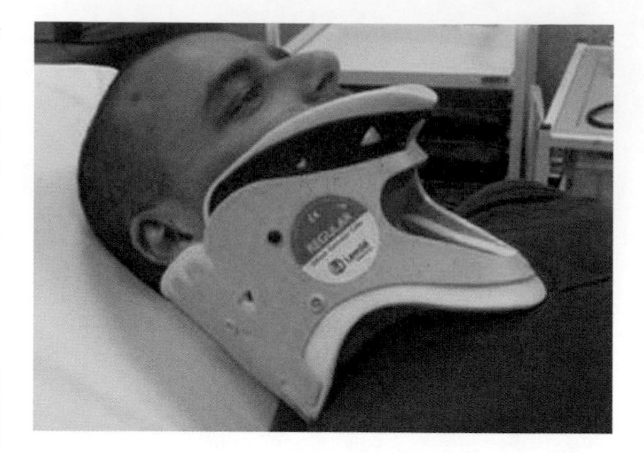

Figure 5.1 A hard collar.

after an injury must be treated as if they have an associated injury of their cervical spine, because abrupt or careless turning may further dislocate or sublux a cervical vertebra and injure the spinal cord when no injury originally existed. It is also possible to convert partial cord damage into a complete transection. *The neck should therefore be immobilized in all unconscious injured patients by in-line longitudinal, manual support and stabilization, ideally using a hard cervical collar (Figure 5.1), sand bags and tape until clinical examination and radiographs have excluded unstable fractures of the cervical spine.*

Conscious patients with threatened airway obstruction will usually find a secure position themselves, often sitting up and leaning forwards if there is significant facial trauma (see Chapter 11).

Airway obstruction in an unconscious patient can usually be relieved by a *jaw thrust*, but it may require the insertion of a *finger into the mouth to extract debris.* Rarely, airway obstruction is associated with a fractured maxilla or mandible, and the jaw or palate may need to be pulled forwards, or the patient rolled into a semi-prone position.

When there is a low suspicion of a cervical spine fracture, the patient may be rolled into the semi-prone ('recovery') position to help maintain the airway, because the absence of a gag reflex in an unconscious patient makes aspiration of saliva, vomitus or blood into the lungs a major hazard. Alternatively, an *oropharyngeal* or *nasopharyngeal airway* (Figure 5.2) should be inserted as soon as possible, and then, in an unconscious patient, replaced by an endotracheal tube inserted by an experienced anaesthetist.

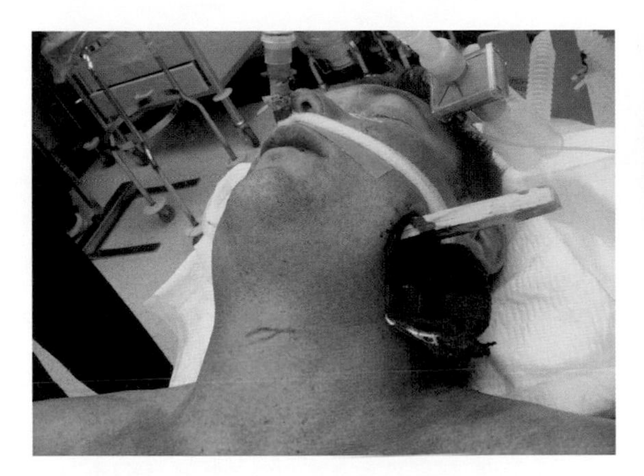

Figure 5.2 A nasopharyngeal airway.

> **NOTE:** The airway must be repeatedly reassessed to ensure that the measures you have taken are effective and secure.

BREATHING AND VENTILATION

Mouth-to-mouth ventilation combined with external cardiac massage may be life saving in patients who have undergone a short period of respiratory arrest. The mouth should be 'swept' with a finger first to ensure there are no physical obstruction to be removed. If possible, a face mask or an Ambu bag and oxygen should be used. If giving cardiopulmonary resuscitation this can be done with a 'hands-only' technique or with chest compressions and rescue breaths.

CIRCULATION

Bleeding remains the most common preventable cause of death after trauma. It is absurd to concentrate on the detailed drills of assessment of the airway and breathing if the patient obviously has a normal airway but is losing vast amounts of blood.

Severe external bleeding at the scene of the accident requires *manual compression directly over the wound or pressure proximal to the point of bleeding,* where the feeding artery can be compressed against an underlying bony point. Direct pressure is usually the most effective technique for controlling blood loss. Remember that if the pressure applied to the outside of the injured blood vessels is greater than the blood pressure, the bleeding will stop.

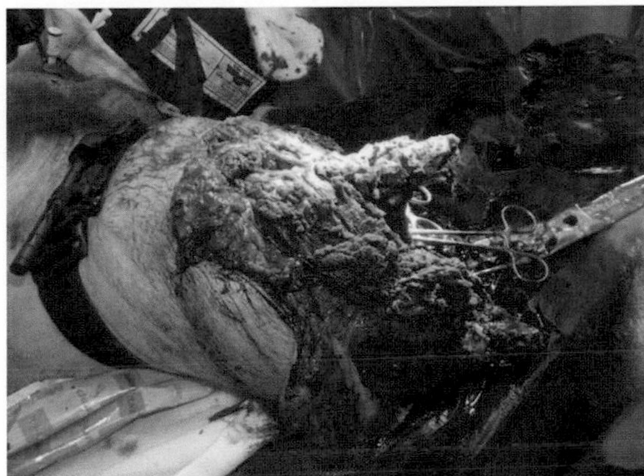

Figure 5.3 Tourniquet used by the armed forces to stop limb bleeding.

Tourniquets should only be used to stop limb bleeding. Improvised tourniquets may exacerbate bleeding by obstructing the venous outflow, while failing to occlude the arterial inflow. Ambulance crews are now often trained and equipped with specially designed tourniquets that have also proved to be effective in military use (Figure 5.3).

An effective tourniquet renders the whole limb ischaemic and will cause permanent muscle and nerve damage if it is kept in place for several hours. Tourniquets can also cause reperfusion injury when released, resulting in *metabolic acidosis, myoglobulinuria* and *hypercalcaemia.*

> **NOTE:** The time of application must be carefully recorded and passed on to ambulance and medical staff.

Direct manual pressure, provided it is achieving its desired effect (i.e. stopping or reducing the blood loss), is usually preferable to a tourniquet.

DISABILITY (NEUROLOGICAL EVALUATION)

A brief note should be made of the patient's level of consciousness using the AVPU scale. Is the patient:

- **A**lert?
- Responding to **V**oice?
- Responding to **P**ain?
- **U**nresponsive?

NOTE: The change in the level of consciousness over time is a very useful indicator of progress or evolving complications.

EXPOSURE AND ENVIRONMENTAL CONSIDERATIONS

An unconscious or immobile patient can rapidly become *hypothermic,* which exacerbates coagulopathy and acidosis. *It is important to keep the patient warm.* In other situations, other environmental hazards need to be considered.

The primary survey in the emergency department

All patients who are unconscious or suspected of having multiple or serious injuries should be admitted directly to the resuscitation area of the emergency department. For medical students to witness assessment and resuscitation in this setting is extremely valuable, as the principles of the process are relevant to many other areas of medical practice.

The clinical assessment (history and examination) and resuscitation must occur simultaneously if lives are to be saved, hence the inclusion of treatment in this chapter. The handover from the paramedics follows a basic scheme:

A – **A**llergies.
M – **M**edication history.
P – **P**ast medical & surgical history.
L – **L**ast meal.
E – mechanism of **E**vent.

The routine 'ABCDE' assessment must be repeated whatever happened before the hospital admission.

AIRWAY AND CERVICAL SPINE CONTROL

The neck must be protected by a collar and immobilized if the patient is unconscious, or if there is any suspicion of a cervical spine injury. An anaesthetist should assess the need for better control of the airway.

Look for the signs of inadequate oxygenation/ventilation (Revision Panel 5.1) (see Chapter 2). These may all indicate the need for endotracheal intubation.

Revision panel 5.1

SIGNS OF INADEQUATE OXYGENATION/ VENTILATION

- Noisy breathing (stridor)
- Respiratory distress
- Apnoea
- Cyanosis
- Loss of consciousness
- The presence of major facial, neck or chest injuries that might obstruct the airway
- Aggressive/confused behaviour

The *neck and jaw should be palpated* to check for deformity. *Insert a finger into the mouth* to extract any foreign bodies, and to check for jaw fractures (see Chapter 11). Occasionally, severe damage to the upper airways or trachea makes intubation impossible. An emergency *cricothyroidotomy* or *tracheostomy* is indicated if the patient's airway is compromised and an endotracheal tube cannot be safely inserted.

BREATHING AND VENTILATION

Assess the condition and function of the thoracic cage (see Chapter 2).

Once you are certain that the airway is patent, assess the adequacy of ventilation by inspecting, palpating, percussing and listening to the chest for *symmetry, movement, dullness and breath sounds.*

Patients with multiple injuries or chest problems causing hypoxia should be given high-flow oxygen through a closed-circuit oxygen mask from the moment of their arrival in the emergency department.

An oxygen saturation monitor is essential for assessing the effectiveness of the patient's ventilation.

INSPECTION AND PALPATION

Examination of the chest must include inspection of the back and sides of the chest wall up into the axillae.

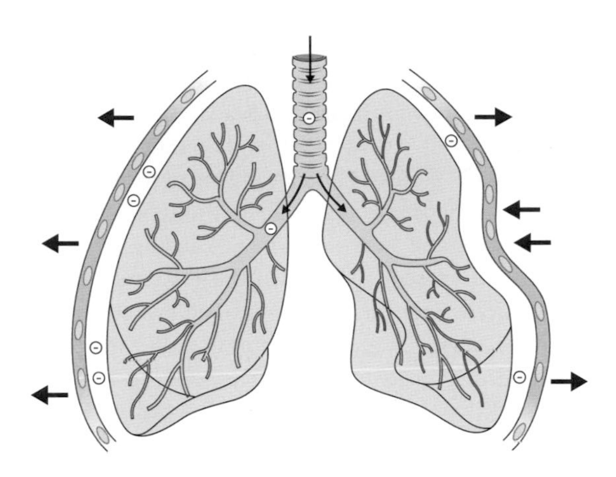

Figure 5.4 A flail segment.

Open chest wounds should be covered with a dressing occluded on three sides to prevent the development of a tension pneumothorax through a 'sucking' chest wound.

Flail segments occur where when several ribs are fractured in two places and the segments sink inwards during inspiration (Figure 5.4). This indicates a high likelihood of a pulmonary contusion, and the patient is likely to need close monitoring to prevent lung collapse and secondary pneumonia.

Bruising over the chest indicates that rib fractures are likely, and the presence of *surgical emphysema* suggests that the pleura has been breached. Surgical emphysema presents as a 'crackling sensation' on palpation of the subcutaneous tissues.

Percussion

Characteristically, a pneumothorax is hyper-resonant to percussion, and a haemothorax is dull to percussion. These signs are, however, easy to miss in a noisy emergency room, and indeed may coexist in a mixed haemo-pneumothorax.

A chest radiograph is an essential adjunct to the primary survey, except in the case of a tension pneumothorax, when clinical suspicion should prompt urgent needle decompression.

Uncomplicated pneumothoraces confirmed on chest radiographs do not necessarily require urgent chest drainage.

A *tension pneumothorax,* in which there is raised intrapleural pressure, must be suspected:

- If breathing is difficult.
- If the trachea is deviated to the contralateral side.
- If there is decreased air entry over the affected lung.

Urgent decompression is indicated if the patient is unstable, ideally with a large bore chest drain.

The rapid insertion of a chest drain that is connected to underwater seal drainage bottles will relieve a tension pneumothorax. *Needle thoracocentesis,* in which a needle is inserted into the pleural cavity through the second intercostal space in the midclavicular line, provides temporary relief while a chest drain is being prepared.

A large haemothorax may also cause respiratory and circulatory problems, which manifest as *reduced breath sounds and a dull percussion note combined with reduced vocal fremitus and vocal resonance.* The diagnosis should be confirmed with an chest radiograph, but a chest drain may occasionally have to be inserted as an emergency measure on the basis of the clinical signs.

The chest drain may occasionally need to be clamped to prevent massive continuing blood loss. Lost blood should be replaced with a crystalloid solution at first, but subsequently with blood as soon as this is available. *Massive* or *ongoing bleeding* from a haemothorax is an indication for thoracotomy.

> **NOTE:** The blood pressure must be carefully and continuously monitored to confirm the adequacy of any blood volume replacement.

CIRCULATION AND HAEMORRHAGE CONTROL

In a clinical setting, assessment and restoration of the circulation can often be performed simultaneously with management of the airway and breathing if an experienced anaesthetist is available to manage ventilation.

There are two major causes of circulatory embarrassment:

- *Haemorrhage.*
- *Cardiac damage/tamponade* (see Chapter 2).

The former is the most common cause of potentially preventable death. The latter is rarer, but also life threatening and easily missed.

Tamponade must therefore be briefly considered in all patients with major injuries, especially in those with penetrating injuries of the chest.

Revealed haemorrhage

Visible arterial bleeding presents as a pulsating stream of bright red blood, whereas venous bleeding is dark and continuous. Arterial haemorrhage from an open wound can usually be controlled by *direct digital pressure* or proximal arterial compression, either manually or by using a medically approved tourniquet or pneumatic cuff.

Deep wounds in junctional areas (the groins, shoulder and neck regions) should not be explored in the emergency department.

Venous bleeding always responds to simple pressure and may be made worse by the application of an inadequate tourniquet.

> **NOTE:** Revealed bleeding should always be assessed and controlled as soon as possible. There is no point in pouring fluid and blood into the circulation through intravenous catheters when an equal amount is rapidly escaping.

Concealed (internal) haemorrhage

This is much harder to diagnose, and therefore must be suspected in all patients with multiple or serious injuries. It always accompanies *major fractures of long bones and displaced pelvic fractures*. It must, if possible, be rapidly diagnosed and treated, as it is an important, potentially reversible, cause of death in an injured patient.

Clinical signs of haemorrhage

The diagnosis of haemorrhage is based on finding the signs of hypovolaemic shock (Revision Panel 5.2).

Revision panel 5.2

SIGNS OF HYPOVOLAEMIC SHOCK

Pale, anxious, sweaty patient with cold extremities
Rapid, thready pulse
Tachypnoea
Hypotension

These signs occur when the body redistributes the circulation in an attempt to maintain the blood flow to the vital organs (heart and brain). Other organs, such as the skin, intestine and kidneys, become inadequately perfused and poorly oxygenated.

This homeostatic response is brought about by the sympathetic nervous system causing a tachycardia and vasoconstriction in the extremities. The skin becomes cool and clammy. The systolic blood pressure is usually maintained at first, but the pulse pressure (the pressure difference between the systolic and diastolic pressures) may be reduced by a rise in the diastolic pressure. The rate of respiration increases to try to improve oxygenation.

Patients who arrive in the emergency department without overt haemorrhage but who exhibit these signs have almost certainly lost 1–2 L of blood.

> **NOTE:** It is important to remember that young, fit patients can often tolerate a considerable blood loss before they develop, often very suddenly, any signs of hypovolaemic shock, whereas elderly patients, especially those on beta-blockers or digitalis, can only tolerate quite small amounts of blood loss.

All seriously injured patients must be continuously monitored for:

- Pulse rate.
- Blood pressure.
- Respiratory rate.
- Level of consciousness.
- Tissue oxygenation.

A *urinary catheter* and the *measurement of central venous pressure* provide additional valuable information for monitoring resuscitation when there are signs of hypovolaemia. An intra-arterial pressure line is also very useful for continuously monitoring the blood pressure, and allows easy sampling of arterial blood for blood gas and acid–base measurement.

Intravenous access should be secured using two wide-bore cannulae inserted into the veins of the cubital fossae or, if ultrasound guidance and appropriate expertise are available, using a central venous catheter.

Blood must be sent for urgent grouping and cross-match.

Clinically stable patients may benefit from a crystalloid (normal saline) infusion, but unstable patients with ongoing bleeding are best resuscitated with red cell concentrate and plasma if this is available. Group O rhesus-negative blood and thawed fresh frozen plasma can be given if there is insufficient time for a cross-match.

Patients who fail to respond to the rapid restoration of their blood volume in the absence of cardiac or major respiratory problems, such as tamponade or tension pneumothorax, probably have severe continuing blood loss. In these circumstances, a blood transfusion should be started while a rapid assessment of the potential sites of concealed blood loss is made.

NOTE: The most common sites of continuing concealed haemorrhage are the *pleural or abdominal cavities.*

Fractures of the pelvis can also cause catastrophic blood loss. The retroperitoneum can also accommodate litres of blood with few external physical signs.

A rapid clinical examination looking for chest dullness, abdominal distension and abdominal tenderness (if the patient is conscious) should be followed by essential primary survey adjuncts including chest radiography and focused assessment with sonography for trauma scan.

The patient should be transferred to an operating theatre or angiography suite once the site of blood loss has been established.

Cardiac tamponade

This occurs when enough blood collects within the pericardial sac around the heart and limits its function (see Chapter 2). The cardiac output is reduced as a consequence, producing a weak pulse and hypotension.

The condition should be suspected:

- If the jugular venous pressure is markedly elevated and rises rather than falls with inspiration (*Kussmaul's sign*); remember, however, that jugular venous distension may not occur in a patient who has lost a large quantity of blood.

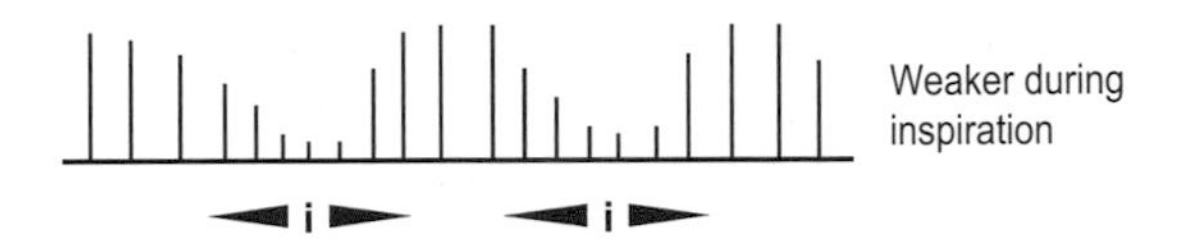

Figure 5.5 Pulsus paradoxus.

- If *pulsus paradoxus* is present, when the pulse volume decreases on inspiration rather than increasing (Figure 5.5).
- If the heart sounds are muffled and poorly heard (which can be difficult to assess in a busy trauma bay).

All of these clinical signs can easily be missed, and the most important thing is to consider the diagnosis. Chest radiographs may show an enlarged cardiac shadow. An *echocardiogram* will confirm the diagnosis.

Definitive surgery is needed through either a left lateral thoracotomy or a sternotomy for life-threatening tamponade.

Echocardiographs and electrocardiographs (ECGs) can be helpful if cardiac injury or coincidental cardiac disease is suspected. The ECG leads should be kept connected to a monitor to detect any dysrhythmias. A cardiac contusional injury should be suspected if there is widespread ST segment elevation or depression.

Very occasionally, a resuscitative or 'clam-shell' thoracotomy in the emergency department may be required to relieve a tamponade, to suture a penetrating wound of the heart or to clamp the hilum of the lung or the descending aorta to prevent massive blood loss. These heroic attempts are often unsuccessful. Rapid transfer to an operating theatre with trained staff, proper instruments and adequate lighting increases the chances of success.

DISABILITY

Following assessment of circulation and control of haemorrhage, a rapid evaluation of central nervous function is performed to establish the patient's level of consciousness, pupillary reflexes and gross motor function. This is performed quickly using *the Glasgow Coma Scale* (shown in Table 3.2). Patients with a Glasgow Coma Scale less than 8 have severe brain injury and cannot protect their airway, therefore require intubation.

At this point it is essential to check the *blood glucose level* as hypoglycaemia can reduce the conscious level and is easily correctable.

EXPOSURE

The final part of the primary survey is to *fully undress* the patient to ensure no injuries are missed. It is also important to cover the patient with warmed blankets and to give warmed intravenous fluids. This helps to prevent hypothermia, which, along with acidosis and hypercoagulability, forms the lethal triad of trauma. The primary survey should be fast, systematic and follow the same steps in all cases (see Revision panel 5.3).

Revision panel 5.3

Systematic assessment of the trauma patient is vital and reproducible. ALWAYS begin with the primary survey:

Airway & cervical spine control
Breathing & ventilation
Circulation & haemorrhage control
Disability (neurological evaluation)
Exposure and environmental control

Do not move onto the next step in the primary survey until all issues with the current step are addressed

The secondary survey

Many injured patients do not deteriorate catastrophically. This provides time to carry out a full secondary survey to assess other systems and body parts that may have been injured and to assess the general fitness of the patient. Continuous monitoring of the patient is essential during the secondary survey to detect any further/new bleeding or chest problems.

The whole patient must be examined from the top of the head to the toes. Other blood tests, investigations and diagnostic procedures should be undertaken as necessary after the secondary survey has been completed. Adequate analgesia may be needed before beginning the secondary survey, especially in fully conscious patients in whom the primary survey and resuscitation have been quickly completed.

History

A detailed history should be taken from a stable, conscious patient at this stage. It is helpful to ask the patient what they remember of the accident, and useful if they can describe what happened. The mechanism of the injury and the possible physical forces involved often give a useful indication of the site and severity of the damage.

It is often helpful to know about:

- The height of a fall.
- The speed of a car.
- The use of guns or knives.
- The presence of an explosion or fire.
- The use of protection devices such as seat belts or airbags.

Obtain the observations and views of family, friends, bystanders or paramedics if the patient is unconscious.

Pain, dysfunction and malfunction

The conscious patient should be asked if they have any localized areas of pain or malfunction, which may indicate particular areas or systems that require more detailed examination.

Conscious patients must also be asked if they experienced any loss of consciousness during or after the injury. Their cognitive function should be quickly tested by asking a few questions about who they are, where they live and their occupation. The history from a third party of a lucid interval is also helpful if the patient is unconscious.

General and previous history

Take a full history of previous illnesses, operations, drugs and allergies (see Chapter 1). The patient's general fitness, occupation and tobacco and alcohol usage should be recorded following a full systematic enquiry.

Record the time that the patient *last ate or drank*. This is very important if the patient is to have a general anaesthetic.

General examination of a conscious patient

THE HEAD

Scalp This must be inspected and palpated for lacerations, swellings, bony depression and distortion.

Orbits Palpate the margins of the orbits for depressions or irregularities.

Eyes Examine the eyes for pupil size, reaction and the red reflex. Test the eye movements and visual acuity (see Chapter 1).

The presence of a large *subconjunctival haemorrhage* (Figure 5.6) that spreads to the full extent of the conjunctival attachment suggests that there is a fracture of the base of the skull.

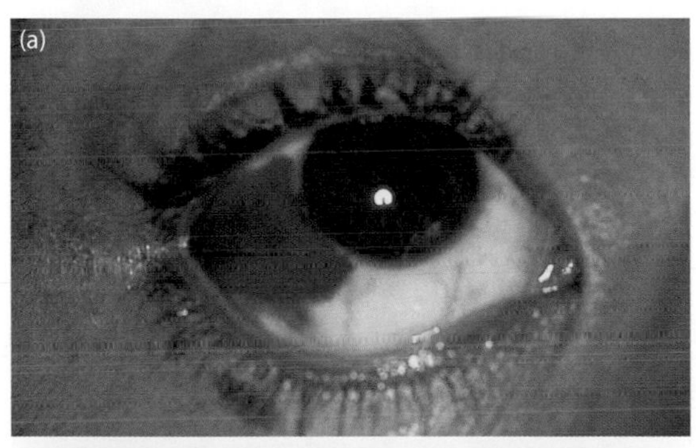

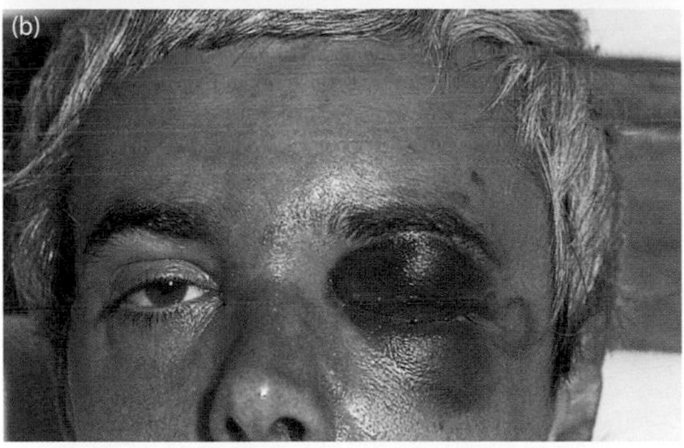

Figure 5.6 SUBCONJUNCTIVAL HAEMORRHAGE. (a) A subconjunctival haemorrhage may arise from a subconjunctival vessel or be blood that has tracked forwards from behind the eye – usually from a fracture of the base of the skull. (b) Extensive bleeding from a fracture of the base of the skull may cause a large periorbital haematoma as well as a subconjunctival haemorrhage.

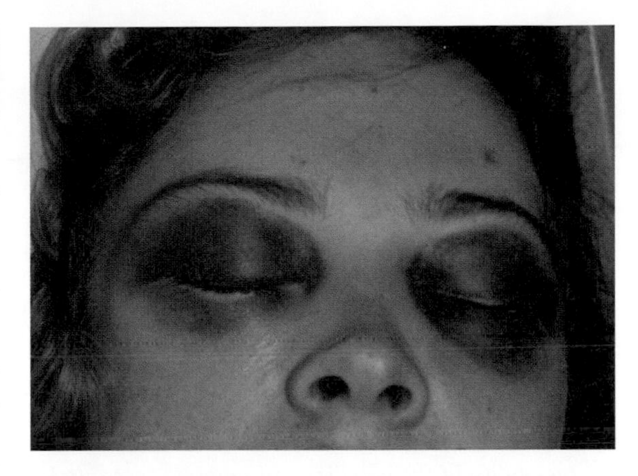

Figure 5.7 Panda eyes. Extensive periorbital extravasation of blood from a fracture of the base of the skull.

Panda eyes (black circumorbital haematomas around one or both eyes) (Figure 5.7) also suggest the presence of a skull base fracture or a fracture of the upper jaw.

Diplopia, especially on looking up, is indicative of a blow-out fracture of the floor of the orbit, which often allows the eyeball to sink inwards, giving the upper face an asymmetrical appearance.

SIGNS OF INTRACRANIAL HAEMORRHAGE (SEE CHAPTER 3)

A fixed dilated pupil indicates IIIrd cranial nerve compression, by a contralateral extradural haemorrhage or a direct injury to the optic nerve.

Deterioration of the patient's Glasgow Coma Scale score and/or agitation indicates increasing cerebral compression.

Loss of upwards gaze, other cranial nerve pareses and the development of contralateral hemiplegia are indicative of a cerebral haemorrhage.

Observations should also be made on the patient's mental state, including whether they are agitated or confused.

A rising blood pressure, a falling pulse (Cushing's reflex) and slowing of respiration suggest coning, a condition in which the swollen brain is forced down into the medullary foramen, with subsequent loss of all vital functions. An urgent CT scan and neurosurgical opinion should be sought.

THE FACE (SEE CHAPTER 11)

Major facial injuries can cause considerable orbital oedema, but it is very important to *retract the lids* carefully, using two people if necessary, to look for any of the features described above.

The *cheek bones should also be palpated* for a 'step', and any asymmetry should be noted.

Fractures of the zygoma and blow-out fractures of the orbit have to be confirmed by CT, but loss of sensation over the cheek from damage to the infraorbital nerve strongly suggests a fracture of the cheek bones.

Instability of the maxillary zygomatic process (a Le Fort-type fracture) is tested by inserting a gloved finger or thumb into the mouth and attempting to pull the upper jaw complex forwards from the base of the skull (Figure 5.8). A fracture is present if rocking occurs.

This needs to be done with care, as forceful rocking may cause a massive pharyngeal bleed, which can only be controlled by pushing the whole bony facial complex backwards to compress the bleeding vessels.

The *lower jaw and its stability on the temporomandibular joints* must also be assessed. Malocclusion and an open-bite deformity suggest a fractured jaw, as does numbness of the lower lip.

Carefully palpate and inspect the mouth, teeth and gums, and record the number of missing or damaged teeth. *Missing teeth indicate the need for a chest X-ray, to exclude the possibility that they have been inhaled and are lodged in the lung.*

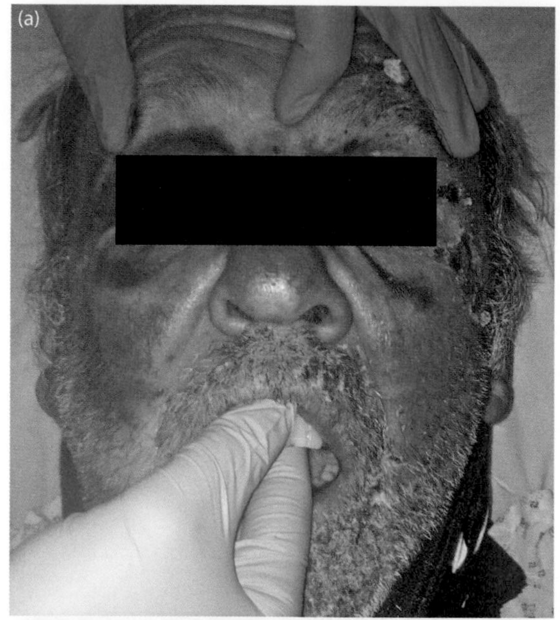

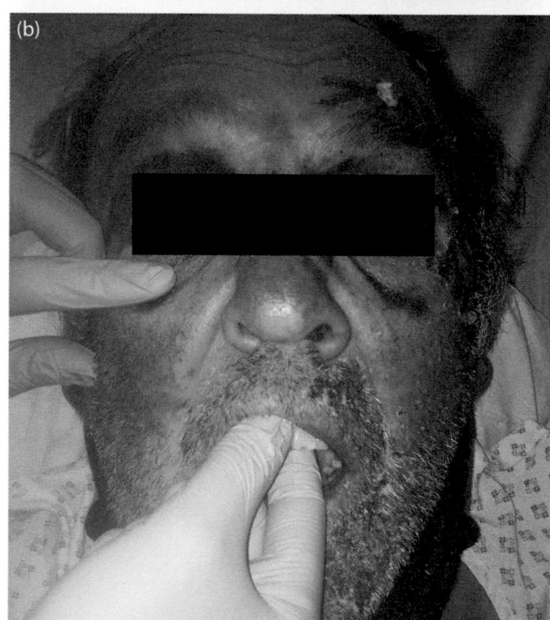

Figure 5.8 LE FORT FRACTURE. (a, b) The maxilla being pulled forwards for the diagnosis of a Le Fort fracture.

THE NOSE AND EARS

The *nose should be palpated* to exclude a fracture and detect the presence of any bloody or clear fluid discharge of *cerebrospinal fluid*, which would suggest the presence of a fracture in the *anterior cranial fossa* (often associated with panda eyes and an extensive subconjunctival haemorrhage).

The facial muscles (VIIth cranial nerve) and auditory acuity should be tested.

Blood or fluid coming from the ear suggests the presence of a posterior fossa fracture.

The tympanic membrane must be examined with an auroscope. Bruising behind the ear (*Battle's sign*) (Figure 5.9) suggests a fracture in the posterior cranial fossa.

CT scans with bone windows are usually required to assess these injuries.

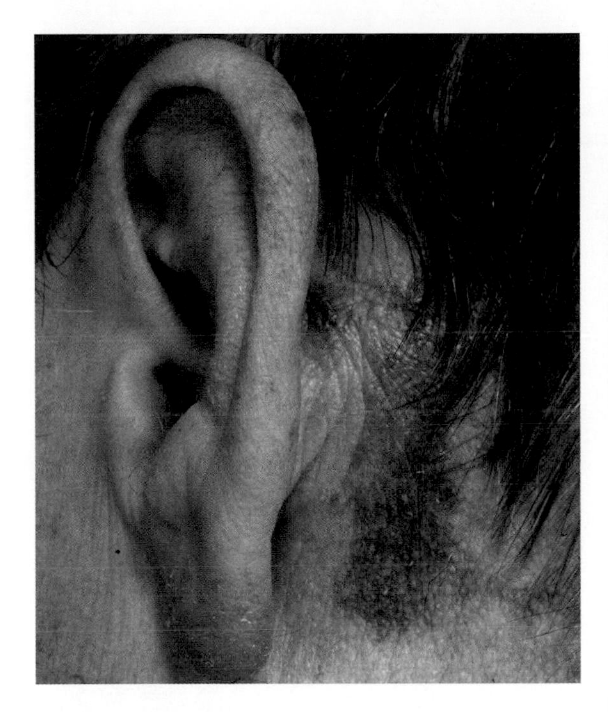

Figure 5.9 Battle's sign. Bruising behind the ear suggests a fracture in the posterior cranial fossa.

THE NECK (SEE CHAPTER 9)

Pain and local tenderness are suggestive of a cervical fracture, but there may be few, if any, physical signs, and further assessment may have to be delayed until the condition of the cervical spine has been established. The importance of *not causing or exacerbating any spinal cord damage*, especially during airway assessment, endotracheal incubation or moving the patient, is now well recognized.

If there are any concerns that the spine may have been damaged, a full radiological assessment of the cervical spine should be carried out as soon as the patient is relatively stable. A CT scan may be necessary if plain radiographic views are inadequate.

The *neck can be carefully palpated for bruising* and *deformity* and inspected for any penetrating wounds if the spine is normal. Gentle palpation should detect the presence of any subcutaneous surgical emphysema in the neck or supraclavicular fossae.

Penetrating descending wounds of the root of the neck can be very dangerous, as they may cause damage to the supra-aortic blood vessels – the carotid, vertebral and subclavian arteries – as well as to the trachea,

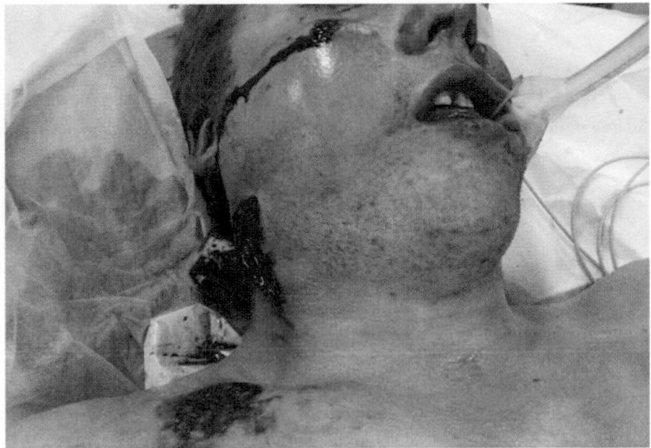

Figure 5.10 An entry wound in the neck.

larynx, pharynx and oesophagus (Figure 5.10). Major structures within the upper chest can also be damaged. The presence of neurological signs or ischaemia of the upper limb suggests a major arterial injury, as does a rapidly expanding haematoma or a machinery murmur.

> **NOTE:** Neck wounds should be explored in the operating theatre.

The *clavicle should be palpated along its course*. Severe compound clavicular injuries are often associated with injuries to the subclavian or axillary vessels, the brachial plexus and the apex of the lung. *Examine the vascular supply and peripheral nerves of both upper limbs* to exclude these possibilities.

THE CHEST (SEE CHAPTER 2)

Although the chest was assessed as part of the primary survey, it should now be carefully reassessed by inspection, palpation, percussion and auscultation to detect any signs that may have been missed at the time of the primary survey, when rapid resuscitation was essential. New signs may have developed, and subtle signs may have been missed. *Remember to check the back and sides of the chest, including into the axillae.*

Test again for rib fractures. A careful inspection may detect a small flail segment. Pain on compression or release indicates the likelihood of rib fractures or costal cartilage separation from the ribs or sternum. Both can then be more accurately localized by detailed palpation. It should be remembered that rib fractures are often associated with injuries of the great vessels, lungs, spleen or liver.

The *sternum must also be inspected and palpated.* Sternal fractures are often associated with cardiac injuries.

Check again for the presence of a haemothorax, pneumothorax and cardiac tamponade, taking particular care to look for small pneumothoraces and an increase in the width of the mediastinum, which may be the only indication of an aortic dissection.

CT of the chest is highly sensitive and specific in detecting cardiothoracic trauma.

THE ABDOMEN (SEE CHAPTER 15)

The primary survey of the abdomen usually detects the signs of major intra-abdominal haemorrhage, but a secondary survey is essential to pick up continuing severe haemorrhage or further bleeding following the restoration of a normal blood pressure.

Increasing abdominal distension, tenderness and guarding are all significant signs, especially when associated with a rising pulse and other signs of hypovolaemia.

The bowel sounds may or may not be abolished by free blood or bowel contents in the peritoneal cavity.

Skin bruising over the abdomen (Figure 5.11), penetrating wounds and associated rib fractures all indicate the possibility of abdominal organ damage.

When doubt persists, CT scanning is indicated. A CT scan can also be very useful if there is an associated pelvic fracture.

Blood coming from the external urethral meatus or frank haematuria suggests kidney, bladder or urethral damage (see Chapters 17 and 18). Rectal and vaginal examination can confirm a high riding and boggy prostate, or associated vaginal injuries. The presence of these injuries must always be excluded before allowing catheterization by inexperienced junior staff or nurses. It may be preferable to insert a suprapubic catheter if palpation or percussion detects a large bladder, especially if the prostate feels abnormal or blood has been seen coming from the urethra.

THE UPPER AND LOWER LIMBS (SEE CHAPTERS 7 AND 8)

All surfaces of the limbs must be fully inspected, taking careful note of the presence of:

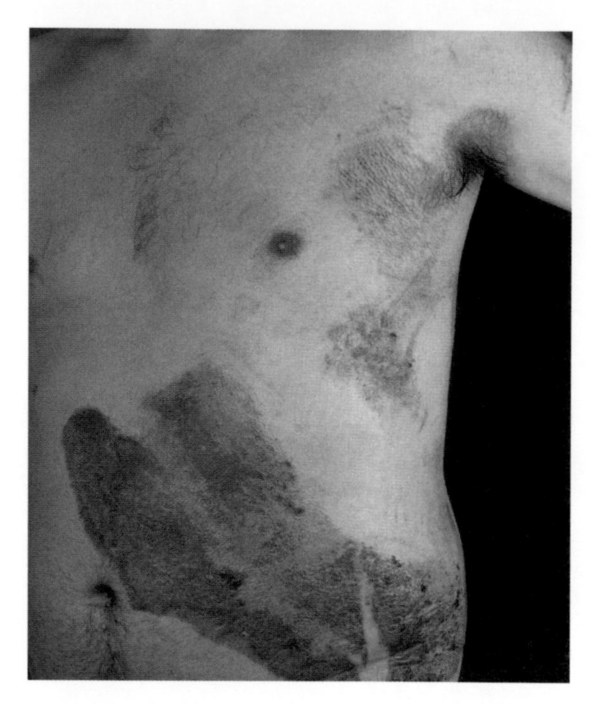

Figure 5.11 Abdominal trauma. This shows the impression and bruising made by a seat-belt, which is often associated with underlying abdominal trauma.

- Bruising.
- Lacerations.
- Instability.
- Deformity.

All the major bones should be carefully palpated along their full length to detect any bony deformity and swelling that were not appreciated by the inspection. The only indication of an undiagnosed, undisplaced fracture may be the detection of a localized point of tenderness. Major fractures are almost always associated with some deformity, together with swelling from the associated bleeding.

The radial and pedal pulses should be felt and compared (see Chapter 10). The presence of equal symmetrical pulses indicates that a major vascular injury in the limbs is unlikely (see Chapter 7). Unfortunately, the peripheral pulses are often difficult to feel in a shocked, cold patient with severe limb bruising and concomitant fractures. When the pulses cannot be felt in an adequately resuscitated patient, it is helpful to measure the arterial pressure with a Doppler flow detector.

Persisting pallor, especially if it only affects one limb, is a sign of severe ischaemia.

> **NOTE:** The presence of a compartment syndrome must always be considered when there are combined orthopaedic and vascular injuries.

This condition may also follow the successful surgical revascularization of an injured limb. Compartment syndromes begin with pain, tenderness and swelling over the anterior shin or calf muscles. The swelling can exacerbate the ischaemia, obliterate the pulses and lead to muscle and nerve death if left untreated.

The peripheral nerves (see Chapter 3)

These must be fully examined in both the upper and lower limbs if the patient is conscious. Test the power, tone, coordination, sensation and reflexes. Test the movement of joints controlled by the major muscle groups. Test sensation by the response to light touch and pinprick. Always test and document an examination of the peripheral nerves beyond any laceration. A more detailed neurological examination should be carried out if abnormal neurological signs are detected, or if the patient is unconscious (see below).

THE BACK (THORACO-LUMBAR SPINE) (SEE CHAPTER 9)

The logroll can be performed in either the primary or secondary survey. The discovery of the paralysis or weakness of several muscles may be the first indication of a spinal cord injury. The patient must then be carefully immobilized to facilitate examination of the spine. Log-rolling allows the patient to be turned in a coordinated manner that keeps the spine immobilized at all times (Figure 5.12).

Palpation down the back over the spinous processes may detect a boggy swelling, a deformity or a 'step' in the regularity of the spinous processes. While the patient is on their side, take the opportunity to inspect and palpate the back of the head, neck, torso and limbs to exclude any major injuries to this surface of the body that may have passed unnoticed at the initial survey.

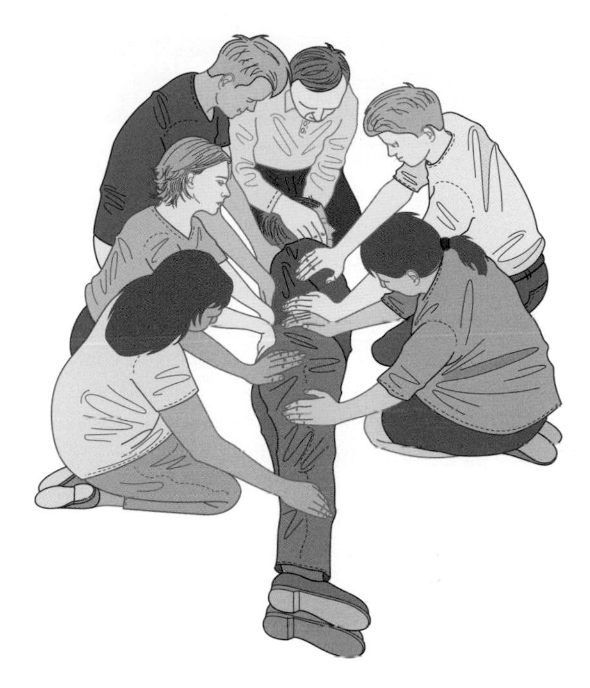

Figure 5.12 The log-rolling technique.

A *rectal examination* should be performed at this stage, and perianal sensation, motor function, sphincter tone and the bulbocavernosus reflex tested.

CT or MRI scans are often required if a spinal fracture or spinal cord injury is suspected. The secondary survey is a comprehensive head to toe assessment performed after life-threatening injuries have been excluded or definitively managed (Revision panel 5.4).

Revision panel 5.4

SECONDARY SURVEY

- The secondary survey is a comprehensive clinical assessment to examine the entire body for injuries ('top to toe examination')
- Smaller injuries (e.g. scaphoid fracture on dominant hand) can easily be missed and have a significant effect on patients in the long term
- Most major trauma centres have secondary survey proformas to minimize the chance of missing smaller injuries

The secondary survey in the unconscious patient

Assessment of the unconscious patient is challenging because of the lack of patient response. The aim of the secondary survey is the same as in the conscious patient, but specific attention needs to be paid to the neurological examination.

Monitoring of the Glasgow Coma Scale score must be carried out at frequent intervals in comatose patients with a score of 8 or less. Patients must be frequently asked to open their eyes and move their limbs. Apply a painful stimulus by pressing hard on the bone of the upper orbit or the manubrium sterni if they do not respond. An ability to localize pain is accepted if the patient moves one or other hand to try to push away the painful stimulus, whereas flexion or, worse still, extension of the upper limbs indicates a severe brain injury.

Verbal responses are impossible to assess in patients who are anaesthetized or intubated, or have suffered severe facial injuries.

> **NOTE:** It must also be remembered that some head-injured patients may have intellectual difficulties, some may have taken an overdose of drugs or alcohol and some be unable to understand your language.

If the brain is shifted to one side by an expanding haematoma, the ipsilateral IIIrd cranial nerve becomes compressed against the rigid free edge of the tentorium cerebelli. At first, this causes slight constriction of the pupil, but then, later, dilatation and eventually a failure to respond to a bright light being shone directly into it.

The haematoma will continue to expand and force the brain down through the tentorium and into the foramen magnum if left untreated (see Chapter 3). The contralateral pupil then becomes dilated and unreactive. Compression of the medulla eventually causes bradycardia, a rising blood pressure and depressed respiration.

Do not forget that optic nerve injuries, previous eye disorders and drugs can also cause the *pupil to be unresponsive*.

Neurological examination of the limb should concentrate on detecting any evidence of *hemiplegia. Unilateral paralysis,* increased muscle tone, brisk reflexes and upgoing plantar reflexes on the contralateral side of the injury all indicate that a haematoma is present.

Intracranial haematomas outside the substance of the brain can be either extradural or intradural.

An *extradural haematoma* is usually the result of haemorrhage from the middle meningeal artery. This is often caused by a linear temporoparietal fracture of the skull. Patients are often briefly knocked unconscious or dazed by the initial injury, but then regain consciousness (*the lucid interval*) before becoming drowsy and eventually losing consciousness. As the intracranial pressure rises, patients may complain of a headache, blurred vision and vomiting. At this time, the localizing signs described above begin to develop.

> **NOTE:** It must be remembered that some patients develop an extradural haematoma without a lucid interval, and without the classic progression of neurological signs.

The certain indicator of deterioration is a progressive reduction in their Glasgow Coma Scale score. A CT scan will confirm the diagnosis.

A *subdural haematoma* can be classified as either acute or chronic. Acute subdural haematomas are invariably associated with a major brain injury when torn vessels on the surface of the brain continue to bleed into the subdural space. Patients are usually deeply unconscious and develop neurological localizing signs.

It is very difficult to clinically differentiate an acute subdural haematoma from:

- An intracerebral haemorrhage.
- Cerebral oedema.
- Diffuse axonal injury.

Chronic subdural haematomas usually occur in elderly patients after a minor injury that tears a vein on the surface of the brain, which bleeds slowly but persistently for days or weeks. They are also common in alcoholics and patients on anticoagulants. Patients often present with fluctuating levels of consciousness, worsening over several days or weeks. The raised intracranial pressure may cause headache, vomiting, blurred vision (papilloedema) (see Figure 1.20), personality change and drowsiness. Pupillary changes and some neurological localizing signs are usually present.

The diagnosis is confirmed by a CT scan of the brain.

Tertiary survey

Following admission to hospital and stabilization after traumatic injury it is essential to perform a tertiary survey, ideally within 24–48 hours of admission. This is because patients with multiple injuries may be distracted from minor injuries that may be missed without thorough, detailed examination.

The tertiary survey should follow the same process as the secondary survey described earlier in this chapter. In addition to detailed clinical examination, it is essential to review all radiological investigations and the reports. Trauma patients often have a multitude of radiological tests and small, occult injuries can be missed without review.

Assessment of multiple casualties

All hospitals should have a major accident plan in which the roles of emergency doctors, other medical staff, nurses, theatre staff, telephone staff, managers and press liaison officers are all clearly defined. These plans should be tested from time to time to assess their effectiveness and encourage familiarity.

Each patient must be carefully assessed by the techniques described above into:

- Those who are dead.
- Those with immediate life-threatening injuries.
- Those with major injuries.
- The 'walking wounded'.

In summary, the management of critically ill trauma patients requires the ability to perform a rapid systematic assessment of life-threatening injuries in a busy trauma bay. Following the ATLS primary and secondary surveys is essential as it facilitates the treatment of life threatening injuries in a systematic way.

In the evaluation of critically injured patients, teamwork is king. Each member of the trauma team is assigned a role by the team leader, thereby not putting any single individual under undue duress. The primary survey is relatively task focused compared to a general examination (e.g. in outpatients) so an experienced team leader is essential to assimilate all the information gathered and to plan for further treatment. When the patient is stable, a detailed secondary survey is required to rule out any distracting injuries (Revision panel 5.5). This comprehensive examination is an excellent opportunity to perform a neurological, orthopaedic, thoracic, cardiovascular and abdominal examination in one sitting. It also regularly yields further injuries that will need to be addressed.

Revision panel 5.5

- A *systematic primary survey* is essential for identifying life-threatening injuries that can be addressed immediately
- A *detailed secondary survey* can alter the management of trauma patients due to the identification of distracting injuries
- *Tertiary surveys* involve a review of radiological investigations as well as clinical examination. This can reveal concurrent pathology (e.g. pancreatic cysts, adrenal incidentalomas) that require further investigation
- *Teamwork is paramount in trauma resuscitation*

Acknowledgements

The contribution of Tom Carrell to this chapter in the 5th edition is gratefully acknowledged.

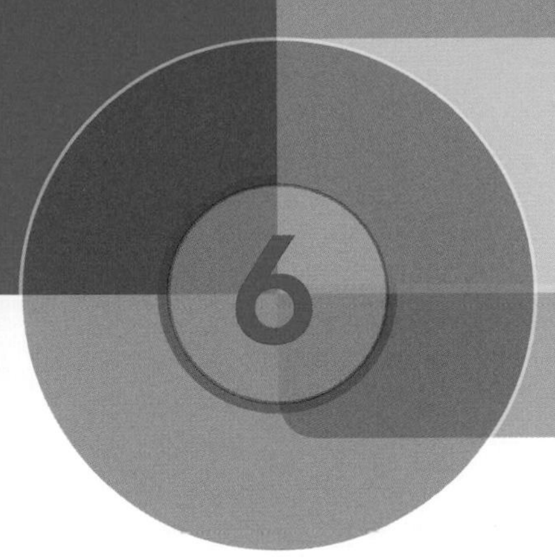

Bones, joints, muscles and tendons

STEVEN A CORBETT, ADIL AJUIED, RICHARD KEEN AND JONATHAN REES

It is essential to learn how to examine the bones and joints properly, which must include an assessment of function, as well as the detection of any structural abnormalities that may be present. This is important because as well as those patients who present to musculoskeletal services, many patients present with musculoskeletal manifestations of systemic disease to other medical services.

Common symptoms

Pain

This is the most common symptom, and pain must be adequately explored and assessed (onset, character, duration, etc.), as has already been discussed in detail in Chapter 1.

It is important to obtain the precise location of 'musculoskeletal pain', which is *usually related to movement*, whereas its severity and character are less helpful in coming to a correct diagnosis. Do not forget that *pain referral* is common; for example, hip pain may be experienced in the knee, and knee pain may be referred to the hip via the obturator nerve. Bone pain and joint pain can be *diffuse* and poorly localized.

Musculoskeletal pain is usually improved by rest and aggravated by movement. The presence of *night pain* is a strong indicator that there is significant disease, and that further assessment and treatment is required to improve the patient's quality of life.

Injury

Any history of problems, especially pain or loss of function after injury, suggests the possibility of bone *fractures* or *joint dislocations*. Soft tissue injuries such as muscle tears or tears of the joint capsules, can also result from trauma, and must be considered. A *pathological* fracture should be excluded when the injury leading to a fracture appears trivial, or radiographs suggest underlying bone abnormality prior to fracture.

Deformity

This may be either congenital or acquired, and the latter may occur following a fracture such as the 'dinner fork' abnormality seen in a Colles-type wrist fracture.

Common congenital abnormalities include club feet (talipes), knock knees (genu valgus) and bow-legs (genu varus).

Contractures of soft tissues and neuropathic damage can lead to deformity, as can large tumours arising from bone, cartilage and soft tissue. Some deformities can disappear with time, while others may progress, with serious consequences.

Stiffness

This may be 'generalized' or 'localized to a single joint or limb'. Early morning generalized stiffness in all joints, especially the hands, is a characteristic of rheumatoid arthritis, while short-lived stiffness of a specific joint, such as the hip, following inactivity, is indicative of osteoarthritis.

'Joint locking'

This occurs most commonly within the knee and elbow, although any joint can be affected. Locking is when there is a sudden inability to 'move' the joint. This is the result of a combination of pain, apprehension and a mechanical block to movement within the joint. This can be followed by 'unlocking' when the structure responsible for the block shifts position.

Swelling

This may arise in a bone, soft tissues or a joint. The swelling may be the result of a congenital deformity, inflammation, fluid or blood accumulation, infection or neoplasm.

Inflammatory or infective swellings are usually painful and associated with pyrexia and malaise, while 'tumours' are commonly painless and progressive. Haematomas are usually sudden in onset, normally follow an injury and then improve, while joint effusions are mostly the result of arthritis and may fluctuate in volume.

Instability

This occurs when a limb 'gives way'. This can be repetitive as a result of ligamentous laxity (patellar dislocation in young females) or following trauma (recurrent dislocation of the shoulder).

Weakness

This is usually the result of disorders of muscles or nerves, although joint disease can also result in muscle weakness. An assessment of which individual muscle groups are weak, combined with a full neurological examination (see Chapter 3), may indicate where the problem lies.

Loss of function

This is a combination of 'symptoms' and their 'effect on the patient'. Examples include an inability to work, run or bend over, which may be the result of disease in the hip, knee or back. The importance of functional loss varies with the occupation and hobbies of the individual.

Alteration in sensation

Numbness or tingling (paraesthesia) is often the result of *nerve damage* (e.g. a prolapsed intervertebral disc), *ischaemia* (e.g. Volkmann's contracture) or *compression* (e.g. carpal tunnel syndrome), although primary neuronal disease must always be considered and excluded. The presence of an upper or lower motor neuron lesion must be established by appropriate examination of limb tone and reflexes (see Chapter 3).

General plan for examining the muscles, bones and joints of a limb

This can be broken down into five components:

- Inspection.
- Palpation.
- Movement.
- Percussion and/or auscultation when indicated.
- Special tests.

Although moving the limb is normally part of inspection and palpation, it is such an important part of the examination that it should be regarded as a separate entity.

> **NOTE:** Percussion, auscultation and special tests are not relevant to all joints or bones.

Examination may be simplified into the four-letter words beloved of the late Alan Apley:

- Look.
- Feel.
- Move.

To these is added X-ray.

Always ask the patient to perform *active movements* before performing *passive movements,* and then remember to check for any *abnormal movements.* Remember that the following is a general plan; the examination of individual joints, bones, tendons and muscles is considered in later chapters.

Remember that the upper and lower limbs should be viewed from both *the front and the back,* which may require the patient to be both standing and supine. The normal limb should always be examined first.

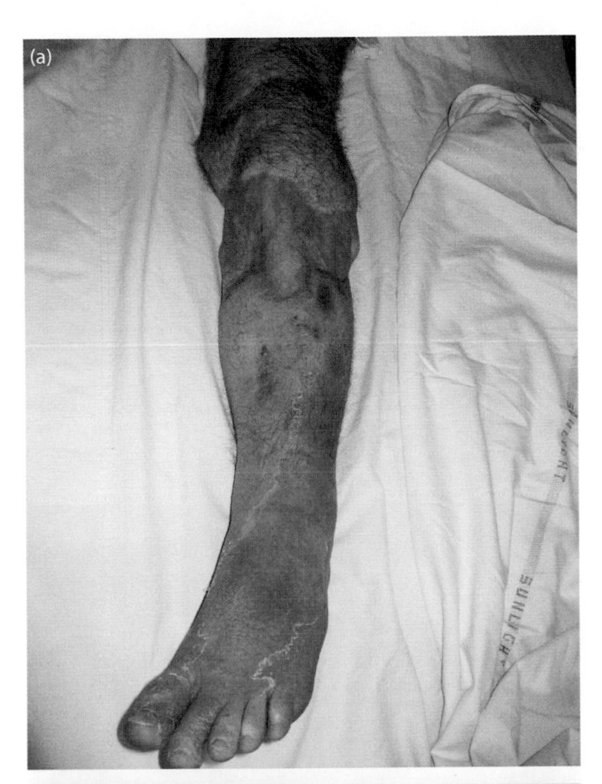

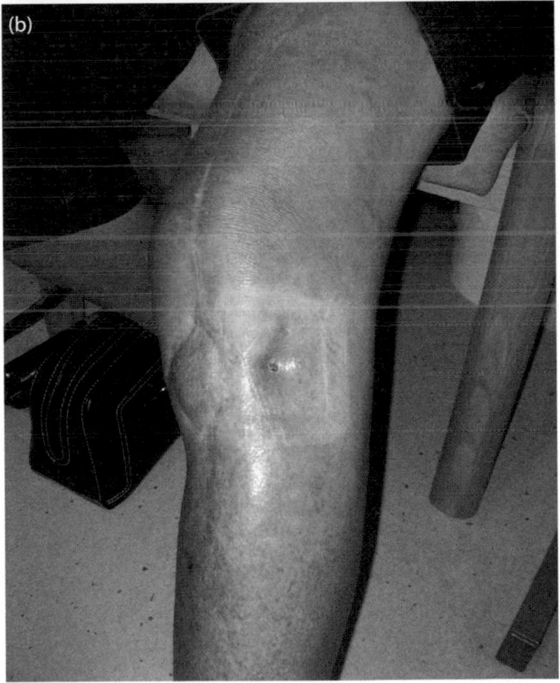

Figure 6.1 (a, b) Sinuses and scars.

INSPECTION

Skin The skin should be assessed for *discolouration, erythema and oedema.* The presence of *bruising* may indicate recent trauma.

Look for *traumatic or surgical scars and sinuses* (Figure 6.1) (see Chapter 4). Observe any *abnormal or asymmetrical skin creases.*

Shape Observe the shape of the limb and consider whether there is a *true deformity* or a *postural alteration* in its appearance. Try to ascertain if the deformity is confined to a single joint (Figure 6.2) or if it is more generalized (Figure 6.3).

Consider whether there is any *swelling* present, and whether this is diffuse or symmetrical or asymmetrical. Symmetrical swelling is more common in rheumatoid arthritis, whilst asymmetrical is more likely in osteoarthritis. Finally, look for *muscular wasting* (Figure 6.4).

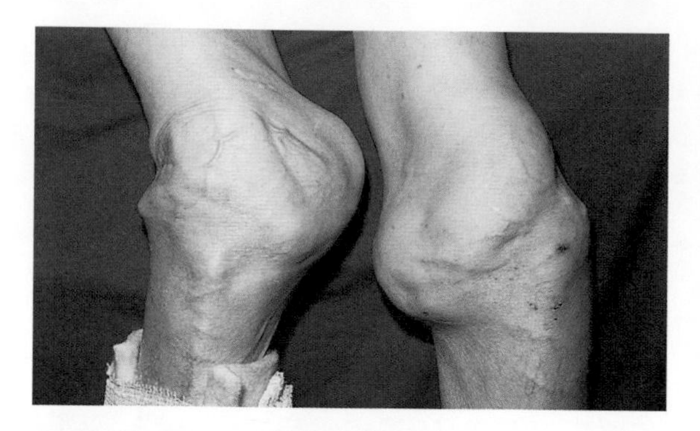

Figure 6.2 Grossly deformed knees that are the results of neuropathic joints.

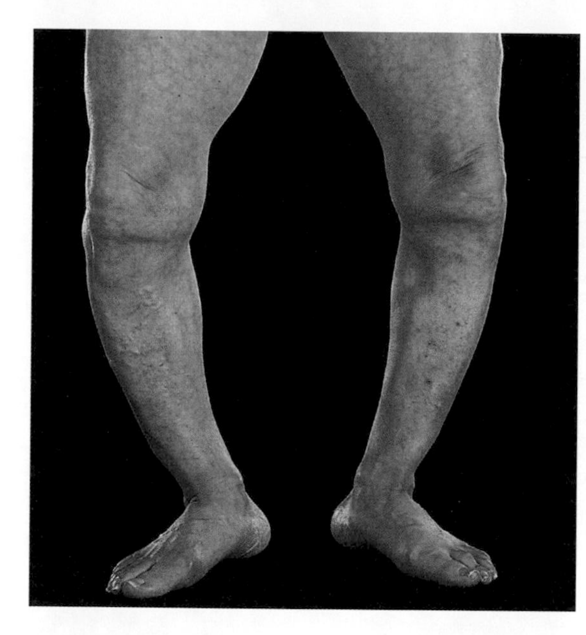

Figure 6.3 Marked deformity of the lower limbs associated with rickets.

Length Make a visual comparison of the length of each part of the limb with the other side.

PALPATION

Skin Assess the *temperature* of the skin.

Palpate for *oedema* and try to decide whether it is local or dependent.

There may be *tenderness* of the limb, which again may be diffuse or localized.

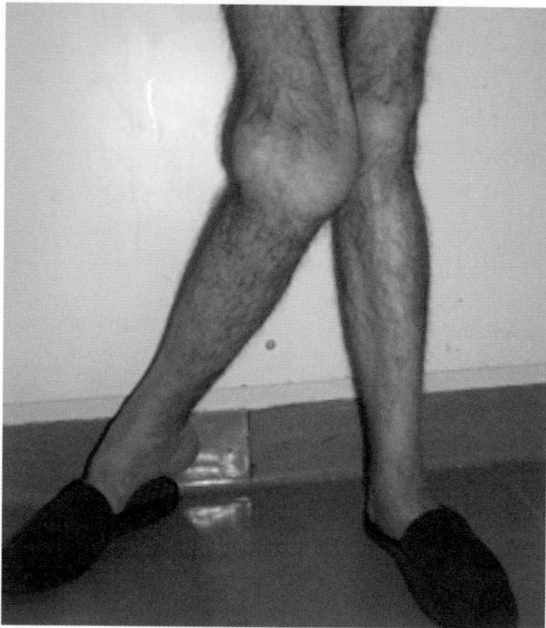

Figure 6.4 Charcot knee in valgus secondary to syphilis with associated quadriceps wasting.

Shape Try to define the cause of any swelling; for example, a swelling confined to a joint may be:

- An effusion.
- Haemarthrosis.
- Pyoarthrosis.
- Thickening of the synovium.

Localized masses may be arising from the muscle or bone.

Note the relation of any swelling to the underlying or neighbouring anatomical structures, and elicit all its physical characteristics, as described in Chapter 1.

Record on a diagram any abnormality and degree of deformity of alignment.

Length Measure the *real and apparent length of each limb* and of each bone (see page 191).

MOVEMENT

Active Ask the patient to move each joint through its full range of movements and show you any tricks or abnormal movements. Watch the limb function on standing, walking, lifting, etc.

Passive Move all the joints of the limb through their full range.

A *complete loss of all movement* of a joint implies either surgical arthrodesis (fixation) or fibrous or bony ankylosis (consolidation or union), as it may be the result of a pathological process, such as infection (see below).

Note *any restriction to movement or fixed deformity*, which may result from contraction of the joint capsule, muscles or tendons. Locking or limitation may also occur as a result of the interposition of soft tissues, bone or loose bodies.

Record as accurately as possible the range of movements in degrees (e.g. 0–90° of flexion).

Test the strength of each movement against resistance (see page 91). Feel and listen for any *clicks or crepitations* (crackling sensations) in the joint on movement.

Abnormal movements Test for these by testing the integrity of the ligaments of each joint.

OTHER TESTS

It is essential to examine the structures that keep the limb alive and make it work – the arteries and nerves.

Arteries Palpate all the pulses (see Chapter 10).

Nerves Peripheral nerves may have **s**ensory, **m**otor, **a**utonomic, **r**eflex and **t**rophic (**SMART**) activity. The objective of the assessment is to identify the nerve root innervation of any pathology (see Chapter 3):

- **Sensory.** Check the appreciation of light touch, pinprick, temperature change, deep pain, vibration sense and position sense.
- **Motor.** During your examination of movement and strength, you will already have obtained some information on the ability of the muscles to contract. If weakness is present, determine which muscles are affected.
- **Reflexes.** Test all the limb's reflexes for reduced or increased activity (see Chapter 3).
- **Trophic/autonomic.** The skin may have an abnormal appearance and may feel hot or cold and sweat excessively.

Examination of the muscles

When a muscle appears to contain a definite lump, begin by examining the lump to ascertain its physical characteristics, as described in Chapter 1. It is better to examine the muscle first and the lump second if there is doubt about the relationship of a lump to the whole muscle.

INSPECTION

Observe the shape of the muscle at rest. Note any:

- Wasting.
- Hypertrophy.
- Irregularity of shape caused by a lump, or displacement of the muscle.

Always compare the abnormal muscle with the normal muscle of the other limb.

Observe the shape of the muscle when it contracts. Alterations in shape that appear when the muscle is contracting are caused by a lump either being concealed or made more obvious by the muscle fibres either closing together or separating.

Look at the adjacent bones and joints.

PALPATION

Place the limb in a comfortable position so that the muscle is relaxed before feeling the muscle at rest.

Try to decide whether any abnormality is caused by:

- A localized swelling.
- An abnormal muscle.

Elicit all the features of any lump (see Chapter 1).

Feel the muscle when it is contracted and record any changes in the position of the mass.

A lump inside or beneath the muscle becomes more difficult to feel when the muscle contracts (Figure 6.5). A lump superficial to the muscle, or breaking through its fibrous sheath, becomes more prominent.

A gap or hollow that appears in the muscle when it contracts usually means that the fibres have ruptured (see below).

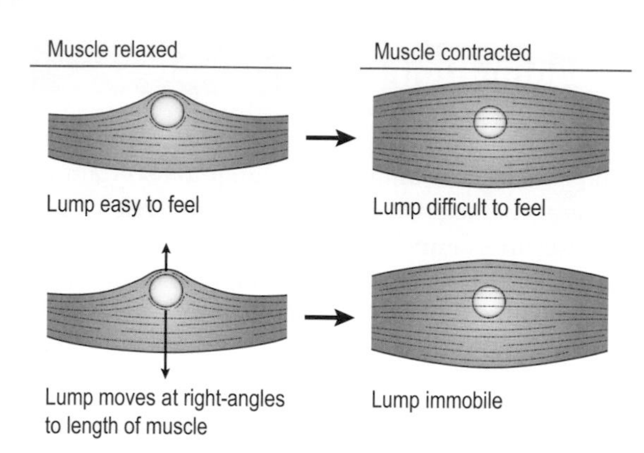

Figure 6.5 Principal features of an intramuscular lump.

STRENGTH

Muscle power can be classified according to the Medical Research Council scale. It is often better not to use numbers but to describe the strength:

- M0: No active contraction is visible.
- M1: Muscle contraction is visible but there is no movement of the joint.
- M2: Active movement is possible if gravity is eliminated.
- M3: Active movement can overcome gravity but not resistance applied by the examiner.
- M4: Active movement can overcome gravity and some resistance applied by the examiner.
- M5: There is full power against resistance.

Remember that muscle strength can be impaired by pain, wasting, denervation or other disease processes.

INNERVATION AND BLOOD SUPPLY

You will know if a muscle is innervated after testing its motor function, but you must also examine the integrity of the whole nerve and the spinal segment supplying the muscle by testing all of its other *motor, sensory and reflex functions* (see Chapter 3). This means that you must know which nerves and which spinal segments innervate the main muscle blocks in the body.

The pulses in the limb must all be palpated (see Chapter 10).

Examination of the bones

The basic plan follows the same format, namely:

- Look.
- Feel.
- Move.

INSPECTION

An old tethered scar or a discharging sinus in the overlying skin is indicative of old or active *osteomyelitis* (see Figure 6.1).

Redness and oedema of the skin are suggestive of underlying infection, inflammation or a malignant growth.

When there is a visible bony deformity, its site and the overall alignment of the limb should be recorded (see Figures 6.2 and 6.3).

PALPATION

Feel the whole length of the bone to assess its shape and compare it with the normal side. If there is a *localized swelling*, all its physical signs must be elicited (see Chapter 1).

The *temperature* of the overlying skin should be assessed, as conditions that increase the bone's blood flow, such as infection, tumours and Paget's disease, may raise the temperature of the surrounding tissues.

MEASUREMENT

There are three measurements that can be made of a limb and its constituent bones:

- The true length of individual bones.
- The apparent length of the whole limb.
- The true length of the whole limb.

The methods and principles of measurement are best described with respect to the lower limb; however, they apply equally to the upper limb, although these are less frequently utilized.

Bone length

Measurement of a single bone is straightforward as the measurement does not cross a joint.

Choose recognizable anatomical points at either end of the bone and measure between them.

Do the same on the other side and compare your findings.

Bony points must be felt through the overlying skin and muscle, and it is difficult to get the end of the tape measure on identical points on both sides. The easiest method is to hold the tape measure between your thumb and index finger, and then press the back of the index finger firmly up against the bony point or edge that you are using as a landmark.

Apparent length of the limb

When a patient lies flat and 'straight' on a couch, the limbs may appear to be of different length (Figure 6.6). This may be caused by a bone or joint abnormality. It is customary to record the *apparent length,* because when it is compared with the *true length,* it gives some indication of the degree to which the skeleton has adapted its position to keep both legs parallel and both feet flat on the ground when the patient stands up, or alternatively an indication of the effect of a joint deformity on the length of the limb.

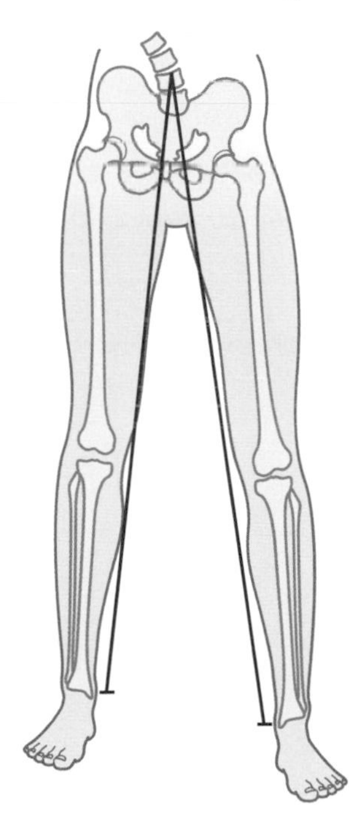

Figure 6.6 The apparent length of the limbs is measured from a central point with the patient lying comfortably straight. It is not possible with this measurement to tell whether any difference in limb length is caused by a bone or a joint abnormality.

Ask the patient to lie straight on the bed. Choose a point in the midline of the trunk – the umbilicus or xiphisternum – and measure from this central point to the tips of both medial malleoli (Figure 6.7). These lengths will be the apparent lengths of the limbs.

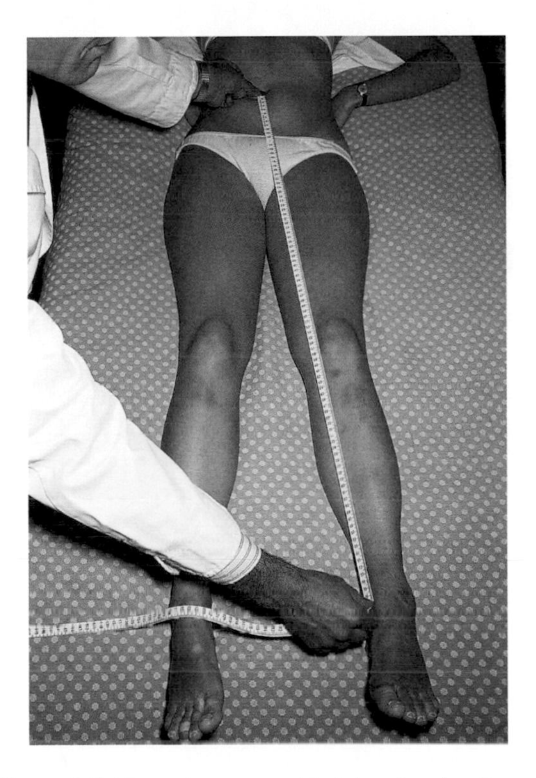

Figure 6.7 Measuring *apparent* limb length using the umbilicus as the measuring point.

Real or true length of the limb

To find out the real length of the limb (i.e. the combined true length of the limb bones and joints, unaffected by the position of the spine, pelvis or hip joints), measure between fixed bony points at each end of the limb with the joints in identical positions. In the leg, the most used points are the anterior superior iliac spine and the tip of the medial malleolus (Figure 6.8).

The position of the joints profoundly affects this measurement. Figure 6.9a shows the measurements between the iliac spines and the medial malleoli in a patient, lying straight in bed, with disease of the left hip that has caused some fixed flexion and

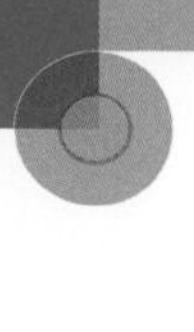

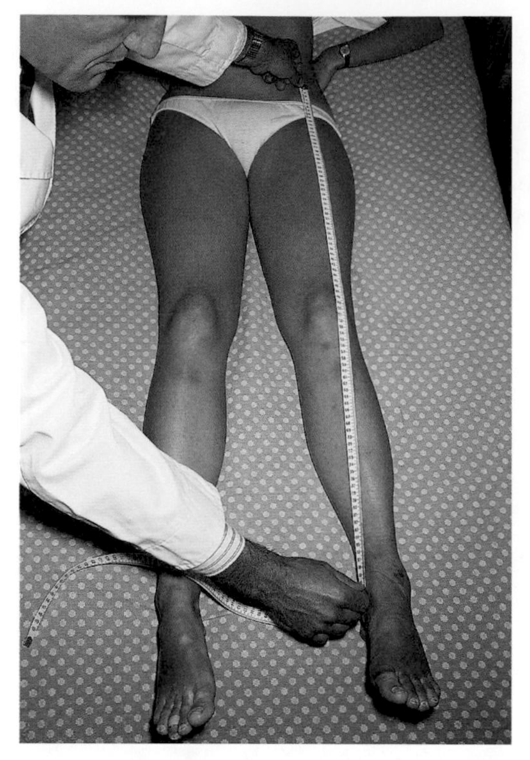

Figure 6.8 Measuring *real* limb length using the anterior superior iliac spine as the measuring point.

abduction. In order to lie straight in the bed, the patient has tilted their pelvis and adducted the other hip. There will be different measurements between the iliac spine and malleolus in this position, because one hip is abducted and the other adducted.

Before measuring the real limb length, the joints of both limbs must be placed in identical positions (Figure 6.9b, c). The pelvis must first be set square to the sagittal plane, by checking that both iliac spines are in the same plane, at a right angle to the line of the spine. This may result in the hip and femur on the diseased side being abducted or adducted. The normal leg must be placed in the same position. Next check that the positions of the knee joints are identical – if one has some fixed flexion, flex the good side to the same degree (Figure 6.10).

Once the positions of the legs are identical, measurements on both sides, from anterior superior iliac spine to medial malleolus, can be made to establish a true comparison of the real leg lengths.

JOINT DEFORMITIES

Record the deformity of a joint in terms of the *angle by which the distal bone is deviated from the*

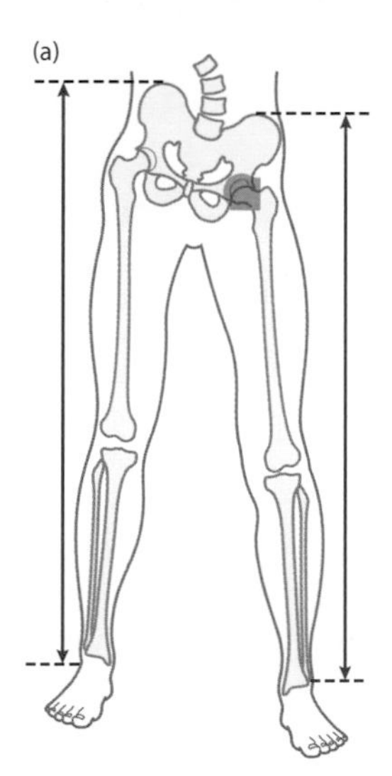

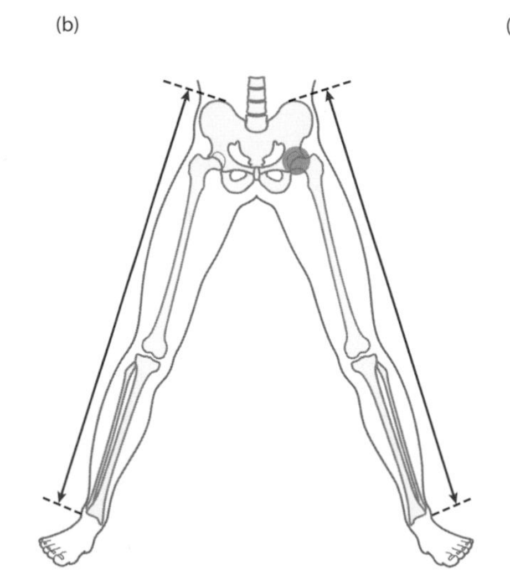

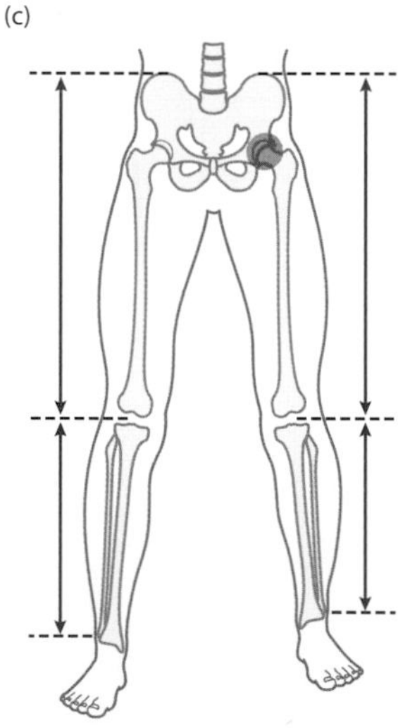

Figure 6.9 Measuring limb length.

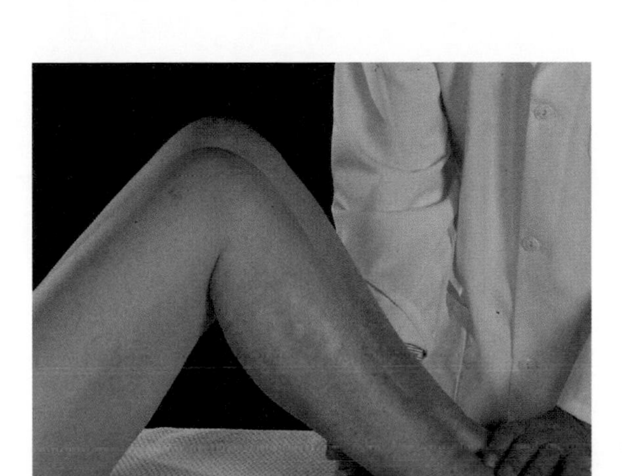

Figure 6.10 A quick method of detecting difference in bone length is to put the patient's heels together, with the knees flexed, and look from the side and the end of the bed. This patient has shortening of the right tibia and femur.

sagittal plane (i.e. the angle of *varus* or *valgus* – see below). Bones may also be rotated on their long axis. Assess the *angle of rotation* from the displacement of the bony protuberances from their normal position.

MOVEMENT

Examine the joints at both ends of the bone. Also make certain that each bone moves as one piece. A fracture will clearly be painful, and it is seldom necessary to confirm the discontinuity. Sometimes a false joint (pseudarthrosis) may develop in the shaft of a long bone as the result of non-union of a fracture and may produce pain-free abnormal movement.

Examination of the joints

The two most common joint abnormalities that you will find are swelling and deformity.

Swelling of a joint must be caused by one or more of:

- Bony enlargement.
- Synovial thickening.
- An effusion.

Deformity of a joint is invariably caused by one or more of:

- Skin contractures (e.g. a scar following burns).
- Fascial contracture (e.g. Dupuytren's contracture).
- Muscle spasm or weakness.
- Tendon division or fixation.
- Capsular fibrosis.
- Bone deformity.

INSPECTION

Observe the colour of the overlying skin, and whether there are any associated sinuses or scars (see Figure 6.1).

Consider the shape of the joint and any obvious deformity (see Figure 6.2).

Malalignment of a joint in the coronal plane, the plane of abduction and adduction, is known as *a valgus* or *a varus deformity*:

- There is a *valgus* deformity if the limb below the joint is angled away from the midline (abducted) (Figure 6.11).
- There is a *varus* deformity if the limb below the joint is angled towards the midline (adducted) (Figure 6.11).

Assess whether there is any general or localized swelling, and whether there is any muscular wasting (see Figure 6.4).

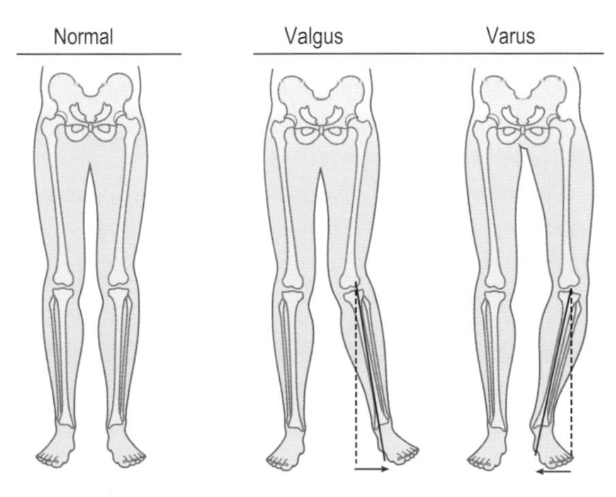

Figure 6.11 The definition of a varus and a valgus deformity. In a valgus deformity, the distal bone forming the joint is abnormally abducted. In a varus deformity, it is abnormally adducted. Remember, knock knees = genu valgum.

Also review the other joints in the limb and note the position in which the patient holds the joint.

PALPATION

Feel the temperature and texture of the skin over the joint. The subcutaneous tissues may be normal or thickened.

Muscles Feel the local muscles for wasting and tone. The muscles may be in spasm if joint movement is painful.

Synovium The synovial membrane or capsule may be *thickened and palpable*. This is unusual, although there may be an *effusion* from excess synovial fluid.

Bones Define the contours of the bones that form the joint. Check that they are in their correct anatomical positions.

MOVEMENT

Active movement Ask the patient to move the joint through its full range of movements. Record the degree of any limitation of movement and any associated discomfort.

Strength of movements Make the patient move the joint against resistance so that you can assess the strength of the muscles producing each movement. Record the power of such movements (see page 91).

Passive movements Move the joint through its full range of movement with the patient's muscles relaxed. Note any *crepitus* (grating sensations) felt during this passive movement, as well as any pain or discomfort.

Ligaments Check the integrity of each ligament associated with the joint by stretching it. This will also reveal any abnormal movements.

General examination of the limb

Examine the arteries, nerves, lymph glands and other joints of the limb.

Examination of specific joints will be presented in the relevant chapters.

Conditions of muscles

RUPTURED MUSCLE FIBRES AND INTRAMUSCULAR HAEMATOMAS

Muscle fibres usually rupture during an excessively strong or unusually sudden contraction. Rupture can also occur following a normal contraction if the muscle is weakened by a pathological process. The rupture may occur in the muscle belly or at the musculotendinous junction. As part of the healing process, an intramuscular haematoma forms within the muscle belly.

History

Age Muscle rupture can occur at all ages, but is most common in young males during exercise, and elderly males performing excessive or unaccustomed physical activity.

Symptoms There is usually pain, swelling and bruising at the time of the rupture.

Site Muscles commonly affected include the *quadriceps, hamstrings and gastrocnemius of the lower limb* and the *biceps of the upper limb.*

Examination

The diagnostic feature of a muscle tear is a depression when the muscle contracts, which is usually associated with a lump on either side from the torn ends of the muscle (Figure 6.12). The lumps cannot be felt when the muscle is relaxed because they have

Relaxed

May be a small depression

Contracted

A lump appears on one or both sides of a sharp depression

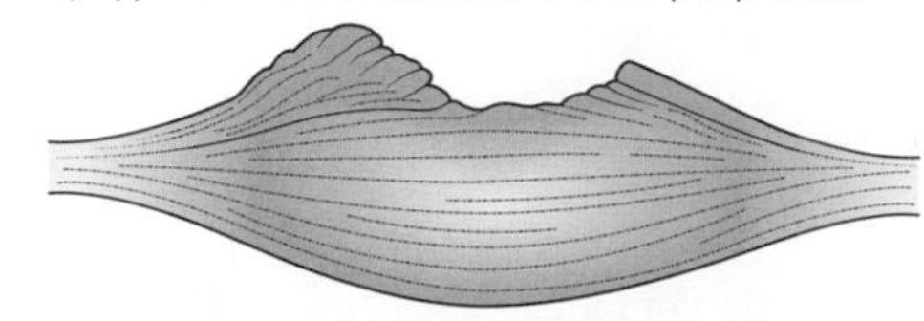

Figure 6.12 The clinical features of ruptured muscle fibres.

the same consistency as the adjacent muscle, but the hollow between the broken fibres may be visible and palpable.

As the muscle fibres try to heal, a haematoma will form, which is tender for a few days, before it is ultimately resorbed.

The local arteries, nerves, bones and joints are normal, as are the adjacent bones and joints.

The strength of the muscle is reduced if a significant number of fibres are ruptured. The muscle action will be lost if all its fibres are ruptured, unless other muscles contribute to its function.

MUSCLE HERNIA

This occurs when a muscle bulges through its surrounding fibrous sheath. The hernia may be visible at rest, but when the muscle contracts, it is likely to become more apparent.

History

Symptoms The patient may notice the lump when looking at or feeling the muscle or experience a slight ache in the muscle and find a lump when trying to pinpoint the source of the discomfort.

Examination

Site Although all muscles are surrounded by a fibrous sheath, only those with a thick covering are likely to cause symptomatic muscle hernias. A common muscle hernia is through the thick fascia that covers the anterior compartment of the lower leg.

Shape and size Muscle hernias can be of any size. Their characteristic feature is that they change in size according to the tension in the muscle. When the muscle contracts, it bulges through the fascial defect. When the muscle is relaxed, there is no lump – just a hole.

These signs are occasionally reversed. The muscle may bulge through the defect when relaxed but be pulled back into its compartment when it retracts. Do not be confused by this variation. Provided the lump comes and goes as the muscle tension changes and there is a palpable defect in its covering fascia, it is a muscle hernia.

INTRAMUSCULAR AND INTERMUSCULAR LIPOMA

Although there is little fat inside a muscle itself, there are often small collections of fat around the nutrient blood vessels and in the loose areolar tissue that separates groups of muscles. Lipomas can develop in this fat. Histologically, they are no different from any other lipomas, but the site gives them some distinctive physical signs.

History

Symptoms An intramuscular or intermuscular lipoma may interfere with the function of the muscle and causes pain when the muscle is being used, but it rarely makes the muscle weak.

The patient may have felt, or seen, a lump appear during exercise. The patient sometimes experiences a sharp pain and notices the sudden appearance of the lump if an intramuscular lipoma suddenly bursts out of a muscle during exercise. They often believe that the exercise caused the lump. The lump may change in size and shape as the muscle contracts.

Muscle lipomas are rarely multiple.

Examination

Site Any muscle can be affected. There is more fat between the flat muscles of the trunk than between the muscles of the limbs; hence lipomas are more common in this region.

Shape and size If there are only a thin layer of muscle or fascia covering the lipoma, its typical multilobular shape may be palpable (see Chapter 4).

These lipomas are often quite large (5–10 cm in diameter) because they grow unnoticed within or between the muscles for many years. They may become larger or smaller, or disappear when the muscle contracts, according to their relation to the main bulk of the muscle.

Edge Their edge is difficult to feel. When a lipoma has herniated through the thick layer of fibrous tissue surrounding the muscle, you may feel a sharp edge, corresponding to the defect in the fascia, but there is usually a lot more of the lipoma deep to this edge that you cannot feel.

Composition The consistency varies with the tension in the muscle. When the muscle is relaxed, the lipoma has its typical soft consistency and may seem to fluctuate. When the muscle contracts, the lipoma becomes hard and tense if it is still palpable.

Relations Intermuscular and intramuscular lipomas are tethered to their site of origin and usually become fixed when the muscle contracts. An

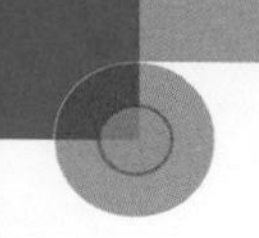

intermuscular lipoma may become impalpable when the muscle overlying it contracts.

MYOSITIS OSSIFICANS

Myositis ossificans is calcification, or ossification, in part of a muscle. It is an uncommon condition that may follow an injury that has caused *extensive intramuscular haemorrhage*, sometimes associated with a fracture of the adjacent bone. Commonly affected muscles are the brachialis, after an elbow fracture, and the quadriceps femoris, after a fracture of the femur or a direct blow to the muscle. The patient often has an associated head injury.

History

Previous injury The patient will describe a recent fracture or previous injury.

Symptoms Stiffness is the principal symptom because the muscle cannot relax and contract normally, and the bone that forms may block movement. Ultimately, any joint that is involved may become fixed. While forced movements may be painful, the condition is usually painless once the original injury has resolved.

Examination

Site, size and shape The common sites for myositis ossificans are the lower part of the brachialis muscle and the lower part of the quadriceps femoris muscle. Its size and shape are very variable. The ossification tends to take the shape of the muscle in which it is occurring. It has an irregular outline.

Tenderness The mass of ossified muscle is not normally tender but forced passive movements may cause pain.

Temperature The mass has a normal temperature.

Composition The mass is bony hard.

Relations The ossification in the muscle may be continuous with callus around an associated fracture, and hence it may be mistaken for a bony swelling.

The muscles over the callus of a healing fracture usually function normally, whereas ossifying muscles cannot work properly and cannot be moved over the callus.

Local tissues There may be other evidence of the previous trauma – bone and joint deformities, or nerve and artery damage – so it is important to examine the whole limb very carefully.

The diagnosis is confirmed by a plain X-ray.

MYOSARCOMA

Primary tumours of muscle are *rare*. There are two types:

- *Leiomyosarcomas* arise from smooth muscle.
- *Rhabdomyosarcomas* arise from striated muscle.

Almost all soft tissue sarcomas developing in the limbs will be *fibrosarcomas*, which arise from the intermuscular and intramuscular fibrous septae or the fibrous tissue at the origin or insertion of the muscles.

True rhabdomyosarcomas are rare, and clinically cannot often be differentiated from fibrosarcomas (Figure 6.13).

The diagnostic features of a tumour arising in or from a muscle are that:

- It moves freely when the muscle is relaxed, especially in a direction at right angles to the length of the muscle.
- It becomes immobile when the muscle contracts, and its physical features may change.

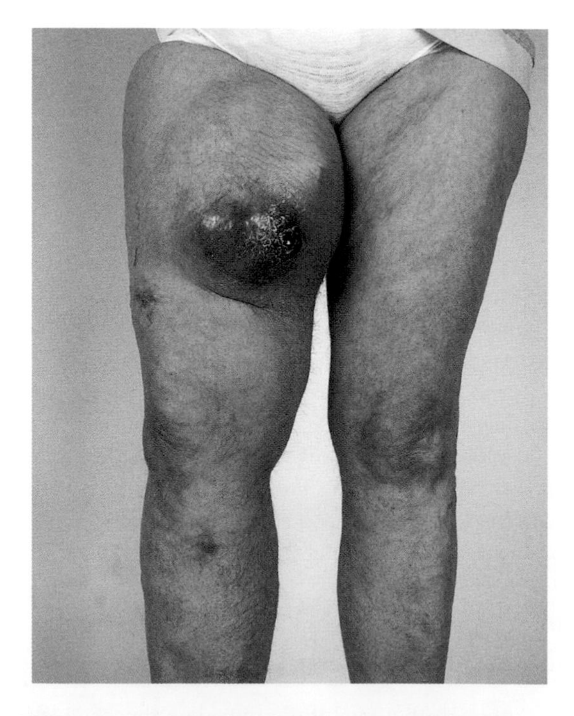

Figure 6.13 A large rhabdomyosarcoma of the thigh arising in the quadriceps muscles.

Conditions of fibrous tissue

Fibrous tissue is tough, durable and stable. It covers muscles and links them to bone as tendons, fibrous insertions or aponeuroses. It generally causes little trouble during life but is sometimes the site of malignant change.

Three tumours can arise from this tissue:

- *Benign fibroma* is very rare.
- *Fibrosarcoma* is a common mesodermal soft tissue malignant tumour.
- *Paget's recurrent desmoid tumour* is less common than fibrosarcoma, locally invasive and often recurrent.

FIBROSARCOMA

This is a malignant tumour of fibrous tissue. It is locally invasive and also spreads via the bloodstream to the lungs and liver. Spread to the lymph glands is uncommon. Distant spread is a late event, and the primary tumour often grows locally for years before metastasizing.

History

Age These tumours are more common in elderly patients, but they can occur at any age.

Duration The patient has often known of the existence of a lump for months – sometimes years – before they present to the doctor.

Symptoms The reasons for complaint include:

- Growth of the lump, causing disfigurement or interference with muscle movements.
- Pain in the lump itself or from invasion of nearby structures.
- Muscle weakness caused by infiltration of nearby muscles.
- General debility, from multiple metastases.

Examination

Site Fibrosarcomas can occur anywhere in the body, but more commonly arise in the limbs.

Colour When a large vascular tumour lies just beneath the skin, it may make the skin shiny and pink. An advanced tumour can ulcerate through the skin.

Temperature Even slow-growing fibrosarcomas have an abnormal blood supply, and usually feel warmer than the surrounding tissue.

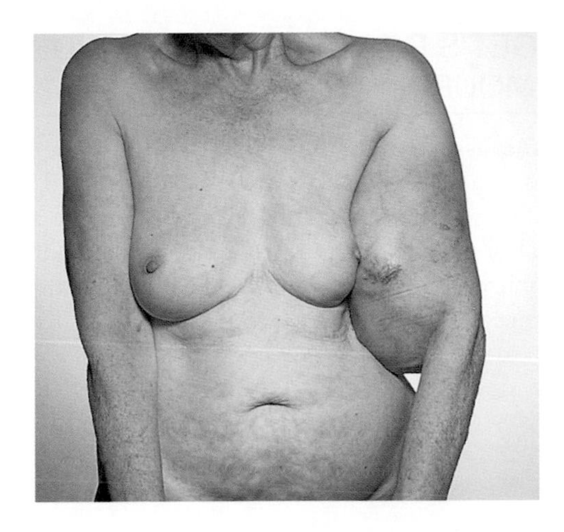

Figure 6.14 A slow-growing fibrosarcoma of the arm. The overlying skin is stretched, and many distended subcutaneous veins are visible. There was no ischaemia or paralysis in the arm or forearm.

Shape Their shape depends upon their site of origin. They are *roughly spherical* if they grow in the middle of a soft tissue. When they arise close to a bone, they tend to be *hemispherical*, with their deep surface fixed to the bone (Figure 6.14).

Surface The surface is usually smooth but may be bosselated (see Chapter 1).

Edge The edge of slow-growing tumours is well defined. Fast-growing and invasive tumours have an indistinct edge.

Composition Their *consistency is firm or hard*. They are rarely stony hard, because they do not ossify, and their marked vascularity tends to keep them soft.

NOTE: They may be so vascular that they can pulsate and have an audible bruit and a palpable thrill.

Relations The relations of the tumour to the surrounding tissues depend entirely on its site of origin, size and invasiveness. *Fibrosarcomas are usually firmly fixed to nearby structures* and often invade neighbouring bones, nerves and arteries.

Lymph glands On rare occasions, the local lymph glands may be enlarged by secondary deposits.

Local tissues Take particular care to test the integrity of any nerves running close to the mass of the tumour. A nerve deficit is more likely to indicate infiltration than stretching of the nerve and is almost diagnostic of a locally malignant lesion.

PAGET'S RECURRENT DESMOID TUMOUR

This is a *rare condition* that has the same features as a fibrosarcoma but is less vascular and very slow growing. It occurs most often in middle-aged females, usually in the fascia covering the abdominal muscles, i.e. the rectus sheath and the external oblique aponeurosis (Figure 6.15).

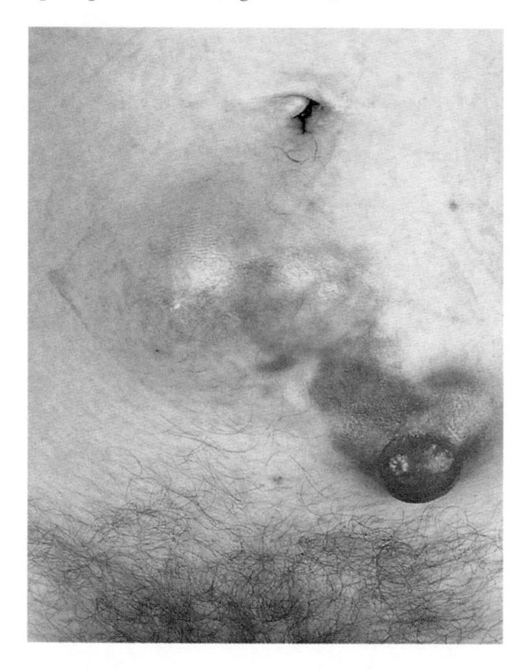

Figure 6.15 A large Paget's recurrent desmoid tumour arising from the anterior sheath of the rectus abdominis muscle.

These tumours can, however, arise in other sites, such as the plantar fascia of the foot or the palmar fascia of the hand. The malignant change affects a wide area. As a result, even after an extensive and apparently adequate excision of the presenting lump, *recurrences may appear years* later in fascia that was apparently healthy at the time of operation.

Conditions of tendons and tendon sheaths

TENDINOPATHY

Tendinopathy is a general term that describes an abnormal tendon. This may be associated with pain, swelling and impairment of function. The most common causes are mechanical overload and ageing. There may also be swelling or inflammation of the surrounding synovial sheath (tenosynovitis) or paratendon (paratendonitis).

RUPTURED TENDONS

When the tendon of a muscle is divided (completely ruptured) the muscle becomes ineffective. To assess the integrity of a tendon, you must know its site of insertion and the movement that contraction of its parent muscle would normally produce.

Tendons can be ruptured by direct trauma and usually occurs in tendons that are already tendinopathic. The tendon of the biceps brachii, the Achilles tendon and various tendons in the hands are most frequently involved. These will be considered in subsequent chapters.

CONDITIONS OF BONES

Fractures

DEFINITIONS AND SUBTYPES

A fracture is a structural discontinuity of a bone and may be:

- Complete or incomplete.
- Open or closed.
- Single or multiple.
- Transverse, spiral, oblique or comminuted.
- Pathological or stress.
- Fracture–dislocation.

Bone is relatively brittle, but easily withstands the stresses of normal life. Most fractures are caused by sudden and excessive direct or indirect force.

An *incomplete fracture* is a crack or splintering of one side of a bone without displacement of the fragments, when it is classified as *complete* and the bone is broken in two (Figure 6.16).

A *'greenstick' fracture* is a type of incomplete fracture that is common in childhood, in which the bone buckles like a bent green twig, but the periosteum and bone ends remain in continuity (Figure 6.16).

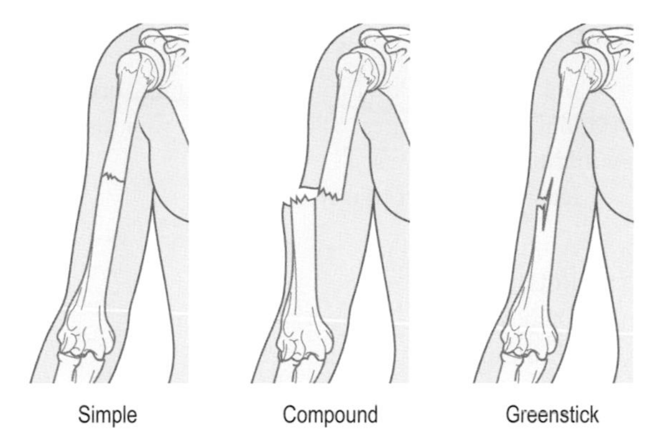

Figure 6.16 A complete and an incomplete fracture, including a greenstick fracture.

Providing the overlying skin remains intact, the fracture is classified as *closed*, but any skin breach or opening of a body cavity makes the fracture 'open', which indicates that it is liable to infection because of potential contamination.

> **NOTE:** Many fractures are confined to a single bone, but patients involved in high-speed accidents, falls from a height or battlefield injuries are liable to sustain multiple fractures (see Chapter 5). The latter are often associated with considerable blood loss and hypovolaemic shock, especially if the pelvis is fractured.

Direct force usually causes the bone to break at the point of impact in a transverse direction (a *transverse fracture*), although *comminution* can occur if the force is considerable. *Comminuted fractures* are defined by the presence of one or more fragments and are usually the result of direct excessive force from, for example, missiles.

Indirect force, which is caused for example by twisting or excessive angulation, results in the bone breaking some distance from the point at which the force was applied. These fractures are often *oblique or spiral*.

Avulsion fractures, in which a fragment of bone is pulled off the main bone by the excessive action of a muscle, tendon or ligament, are also caused by indirect force.

Pathological fractures occur through diseased areas of bone and are often spontaneous or caused by trivial force. Well-recognized causes of pathological fractures include *osteoporosis* (see page 205), *Paget's disease* (see page 204), *infections* (see page 206) and *bone tumours* (see page 209).

Stress fractures occur in bones that are subjected to repetitive trauma (like a plane's fuselage) and low levels of stress. These fractures often develop in dancers, athletes and young soldiers sent on forced marches, and commonly occur in the *vertebral bodies, metatarsals, tibia* and *fibula*.

Fractures that involve a joint that can quite commonly become complexly or partially displaced. This is called *subluxation* (partial) or *dislocation* (complete) (Figure 6.17). The injury can result in a combination of bone and joint injury when a 'fracture–dislocation' occurs (Figure 6.17). This can damage the articular cartilage, the metaphysis or the epiphysis, which will result in disordered bone growth.

Always remember that, although the fracture of the bone appears to be the major injury, the soft tissues in the region are also severely damaged, and

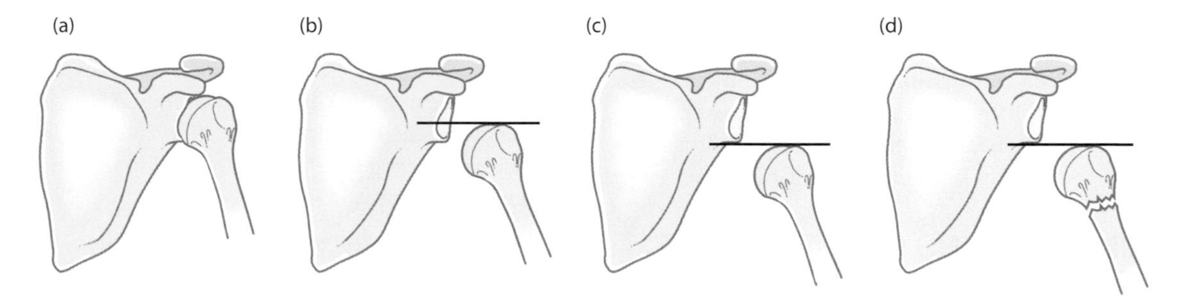

Figure 6.17 SHOULDER GLENOHUMERAL JOINT (USED AS EXAMPLE). (a) Normal joint; (b) subluxation; (c) dislocation; (d) fracture–dislocation.

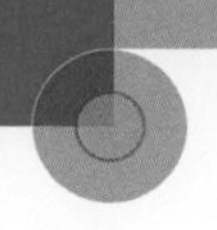

the nerves and blood vessels must always be carefully assessed.

FRACTURE DISPLACEMENT

The fragments of a complete fracture are displaced by the external force, by gravity and by the pull of the muscles attached to either side of the fracture line. The following need to be considered:

- **Shift.** The fragments can be shifted sideways, backwards or forwards, but will usually unite.
- **Angulation.** The fragments are tilted from one another, causing malalignment.
- **Rotation.** One fragment is twisted over the other, causing a torsional deformity of the limb.
- **Length.** The fragments may overlap or be separated. This can result in shortening of the limb.

SYMPTOMS

It is important to obtain a careful history of the injury, including the mechanisms and likely forces involved. It should, however, always be remembered that fractures can occur some distance from the point of impact.

Pain, bruising and swelling are the common symptoms, but do not differentiate 'a fracture' from 'a soft tissue injury'.

The presence of a fracture is suggested by a history of *continuing pain especially on movement* or *'an inability' to use the injured limb.*

The presence of a *deformity* is highly suggestive of a fracture, but in impacted fractures and greenstick fractures this may not be present and pain is often minimal.

Symptoms of associated injuries such as numbness, abdominal or chest pain, and loss of consciousness must always be enquired about (see Chapter 5), and a full history of past illnesses, family history, drugs and allergies must also be obtained (see Chapter 1).

CLINICAL SIGNS OF A FRACTURE

The injured tissues must be carefully handled, and the general effects of trauma must be treated (see Chapter 5).

Inspection

Look for the following signs. Swelling, bruising and deformity (Figure 6.18) may be obvious and should be recorded.

Measure and record any:

- Angulation.
- Rotation.
- Displacement.
- Shortening.

This can sometimes be assessed clinically, but X-rays usually provide this valuable information.

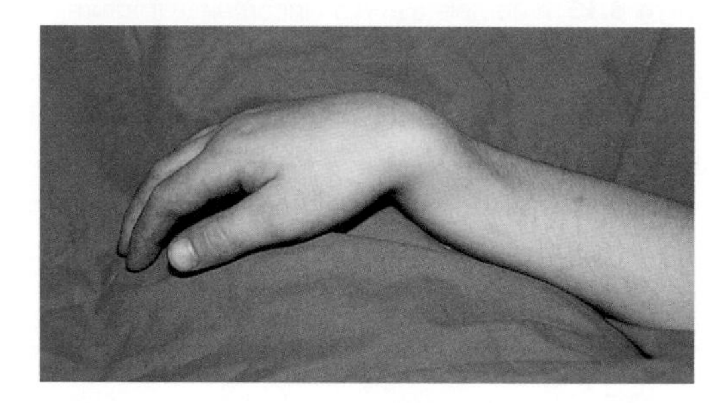

Figure 6.18 The classic dinner fork deformity of a Colles fracture.

Soft tissue swelling and injury must be assessed. This should be graded by the *Tscherne classification*:

- Grade 0: negligible soft tissue injury.
- Grade I: superficial abrasion or contusion of the soft tissues overlying the fracture.
- Grade II: significant contusion of the muscle with contaminated skin abrasions or both. The bone injury is usually severe.
- Grade III: significant injury to the soft tissues with significant degloving, crushing, compartment syndrome or vascular injury.

The presence of a *compound wound* should always be specifically looked for. This should be assessed and recorded using the *Gustilo classification*. There is a tendency for the Gustilo classification category to 'increase' with time as the patient moves through the management pathway:

- Type I: open fractures with a small, less than 1 cm clean wound with minimal injury to the musculature and no significant stripping of the periosteum from the bone. The bone injury is simple with minimal comminution.

- Type II: open fractures with 1–10 cm wounds but no significant soft tissue damage or avulsion. The fracture contains moderate comminution.
- Type III: open fractures with larger wounds and associated extensive injury to the muscle, periosteum and bone that is often associated with significant contamination of the wound. The fracture may be segmental. Such injuries can be subdivided into:
  - IIIa: extensive contamination or injury to the underlying soft tissues, but adequate viable soft tissue is present to cover the bone and neurovascular structures without muscle transfer.
  - IIIb: extensive injury to the soft tissues requiring a rotational or free muscle transfer to achieve coverage of the bone and neurovascular structures. These usually have massive contamination.
  - IIIc: open fractures with associated vascular injuries that require arterial repair.

Palpation

The site of the fracture is almost always tender.

Crepitus may be demonstrated if the patient is unconscious. This is a 'grating' sensation from the two sides of the fracture rubbing together. This can cause considerable pain in a conscious patient and should not be specifically elicited!

Movement

Movement is often very painful and is seldom required to prove a fracture. Remember that encouragement of abnormal movement may cause further soft tissue damage and further periosteal stripping.

Obtain an X-ray if a fracture is suspected.

X-rays

When ordering an X-ray, obtain the appropriate views, and follow the *rule of twos*:

- *Two views*: usually an anterior–posterior view and a lateral view.
- *Two joints:* include the joint above and the joint below the bone under consideration.
- *Two sides:* which is useful for comparison, particularly in children, because it allows a comparison of the epiphyseal lines in immature bones and distinguishes them from the fracture line.
- *Two injuries:* one at a higher or lower level, for example the calcaneum with the pelvis or spine.
- *Two occasions:* another X-ray if the symptoms persist, for example a scaphoid fracture.

General examination

The *peripheral pulses* must be felt and recorded, and the skin circulation assessed (see Chapter 10).

The peripheral nerves must also be examined, and defects recorded. Associated visceral injuries and any distal injuries must be excluded (see Chapter 3).

Remember that:

- *Heart and lung injuries* are associated with *fractures of the ribs and sternum* (see Chapter 2).
- *The spinal cord* may be injured in patients with *spinal fractures* (see Chapter 9).
- *Pelvic fractures* are associated with *abdominal visceral and urinary tract injuries* (see Chapters 9, 15 and 17).
- *Pectoral girdle injuries* are often associated with *brachial plexus and subclavian vascular injuries* (see Chapters 3 and 10).

JOINT INJURIES (FIGURE 6.17)

A joint can be injured by either being:

- Dislocated, where there is complete discontinuity.
- Subluxed, where there is partial discontinuity.
- Dislocated with an associated fracture.

If a joint dislocates, injuries to other structures can also occur. These include:

- Soft tissue damage – ligaments, tendons and intra-articular structures.
- Joint surface damage with chondral defects.

- Neurovascular injury.
- Chronic instability of the joint.
- Recurrent dislocation.
- Aseptic necrosis.

A dislocation may present with *pain, loss of function* or *abnormal mobility*.

The most affected joints are the shoulder glenohumeral joint, the acromioclavicular joint and the elbow, finger, hip and knee joints. Dislocations and subluxations of specific joints are discussed in Chapters 7 and 8.

Complications are listed in Revision panel 6.1.

Revision panel 6.1

COMPLICATIONS OF FRACTURES

General

Blood loss
Deep vein thrombosis
Pulmonary embolism
Fat embolism
Acute respiratory distress

Immediate local

Bleeding
Vascular injury
Nerve injury
Visceral injury

Early complications

Local infection
Septicaemia
Gas gangrene
Compartment syndrome
Haemarthrosis
Fracture blisters/sores
Plaster sores
Nerve entrapment

Late complications

Malunion
Delayed union
Non-union
Myositis ossificans
Avascular necrosis
Joint instability
Joint stiffness
Algodystrophy
Osteoarthritis
Volkmann's ischaemic contracture
Complex regional pain syndrome

Bone diseases and deformities

It is vital to make an accurate diagnosis of any bony lump, as bony swellings can be entirely benign or highly malignant. The clinical presentation may provide some useful hints on the underlying nature of the pathological process, although radiological assistance is usually required. The actual site of a tumour in a long bone may give some clue as to its underlying pathology.

EXOSTOSIS

This is a lump that sticks out from the bone. An exostosis is mainly cancellous bone, with a covering of cortical bone and a cartilaginous cap (Figure 6.19). Exostoses are usually single but may be congenital and multiple (see below).

Solitary (diaphyseal) exostosis

These are derived from small pieces of metaphyseal cartilage that were not remodelled during the growth of the bone and have become separated from the main cartilaginous epiphyseal plate. Although isolated on the side of the bone shaft (diaphysis), they continue to grow and ossify, and so produce a bony lump just above the epiphyseal line (Figure 6.19).

They sometimes have an adventitious bursa over their cap, and *they are not neoplasms*.

History

Age Exostoses present when they are large enough to cause symptoms – usually in teenage and early adult life.

Symptoms The patient may have felt the lump, or it may have become noticeable and cosmetically disfiguring.

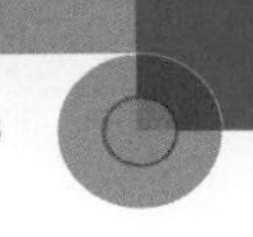

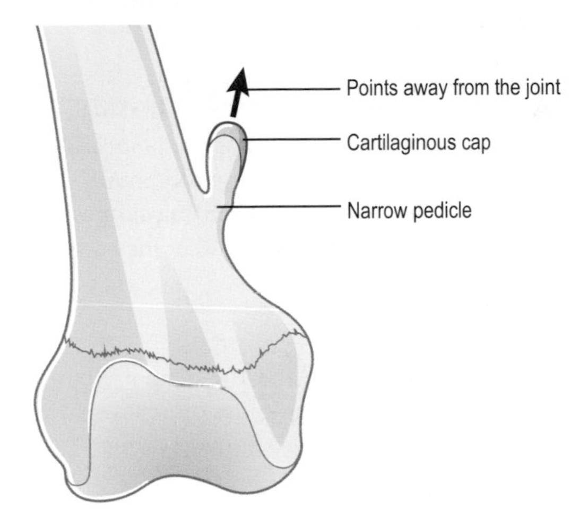

Figure 6.19 The features of a solitary exostosis.

They sometimes interfere with the movement of the joint and its tendons because they arise near joints. Patients may find the movements of the joint limited or associated with 'clicks' or 'jumps' as the tendons slip over the lump.

The overlying bursa, if present, may become enlarged and inflamed.

Examination

Position They are usually found adjacent to the epiphyseal line of the bone, just on the diaphyseal side. The majority occur at the lower end of the femur and upper end of the tibia.

Shape and size Initial palpation gives the impression of a *sessile, smooth, hemispherical protuberance*, but with careful palpation it is often possible to feel that the base is quite narrow, and that the exostosis leans away from the joint.

Exostoses are usually 1–2 cm in diameter when they are first noticed. As the cartilaginous cap ossifies, they may enlarge (4–5 cm across) and then interfere with joint movement.

Surface Their surface is smooth.

Composition They are *bony hard*, but their consistency may be masked by a soft, fluctuant bursa overlying their cap.

Relations They are *fixed to the underlying bone*. It is important to palpate the lump while the adjacent joint is moving to feel which muscles and tendons lie close to the lump, and to measure the range of joint movement.

Local tissues The rest of the bone and the nearby joint should be normal.

Multiple exostoses (diaphyseal aclasis)

This is an *autosomal dominant hereditary condition*, in which one-half of the patient's children can be expected to have the abnormality. It is more common in males. All the bones that ossify in cartilage can be affected, with the exception of the spine and skull. The long bones may be a little shorter than normal because this condition is caused by a widespread generalized abnormality of bone remodelling at the epiphyseal line, as opposed to the sporadic event that produces a solitary exostosis.

The clinical features of each exostosis are similar to those described for the solitary variety. They are multiple and especially common on the limb bones. They can grow to a considerable size of up to 5–10 cm in diameter.

CALLUS

Perhaps the most common cause of thickening of a bone is callus. Callus is the buttress of new bone formed around a fracture site to unite and strengthen it while the cortical bone is being slowly repaired.

History

In most cases, the patient knows of the injury and the subsequent discomfort associated with the fracture that caused the callus, but this is not always the case. Some fractures are caused by repetitive stress. Furthermore, not every fracture causes severe pain, so the absence of a history of trauma or pain does not necessarily exclude the possibility that the lump might be callus. Clearly, however, this is unlikely.

Examination

Position The thickening of a bone by callus should be greatest at the site of the fracture, but it may be asymmetrical.

Tenderness Mature callus is not tender. Once a fracture has united, there is no local tenderness, and if an area of thickening in a bone is tender, it is

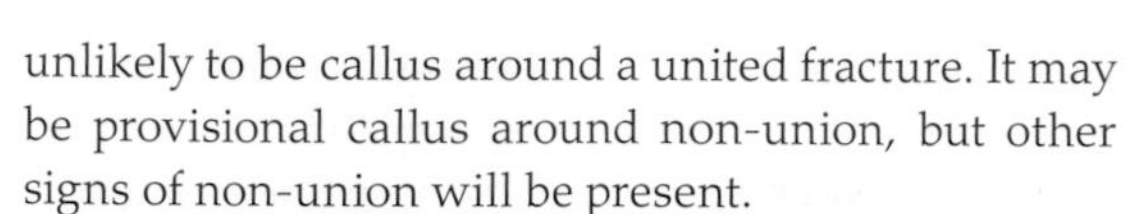

unlikely to be callus around a united fracture. It may be provisional callus around non-union, but other signs of non-union will be present.

Shape Callus usually causes a fusiform enlargement of the whole bone – thickest at the site of the fracture.

Surface Callus becomes smooth as time passes. In young people, callus can be completely resorbed and remodelled.

Abnormalities of bone metabolism

PAGET'S DISEASE OF BONE (OSTEITIS DEFORMANS)

Bone is usually continually repaired and replaced throughout life. This process follows the same pattern as the original ossification. The ossified cartilage that is reorganized into mature bone is called osteoid bone.

In Paget's disease, the *repair process stops at the osteoid bone stage*, with the healthy, mature bone being gradually replaced by thick, bulky, very vascular *osteoid bone*. The old bone, which is absorbed by the osteoclasts, is replaced by fibrous tissue. If the repair process stops a stage earlier, the bone is very weak. *The underlying cause of Paget's disease is still not known.*

Paget's disease occurs in later life and usually affects multiple bones but can occasionally affect just one bone in the whole skeleton (monostotic Paget's disease). There is the potential for malignant change in the bone, and *osteogenic sarcoma* complicates 1% of cases.

History

Age The patient is rarely under 50 years of age, often much older, and can be of either gender.

Symptoms *Pain* is the most common symptom, although patients may be symptomless. As the bones enlarge and become more vascular, the patient feels a deep-seated aching, gnawing pain in the bone. *The back is the most common source of pain.* Make a careful note of any change in the nature and severity of the pain. This may indicate malignant change. Headache may be the result of the increased vascularity of the bones.

Deformity The bone grows bigger and bends. The typical complaints are:

- *Enlargement of the skull*, with the frontal bones becoming prominent (see Chapter 3, Figure 3.3).
- Curvature of the spine, causing a kyphosis and increasing difficulty with fitting clothes; patients occasionally complain that they are getting shorter.
- Bowing of the legs.

Deafness Paget's disease in the temporal bones may affect the middle ear and cause otosclerosis and deafness. The patient may also develop vertigo.

Examination

General appearance The patient with generalized disease has a large head, a bent back, arms that seem too long (because of the kyphosis) and bowlegs.

Cardiovascular system Examine the cardiovascular system with care. The increased bone blood flow causes an increased cardiac output. The heart may be enlarged, there may be an aortic ejection murmur and the blood pressure may be elevated. Paget's disease can cause a *high-output heart failure*, but this is very uncommon (see Chapter 2). The exacerbation of any myocardial ischaemia, secondary to coronary vessel disease, by the extra demands placed upon the heart of an elderly person is well recognized.

Respiratory system Rales and rhonchi may be present at both lung bases if the kyphosis is severe enough to interfere with movements of the chest wall.

Skeleton

- **Skull.** The enlargement occurs in the vault. The dome looks swollen, and the enlarged frontal bones make the forehead bulge forwards (see Chapter 3, Figure 3.3). Deafness is common.
- **Spine.** The disease usually affects the whole skeleton, producing an even kyphosis. The shoulders are rounded, and the head and neck protrude anteriorly.
- **Legs.** The femur and the tibia may bow in both anterior/posterior and lateral directions.

The sharp anterior edge of the tibia becomes so prominent that the description 'sabre tibiae' is apt (Figure 6.20), although this expression is usually reserved for bowing caused by syphilis and yaws.

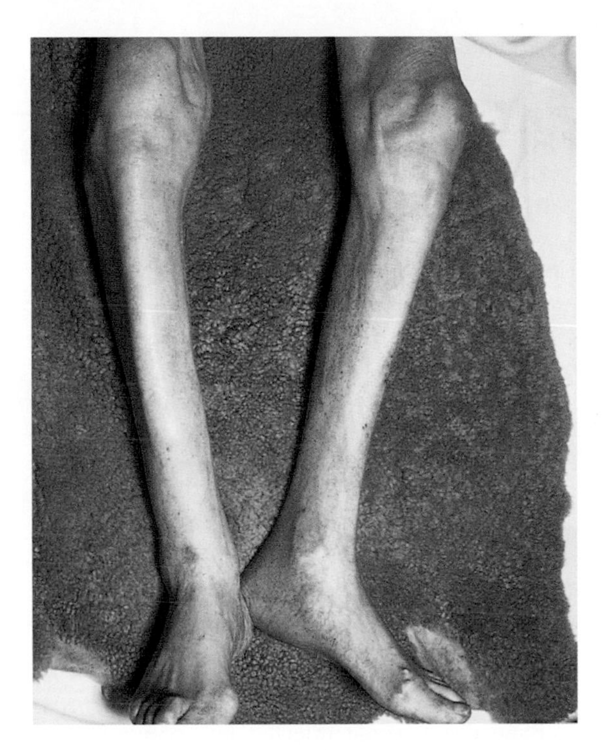

Figure 6.20 'Sabre tibiae'. The anterior edge of the tibia is normally straight and sharp. In this patient, Paget's disease has made these edges thick and curved.

When examining the skeleton, look for any localized bony enlargement, especially in the areas where the pain is severe or has changed. A swelling of the bone that is painful, a little tender and warm to the touch suggests the presence of *sarcomatous change*.

Central nervous system The patient may have a *conduction deafness* and difficulty when standing, caused by middle ear and vestibular apparatus damage (Chapter 3, page 104).

The function of other cranial nerves can be affected if the thickening of the bones reduces the size of the foramina in the base of the skull. *Blindness* can occur if the optic nerves are compressed.

Spinal nerves may also be damaged by collapse of the vertebrae.

Osteoporosis

In this disease, the bone mineral density is reduced, because *the balance of bone formation and resorption is disturbed*. This causes defects in the bone architecture in which the cortex is thinned with fewer trabeculae, and this leads to a *greater risk of fracture*.

Osteoporosis may be primary or secondary.

Risk factors for primary osteoporosis include:

- Female sex.
- Increasing age.
- Early onset menopause (before 45), oophorectomy or other causes of amenorrhea (including anorexia).
- Family history.
- Certain racial groups are at more risk of osteoporosis such as Caucasians and Asians.

Risk factors for secondary causes of osteoporosis include:

- Chronic diseases such as rheumatoid arthritis, thyrotoxicosis and coeliac disease.
- Medications including corticosteroids and long-term unfractionated heparin.
- Smoking.
- Alcohol consumption.

History

Age Females are usually perimenopausal or postmenopausal, usually between the ages of 45 and 50 years.

Symptoms In the early stages, it is symptomless, but symptoms arise from the development of *fragility fractures* or secondary to *pathological fractures*. Principal fracture sites include the vertebral body, wrist and hip.

Deformity Fragility fractures in the spine can result in decreased height and increased *thoracic kyphosis* from wedging or compression of the vertebral bodies.

Examination

Loss of height may be recorded secondary to vertebral fractures. Other than the presence of a fracture, and its possible sequelae, the examination is normal.

RICKETS/OSTEOMALACIA

These conditions are the result of an *inadequate mineralization of bone caused by inadequate absorption or utilization of calcium*.

Osteomalacia is 'softening of the bones' in which thin bony trabeculae are covered by wide osteoid seams. The incomplete ossification process in children that occurs in *rickets* affects the physeal growth plate, leading to skeletal deformities.

In the past, the principal cause was often *lack of dietary vitamin D* or *insufficient exposure to sunlight*. Other vitamin D metabolism problems have been recognized including some forms of *renal and liver disease*.

Calcium deficiency and hypophosphataemia can result in similar mineralization defects.

History

Age Rickets occurs in children, while osteomalacia occurs in later life, and its effects become more apparent over a longer period.

Symptoms Adults present with *bone pain, muscle weakness* and even occasionally *tetany*.

Children may be *listless and have a 'failure to thrive'*.

Deformity In rickets, early bone changes include:

- Deformity of the skull (craniotabes).
- Thickening of the bones of the wrist.
- Enlargement of the costochondral junction (rickety rosary; Figure 6.21).
- Indentation of the chest (Harrison's sulcus).
- Tibial bowing (coxa vara).
- Increasing spinal curvature.

In osteomalacia, fragility fractures in the spine can result in increased *thoracic kyphosis*. There is also increased risk of *traumatic fractures* of the long bones.

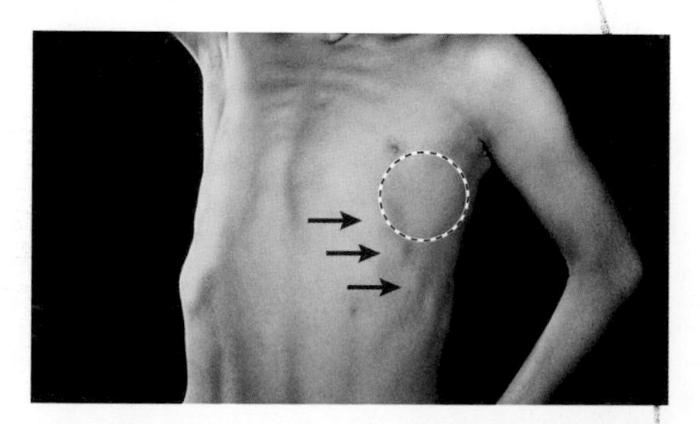

Figure 6.21 A rickety rosary. Enlargement of the costochondral junctions and presence of Harrison's sulcus.

Examination

Children may be small for their age because bone growth is stunted. Once the child stands, any deformity, particularly in the lower limbs, will increase. In adults, vertebral collapse can also cause loss of height, with mild deformities becoming more pronounced.

HYPERPARATHYROIDISM

This is discussed in Chapter 12. The *osteoclastic resorption of bone*.

Brown tumour-like masses develop in the bones that liquefy and become cystic. Less than 10%, however, present with bone pains and pathological fractures.

Infections of bone

ACUTE OSTEOMYELITIS

Bone can become infected by organisms that reach it through the *bloodstream* or *directly through a wound*. Blood-borne organisms are probably trapped in thrombi or haematomas caused by minor trauma, usually in the capillary loops in the shaft adjacent to the epiphyseal line known as the metaphysis. The common infecting organisms are *Staphylococcus aureus* and *Streptococcus pyogenes*.

History

Age Patients with acute osteomyelitis are usually between 1 and 12 years old. When adults are affected, infection is often associated with immune suppression.

Symptoms The site of infection is *painful*, although in the early stages this is only a deep-seated ache. When pus forms and intramedullary tension increases, the pain becomes intense and throbbing.

A child will *refuse to use a limb or allow it to be touched*. Some swelling may be noted around the painful area, but this is not marked as it is caused by diffuse oedema of the overlying tissues, rather than swelling of the bone. The adjacent joint is often swollen and stiff.

Systemically, the infection causes a loss of appetite and general debility. Most patients feel hot and sweaty, and they may suffer from rigors.

Examination

Site The tibia, femur, humerus, radius and ulna are the most affected bones.

Colour The skin over the painful area may be red or reddish-brown.

Temperature The skin becomes *palpably hot* when the infection has spread through the bone into the subperiosteal layer.

Tenderness The swollen area is *tender*, and the whole bone is sensitive.

Consistency Any swelling is soft and indistinct because it is caused by oedema of the overlying structures. There may be an area that fluctuates when there is pus near the surface.

Lymph glands The local lymph glands are only enlarged if the infection has spread outside the bone.

Local tissues The overlying skin may be oedematous. The adjacent joint may be swollen by an effusion, and its movements limited and slightly painful. The infection has probably spread into the joint and caused a *septic arthritis* if the joint movements are very restricted and painful (see below).

The subcutaneous veins of the limb are often dilated.

General examination The patient looks ill and feverish. Their face may be *flushed*, and their *temperature raised*. They may be hypotensive, sweating and possibly shaking, with a dry tongue and oliguria, if septicaemia has developed.

CHRONIC OSTEOMYELITIS

This often follows an *open fracture* or a *surgical procedure* or *implant* and can also develop from acute osteomyelitis.

The common infecting organisms are again *Staphylococcus aureus* and *streptococci* (especially *Streptococcus pyogenes*). *Staphylococcus epidermidis* is frequently isolated if there is associated metalwork from previous surgery. In children or patients with sickle-cell disease, chronic osteomyelitis can be caused by *Escherichia coli*.

As a result of the infection, bone is destroyed in areas around the focus of the infection or around a foreign implant. Cavities containing pus and dead bone (*sequestra*) become surrounded by vascular tissue and by areas of sclerosis. This may form an *involucrum* or bony sheath.

History

Age Patients can present at any age. It is more common in those who have either been inadequately treated or have *immune suppression*, for example elderly patients, those with diabetes or malnutrition and those on steroid medication.

Symptoms Patients often present with *recurrent bouts of pain* around the infected area. They *avoid using the limb.*

Systemic features of infection include feeling feverish from a raised temperature, associated with nausea and malaise. Episodes of infection are often interspersed with periods of quiescence.

Examination

Site The long bones of both the upper and lower limbs are most affected. The spine may also be involved particularly after previous operations (see Chapter 9).

Colour The skin may appear red, with a flare.

Temperature This may be increased, but it may also be normal.

Tenderness The area is normally tender, and the bone is often very sensitive.

Local tissues A surgical scar may be present. *Sinuses* may also be noted in the skin, with discharging pus (Figure 6.22). The skin itself is often thickened and puckered.

There may be deformity of the bone secondary to previous trauma. Despite surgical intervention, the bone itself may not have healed because of the infection. This can lead to further deformity.

The sinuses may wall off over time, which suggests that they may have healed only to reopen again, either in the same place or elsewhere. The bone becomes brittle, and this can result in a pathological fracture.

TUBERCULOSIS

Where pulmonary disease is endemic, the bones and joints of children and young adults may become infected. Elsewhere in the world, it tends to develop in elderly adults with debilitating disorders or patients with immunodeficiency (AIDS).

It reaches the skeleton by *haematogenous spread*, and the *acid-fast bacilli* often lodge in the *bone metaphysis*, which has the greatest blood supply. Initially, there is a chronic inflammatory reaction with *granuloma*

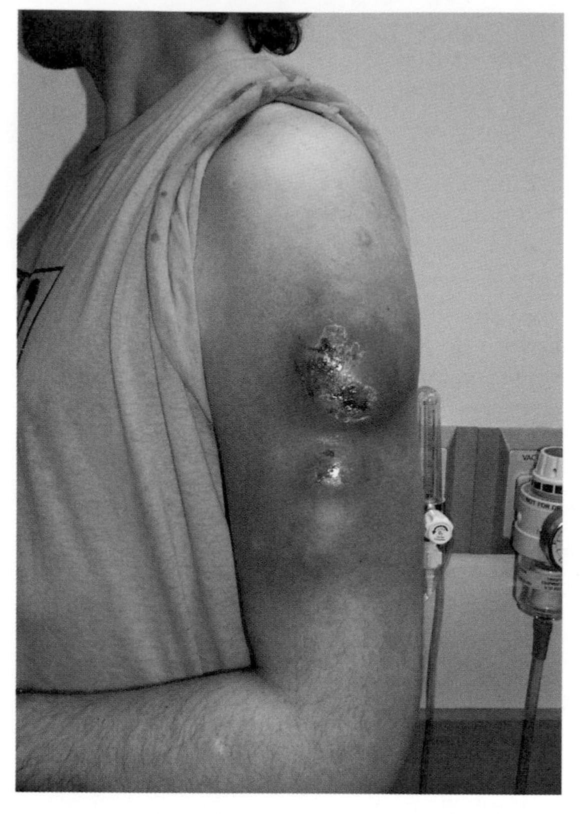

Figure 6.22 A sinus discharging pus associated with chronic osteomyelitis.

formation and caseation, which spreads into the soft tissues, where it liquefies to form a 'cold abscess'. This can point some distance away, having tracked down through the tissue planes (Figure 6.23).

It arises quite commonly in the anterior part of the vertebral body near the disc and can spread to the adjacent vertebra, which can lead to collapse and sharp angulation (a *kyphus*) (see Chapter 9).

Tuberculous arthritis is discussed on page 219.

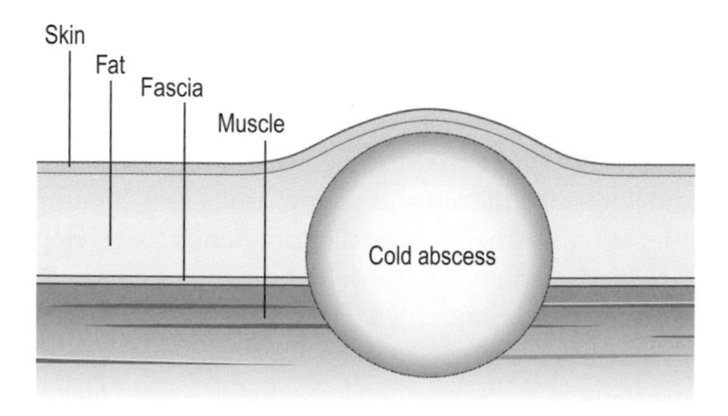

Figure 6.23 A cold abscess.

Miscellaneous conditions of bone

OSTEONECROSIS (AVASCULAR NECROSIS)

Osteonecrosis occurs when the blood supply to a bone is disrupted. This may be caused by:

- Severance of the blood supply, or pathology in the lumen of the vessel or the vessel wall.
- External compressive forces causing occlusion of the blood flow (Revision panel 6.2).

As a result, the bone cells die, but on reperfusion of the bone, there is attempted repair of the ischaemic areas. The necrotic bone collapses, and reactive new bone forms in the ischaemic boundary, with accompanying sclerosis.

History

Age Patients can present at any age, depending on the underlying cause.

Patients with *sickle-cell disease* present initially with an acutely painful crisis. Once vascular necrosis becomes established, they generally re-present

Revision panel 6.2

CAUSES OF AVASCULAR NECROSIS

Trauma
Sickle-cell disease
Caisson disease (decompression sickness)
Coagulation disorders
Vasculitis
Gaucher's disease
Septic arthritis
Osteomyelitis
Corticosteroids
Excessive alcohol
Systemic lupus erythematosus
Ionizing radiation

in young adulthood, either from the pain associated with the condition or as the result of secondary joint changes.

Similar presentations occur following traumatic injury.

Symptoms *Pain* is the common feature, although the early stages of cell death may be symptomless.

Examination

Site The shoulder, hip and knee are most often affected. The hip, talus and scaphoid may all develop osteonecrosis after a fracture.

Colour The skin appears normal.

Temperature The temperature is normal.

Tenderness The area may be tender, with sensitivity of the bone.

Movements There may be restriction in movement secondary to pain, with muscle wasting from disuse. Deformities of the joint may arise.

The diagnosis is dependent on finding the typical changes on X-ray and MRI scan.

OSTEOCHONDRITIS

In this group of conditions, the *bone is usually compressed, fragmented or separated* near the bone ends or articular surfaces. The sclerosis and increased vascularity that occurs is very similar to the changes found in avascular necrosis.

The individual entities are dealt with in the chapters on the areas where they occur, for example *Perthes' disease* in the hip section of Chapter 8.

BENIGN TUMOURS OF BONE

Benign tumours of bone fall into two categories:

- Those arising from cortical bone (so-called *'ivory' osteomas*).
- Those which are primarily cartilaginous tumours that arise within or on the surface of long bones (*enchondromas and ecchondromas*).

Osteoma

History

The patient complains of a lump that they have either felt or had drawn to their attention. These lumps are not painful, and they rarely occur in a site that interferes with joint or tendon movements.

Examination

Site Osteomas are common on the surface of the vault of the skull, frequently the forehead (Figure 6.24).

Shape and size They are sessile, flattened mounds with a smooth surface.

Consistency Osteomas are *bony hard* – hence the name 'ivory' osteoma.

Relations Nearby muscles and fascia move freely over the lump, which is obviously fixed to and an integral part of the underlying bone.

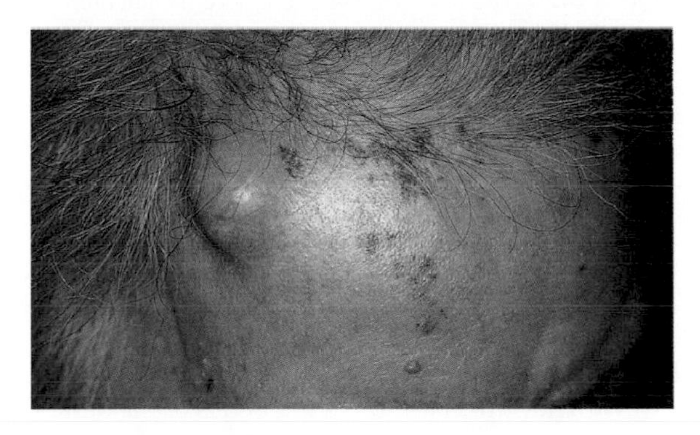

Figure 6.24 An osteoma of cortical bone – an 'ivory' osteoma on the forehead, which has been present for 40 years.

Chondroma

A chondroma can grow inside a long bone only if a piece of the cartilage from which the bone developed fails to become converted to bone:

- An *enchondroma* is a chondroma growing in the centre of the bone (Figure 6.25).
- An *ecchondroma* is a chondroma growing on the surface of the bone (Figure 6.25).

There is no pathological difference between these two varieties of chondroma.

When the chondromas are multiple and congenital (but not familial), the condition is called *dyschondroplasia* or *Ollier's disease*.

History

Age Patients usually present in teenage or early adult life.

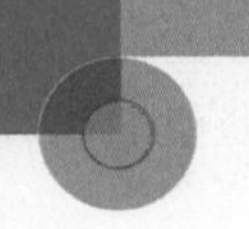

Enchondroma

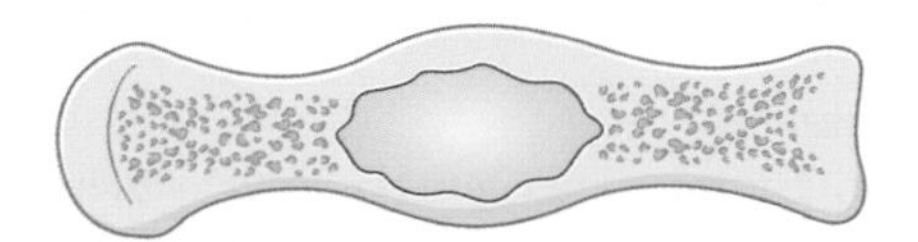

Ecchondroma

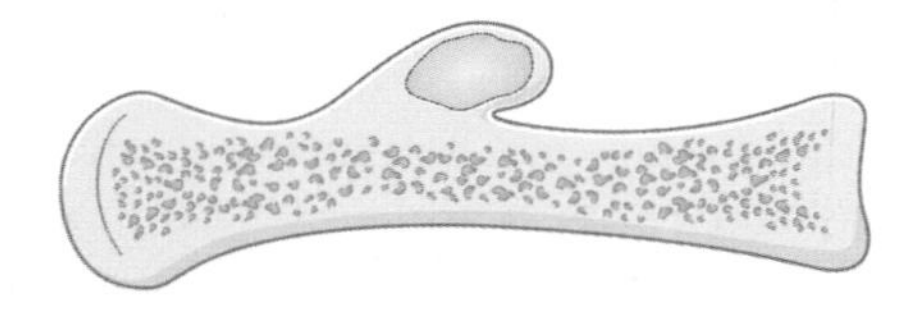

Figure 6.25 The two varieties of chondroma that are found in long bones.

Symptoms The patient notices either that a bone is gradually expanding or that a lump is appearing on the side of a bone.

Neither type of chondroma is painful, but an ecchondroma may interfere with joint and tendon movement.

Examination

Site They are common in the bones of the hands and feet but may occur anywhere. Large, long bones are rarely affected, except when the patient has congenital and multiple chondromas (Ollier's disease).

Temperature The overlying skin has a normal temperature.

Shape *Enchondromas cause a fusiform enlargement* of the shaft of the bone.

Ecchondromas form a sessile lump on the surface of the bone (Figure 6.26).

Surface The surface of both varieties is smooth.

Consistency They feel hard as they are usually covered by a thin layer of cortical bone.

Osteoid osteoma

This is a very small bone tumour that can occur in any bone except the skull. It is usually less than 1 cm in diameter, and accounts for approximately 10% of all benign bone tumours.

History

Age Patients usually present in teenage or early adult life. There is an increased incidence in males.

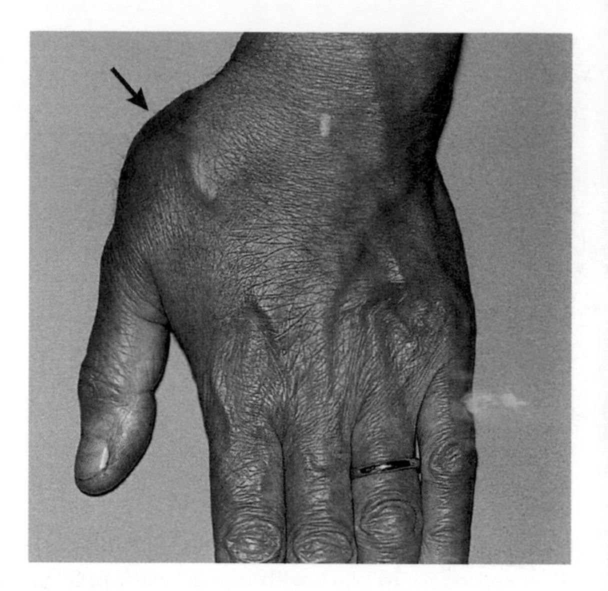

Figure 6.26 A large ecchondroma of the metacarpal bone of the thumb (arrow).

Symptoms The patient usually presents with *significant localized pain* in the bone. They do not want to use the limb or affected region, which can lead to wasting and weakness. Pain is typically *severe at night*, with a dull ache during the day, and is typically *relieved by salicylates*.

Examination

Site The most affected bones are the tibia and femur.

Signs The patient may develop a limp with muscular atrophy.

Temperature The overlying skin has a normal temperature.

Shape The bone itself usually maintains its normal shape, as the tumour is located within the bone itself.

X-rays show the tumour as a radiolucent area known as *a nidus*, surrounded by a distinct *zone of necrosis*.

CONDITIONS THAT PRESENT LIKE BENIGN TUMOURS

Fibrous dysplasia

In this condition, normal bone is replaced by fibrous bone tissue. It can occur in childhood or early adulthood, and can affect one bone (*monostotic*), one limb (*monomelic*) or many bones (*polyostotic*).

Males and females are equally affected.

Symptoms In many cases, fibrous dysplasia is *symptomless*, and is an incidental finding when an X-ray is taken.

Bone expansion can cause pain, most often in the femur, tibia, humerus and ribs, and the patient may develop a limp.

Signs There may be *palpable tenderness* but no changes in temperature. There may be *bowing* of the upper femur or weight-bearing bones. *Pathological fracture* may occur.

Non-ossifying fibroma (fibrous cortical defect)

This is the most common benign lesion of a bone, in which fibrous tissue appears and persists for some years before ossifying. It is almost always symptomless and is common in children, presenting as an incidental finding within the metaphyses of long bones.

Simple bone cyst

This is also known as a *solitary cyst* or *unicameral bone cyst*. It generally appears in childhood, usually in the *metaphysis of a long bone*, commonly in the proximal humerus or femur. It does not expand the bone.

It is usually *symptomless* and is an incidental finding on an X-ray, although it can present with a *pathological fracture*.

Aneurysmal bone cyst

This benign bone neoplasm can arise *de novo* or secondary to a pre-existing bone tumour. It may be intraosseous, *blood-filled spaces separated by fibrous septa*, or extraosseous.

The tumour can arise at any position, but is most commonly found in the upper extremity, lower leg and femur. Initially it is *painless*, but as it expands it often causes *discomfort of increasing severity*. A large cyst may become visible or palpable. The skin temperature around the bone may increase. There may be a restriction of movement in the adjacent joints.

MALIGNANT TUMOURS OF BONE

These are either *primary* or *secondary*. A *metastasis* (a secondary deposit) is much the more common (see below).

There are five principal primary tumours of bone:

- Osteosarcoma.
- Chondrosarcoma.
- Reticulum cell sarcoma (Ewing's tumour).
- Giant cell tumour (osteoclastoma).
- Multiple myeloma.

The five primary carcinomas that commonly metastasize to bone, producing secondary metastatic tumours, originate in the:

- Lung.
- Breast.
- Kidney.
- Thyroid.
- Prostate.

Although these are the most common primary sites for bone metastases to originate, remember that *any tumour can metastasize to bone*.

The first four tend to produce *lytic* (dissolution of bone) metastases, while prostatic 'secondaries' are often *sclerotic* (hard).

The *bones* that most often contain secondary deposits are:

- The vertebral bodies.
- The pelvic bones.
- The ribs.
- The upper ends of the femur and the humerus.

These bones all contain red bone marrow and have a good blood supply.

History

General features Patients often give a history of previous malignancy (e.g. a mastectomy for a lump in the breast). They may also have symptoms related to the primary growth, such as a cough with haemoptysis, or difficulty with micturition.

> **NOTE:** Some patients develop bony secondary deposits with no signs or symptoms to indicate the site of the primary tumour.

Symptoms The most common symptom is *pain*. Low back pain or pain in the pelvis and hip is often the first indication of the existence of secondary deposits.

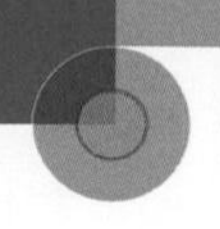

Acute pain will occur if there is a *pathological fracture,* such as the collapse of a vertebral body or a fracture of the femur.

Noticeable swelling at the site of a metastasis is very unusual unless it is in a superficial bone such as the vault of the skull, the clavicle or a rib.

Examination

Deep-seated bony metastases rarely produce any physical signs except pain on movement and tenderness on percussion.

When superficial, they may cause a swelling of the bone that appears rapidly and grows steadily.

The consistency of a secondary deposit in a bone may vary from hard and bone-like to soft and compressive.

OSTEOSARCOMA

This is a malignant sarcoma of bone. It is seen in two groups of patients:

- The young.
- Elderly patients with Paget's disease.

Sarcoma complicating Paget's disease has already been described (see page 204).

Osteosarcoma is a *highly malignant spindle-cell tumour.* It spreads locally into the surrounding soft tissues, and early and rapidly by the bloodstream.

History

Age It occurs in childhood and the teenage years.

Symptoms *Pain* is the predominant symptom. It usually begins before the patient notices a lump and is a persistent ache or throb.

Swelling of the bone may be noticed, and in some instances this increases rapidly.

The development of *general malaise, cachexia* and *loss of weight* may precede or coincide with the appearance of local symptoms.

Pulmonary metastases may cause a cough and haemoptysis.

Abdominal discomfort and jaundice may follow the enlargement and destruction of the liver by metastases.

Patients often relate the onset of their symptoms to an injury, but there is no evidence that trauma causes sarcoma. The injury simply focuses their attention on symptoms that they had previously dismissed as trivial and insignificant.

Examination

Site The most common places to find an osteosarcoma (Figure 6.27) are:

- The lower end of the femur.
- The upper end of the tibia.
- The upper end of the humerus.

Colour The overlying skin may be reddened, and the subcutaneous veins visibly distended.

Tenderness The swelling may be slightly tender but not exquisitely painful like osteomyelitis (see page 206).

> **NOTE:** Any red, warm, non-tender bony swelling should, in the first instance, be considered to be a tumour and not an infection.

Temperature The skin over the swelling is usually warm and sometimes quite hot.

Shape The swelling tends to appear on one side of the lower end of the bone, making it asymmetrical.

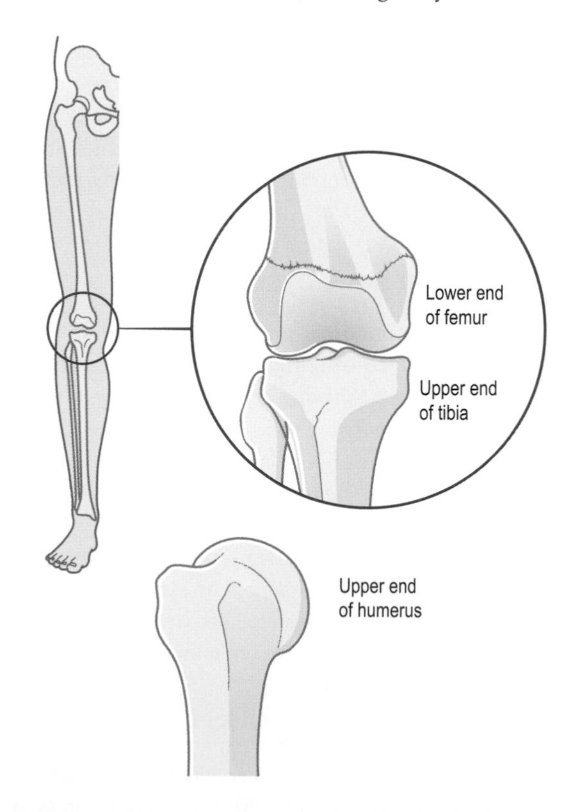

Figure 6.27 The common sites to find osteosarcomas.

Surface Its surface is smooth unless it has spread into the surrounding tissues when it becomes irregular.

Consistency Bony sarcomas feel firm but not bony hard.

> **NOTE:** It is a clinical aphorism that benign tumours of bone feel hard, whereas malignant tumours of bone feel soft.

A very vascular tumour may pulsate.

Relations The structures overlying a small osteosarcoma are mobile but become fixed to it if the tumour spreads locally beyond the bone.

Lymph glands The draining lymph glands are not enlarged in the early stages of the disease, which may be another indication that the red, warm swelling is not an infection. When the tumour invades the surrounding soft tissues, it may then spread to the local lymph glands.

Local tissues The nearby joint often becomes stiff and develops an effusion. The adjacent artery and nerves are only involved in advanced local disease.

General examination Take particular care to examine the chest and the abdomen, because the lungs and the liver are common sites for metastases. There may be generalized wasting, or isolated wasting of the muscles of the affected limb.

CHONDROSARCOMA

This is one of the most common malignant tumours originating in bone. It may arise centrally in *the medullary cavity* or peripherally from *the cortex*. It may develop *de novo* or *by malignant change in a pre-existing benign lesion* (secondary chondrosarcoma).

History

Age The incidence is greatest in the fourth to fifth decades, with males more commonly affected than females.

Symptoms The tumour is often *symptomless* in the initial stages. As it grows, the patient may become aware of a *dull ache* or a *gradually increasing lump*. Acute pain is associated with a *pathological fracture*.

Examination

Site These tumours most commonly arise in the metaphyses of the long bones of the lower limb. They can also occur in the pelvis, ribs and upper limbs.

Colour The overlying skin is normal.

Tenderness There may be tenderness of the bone.

Temperature This is usually normal.

Shape The tumour may cause a swelling and enlargement of the bone with a smooth surface.

Lymph glands The lymph glands are not usually palpable as most chondrosarcomas are slow growing and metastasize late.

RETICULUM CELL SARCOMA (EWING'S TUMOUR)

This is a tumour that arises most often in the *centre of long bones* – a feature that helps to distinguish it from osteosarcoma and osteomyelitis.

This tumour occurs as large sheets of polyhedral cells that have a distinct reticulate staining and can be mistaken for a secondary deposit from an adrenal neuroblastoma.

The cell of origin is not known, but it may arise from the *endothelial cells* of the bone marrow.

History

Age This tumour occurs in *childhood* and the *teenage years*.

Symptoms The most common symptom is a *persistent ache or pain* made worse by movement.

Patients may also notice a *swelling* as the tumour enlarges, and many children with a tumour in the femur present with a *limp*.

These tumours can sometimes present as a *pyrexia of unknown origin* and cause rigors and night sweats.

There may be *weight loss and malaise*, especially if the lesion is a metastasis from a neuroblastoma.

Examination

Site The mid-shaft of the femur is the most common site to find these tumours, but the tibia and the humerus can also be affected.

Colour The overlying skin may be reddened.

Tenderness The swelling is usually a little tender.

Temperature The increased vascularity makes the whole area feel warm.

Shape The tumour causes a symmetrical fusiform enlargement of the *shaft of the bone*, the upper and lower limits of which are indistinct.

Surface The surface of the swelling is smooth.

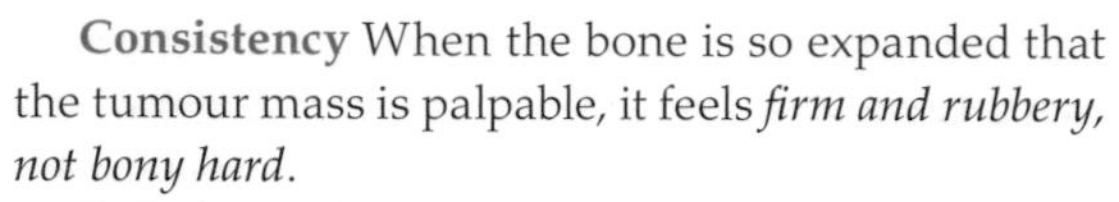

Consistency When the bone is so expanded that the tumour mass is palpable, it feels *firm and rubbery, not bony hard*.

Relations The overlying structures can be moved over the mass because, although they are displaced, they are not usually infiltrated.

Lymph glands The lymph glands should not be palpable.

Local tissues The arteries and nerves of the limb are rarely involved.

General examination There may be pyrexia and weight loss.

Examination of the lungs and liver may reveal evidence of secondary deposits.

Very rarely, a primary neuroblastoma may be palpable in the abdomen. This is palpable as a lobulated mass in the upper part of the abdomen, which may cross the midline (see Chapter 15).

GIANT CELL TUMOUR (OSTEOCLASTOMA)

These tumours are sometimes classified as having a *variable malignant potential* because approximately one-third are entirely benign, one-third invade nearby tissues, and one-third metastasize. The tumour has a red fleshy appearance and consists of multinucleate giant cells in a background of stromal cells that extend into the surrounding bone.

History

Age The patient is usually between 20 and 40 years old.

Symptoms The usual presenting symptom is *pain*. The pain is a dull ache, but it may become acute if there is a *pathological fracture*.

The patient may also notice *swelling of the lower end of the femur or the upper end of the tibia*.

The nearby joint may get stiff if the swelling disturbs the tendons around it, or if the tumour invades the bone just beneath the articular cartilage.

Examination

Site The common sites to find giant cell tumours are the *lower end of the femur and upper end of the tibia* (i.e. either side of the knee), and *the upper end of the humerus and lower end of the radius* (i.e. away from the elbow).

Colour The colour of the skin is normal.

Tenderness The swelling may be tender.

Temperature These tumours are not usually vascular, and the temperature of the overlying skin should be normal.

Shape Giant cell tumours usually cause a diffuse expansion of the end of a bone, but it may be asymmetrical and noticeable only on one side. *Surface* Their surface is smooth.

Consistency The lump feels *bony hard* provided the outer layer of bone is reasonably thick. It may feel firm and slightly pliable if it is thin, and when it is very thin it crackles and bends when touched and feels like *a broken eggshell*.

It does not pulsate unless very thin walled and malignant.

Relations The surrounding structures are usually freely mobile over the swelling.

Lymph glands The local lymph glands should not be enlarged.

MULTIPLE MYELOMA (PLASMACYTOMA)

This is a malignant B-cell lymphoproliferative disease of the bone marrow with multiple deposits of plasma cells. These cells have a large, eccentric 'cartwheel' nucleus.

The vertebral bodies, ribs, pelvis, skull and proximal ends of the femur and the humerus are the most commonly affected, and usually contain multiple lytic deposits.

History

The patient is usually aged 45–60 years and presents with *general malaise, loss of weight* and *intractable pain in the skeleton* – mostly in the back and chest wall.

Pathological fractures can occur and cause even more *severe acute pain*.

Hypercalcaemia may cause *polyuria, thirst* and *abdominal pain*.

A large single deposit (*plasmacytoma*) may become obvious as a bony 'lump'.

Examination

A *plasmacytoma may be palpable as a single bony lump*.

There may be signs of involvement of other parts of the blood-forming tissues – enlarged lymph glands, hepatomegaly and splenomegaly.

The presence of *Bence-Jones protein* in the urine is diagnostic, and an abnormal band of protein is usually present on the electrophoretic strip.

Conditions of joints

OSTEOARTHRITIS

This common condition can affect any joint. It is believed to be caused by asymmetrical wear and tear, often exacerbated by injury and a disturbance of the normal stresses and strains associated with the transfer of weight across the joint. There may be an inherited genetic defect in the structure of type IV collagen that weakens the strength of articular cartilage.

The accepted causative factors are:

- Age.
- Previous fractures involving the articular surface and cartilage.
- Previous joint diseases.
- Malalignment of the skeleton following trauma or bone disease.

The *articular cartilage* becomes thin and softened, before it ultimately disintegrates and wears through.

This leads to joint space narrowing, with *subchondral cysts* and *sclerosis* developing in the subarticular bone.

The joint synovium becomes inflamed, and the joint capsule becomes fibrotic.

This is accompanied by new growth of bone at the edges of the cartilage, causing *osteophyte formation*.

History

Age Most patients with osteoarthritis are over 50 years old, but secondary osteoarthritis following trauma or disease may begin in early adult life.

Symptoms The principal symptom is *pain*, which comes on gradually, but steadily increases until all movements of the joint are very painful. This is a very slow process. Associated with the pain is an *increasing stiffness* that may precede the onset of the pain.

Weakness The stiffness and pain lead to disuse atrophy, so the muscles controlling the joint become weak and wasted.

Deformity As the stiffness increases, the joint often develops a degree of *fixed flexion*, and the limb may lie with a degree of *abnormal abduction* or *adduction*.

Limping Pain, stiffness, weakness and deformity of the joints in the lower limb interfere with walking.

Swelling The whole joint is often swollen by bony osteophytes and an effusion. The synovium is not usually thickened.

Examination

Inspection

Colour The skin should not be reddened or discoloured.

Contour The joint is usually swollen (see Figure 8.28).

Deformity The joint may be fixed in an abnormal position. Nearby muscles are wasted (see also Figure 6.4).

Relations Other joints in the same limb, and the same joint in the other limb, may be similarly diseased.

Palpation

Skin The skin temperature is normal, not hot.

Tenderness Pressure on the joint, especially if it is swollen, may cause pain, but local tenderness is uncommon except during an acute exacerbation when there is an effusion.

Synovium The synovium is not normally palpable.

Muscle bulk The bulk of the muscles that control the joint is reduced (see Figure 6.4).

Bony contours The bone at the edge of the articular cartilage may feel irregular and protuberant.

Movement

All movements of the joint are painful at their extremes, and some movements are reduced. Affected joints may eventually become unstable.

Not all movements of the joint will be equally affected. For example, early osteoarthritis of the hip may cause limitation of abduction and medial rotation long before it affects flexion, extension, adduction and lateral rotation.

NOTE: Make sure that you assess the limitation of movement accurately by asking the patient to do active movements before you perform passive movements.

Crepitus The joint often crackles and clicks during movement. Although the patient can feel a grating sensation associated with the crepitus, it is not usually painful.

Abnormal movements There should be no abnormal movements because all the ligaments should be intact.

Arteries and nerves in the limb

These structures should all be normal.

Other joints

Osteoarthritis is often bilateral and symmetrical. The joints most often affected are the hip, knee, spine and fingers.

General examination

Osteoarthritis is not associated with any other generalized disease, so the rest of the examination should be normal.

> **NOTE:** As many of the patients with osteoarthritis are old and overweight, they frequently have unrelated diseases such as coronary, cerebral and peripheral artery disease. The detection of these diseases is important because their existence may alter the patient's management.

RHEUMATOID ARTHRITIS

Rheumatoid arthritis is a chronic, systemic inflammatory autoimmune disorder that affects the *synovium* and can affect *multiple organ systems*. The precise cause is unknown although a genetic predisposition and environmental cause (such as some viral infections) are believed to be important factors. It especially affects the joints of the hands and feet.

The *synovial membrane* becomes inflamed thickened by hyperaemia and inflammatory cell infiltration. Left untreated the cartilage becomes damaged and eroded, and eventually the joint is destroyed, with progressive instability and deformity. There may be an *associated effusion*. Near the joints, there may be *nodules* consisting of necrotic collagen surrounded by fibroblasts.

History

Age It may appear in patients of all ages, but the common time of onset is between the ages of 30 and 40 years.

Sex Females are affected three times more often than males.

Symptoms The first complaint is often of *early morning swollen and stiff fingers and toes.* The main symptoms are *pain and swelling* of multiple joints. Occasionally, the condition can begin in a single large joint. The disease usually fluctuates between *remissions and 'flare-ups'*. Left untreated the condition is almost always progressive.

Wasting As the disease progresses, the joint movements become restricted, and the muscles that control the joint waste away and become weak.

General malaise The patient may be *fatigued and generally unwell.*

Examination

Inspection

The disease, which is an *asymmetrical polyarthritis*, usually *starts in the small joints* at the end of the limbs – fingers, wrists, toes and ankles – before it moves to the larger joints of the limb, and ultimately to the joints of the trunk. The manifestations of the disease in the hands are described in Chapter 7.

Contour The joints are evenly enlarged. The finger joints become fusiform (Figure 6.28).

Colour The skin overlying the joint may be red and, if there is much swelling, shiny and taut.

Deformity As the disease advances, it affects the ligaments and tendons around the joint as well as the articular surfaces, causing a variety of joint deformities. For example, there is often *ulnar deviation at the wrist joint* and *hyperextension of the proximal interphalangeal joints* (Figures 6.28a, b) (see Figure 7.34). There may also be subluxation or dislocation of the metacarpal joints, with the development of *swan neck and boutonnière deformities.*

Wasting The muscles that control the affected joints are wasted.

Other joints Many joints are affected, and the condition is frequently symmetrical.

Palpation

Temperature The skin over the joint is warm.

Tenderness In the acute stage of the disease, the joint is tender to light palpation. The tenderness subsides as the condition progresses, but the pain during movement persists.

Synovium Soft tissue thickening can often be felt around the joint. It is only possible to be certain that there is thickened synovium in those joints where

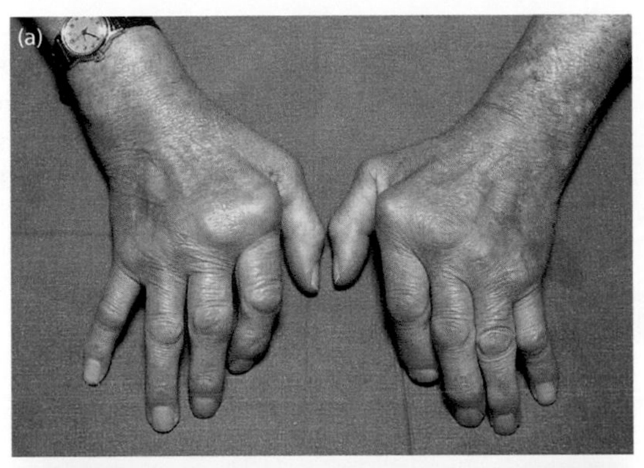

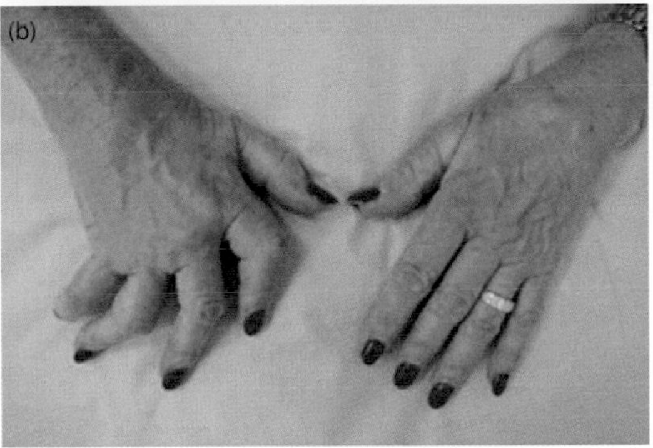

Figure 6.28 RHEUMATOID HANDS. (a, b) Both show the typical features of fusiform swelling of the finger, muscle wasting and ulna deviation.

it has a clearly palpable edge beyond the joint line. There may also be an *effusion* in the joint.

Muscle bulk The muscles that control the joint feel thin and atrophic.

Bony contours Until the joint surfaces are destroyed and *pathological dislocations* occur, the general bony contour of the joint remains normal, but it is often obscured by the synovial thickening.

Movement

- Active movements are limited by pain and reduced in power.
- Passive movements are limited by pain and fibrous contractures.
- Abnormal movements appear when the disease has weakened the ligaments, or tendons have ruptured.

Arteries and nerves in the limb

The other structures in the limb should be normal. Patients with long-standing rheumatoid arthritis sometimes get a peripheral arteritis, which causes gangrene of the tips of the toes and fingers, and ulceration of the skin of the lower third of the leg. In countries with good access to healthcare, this is now less common because of disease modifying medication. Swelling of the joints around the wrist may cause a *carpal tunnel syndrome* (see Chapter 7), and peripheral neuritis can develop.

General examination

Apart from other joint involvement, there may be generalized wasting and anaemia. Three systemic diseases are associated with rheumatoid joint disease:

- *Still's disease*, a disease in which adults develop arthritis, splenomegaly and lymphadenopathy.
- *Reiter's syndrome*, in which there is urethritis, conjunctivitis, skin rashes and arthritis.
- *Systemic lupus erythematosus*, a collagen disease in which there is a scaly, red rash on the face, debility and manifestations in all tissues of a small vessel arteritis (see Chapter 3).

Other conditions that may also present in a similar fashion to rheumatoid arthritis include:

- *Juvenile idiopathic arthritis*, which is an inflammatory arthritis occurring in patients under the age of 16 years.
- *Reactive arthritis*, when joint pain and swelling is triggered by an infection in another part of the body – most often the intestines, genitals or urinary tract. This usually targets the knees and the joints of the ankles and feet.
- *Lyme disease*, which is an infectious disease caused by the *Borrelia bacterium*, which is spread by ticks, and associated with joint inflammation.

GOUT AND PSEUDOGOUT (PYROPHOSPHATE CRYSTAL DEPOSITION)

These two conditions are considered together as their symptoms are very similar. Gout is the result of deposition of *uric acid crystals*, while in pseudogout, *calcium pyrophosphate crystals* are deposited.

A disorder of *purine metabolism* is responsible for gout, in which there is often hyperuricaemia, deposition of urate crystals in the joints causing acute synovitis, and the formation of renal stones (see Chapter 17).

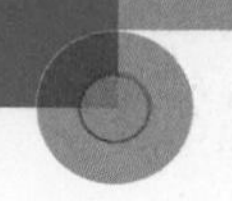

Revision panel 6.3

DIFFERENTIAL DIAGNOSIS OF RHEUMATOID ARTHRITIS

- Seronegative polyarthritis
- Systemic lupus erythematosus
- Gout and pseudogout
- Ankylosing spondylitis
- Reactive arthritis
- Polyarticular osteoarthritis
- Polymyalgia rheumatica
- Juvenile idiopathic arthritis
- Still's disease
- Lyme disease
- Psoriatic arthitis

Secondary gout can be caused by *renal failure* and *cytotoxic treatment of malignancy*, with massive cell death resulting in an increased purine load.

Pyrophosphate is generated in cartilage, where it combines with calcium to form crystals in the collagen. These are extruded into the joint from time to time, where they cause an acute local inflammatory reaction that is almost identical to gout.

History

Age *Gout* usually occurs in middle-aged or elderly males, often with a family history of the disorder.

Pseudogout tends to occur in middle-aged females.

Symptoms The onset of gout is often heralded by the development of an *acute painful red first metacarpal joint*. The attack begins spontaneously, but can follow an *alcoholic binge*, a *minor injury* or *excessive exercise*, and usually takes several days or a week to abate. It can also arise in the ankles, knees, finger joints and bursae, and can occasionally present with acute pain in the heel or sole of the foot.

Patients may notice *tophi*, which are clumps of crystals in tendons, in bursae and 'classically' in the subcutaneous tissues of the pinnae of the ears. They may also present with *colic* from renal calculi (see Chapter 17). The condition can become chronic, with recurrent bouts of acute pain that may become continuous, leading to stiffness of many joints. Large tophi may form, which may ulcerate.

The onset of pseudogout is also usually heralded by sudden pain and swelling in a joint, but this is *usually in the knee rather than the foot* and is seldom as severe. Other conditions may also present in similar fashion to gout, especially involving the first metatarsal phalangeal joint (Revision panel 6.4).

Revision panel 6.4

DIFFERENTIAL DIAGNOSIS OF GOUT/ PSEUDOGOUT

- Septic arthritis
- Rheumatoid arthritis
- Osteoarthritis

Examination

Colour The gouty joint is red (Figure 6.29), but the joint affected by pseudogout is not.

Contour Both conditions cause joint swelling.

Tenderness The joint feels tender and hot in both conditions.

All joint movements are painful and restricted. Gout makes weight-bearing and walking very difficult.

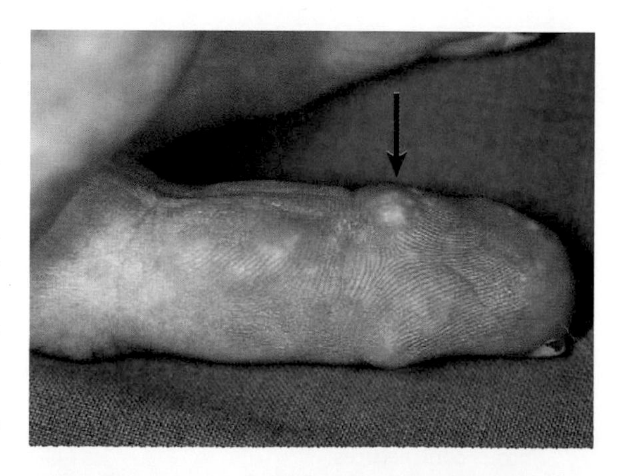

Figure 6.29 Gouty tophi occurring in a thumb (arrow).

NOTE: The diagnosis of both conditions is confirmed by identifying their characteristic crystals on joint aspirates.

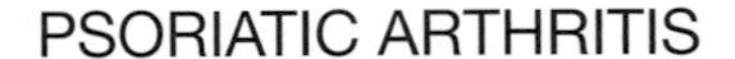

PSORIATIC ARTHRITIS

This type of arthritis develops in some people with the skin condition known as *psoriasis* (see Chapter 4, page 163). It causes joints to become inflamed, swollen and painful. The most affected joints are the hands, feet, knees, neck, spine and elbows. Over a period of time, the symptoms can get worse, though there can be periods of improvement, known as remission.

History

Age Psoriatic arthritis can start at any age, but often appears between ages 30 and 50. For most people, it starts about 10 years after psoriasis is first recognized. While it is less common, people can develop psoriatic arthritis without having psoriasis.

Symptoms The common joint symptoms are *pain and swelling over tendons, with swollen fingers and toes*. The joints affected may be *symmetrical* or *asymmetrical*.

The pain *limits movement of the joint* and is associated with stiffness.

Morning stiffness and tiredness are common associated non-specific symptoms.

Examination

Contour The affected joints are diffusely swollen, and the digits can appear sausage-like.

Colour The colour of the skin over the joint is normal.

Muscle wasting There can be muscle wasting due to disuse.

Skin and nails The nails may be pitted or fall off (*onycholysis*).

Eyes People with psoriatic arthritis may experience eye problems, such as inflammation and redness.

Skin Depending on the extent of the underlying inflammatory process, the skin over the joint may be warmer. There may be signs of psoriatic skin plaques (see Chapter 4, page 163)

Tenderness The joint may be tender.

Movement is limited because of the stiffness that develops with the condition.

TUBERCULOUS ARTHRITIS

Any joint can become infected with the human or bovine tubercle bacillus, either directly from the bloodstream or more commonly from the adjacent bone (see page 206).

The infection produces typical pathological changes in the synovium, with *granulomas* containing giant cells, lymphocytes and macrophages, before caseation occurs. The articular cartilage and bone are destroyed as the disease progresses.

The joints of the *vertebral column* are most often affected, but it can also occur in the hip or knee, and occasionally in the joints of the upper limb.

History

Age Tuberculous arthritis tends to occur in young adults and children. Mild symptoms may be present for many years before the patient complains or seeks advice.

Symptoms The common joint symptoms of *pain* and *swelling* usually begin simultaneously, but in the hip or the spine where the swelling is not apparent, pain is the presenting feature.

The pain limits movement of the joint, and this usually interferes with *walking, bending* and *stooping.*

An abscess can form in the joint, which may point onto the skin and then discharge. The resulting *chronic sinus* (see Figure 6.1), with a sero-purulent discharge, persists until the disease is cured or dies out.

General malaise and *loss of weight* are common associated non-specific symptoms.

Social history It is important to enquire about social conditions, such as diet, housing and international travel, as well as the existence of any family history of tuberculosis.

Examination

Contour The joint (especially the knee) is diffusely swollen.

Colour The colour of the skin over the joint is normal.

Sinuses There may be a *discharging sinus near the joint, or the scars of healed sinuses* (see Figure 6.1).

Muscle wasting There is usually marked muscle wasting, especially of the quadriceps femoris muscles when the knee joint is diseased (see Figure 6.4).

Skin The skin over the joint is not hot, but the inflammatory hyperaemia in the underlying synovium may make it slightly warmer than normal.

Tenderness The joint may be tender for a short period in the early acute phase of the disease, but once the infection is established, the joint is not usually painful.

Synovium The swelling around the joint feels soft and pliable – something like unbaked dough. There is always an effusion in the joint.

Bony contour The bones are only deformed or destroyed in long-standing severe disease.

Movement is only limited if the joints are painful, usually because of pronounced protective muscle spasm.

There should be no abnormal movements.

When the disease is advanced and has destroyed the joint, it becomes fixed by a *fibrous ankylosis* (Figure 6.30).

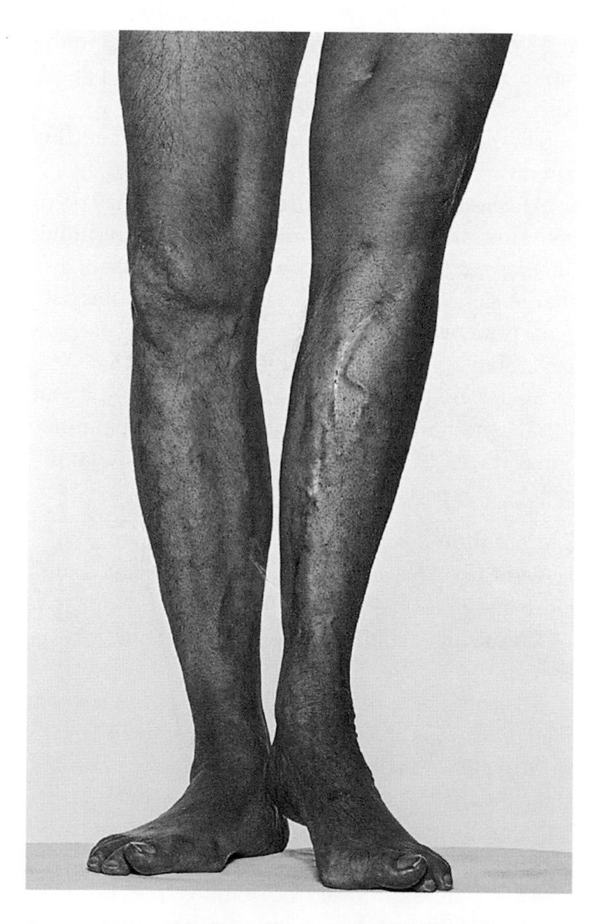

Figure 6.30 The end result of severe tuberculosis of the left knee joint: a fibrous ankylosis, shortening and wasting of the limb and healed sinuses.

General examination

There may be evidence of tuberculosis elsewhere, such as in the lungs or the kidneys, so the general examination must be thorough and complete.

HAEMOPHILIC ARTHRITIS

Intra-articular haemorrhage is a common complication in patients with deficiency of clotting factor VIII (*haemophilia*) or of factor IX (*Christmas disease*). These are *X-linked recessive disorders* and are therefore manifest in males, although females are the carriers of the conditions.

Recurrent episodes of bleeding leads to progressive articular cartilage destruction, with subchondral bone changes, including cyst formation.

History

Age Initial bleeding into the joint usually starts when the child begins to stand and walk. The arthritis usually develops in young adults.

Symptoms *Pain and swelling of the joints* occurs often after relatively trivial trauma, although the degree of bleeding also depends on the severity of the disorder.

The most affected joints are the ankles, knees, shoulders, elbows and hips.

Bleeding can also occur into muscles, causing a painful swelling, with restriction of movement in the joints adjacent to the muscle.

Secondary compression of a peripheral nerve can cause neurological symptoms if the swelling is large. Bleeding into the nerve can also cause intense pain.

Examination

Contour The joint is diffusely swollen.

Colour The colour of the skin over the joint may be normal, or *bruising* may be apparent.

Muscles There may be muscle wasting when arthritis has become established. In an acute bleed, the muscles may contain a lump or become swollen.

Skin The skin over the joint will be warm when bruising is present, and slightly warmer than normal in established chronic synovitis.

Tenderness The joint is painful following a bleed and becomes progressively more tender, as cartilage degeneration follows recurrent episodes.

Movements are limited by pain. When the disease is advanced and has destroyed the joint, it may become ankylosed.

NEUROPATHIC JOINTS (CHARCOT'S JOINT)

The brain is unable to protect a joint that has lost its 'pain and position sense' from harmful stresses and strains. The frequent minor injuries that result ultimately destroy the bones and the ligaments of the joint.

A neuropathic joint is therefore a *painless, disorganized joint.*

The possible causes of loss of joint sensation are:

- Diabetic neuropathy (the most common cause nowadays).
- Tabes dorsalis (rare today).
- Syringomyelia.
- Leprosy.
- Cauda equina lesions such as a myelomeningocele.

History

Age Neuropathic joints usually occur in middle and old age. In syringomyelia, the condition often dates from an earlier age, and there is often dissociation of sensory loss, with loss of pain and temperature sense, but not of touch.

Symptoms The patient notices that the joint is becoming *swollen and deformed* and *gives way frequently but is not painful.*

The mechanical weakness of the joint together with the sensory defects of the neuropathy make the patient's *gait unstable.*

Previous illness The patient will probably know if they have had *diabetes* for many years but may not know if they have had syphilis.

Other neurological conditions may be present.

Examination

Colour The colour of the skin over the joint is normal.

Contour The joint is usually *swollen and obviously deformed* (Figures 6.4, 6.31). There is no common pattern of deformity for any particular joint.

Palpation

Tenderness The joint is not tender, and movements in any direction do not usually cause pain.

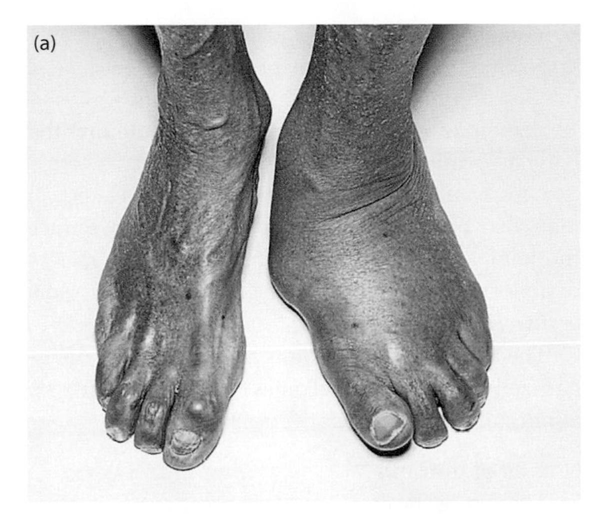

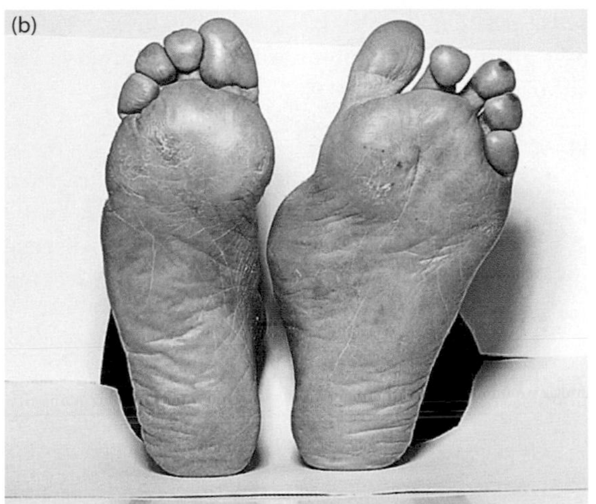

Figure 6.31 TWO VIEWS OF A CHARCOT JOINT. (a, b) A totally disorganized, but painless, left ankle and foot. This Charcot ankle and foot was caused by diabetic peripheral neuropathy.

Synovium The synovium is not thickened, but there is always an effusion.

Bony contours The bones are *displaced and deformed.* The normal shape of the bones forming the joint may completely disappear as a result of a combination of bone destruction in some areas, and new bone formation and hypertrophy in others.

The joint may be *subluxed* or *dislocated,* and there is gross bone erosion with irregular calcified masses in the capsule.

Movement

Normal movements may be impossible because of the destruction of the joints and ligaments.

Some passive movements may be limited by the bony deformities.

Grossly abnormal movements may be possible. It may also be possible to dislocate and then reduce the joint, which can usually be moved in a variety of abnormal ways *without the patient feeling any pain or discomfort.*

The knee and elbow joints may become so disorganized that the limb becomes *flail-like,* with grossly abnormal but painless movements.

Nerves of the limb

These must be examined with great care. *Vibration sense, position sense* and *deep pain sensitivity* are usually all reduced or absent. The motor innervation should be normal.

General examination

Look for the signs of diabetes and syphilis. Take particular care to examine the whole of the nervous system for evidence of any other neurological disease processes, such as syringomyelia, and test the urine for sugar.

ACUTE SEPTIC ARTHRITIS

This is usually caused by *Staphylococcus aureus* (like osteomyelitis; see page 206), but *Haemophilus influenzae* (see Figure 6.22) can also cause joint infection in young children. The organisms obtain access to the joint from the bloodstream, from a penetrating joint injury or from direct spread from an infected bone (*osteomyelitis*).

The infection destroys the joint, and the pus may then track into the soft tissues before discharging onto the skin as one or more *sinuses*.

The infection will eventually settle, and a *fibrous* or *bony ankylosis* will occur (see below).

History

Age Children of both sexes are most commonly infected, but septic arthritis is also seen in adults of all ages.

Symptoms *Acute pain and joint swelling* are the two most common symptoms, and limit joint movement, leading to immobility and loss of function.

The patient will feel hot and sweaty, which may be accompanied by loss of appetite, general malaise and sometimes even rigors.

In neonates, the symptoms of sepsis predominate – irritability and failure to feed. Likely portals of entry include the umbilical cord and intravenous access sites.

Examination

Inspection

Colour The overlying skin may be red.

Contour The joint will usually appear swollen, and the limb may be held in flexion.

Overlying skin One or more discharging or healed sinuses may be present depending on the stage of the disease.

Palpation

Skin This may feel warm.

Tenderness This will be present over the joint, and there may be fluctuation if an abscess has formed.

Movement

Both active and passive movements will be *severely restricted and very painful.*

ANKYLOSIS

An ankylosed joint is a fixed joint.

A *bony* ankylosis is present if the bones that form the joint are fixed together by bone. This is absolutely fixed and painless even when stressed.

A *fibrous* ankylosis occurs when the bones are fixed by dense fibrous tissue. This moves a little and forced movement causes pain.

Congenital/genetic disorders of bones and joints

There are numerous disorders of cartilage and bone development, most of which cannot be discussed in a book of this type. Some (e.g. Marfan's syndrome) are the result of single defective genes, others are probably polygenomic, and some result from damage to the fetus in utero (e.g. phocomelia from thalidomide). The common conditions are covered in different anatomical sections of this book but are summarized in Revision panel 6.5.

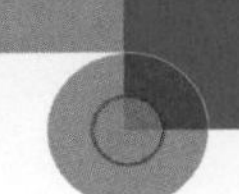

Revision panel 6.5

GENETIC SKELETAL DISORDERS

- Multiple exostoses (see above)
- Dyschondroplasia (see above)
- Achondroplasia (see Chapter 1)
- Multiple epithelial dysplasia (abnormal metaphyses of long bones)
- Osteopetrosis (marble bone disease)
- Candle/spotted or striped bones
- Osteogenesis imperfecta (brittle bones)
- Extra/absent/hypoplastic or fused bones
- Hemi- or fused vertebrae (see Chapter 9)
- Congenital pseudo-arthrosis
- Ehlers–Danlos syndrome (joint laxity and aneurysms)
- Marfan's syndrome (see Chapters 1 and 9)
- Hurler's syndrome (gargoylism)
- Gaucher's disease (mucopolysaccharidoses/ excessive storage of glycosaminoglycans)
- Neurofibromatosis (see Chapter 3)
- Down's syndrome (see Chapter 1)
- Sprengel's deformity (see Chapter 7)
- Phocomelia (hypoplastic/absent limb)

Upper limb

STEVEN A CORBETT, W JAMES WHITE AND DONALD SAMMUT

THE SHOULDER

The shoulder is one of the most mobile joints in the human body, and therefore also one of the least stable. This allows the arm and hand to be orientated in space. There are three principal joints of the shoulder:

- The glenohumeral joint.
- The acromioclavicular joint.
- The sternoclavicular joint.

The scapulothoracic articulation, together with a pseudo-joint between the humerus and the coracoacromial arch, is also required to facilitate movement and versatility.

The shoulder is made up of three principal bones:

- The clavicle (collar bone).
- The scapula (shoulder blade).
- The humerus (upper arm bone).

The principles of examination of the shoulder joint are the same as for any other joint:

- Look.
- Feel.
- Move.

Additionally, one may use special tests for anatomical structures and pathological conditions. As in any orthopaedic examination, it is important to assess the joint proximal and distal to that being examined, in this case the cervical spine and the elbow.

The symptoms most commonly encountered are:

- *Pain*, which may be located to a particular region of the upper limb such as the shoulder, elbow or hand, or may be referred into the upper limb from the neck (see Chapter 9); the pain may be present at rest, night time or on movement.
- *Deformity*, which is the result of congenital anatomical abnormalities, tumours, trauma or wasting.
- *Disability*, caused by loss of function and stiffness, which may result from joint pathology, nerve damage or muscular weakness.

Plan for examination of the shoulder

INSPECTION

The patient should be adequately exposed to the waist and examined from both the front and the back. The upper torso, neck, shoulder, scapula and both upper limbs should be examined and compared.

The skin should be inspected for evidence of *scars, sinuses* and *discolouration*.

Arthroscopic surgical scars are small and are easily missed. Arthroscopy of the shoulder is carried out through a scar positioned approximately 1 cm medial to and below the posterior lateral border of the acromion, i.e. on the posterior aspect of the shoulder joint. Further arthroscopic portals can be positioned laterally and anteriorly. Open surgical procedures usually involve an incision placed in the deltopectoral groove; however, lateral approaches are also used for certain procedures.

Shape

The muscles of the shoulder girdle may be wasted.

- *Deltoid* wasting can occur secondary to an axillary nerve palsy.
- Wasting of the *rotator cuff muscles* – supraspinatus, infraspinatus, teres minor and subscapularis – can be associated with nerve palsy, for example of the suprascapular nerve affecting supraspinatus and infraspinatus, or with tendon tears.
- Wasting of the *trapezius muscle* can be seen following injury to the spinal accessory nerve during surgery to the neck or following blunt trauma or traction injury (see Chapter 4).

A 'Popeye sign' is associated with a rupture of the long head of biceps (see Figure 7.17).

In addition, the overall shape of the shoulder may be altered by a rupture of the pectoralis major tendon (Figure 7.1).

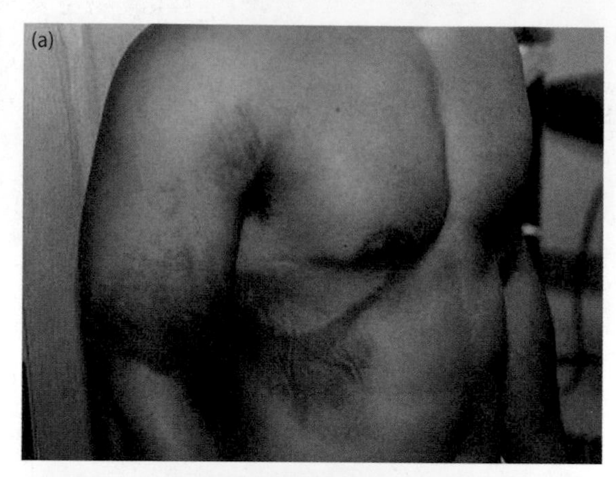

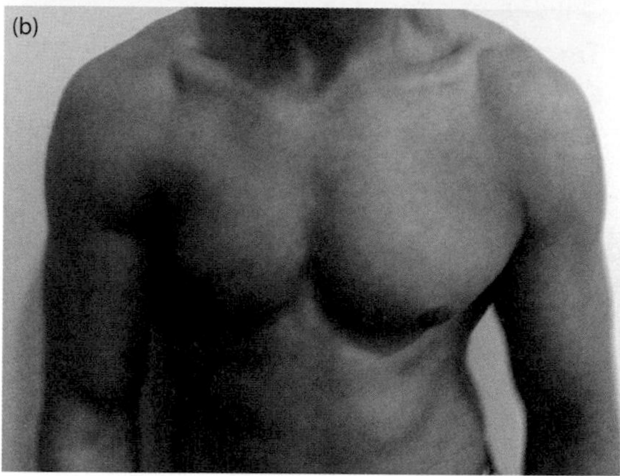

Figure 7.1 RUPTURE OF PECTORALIS MAJOR. (a) Acute rupture. (b) Chronic rupture.

The shape of the shoulder can also be significantly altered by the size, shape and position of the scapula. The scapulae should be symmetrical.

Failure of descent of the scapula during development can result in the scapula remaining elevated, smaller than usual and more prominent (*Sprengel's deformity*). This is associated with a shorter neck, and often a kyphosis or scoliosis of the thoracic spine (Figure 7.2).

More commonly, both scapulae fail to descend (*Klippel–Feil syndrome*). Patients appear to have no neck with associated low hairline, bilateral neck webbing and limitation of neck movement.

Lateral winging of the scapula can occur in association with *long thoracic nerve palsy*, resulting in *wasting of serratus anterior*. This can be demonstrated

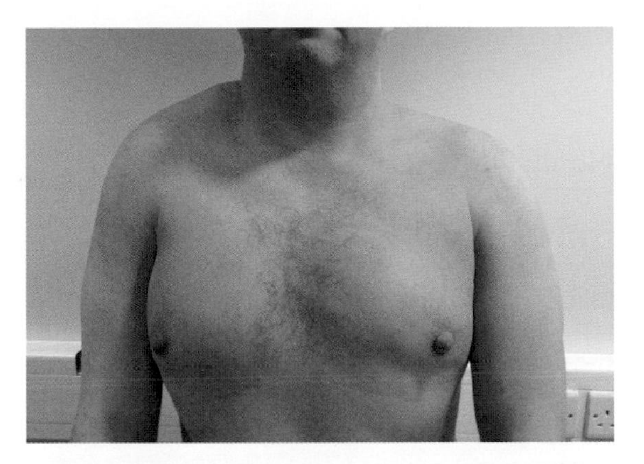

Figure 7.2 Sprengel's deformity.

by asking the patient to raise both arms to shoulder height and press into a wall (Figure 7.3).

Abnormalities of the acromioclavicular joint can alter the shape of the shoulder. Degenerative change or previous trauma resulting in dislocation makes the joint more prominent, with the appearance of a raised bump at the outer end of the clavicle.

Occasionally, a glenohumeral joint effusion can be observed as an anterior swelling that rarely extends into the axilla.

Other soft tissue masses may be visible, particularly lipomas in the region of the deltoid and scapula. Cystic swellings of the superior aspect of the shoulder are also common, particularly in relation to the acromioclavicular joint, and in association with significant rotator cuff tears.

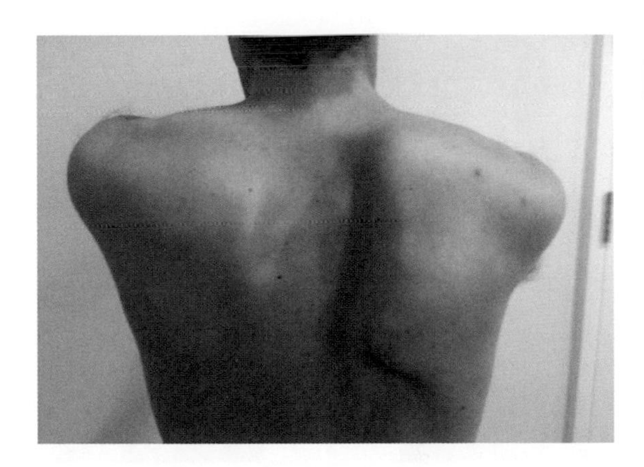

Figure 7.3 Winging of the right scapula.

PALPATION

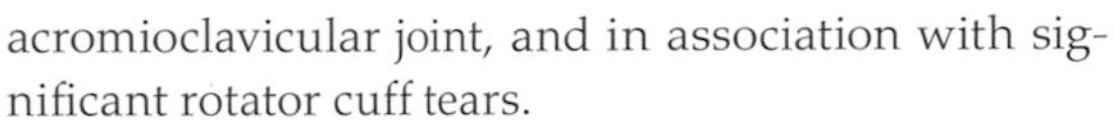

Palpation should begin at the sternoclavicular joint and proceed laterally along the clavicle. Clavicular irregularity may follow a fracture or sternoclavicular dislocation. The acromioclavicular joint and acromion should both be examined. The acromion passes laterally and posteriorly to the spine of the scapula. The anterior and posterior glenohumeral joint should be assessed.

Palpation of the greater tuberosity may reveal problems associated with the supraspinatus tendon at the site of its insertion, while palpation of the biceps anteriorly in the bicipital groove may also reveal pathology. Palpation is principally to elicit tenderness rather than to assess a temperature change associated with inflammation, which is generally difficult to identify.

MOVEMENT

This can be divided into active and passive. The normal range of shoulder movement is shown in Revision panel 7.1. The range of movement in the shoulder may be restricted because of stiffness or increased as the result of laxity of the joints.

Revision panel 7.1

NORMAL RANGE OF SHOULDER MOVEMENT

0–175° forward elevation
0–175° abduction
Less than 80° external rotation with the elbows at the sides
90° external rotation in 90° abduction
70° internal rotation in 90° abduction
Internal rotation assessed by the patient reaching up the back to thoracic vertebrae 7–10

Active movements may be limited by pain or weakness, and hence passive movement must always be assessed.

Movements should be observed from in front of the patient and from behind.

As well as the range of movement, the rhythm of movement also warrants consideration.

When assessing movement, the plane of the scapula is strictly 30° anterior to the frontal plane. It is, however, generally accepted that forward elevation is in the sagittal plane, and abduction is in the coronal plane.

The glenohumeral joint does not account for all the movement of the shoulder and shoulder girdle, as some movement also occurs at the *scapulothoracic joint*. To assess this, the scapula should be fixed by placing the hand on the top of the shoulder. Early movement takes place almost entirely at the glenohumeral joint, but as the arm is raised, the scapula begins to rotate on the thorax. The final one-third of movement is almost entirely scapulothoracic. In abduction, approximately 100° of movement arises from the glenohumeral joint, and 60° at the scapulothoracic joint.

When there is pathology around the shoulder, this movement may become disturbed. Patients 'hitch' to gain increased range, by using their trapezius muscle to help raise their arm. During forward elevation and abduction, patients may experience a *painful arc* suggestive of rotator cuff pathology.

POWER

This should be assessed in the principal muscles around the shoulder girdle:

- The *deltoid* is assessed by abduction against resistance.
- The *serratus anterior* is assessed by asking the patient to push against a wall with both hands. The scapula should remain close to the thorax, but if there is weakness it becomes more prominent.
- *Pectoralis major* may be assessed by asking the patient to push both hands into their waist.

Specific tests for the rotator cuff complex will be described below.

NEUROLOGICAL EXAMINATION

A formal neurological examination should be performed, including for sensation (see Chapter 3). The most common abnormality is altered skin sensation in the axillary nerve distribution overlying the deltoid. This region is known as the *regimental patch*. Birth trauma palsies such as *Erb's* (C5/6) and *Klumpke's* (C8/T1) neurological deficits may also be apparent.

SPECIAL TESTS

Several special tests have been developed to assess the anatomy and function of the shoulder.

Rotator cuff tendons

Supraspinatus – the empty can test

The arm is placed with the thumb pointing to the floor in the plane of the scapula with 90° of elevation, as if 'emptying a can' (Figure 7.4). Patients are assessed for pain and weakness as the examiner applies downward pressure on the arms.

Infraspinatus/teres minor

The elbows are placed at the sides in 90° of flexion. The patient is then asked to externally rotate against

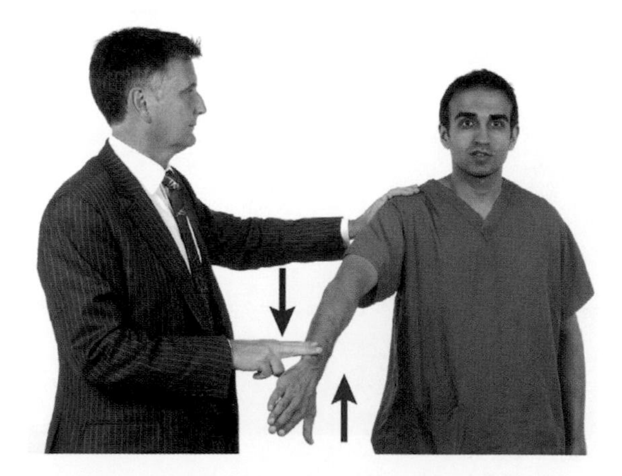

Figure 7.4 The supraspinatus empty can test.

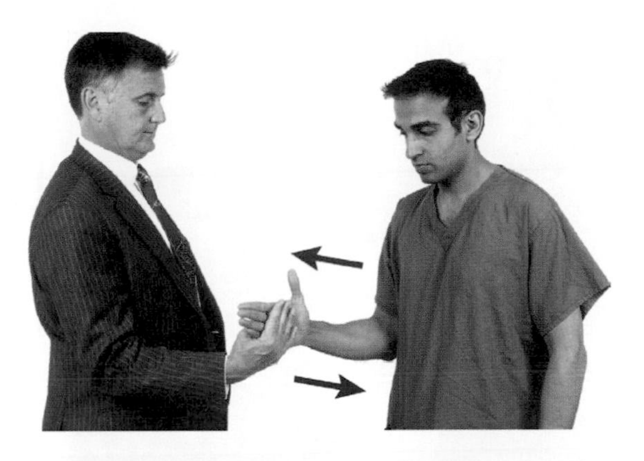

Figure 7.5 The infraspinatus external rotation test.

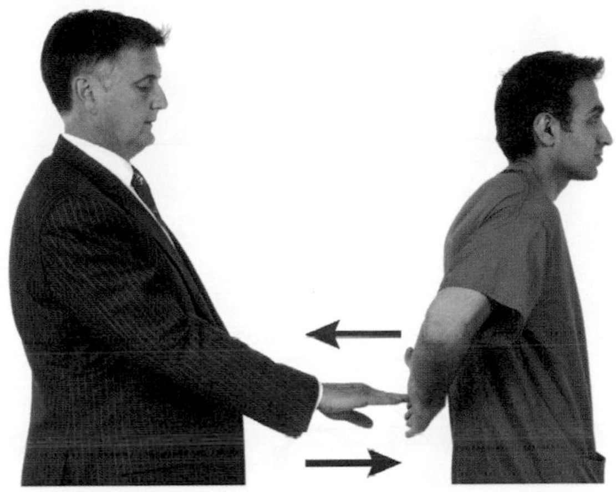

Figure 7.7 The subscapularis Gerber lift-off test.

resistance. If weakness is perceived, the elbow is then placed in maximum external rotation, and the patient is asked to maintain this position (Figure 7.5). When there is a major tear in these tendons, this position cannot be maintained, and the arm drifts back towards the midline (the *lag sign*).

Patients with massive cuff tears cannot externally rotate the elevated abducted arm (*Hornblower's sign*).

Subscapularis

The patient is asked to stand with their hands in front of their belly, with their elbows forward in the coronal plane. The examiner pushes against the patient's elbow to elicit pain and weakness (the *belly press test*) (Figure 7.6).

Alternatively, the patient places their arm behind their back in the mid-lumbar spine region. The examiner then lifts the patient's hand away from their back, and the patient is asked to maintain this position. This is impossible if there is pain or weakness from a tear (*Gerber's lift-off test*) (Figure 7.7).

Long head of biceps

The arm is placed in 90° of forward elevation and external rotation. The patient is asked to resist flexion (*Speed's test*) (Figure 7.8).

Alternatively, the elbow is flexed at 90°, and the patient is asked to supinate actively against resistance from a pronated position (*Yergason's test*) (Figure 7.9).

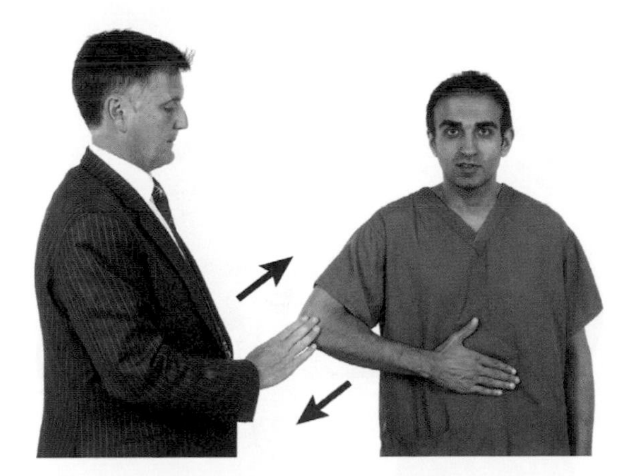

Figure 7.6 The subscapularis belly press test.

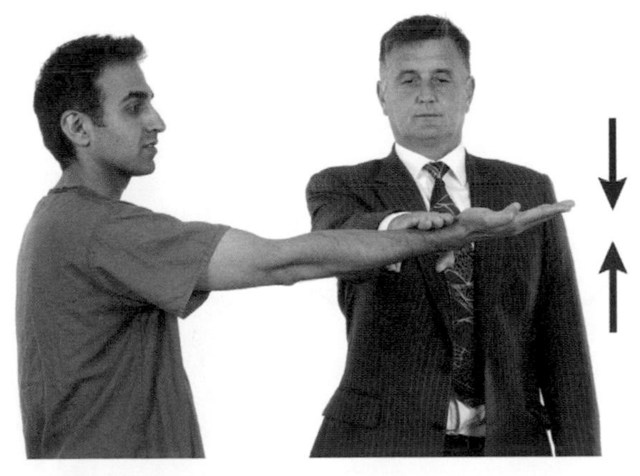

Figure 7.8 Speed's test for the biceps.

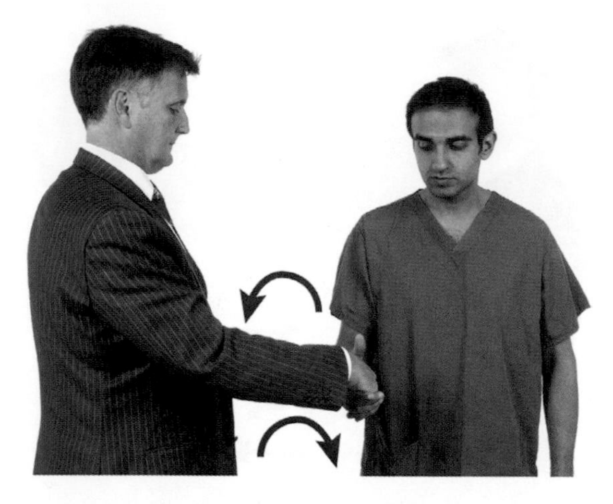

Figure 7.9 Yergason's test for the biceps.

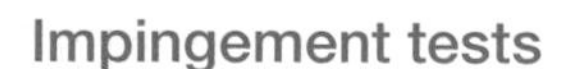

Impingement tests

There are several tests that can be used to assess for impingement, which occurs when the patient experiences pain, usually in the anterolateral aspect of the shoulder, from compression of the subacromial bursa and rotator cuff tendons as they pass under the coracoacromial arch.

The painful arc

When moving the arm in abduction, the patient classically experiences pain between 60° and 120° (Figure 7.10).

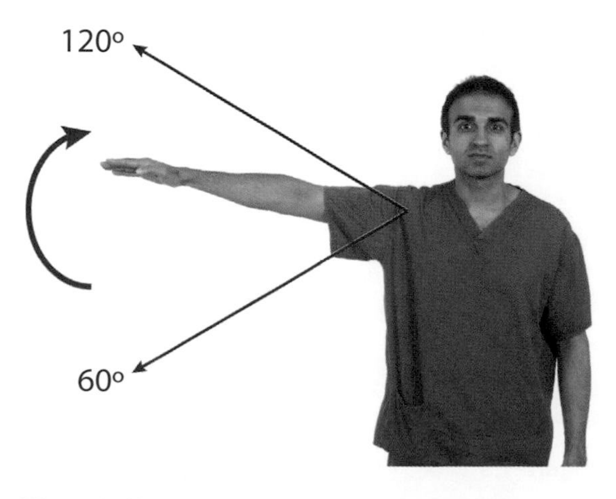

Figure 7.10 The painful arc.

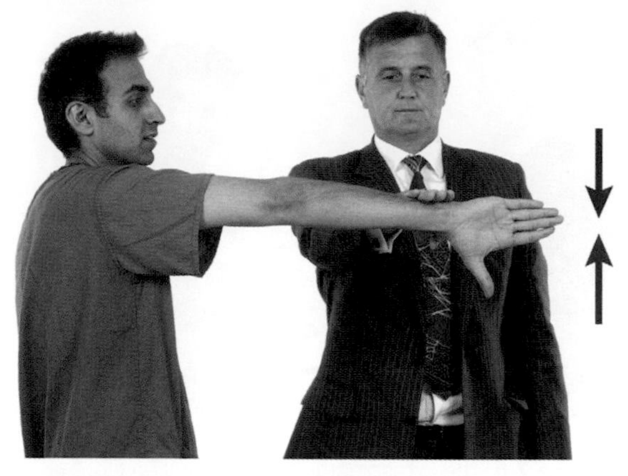

Figure 7.11 Neer's impingement test.

Neer's impingement sign

The scapula is stabilized, and the affected arm is raised and placed in flexion, abduction and internal rotation (Figure 7.11). The test is positive when pain is elicited as the greater tuberosity passes under the coracoclavicular arch.

Local anaesthetic may be injected into the subacromial space as a diagnostic test, which is considered positive if it relieves the patient of their symptoms.

Hawkin's test

The arm is placed in 90° of forward flexion with the elbow flexed to 90°, and the arm is then rotated internally. A positive test occurs when pain is elicited and is experienced in the anterolateral aspect of the shoulder (Figure 7.12).

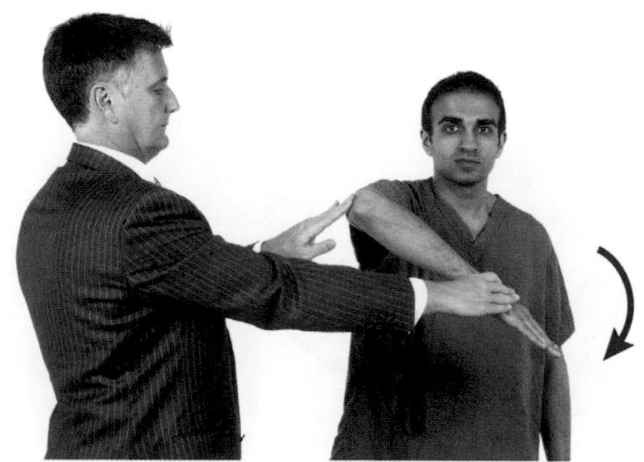

Figure 7.12 Hawkin's test for impingement.

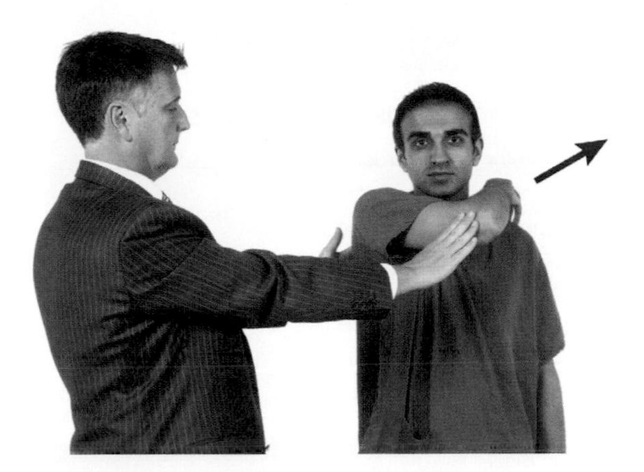

Figure 7.13 The scarf test.

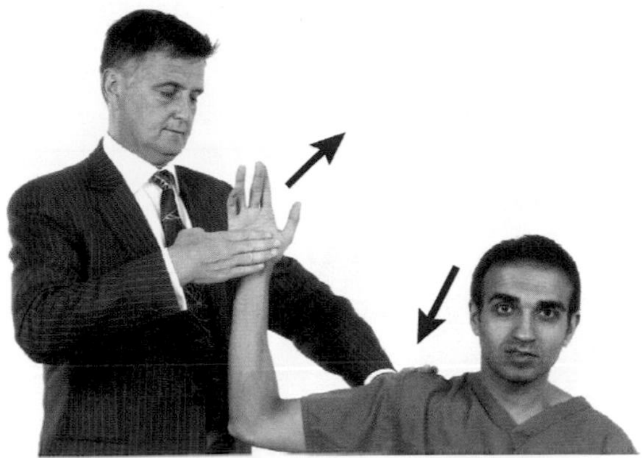

Figure 7.14 The apprehension test.

Acromioclavicular joint

The arm is placed in maximum adduction and pulled forcibly across the chest. This is a screening test for acromioclavicular joint pathology (the *scarf test*) (Figure 7.13).

Instability tests

The three major causes of shoulder glenohumeral joint instability are:

- Trauma.
- Hyperlaxity.
- Muscle patterning disorders, either in isolation or in combination.

These can result in anterior, posterior or multidirectional instability.

The tests described below aim to qualify the degree and nature of the instability.

General instability: the load shift test

The examiner places one hand over the shoulder and the scapula to stabilize the shoulder girdle and uses the other hand to grasp the humeral head. The humerus is then loaded into the glenoid and pulled (translated) anteriorly and posteriorly. The humeral head may be felt to ride up on the glenoid rim.

The patient is placed in different positions to assess different components of the shoulder stabilizing structures. Grading is based on the position:

- Mild: 0–1 cm translation.
- Moderate: 1–2 cm translation.
- Severe: Greater than 2 cm translation up to the glenoid rim.

Anterior instability: the anterior apprehension test

The patient is asked to lie on the examination couch. The arm is placed in 90° of abduction. External rotation is then performed from the neutral position. The examiner observes the 'apprehension' of the patient, i.e. the patient becomes worried that the shoulder is unstable and may dislocate (Figure 7.14).

Anterior instability: Jobe relocation test

The examiner repeats the apprehension tests and then returns to the start position, having noted the degree of external rotation. This is then repeated, and a posterior stress is applied over the humeral head, so that the escaping humeral head is pushed back into the joint. An increase in the external range before symptoms of apprehension are reproduced indicates a positive result (Figure 7.15).

Posterior instability

Posterior labral shift tests are assessed in the same manner as the anterior load and shift.

Posterior instability: the posterior apprehension test

The arm is held in an adducted and flexed position. The examiner pushes posteriorly to elicit apprehension.

Inferior laxity: the sulcus sign

The patient sits or stands with the shoulder in the neutral position. An inferior traction is applied by

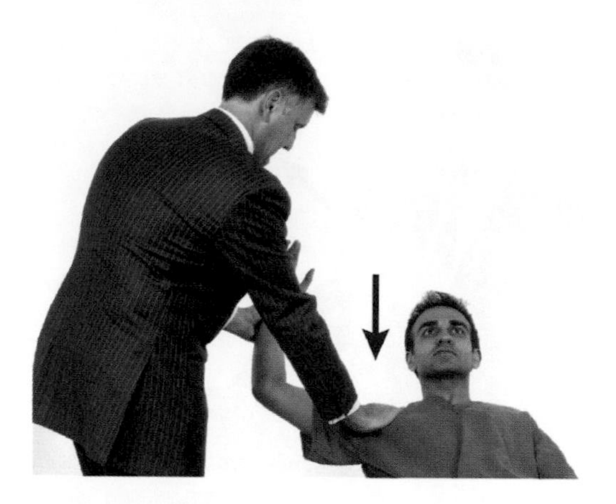

Figure 7.15 The Jobe relocation test.

grasping the arm. The examiner observes for dimpling of the skin below the acromion, which indicates a widening of the subacromial space between the acromion and the humeral head. This may be graded I, II, or III depending on the degree of laxity.

Revision panel 7.2

Shoulder examination summary

- Inspection
- Palpation
- Movement
- Power
- Neurology
- Special tests
  - Stability tests
  - Rotator cuff tests
  - Impingement tests
  - Acromioclavicular joint tests
  - Biceps tests

Revision panel 7.3

COMMON CAUSES OF SHOULDER PAIN

Rotator cuff disorders
Impingement syndrome
Supraspinatus tendinitis
Subacromial bursitis
Tendon tears: partial or complete
Calcific tendinitis
Biceps tendinitis
Adhesive capsulitis (frozen shoulder)

Arthritis

Glenohumeral joint
Acromioclavicular joint

Bone lesions

Infection
Tumour
Avascular necrosis

Instability

Dislocation
Subluxation

Trauma

Fracture

Neurological pain

Brachial plexus neuritis
Suprascapular nerve compression

Referred pain

Cervical spondylosis
Cardiac ischaemia
Mediastinal pathology

CAUSES OF SHOULDER PAIN

The most common causes of shoulder pain are listed in Revision panel 7.3.

Impingement syndrome

This is pain in the subacromial space when the humerus is elevated or internally rotated and is classically seen between 60° and 120° in abduction. This is generally considered synonymous with supraspinatus tendinitis or subacromial bursitis.

History

Age and sex Usually seen in middle-aged patients, from 30 to 55 years of age. Both males and females can be affected. Instability should be considered as an associated factor when the syndrome is present in patients under 30 years.

Cause Often no cause is elicited, although it may be because of recurrent or unaccustomed activity, for example, decorating or exercising at the gym. Symptoms can also arise and persist following an injury.

Symptoms *Pain and weakness* are noted during shoulder movement. The pain may be related to activity or may occur at rest and is usually centred on the anterior and lateral aspects of the shoulder, radiating to the deltoid insertion.

Night pain can occur, particularly when lying on the shoulder.

Activities of daily living become inhibited, with difficulty reaching high (e.g. into a wardrobe) and behind the body.

Examination

The patient exhibits a *painful arc in abduction*, particularly in the mid-range. This may be associated with weakness of the rotator cuff, particularly the supraspinatus and, to a lesser extent, infraspinatus muscles. The patient has *a positive impingement sign*, and a positive *Hawkin's test* (see above).

The pain is often relieved by injection of local anaesthetic into the subacromial space.

Primary impingement is *uncommon in patients under the age of 25* and may be a secondary symptom to an alternative diagnosis, for example instability. This should be considered in this age range.

Rotator cuff tears

These occur in one or more of the four rotator cuff tendons, which attach to the supraspinatus, infraspinatus, subscapularis and teres minor muscles. The supraspinatus is the most commonly affected tendon, with a tear occurring at its insertion on the greater tuberosity of the humeral head.

The tears may be partial or complete. They can be caused by trauma, or more commonly are the result of degenerative age-related changes to the tendon; hence they may be either acute or chronic.

History

Rotator cuff tears are usually characterized by the *acute onset of pain following trauma*, or *gradual persistent pain (chronic)* with weakness.

Age and sex Patients are usually over the age of 40 years. Partial tears are more common initially, but full-thickness tears become increasingly common with age, especially after the age of 65 years. Tears can occur in both males and females.

Symptoms These usually consist of *pain* and and *reduced function*, particularly when lying on the shoulder and reaching forwards trying to lift a weight.

Weakness eventually leads to *difficulty in raising the arm*, and *muscular wasting* can occur (Figure 7.16).

Rotator cuff tears may also be symptomless.

Examination

Movement is restricted by pain and there is weakness in all planes, particularly forward elevation and abduction (supraspinatus). *Passive movements are, however, largely preserved*. Rotation may also be compromised by involvement of the infraspinatus and teres minor (external rotation) and subscapularis (internal rotation). Each tendon can be assessed by

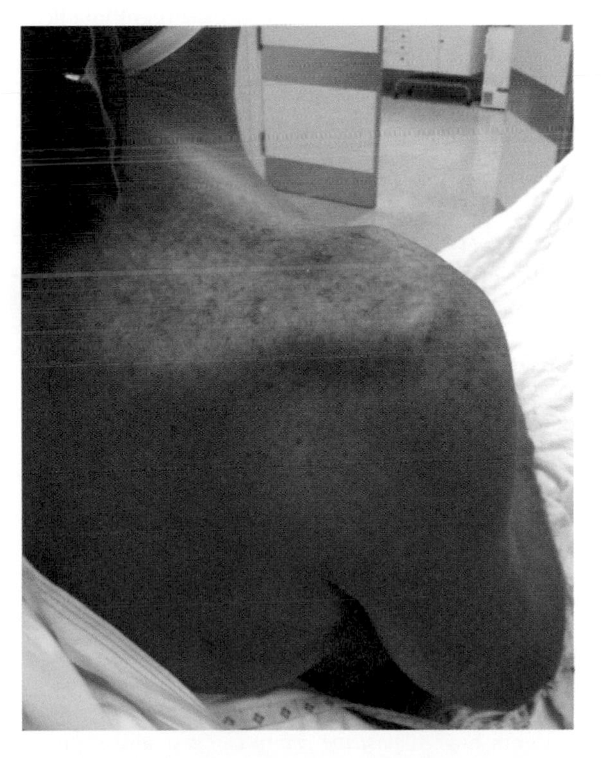

Figure 7.16 Rotator cuff wasting of supraspinatus and infraspinatus.

the special tests described above. Patients may also have positive impingement signs.

Patients may clinically have *good function*, despite significant full thickness rotator cuff tears, particularly if the tear is a degenerative tear with progressive onset. Therefore, patients should be treated based on function and symptoms rather than radiological appearance.

CALCIFIC TENDINITIS

This is the result of a deposition of calcium hydroxyapatite in the tendons of the rotator cuff causing pain and inflammation. The *most affected tendon is the supraspinatus tendon*. The cause is unknown. It may occur in an acute or a chronic form.

History

Age and sex The majority of patients will be aged 30–50 years. The condition can affect both males and females.

Symptoms In the acute disorder, the patient develops *severe pain* over a period of a few hours, which often causes them to seek urgent medical advice. The pain usually lasts 7–10 days, and then the shoulder generally returns to normal over a 6-week period.

In chronic calcific tendinitis, the patient may be symptomless, and the calcification may be an incidental finding on a shoulder X-ray. When the calcification is painful, it is generally less marked than in acute calcific tendinitis and is more consistent with the presentation of an impingement.

Examination

The arm is often held immobile in an acute presentation because the pain causes limitation of movement. Even passive movements are likely to cause great pain.

Palpation 'about the shoulder' may reveal generalized tenderness, which is usually most marked over the greater tuberosity.

In chronic calcific tendinitis, patients have pain on movement, but this is generally relatively well preserved, often with an impingement arc. When the calcification is within the supraspinatus tendon, patients have a *positive empty can test* and *signs of impingement* (see above).

ADHESIVE CAPSULITIS (FROZEN SHOULDER)

This condition is caused by the capsule of the shoulder joint becoming contracted, thickened and inflamed secondary to an ill-defined process that appears to involve fibroblastic proliferation, similar to Dupuytren's disease of the hand (see below).

History

Age and sex This condition occurs mainly in patients aged 40–60 years and is seen more frequently in females.

Cause There is often no obvious cause for the development of adhesive capsulitis. There is, however, an association with diabetes mellitus and possibly thyroid disease. The condition can also occur following a stroke or arterial or cardiac catheterization, and after trauma or surgery to the shoulder.

Symptoms The condition is characterized by an *initial phase of increasing severity of pain*, leading to difficulty in lying on the shoulder and marked sleep disturbance. Even at rest, there is a 'toothache-like' discomfort with significant positional exacerbation, particularly if a sudden movement is attempted.

Examination

The shoulder becomes increasingly stiff, with a *restricted range of both active and passive movement*, classically below 90° of forward elevation and 90° of abduction. Additionally, rotation is reduced, with external rotation of 0° and limited internal rotation, the arm often only reaching to as high as the buttock – indeed, *the loss of rotation is the key feature*.

The condition is generally self-limiting. The initial painful and stiff (freezing) phase progresses through to a stiff but relatively painless (frozen) phase, before finally there is a recovery of movement (thawing) phase. *The whole process can take 18 months or more*. During these periods, the signs can vary, but the characteristic of reduced passive movement, especially of external rotation, remains the key feature.

In the early stages of adhesive capsulitis, the history and examination may be very similar to patients presenting with *subacromial bursitis alone*.

BICEPS TENDINITIS

The long head of biceps is often considered to be part of the rotator cuff and can become inflamed as part of an impingement syndrome. It can also be present as an isolated inflammation, particularly in association with lifting heavy weights or gym activity. In most cases, the tendon remains constrained in the bicipital groove, but if the supporting structures on either side are deficient, the tendon may become unstable.

History

Age and sex The patient is usually 30–55 years of age. It can occur in both sexes, although it is slightly more common in males.

Symptoms The patient presents with *pain on activity* and will often trace a line of pain along the course of the biceps tendon, into the muscle belly. The symptoms are similar to those of impingement syndrome.

Examination

There may be localized tenderness along the bicipital groove.

The patient may have *positive Speed's* and *Yergason's tests* (see above).

They are likely to have positive impingement signs (see above).

LONG HEAD OF BICEPS TENDON RUPTURE

Occasionally, a patient presents with chronic symptoms of bicipital tendinitis, prior to a rupture of the long head tendon. The tendon arises from the superior glenoid tubercle, where it attaches to the glenoid labrum.

History

Age and sex Patients are usually aged over 50 years, and the condition is more common in males.

Cause The injury can occur spontaneously but can also be related to lifting a heavy object.

Symptoms The patient may have *chronic pain* in the proximal biceps region, which may be alleviated by the rupture. There is often a *snapping sensation*, particularly if the rupture occurs when lifting a heavy weight. Sometimes, however, the rupture is relatively painless, and the patient is unaware of its occurrence.

Examination

The patient develops a lump in the lower part of the upper arm, which is particularly prominent when the elbow is flexed (Figure 7.17). This is commonly known as the *Popeye sign* and may, in the initial stages, be associated with bruising.

Unless there are other pathological conditions, such as impingement syndrome or rotator cuff tears, the remainder of the examination is usually unremarkable.

During surgery on elderly patients, a biceps tenotomy (deliberate cutting of the tendon) is occasionally performed to relieve the symptoms.

The biceps tendon can sometimes hypertrophy and enlarge, making it unable to slide in and out of the bicipital groove. The tendon becomes trapped between the humeral glenoid when the arm is elevated. This can lead to pain and a loss of the end range of movement, particularly in forward elevation. The condition is sometimes called the 'hourglass' biceps.

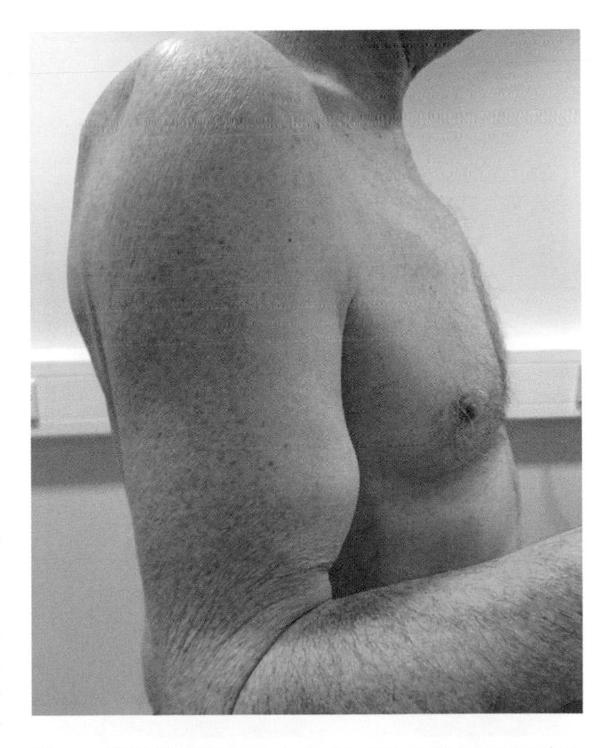

Figure 7.17 The 'Popeye sign' of a ruptured biceps tendon.

OSTEOARTHRITIS OF THE GLENOHUMERAL JOINT

This is a well-recognized cause of shoulder pain. This can be primary arthritis secondary to osteoarthritis or inflammatory arthritis, or can occur secondary to previous trauma, instability or longstanding rotator cuff lesions. It may also occur after avascular necrosis of the proximal humerus (see Chapter 6).

History

Age and sex The patient can be of either sex, and is usually over the age of 50 years.

Symptoms The patient complains of *progressive pain and stiffness in the shoulder*, particularly in abduction and forward elevation. Rotational movements may also become reduced.

Occasionally, a more aggressive and destructive form of osteoarthritis may develop in the presence of long-standing or massive rotator cuff tears, leading to severe erosion of the glenohumeral joint. The humeral head migrates to lie directly beneath the acromion, where further erosion occurs. A rapidly destructive arthropathy with hydroxyapatite crystal formation has been called 'Milwaukee shoulder' (Figure 7.18).

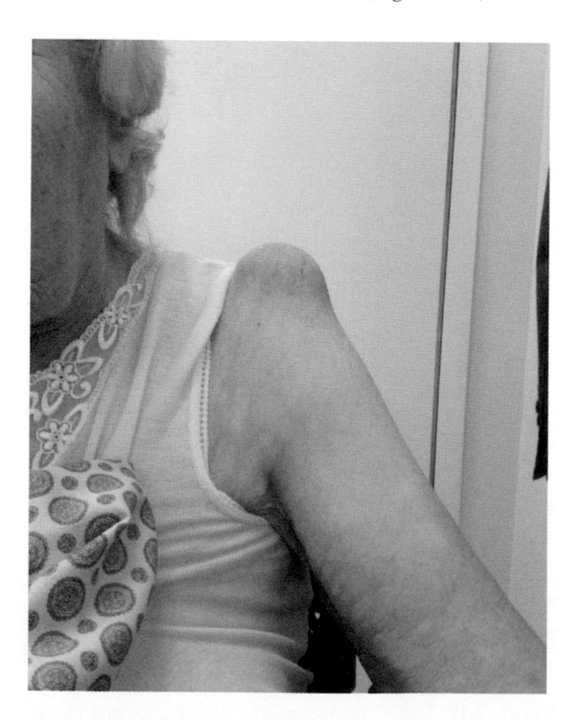

Figure 7.18 Milwaukee shoulder.

Examination

Active and passive movements become progressively more limited, although the speed of the restriction is slower than for adhesive capsulitis, and the pain is comparatively less in the early stages. Other tests are likely to be normal, unless there is associated rotator cuff pathology.

OSTEOARTHRITIS OF THE ACROMIOCLAVICULAR JOINT

This is a relatively common problem but should not be confused with age-related changes in the acromioclavicular joint. These occur from the age of 20 because of an alteration in the structure of the fibrocartilaginous disc. The latter can result in expansion of the joint, with a symptomless lump developing.

History

Age and sex Both sexes can develop the condition over the age of 40 years.

Symptoms They present with *pain and tenderness directly over the acromioclavicular joint*. There may be associated bony or soft tissue swelling. The pain may radiate into the neck muscles or into the upper arm.

Examination

Movements of the shoulder become painful, particularly in the end range, but the passive range should be maintained. Most notably, there is pain and restriction in cross-arm activity (adduction).

A bony/soft tissue swelling may be palpable over the joint.

> **NOTE:** Patients commonly have degenerative changes on X-ray but are often symptomless on testing. It is important to search for other sources of shoulder pain.

RHEUMATOID ARTHRITIS OF THE SHOULDER JOINT

This can affect both the glenohumeral and acromioclavicular joints. Previously, this was suggested to be the most common arthropathy to affect the shoulder joint, but because of advances in the medical management of rheumatoid arthritis, it is now much less common.

A severe synovitis within the glenohumeral joint can cause rupture of the rotator cuff with secondary migration of the humeral head, leading to the development of a rotator cuff arthropathy. The acromioclavicular joint can also develop erosive changes.

History

Age and sex Rheumatoid arthritis can arise in patients of all ages, but most commonly between 30 and 40 years. Females are more commonly affected than men (see Chapter 6).

Symptoms Patients present with *pain* and *restricted function* from loss of movement.

There may be *swelling around the joint*, particularly anteriorly, and the swelling may also extend into the axilla.

Examination

The patient may be known to have generalized rheumatoid arthritis affecting other joints.

Active movement becomes progressively more restricted, and while greater passive movement may be maintained initially, this also eventually becomes restricted. Impingement signs and special tests of rotator cuff function are positive if the rotator cuff tendons are involved (see above).

SHOULDER INSTABILITY

Glenohumeral joint stability is provided by static and dynamic stabilizers. The static stabilizers consist of the glenoid and the capsular ligaments, while the dynamic stabilizers are principally the muscles of the rotator cuff, but also include the shoulder ligaments. The negative intra-articular pressure within the joint also helps to maintain stability.

Instability of the joint may occur because of trauma, hyperlaxity or muscle patterning conditions, and all these may contribute independently to the problem. The instability may be acute, chronic or recurrent.

The joint is considered to have *dislocated* if there is complete separation of the articular surfaces, while a partial disruption of the joint alignment produces *subluxation* (see Chapter 6).

History

Age and sex The most common type of shoulder instability is *traumatic anterior instability*. This develops after an injury when the arm is in an abducted and externally rotated position. This is most common in males aged 16–25 years and is often related to sporting activity.

Symptoms The patient may have *a single dislocation* or develop *recurrent problems* because of a tear of the anterior labrum (a *Bankart lesion*) around the glenoid, together with a bony injury to the posterior superior humeral head (a *Hill–Sachs lesion*). Patients with recurrent dislocations may also develop glenoid bone loss adding to their instability.

The patient may also develop episodes of subluxation (partial dislocation). Even after the joint has been reduced and made congruent, these episodes may be associated with a period of pain and reduced movement before normal function is restored.

Patients often complain of *a lack of confidence* and are apprehensive of placing the shoulder in certain positions, particularly abduction and external rotation. As a consequence, they often avoid certain activities, for example throwing a ball or serving at tennis.

Examination

The special tests for shoulder instability, described above, are utilized to assess for increased movement of the humeral head in the glenoid (*anterior draw test*) and evidence of apprehension (the *anterior apprehension* and *Jobe relocation tests*) (see above).

Posterior instability of the glenohumeral joint is far less common but may be demonstrated by special tests (the *posterior draw* and *posterior apprehension tests*).

The patient should be assessed for signs of generalized ligamentous laxity, which may be contributing to the problem.

SUPERIOR LABRUM ANTERIOR POSTERIOR TEAR LESION

The labrum that surrounds the glenoid in the glenohumeral joint can be damaged not only by a dislocation, but also from loading of the arm in a flexed and abducted position, for example falling with the arm outstretched. This can cause a tear of the superior aspect of the labrum at the insertion of the long head of biceps tendon: a superior labrum anterior posterior tear. Different configurations of the tear can occur, but generally all present in a similar manner.

History

Age and sex The patient is usually less than 30 years old, and the condition is more commonly seen in males involved in sporting activity.

Symptoms After the initial pain of the injury subsides, the patient continues to have discomfort when *lifting the arm above shoulder height*. There is also a functional restriction from loss of power, particularly when trying to throw an object.

Examination

Pain may be elicited by stressing the biceps tendon.

O'Brien's test should be carried out. In this, the arm is adducted medial to the sagittal plane with the elbow extended and the arm flexed to 90°. The patient is then asked to resist the downward force with the arm internally rotated, before this is repeated in supination. Pain is usually elicited with the first manoeuvre, but reduced or eliminated by the second.

Revision panel 7.4

CAUSES OF REDUCED EXTERNAL ROTATION

There are three main causes of significantly reduced external rotation on examination:

- Posterior dislocation (must be excluded).
- Adhesive capsulitis.
- Osteoarthritis.

THE ELBOW JOINT

This is a synovial hinge joint between the humerus in the upper arm, and the radius and ulna in the forearm. This allows the hand to be moved towards and away from the body. The proximal radioulnar joint also lies within the capsule of the elbow joint.

Plan for examination of the elbow

INSPECTION

Both upper limbs should be exposed. The elbows should be viewed front and back.

The joint above (the shoulder) and below (the hand and wrist) the elbow should also be examined.

The skin should be inspected for *scars and sinuses*, including small arthroscopic portal incisions, which are usually sited on the medial and lateral aspects of the joint.

Look for *generalized swelling* of the joint or *muscular wasting*, which may be associated with arthritis.

Swelling may be caused by an effusion filling out the hollows seen in the flexed elbow above the olecranon, or swelling about the radiohumeral joint.

Localized swellings may also be associated with olecranon bursitis, gouty tophi and rheumatoid nodules (see below).

Shape

The two elbows should be compared. In the normal elbow, if the elbows are extended with the palms facing forwards or up, the bones of the humerus and forearm are not perfectly aligned. This deviation at the elbow, away from the body, is called the *carrying angle*. The normal carrying angle is approximately 5–15° of valgus.

The carrying angle may be increased, commonly from a previous fracture of the lateral humeral condyle (see page 259). This is known as *cubitus valgus* (see Figure 6.11). The ulnar nerve is applied to the medial aspect of the elbow and can be stretched by valgus, resulting in ulnar palsy. If the carrying angle is less than 5–15°, such that the elbow is more angulated towards the midline, this is known as *cubitus varus* (a *gunstock deformity*). The most common cause is malunion of a previous supracondylar fracture (Figure 7.19).

PALPATION

The joint should be *palpated along the bony landmarks*, starting at the olecranon process posteriorly, and proceeding to the medial and lateral epicondyles, the head of the radius and the joint line. The *bony*

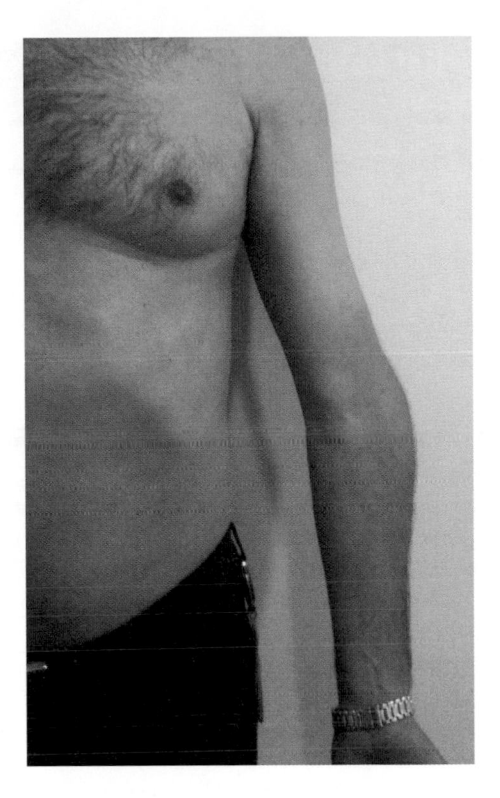

Figure 7.19 Cubitus varus.

landmarks of the epicondyles and the olecranon should form an equilateral triangle; previous elbow trauma may disturb these landmarks.

The *soft tissues* should also be assessed, including the *olecranon bursa*. The anterior joint line, extending about the biceps tendon in the antecubital fossa and radiohumeral joint, should be palpated during movement. The *ulnar nerve* can be palpated behind the medial epicondyle.

MOVEMENT

Both elbows should be compared for active and passive movement. Normal extension of the elbow is to 0°. Patients with generalized ligamentous laxity may hyperextend beyond this.

Normal flexion of the elbow is approximately 140°. The functional range of movement at the elbow joint, without a significant restriction in the ability to perform tasks, is generally accepted to be 30–120°. Restriction of movement may signify either a bony block or soft tissue contraction.

Pronation occurs when the elbow is flexed to 90° and the palm maximally rotated towards the ground, with a normal range of 75°. Supination occurs with the elbow flexed to 90° and the palm facing maximally upwards, with a normal range of 80°.

Loss of supination and pronation can be associated with fusion when there is a bony connection between the radius and ulna (*proximal radioulnar synostosis*). This can be congenital or acquired secondary to trauma. The radial head can also be displaced as the result of a congenital dislocation or subluxation, as a consequence of other bone dysplasia or following an unreduced dislocation.

INSTABILITY

This can arise following a previous dislocation or injury to the medial or lateral collateral ligaments, which can be stretched or ruptured. An apprehension response can be obtained by supinating the forearm while applying a valgus or varus force during flexion or asking the patient to weight bear on the arm and perform a triceps dip.

POWER

Power is assessed during *elbow flexion*, which is performed by the biceps brachii, brachialis and brachioradialis.

The action of elbow *extension* is performed by the triceps brachii.

Supination is achieved by the supinator muscle, together with a contribution from the biceps brachii and to a lesser extent brachioradialis.

Pronation is performed by pronator teres, pronator quadratus and brachioradialis.

Revision panel 7.5

ELBOW EXAMINATION SUMMARY

Inspection
Shape
Palpation
Movement
Power
Instability
Neurology

CAUSES OF ELBOW PAIN

Lateral epicondylitis (tennis elbow)

This is a common tendinopathy that occurs at the common extensor origin on the lateral epicondyle of the elbow. Small interstitial tears can develop within the tendon, associated with neovascularization. Localized inflammation may also occur. While it can occur in tennis players, it is also seen in patients not involved in sporting activity.

History

Age and sex The condition is seen in middle age and can occur in both sexes. The cause is unknown. It may be associated with everyday activities such as gardening and the repetitive lifting of heavy objects.

Symptoms The patient complains of *pain and tenderness over the lateral aspect of the elbow*. This is made worse when the common extensor origin is stressed during strong grip or even shaking hands. The patient may occasionally complain of a *localized swelling* over the lateral epicondyle.

Examination

There is *localized tenderness just below the lateral epicondyle*.

There may be a minor restriction in elbow extension.

The patient may have *a positive finger extension test*, in which the elbow, wrist and fingers are extended, and pressure is then applied to the extended fingers by the examiner. The patient is asked to resist the downward force, and pain is felt about the lateral epicondyle.

Radial tunnel syndrome from compression of the radial nerve in the region of the elbow and can mimic the symptoms of tennis elbow. Extension tests involving all the fingers simultaneously are, however, less positive, while single stressing of the middle finger is usually comparatively worse. Tenderness is localized to just distal to the radial neck.

NOTE: Nerve conduction studies may be normal in radial tunnel syndrome.

Medial epicondylitis (golfer's elbow)

This condition is comparable to tennis elbow, except that it affects the *common flexor tendon origin*, which originates from medial epicondyle of the humerus. The same pathological processes occur as those seen in other tendinopathies. Although it is common in golfers, it can also occur in all situations needing a strong and prolonged grip.

History

Age and sex The condition usually occurs in middle age in both males and females.

Symptoms *Progressive pain is experienced around the medial epicondyle*. The patient has difficulty in lifting heavy objects because this causes pain. The patient may complain of ulnar nerve symptoms if there is associated inflammation irritating the nerve.

In javelin throwers or other sportsmen performing similar repetitive throwing activities, pain can occur on the medial aspect of the elbow that is similar to golfer's elbow. This is usually because of an injury of the medial collateral ligament.

Examination

Pain is reproduced by *flexing of the fingers against resistance and/or by passive extension of the wrist*. There may be some localized swelling around the medial epicondyle, and tenderness on palpation.

Olecranon bursitis

This occurs on the posterior aspect of the elbow overlying the olecranon (Figure 7.20). The bursa can become enlarged from an accumulation of inflammatory tissue. The serum uric acid levels may be raised, and urate crystals may be seen in any aspirate if the bursa is swollen by gout.

History

Age and sex This is normally seen in middle-aged and elderly males.

Cause It may be the result of recurrent trauma. Bursitis is also associated with *gout and pseudogout*, or *rheumatoid arthritis*. Infection is unusual but can occur. Minor trauma can cause bursitis (inflammation).

Symptoms The patient complains of *pain at the elbow*. They may have an associated systemic illness.

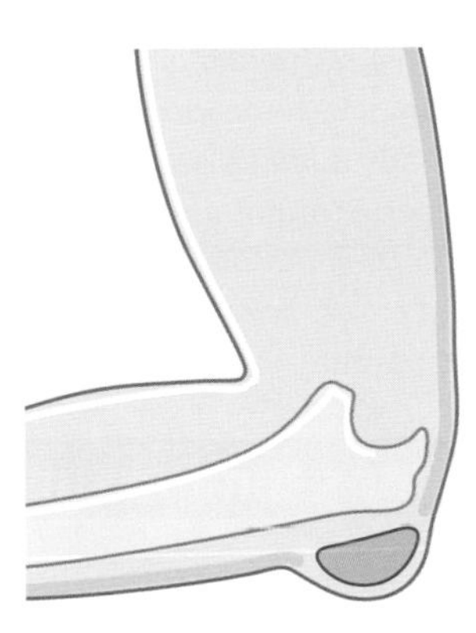

Figure 7.20 Olecranon bursa (student's elbow) (see also Figure 4.65).

They may also complain of *stiffness* and some *restriction in movement*.

Examination

There is a large *swelling on the posterior aspect of the elbow*, with associated erythema and localized tenderness (Figure 7.21). The swelling may be hot, and the condition may be bilateral.

> **NOTE:** The swelling of the elbow due to olecranon bursitis often settles over a period of 6–8 weeks without intervention.

Loose bodies

These can occur in the elbow joint and present with both pain and mechanical locking. The loose bodies may be a consequence of *trauma*, *osteochondritis dissecans*, *synovial chondromatosis* or *osteoarthritis*.

History

Age and sex Loose bodies can occur in both males and females, with the age of presentation dependent on the underlying cause.

Symptoms The elbow becomes *painful* and *locked in a specific position*. Depending on the position of the loose body in the joint, there may be a limitation of extension, flexion, supination and pronation or a combination of movements. The elbow then frees itself, and the range of movement is gradually restored. This, however, can take several days depending on any swelling that might arise.

Examination

There may be joint swelling in the acute phase, but there may be few signs after the acute episode. Very occasionally, permanent restrictions in movement can develop. Loose bodies are almost never palpable.

OSTEOCHONDRITIS DISSECANS

This is a condition in which the cartilage–bone interface is altered, with separation and necrosis of these structures, often as the result of an ischaemic cause (see Chapter 6). The capitellum is one of the common sites for this process to occur.

History

Age and sex The condition is common in adolescents and young male adults.

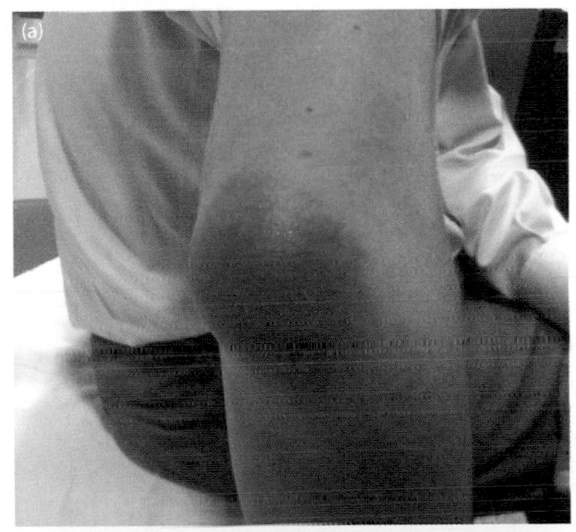

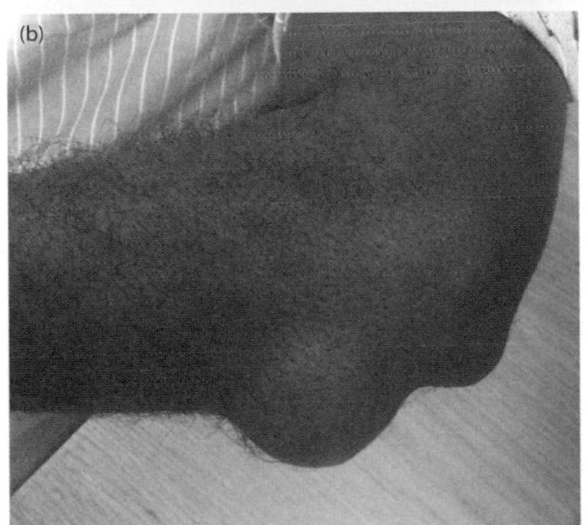

Figure 7.21 OLECRANON BURSA. (a) Inflamed bursa. (b) Chronic bursa.

Symptoms The patient complains of a *generalized ache* in and around the elbow, which is made worse by activity and relieved by rest.

Examination

Occasionally, there is some *localized tenderness* on the lateral aspect of the elbow, with *mild stiffness* of the joint with some *associated swelling and an effusion*.

Locking of the joint can occur if a cartilage fragment becomes detached and forms a loose body within the joint.

Osteoarthritis

This is relatively uncommon in the elbow joint. It can follow a previous injury or fracture and may be the result of long-term occupational demands on the elbow joint.

History

Age and sex The condition can occur in both middle-aged and elderly males and females.

Symptoms Patients complain of *pain and stiffness of the elbow*, worse following inactivity.

They may also complain of *locking of the elbow* if loose bodies have formed.

Examination

There is often *localized tenderness* around the joint line, *crepitus* and *restricted movement*.

Rheumatoid arthritis

Although joint manifestations of rheumatoid arthritis have been significantly reduced with the advent of new medical treatments, it can still affect the elbow and superior radioulnar joint. In many cases, the condition is bilateral.

History

Age and sex It is more common in females, and usually presents in the fourth or fifth decade.

Symptoms Patients usually complain of an *insidious onset of progressive pain*. They may also complain of *swelling about the elbow* and *stiffness*. Other joints are often involved, and systemic pathology may be present (see Chapter 6).

Examination

There is usually *swelling* of the elbow joint, with tenderness along the joint line.

There may be *a restriction of flexion and extension*, and the elbow may become *unstable*.

There is usually a *limitation of supination and pronation* if the superior radiohumeral and/or radioulnar joint is involved.

In advanced cases, *deformity of the joint* becomes increasingly apparent.

Distal biceps tendon rupture

The distal biceps can separate from its insertion into the radial tuberosity, or the tendon can rupture, causing a painful swollen tendon with bulging of the biceps muscle belly. This usually occurs following a traumatic incident when the elbow is flexed against resistance.

History

Age and sex Injury is more common in males in middle age.

Symptoms The patient experiences *sudden pain in the arm* and complains of *weakness in flexion*.

Examination

The biceps tendon and the bicipital aponeurosis can usually be felt as cordlike structures crossing the joint when the patient is asked to flex the elbow against resistance. When the tendon has ruptured, it cannot be felt, and the biceps muscle belly usually retracts superiorly (Figure 7.22). *A palpable gap can often be felt.*

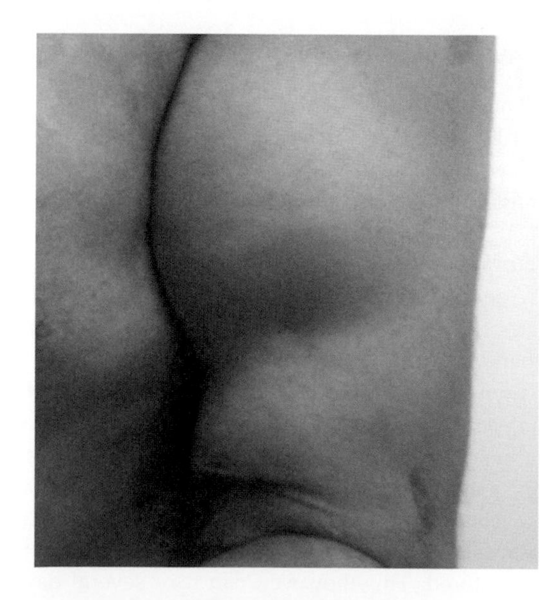

Figure 7.22 Distal biceps rupture.

There is a *partial reduction in the patient's flexion strength*; but, the most significant deficit is in *supination power*. Flexion and supination are still possible even in the presence of a biceps tendon rupture because of the action of the brachialis and supinator muscles.

Triceps tendon avulsions can also occur, but these are far less common, and are likely to be associated with weight training and steroid abuse.

Congenital dislocation of the radial head

In this condition, the radial head is dislocated anteriorly, posteriorly or laterally to the capitellum. It is usually bilateral and can be associated with the rare nail–patella syndrome.

History

Age and sex Both males and females are affected. Patients usually present in early childhood or adolescence. The dislocation is sometimes recognized following a minor injury when an X-ray is taken.

Symptoms The patient is often *symptomless* but often notices *a lump* at the elbow joint (the radial head). *Pain is unusual.*

Examination

There may be slight loss of extension and supination. Examination is often unremarkable.

Pulled elbow

This is a separation of the head of the radius from the annular ligament and often occurs when a child's elbow is 'jerked' by a parent pulling on the arm. This common condition is sometimes called 'nursemaid's' or *temper-tantrum* elbow.

History

Age and sex It can affect both males and females, usually below the age of 6 years.

Symptoms The elbow is painful, and movements are restricted.

Examination

There is an inability to use the elbow, which is *held immobile in extension with the forearm pronated. Attempted supination increases the pain.* Supination combined with flexion of the elbow may cause the radial head to relocate within the annular ligament.

Ulnar nerve compression

The ulnar nerve passes behind the medial condyle of the humerus through the cubital tunnel. It can become trapped or compressed at various levels including: its passage through the intermuscular septum; entrapment in a hypertrophied triceps, the cubital tunnel, particularly in the presence of arthritic change or valgus deformity; or in the passage beneath the arch of origin of the flexor carpi ulnaris. All of these points must be released at surgery (see Chapter 3).

History

Age and sex The condition can affect both male and female patients, usually in middle age.

Symptoms The patient complains of *pain, numbness and tingling in the little finger and ulnar half of the ring finger.* The pain may extend from the forearm into the hand.

The symptoms may be exacerbated when the elbow is flexed or held in position for a long period.

In the later stages, *weakness of grip and clawing of the fingers, together with intrinsic muscle wasting*, may be observed.

Examination

A *bony abnormality* or *soft tissue swelling* may be apparent.

A *Tinel's sign* may be elicited by percussing over the ulnar nerve. This elicits tingling along the course of the nerve.

The patient may demonstrate *Froment's sign* if there is motor weakness, causing weakness of the adductor pollicis (see Chapter 3). A simple test is to ask the patient to cross their fingers. This tests abduction/adduction.

Radial nerve compression

The radial nerve can be compressed at different points along its course through the elbow and into the forearm. Around the elbow, it divides into the superficial branch and the posterior interosseus nerve. The superficial branch provides sensation to the skin over the radial half of the back of the hand. The posterior interosseus nerve passes between the two heads of supinator, and supplies motor branches to all the extensors below the elbow (see Chapter 3).

HISTORY

Age and sex The condition affects both males and females, usually in middle age.

Symptoms The patient may experience pain if there is compression at the radial tunnel, similar to tennis elbow. This is generally worse at night or related to activity.

There is a motor weakness of the wrist and finger extensors if the posterior interosseous nerve is compressed (see Chapter 3). As extension is essential to full grip, the hand is weakened.

NOTE: When patients present with neural symptoms affecting the upper limb, the neck should also be considered as the site of the pathology and examined.

THE HAND

The hand is mankind's greatest physical asset and, anatomically, one of its most distinctive features. Everything that the doctor does to the hand should be aimed at restoring or maintaining its function.

Plan for the examination of the hand

This 'Plan for examination' is, to some extent, an artificial exercise since a patient does not present asking *'please examine my hand'*. The patient presents with a history and a set of symptoms. Examination is directed primarily at those symptoms along with some general principles.

Examine each system in turn, based on the principles of:

- Look.
- Feel.
- Move.

INSPECTION

Look for any abnormality of the *shape, size* and *contour* of the hand. Look for local discolouration, *scars, lumps/cords* and *sinuses*. Look for *muscle wasting* by assessing the size of the thenar and hypothenar eminences, and the bulk of the muscles between the metacarpal bones (the interossei). Look at the wrist joint.

PALPATION

Feel the bony contours, the tender areas and any localized swellings. Feel the finger joints to assess whether there is any swelling of these joints.

MOVEMENT

Check the range and ease of movement of all the joints:

- The *carpometacarpal joint of the thumb* (flexion, extension, abduction, adduction and opposition).
- The *metacarpophalangeal joints* of the fingers (flexion, extension, abduction and adduction in extension; stability in flexion).
- The *interphalangeal joints* (flexion and extension).

An inability to move these joints may be caused by joint disease, soft-tissue thickening, divided tendons or paralysed muscles.

THE CIRCULATION

Inspection

Pallor of the fingers indicates arterial insufficiency or anaemia. During an episode of vasospasm, the fingers may be white or blue (see Chapter 10). Observe the degree of filling of the veins on the back of the hands. Ischaemic atrophy of the pulps of the fingers makes the fingers thin and pointed ('pencilling'). Ischaemic ulcers, small abscesses and even frank gangrene may be visible (see Chapter 10). Calluses indicate active use and may/may not correlate with symptoms.

Palpation

Feel the temperature of the skin of each finger. Feel both pulses (radial and ulnar) at the wrist (see

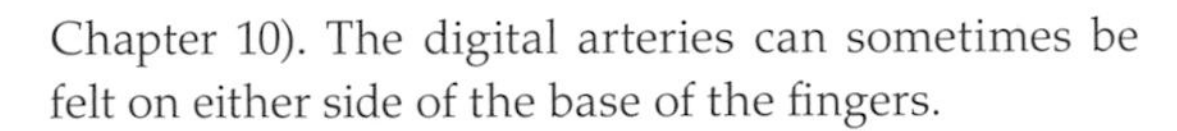

Chapter 10). The digital arteries can sometimes be felt on either side of the base of the fingers.

Capillary return

A crude indication of the arterial inflow to the fingers can be obtained from watching the rate of filling of the vessels beneath the nail after blanching by pressure on the tip of the nail (see Chapter 10).

Allen's test

Ask the patient to clench one fist tightly, and then compress the ulnar and radial arteries at the wrist with your thumbs. After 10 seconds, ask the patient to open their hand. The palm will be white. Release the compression on the radial artery, then watch the blood flow into the hand. Repeat this with the ulnar artery.

Slow flow into one finger will be apparent from the rate at which that finger turns pink.

Auscultation

Listen with the bell of your stethoscope over any abnormal areas. Vascular tumours and arteriovenous fistulas may produce a bruit, and sometimes a palpable thrill (see Chapter 10).

Measure the blood pressure in both arms.

THE NERVES

The nerves should be examined in accordance with their anatomical distribution, remembering that each nerve has **s**ensory, **m**otor, **a**utonomic, **r**eflex and **t**rophic (**SMART**) function (see Chapter 3). It is always best to compare sensation in two territories 'Do these feel equally clear?' rather than 'Can you feel this?' Test for skin moisture by running a plastic ballpoint pen along the skin – moist skin produces a drag; dry skin has no drag. The nerves supply the sweat glands and this test is a useful corroboration of reported alteration in sensation and in children.

THE SKIN AND CONNECTIVE TISSUES

Much will have been learnt about the skin after studying its circulation and innervation. Be careful to note any colour changes and any inflammatory processes.

If the fingers cannot extend fully, palpate the palm for firm nodules or cords caused by contracture of the palmar fascia (*Dupuytren's contracture*).

Also note any change in the shape or configuration of the hand and digits, and any abnormal skin creases. Faint or absent creases indicate poor or absent movement of the underlying joint.

Hyperextensibility of the joints may indicate hypermobility (a normal variant particularly in young females) or a connective tissue disorder such as Ehlers–Danlos syndrome.

THE WRIST, ELBOW, SHOULDER, THORACIC OUTLET AND NECK

Examine the wrist, elbow, shoulder, thoracic outlet and neck because abnormalities at these sites can cause symptoms in the hand. This is particularly the case when there are widespread, bilateral, vague or changing symptoms and may also suggest more proximal nerve compression or irritation. Nerve stretch provocation tests may reveal a significant radiculopathy (compression at the nerve roots).

RECORDING DATA ABOUT THE HAND

Inadequate or misleading records of hand pathology can lead to serious errors. It is imperative to state which hand you are describing and record in words: RIGHT or LEFT. A bad R can easily be confused with an L. Angles of joints should be measured (a goniometer) and recorded. It is insufficient to state 'Reduced range' or 'Movement reasonable'.

Name the digits

Some people prefer to number rather than name the digits, the first digit being the thumb, the second digit the index finger and so on. But unless you remember to write the word 'digit' every time, you will eventually make a mistake because the first finger, which is the index finger, is the second digit.

If you are marking a patient for surgery, ensure the arrow is directed to the digit involved. In addition, mark the radial or ulnar aspect of the digit if one side or the other is to be operated. If the local anaesthetic is to be administered from a dorsal approach, mark the front *and* back of the digit.

NOTE: Description of the digits of the hand must be universally recognized and able to be communicated accurately to prevent mistakes arising.

ABNORMALITIES AND CONDITIONS OF THE HAND

Congenital abnormalities

There are three common congenital skeletal abnormalities in the hand:

- Part of the hand (usually a digit) may be absent (*hypoplasia/aplasia*).
- There may be an extra digit/s (*polydactyly*) (Figure 7.23).
- The digits may be fused (*syndactyly*) (Figure 7.24).

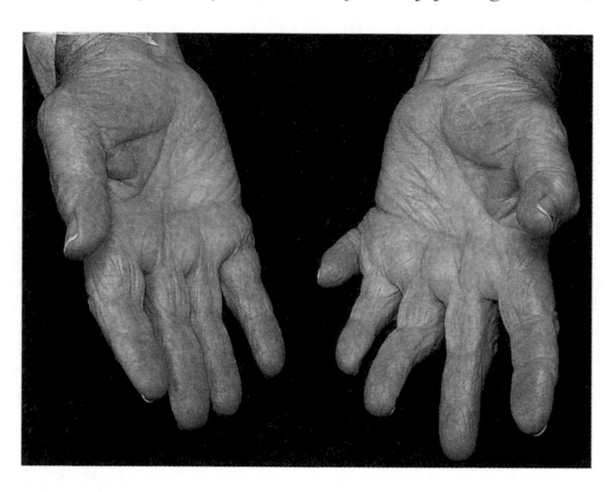

Figure 7.23 Polydactyly.

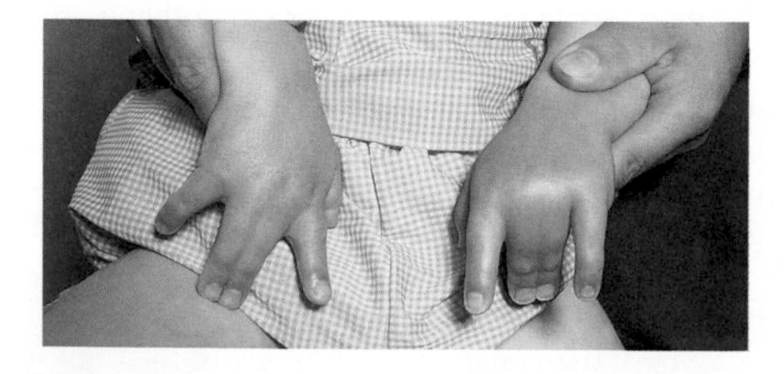

Figure 7.24 Syndactyly.

All these abnormalities are uncommon, but immediately recognizable. Syn/polydactyly has an overall incidence of 1:1500/2000. Polydactyly is 10 times more common in the Afro-Caribbean population.

Dupuytren's contracture

This is a *thickening and shortening of the palmar fascia* and the adjacent connective tissues that lie deep to the subcutaneous tissue of the hand and superficial to the flexor tendons. The cause of this change in the fascia is not certain. As the thickening increases, the fascia may become attached to the skin of the palm, causing pits.

The condition is linked to genetic make-up and is most prevalent in Celtic and Nordic bloodlines. It is known to be provoked earlier by *local trauma* and to manifest earlier in that hand if the individual is predisposed.

History

Age Dupuytren's contracture usually begins in middle age; but, its progression and distribution is very variable.

Sex Males are affected 10 times more often than females.

Symptoms In the early phases, there is a *nodule in the palm*. The patient may notice a thickening in the tissues in the palm of the hand, near the base of the ulnar fingers, long before the contractures develop (Figure 7.25).

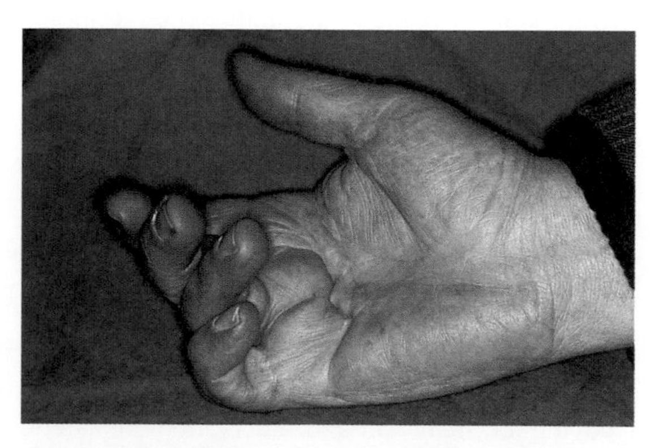

Figure 7.25 Dupuytren's contracture, showing puckering of the skin.

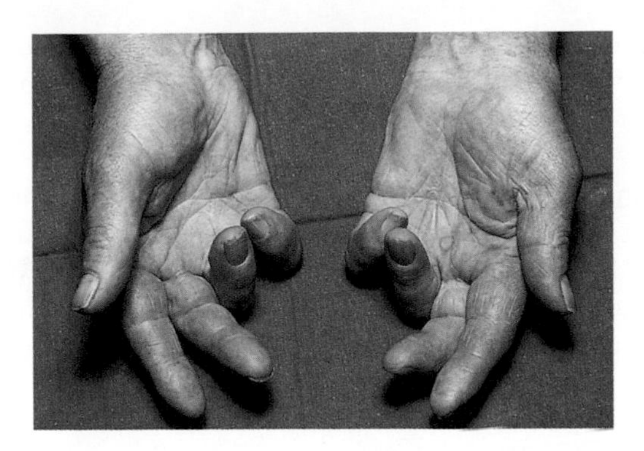

Figure 7.26 Dupuytren's contracture – anterior view.

Contraction deformities occur. The patient notices an *inability to fully extend the ring and/or little finger*. Longstanding contracture involving the proximal interphalangeal joint can cause secondary irreversible *fixed* flexion. (Figure 7.26). Involvement of the first webspace can cause limitation in thumb movement and span.

There is usually no pain associated with this condition, except temporarily at the outset. This usually settles and is not an indication for surgery.

Development The nodule gradually enlarges, and the strands of contracting fascia become prominent. Deep creases form where the skin becomes tethered to the fascial thickening, and the skin in these pits may get soggy and excoriated. The deformity of the fingers slowly increases. Surgery does not cure the condition – it restores range of movement. It follows that surgery is only indicated if the patient is unable to lay the hand flat on a tabletop (*Hueston's tabletop test*). The metacarpophalangeal joint is more forgiving than the proximal interphalangeal joint. Surgery should be considered early if the proximal interphalangeal joint is involved to avoid secondary fixed contracture.

Multiplicity Dupuytren's contracture is commonly (eventually) *bilateral and can also occur in the feet*.

Cause The cause is usually genetic and it is most prevalent and most severe in those with a strong Celtic or Nordic bloodline. Many other factors have been implicated, with varying levels of evidence. Trauma can provoke presentation in those who are predisposed to develop the condition.

Systemic disease There is a higher incidence of *epilepsy* and *alcoholism* in patients suffering from these diseases. The reasons for these associations are unexplained (Revision panel 7.6).

Revision panel 7.6

FACTORS THAT *MAY* BE ASSOCIATED WITH DUPUYTREN'S CONTRACTURE

- Alcoholism
- Epilepsy
- Diabetes
- Repeated trauma
- Family history

Examination

In the early stages, palpation of the palm of the hand reveals *a firm, irregularly shaped nodule with indistinct edges* at any level of the palm or digit. *Taut strands* can be felt running from the nodule to the sides of the base of the ring and little fingers, and proximally towards the centre of the flexor retinaculum. These bands get tighter if you try to extend the fingers.

The skin may be *puckered and creased* and *tethered* to the underlying nodule.

The deformity The metacarpophalangeal joint and/or the proximal interphalangeal joint are flexed. The ring and little fingers are most affected and may eventually be pulled down so far that the nail digs into the palm of the hand (Figure 7.26).

The flexion deformity is not lessened by flexing the wrist joint. If both metacarpophalangeal joint and proximal interphalangeal joint are flexed, test for improved extension of the proximal interphalangeal joint with the metacarpophalangeal joint flexed. This assesses the contracture of the proximal interphalangeal joint to discover whether it is fixed or flexible.

Local tissues The rest of the hand is normal. There may be some thickening of the subcutaneous tissue on the back of the proximal phalanges of the affected fingers, sometimes called *Garrod's pads*.

The condition may be present in the feet (*Ledderhose disease*) or penis (*Peyronie's disease*) (see Chapter 18).

NOTE: The rate of progression of deformity in the hand due to Dupuytren's contracture can be very variable between individuals.

The patient is rarely aware of the fact that they have a deformity, accepting it as the normal shape of their little finger.

It is mentioned here because the student who is unaware of its existence may misdiagnose it. It is best to diagnose and treat this early and before there are secondary joint deformities. Late presentation usually cannot be treated or is treated with fusion of the joint in a more useful position.

It is mentioned here because the student who is unaware of its existence may misdiagnose it.

Pick up a teacup with your thumb and index finger and hook your little finger in the manner of the affected individual at a tea party. You will find that you have extended your metacarpophalangeal joint and flexed both interphalangeal joints. Someone with a congenital contracture of the little finger has this deformity all the time and cannot straighten the finger (Figure 7.27).

Occasionally, a patient will present with a sideways deformity, usually of the little finger in an ulnar direction. This is known as Clinodactyly and is usually the result of a skeletal abnormality; an asymmetric growth plate.

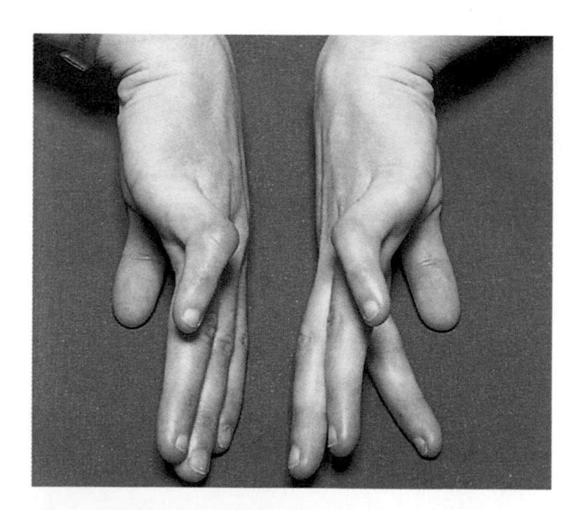

Figure 7.27 Congenital contracture of the little finger.

Compartment syndrome and Volkmann's ischaemic contracture

Compartment syndrome is defined as: a rise in pressure in a muscular compartment sufficient to impair blood supply. It is best diagnosed early and relieved rapidly to prevent the development of an irreversible contracture.

Volkmann's contracture is the late outcome of an unrecognized or unrelieved compartment syndrome. This is an irreversible shortening of the long flexor muscles of the forearm, caused by fibrosis of the muscles, secondary to ischaemia. The common causes of the ischaemia are direct arterial damage at the time of a fracture near the elbow (most often a supracondylar fracture (see below), or an undiagnosed, or late treated, compartment syndrome in the forearm, most commonly from an overtight plaster. It is a condition relatively easy to prevent but very difficult to treat.

History

Age Supracondylar fractures are common in children and young adults (see page 248), so Volkmann's contracture is most likely to begin between the ages of 5 and 25 years.

Cause The patient usually knows the cause of the deformity because they can clearly relate the loss of finger extension to their injury. Indeed, the loss of finger movements frequently begins while the arm is immobilized for the treatment of the fracture.

Symptoms *In the acute situation:* Suspect compartment syndrome in the presence of disproportionate pain, unrelieved swelling of a limb, especially beneath plaster. *Gentle stretching* – Ischaemic muscle is painful and it is acutely painful when stretched. Pain, for instance, in the flexors when the wrist is gently extended, should raise the index of suspicion of compartment syndrome and steps should be taken to relieve pressure.

Movements of the fingers, especially extension, become painful and then limited. This is more noticeable if there is no restriction of movement caused by a coexisting fracture. The patient soon discovers that they can extend their fingers if they flex their wrist when the forearm is not in a plaster cast.

In the late stages, skin of the hand will be cold and pale as the blood supply of the hand is also diminished, but this is a late sign. The pulse is often maintained and palpable and is not a reassuring feature.

Ischaemia of the nerves in the anterior compartment (the median and anterior interosseous nerves) often causes 'pins and needles' *(paraesthesia) in the distribution of the median nerve,* and sometimes the severe burning pain of ischaemic neuritis. Nerve changes are also late.

Development As the acute phase passes, the pain slowly fades away, but the restriction of finger extension increases, and the hand becomes claw-like as the secondary changes of muscle ischaemia become irreversible. The patient may present late with a painless, fully developed contracture.

Examination

Inspection The hand often looks wasted and underused. *All the finger joints are flexed,* and the anterior aspect of the forearm is thin and wasted. At this stage, the flexor compartment has a 'fixed flexion contracture' (Figure 7.28).

Palpation In the acute phase, the forearm is swollen and tense, but once this has resolved the forearm atrophies, the hand is cool and the pulses at the wrist may be absent. In the later stages, the fibrosis and shortening make the forearm muscles hard and taut.

Movement *Extension of the fingers is limited but improves as the wrist is flexed.* This is an important sign, as it differentiates Volkmann's ischaemic contracture from Dupuytren's contracture.

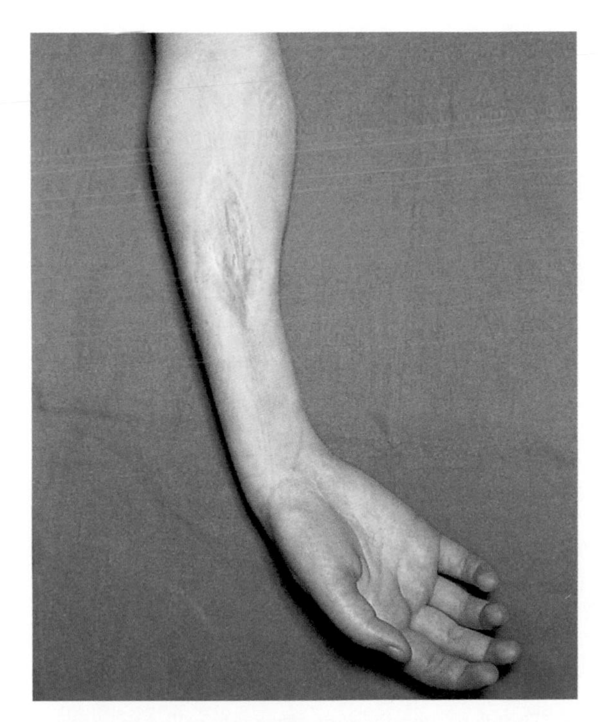

Figure 7.28 Volkmann's ischaemic contracture.

Further flexion of the fingers (beyond the deformity) can occur, but the grip is weak. All other hand movements are present but may be difficult to perform with the fingers fixed in an acutely flexed position.

Passive forced extension of the fingers is painful in the acute stage and uncomfortable in the established condition.

Local tissues The abnormalities in the arteries and nerves of the forearm and hand have already been described. The vessels and nerves above the level of the fracture should be normal if the contracture follows a fracture.

The heart, great vessels, subclavian and axillary arteries must be examined carefully in case they are the source of an arterial embolus.

Palpate the supraclavicular fossa for a cervical rib (see Chapter 9) or subclavian artery aneurysm (see Chapter 10).

Carpal tunnel syndrome

This is a condition in which the median nerve is compressed as it passes through the carpal tunnel – the space between the carpal bones and the flexor retinaculum. The compression can be caused by skeletal abnormalities, swelling of other tissues within the tunnel, or thickening of the retinaculum.

It can be associated with:

- Pregnancy.
- Rheumatoid arthritis.
- Diabetes
- Myxoedema.
- Previous trauma.
- Osteoarthritis.
- Growth hormone disturbance.

all of which alter the relationship between volume of tunnel and volume of contents. In most cases, there is no identifiable cause.

History

Age and sex Carpal tunnel syndrome is commoner in middle-aged females, especially at the menopause.

Local symptoms *Pins and needles in the fingers in the median nerve territory, thumb, index and middle, is the common presenting symptom.*

Theoretically, the little finger should never be affected, as it is innervated by the ulnar nerve, but occasionally patients complain that the whole of their hand tingles.

Pain in the forearm may also occur. This is likely due to altered proprioception in the hand, which alters the fluid and precisely controlled action of the hand, particularly grip. This is usually an aching pain, not a sharp pain.

There may be an associated *loss of hand function*. As the compression increases, the axons in the nerve are killed, and objective signs of nerve damage appear. Because the sensitivity of the skin supplied by the median nerve is reduced, the patient notices that they drop small articles and cannot carry out delicate movements. Note that this is *not caused by a loss of muscle power*, but by the loss of fine discriminatory sensation.

Ultimately, if the nerve damage is severe, there may be a loss of motor function, which presents as *weakness and paralysis of the muscles of the thenar eminence, particularly the abductor of the thumb* (see median nerve palsy in Chapter 3, page 107).

Patients are often woken in the middle of the night by their symptoms. This is because the pressure in the carpal tunnel rises with flexion or extension of the wrist (this the basis of the *Phalen test*). Most will sleep with their wrist flexed or extended or wake with a numb hand and hang their arm out of the bed (which straightens the wrist).

General symptoms An increase in weight commonly exacerbates the symptoms of carpal tunnel syndrome. A change in weight may be secondary to another disease such as myxoedema, diabetes or steroid therapy, or to physiological water retention, as in pregnancy.

The patient may have symptoms of arthritis in the wrist and other joints, particularly osteoarthritis of the basal joint (carpometacarpal joint) of the thumb.

Examination

Inspection The hand usually looks quite normal, except in advanced cases, where there may be visible *wasting of the muscles forming the thenar eminence* (Figure 7.29).

Palpation Pressure on the flexor retinaculum does not produce the symptoms in the hand, but holding the wrist fully flexed for 1 minute may induce symptoms *(Phalen test)*. Light-touch sensitivity and two-point discrimination may be reduced in the skin innervated by the median nerve (palm, thumb, index and middle finger). Sweating is reduced in this territory (ballpoint drag test). The *loss of muscle bulk in the thenar eminence* may be easier to feel when these muscles are contracting.

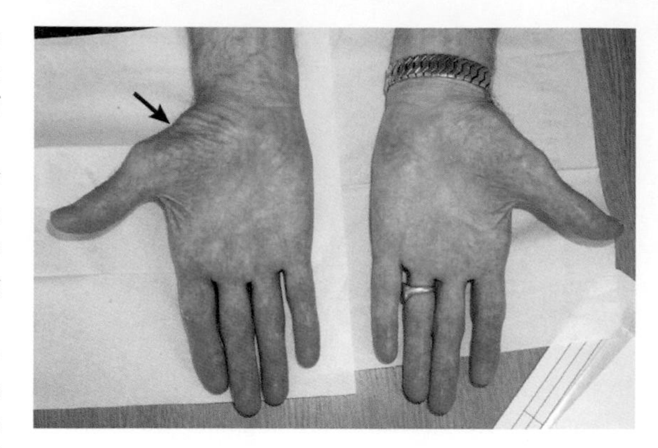

Figure 7.29 Wasting of the thenar eminence.

The wrist pulses and the colour and temperature of the skin should be normal.

Movement All movements of the joints of the hand, active and passive, should be present.

Abduction of the thumb (moving the thumb at right angles to the palm) is the commonest reduced or lost function since the abductor is purely median nerve innervated while the other thenar muscles share innervation with the ulnar nerve.

General examination There are two important aspects of the general examination.

First, you must exclude other causes of paraesthesia in the hand, such as *cervical spondylosis, cervical rib, peripheral neuritis* and *rare neurological disease*. This requires a detailed examination of the head, neck and arm. Changing, vague, ill-defined, and bilateral symptoms suggest a cause arising in the neck.

Also, check on proximal compression of the median nerve, such as anterior interosseous compression – this will weaken Flexor pollicis longus, tested by resisted flexion of the thumb interphalangeal joint.

Second, you must look for *evidence of the cause* of the carpal tunnel syndrome, such as pregnancy, rheumatoid arthritis, osteoarthritis or myxoedema.

Claw hand

The 'claw' hand is more correctly called the 'intrinsic minus hand' because it results from paralysis of the intrinsic muscles. The essential feature is a hyperextension instability of the metacarpophalangeal joints, which buckle backwards. Flexion of the interphalangeal joints follows since the main extensors of the interphalangeal joints are the interossei and lumbricals, which are paralysed. It mainly affects the ulnar innervated fingers, ring and little, but also the thumb since the stabilising thenar muscles (Adductor Pollicis, and Flexor Pollicis Brevis) are also paralysed (Figure 7.30).

Neurological causes

Remember these causes by thinking of the course of the nerve fibres from the spinal cord through the brachial plexus into the peripheral nerves. Although the deformity is caused by a loss of motor function, there is often an associated sensory loss:

- Spinal cord – poliomyelitis, syringomyelia, amyotrophic lateral sclerosis.
- Brachial plexus – trauma to the medial roots and cords, especially birth injuries of the lower cord, as in Klumpke's paralysis; infiltration of the brachial plexus by malignant disease.
- Peripheral nerves – traumatic division or compression of the ulnar nerves; peripheral neuritis, leprosy.

See Chapter 3.

Trigger finger

This is a condition in which a finger *clicks painfully as it flexes* and eventually starts to *lock in flexion* when it will only extend after excessive voluntary effort, or with help from the other hand. *When extension begins, it does so suddenly and with a click* – hence the name trigger finger. The condition is caused by a thickening of the flexor tendon or paratenon, impairing movement of the tendon through a narrow pulley in the sheath wall.

History

Age and sex There are two groups of patients affected by this condition – middle-aged females and very young children. The thumb can be affected in neonates and infants, but this is a relatively rare condition.

Symptoms The patient complains that the finger clicks and jumps as it moves or gets stuck in a flexed position.

A trigger finger is not always a painful condition, even when force is required to extend it. The impact at the pulley site causes a localized synovitis and this can be painful and tender. Occasionally the synovitis is the primary cause of triggering.

The disability gradually gets more severe, but a fixed, immovable flexed finger is uncommon.

Cause In most cases there is no indication of the cause. It is commoner in diabetics and increasingly common with age.

Examination

Inspection The patient will show you how the finger gets stuck and how it snaps out into extension. The finger looks quite normal.

Palpation and movement The thickening of the tendon can be felt at the level of the head of the metacarpal bone. During movement, a nodule can be felt in the tendon as it moves in the sheath.

General examination Trigger finger is not associated with any systemic musculoskeletal disease.

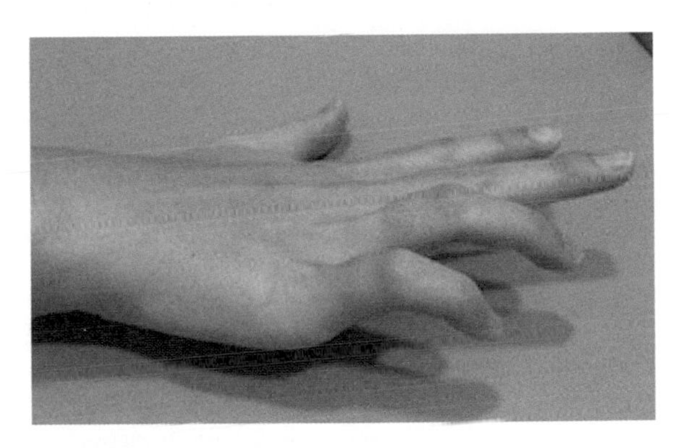

Figure 7.30 Ulnar claw hand.

Mallet finger

This is an *inability to extend the distal interphalangeal joint of a finger*, caused by an interruption of the extensor mechanism, either by a rupture of the extensor tendon, or by an avulsion fracture of its insertion. It is also known as *'baseball' finger* because the most common cause of the injury is a blow on the tip of the finger by a ball or hard object that forcibly flexes it against the pull of the extensor tendon, which ruptures or pulls off the bone.

History

The patient usually remembers the original injury but, if the finger is not painful, may not complain about it until the deformity is established and a nuisance.

Symptoms The inability to extend the tip of a finger is not a great disability, but for a person with an occupation that requires fine finger movements, including full extension of the distal interphalangeal joints, the deformity can be a serious handicap. Some patients complain that the deformity is disfiguring.

Examination

When the patient holds out their hand, with the fingers extended, the distal phalanx of the affected finger remains flexed to 15–20° (Figure 7.31). If you flex the distal interphalangeal joint to 90°, the patient can extend it back to the 20° position but cannot get it straight. The joint can be passively extended straight.

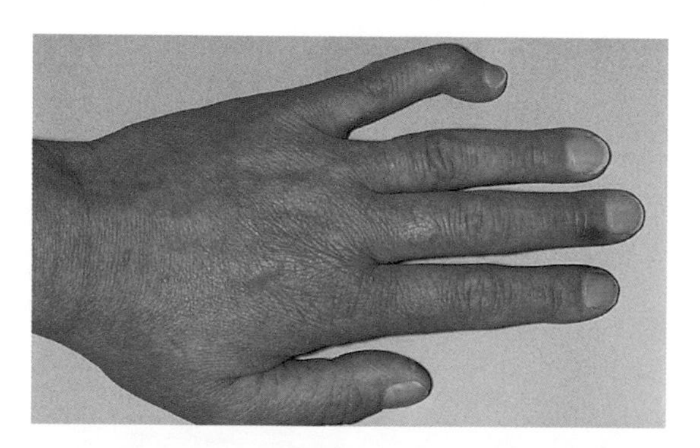

Figure 7.31 Mallet finger.

Ganglion

A ganglion is an encapsulated myxomatous degeneration of fibrous tissue. When a ganglion occurs on the anterior aspect of a flexor sheath, it can interfere with grip, and may cause pain and disability out of proportion to its size. It arises from any synovial space including joints and tendon sheaths. The commonest origin is from the wrist joint (see Chapter 4).

History

Age and sex Flexor sheath ganglia are most common in middle-aged males. Wrist ganglia are commoner in females.

Symptoms The commonest presenting symptom is a lump. Occasionally the patient complains of an ache in the ganglion or a sharp pain, particularly with flexor sheath ganglia. The cause of an ache is the degeneration that caused the ganglion, not the ganglion itself. Removing it may not resolve the ache.

Examination

Colour and temperature These are normal.

Site A small, tender nodule can be felt on the palmar surface of the base of a finger, superficial to the flexor sheath. A lump can be visible around the wrist.

Tenderness Direct pressure on the lump is often painful.

Shape The nodule is spherical or hemispherical (Figure 7.32).

Size Flexor sheath ganglia are usually quite small; some cause symptoms when they are only 2–3 mm in diameter.

Surface and edge The surface of the nodule is smooth, and the edge sharply defined.

Composition The cyst is tense and can be bony hard and even mistaken for bone by the patient and/or examiner. Flexor sheath ganglia are too small to permit the assessment of any other features such as fluctuation or translucency.

Lymph glands The local lymph glands are not enlarged.

Local tissues The rest of the hand is normal.

Comment Benign giant cell tumours of the flexor sheath present in an identical manner and are indistinguishable from flexor sheath ganglia.

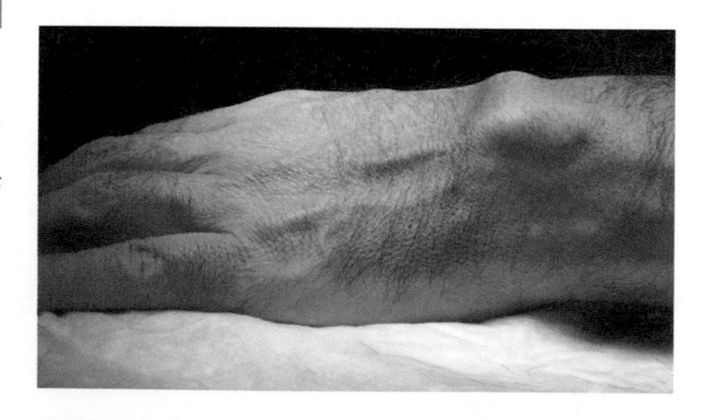

Figure 7.32 Soft multilocular ganglion on the back of the wrist.

Heberden's nodes

Heberden's nodes are bony swellings close to the distal finger joints. They are non-specific, and do not indicate any particular disease but are associated with osteoarthritis.

History

The patient complains of *swelling and deformity of* the back of hand joints. There may be a history of an old injury to the finger, or aching pains in both the lumps and the joints.

Examination

They are commonly found on the dorsal surface of the fingers just distal to the distal interphalangeal joint. They are not mobile and can be easily recognized as part of the underlying bone (Figure 7.33).

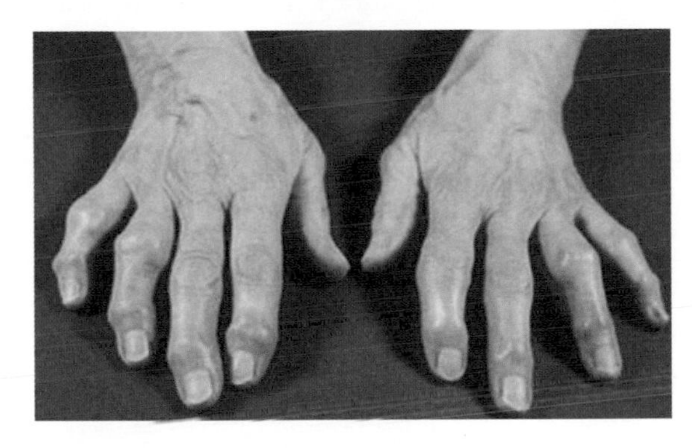

Figure 7.33 Heberden's nodes.

The joint movements may be slightly restricted by osteoarthritis, and there may be deviation of the distal phalanx. The index finger is most often affected. Small adventitious bursae may develop between the skin and the nodes. Similar nodes may appear near the proximal interphalangeal joint.

> **NOTE:** Heberden's nodes are associated with osteoarthritis of the affected joints. They should not be confused with rheumatoid nodules, which are areas of necrosis surrounded by fibroblasts and chronic inflammatory cells and are found in all types of connective tissue. Patients with rheumatoid nodules invariably have other evidence of rheumatoid arthritis.

Rheumatoid arthritis in the hand

The symptoms and signs of rheumatoid arthritis are described in Chapter 6, but, as it so often affects the hand, its manifestations are described again here. All the deformities result from the combination of an uneven pull by the tendons and destruction of the joint surfaces. Gross deformities from rheumatoid arthritis are becoming rarer, as a result of increasingly successful medical therapy.

Thickening of the joints

The joints most affected are the metacarpophalangeal joints and the proximal interphalangeal joints. Swelling of these joints gives the finger a fusiform, spindle shape.

Ulnar deviation of the fingers

The fingers drift towards the ulnar side of the hand, causing a varus deformity at the metacarpophalangeal joints. In advanced disease, the varus deformity can be as much as 45–60°.

Flexion of the wrist

The wrist joint develops a flexion deformity and usually some radial ulnar deviation (Figure 7.34).

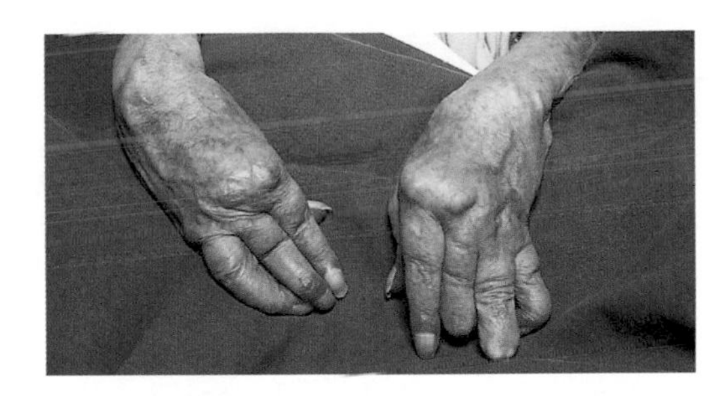

Figure 7.34 Rheumatoid arthritis of the hands.

'Swan neck' deformity of the fingers

This deformity is caused primarily by hyperextension instability of the proximal interphalangeal joint; flexion of the distal interphalangeal joint follows. It is caused by a variety of causes including volar plate laxity, loss of flexor digitorum superficialis integrity, mallet finger (Figure 7.35). It can also be caused by

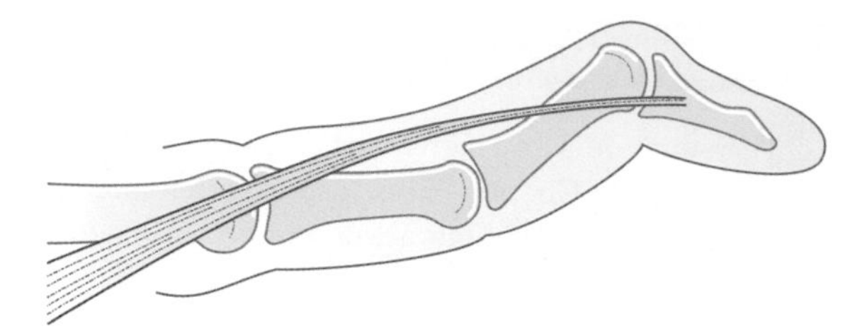

Figure 7.35 Swan neck deformity.

the patient habitually hyperextending the proximal interphalangeal joint in the formative years. It is not always pathological and a patient may seek treatment only when there is a noticeable or painful click as flexion is initiated.

Boutonnière deformity

The joint deformities of this abnormality are the opposite of those of the 'swan neck' deformity: flexion of the proximal interphalangeal joint, and hyperextension of the distal interphalangeal joint (Figure 7.36).

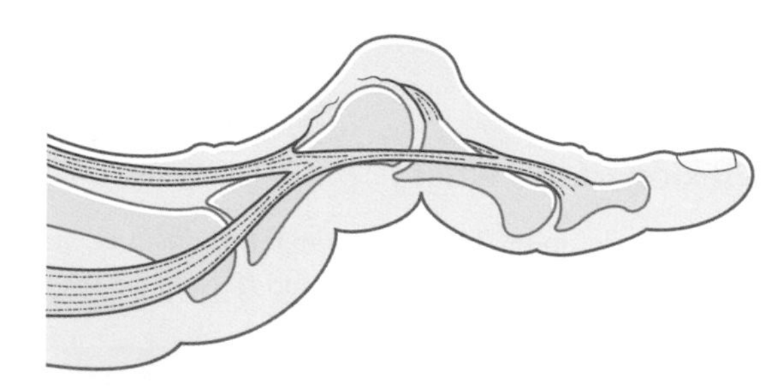

Figure 7.36 Boutonnière deformity.

It is caused by the interruption of the central portion of the extensor tendon that gradually causes the proximal interphalangeal joint to 'buttonhole' through the tendon and this rapidly becomes fixed in flexion. This is another condition which is easier to prevent than it is treat. It should be recognized early.

Tendon ruptures

Any tendon may undergo attrition (damage from friction) and rupture. This may be caused by severe rheumatoid arthritis or by other causes of attrition, for example, a wrist fracture or fixation plate. This causes variable deformities. The most common tendons to rupture are the long extensor tendons of the fingers and thumb.

Compound palmar 'ganglion'

This is a term that is applied to an effusion in the synovial sheath that surrounds the flexor tendons. It is not a ganglion. In the UK, it is now almost invariably secondary to rheumatoid arthritis or prolonged trauma, but in many other parts of the world it is often caused by a *tuberculous synovitis*.

History

The most common presenting symptom is *swelling on the anterior aspect of the wrist* and sometimes in the palm of the hand. *Pain is uncommon*.

The patient may notice crepitus during movements of the fingers.

Paraesthesia may occur in the distribution of the median nerve.

Examination

Distension of the flexor tendon synovial sheath produces a *soft, fluctuant swelling* that can be felt *on the anterior aspect of the wrist and lower forearm*, and in the *palm of the hand*. Because the swelling passes beneath the flexor retinaculum, compression of the lump on one side of the retinaculum makes it distend on the other side.

Crepitus may be felt during palpation and when the patient moves their fingers. This is caused by the presence of fibrin bodies within the synovial sheath – commonly called 'melon seed bodies'.

There are no local signs of inflammation.

General examination All the joints should be examined to exclude rheumatoid arthritis, and the chest should be examined (and X-rayed) to exclude tuberculosis.

THE NAILS

Inspection of the nails often yields useful information about the patient's general health. Conditions of the nails are described in Chapter 4.

FRACTURES AND DISLOCATIONS OF THE UPPER LIMB

Fractures of the upper limb occur at all ages, the most common cause being a *fall onto the outstretched hand*. A history of the mechanism of injury suggests which bones and joints are likely to have been injured – a fall forwards tends to cause injury to the radial structures; a fall backwards tends to cause injury to ulnar structures. High-energy trauma can lead to more significant injuries including soft tissue injuries, it also should raise the suspicion for concomitant injuries. Patients with multiple injuries should have their upper limbs examined as part of the secondary survey (see Chapter 5).

Fractures of the clavicle

These common injuries can occur in children and adults. Most are the result of a fall directly onto the shoulder, although some result from a direct blow and less commonly a fall onto the outstretched hand.

The site can be the:

- Middle third (80%).
- Lateral third (15%).
- Medial third (5%).

History

There is pain and arm movements hurt, especially *cross-arm abduction*.

Examination

Distortion and swelling are apparent at the fracture site (Figure 7.37).

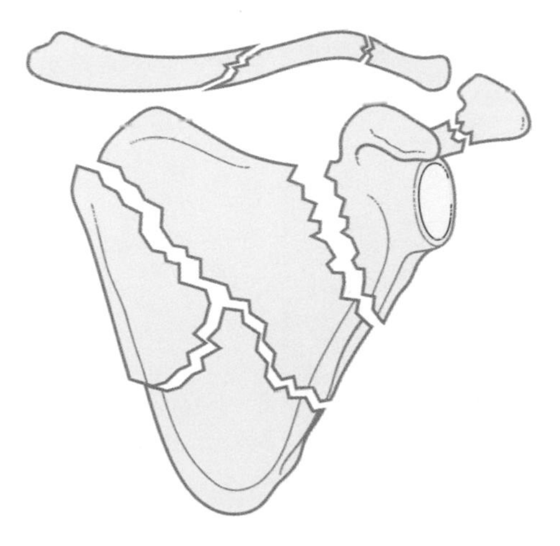

Figure 7.37 Fractures of the clavicle and scapula.

The overlying skin may be lifted and give the appearance that it will be pierced by a spike of bone, although this is event is very unusual.

The *shoulder is rotated anteriorly and inferiorly,* and *the arm is often held supported by the other hand.*

Associated injuries of the *brachial plexus* and *blood vessels* (see Chapters 3 and 10) must be excluded in all cases.

Fractures of the scapula

Considerable direct force (such as a blow on the back of the shoulder from a fall) is required to cause a scapular fracture as the bulky surrounding muscles protect the bone. Additional injuries to the ribs and chest are common.

Scapular fractures can be subdivided into those of the body, spine, neck, glenoid, acromion and coracoid process:

- Fractures of the *body and spine* cause pain and bruising. The arm is held adducted, and all shoulder movements are restricted.
- Fractures of the *neck* are often associated with fractures of the humerus or clavicle. The glenoid, which is effectively lying free, is usually displaced inferiorly by the weight of the arm.
- Fractures of the *glenoid* may be minor and associated with shoulder dislocation (see below), or more severe and comminuted, when there is severe bruising and swelling with restriction of all shoulder movements.
- Fractures of the *acromion* and *coracoid* are caused by direct blows and produce local pain and tenderness with restricted shoulder movements.

Injuries of the acromioclavicular joint

Dislocation and subluxation of this joint is a common sports injury from a fall onto the shoulder or, less commonly, the outstretched hand. The acromioclavicular and strong coracoclavicular ligaments are disrupted to a varying extent.

This may be a simple sprain involving only the acromioclavicular ligaments or involve a total disruption of all the ligaments. The position of the clavicle varies accordingly, and may be relatively well aligned, or severely displaced upwards, backwards or very rarely downwards (Figure 7.38).

History

There is always *pain and swelling over the joint*. All shoulder movements are restricted and painful.

Examination

The joint appears swollen and is tender to palpation. The arm is held adducted.

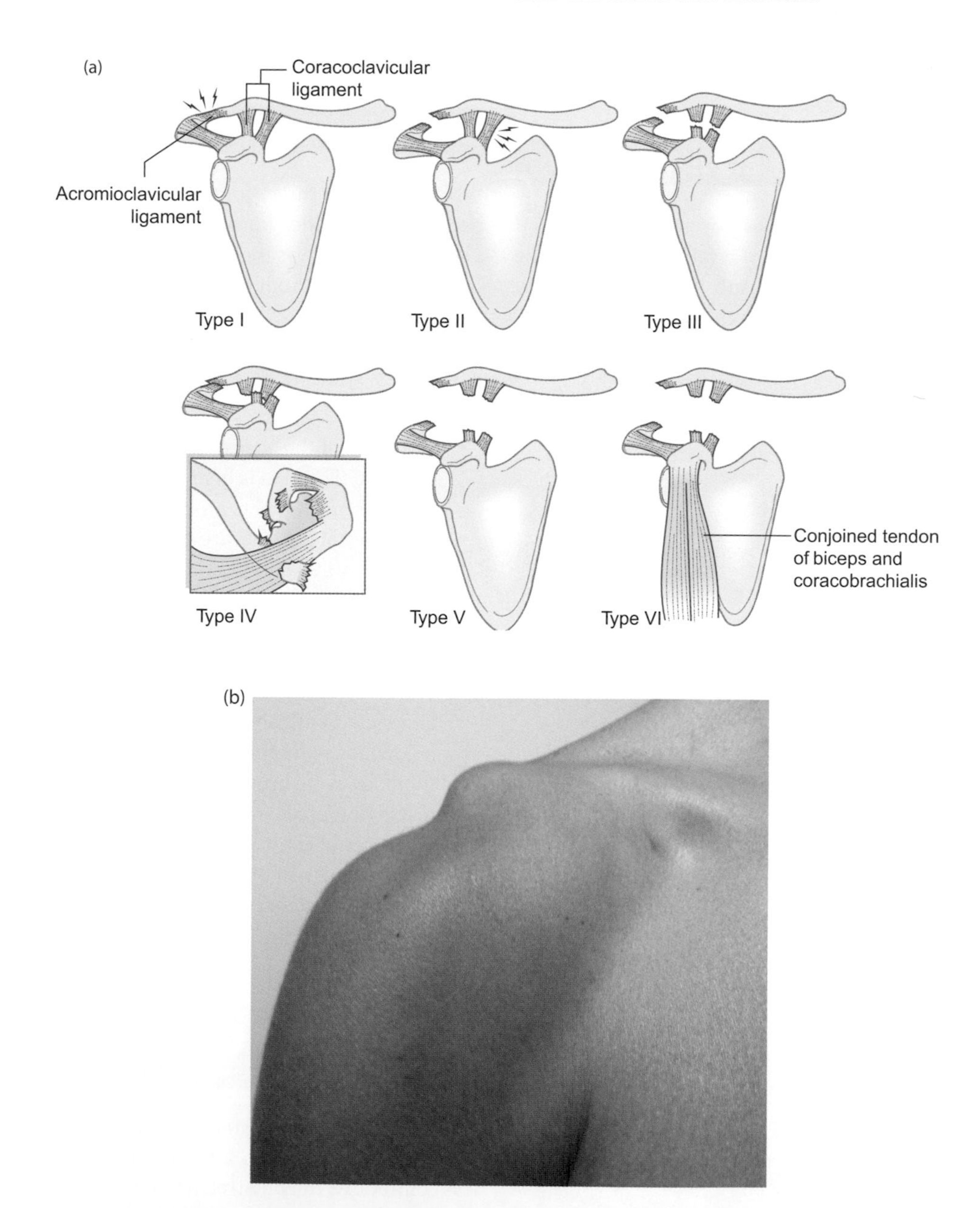

Figure 7.38 DISLOCATION OF THE ACROMIOCLAVICULAR JOINT (ACJ). (a) Types of ACJ injury. (b) Clinical appearance of a type V acromioclavicular joint injury.

> **NOTE:** The lateral end of the clavicle is usually displaced upwards relative to the downwards displacement of the shoulder; hence there is an altered contour.

It may be reduced back into place, but springs back when the pressure is released.

Injuries of the sternoclavicular joint

This joint is injured much less commonly and can be damaged without a history of trauma.

The grade of injury again varies between a partial ligamentous tear (a sprain) to total disruption with anterior, or less commonly posterior, displacement of the medial end of the clavicle.

A direct blow in a road traffic or sporting accident applies medial force to the lateral aspect of the shoulder.

The injury can also occur from a fall onto an outstretched hand.

History

The pain is made worse by shoulder abduction and adduction.

Examination

There is *localized tenderness* over the swollen joint. The *medial end of the clavicle is prominent* with an anterior dislocation and lies downwards and forwards.

With *posterior dislocation,* the normal anterior bony clavicular contour is lost.

Associated injuries Venous congestion and arterial damage to major blood vessels, or dyspnoea from a pneumothorax or tracheal injury, can all occur.

Dislocation of the glenohumeral joint

The shoulder is the most mobile joint in the body, but with the least bony stability. This makes it very likely to dislocate.

There are two peaks of incidence, the first between 16 and 25 years, associated with trauma, and the second much later in the elderly, when the stability is impaired by muscle weakness and falls become more frequent.

ANTERIOR DISLOCATION

This is far more common, usually caused by a fall with the shoulder in an abducted and externally rotated position.

There is *severe pain* and *loss of shoulder movements.*

On examination, the *shoulder contour is flattened or lost*, and the arm, often supported by the opposite hand, is held in slight abduction and internal rotation. The acromion and humeral head appear prominent (Figure 7.39), and *all movements are limited and painful.*

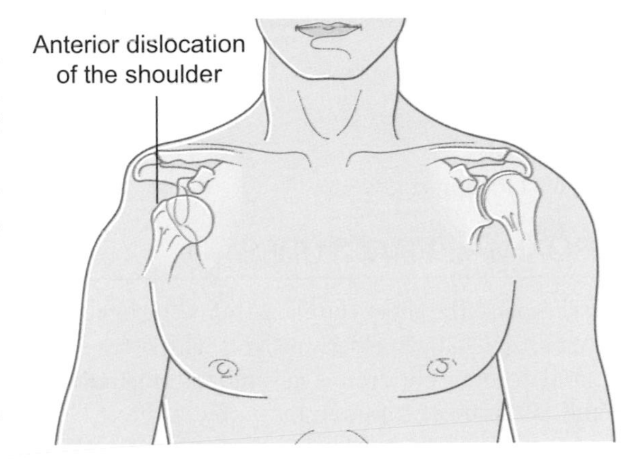

Figure 7.39 Anterior dislocation of the shoulder.

POSTERIOR DISLOCATION

This is less common. It is caused by a fall onto an outstretched internally rotated arm. This can also occur during an epileptic fit or can follow a direct blow on the front of the shoulder.

On examination, the shoulder appears normal in contour, but the *arm is held adducted* and *internally rotated.* Abduction is limited, and external rotation beyond the neutral position is very difficult.

INFERIOR DISLOCATION (LUXATIO ERECTA)

This is rare. The patient is in great pain, and the arm is held above the head. The humeral head may be palpable over the lateral chest wall. There is a high incidence of associated neurovascular injury.

COMPLICATIONS

There is a high rate of recurrent shoulder dislocation, particularly in the younger population. Associated humeral fractures can occur. The *axillary nerve is injured in 10–20% of cases* and can be assessed by testing pinprick sensation over the 'regimental patch' area on the lateral aspect of the proximal humerus. Other brachial plexus injuries occur less frequently. The rotator cuff tendons can be torn during the injury, especially in the elderly.

Fractures of the humerus

The site can be:

- Proximal.
- Shaft.
- Distal/supracondylar.

PROXIMAL FRACTURES

These are the most common and occur in all age groups, especially in elderly patients with osteoporosis and in young children. A fall onto the outstretched hand is the most common cause, but a direct blow on the outer arm can also be responsible. Fractures may involve the surgical neck, the anatomical neck, the greater tuberosity, the lesser tuberosity or a combination, whereby they are described as two-part, three-part or four-part fractures.

History

Pain, swelling and restriction of shoulder movement suggest a fracture.

Examination

There is *tenderness, swelling* and *restricted arm movement with crepitus*. Significant bruising may develop down the arm. There may be an associated neurovascular injury, especially to the axillary nerve, and shoulder dislocation.

HUMERAL SHAFT FRACTURES

These occur at all ages, usually caused by a direct blow from a motor car accident or a fall. They can also follow a fall onto the elbow or outstretched hand. Twisting injuries, caused by arm wrestling, can result in spiral fractures.

History

There is pain and loss of use of the arm.

Examination

Tenderness, swelling/bruising and *deformity with crepitus* are seen. The deformity depends upon the force applied and the relationship of the muscle insertions to the site and direction of the fracture (spiral or transverse).

In upper third fractures, the proximal fragment is pulled into adduction by the action of the pectoralis major muscle, while in the middle third the proximal fragment is abducted by the deltoid.

> **NOTE:** A radial nerve injury complicates 20% of humeral shaft fractures and results in a wrist drop.

DISTAL/SUPRACONDYLAR FRACTURES

In children, fractures around the elbow are common. Supracondylar fractures have a peak incidence at 8 years and result from a hyperextension of the elbow, with the olecranon levering on the back of the humerus, during a fall onto an outstretched hand.

History

A *painful swollen elbow* occurs, with *restricted movement*.

Examination

The inferior fragment is *usually displaced backwards*, and the humeral shaft appears prominent and may tent the overlying skin. The *olecranon is palpable posteriorly* and appears displaced upwards (Figure 7.40). Occasionally, the distal fragment is displaced anteriorly.

Neurovascular injuries are commonly associated. The radial, median and ulnar nerves may all be damaged, but *injury to the brachial artery is especially important*. The vessel may be torn, stretched, lacerated or trapped in the fracture fragments. It may be transected or thrombosed, or the intima may be torn.

> **NOTE:** Look carefully for the radial pulse and signs of arterial compromise (pain, pallor, paraesthesia, paralysis and perishing cold).

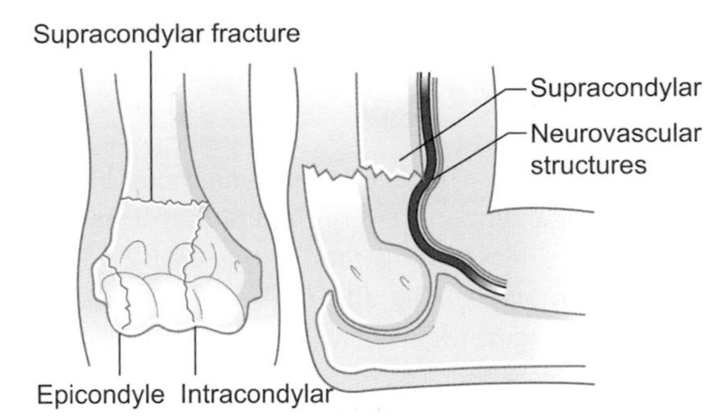

Figure 7.40 Supracondylar and intracondylar fracture of the humerus.

FRACTURES OF THE MEDIAL EPICONDYLE

These are much more common in children than adults, and are caused by a direct blow, a fall onto the outstretched hand with the wrist hyperextended, or avulsion by the ulnar collateral ligament during elbow dislocation. The pain is made worse by elbow flexion, and the medial epicondyle is tender, swollen and bruised.

Fractures of the lateral epicondyle are less common but present in a similar manner to medial epicondyle fractures, although they involve the outer aspect of the joint.

In the adult, *distal humeral fractures* occur following a fall on the outstretched hand. The clinical features are as for children, but there may be more comminution and angulation of the fracture fragments.

INTRACONDYLAR FRACTURES

Intracondylar fractures, which are T- or Y-shaped fractures extending into the articular surface, can also occur (Figure 7.40). They cannot be differentiated clinically from supracondylar fractures.

Dislocation of the elbow

The elbow is the second most common large joint to dislocate, and this can occur in children and adults. It can be confused with a supracondylar fracture.

The majority of dislocations are in a posterior direction. Disruption of the medial and lateral ulnar collateral ligament or fracture of the medial epicondyle allows the radial head and olecranon to displace backwards behind the lower end of the humerus.

Anterior dislocation can occasionally occur following a blow on the back of the elbow.

History

A fall onto the outstretched hand in a teenager or young adult is the usual cause.

Examination

In posterior dislocation, the elbow is swollen and held in 45° of flexion. The olecranon appears very prominent, and its relationship with the medial and lateral epicondyles is disrupted, unlike in supracondylar fractures, where the relationship is maintained (Figure 7.41).

In *anterior dislocation*, the elbow is extended, and the olecranon cannot be felt in its usual position. The forearm appears elongated and is held supine.

> **NOTE:** Neurovascular injuries of the median and ulnar nerves and brachial artery must be carefully excluded in all patients with elbow dislocations. The same thorough neurovascular assessment should be repeated and documented following reduction of the elbow joint.

Associated fractures are common, especially of the medial epicondyle, radial head and coronoid process.

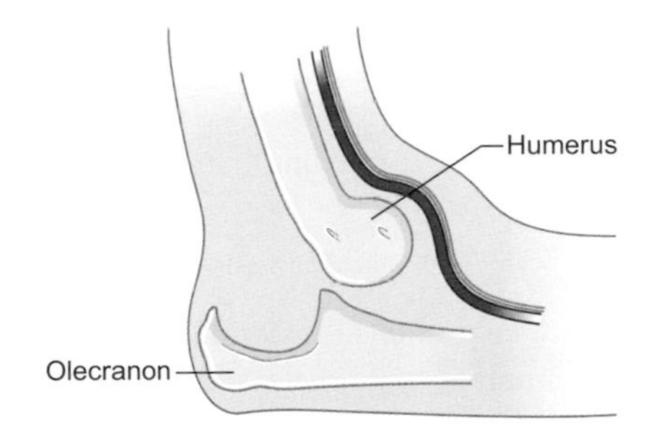

Figure 7.41 Posterior dislocation of the elbow.

Fractures of head and neck of radius

These occur at all ages, in isolation or with other fractures and elbow dislocation. They may be displaced or undisplaced, comminuted or simple, and may involve the articular surface. A transverse fracture across the neck of the radius can lead to the radial head lying free from the shaft. The fracture line may alternatively run through the head itself.

The mechanism of injury is usually a fall onto the outstretched hand, which causes the radial head to impact against the capitellum, disrupting the distal radioulnar joint and the interosseous membrane and fracturing the radial head.

History

The elbow joint is swollen and painful.

Examination

The joint is swollen by haemarthrosis, and there is localized tenderness over the head of the radius. Elbow movements and forearm rotation are painful and diminished. During recovery, elbow extension is usually the last movement to be restored. The distal radioulnar joint and interosseous membrane may also be injured and therefore tender, with subluxation of the distal end of the ulna (an *Essex–Lopresti fracture–dislocation*).

Fractures of the olecranon

Rare in children, the fracture can be displaced or undisplaced, transverse, oblique or comminuted. The mechanisms of injury may be a direct blow, or a fall onto the elbow or outstretched hand when the elbow is flexed, and the triceps is forcefully contracted.

History

There is pain and swelling over the back of the elbow.

Examination

It may not be possible to extend the elbow against gravity and there is tenderness and a palpable swelling over the point of the elbow. A gap can sometimes be felt between the bone fragments.

COMPLICATIONS

The ulnar nerve is at risk and must be tested (see Chapter 3).

Fractures of the shafts of the radius and ulna

These bones articulate at each end, bound by the annular ligament and inferior radioulnar ligaments, and are further held together by the strong interosseous membrane. This allows the radius to rotate around the static ulna, such that they act as a single unit. It means that fractures or dislocations of the shafts of either bone are often accompanied by similar injuries in the other.

A *Galeazzi fracture* occurs when there is a fracture between the middle and distal thirds of the radius, accompanied by a subluxation/dislocation of the distal radioulnar joint (Figure 7.42a).

A *Monteggia fracture* occurs when there is a fracture of the proximal third of the ulna, accompanied by a dislocation of the radial head (Figure 7.42b).

These injuries commonly result from a fall onto the front or back of an outstretched hand. Direct

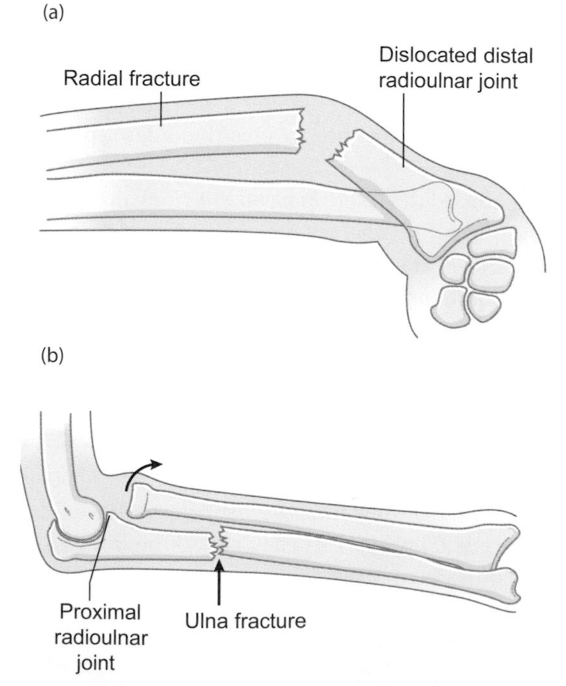

Figure 7.42 FRACTURES OF THE SHAFTS OF THE RADIUS AND ULNA. (a) A Galeazzi fracture. (b) A Monteggia fracture.

trauma can also fracture both bones, such as in road traffic accidents. In a Monteggia fracture dislocation, there may be forced pronation of the arm at the moment of impact.

When the arm is raised to protect the head from attack, a direct blow from a blunt instrument can cause an isolated ulnar fracture (a *nightstick fracture*).

In children, greenstick fractures are very common, and displacement is often minimal.

History

There is *pain, swelling, deformity and an inability to rotate the forearm*. Associated injuries may interfere with movement of the wrist or elbow.

Examination

There is an *obvious deformity* if both bones are broken, with localized tenderness and swelling over the fracture lines. Examine the elbow and wrist to exclude dislocation of the radial head (see above) and distal radioulnar joints. *Pronation and supination are prevented by severe pain*.

COMPLICATIONS

Open fractures are not uncommon, but they are often associated with nerve injury (especially the posterior interosseous nerve) and other soft tissue damage. It is crucial to exclude a compartment syndrome.

Fractures of the distal radius and ulna

These are the most common fractures in both adults and children, with age peaks at 5–10 and over 50 years of age.

A *Colles' fracture* is an impaction fracture through the distal radial metaphysis within 2.5 cm of the wrist joint, with *dorsal angulation, dorsal displacement, radial angulation* and *radial displacement*. It was originally common in elderly patients but is now recognized in all ages. It can be accompanied by a fracture of the ulnar styloid in 60% of cases (Figure 7.43a).

A *Smith's fracture* is also through the distal radius, but with *volar displacement of the distal fragment*. The fracture can extend into the joint (Figure 7.43b). Smith's fractures are less common than Colles' fractures.

A *Barton's fracture* is subluxation or fracture–dislocation of the wrist accompanied by an intra-articular fracture of the distal radius. This causes the carpus and hand to displace backwards or forwards (Figure 7.43c).

Fractures in children occur through either the metaphysis or the epiphysis. They can be minimally displaced greenstick fractures, where there is only slight buckling of the cortex (see Chapter 6), although complete fractures do occur.

(a)

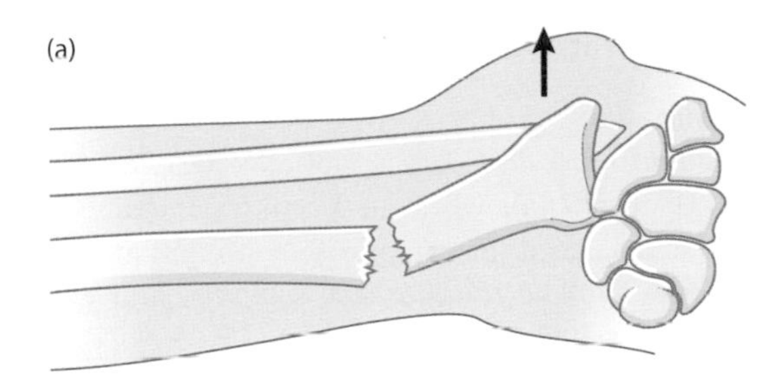

(b)

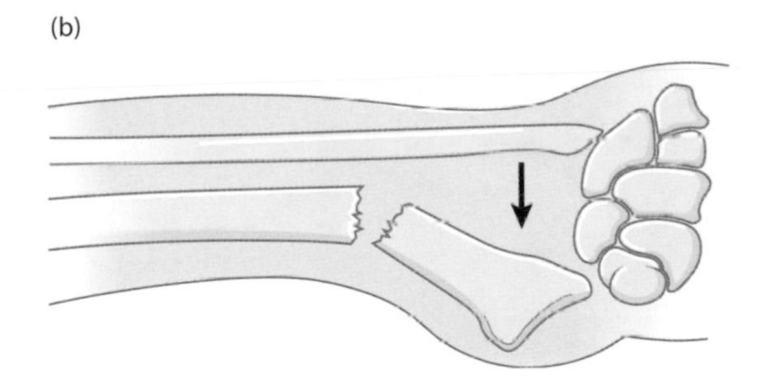

(c)

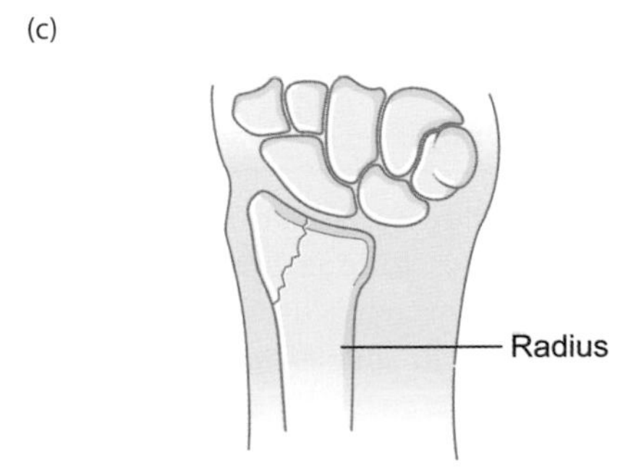

Figure 7.43 FRACTURES OF THE DISTAL RADIUS AND ULNA. (a) A Colles' fracture. (b) A Smith's fracture. (c) A Barton's fracture.

MECHANISM

Wrist fractures usually result from a fall onto the outstretched hand, common in snowy and icy conditions. Direct blows and motorcycle injuries are other causes. The direction of force often determines the type of fracture.

A Colles' fracture usually occurs when there is a fall onto an outstretched arm with the wrist in extension. In a Smith's fracture, the wrist is flexed on impact.

History

There is *pain, deformity* and *an inability to move the wrist* following a fall or injury.

Examination

A *dinner fork deformity* is typical of a Colles' fracture (Figure 7.44), while in a Smith's fracture the hand is displaced forwards, with a swelling in front of the wrist. The fracture site is tender, and wrist movements are restricted.

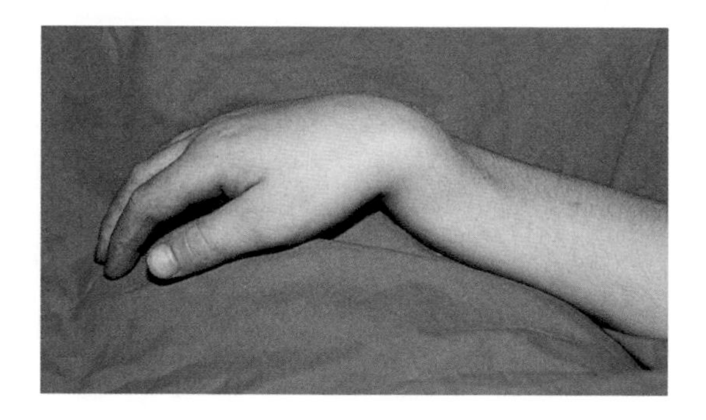

Figure 7.44 Dinner fork deformity from a distal radial fracture.

COMPLICATIONS

Open fractures following falls are rare. They happen when considerable force is involved, and the bones puncture the skin from within.

Injury to the *median* and *ulnar nerves* should always be excluded.

Forearm *compartment* and acute *carpal tunnel syndromes* can occur acutely, while carpal tunnel syndrome can also develop late.

Complex regional pain syndrome Type 1 (previously known as reflex sympathetic dystrophy) complicates up to 40% of wrist fractures, causing pain, swelling, loss of joint mobility and vasomotor instability.

Rupture of the extensor pollicis tendon and osteoarthritis of the wrist joint are late complications.

Fractures of the scaphoid bone

The scaphoid is the largest bone of the proximal carpal row, linking the two rows of carpal bones and the radiocarpal joint; 80% of its surface is articular, and 80% of its blood supply enters the middle portion, or 'waist', so that fractures can cause devascularization of the proximal fragment.

The most common site for a fracture is through the waist of the bone (50%), followed by the proximal half (38%) and the distal half (12%).

MECHANISM

Fractures of the scaphoid account for three-quarters of all carpal injuries. They are usually caused by a fall forwards onto the outstretched hand with the wrist hyperextended. The scaphoid is compressed by the distal radius.

The fracture may be complete or incomplete, angulated or rotated, displaced or undisplaced and occasionally comminuted.

History

The *pain may be mild*, and patients often think that they have only sprained their wrist.

Examination

The *signs may be minimal*. There is often some subtle swelling and *localized tenderness in the anatomical snuff box* (Figure 7.45). Maximal passive radial and ulnar deviation of the wrist produces pain in the radial side of the wrist. Thumb compression may also induce pain.

COMPLICATIONS

Avascular necrosis of the proximal fragment is an important and not infrequent complication that leads to progressive bony collapse and late osteoarthritis.

Non-union of the fracture is also a common complication and may follow a missed fracture with normal

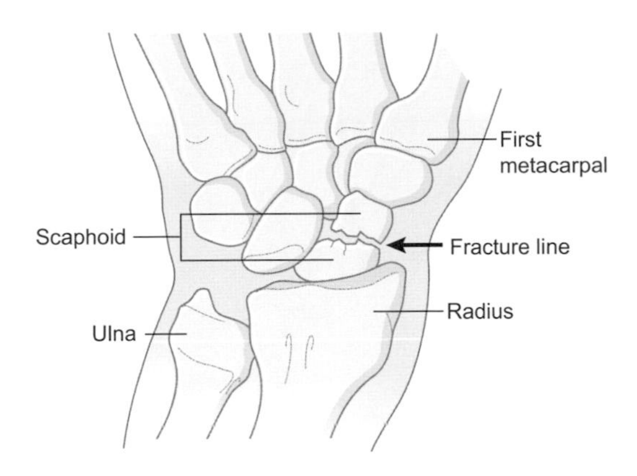

Figure 7.45 Fracture of the scaphoid: tenderness in the anatomical snuff box.

X-ray. It is important to re-examine for tenderness 2 weeks after injury.

Additionally, injury to wrist soft tissues should be considered, for example, the scapholunate ligament.

Perilunate and lunate and dislocation of the wrist

Dislocations of the carpus are an uncommon group of injuries. A perilunate dislocation occurs when the metacarpals, distal carpal row and part of the proximal row are dislocated (Figure 7.46a). The term 'peri' is used to describe the bones that remain undisplaced in the proximal row. The lunate remains attached to the radius through a strong volar ligament, while the rest of the carpus dislocates posteriorly. These injuries may be associated with fracture of the scaphoid.

The distal row may alternatively realign with the radius, and part of the proximal row is extruded, causing a lunate dislocation (Figure 7.46b). This is the most common carpal dislocation.

The injuries are usually caused by a fall onto an outstretched hand, or a road traffic accident causing extreme dorsiflexion of a radially deviated wrist.

History

Pain is often surprisingly mild, but wrist movements are uncomfortable.

Examination

Physical signs are subtle and *the diagnosis, like that of a scaphoid fracture, is easily missed*. There is usually some swelling, diffuse tenderness and discomfort on wrist movement. The median and ulnar nerves and wrist tendons may be damaged.

Metacarpal fractures and dislocations

These bones can fracture at the shaft, base or neck The usual mechanism is punching a hard object, either deliberately or in a fall. A direct blow on the back of the hand may also be responsible. Deformity is often minor, as the metacarpals are splinted by

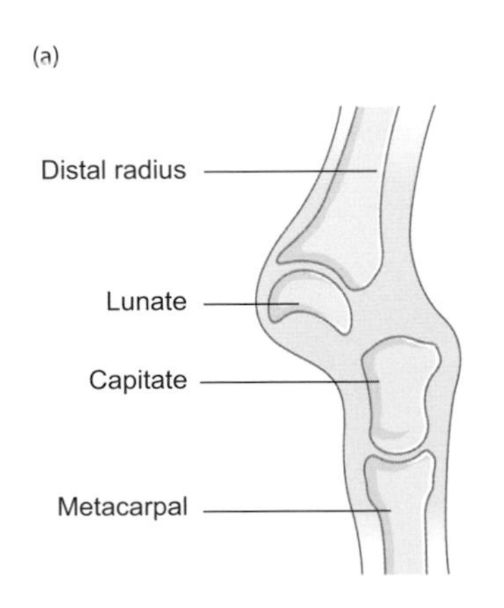

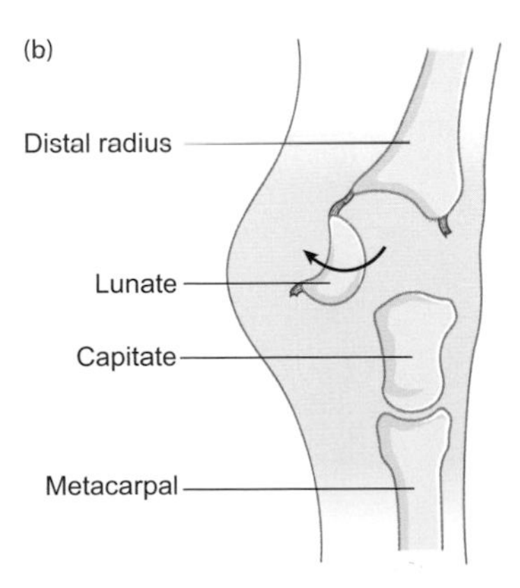

Figure 7.46 DISLOCATIONS OF THE WRIST. (a) Perilunate. (b) Lunate.

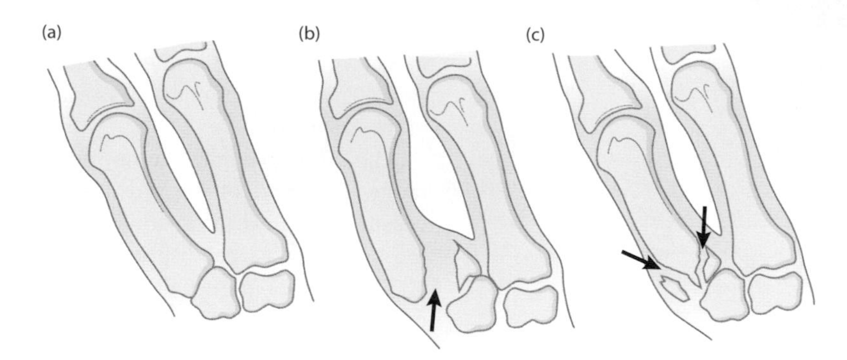

Figure 7.47 TYPES OF FIRST METACARPAL FRACTURES. (a) Normal metacarpal bones. (b) A Bennett's fracture. (c) A Rolando's fracture.

their fellows and surrounding muscles. Rotational deformity can interfere with hand function by causing 'scissoring' of the path of one finger across that of another. The most common fracture is to the neck of the little finger (fifth) metacarpal (a *boxer's fracture*).

History

There is local pain, swelling and loss of hand function.

Examination

Local tenderness and swelling are seen.

A fracture of the neck of a metacarpal results in a drop of the head of the bone and a flattened knuckle. There may be rotational deformity due to 'scissoring' of one digit across the path of another.

Bennett's fracture–dislocation is an oblique fracture at the base of the first metacarpal bone extending into the carpometacarpal joint. The loss of continuity of metacarpal with volar beak ligament makes the joint unstable, with proximal and lateral subluxation of the thumb (Figure 7.47b). The usual cause is a punch or forcible abduction/extension of the thumb column, as in a rugby tackle. The thumb is shortened because of posterior subluxation and is swollen around its base.

In a *Rolando fracture*, there is a fracture at the base of the thumb metacarpal with a T- or Y-shaped extension (Figure 7.47c). Its presentation and signs are similar to those of a Bennett's fracture.

Fractures and dislocations of the phalanges

Direct trauma, often in sport, is the most common cause, and fractures may often be compound.

There is pain, loss of function, swelling, deformity and local tenderness.

Dislocations of finger joints are usually obvious from the deformity and loss of function. In the presence of significant swelling, however, they can be missed. They are often reduced on the sports field and present late.

8 Lower limb

STEVEN A CORBETT, IAN P HOLLOWAY, DAVID HOULIHAN-BURNE AND ANDREW ROCHE

THE HIP

This is a mobile ball and socket joint that articulates between the lower limb and the pelvis, supporting the weight of the body for both static and dynamic functions. It comprises:

- The head of the femur.
- The three bones that form the pelvis and acetabulum: the ilium, ischium and pubis.
- A tough membranous capsule lined by synovium.
- A labrum surrounding the socket.
- Synovial fluid, which lubricates the joint.
- Muscles and tendons, which stabilize the joint and assist in movement.

As with any joint, examination is based on the principles of:

- Look.
- Feel.
- Move.

These principles are followed using specific tests of anatomical structure and for pathological conditions.

Remember that the examination of the hip is not complete until the joints below and above have also been assessed, namely *the knee* and *lower back*.

Symptoms

The main symptoms caused by hip diseases are *pain* and *stiffness*.

Pain is classically experienced in the groin region, and the patient often points to or places their hand in this region.

> **NOTE:** Pain from the hip joint can be referred to the knee, and hip pathology can sometimes cause pain only in the knee.

Equally, pain from the lower lumbar spine and sacroiliac joints can be experienced in the hip region, which is a consequence of their shared nerve supply from the L2, L3 and L4 nerve roots. Spinal pain tends to be referred to the buttock or lateral hip. This highlights the importance of always examining the joints above and below the joint under investigation.

NOTE: Initially, hip pain may be present only on activity. As the pathology progresses, the pain may be felt at rest, including at night, causing sleep disturbance.

In the degenerate hip, stiffness in the morning is a common complaint, coupled with restriction of movement during the day. This results in disability and loss of functional capacity, such as the ability to put on socks and shoes. The patient may walk with a limp, using a walking stick for support.

Deformity of the hip can arise from congenital or acquired conditions, including trauma, infection and degenerative, neurological and neoplastic conditions, which affect the anatomical structures (Revision panel 8.1).

Revision panel 8.1

CAUSES OF JOINT DEFORMITIES

Skin – contractures
Fascia – contractures
Muscle – paralysis, fibrosis, spasm
Tendon – division, adhesion
Ligament – rupture, stretching
Capsule – rupture, fibrosis
Synovium – inflammation
Bone – changes in shape, trauma, pressure atrophy

Plan for examination of the hip joint

Inspect the patient's surroundings, paying particular attention to any walking aids and shoe raises, which can alert you to a limb length discrepancy.

First examine the patient standing up if possible. This gives you the opportunity to inspect the patient from the front, the side and then the back.

Next perform Trendelenburg's test and assess the patient's gait (see below). Then ask the patient to lie flat and straight on the couch, and check that the pelvis is square to the midline by feeling the positions of the anterior superior iliac spines. By examining a hip in this manner, unnecessary position changes are avoided during the examination.

INSPECTION

Skin

Remember that sinuses and scars from the hip joint are often found on the buttock and posterior aspect of the upper thigh, so look at the skin over the back of the joint as well as the front.

Shape

Check the contours of the thigh and buttock. Asymmetrical skin creases indicate joint displacement. Note any muscle wasting or rotational deformity. Also observe any increased lumbar lordosis or scoliosis (see Chapter 9).

Position

When the hip joint is painful or distended by an effusion, it is held slightly flexed, abducted and externally rotated. These deformities may be fixed. In cases of true shortening, once the anterior superior iliac spines are level, a degree of shortening may be apparent by noting that the heels are not level. This should stimulate an accurate assessment of shortening and limb length measurement (see Chapter 6).

PALPATION

The capsule and synovium of the hip joint cannot be felt, but the bony contours of the pelvis and trochanter can be. It is important to note any tenderness over the greater trochanter as this is indicative of trochanteric bursitis, which can be confused with hip joint pathology.

Relationship between the pelvis and femur

In cases of shortening, the position of the greater trochanter with respect to the pelvis (i.e. acetabulum) can be checked in three ways:

- **Bilateral palpation.** To compare the two sides, put your thumbs on the anterior superior iliac spines and your fingers on the tips of the greater trochanters. You will appreciate any difference

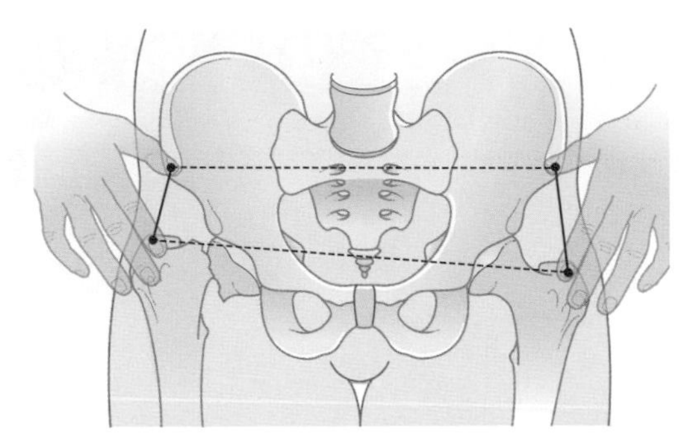

Figure 8.1 Bilateral palpation. Thumbs placed on the anterior superior iliac spines, index finger on the greater trochanters. Length differences indicate pathology in the femoral head or neck, e.g. developmental dysplasia of the hip or fractures of the femoral neck.

in the distance between these points through the position of your fingers (Figure 8.1).

- **Nélaton's line.** Turn the patient on their side, and imagine a line drawn from the anterior superior iliac spine to the ischial tuberosity (Figure 8.2). The top of the greater trochanter should just touch this line. If it lies above the line, there is shortening of the neck of the femur or a dislocation of the hip.
- **Bryant's triangle.** This gives a measurement of the distance between the top of the greater trochanter and the coronal plane of the iliac spine. Lie the patient supine. Imagine a horizontal line passing through the anterior superior iliac spine. Measure the vertical distance between this line and the top of the greater trochanter (Figure 8.3). This should form an isosceles triangle.

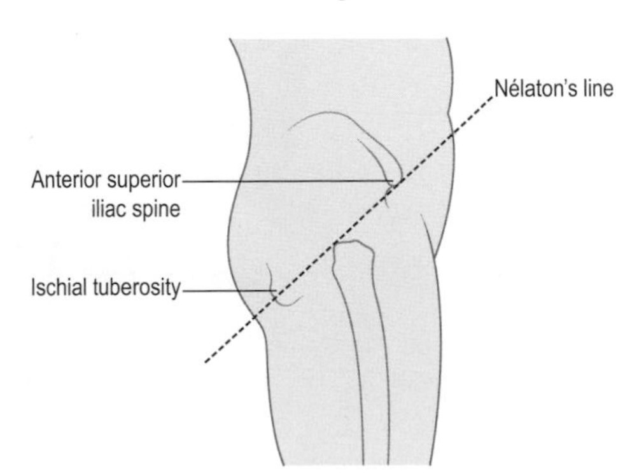

Figure 8.2 Nélaton's line is a line drawn through the anterior superior iliac spine and the ischial tuberosity. It should just touch the top of the greater trochanter.

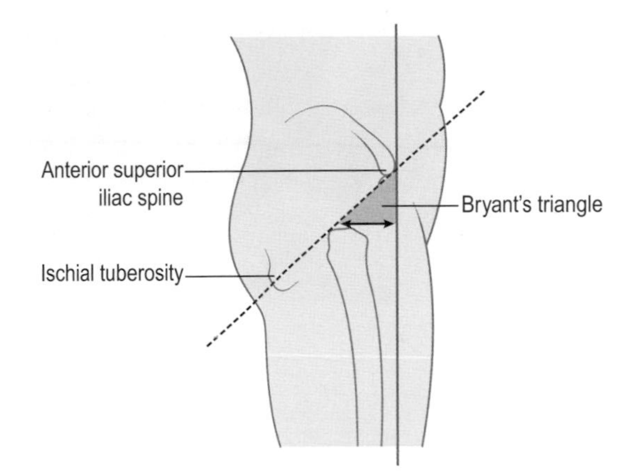

Figure 8.3 Bryant's triangle measures the vertical distance from the anterior superior iliac spine to the greater trochanter, and the horizontal distance between the coronal planes of the iliac spine and the trochanter.

Nélaton's line and Bryant's triangle are now very rarely used clinically (as radiographs are much more accurate), but they are useful ways of remembering the normal relationships of the bony landmarks.

MOVEMENT

This can be divided into active and passive. The passive range is generally more useful in determining pathology in the hip joint.

The *normal range of hip movement* is:

- Flexion 0–130°.
- Extension 0–10°.
- Internal rotation 45°.
- External rotation 45°.
- Abduction 45°.
- Adduction 30°.

The range of movement in the hip can be restricted by stiffness, such as fixed flexion.

Thomas' test for fixed flexion

When the hip joint is stiff, the range of movement may appear to be preserved by compensation from the surrounding joints. Fixed deformities of adduction and abduction will be clearly visible from the position of the thigh when you set the pelvis square with the spine, *but fixed flexion can be masked by a lumbar lordosis.*

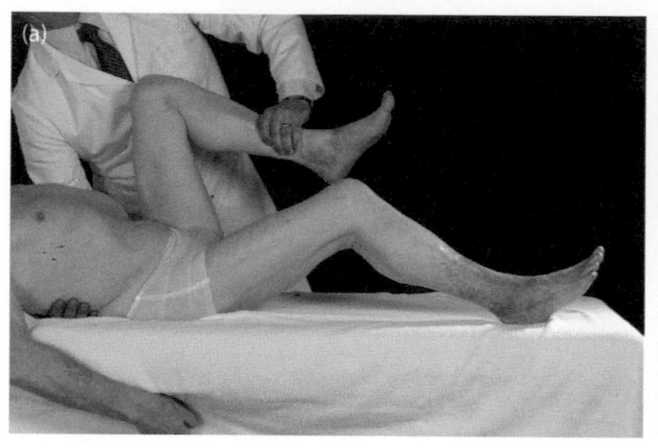

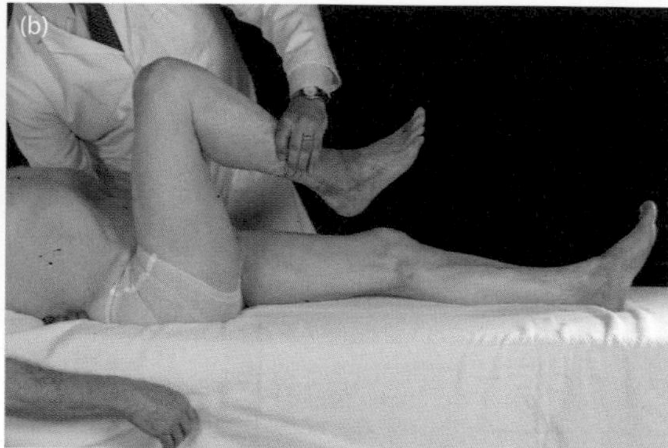

Figure 8.4 THOMAS' TEST FOR FIXED FLEXION. Measure the degree of fixed flexion by flexing the good hip until the lumbar spine straightens and presses on your other hand placed beneath the lumbar spine. There is no fixed flexion in the left hip (a) but there is 25° of fixed flexion in the right hip (b).

To assess for fixed flexion, place your left hand underneath the hollow of the lumbar spine. Ask the patient to bring both knees up to their chest as far as possible. At this point, you can assess hip flexion of both hips and note any discrepancies between the limbs. The lumbar lordosis should be obliterated at this point.

Next ask the patient to let one leg lie back on the couch. The thigh on that side will remain flat on the couch if the hip joint is normal. If the hip lifts off the couch, this indicates a loss of extension in that hip, which is referred to as a *fixed flexion deformity* (Figure 8.4), and the angle of elevation, or fixed flexion, should be recorded. This is called *Thomas' test* for fixed flexion. Now flex the other leg to check the opposite joint.

Passive movements

You can only test the movements of a joint by keeping one of the bones that forms the joint still, whilst moving the other bone. A false impression of hip movement may be obtained if the pelvis moves during the examination. Therefore, during all passive movements of the hip, you must continually check that the pelvis is not moving by keeping the thumb and little finger of one hand resting upon the two anterior superior iliac spines.

Flexion Flex the good hip and knee until the thigh presses against the abdomen, then ask the patient to hold the leg in this position. Next flex the hip under consideration, using your other hand to check that no further pelvic movement takes place. Record the degree of flexion, and any fixed flexion deformity that is present (Figure 8.5).

Abduction and adduction Keeping one hand firmly on the anterior superior iliac spines, abduct or adduct each leg until the pelvis begins to move, and record the range of movement (Figure 8.6).

Rotation Both internal and external rotation can be assessed by rolling the whole limb, but the best way is to flex the hip and knee to 90°. The foot can then be moved laterally to assess internal rotation, and medially to assess external rotation (Figure 8.7). The range of movement can then be measured by comparing the position of the leg to the midline.

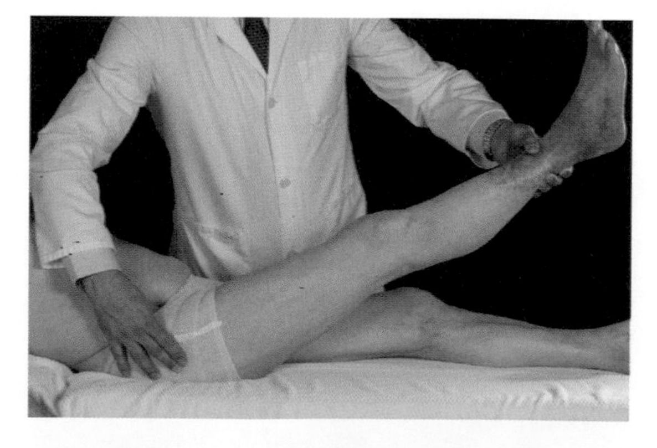

Figure 8.5 When testing hip movements such as flexion, place your fingers on the greater trochanter and your thumb on the iliac spine so that you detect any tilting of the pelvis.

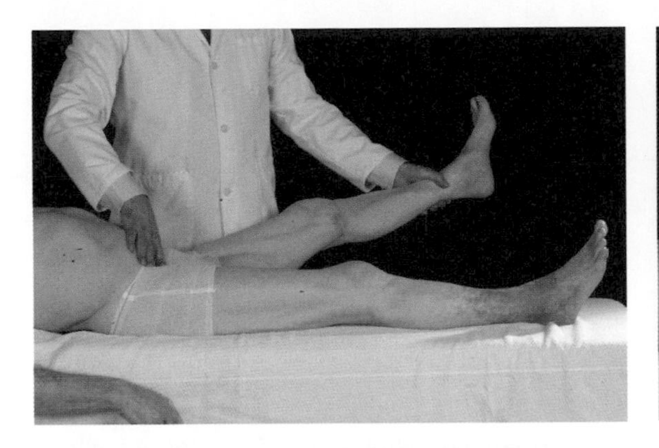

Figure 8.6 Keep your fingers and thumb stretched across the iliac spines when testing abduction and adduction to detect any movement of the pelvis.

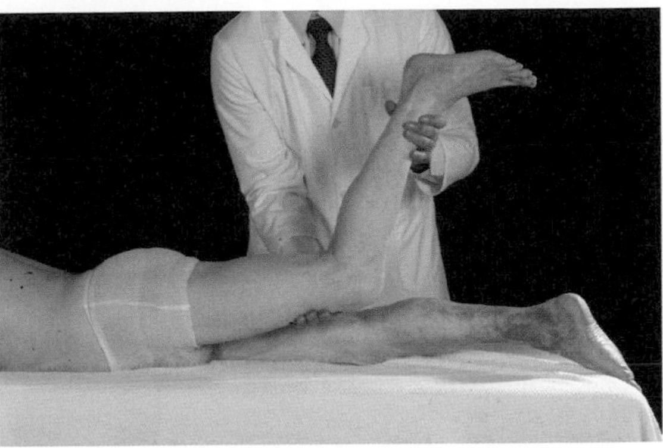

Figure 8.8 With the patient lying on their front, lift each thigh and assess hip extension.

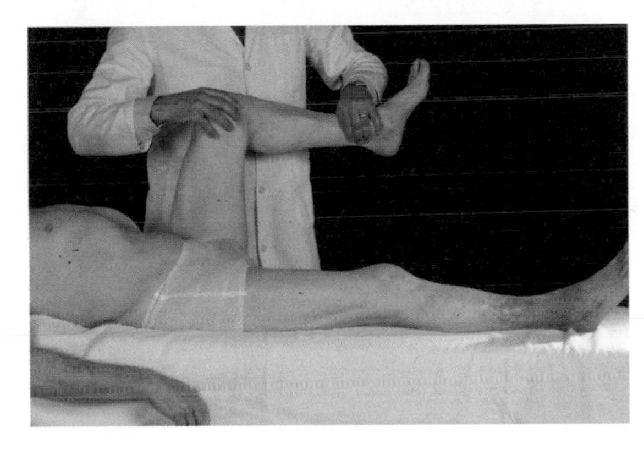

Figure 8.7 Rotation is measured by flexing the hip and the knee to 90° and rotating the femur by moving the foot back and forth across the line of the limb.

Abnormal movements The only abnormal movement you are likely to meet, except those caused by acute trauma, is *telescoping* of the joint, caused by a dislocated head of the femur sliding up and down the outer aspect of the ilium. This abnormal movement is detected by pushing and pulling the femur along its long axis while steadying the pelvis and feeling the top of the greater trochanter. It is sometimes easier to do this by flexing the hip to 90° and pulling the thigh upwards.

Extension Do this last, as you need to turn the patient onto their face. Put your hand under the knee and lift the thigh, again steadying the pelvis with your other hand (Figure 8.8). A normal hip extends up to 10°.

NOTE: Other joints can compensate for stiffness in the hip and this must be corrected before an accurate assessment can be made for hip movements.

With the patient standing

Look for deformities and abnormal skin creases from the front side and back if this has not already been done.

Trendelenburg test

With the patient standing, ask the patient to hold onto your forearms to provide support. Now ask the patient to stand on one leg, ensuring they do not flex the hip on the raised leg. The unsupported side of the pelvis should rise to help balance the trunk on the standing leg by bringing the centre of gravity over the weight-bearing foot (Figure 8.9). This involves the use of the hip abductors – gluteus medius and minimus. The *test is positive if the unsupported side of the pelvis falls* and the patient has difficulty standing and leans on one of your forearms. A positive test means one of the following:

- The abductor muscles are paralysed.
- The joint is unstable (e.g. a congenital dislocation of the hip or a fracture of the neck of the femur).
- The abductor tendons are damaged.

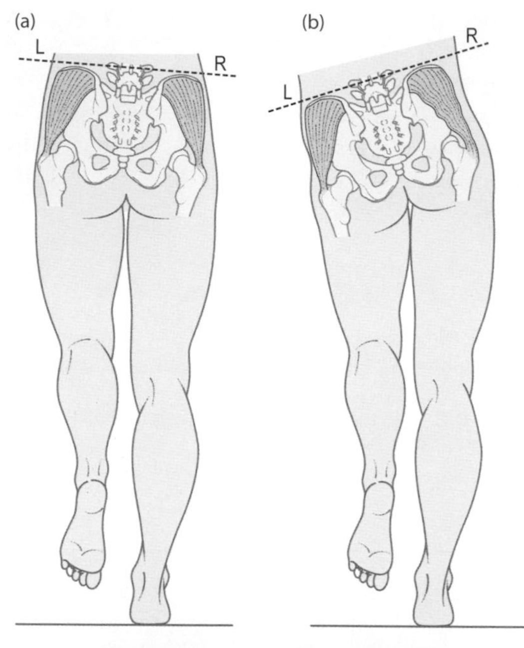

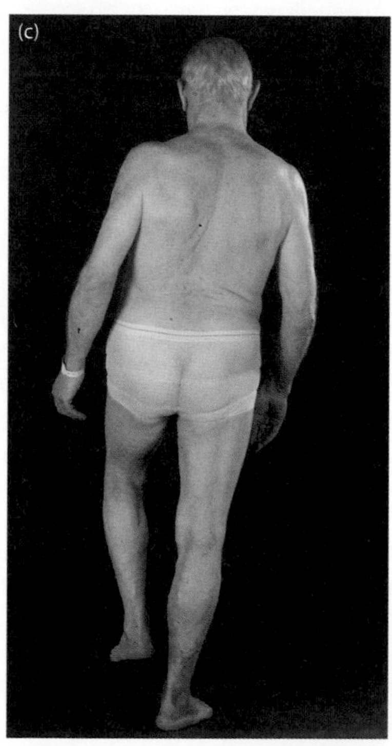

Figure 8.9 TRENDELENBURG'S TEST. (a) Ask the patient to stand on one leg. There should be a raising of the pelvis on the opposite side, a negative Trendelenburg test. (b) When the pelvis drops, the sign is positive. (c) The pelvis remains parallel to the floor as the leg is raised, hence this is a negative test for pathology.

- The insertion and origin of the abductor muscles are approximated, preventing their proper function, which is produced by femoral neck shortening or a dislocation of the hip.

Assessment of the gait

Ask the patient to walk. Observe their gait from the front, the rear and the side. Different patterns of gait can be recognized depending on the underlying pathology. An *antalgic (painful) gait* occurs when there is a shortened stance phase and a lurch of the trunk towards the painful side during the stance phase.

This is different from a *Trendelenburg gait*, which arises for the reasons outlined above, most commonly from abductor insufficiency. The weakened glutei allow the opposite side of the pelvis to tilt downwards during the stance phase on the weakened side. In an effort to compensate, the trunk lurches towards the weakened side (an abductor lurch) during the stance phase. In moving the centre of gravity towards the hip joint, there is a reduction in the effort that is required of the adductors.

Examination of the nerves and arteries of the limb

See Chapters 3 and 10.

Joint disease is often secondary to neurological abnormalities.

Conditions causing pain in the hip

TROCHANTERIC BURSITIS

There are two bursae that lie between the gluteus medius, gluteus minimus and tensor fascia lata muscles and their attachments to the greater tuberosity. These bursae can become inflamed, resulting in pain and disability.

History

Age and sex Trochanteric bursitis is usually seen in middle-aged patients, from 30 to 55 years. It is more common in females.

Cause Often no cause is elicited, although it may occur because of recurrent or unaccustomed activity, for example exercising at the gym or running. Symptoms can also arise and persist following an injury. Patients may have a previous history of other sites of bursal inflammation, such as the shoulder or knee.

Symptoms *Pain and weakness* are noted during hip movement. The pain may be activity related or occurs at rest and is usually centred over the lateral aspect of the hip joint. Patients are unable to lie on the affected side and have difficulty getting out of a chair and going up stairs.

Examination

There is usually no visible swelling because the trochanteric bursa lies deep to the iliotibial band. *Palpation is often painful,* and *tenderness is localized over the greater trochanter.*

Movements of the hip, particularly passive adduction, may reproduce the pain. A clicking sound may be present if the iliotibial band is also inflamed, as it moves over the greater tuberosity.

ADDUCTOR TENDINITIS

Inflammation of the principal adductor muscles – pectineus, adductor magnus, adductor longus and adductor brevis – can occur.

History

Age and sex The majority of patients will be aged 30–50 years. The condition can affect both males and females. It is common in athletes, especially horse riders.

Symptoms *Pain* is classically centred in the groin in the region of the adductor muscles and is exacerbated by exercise.

Examination

There are no visible manifestations of the inflammation, but palpation reveals *tenderness over the insertion of the adductor muscles and down the inside of the thigh.* Adduction of the hip causes localized pain in the groin and around the adductor tendon insertions on the medial aspect of the femoral shaft.

ILIOPSOAS TENDINITIS

The iliopsoas comprises two muscles that merge to form a single large tendon that inserts into the lesser trochanter. The iliacus arises from the ischium, and the psoas originates from the first to the fifth lumbar vertebrae.

History

Age and sex The condition arises in both males and females, most commonly from 20 to 50 years of age.

Symptoms *Pain is experienced in the groin* and can extend down the leg, sometimes to the knee. It increases with activity, and stiffness of the hip may develop. Some patients complain of clicking *in the groin.*

Examination

Tenderness is felt on palpation of the groin, and resisted flexion of the hip increases the pain. As the hip is flexed and then extended, the psoas tendon may, if it is inflamed and thickened, catch on the front of the pelvis, *giving a clicking sound.*

DEVELOPMENTAL DYSPLASIA OF THE HIP

Congenital dislocation of the hip is now known as developmental dysplasia of the hip. This describes the abnormal development of the acetabulum, encompassing a spectrum of disorders of acetabular dysplasia and femoral head subluxation and dislocation. In mild cases, the acetabulum is shallow, but may never cause pathology, in severe cases the acetabulum can be so shallow that the femoral head dislocates at birth.

History

Age and sex The condition occurs in 1.5 per 1000 live births, and usually presents from 0 to 4 years of age. It is more common in females than males (7 to 1). The left hip is more commonly affected. Other risk factors include being:

- A first born.
- Breech presentation.
- Caesarean section.
- Oligohydramnios.
- A positive family history.

Geography It is more common in the North and Eastern Mediterranean, because of a genetic predisposition. It is also more common in Lapp and North American Indian populations, who swaddle their babies with their legs together.

Examination

Every newborn child should be screened for hip instability. In *Ortolani's test,* the baby's thighs are held with the thumbs medially and the fingers resting on the greater trochanters; the hips are then flexed to 90°, which should normally be a smooth movement (Figure 8.10). In the presence of dysplasia or dislocation, the hips are abducted, and the joints are pushed forwards to demonstrate *dislocation click;* there is resistance that is overcome when pressure is applied to the greater trochanter. There is a *soft clunk* as the hip is reduced.

Barlow's test is performed in a similar manner, but in this instance the examiner's thumb is placed in the groin and the thigh is then held (Figure 8.11).

(a)

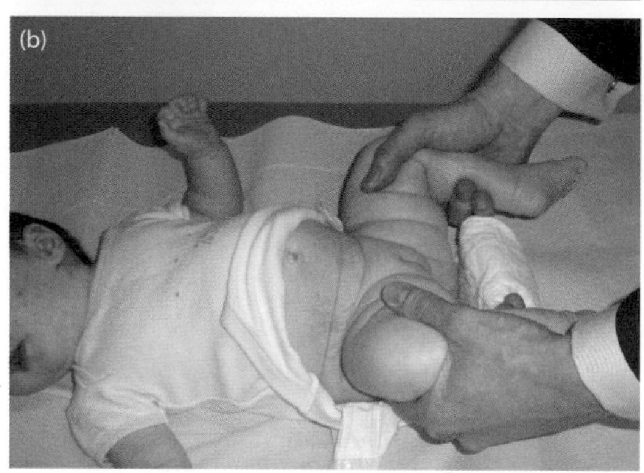

(c)

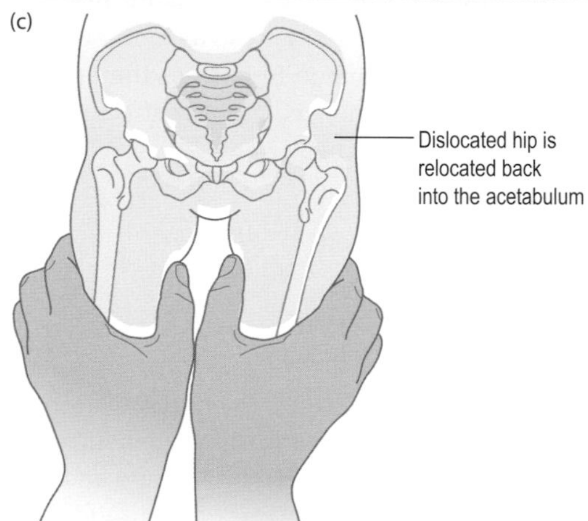

Figure 8.10 ORTOLANI TEST. (a) The hips are abducted and the joints are pushed forwards to demonstrate 'dislocation click'. (b) The dislocation is reduced. (c) The lower limbs are pushed together and apart by the examiner.

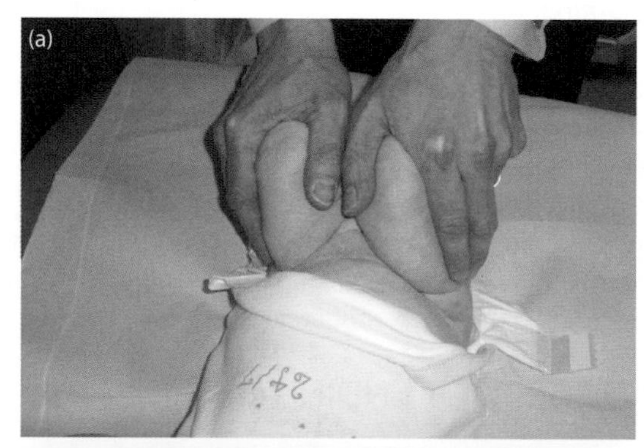

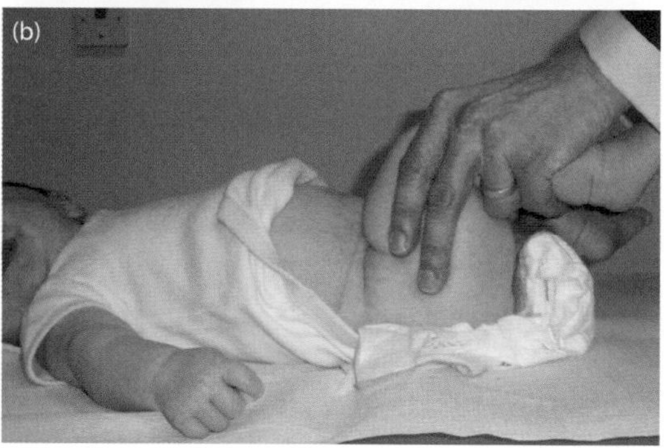

(c)

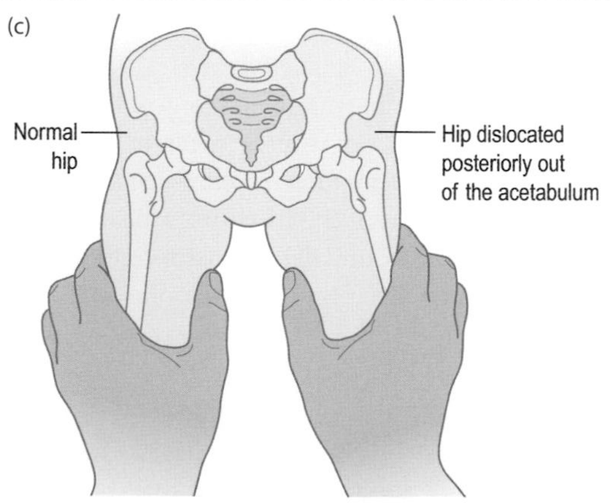

Figure 8.11 BARLOW'S TEST. (a) Forced adduction. (b) Forced abduction. (c) Forced abduction and adduction applied. Hip on left dislocates.

By applying pressure with adduction and abduction, the examiner tries to dislocate the femoral head from the acetabulum.

A child may present later in life if the diagnosis was missed when he or she was newborn. Symptoms include clicking and gait disturbance because of a shortened leg and limitation of abduction. Affected individuals may have asymmetrical buttock skin creases.

LEGG–CALVE–PERTHES' DISEASE

This is an *osteochondritis of the proximal femoral epiphysis caused by a vascular disturbance* (see Chapter 6). The femoral head undergoes a form of avascular necrosis with remodelling.

History

Age and sex This occurs in 1 in 10,000 children and usually presents from 4 to 9 years of age. It is more common in males than females (4 to 1) and it is bilateral in 15% of cases. There may be a family history.

Geography The condition is more common in Japanese and central European individuals. It is less common in native Australians, native Americans, Polynesians and black races.

Symptoms The child complains of *pain in the hip*, which is worse on activity. Although the pain is centred in the groin, it can radiate to the knee and cause a *limp*.

Examination

There is often little to find on examination, especially in the early stages, but the *hip may be irritable with all movements*. When the child is seen late in the progression of the condition, abduction is limited, and this is often associated with a *restriction of internal rotation*. The older the child at the time of onset, the worse the prognosis.

SLIPPED UPPER FEMORAL EPIPHYSIS

This occurs because of a *slip in the hypertrophic zone of the cartilaginous growth plate of the upper femoral epiphysis*. The head of the femur remains in the acetabulum, but the femoral shaft displaces anteriorly and rotates externally.

History

Age and sex This occurs in 1 in 10,000 children, and the condition usually develops between 10 and 14 years of age. Males are more affected than females, and generally present 2–3 years later than females. The left hip is more commonly affected, and 35% of cases are bilateral.

Symptoms The child presents with *pain in the groin radiating to the knee*, that is made worse by exercise, and begins to limp. There are often a series of minor episodes of pain rather than a single event, although 'acute-on-chronic' and isolated acute slips can occur. Half the cases are associated with some form of trauma.

Examination

The child may become aware that the leg is turning outwards, and examination reveals that the *leg is externally rotated and shortened by 1–2 cm*. As the hip is flexed, it rotates into further external rotation.

The hip is painful on movement if there has been a recent acute slip.

> **NOTE:** Many of the children are overweight or skeletally immature, and they may have an underlying hormonal imbalance, such as hypogonadism (Fröhlich child) or hypothyroidism.

COXA VARA

This condition may be congenital (noted at birth), developmental or acquired. It is usually the result of a *defect in an ossification centre in the femoral neck*, which leads to a decreased angle between the femoral head and neck. It is bilateral in 33% of cases and occurs in 1 in 25,000 births.

Acquired causes include *trauma, slipped upper femoral epiphysis and Perthes' disease* (see above).

History

Symptoms The child usually presents aged 2–6 years with an *altered gait*, but otherwise they are relatively free of symptoms.

Examination

The gait may be waddling when the condition is bilateral, or a painless limp when the condition is unilateral.

The *affected leg is shortened*.

Movements of the hip are restricted in all directions, especially abduction and internal rotation.

IRRITABLE HIP (TRANSIENT SYNOVITIS)

This is a condition in which there is a *short-lived, non-specific synovitis* in the hip joint. The cause is often unknown, but it may follow a recent viral infection. A synovial effusion develops in the hip joint, and the condition usually resolves within 7 days.

History

Age and sex It occurs in 14 per 1000 children and is more common in males than females (2 to 1). It usually occurs in 3–8-year-olds, and in 5% of cases can affect both hips.

Symptoms The child presents with *acute pain in the hip, difficulty weight-bearing* and *a limp*. The pain may radiate to the knee and is worse on activity.

Examination

All movements are painful and may be restricted.

SEPTIC ARTHRITIS OF THE HIP

Infection in the hip joint is relatively uncommon in adults, unless it is associated with a previous hip replacement.

History

It is more common in children, usually under the age of 2 years. Up to 50% of neonates with the condition have adjacent infection in the bone metaphysis. The usual infecting organism is *Staphylococcus* spp.

Symptoms The child usually complains of localized pain in the groin and the medial aspect of the thigh. The pain is normally progressive and severe.

Examination

The child lies still with the *hip flexed, abducted and externally rotated*. All movements, especially internal rotation, are painful and resisted. The child does not want to weight bear.

Palpation of the hip and groin is tender.

> **NOTE:** Pyrexia, loss of appetite and sweating are usually present, and indicate the presence of systemic infection.

OSTEOARTHRITIS OF THE HIP

The hip is one of the most common joints to be affected by osteoarthritis, which can be either primary or secondary (see Chapter 6).

History

Age and sex *Primary osteoarthritis* usually presents in patients over 50 years of age. The exact aetiology is unknown. It occurs in both males and females.

Secondary osteoarthritis can be predisposed to by

- Developmental dysplasia of the hip.
- Perthes' disease.
- Slipped upper femoral epiphysis.
- Avascular necrosis.
- Previous fracture.
- Previous infection.
- Femoroacetabular impingement.
- Abnormal biomechanics.

It often presents in a younger age group, with both males and females equally affected.

Symptoms Patients complain of *groin pain*, which is often accompanied by *pain in the knee*. Severe pain may cause *sleep disturbance*. Patients are usually *stiff in the morning* and often have *difficulty getting out of a chair*. They have *a reduced walking distance* and must *stop walking frequently*. They complain of having *a limp* and may be helped by using a stick for support.

> **NOTE:** Dressing and washing becomes difficult, and they struggle to put their shoes and socks on and wash their feet.

Examination

Deep palpation of the hip may elicit tenderness.

Hip movement produces variable pain. There may be a limited painless range of movement, followed by pain at the end of range.

There is often *reduced flexion* of the affected hip, and a *positive Thomas'* test. *Abduction* and *adduction are also often restricted, with a loss of internal and external rotation*.

The leg often lies in *external rotation and adduction*, and hence it may appear short. While there may be a true leg length discrepancy, you must measure both the true and apparent leg lengths to establish this. If the shortening is real, you must determine whether it is occurring above or below the hip joint (see Figure 8.1). In severe cases, cysts in the femoral head may collapse, causing shortening.

When asked to walk, the patient will often have an *antalgic gait* and may have a *positive Trendelenburg test*.

RHEUMATOID ARTHRITIS OF THE HIP

As elsewhere in the body, rheumatoid arthritis attacks the synovium causing tissue destruction, articular cartilage erosion and progressive changes in the bones on either side of the hip joint, without osteophyte formation (see Chapter 6).

The signs and symptoms are similar to those of osteoarthritis, but the patient may also have other joints affected by the condition, especially in the hands (see Chapter 7).

FEMOROACETABULAR IMPINGEMENT

This is a relatively newly recognized condition, which is caused by a *pinching mechanism* in the hip joint. This may be the result of a pincer movement where the femoral head is over-covered by an acetabular rim prominence. During rotation, the femoral neck abuts against this prominence and the acetabular labrum, causing pain. The condition may also occur from a *cam* (projection) mechanism that is the result of a bump at the junction between the femoral head and neck, which causes impingement of the femoral neck against the acetabulum.

History

Age and sex The pincer type is more common in females and presents at age 30–40 years. The cam type is more common in athletic males between 20 and 30 years of age.

Symptoms *Intermittent groin pain* and *limited movement* are the usual presenting symptoms. The patient classically demonstrates a C-shaped distribution of pain around their hip (*the C sign*). The pain may be exacerbated by periods of prolonged sitting or be related to activity. It then can extend into the thigh, buttock and lower back. Patients may complain of a sudden catching and the hip giving way.

Examination

There is usually a *painful restriction of internal rotation in flexion and adduction*, known as a *positive hip impingement sign*.

SNAPPING HIP

This is a snapping sensation experienced in the hip. It usually occurs in males aged 15–40 years and is more common in athletes of both genders.

It can be caused by *extrinsic causes* outside the hip, such as the iliotibial band of the tensor fascia lata sliding back and forth across the greater trochanter. It can also occur if the iliopsoas tendon catches on the front of the acetabulum.

Intrinsic (intra-articular) causes include loose bodies, acetabular labral defects and articular damage.

History

Symptoms Patients complain of a *pop or snap* when they move their hip, which may be associated with pain if the surrounding tissues become inflamed. The pain is usually relieved by rest and aggravated by activity.

Examination

When the hip is flexed and extended, the affected structures can be felt to snap across the bony prominence.

AVASCULAR NECROSIS OF THE FEMORAL HEAD

This is also sometimes called 'osteonecrosis' or 'aseptic necrosis' and is *caused by an occlusion of the microcirculation of the femoral head*. This causes the bone and overlying articular cartilage to die, with subsequent collapse of the avascular portion, eventually leading to osteoarthritis (see above).

History

Age and sex Males aged around 40 years are most commonly affected, and in one-half the condition is bilateral.

Symptoms Deep pain in the groin is the usual presenting symptom, and patients may develop a limp.

Revision panel 8.2

CAUSES OF OSTEONECROSIS

Trauma

- fractures of femoral neck
- acetabular fractures
- hip dislocations

Systemic disorders

- sickle-cell disease
- decompression sickness
- fat emboli

Other factors

- steroid treatment
- excessive alcohol intake4
- radiation treatment
- pregnancy
- Perthes' disease
- systemic lupus erythematosus
- Gaucher's disease (see Chapter 6)

Examination

All movements of the joint are painful, but they only become limited at a late stage in the disease.

THE KNEE JOINT

The joint is a synovial hinge joint between the femur and the tibia and is the largest joint in the body. It has two articulations, one between the femur and the tibia, and the other between the femur and the patella. This allows flexion and extension of the lower leg with some rotation, and facilitates the transmission of loads when running, walking and jumping. Stability of the joint is provided by tendons, ligaments and muscles rather than bones.

Symptoms

Adults with knee problems may present with *pain, swelling, instability, locking or deformity.* The patient may point to a specific area of the knee or experience more diffuse symptoms.

> **NOTE:** Remember that pain felt about the knee can be referred pain arising from hip and spinal pathology.

Knee pain can occur at rest or during movement and exercise. It can become debilitating and cause sleep disturbance.

In the degenerate knee, *stiffness in the morning* is a common complaint, coupled with restriction in movement during the day. The patient may walk with a *limp.*

If the patient has injured the knee, they may state that the knee feels unstable and that it *gives way.* This is usually caused by disruption of the stabilizing ligaments. This is particularly common when ascending or descending stairs, or suddenly changing direction of travel.

The knee may also become *locked* in a position or significantly restricted in its range of movement; for example, the patient may state that they are unable to fully extend the knee. This may be a symptom of meniscal pathology.

Plan for examination of the knee joint

INSPECTION

Gait

Ask the patient to stand up and walk about. Observe the gait carefully. Look for a limp, use of a walking stick or shoe raise.

Alignment of the knees

The normal alignment of the knee is 5–7° of valgus and is best observed when standing. *Genu varus (bowlegs)* is diagnosed by measuring the distance between the knees with the malleoli placed together. This is usually less than 6 cm. In children, this can be a normal finding and corrects itself as the child grows. It may, however, also be associated with bone dysplasia or rickets. In adults the distance between the knees increases if the deformity is progressive such as in degenerative disease.

Genu valgum (knock knees) can be estimated by placing the knees together and measuring the distance between the malleoli. Again, this can be a normal developmental finding in children.

If abnormal alignment of the knees develops in adulthood, this is usually secondary to trauma or underlying degenerative change. Varus deformity is commonly associated with osteoarthritis, while valgus deformity is more commonly seen in rheumatoid arthritis.

Skin

Look at the skin all around the joint – front and back – for *discolouration, scars, swellings* and sinuses (see Figure 6.1). Erythema may be associated with inflammation and infection, whereas bruising may indicate trauma. Note any skin conditions that are often associated with joint problems, such as psoriasis.

Shape

The contours of the knee joint are easy to see, and any bony or joint swelling distorts them at an early stage.

> **NOTE:** The size of the whole joint should be compared with that on the other side. A swelling in the knee joint is usually first seen in the hollows either side of the patella.

Assess any swelling to determine whether it is confined to the limits of the synovial cavity or extends beyond the joint boundaries, which would suggest infection, tumour or injury.

Note any localized swellings that may indicate bursitis, a meniscal cyst or 'tumours' such as exostoses. *Look for any evidence of muscle wasting, particularly of the quadriceps muscle* (see Figure 6.4).

Position

A knee joint that is swollen and painful is most comfortable when *slightly flexed*. Stand the patient up and look for any degree of genu valgus or varus (Figure 8.12; see also Figure 6.11).

PALPATION

Skin

Note any increase in temperature that may indicate active arthritis or infection.

Synovium

The synovium of the knee joint can be felt on either side of the patella and in the suprapatellar pouch. In some diseases, it becomes thickened and

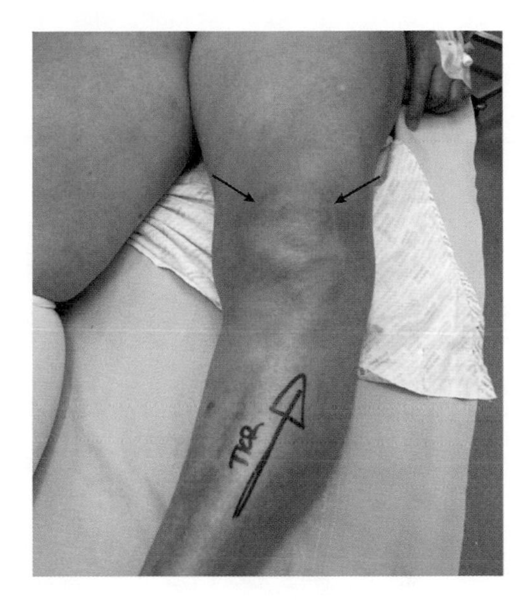

Figure 8.12 Knee effusion seen as a fullness on either side of the patella.

rubbery, or 'boggy'. A thickened synovium is usually hyperaemic and makes the overlying skin warm.

Bony Contour

Check the position of the patella. It should be in the patellar groove of the femur, but it may be displaced laterally or superiorly if there is lengthening or rupture of the patellar ligament. The size, shape and position of the patella should be noted. The bone should also be felt on its anterior surface, at its edges and at the sites of attachment of the quadriceps and patellar tendons.

Check the position of the knee joint..

> **NOTE:** When students are asked to put their index finger on the line of the knee joint, they invariably point to a spot 2.5–5 cm above the joint.

Remember that the main bulge of the knee is formed by the lower end of the femur. The easiest way to find the joint line is to flex the knee until you can feel the anterior curved edge of the femoral condyles and can slide your finger downwards over this edge until you reach the tibial plateau.

It is important to relate areas of tenderness to the joint line (Figure 8.13a) and the points of attachment of the collateral ligaments.

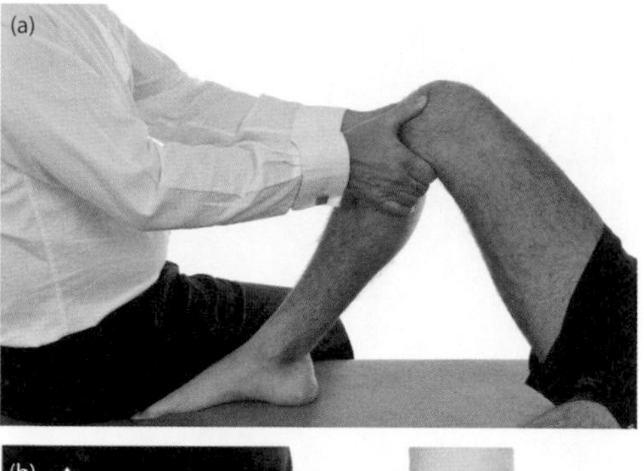

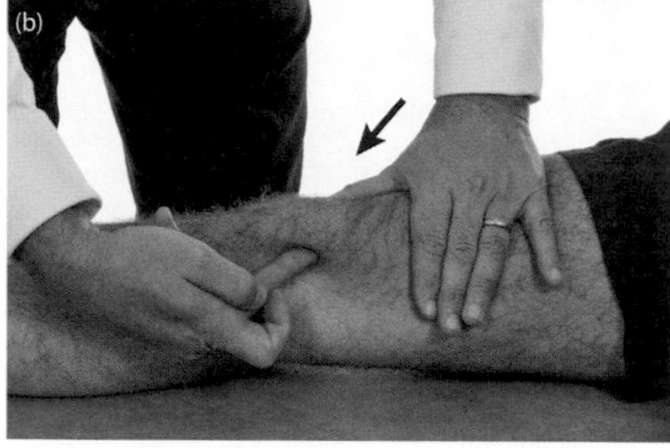

Figure 8.13 PALPATION FOR TENDERNESS ABOUT THE KNEE. (a) Joint line tenderness. (b) Patellar tenderness.

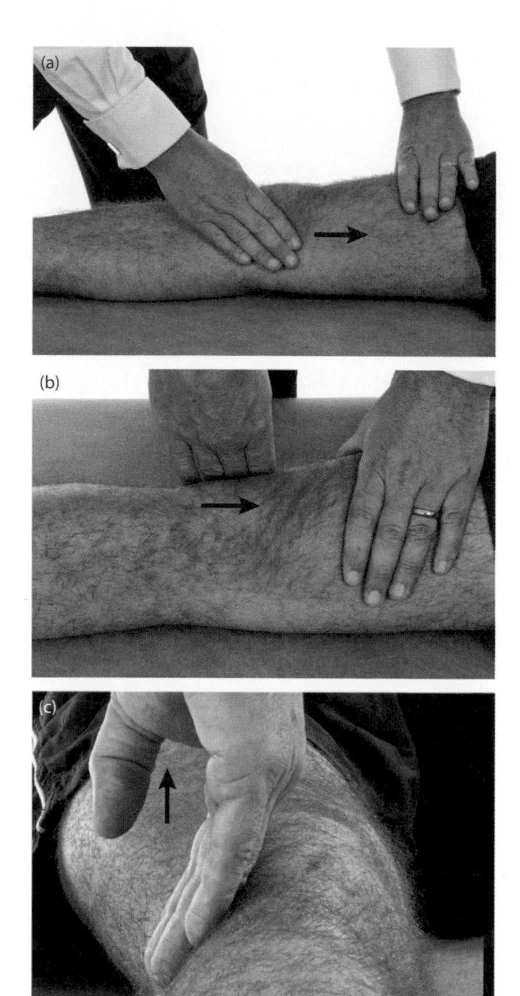

Figure 8.14 TESTING FOR A KNEE EFFUSION. Milking of fluid on the medial side of the knee. The *fluid displacement test*: compress one side of the knee and note the joint distending on the opposite side. Empty the supra-patella pouch and then sweep or milk the fluid from the lateral side of the knee and note the joint distending on the opposite side.

Effusions

Effusions of the knee joint are common and easy to detect because the excess synovial fluid collects in the front of the joint where it can be seen and felt. There are three tests for detecting an effusion in the knee joint:

- **Visible fluctuation.** A small quantity of fluid does not make the whole joint look swollen, but if you sweep gently down one side of the joint, the other side may bulge outwards (Figure 8.14a). Position the leg in a good oblique light so the hollows on either side of the patella are visible. Stroke the joint just to one side of the patella and watch the hollow on the other side of the patella to see if it gradually fills out as the effusion is pushed into it. This is the most sensitive way of detecting a small effusion (Figure 8.14c). It cannot be used if the joint is full and tense.
- **Palpable fluctuation.** When the knee joint is full of fluid, it is possible to press on one side and feel the increase in pressure transmitted over to the other side. Place the palm of the left hand above the patella, and the thumb and index finger either side of it (Figure 8.14b). Press posteriorly and distally to squeeze any fluid in the suprapatellar pouch down into the joint behind and either side of the patella. Place the thumb and index finger of the right hand either side of the patella and see if you can feel expansion or fluid displacement between your thumb and finger.
- **Patellar tap.** When the joint is full of fluid, the patella is lifted off the femur. If it is

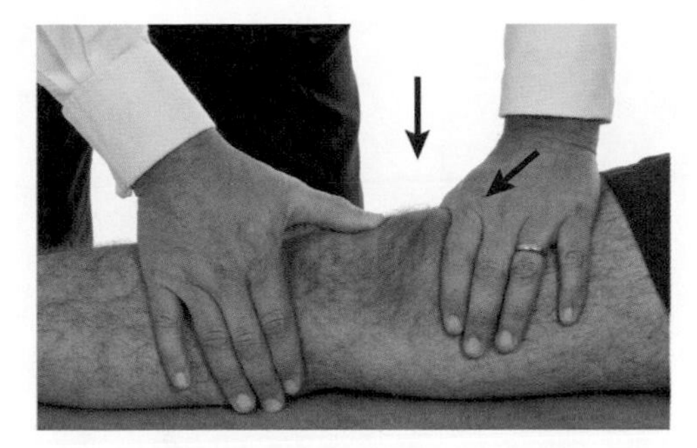

Figure 8.15 The patellar tap test: squeeze any fluid out of the suprapatellar pouch using the right hand and then press down on the patella. A tap or click will indicate an effusion.

pressed or tapped, it can be felt to move backwards and hit the femur (Figure 8.15). This test is also helped by emptying the suprapatellar pouch into the space behind the patella with the left hand.

Surrounding tissues

Pay particular attention to the bulk and strength of the quadriceps muscle and remember that the quadriceps of the patient's dominant leg will always be slightly bulkier. Any substantial wasting can be measured by comparing the circumference of the thighs at the same distance above the joint line (Figure 8.16).

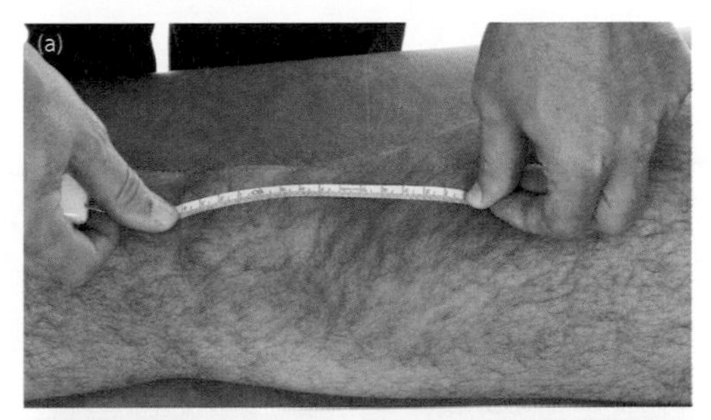

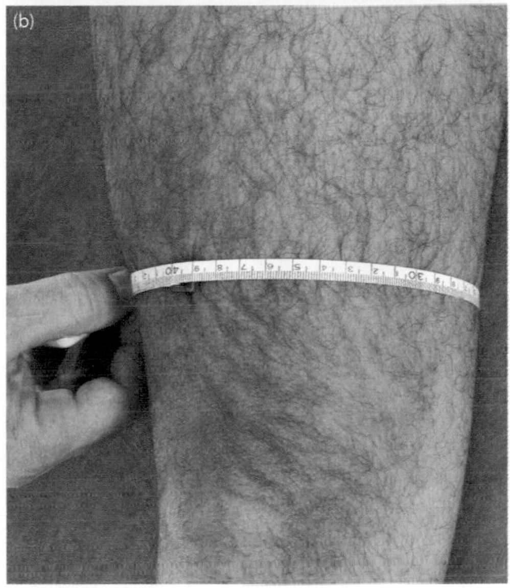

Figure 8.16 QUADRICEPS MEASUREMENT. (a, b) Measurement of quadriceps muscle bulk for wasting from a fixed measurable distance from the tibial tubercle.

MOVEMENT

Ask the patient to move the joint unaided before checking passive movement. Record the extent of the active knee movements in degrees. Remember that when the leg is straight, the angle between the femur and tibia is 0°. The angle is usually 135–150° in full flexion, and between 0° and –10° in full extension.

Flexion

Bend the knee as much as possible (Figure 8.17). When there is disease of the hip joint, you may have to turn the patient on to their side to see the full extent of knee flexion. Record the degrees of flexion from the zero position of normal extension.

Extension

Lift the leg off the bed by the heel and ask the patient to relax (Figure 8.18). Record any limitation of extension as well as any excess of extension. In females, the knee joint often hyperextends several degrees past the 0° mark.

Rotation

There are small degrees of rotation of the tibia on the femur, but these are not easy to detect unless the knee is slightly flexed.

Crepitus

This can be felt during movement and usually signifies patellofemoral pathology.

Abnormal movements

Abnormal movement can occur if the ligaments are ruptured or stretched, because the knee joint is a hinge joint that depends entirely on muscles and ligaments for its stability. Thus, by testing for abnormal

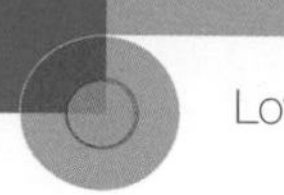

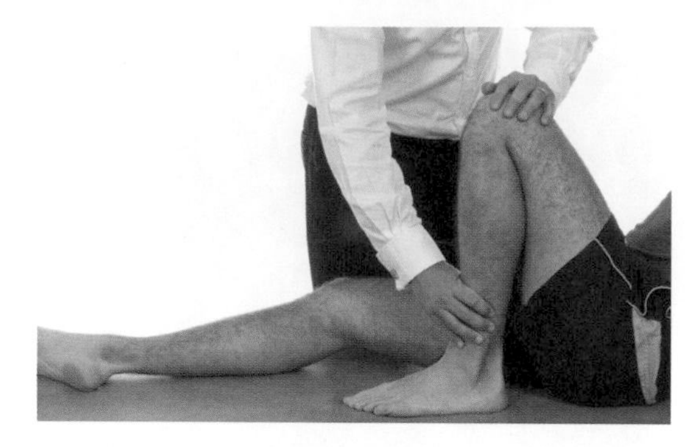

Figure 8.17 Testing knee flexion.

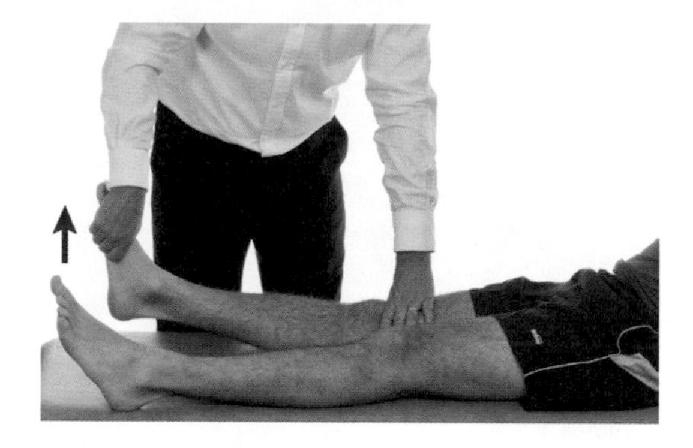

Figure 8.18 Testing knee extension.

movements such as abduction and adduction, and anteroposterior glide or sliding of the tibia on the femur, you are really checking the stability of the knee and the integrity of its ligaments.

Medial and lateral collateral ligaments Let the leg rest extended on the couch. Standing on the patient's left side, cradle the back of thigh in the palm of your right hand, and the gently grasp the calf of the leg. Keep this hand firm and use it as a fulcrum to try to abduct the knee joint by pulling the leg towards you with your left hand (Figure 8.19). There should be only the slightest movement in the joint. If it moves easily, the medial collateral ligament is lax. If you stay on the same side of the patient, the same action on the other leg will abduct the joint and test the lateral collateral ligament.

To test the ligaments on the opposite side of the joint, keep your hand in the same position and gently abduct the lower leg. This will test the lateral collateral ligament.

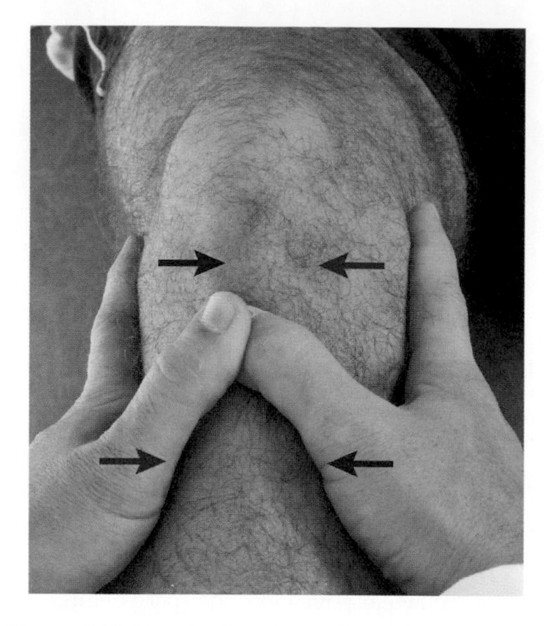

Figure 8.19 Examination of the collateral ligaments. The blue arrows show forces applied to assess the medial collateral ligament, whilst the red arrows show forces applied to assess the lateral collateral ligament.

These movements should be done in full extension and at 30° flexion, to examine for natural laxity with the two knees compared.

An alternative method is to tuck the patient's leg under your arm and then, with your hands on each side of the knee joint to detect movement, move the tibia from side to side with your body (Figure 8.20).

Anterior and posterior cruciate ligaments Remember that the anterior cruciate ligament stops the tibia rotating and sliding anteriorly. The posterior ligament stops the tibia sliding posteriorly.

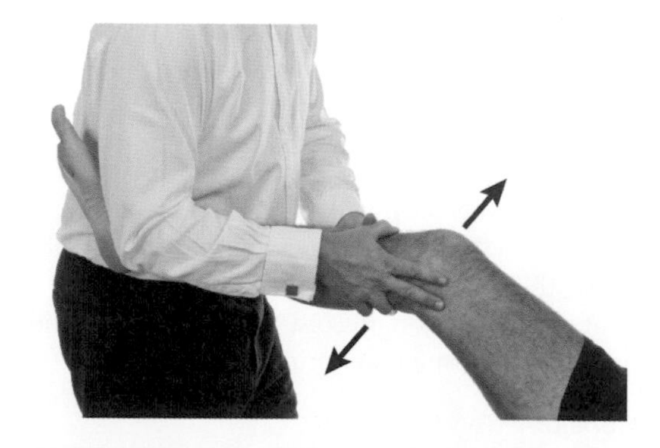

Figure 8.20 Varus (red arrow) and valgus stress (blue arrow) of the knee with the leg supported.

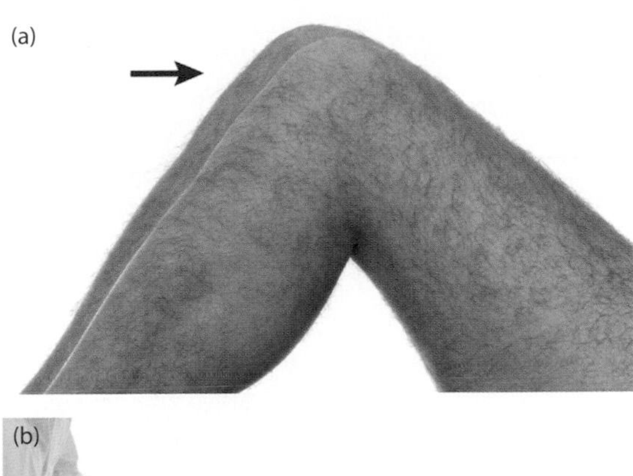

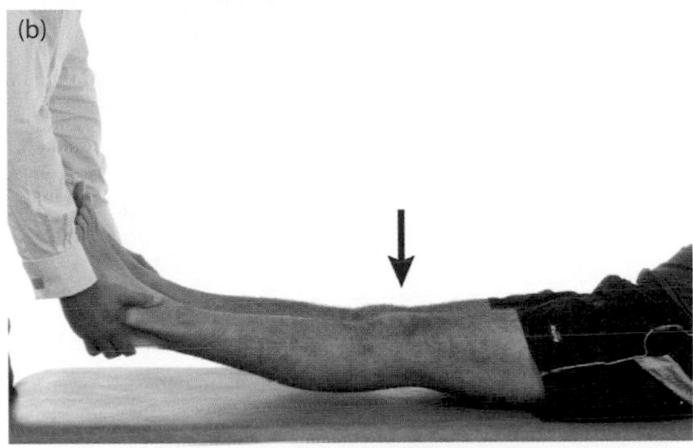

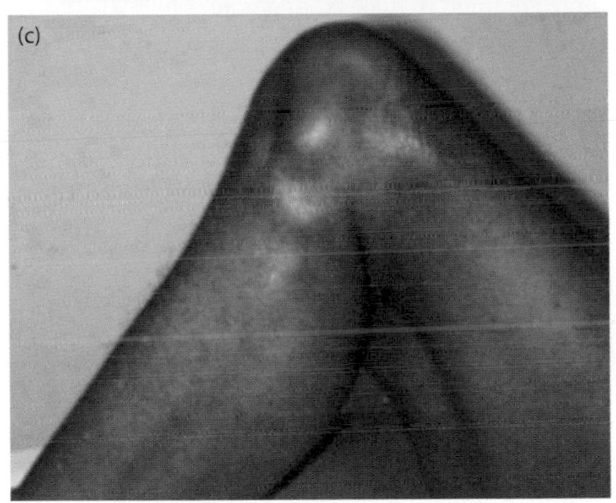

Figure 8.21 POSTERIOR SAG. (a–c) Posterior sag of the knee occurs when the upper end of the tibia falls backwards from the normal contour.

Assess the resting position with both patient's knees flexed to 90° and their heels placed together on the couch. Observe the upper tibia from the side. If the upper end has dropped back, it can indicate a tear of the posterior cruciate (*the sag sign*) (Figure 8.21).

Then gently grasp the upper end of the tibia with both hands and pull it towards you. This is the *anterior draw test*, and any significant movement suggests a torn anterior cruciate, possibly associated with damage to the lateral ligaments as well (Figure 8.22).

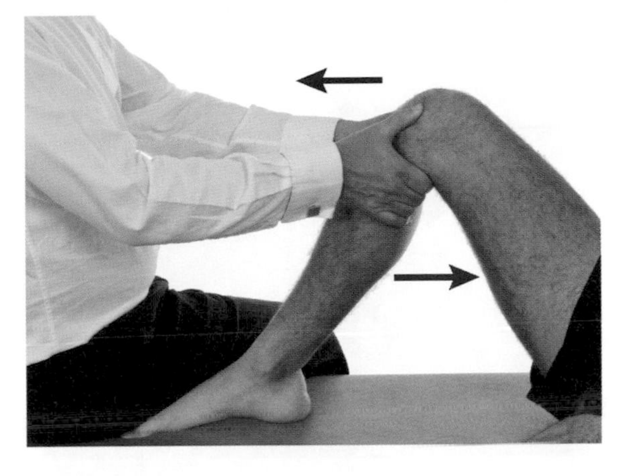

Figure 8.22 Anterior draw test (blue arrow) for the anterior cruciate ligament and posterior draw test (red arrow) for the posterior cruciate ligament.

Now repeat the test, but this time pushing the tibia backwards – the *posterior draw test*. Any significant displacement indicates rupture of the posterior cruciate. Always compare the degree of movement between the two sides.

The *Lachman test* is difficult to perform if the patient has large thighs, but an easier modified test is used to assess the cruciate ligaments. The knee is flexed to 20° by draping the knee over your thigh on the couch. Stabilize the patient's thigh with one hand and by placing the other hand behind the calf, gently pull the tibia forwards (Figure 8.23). The knee is unstable if the joint surfaces excessively glide over each other. The aim is to observe a difference between the two knees

The knee may have rotational instability if there are combined injuries of the collateral and cruciate ligaments. This can be assessed by the *pivot shift test*. Lift the leg in full extension and internally rotate the tibia. Then apply a valgus force to the joint as the

NOTE: It is not necessary to sit on the patient's foot and crush their toes to death to perform some of these procedures, but it does help if the foot is fixed by the pressure of your buttock as you sit beside the leg, facing the patient's head, so that both of your arms are in front of you and in line with the leg.

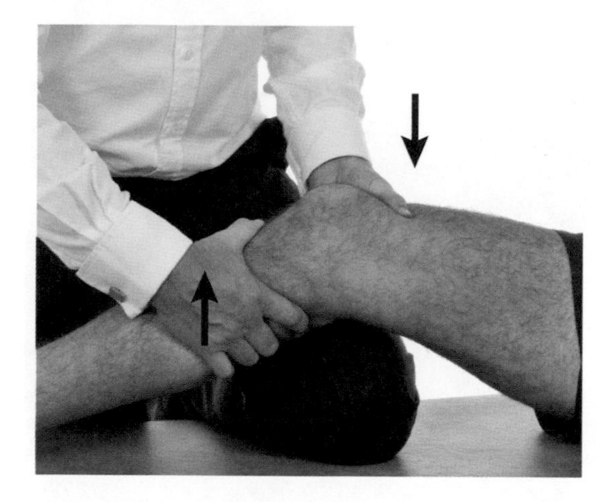

Figure 8.23 The Lachman test for cruciate insufficiency.

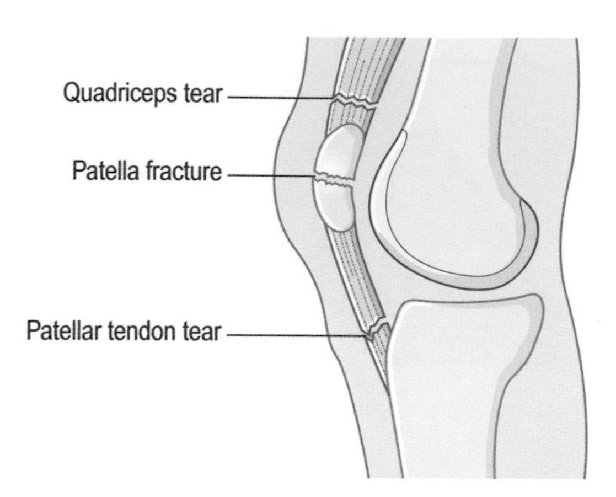

Figure 8.24 The quadriceps mechanism will fail with a quadriceps tear, patella fracture or patellar tendon tear.

knee is flexed. If there is instability, the lateral tibia will suddenly slide or jump posteriorly as the joint relocates.

Clicks

> **NOTE:** There are some special tests that make the joint click if there is a torn cartilage. Do not try these tests. They are difficult to perform and to interpret.

Normal joints sometimes click. If the patient is complaining of clicking, find out exactly when it occurs, and whether it is painful. Then ask the patient to reproduce it for you, but do not indulge in excessive manipulation just to hear it.

Conditions causing knee pain

TENDON RUPTURES

The quadriceps and patellar tendons form part of the knee extensor mechanism on either side of the patella. Tears can occur when there is resisted extension of the knee. This usually occurs during sporting activity or falls.

History

Age and sex The age of the patient has significant bearing on the level of injury. In the elderly, the injury is usually above the patella, either in the rectus femoris muscle or as an avulsion of the quadriceps tendon from the upper pole of the patella (Figure 8.24). It is more common in males than females (8 to 1).

In middle age, fractures of the patella are more common (see below).

In the young, the patellar tendon is ruptured or avulsed from the inferior pole of the patella.

Symptoms The patient is likely to present with *severe pain, swelling* and an *inability to walk*.

Examination

There will often be a haemarthrosis of the knee joint. There is usually a palpable gap in either the quadriceps or the patellar tendon. The patella will migrate proximally (a *high-riding patella*) if the patellar tendon is torn. The patient is usually unable to perform a straight leg raise.

RECURRENT DISLOCATION OF THE PATELLA

The patella can dislocate acutely as the result of trauma (see below), resulting in chronic instability in 15–20% of cases. In rare cases, the patella can dislocate spontaneously, when the quadriceps contracts with the knee in flexion (Revision panel 8.3).

History

Age and sex *Atraumatic rupture* occurs commonly between 10 to 30 years of age and is more common in females. The condition may be bilateral.

Symptoms There is *acute pain* and the *knee becomes stuck in flexion*. The patient is unable to weight bear.

Revision panel 8.3

PREDISPOSING FACTORS

- generalized ligamentous laxity
- underdevelopment of the lateral femoral condyle
- maldevelopment of the patella
- valgus deformity of the knee
- external tibial torsion
- sickle-cell disease

Examination

The patella is dislocated laterally, exposing the medial femoral condyle and causing a *flattening of the front of the knee* (Figure 8.25). A haemarthrosis develops. Once the patella has been reduced, the patient may have a positive *patellar apprehension sign*. Place pressure on the medial aspect of the patella while flexing the knee. This causes the patient to worry that it is going to dislocate.

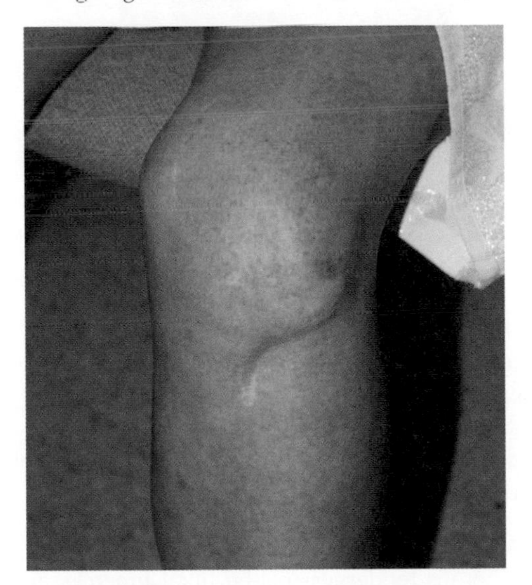

Figure 8.25 Flattening of the front of the knee in patellar dislocation.

PATELLOFEMORAL PAIN SYNDROME

This was previous known as *chondromalacia patella* and thought to be the result of softening of the cartilage on the articular surface of the patella.

History

Age and sex This is very common in adolescents and in athletic young adults. It is especially common in teenage females. It can be bilateral.

Symptoms There is diffuse *anterior knee pain*, which is worse on walking up stairs and after sitting with the knee flexed for prolonged periods. The patient often complains that the pain is centered 'underneath the kneecap'. There is no swelling and rarely instability.

Examination

Look for evidence of disuse and *quadriceps wasting* (see Figure 6.4). The is often diffuse tenderness and the *patella may appear laterally placed, tilted or high riding*.

Crepitus of the patella femoral joint may be felt on flexing and extending the knee, and also by compressing the patella into the femoral trochlea.

PATELLAR TENDINITIS (JUMPER'S KNEE)

This is part of the family of tendinopathies that can occur around the body.

History

Symptoms *Anterior knee pain* occurs principally over the patellar tendon and the inferior pole of the patella, particularly during running and jumping.

Examination

There is localized tenderness on palpation of the patellar tendon, and pain on extending the lower leg against resistance. The tendon may appear thickened.

PLICA SYNDROME

This is caused by an embryonic remnant of a synovial partition that persists into adult life. It is usually found as a *medial infrapatellar fold*. It only becomes pathologically significant if there is an acute injury or repetitive activity that causes it to become inflamed, when it acts like a bowstring, causing further inflammation in the joint.

History

Age and sex It can occur in both males and females, usually in adolescence or young adulthood.

Symptoms It presents as *anteriomedial knee pain,* worse after activity or prolonged periods of inactivity. The pain may be an ache, or more acute when the knee is stressed. The patient may complain of *clicking.*

Examination

There may be *muscle wasting* (see Figure 6.4) caused by disuse.

Palpation reveals *localized tenderness near the upper medial pole of the patella* and over the femoral condyle. A thickened band of tissue can occasionally be felt, which snaps during movement of the knee.

OSTEOCHONDRITIS DISSECANS

A segment of bone undergoes avascular necrosis (see Chapter 6) and separates from one of the femoral condyles, often appearing as a loose body in the joint. The aetiology is poorly understood but it often occurs in athletic individuals. It is most frequently observed on the lateral part of the medial femoral condyle. Less commonly, the lateral femoral condyle or patella is involved.

History

Age and sex This is more common in males and presents between 10 and 25 years of age. Its incidence has increased in recent years, probably because of greater participation in sports. It can be bilateral in 25% of cases.

Symptoms There is an *aching pain on the anterior aspect of the knee.*

The knee may *lock* or *give way.*

Examination

It is usually possible to observe *wasting of the quadriceps* and a *small effusion* in the joint. It may be possible to elicit tenderness of the femoral condyle.

OSGOOD–SCHLATTER DISEASE

This is a *traction apophysitis (inflammation) of the tibial tubercle,* where the patellar tendon inserts into the tibia.

(a)

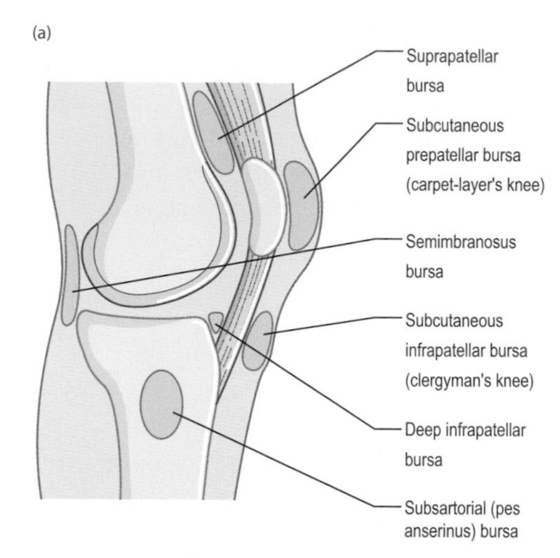

(b)

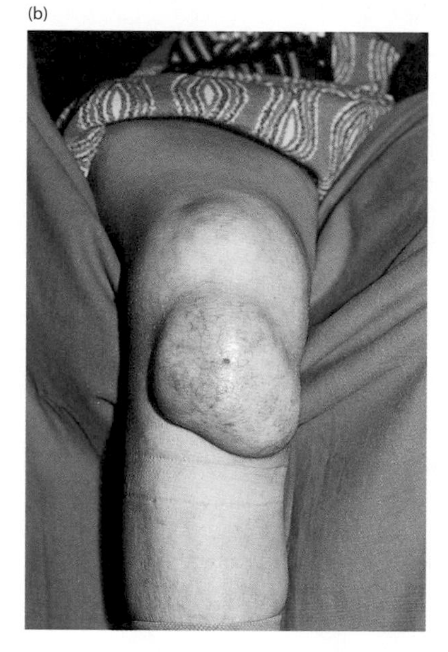

Figure 8.26 KNEE BURSITIS OR 'CARPET-LAYER'S KNEE'.

History

Age and sex This is a common disorder of teenagers, most often seen in males.

Symptoms *Pain* mainly occurs during activity such as running, football and cycling but can develop into discomfort at rest.

Examination

There is tenderness of the tibial tubercle, and a lump is felt on palpation. Active knee extension against resistance can be painful.

BURSITIS AROUND THE KNEE

Fluid can collect in and distend the prepatellar (carpetlayer's knee [Figures 8.26a, b]), infrapatellar (clergyman's knee) and semimembranosus bursae (Figure 8.26, see Figure 4.65).

The *prepatellar bursa* (Figure 8.26a) is a normal structure that allows the skin to slide over the patella as the knee is flexed. It can become inflamed when there is prolonged kneeling on the knee. It is associated with occupations such as carpet fitting, tiling and roofing.

The *infrapatellar bursa* (Figure 8.26b) lies in front of the tibial tubercle and can become inflamed when load is taken through this region rather than the patella.

The *semimembranosus bursa* lies at the back of the knee, medial to the joint line, and can become swollen in children and adults.

History

Symptoms The knee may be painful on movement, although the range of movement is preserved.

Examination

Prepatellar and infrapatellar bursitis presents with localized swelling of the bursae, which may feel warm. The skin may become erythematous if there is associated infection. Swelling of the semimembranosus bursa is not usually tender.

BAKER'S CYST (POPLITEAL CYST)

This results from the passage of fluid through the posterior joint capsule. It is associated with degenerative joint disease and meniscal tears.

History

Symptoms The lump is usually painless, but if it ruptures there is significant pain behind the knee, radiating into the calf, with marked swelling. It can then be mistaken for a deep vein thrombosis.

Examination

The swelling is usually in the popliteal fossa, either at the level of or just below the joint line. It is usually non-tender.

HAEMARTHROSIS

This is caused by a bleed into the joint and can occur spontaneously, in patients with a bleeding disorder such as haemophilia, or when a patient is taking anticoagulation, for example warfarin.

More commonly, it is associated with a traumatic injury.

There has usually been either been an associated fracture, or an anterior cruciate or meniscal tear if the swelling occurs almost immediately after injury.

History

Symptoms The joint is often painful and feels tense.

Examination

The knee is warm and tender to the touch. All movements are restricted.

MENISCAL TEARS

These can occur as a result of trauma, or from degenerative changes with increasing age. The menisci are important as they distribute the load across the joint, help lubricate and facilitate the rolling and gliding actions of the joint, and provide proprioception leading to improved stability of the knee.

Both menisci are C shaped. The medial meniscus is larger and less mobile, and consequently tears of it are more common. Tears can be *longitudinal*, with the fragment remaining attached at the front and back, called a *bucket handle* tear (Figure 8.27). Where

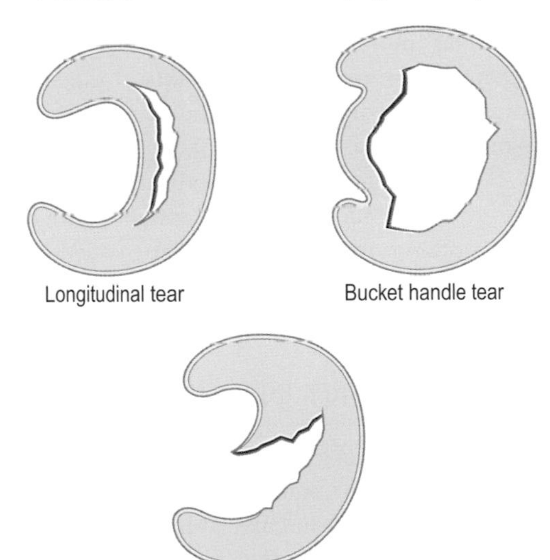

Figure 8.27 Line diagram of types of meniscal tear.
There is usually initial difficulty in weight-bearing, but this will improve in the absence of locking.

the tear emerges at a free edge, it is either an *anterior horn* or a *posterior horn* radial tear. Horizontal tears are more frequent in the degenerative knee. Tears can occur in combination with ligamentous injuries.

History

Age and sex Traumatic tears are common in the young athletic person and are often associated with a *twisting injury*. Degenerative tears become increasingly common from 40 years onwards.

Symptoms In an acute traumatic tear, the knee is *painful* and *may be locked in a flexed position*.

Degenerative tears may become slowly painful. These patients usually complain of the knee *locking* or *giving way*.

Examination

The knee *swells* within a few hours of the injury. It is often *held in flexion*. Full flexion is not usually possible because of pain.

Joint line palpation elicits *localized tenderness over the meniscus*, usually on the medial side.

> **NOTE:** There are specific tests for meniscal pathology, such as *McMurray's test*, but these are painful and not considered useful.

Meniscal cysts can occasionally develop at the site of a tear, most commonly of the lateral meniscus. Examination reveals a *small lump* at the side of the joint, most easily seen with the knee flexed. The lump may be tender.

In 3% of patients, the lateral meniscus may be disc shaped (a *discoid lateral meniscus*) rather than semilunar. It is often symptomless, but young patients may complain that the *knee gives way and clunks*, typically at 110° of flexion and 10° from full extension.

KNEE LIGAMENT INJURIES

There are four principal ligaments around the knee joint, namely the anterior and posterior cruciate ligaments, and the medial and lateral collateral ligaments. These provide support for the joint because the bony structures are inherently unstable.

All the ligaments are usually injured during sporting activity, and therefore they are more common in the younger, usually male population.

Anterior cruciate ligament injury

This ligament is intra-articular and *prevents anterior translation and external rotation of the tibia on the femur*. It has two bundles: the anteromedial bundle resists excess translation (forward–backward movement) in flexion, while the posterolateral bundle tightens as the knee is extended.

A tear of this ligament is often sustained when there is a *sudden change in direction* about an implanted foot, with a twisting motion. It can also occur after jumping and landing on a flexed knee. Injury is often associated with a lateral meniscal tear.

History

Symptoms The knee is *immediately painful* and there is *difficulty weight-bearing*. The patient may have a heard a 'pop' as the tear happens. As the acute event settles, the patient feels the *knee is unstable*, and they have difficulty changing direction with the *knee collapsing*.

Examination

There usually a *large haemarthrosis* almost immediately after the injury. All movements are painful in the initial phase. The diagnosis is made from the history and confirmed, once the acute pain has settled, by a *positive anterior draw test, positive Lachman's test* and possibly a *positive pivot shift test* (see above),

In the chronic case, movements may be painless, but the special tests remain positive.

Posterior cruciate ligament injury

This ligament *prevents posterior 'sliding' of the tibia on the femur*. It has two bundles: the anterolateral bundle, which stabilizes the knee in 90° of flexion, and the posteromedial bundle, which stabilizes the knee when straight.

Injuries are usually caused by a *blow to the knee while it is bent*, for example when striking the dashboard in a road traffic accident or falling directly onto the knee while it is flexed. The posterior ligament is stronger than the anterior and is less frequently injured.

History

Symptoms There is usually *initial pain and swelling*, but this often settles, and unless examined carefully these injuries can be missed. In time, the patient will complain of the knee *feeling unstable coming down slopes and stairs.*

Examination

There is often a small effusion a *positive posterior sag sign* and a *positive posterior draw test.*

Medial collateral ligament injury

This prevents the knee from opening into a valgus position. Tears occur when the knee is forced into valgus, commonly in rugby, football or skiing. They are commonly isolated but can be associated with a cruciate tear.

History

Symptoms The *knee is very painful*, and there may be initial *difficulty in weight-bearing*. The knee may feel *unstable*.

Examination

Tenderness can usually be elicited along the course of the ligament from the medial epicondyle of the femur to the medial tibial condyle. As this is extra-articular, there is normally no haemarthrosis, but there may be some *localized swelling*. Movements will be relatively uncomfortable.

Tests for disruption of the ligament by *applying a valgus strain* cause pain and opening of the joint as the result of joint.

Lateral collateral ligament injury

This is seldom injured in isolation and it is usually part of a pattern of injury that results in posterolateral instability.

OSTEOARTHRITIS OF THE KNEE

The knee is the most common of the large joints to be affected by osteoarthritis. Several predisposing factors are recognized, including previous fracture, meniscal pathology and abnormal biomechanics caused by instability or deformity.

History

Age and sex Patients are usually over 50 years old. In white populations, there is an equal male to female distribution. Black African females are, however, more commonly affected than their male counterparts.

Symptoms This condition usually has a slow insidious onset, with patients complaining of *pain on weight-bearing* that is made worse by walking and exercise.

Subsequently, they develop *night pain* and often sleep with a pillow between their legs. The knee becomes *stiff* when they awake in the morning or after prolonged immobilization. The knee *may lock* or *give way*.

Examination

There may be *wasting of the quadriceps* from disuse (see Figure 6.4), with an obvious deformity, usually *varus and fixed flexion* (Figure 8.28).

An effusion may be present. Crepitus may be felt and heard, and the joint line is occasionally tender on palpation. The range of movement may be reduced, with *loss of extension* and pain elicited on all movements.

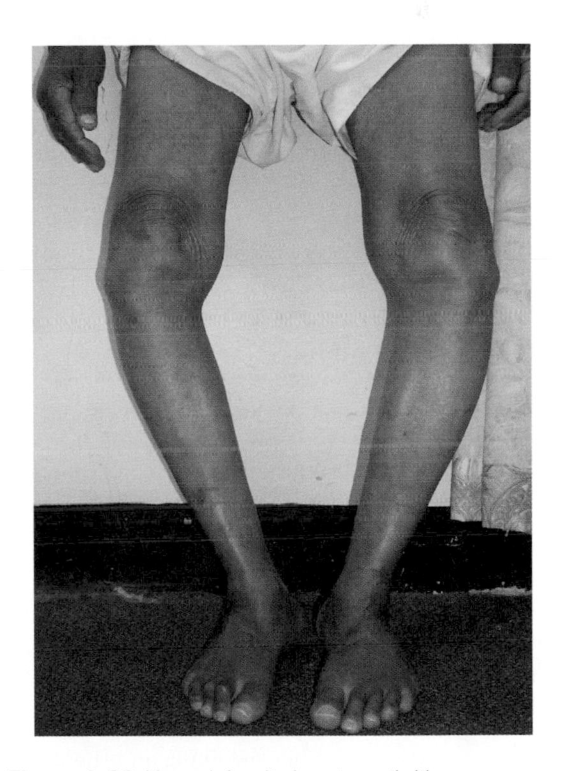

Figure 8.28 Knee deformity in osteoarthritis.

RHEUMATOID ARTHRITIS

This can occur in the knee joint but, as in other joints, the presentation of significant pathology is now much less common as a result of advances in medical management.

Symptoms While the synovitis develops, the knee is *painful* and *swollen*. As the disease progresses, the knee becomes increasing unstable, with progressive pain. The patient has *difficulty mobilizing*, using the stairs and standing from a sitting position.

Examination

On inspection, there may be *quadriceps wasting* and *valgus deformity* of the joint. Palpation reveals a palpable *effusion* and *thickened synovium*. *Movements become increasingly restricted*. Examination of the supporting ligaments may demonstrate instability.

SEPTIC ARTHRITIS AND TUBERCULOSIS

History

These can both cause infection in the knee joint but are uncommon. They present in much the same way as the same infections of the hip joint with pain, loss of movement, swelling and signs of systemic infection.

Examination

The knee joint is swollen and tender, and its movements are restricted.

BONY SWELLINGS

These are common around the knee and vary from benign osteomas/diaphyseal achalasia through osteoclastomas to highly malignant osteosarcomas (see Chapter 6).

THE FOOT AND ANKLE

The ankle joint

The ankle joint is a synovial hinge joint between the lower ends of the tibia and fibula and the upper part of the talus. The proximal articular surface comprises the distal end of the tibia, which includes the medial malleolus and the lateral malleolus and the distal part of the fibula, which together form a mortise socket for the talus. The socket is wider anteriorly than posteriorly, and articulates with the upper part of the talus, which is reciprocally wedge shaped. The lateral side of the talus is larger than the medial side.

The ankle joint is supported by:

- The lateral ligaments.
- The anterior and posterior talofibular and calcaneal fibular ligaments.
- The medial deltoid ligament.
- The transverse tibiofibular ligament.
- The syndesmosis ligaments between the tibia–fibula.
- A fibrous capsule.

The movements are primarily extension (*dorsiflexion*) and flexion (*plantar flexion*). The ankle is more stable in dorsiflexion than plantar flexion.

Distal to the ankle joint is the *subtalar joint*, which is the articulation between the talus and the calcaneum. This joint allows a complex movement in three planes, the transverse, frontal and sagittal planes. This motion is commonly referred to as inversion and eversion of the foot. The other joints of the foot include those between the tarsal bones, the metatarsals and the phalanges. They are all synovial joints, and have shapes related to their movement.

The foot arches

The *medial arch* is higher and forms the instep of the foot. It comprises the calcaneum, the talus, the navicular, the cuneiforms and the medial three metatarsals.

The *transverse arch* runs in a medial to lateral direction on the plantar surface of the foot (concave). The distal tarsal joints make up the arch. The arch/bones provide stability across the midfoot.

These arches are important in promoting forward propulsion by helping the foot form into a rigid, efficient lever during stance and forward movement. Each arch is supported by ligaments, muscles and tendons.

Symptoms

Adults with foot and ankle problems generally present with *pain*, *swelling*, *deformity* and *impaired function*. Simple screening questions to begin a history, that are very useful are

- Have you noticed any change in the shape of the foot/ankle?
- Have you changed your shoe wear that may account for the symptoms?
- Have you changed your activity profile that may account for the symptoms?

Pain is usually referenced to a well-localized structure, therefore a good working knowledge of the surface anatomy is important, but pain symptoms are sometimes vague; for example, *metatarsalgia* is a poorly localized pain in the forefoot that has many causes (Revision panel 8.4).

Pain may be present at rest or be 'activity related' (Revision panel 8.5). It may also be associated with the wearing of shoes. The foot and ankle can often be *stiff in the morning*. This can result in *difficulty weight bearing*. Ascending and descending the stairs can be problematic.

Deformities of the foot and ankle can be caused by either congenital or acquired conditions. Deformity may or may not coexist with *pain*.

The ankle or subtalar joints *can become unstable*, leading to episodes of the joint giving way.

Revision panel 8.4

CAUSES OF PAIN IN THE ANKLE REGION

Common causes

Ankle osteoarthritis
Ankle osteochondral defects
Ankle impingement – anterior or posterior
Achilles tendinosis
Tenosynovitis
Inflammatory arthritis
Tibialis posterior tendon dysfunction
Peroneal tendinopathy

Rare causes

Acute and chronic osteomyelitis
Septic arthritis
Haemophilic arthritis

Revision panel 8.5

THE PAINFUL FOOT

Heel

Achilles tendinopathy
Retrocalcaneal bursitis
Plantar fasciitis
Stress fracture of the calcaneus

Midfoot

Osteochondritis of the navicular bone (Köhler's disease)
Midfoot osteoarthritis
Stress fracture of the navicular
Tibialis anterior tendinosis
Charcot arthropathy (late stages)

Forefoot

Stress fracture of a metatarsal
Morton's neuroma
Osteochondritis of the second metatarsal head (*Freiberg's disease*)
Hallux valgus
Hallux rigidus
Claw toes/hammer toes/mallet toes
Pes cavus metatarsalgia
Gout
Inflammatory arthropathy
Neoplasms – benign and malignant – of the bones of the foot

Plan for examination of the foot and ankle

This follows the usual principles of look, feel and move. The examination includes the joints above and below the principle area of assessment, together with a neurovascular examination (see Chapters 3 and 10).

Observe for walking aids or supports/insoles. Ask to see the patient's footwear, the shape of which may be altered because of an underlying deformity. Observe the heel and sole for patterns of wear that may be altered as a result of changes in gait.

Ask the patient to stand and expose the lower limbs from the thighs down.

Ask the patient to walk, paying attention to all the phases of the walking cycle: *heel strike, foot-flat, mid-stance to heel off* and *heel off to toe off*.

Patients may have an antalgic gait secondary to pain. Their gait may also be disturbed by muscular weakness, deformity or stiffness or leg length discrepancies.

Patients may have a *foot drop* when the ankle dorsiflexors are weak, causing a slapping foot strike. The leg may be lifted higher than usual so the weak foot can clear the ground (a *high-stepping gait*), usually because of neurological conditions.

Patients may also walk on the inner or outer border of the foot because of valgus or varus deformity respectively.

Push-off from the ground involves the first metatarsal joint and can be altered by joint pain or stiffness involving the great toe.

INSPECTION

During standing, the heels are normally in slight valgus alignment related to the tibial shaft. When a person is on tip toes, there is inversion because of movement at the subtalar joint (Figure 8.29).

Skin

Look all around the joints from front and back for scars, and for callosities caused by pressure from footwear or abnormal transmission of load. Don't forget to inspect the sole of the foot as it can be easily overlooked.

Shape

Deformity may occur in the ankle, foot or toes. Common deformities include:

- Flat foot (*pes planus*).
- High instep (*pes cavus*).
- Lateral deviation of the great toe (*hallux valgus*).
- Toe deformity:
  - Flexed proximal interphalangeal joint in isolation (*hammer toe*).
  - Flexed proximal interphalangeal joint and distal interphalangeal joint with hyperextension at the metatarsophalangeal joint (*claw toe*).
  - Flexed distal interphalangeal joint in isolation (*mallet toe*).

PALPATION

Any increased temperature of the skin may be indicative of an inflammatory change or infective process.

Feel for any localized tenderness, swelling and oedema of soft tissue or bone.

Ensure an assessment of sensation and motor function is performed (see Chapter 3).

MOVEMENT

Ask the patient to move their joints themselves before checking the passive range.

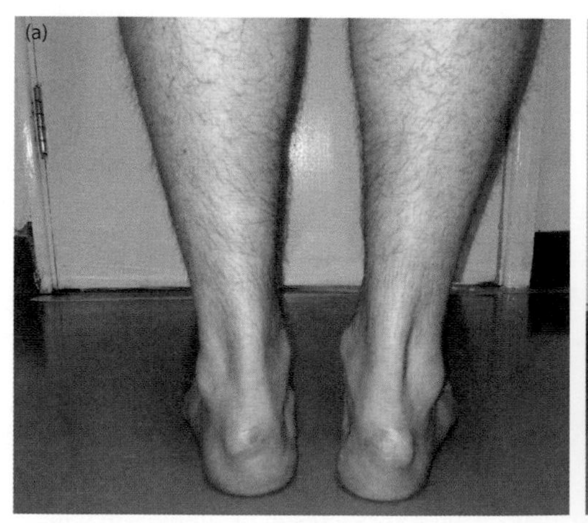

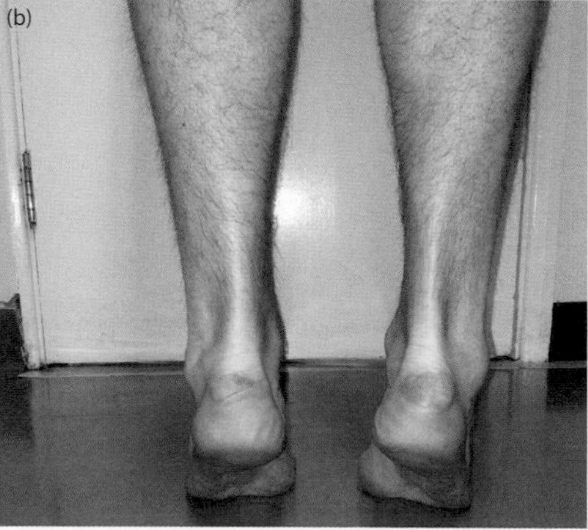

Figure 8.29 ANKLE INSPECTION. (a) The heel is in valgus when viewed from behind. (b) As the patient goes onto tip toes, the heel swings inwards into varus.

Ankle joint

Hold the heel in the left hand and the midfoot in the right hand (Figure 8.30). Assess plantar flexion (0–40°) and dorsiflexion (usually 0–15°).

Subtalar joint

In order to assess inversion and eversion, the ankle joint should be held locked in the plantigrade position. It can be easier to accurately assess this with the patient prone. Eversion is usually around 0–15°, and inversion greater, at around 0–30°.

Mid-tarsal joint

Firmly hold the heel to stabilize the hindfoot and assess movement of the forefoot in both the vertical and horizontal planes.

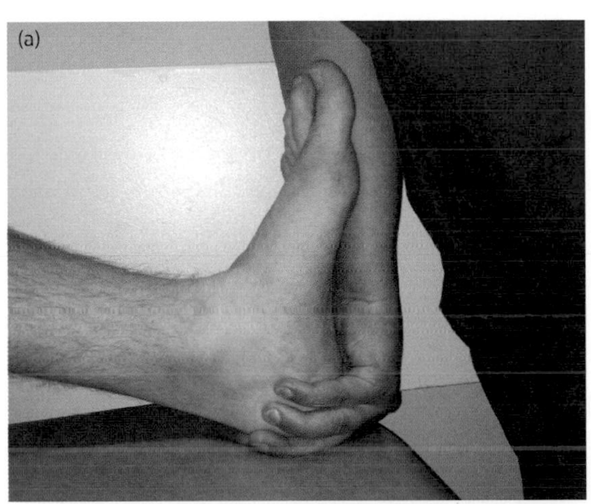

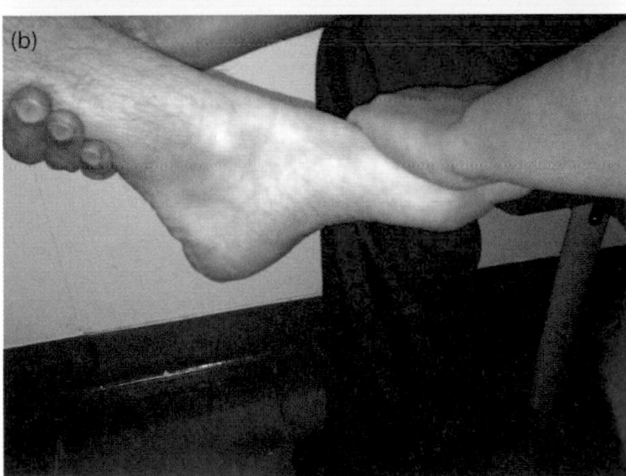

Figure 8.30 ANKLE JOINT INSPECTION. (a) Ankle dorsiflexion. (b) Ankle plantar flexion.

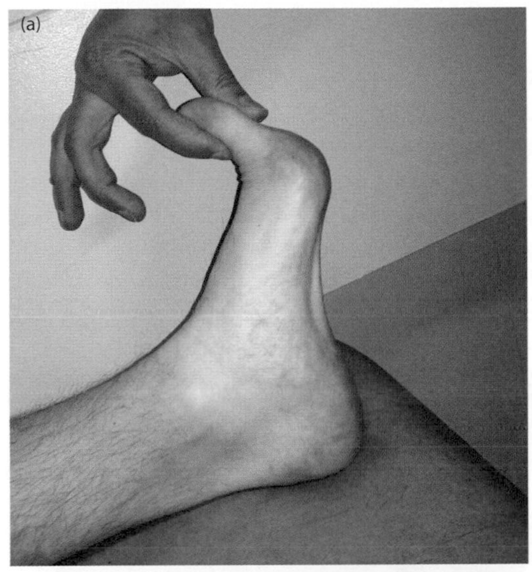

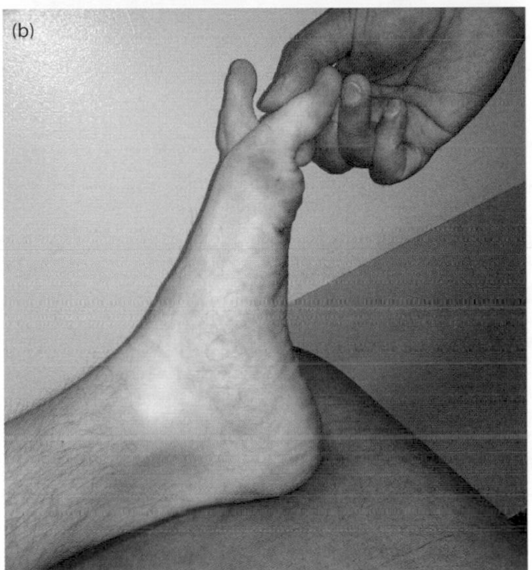

Figure 8.31 EXTENSION AND FLEXION OF THE TOES. (a) Great toe dorsiflexion. (b) Great toe plantar flexion.

Toes

Extension and flexion of the toes, in particular the great toe, should be assessed (Figure 8.31).

Abnormal movements

To maintain stability, the ankle joint is reinforced by muscles and ligaments. Abnormal movement and instability can occur if the ligaments are injured.

Stability in the anterior and posterior plane is tested with the patient sitting on the couch with the leg over the edge flexed at the knee. One hand holds the distal whilst the other firmly holds around the hindfoot grasping the calcaneus and talar neck, whilst pulling and pushing smoothly backwards and forwards moving the foot on the distal tibia. In normal ankle joints, there should be little or no movement. Stability to varus stress by moving the heel is a useful test for integrity of the calcaneofibular ligament (Figure 8.32).

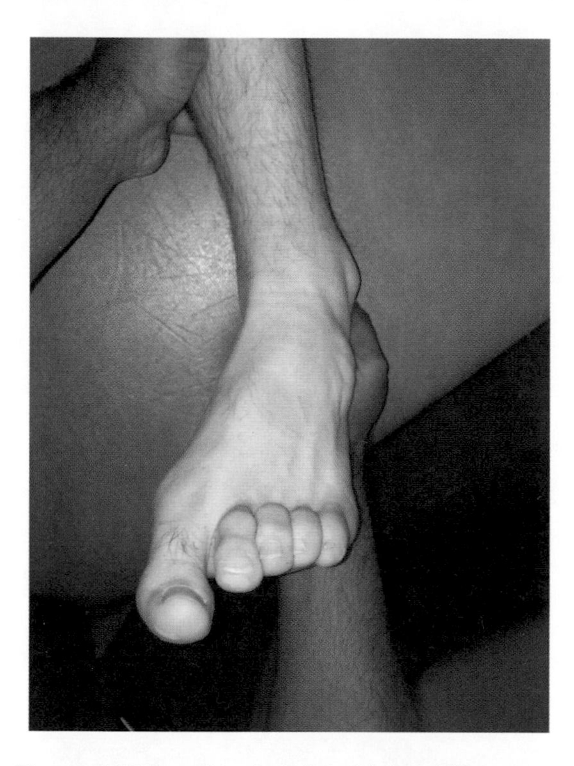

Figure 8.32 Inversion stress for ankle instability.

Congenital and acquired conditions of the foot and ankle

There are many congenital abnormalities of the foot, such as polydactyly (too many toes) (Figure 8.33), but the most important is club foot.

CLUB FOOT (CONGENITAL TALIPES EQUINOVARUS)

These deformities of the foot and ankle develop in utero and are usually present at birth. They are classified according to the skeletal deformity but are collectively known as talipes or club foot. Similar deformities can also develop in adult life after injury, paralysis and other musculoskeletal disorders.

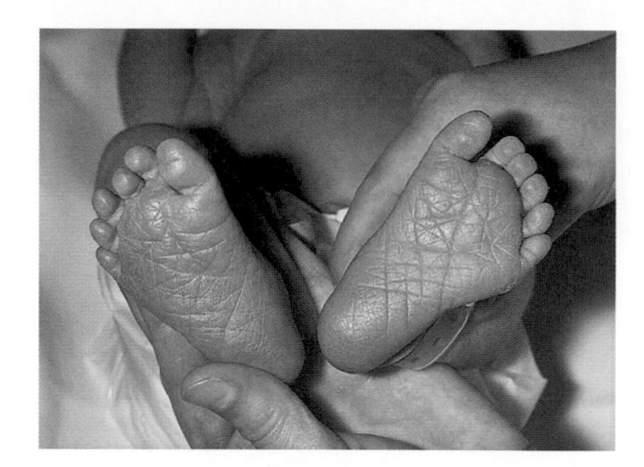

Figure 8.33 An infant demonstrating polydactyly of both feet.

The incidence is 1–2 per 1000 births, with males more often affected than females (2 to 1).

The condition is bilateral in one-third of cases.

When a club foot abnormality is present, the infant must be examined for other associated disorders, especially *developmental displacement of the hip* and *spina bifida* (see Chapter 9) or arthrogryposis.

There are two main types of deformity (Figure 8.34):

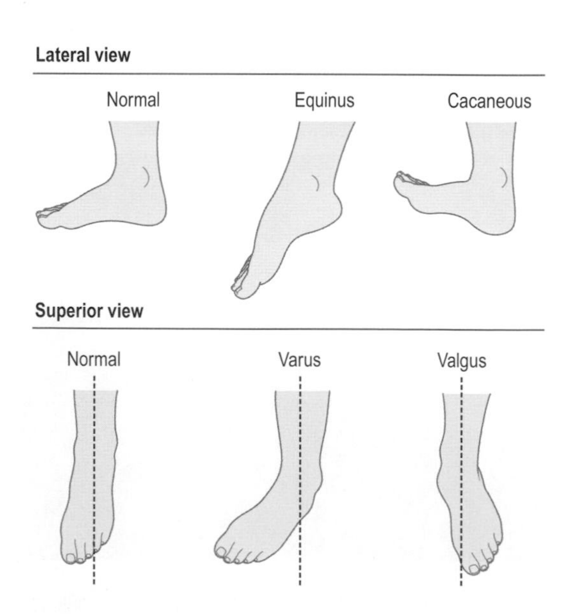

Figure 8.34 Deformities of the foot.

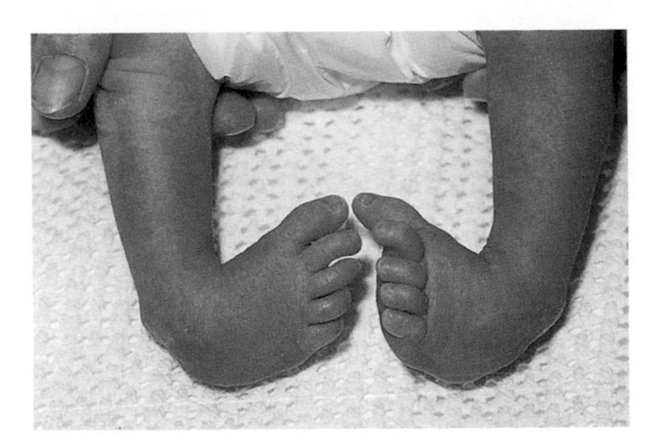

Figure 8.35 Severe bilateral clubbed feet. The varus deformity is so severe that the feet are pulled upwards as well as inwards, making this a talipes calcaneovarus.

- The ankle may be abnormally extended so the weight-bearing is on the toes – an equinus deformity; or abnormally dorsiflexed so that the weight-bearing is on the heel – a calcaneous deformity.
- The foot may be deviated into a varus or valgus position, which usually means there is some associated inversion and eversion, respectively.

Of these eight variations, only two are common: *talipes equinus,* caused by a short Achilles tendon, and *talipes equinovarus – the true club foot* (Figure 8.35).

The obvious deformities of the true club foot would be equinus at the ankle, so the ankle keeps pointing downwards, and varus or inward pointing of the heels. There is also supination in the subtalar joint and adduction of the forefoot. The joint movements are limited, and the muscles that affect the joint are wasted. The calf muscle is smaller. These result in the foot having a bean-shaped appearance.

FLAT FEET (PES PLANUS)

The foot has a longitudinal and a transverse arch. The patient has a flat foot if the longitudinal arch flattens to the extent that the medial border of the foot rests on the ground. It is usually associated with a mild valgus deformity of the hindfoot, which results in pronation of the forefoot and subsequent loss of the medial arch (Figure 8.36).

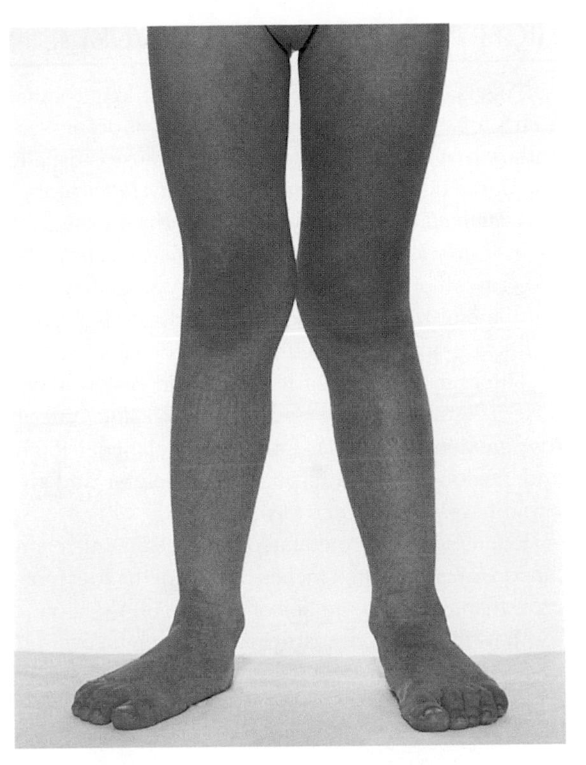

Figure 8.36 Flat feet (pes planus). The medial border of the foot rests on the ground. There is also mild genu valgum (knock knees).

All children are flat-footed when they start walking, but the arch develops as they grow more active. The infantile pattern may persist into adult life, and the deformity may become fixed by secondary contractures or excessive laxity in the joints.

When assessing for flat feet, it is important to check for symmetry in the arches of both feet. *Ask the patient to go onto tip toe.* With normal feet, the heel moves inwards or into varus.

Tarsal coalition, in which there is an abnormal congenital connection in the bones, is a possibility in the younger patient if the heel does not move. In older patients, it may be the result of dysfunction and tendinosis of the tibialis posterior tendon, which assists in stabilizing the arch.

Contrary to popular opinion, *flat feet rarely cause trouble in adult life* as the body weight is spread over a large flat area. A flat foot is a normal foot in most cases, simply a variation of foot shape. The fastest runners often have flat feet!

HIGH-ARCH FOOT (PES CAVUS)

This is the opposite of a flat foot; the longitudinal arch is accentuated (Figure 8.37). Pes cavus occurs secondary to *muscle imbalance*. A specific cause is usually not found, but *it is important to carry out a full neurological examination* as peripheral neuropathies, especially *Charcot–Marie–Tooth disease, spina bifida* and *poliomyelitis* can all present with pes cavus. Asymmetry with a unilateral high-arch foot is a 'red flag' suggesting significant underlying neurological problems.

The high arch is clearly visible and easy to diagnose (Figure 8.38). The *toes are usually 'clawed'* (hyperextension of the metatarsophalangeal joints and flexion of the interphalangeal joints) and the patient *cannot straighten their toes.*

Extension of the metatarsophalangeal joints combined with a high arch makes the ball of the foot more prominent and lifts the tips of the toes off the ground so that they do not participate in weight-bearing.

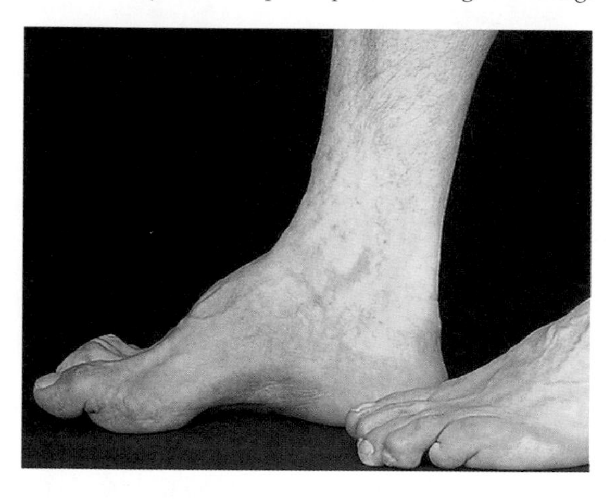

Figure 8.37 A high-arched foot (pes cavus).

Consequently, *callosities develop* on the ball of the foot beneath the heads of the metatarsal bones and on the dorsal aspect of the toes where they rub against the shoes.

HALLUX VALGUS (BUNION)

A *valgus deformity at the metatarsophalangeal joint of the great toe* is a common abnormality. It can be congenital or acquired, with the latter far more common in females, the reason postulated to be poorly fitting footwear. The *bunion* is the name given to the bursa that forms over the medial aspect of the prominent head of the first metatarsal. It often swells up. The local sensory nerve can get stretched by the bunion and compressed between the bunion and the shoe. The patient has difficulty finding comfortable shoes as the *bunion is painful when rubbed or touched.* The fluctuant subcutaneous swelling or bursa is often easy to feel and distinguish from the underlying bony prominence and can get very inflamed and erythematous.

Osteoarthritis can develop as a result of prolonged abnormal stresses in the first metatarsophalangeal joint. This causes pain in the joint during movement and weight-bearing.

Clinical examination should start with inspection of the arch as hallux valgus is more common in patients with flat feet. There is a valgus deformity of the first metatarsal phalyngeal joint (Figure 8.39) with an apparent fluctuant swelling (*bunion*). There may also be lesser toe abnormalities. Look for evidence of abnormal loading in the sole of the foot with *callus formation* under the lesser metatarsals' heads.

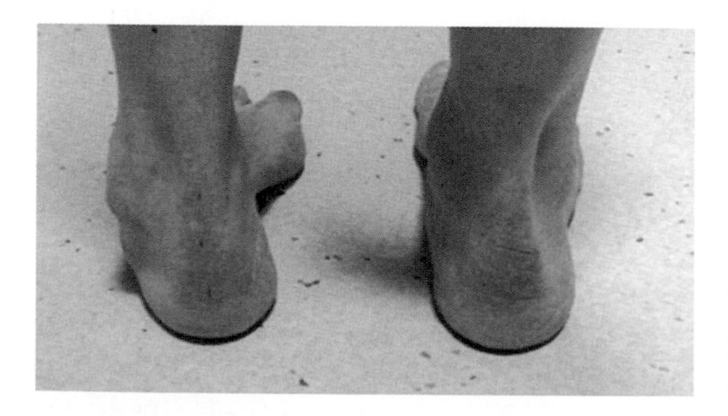

Figure 8.38 A unilateral high-arch (cavus) left foot.

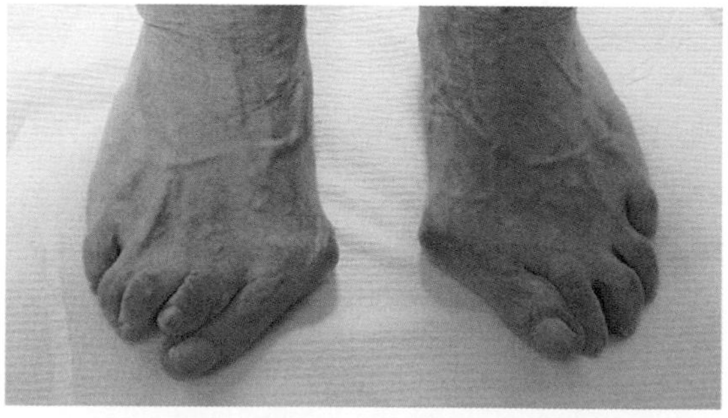

Figure 8.39 Bilateral hallux valgus.

Check for *tenderness* over the actual bunion. Check the *range of movement in the joint* and *whether the deformity is passively correctable* to a straight toe.

HALLUX RIGIDUS

The first metatarsophalangeal joint is a joint that is commonly affected by osteoarthritis even when it is in normal alignment. This can cause *pain, sometimes erythema, swelling* and a *progressive reduction of joint movement.*

Clinical examination may reveal a *bony prominence on the top of the joint,* produced by the underlying bony osteophytes. These osteophytes can block dorsiflexion and plantar flexion of the great toe can also be significantly reduced.

GOUTY ARTHRITIS

This has been discussed in Chapter 6 and is mentioned here as it is an important cause of arthritis in the first metatarsophalangeal joint.

History

Severe acute *pain, redness* and *swelling* usually develop in the first metatarsophalangeal joint. The ankles and knees and other toes can also be affected, most commonly in a middle-aged or elderly male.

Examination

The joint is *red, swollen* and *exquisitely tender. Septic arthritis must be considered,* but the absence of systemic symptoms combined with the presence of tophi and a raised serum urate can help differentiate and confirm the diagnosis.

MALLET AND HAMMER TOES

In a mallet toe, the contracture is at the level of the distal interphalangeal joint, and in a hammer toe, which is more common, it is at the level of the proximal interphalangeal joint.

Patients often *present with pain* and *notice the deformity.* There may be hard skin over the affected joint (Figure 8.40), which can also be painful.

Clinical assessment involves checking for other associated conditions such as a *bunion,* which is very common and can actually cause the hammer toe (often to the patients surprise as the bunion may be pain free!), or hard skin on the sole of the foot. It is not always easy to say if it is a classic mallet toe, hammer toe or both. Sometimes it is just easier to call it what you see, that is, a flexion deformity of the lesser toe.

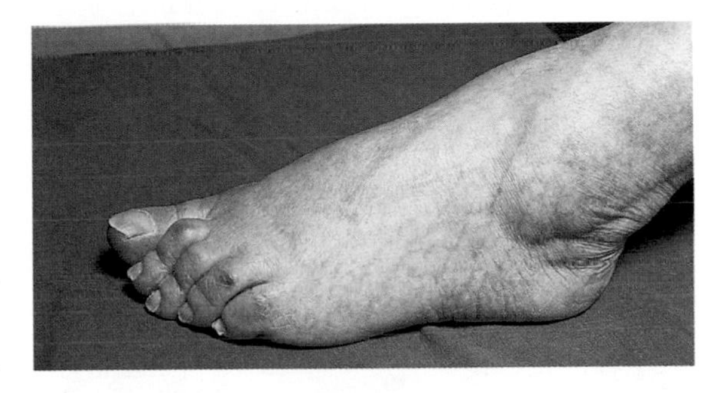

Figure 8.40 A row of hammer toes. The tips of some of the toes are off the ground, and there are callosities over the flexed proximal interphalangeal joints. The distal interphalangeal joints of the second and third toes are only slightly hyperextended.

CLAW TOES AND THE NEUROLOGICAL FOOT

There is sometimes a neurological basis to a claw toe. In a claw toe, there is hyperextension of the joint at the level of the metatarsophalangeal joint, with flexion at the interphalangeal joints and distal interphalangeal joints.

Check for a high arch or cavus foot as a claw toe is often associated with this deformity (see above). Look for symmetry in the arch. The great toe may also be clawed. Note whether there are any *calluses* on the tops of the toes and assess the correctability of the joints. If they cannot be passively corrected, this affects treatment options.

MORTON'S NEUROMA

This is a *swelling around a digital nerve* called a neuroma, most commonly found between the *3rd and 4th toes*. It may be caused by repetitive trauma of the intermetatarsal space, possibly by tight-fitting shoes. It usually causes *pain* or *parasthesia on weight-bearing* over the ball of the foot (metatarsalgia) or into the toes.

Externally, there may be no visible signs of this condition. Squeezing the web space can recreate the pain. Lateral compression at the same time makes the pain worse as you are now compressing the enlarged digital nerve between your fingers and the metatarsal neck. This is painful, and a soft click can sometimes be heard, the so-called *Mulder's click* (Figure 8.41).

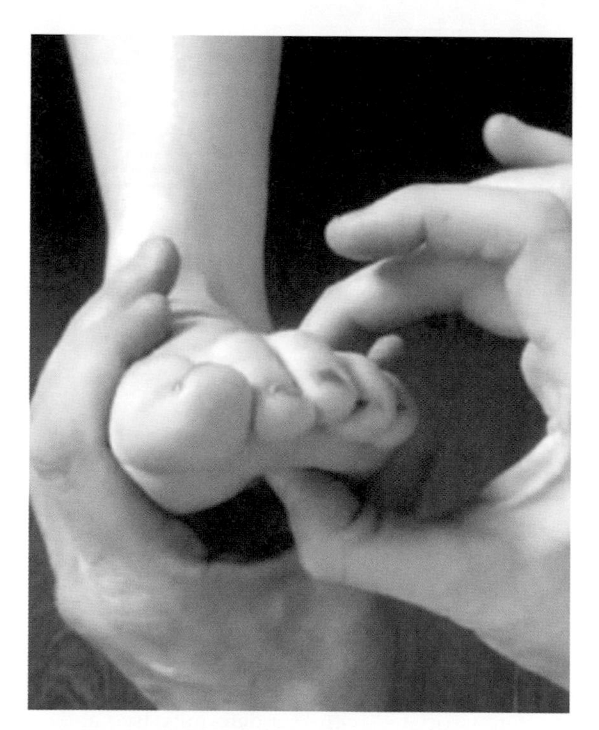

Figure 8.41 Technique to elicit a Mulder's click.

BUNIONETTE

This is a prominence on the outer aspect of the foot – a bunion of the fifth toe – just like a bunion of the great toe. There may be hard skin or an inflamed bursa over it. The foot is wider, and finding comfortable shoes is more difficult.

OSTEOARTHRITIS OF THE ANKLE

History

This is less common than osteoarthritis of the hip or knee, and unlike hip arthritis, it is usually post-traumatic, as a consequence of either previous sprains or fractures. It therefore can more commonly develop in a younger patient population than is usually seen with hip or knee arthritis.

It causes *pain and swelling* and can *limit walking* and *load-bearing activities*.

Examination

There may be *visible malalignment* of the joint. When the patient stands, the heel may be in *valgus* or *varus*, with the whole ankle joint tilted. The joint can be bulky because of joint swelling and new bone formation (Figure 8.42).

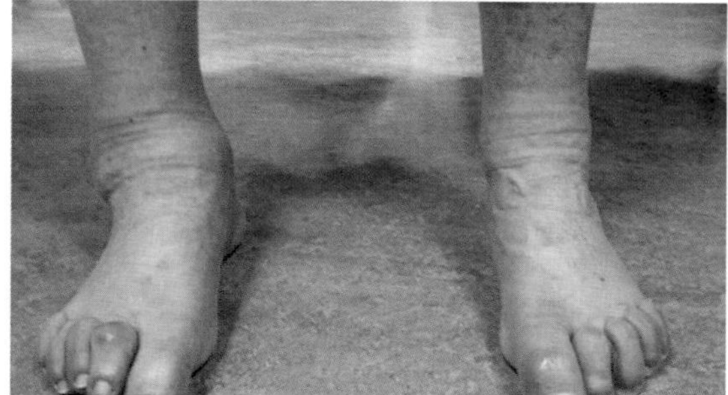

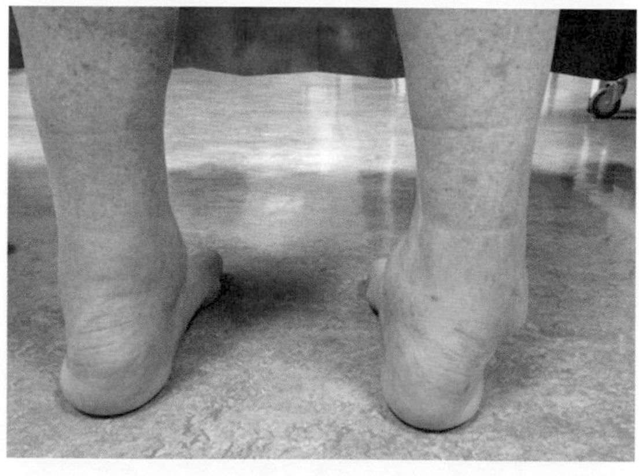

Figure 8.42 Varus malalignment of the ankle secondary to osteoarthritis.

The most striking abnormality is *tenderness along the joint line with pain on movement of the joint,* usually associated with a reduction in movement when compared with the normal side. Sometimes there is no movement at all, and the ankle may be stiff.

RHEUMATOID ARTHRITIS OF THE FOOT AND ANKLE

This has been already covered in Chapter 6 and discussed with the upper limb, where it commonly affects the joints of the hand (see Chapter 7). It is, however, nearly as common in the joints of the foot and ankle. It starts as a synovitis in the metatarsophalangeal joint, tarsal and ankle joints and also involves the tendons. It is increasingly less common because of the relative success of medical treatments for the condition.

History

It presents with pain, swelling and deformity in the foot, which interferes with mobility.

Examination

There is often *swelling of the ankle and the small joints of the foot.* Ankle movements, especially *inversion and eversion, are reduced,* and the ankle may eventually develop, for example, a valgus malalignment. The forefoot often has a hallux valgus deformity of the great toe. Lesser toes develop multiple hammer or claw type deformities and there may be dislocation of the lesser metatarsophalangeal joints. This is caused by stretching of the joint capsules and tendon dislocation, which are damaged by the inflammatory process.

It is essential to examine the plantar aspect of the foot where the metatarsal heads are more prominent following subluxation of the fat pad.

ACHILLES TENDINOSIS

An acute tendinitis presentation of the Achilles area is much less common than chronic Achilles tendinosis. This can occur in both active and sedentary populations and is characterized by an initial local inflammatory process followed by a chronic degenerate process within the tendon. The paratenon or

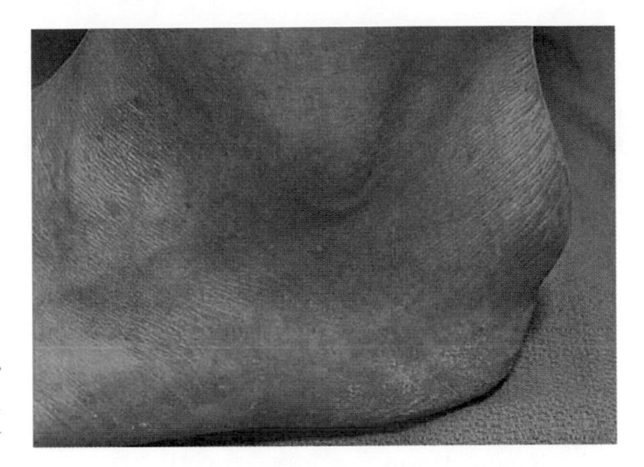

Figure 8.43 A Haglund bump.

sheath of the tendon can also be affected with an acute paratendinitis.

It is important to delineate whether the pain is in the middle of the Achilles tendon (*non-insertional tendinopathy*) or is present where the tendon joins the bone (*insertional tendinopathy*).

History

It typically causes *pain in the tendon,* which is experienced during activity.

Non-insertional tendinopathy is associated with a tendon that is very tender to palpate and may be thicker as a consequence of repeated small tears in the tendon, healing with degenerate infiltrate and scar tissue. It is essential to assess whether the tendon is in continuity. Also compare its thickness with that of the normal side.

Insertional tendinopathy often presents with an enlargement at the back of the heel from a bony prominence (a *Haglund bump*) or from ossification of the tendon insertion itself (Figure 8.43).

ACHILLES TENDON RUPTURE

It is important not to miss this diagnosis as the consequences of loss of function from a missed tear are severe.

History

Patients typically feel a *searing pain* or *hear a loud pop* or *bang* as they push off. Typical activities in which this happens are tennis, badminton, squash and football. The pop is often so loud that others can hear it. *They often think that they have been kicked or 'shot' in the leg.*

Examination

The diagnosis can often be made based on the history and simply looking at the tendon for characteristic features. There is usually *bruising and tenderness* at the site of the rupture. Surprisingly, it *may not be painful*, but the patient will *limp* and *step high* to clear the foot. The patient should be examined prone on the couch. A *palpable gap* can be felt in the tendon, and the foot has an abnormal lie being more dorsiflexed because of a lack of the downward pull from the calf musculature.

Squeezing the calf muscles normally causes plantar flexion of the ankle, but a *calf squeeze test* does not produce plantar flexion of the ankle if the Achilles tendon is ruptured. This is very easy to see when this is compared with the normal side (Figures 8.44, 8.45) but this test must not be relied upon in each case.

PLANTAR FASCIITIS

This is caused by inflammation of the plantar fascia.

History

This is the most common disorder of the foot.

Pain is experienced in the heel. The condition can be brought on by a change of footwear, walking barefoot or high-impact exercise, or it can just arise without an obvious cause. The complaint is of *startup pain,* which is pain that is experienced first thing in the morning or when getting up having been static for a long time at a desk. After a few minutes, the pain gets a little better. The foot often again becomes sore at the end of the day.

Examination

Check for the alignment of the heel with varus or valgus as the condition can be associated with deformity. There is *invariably severe point tenderness*

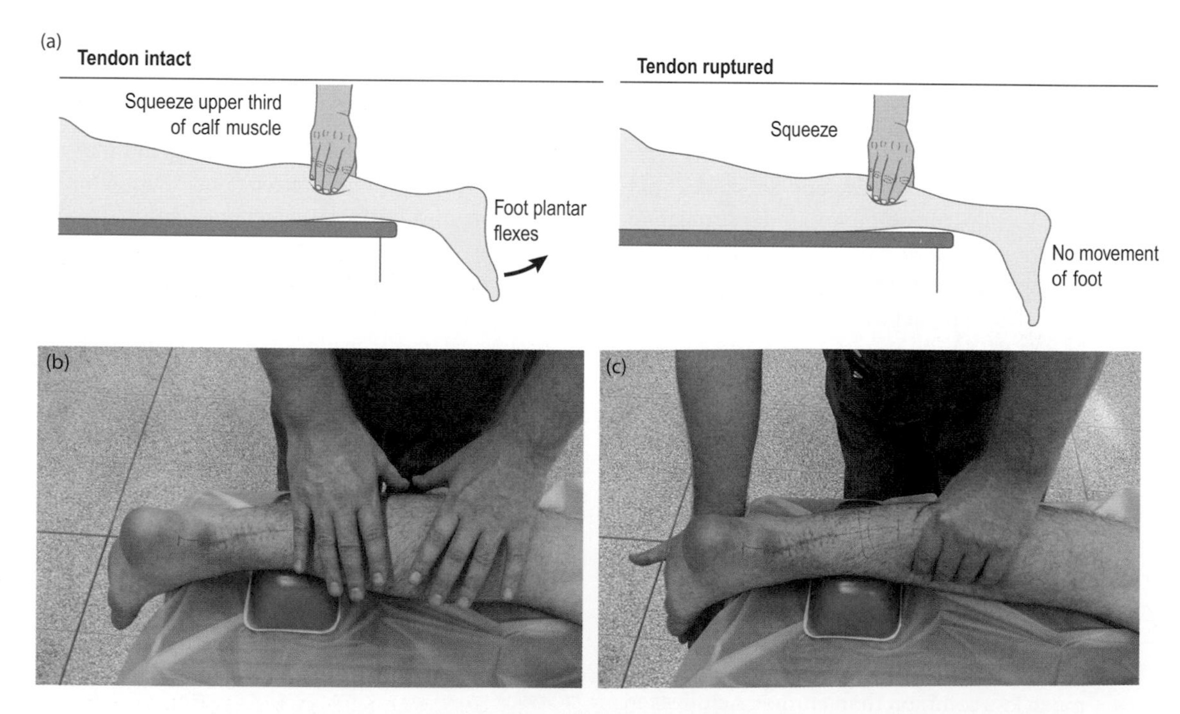

Figure 8.44 THE SQUEEZE TEST FOR ACHILLES TENDON DYSFUNCTION. (a) Place the patient prone with the feet hanging freely over the end of the couch. Squeeze the calf muscles. If the Achilles tendon is intact, the foot will plantar flex. (b) This patient has re-ruptured his Achilles tendon. Note the position of the ankle before the calf is squeezed. (c) The ankle remains in the same position despite firm squeezing of the calf muscle. The calf tendon complex is not in continuity.

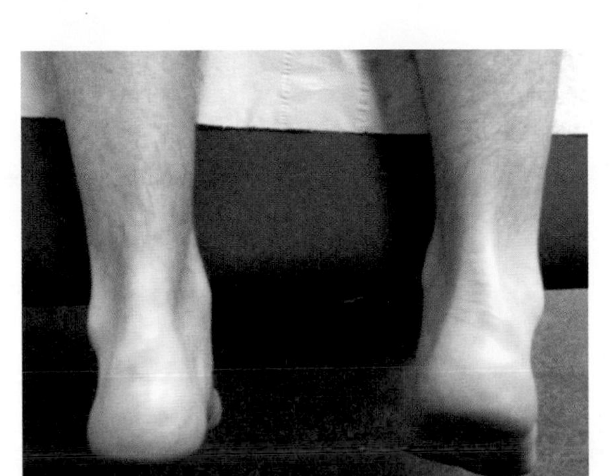

Figure 8.45 Achilles rupture on the left side with relative ankle dorsiflexion on this side.

where the plantar fascia inserts onto the heel, usually the medial aspect. Ankle dorsiflexion is often reduced because of associated calf tightness. The great toe may be stiff. Thickened nodules appear on the plantar surface of the foot and may attach to the skin in a condition called plantar fibromatosis, much less common than plantar fasciitis in isolation (Figure 8.46).

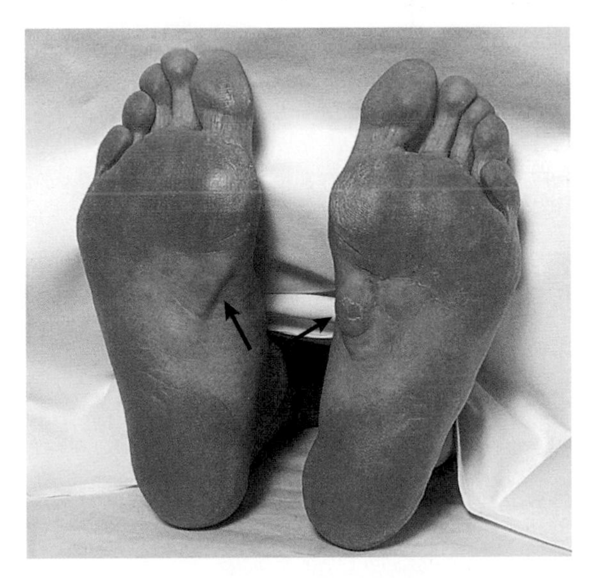

Figure 8.46 Plantar fibromatosis of the feet. There are bilateral thick nodules in the plantar fascia but no flexion deformities of the toes.

Plantar fibromatosis (Ledderhose disease)

This condition is very similar in aetiology to the more common Dupuytren's disease of the hand.

CALLOSITIES AND CORNS

Continual pressure and *friction* on small areas of the skin of the foot caused by poor-fitting shoes or skeletal deformities stimulate thickening of the skin with overload of repetitive stress on a particular bony prominence. A patch of thickened hyperkeratotic skin is called a *callosity*. It is often called a *corn* if it is pushed into the skin so that it appears to have a deep central core. These can also be painful when squeezed, making the differential diagnosis from a plantar wart difficult.

FRIEBERG'S DISEASE

This is an *osteochondritis of the second* and *sometimes third metatarsal head*. It is most often seen in young females and presents with *metatarsalgia*. The metatarsal head area can gradually enlarge with osteophytes and synovitis and become palpable as a dorsal lump in the forefoot especially in later presentation in older adults, and is tender on movement or pressure.

FRACTURES OF THE LOWER LIMB

Proximal femoral fractures

Proximal femoral fractures can occur proximal or distal to the intertrochanteric line.

There are broadly two principal fracture patterns about the femoral neck:

- *Intracapsular:* subcapital and transcervical.
- *Extracapsular:* intertrochanteric and subtrochanteric.

> **NOTE:** Intracapsular fractures have the greatest risk of avascular necrosis and non-union.

These fractures may be described as incomplete, complete or slightly or significantly displaced,

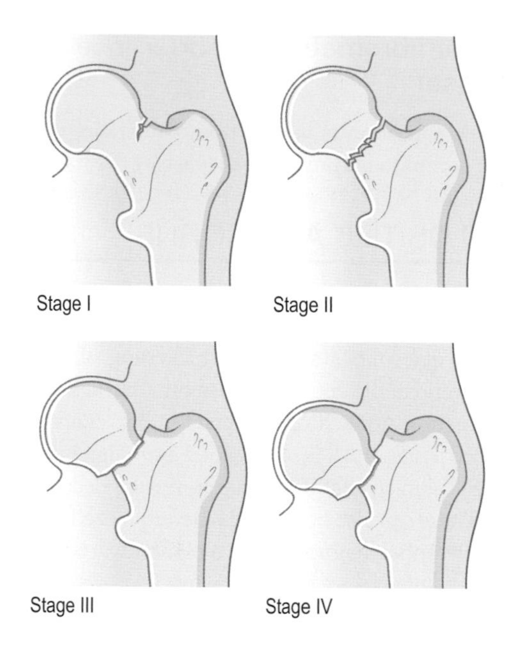

Figure 8.47 Garden's classification of fracture.

according to the *Garden classification* (Figure 8.47). Displaced fractures carry the worst prognosis.

Mechanism of injury This is usually a *simple fall* on to the greater trochanter, a *direct blow* in a road traffic injury or *fall from a height*. The latter is often associated with other injuries.

Elderly patients with extracapsular or intracapsular injuries may have reduced bone density as a result of *osteoporosis*. These fractures occur more commonly in females.

Occasionally, the patient may have a *pathological fracture* from osteomalacia, Paget's disease or bony metastases.

History

After a *minor fall or accident*, an elderly patient complains of *persistent pain in the hip*, often radiating to the thigh. *Standing and walking are impossible if the fracture is unimpacted and displaced. The patient may still, however, be able to weight bear if the fracture is impacted.* The injury will be higher energy. In younger patients with normal bones, such injuries are more common in males.

Examination

In patients with femoral neck fractures, the limb is usually *shortened, adducted and externally rotated*, because of the unopposed action of the iliopsoas. The presence or absence of external rotation varies depending on the level of the fracture and the amount of displacement. The joint may be tender over the femoral neck anteriorly, and hip movements, particularly flexion and internal rotation, are very painful. The thigh may be swollen.

General complications are shown in Revision panel 8.6.

Revision panel 8.6

GENERAL COMPLICATIONS OF PROXIMAL FEMORAL FRACTURES

- Venous thromboembolism: deep vein thrombosis or pulmonary embolus
- Fat embolus
- Adult respiratory distress syndrome
- Pneumonia
- Blisters or pressure sores
- Local complications include:
  - Infection
  - Avascular necrosis of the femoral head
  - Heterotopic ossification
  - Malunion
  - Non-union
  - Osteoarthritis of the hip joint

Dislocations of the hip

These are *usually the result of road traffic accidents*, where force is transmitted up the femoral shaft. They can also result from *falls from a height*. The most common is a posterior dislocation, but anterior and central dislocations can also occur.

POSTERIOR DISLOCATION

This often occurs when a vehicle passenger or driver is thrown forwards and hits their bent knee against a rigid structure, such as the dashboard. The femoral head is forced backwards, often fracturing the posterior acetabulum.

History

Pain in the hip is severe, the limb is shortened, and patients cannot weight bear or walk.

Examination

The *limb is shortened, internally rotated, adducted* and *flexed*. All movements of the hip are restricted and painful. The greater trochanter may appear prominent, and the buttock appears swollen.

> **NOTE:** There may be an associated femoral shaft fracture, which may mask the signs of the hip dislocation (see Fractures of the Femoral Shift).

Complications

There may be other *associated fractures* of the femoral head, neck and shaft, and these must not be missed if an attempt is to be made to reduce the dislocation. *Sciatic nerve injury* (see Chapter 3) complicates over 10% of dislocations, although fortunately most recover.

Avascular necrosis of the femoral head is common, appearing within 12 months of the injury in 10% of cases. Heterotopic ossification can also occur.

Osteoarthritis is a late complication.

ANTERIOR DISLOCATION

The history is similar, but the limb lies *abducted, externally rotated* and *slightly flexed*. The femoral head is usually seen and felt bulging anteriorly.

Complications

Femoral vein thrombosis, arterial injury and femoral nerve damage are associated complications.

CENTRAL DISLOCATION

This occurs when a fall or blow on the greater trochanter drives the femoral head through the acetabular floor, causing a pelvic fracture (see Chapter 9).

Fractures of the femoral shaft

These are usually caused by high-energy injuries such as road traffic accidents and are most common in young male adults. In elderly individuals, a pathological fracture must always be considered, especially if the force involved seems insignificant. Fractures can also occur around the prosthesis of hip and knee replacements in this age group. Open fractures occur when the skin is breached by sharpened bone ends or by penetrating injuries.

History

There is severe *thigh pain* and an *inability to weight bear.*

Examination

The thigh is very *swollen*, and *all movements are painful*. The leg is often *shortened, abducted* and *externally rotated.* There may be significant blood loss into the thigh, and there may be signs of *hypovolaemic shock.*

Complications

Complications are shown in the Revision panel 8.7.

Revision panel 8.7

COMPLICATION OF FRACTURES OF THE FEMORAL SHAFT

- Neurovascular injury
- Infection
- Fat embolus
- Venous thromboembolism
- Joint stiffness
- Delayed union
- Malunion
- Non-union

Supracondylar fractures of the femur

These follow falls in elderly osteoporotic females and direct injury in young males involved in high-speed traffic accidents. A previous knee arthroplasty is also a risk factor.

The fracture can be extra- or intracapsular and may involve one or both condyles.

History

The knee is painful, and the patient notices swelling and deformity in and around the knee.

Examination

The knee is tender and swollen, and all movements are painful and restricted. Weight-bearing is usually impossible. The distal pulses must be carefully palpated as injuries to the popliteal artery are common (see Chapter 10).

Fractures of the knee, ankle and foot

FRACTURES OF THE SHAFTS OF THE TIBIA AND FIBULA

Fractures of the tibia shaft are often associated with high-energy trauma such as road traffic collisions but can also be frequently seen in lower-energy mechanisms, for example field sports. It is very subcutaneous, which increases the risk of associated skin damage, leading to an open fracture.

The mechanisms of injury can include twisting, for example in football or skiing (spiral fractures of both tibia and fibula), or direct blows with angulation (transverse, segmental, comminuted or oblique fractures) in road traffic collisions or falls from heights.

History

This is of pain, deformity and an inability to weight bear or walk.

Examination

Bruising, local tenderness, swelling and angulation or rotational deformity are all possibly present. The skin, nerves and pulses must all be very carefully examined.

Complications

Compartment syndrome is the commonest most serious early complication of this injury and must always be examined for repetitively over the course of the peri-injury period.

Vascular and nerve injuries are less commonly encountered but must be examined for.

Infection is clearly more likely if the fracture was initially an open fracture. Malunion and delayed union can also occur.

FRACTURES OF AND AROUND THE ANKLE

These are common injuries in children, skiers, footballers and rugby players, and are often associated with sprains and dislocations.

They are usually caused by the ankle twisting and the talus rotating within the tibiofibular mortise, resulting in fractures of the ankle bones. The pattern of the fracture depends on two things, the position of the foot at the time of the injury and the direction of the force applied to the ankle. The commonest mechanism is a classic ankle sprain or inversion injury, which commonly sees the distal fibula fractured and, depending on the severity, an associated medial sided injury, with deltoid ligament injury or malleolus fracture. The *Weber classification* is a useful radiological classification depending on the level of the fibular fracture and can also be a guide to the mechanism of injury. Distal to the syndesmosis is type A, usually with ankle inversion; level with the syndesmosis is type B and above the syndesmosis is type C, usually with ankle eversion (Figure 8.48).

Occasionally, a more complex fracture of the ankle can occur with a high-energy mechanism of a twist, impact or fall and causes a pilon (hammer) fracture, in which the articular surface of the tibia and fibula possibly, becomes comminuted.

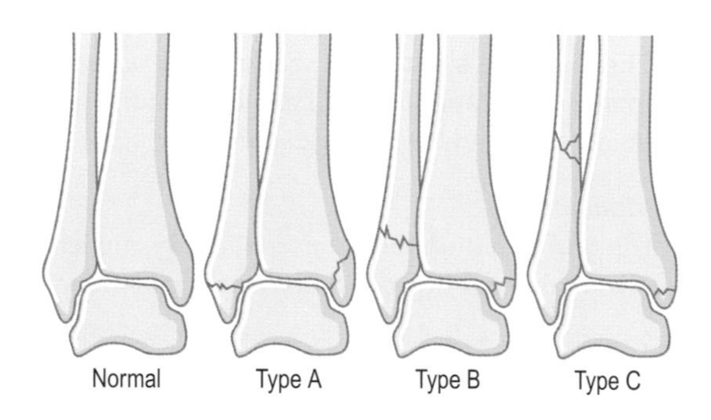

Figure 8.48 The Weber classification of fractures around the ankle.

History

Pain and inability to weight bear follow an ankle injury.

Examination

The ankle is swollen and very tender. Deformity suggests that there is a fracture or dislocation. In a dislocation it is important to ensure the skin around the ankle does not have a compromised blood flow due to pressure on the skin from the underlying bone. Tenderness is maximal over the fracture sites at the ankle. However, tenderness may also be felt higher up the fibula because of a further fracture (*Maisonneuve fracture*), indicating a likely eversion mechanism of injury.

Complications

These include pain, instability, stiffness, malunion and late OA.

ANKLE DISLOCATION

This is usually invariably associated with an ankle fracture. Pure dislocation of the ankle in the absence of a bony injury is exceedingly unusual.

FRACTURES OF THE TALUS AND CALCANEUM

These fractures are often associated with other foot injuries or fractures, and the whole of the foot, its nerves and its blood vessels must always be carefully examined.

Fractures of these bones are often caused by falls from a height or other high-energy mechanisms, for example road traffic collisions, where the foot is traumatized in vehicle footwell at the time of impact. Other fractures of the spine, pelvis or hip may be an association in a polytrauma victim.

Calcaneal fractures are more common than talar fractures.

As the talus articulates in three joints – the ankle joint (tibia/fibula), the subtalar joint (calcaneus) and the talonavicular joint (navicular bone) – injuries can have significant long-term implications.

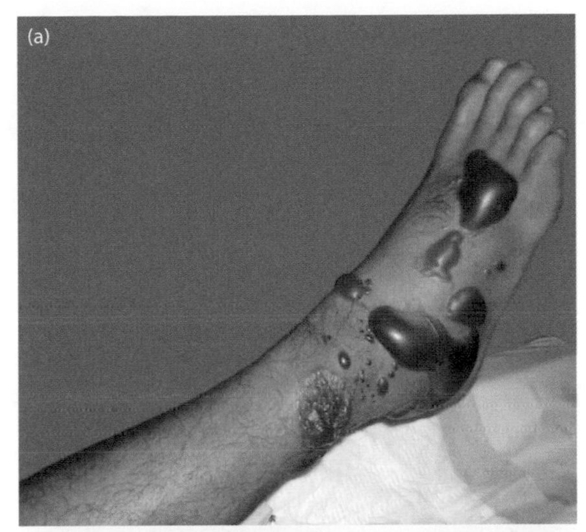

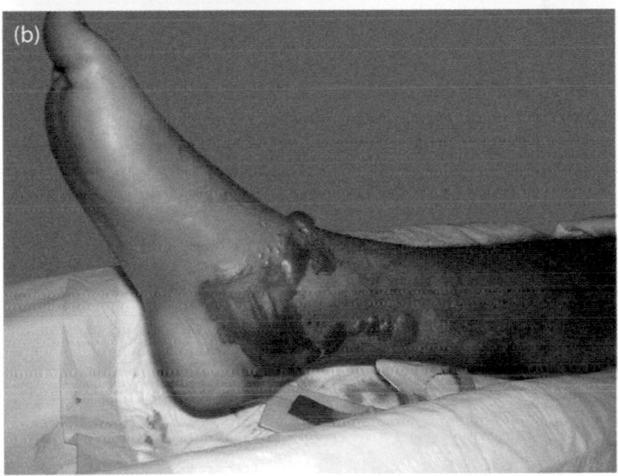

Figure 8.49 Heel deformities caused by calcaneal fractures with associated fracture blisters.

History

The history of the accident may be suggestive, and the ankle and foot are usually painful and swollen. Weight-bearing is painful and often impossible.

Examination

The foot is usually very swollen and bruised and may be deformed, with the heel appearing broad and squat (Figure 8.49). Movements at the subtalar joint are impossible. The relevant bone is tender.

Complications

These include hindfoot stiffness and pain with avascular necrosis in severe cases and OA. There may be an associated talar or subtalar dislocation but marked swelling often masks the deformity. Skin damage and eventual necrosis may occur over the extruded, displaced talus, hence the need for early manipulation and reduction of the joint.

MID-TARSAL FRACTURES

Fractures of other individual tarsal bones are rare, and when they occur are often associated with a combination of other fractures and dislocations in the foot. One exception to this are stress injuries and fractures of the midtarsal bones, especially the navicular bone in the more athletic population.

History

There is usually a history of severe blunt trauma or crush injury to the foot, which is swollen, bruised and painful.

Examination

A deformity is often present with severe swelling, poor demarcation of normal bony contour and bruising including on the sole of the foot. The whole midfoot is usually extremely tender.

METATARSAL FRACTURES

These can be caused by a direct blow or a twisting force. They are also a common site for stress fractures in army recruits and professional sportsmen, commonly the base of the 5th metatarsal or the shaft of the 2nd metatarsal.

The metatarsal bones as they articulate with the midfoot is also a common site of injury. A fracture at the base of the second metatarsal associated with subluxation or dislocation of the tarsometatarsal joint is known as a *Lisfranc fracture*.

History

There is pain and swelling in the forefoot.

Examination

Localized tenderness over the fracture may be the only sign as the fractures are usually undisplaced. There may be marked swelling. Compartment syndrome may occur. Lisfranc fractures should be carefully examined utilizing clinical assessment and weight-bearing (when possible) radiography, comparing the injured foot to the uninjured foot. Missed Lisfranc injuries are a common cause of post-traumatic foot morbidity.

FRACTURED TOES

These are caused by stubbing, stamping or heavy objects falling on the toes.

Pain, swelling, deformity and local tenderness are suggestive and fractures may be associated with subluxations and dislocations.

FRACTURED SESAMOID BONES

These can be fractured directly, or most commonly by traction with hyperdorsiflexion of the hallux or by a stress phenomenon. Pain is experienced over the bone and is reproduced by digital pressure or hyperextending the great toe. In the acute setting, swelling and bruising can be marked.

Acknowledgements

The contributions of Sam Singh, Diane Back and Jay Smith to this chapter in the fifth edition are gratefully acknowledged.

Spine and pelvis

JASON R HARVEY, GLYN TOWLERTON AND STEVEN A CORBETT

SYMPTOMS OF SPINAL DISORDERS

Spinal problems present with symptoms that fall into two main categories:

- Axial spinal pain, which may be associated with other symptoms such as stiffness.
- Pain and/or neurological dysfunction from compression of neural structures.

Pain can also occur in the absence of compression from inflammation affecting the nerve.

Patients may present with a mixture of axial symptoms and neural symptoms.

Conditions in which these symptoms arise include:

- Mechanical type neck or low back pain.
- Neural compression with radiation to the arm (radicular pain).
- Neural compression with radiation to the leg (radicular pain).
- Cauda equina syndrome.
- Spinal cord compression.

Axial pain can occur throughout the spine; however, this presents more frequently in the lumbar and cervical spine, rather than the thoracic spine. The pain that is generated may be the result of underlying degenerative changes in the bone and joints or arise from the adjacent muscles or ligaments.

The typical features of mechanical back pain are:

- Activity related pain.
- Relieved by rest.
- Absence of systemic symptoms.

On occasion, axial symptoms may be caused by a more serious pathology, which may include:

- Tumours within the spine: benign or malignant; primary or secondary.
- Infection.
- Fracture.

Under these circumstances, the pain may be non-mechanical in nature, such that the patient presents with pain that is:

- Constant and unrelated to movement.
- Not relieved by rest.
- Associated with night pain.
- Associated with systemic symptoms including fever, weight loss or general malaise.

When *neural compression* arises in the cervical spine, pain may radiate into the arm (*brachalgia*), caused by pressure on the nerve root. The pain is experienced in the area supplied by the nerve root and radiates from the neck to that area (*radicular pain*).

If neural compression occurs in the lumbar spine, radicular pain may arise in the lower limbs (*sciatica damage*). Again, the pain is experienced in the area supplied by the nerve root.

Cauda equina can occur when the nerves of the lower spine become compressed. The spinal cord usually terminates at the L1 level in the adult, beneath which is a transitional area known as the *conus medullaris*, where there is a mixture of upper and lower motor neurons. Below this region is the *cauda equina*, consisting of *lower motor neuron nerves*, which carries the nerves to the lower limbs and nerves controlling bladder, bowel and sexual function. The nerves supplying the bladder and bowel function are particularly vulnerable to compressive damage.

Spinal cord compression may cause significant neurological symptoms and signs that vary in severity and rapidity of progression (see Chapter 4). Commonly the compression is caused by degenerative changes in the neck, spondylolytic cervical myelopathy, but other causes include infection or tumours of the spine (see Cervical myelopathy).

Psychosocial elements are known to contribute to disability and pain, and these should always be assessed. These are referred to as yellow flags.

ASSESSMENT OF SPINAL PROBLEMS

The majority of spinal problems are not caused by serious pathology.

Assessment of spinal problems falls into three categories:

- **Emergency** – requiring immediate assessment and investigation.
- **Urgent** – concerning symptoms that do not warrant emergency treatment but cannot wait for routine assessment.
- **Routine assessment.**

The history of the presenting problem should reference pain, stiffness and loss of function. The presence or absence of neurological symptoms is also very important, particularly the degree of any deficit and progressive change.

- *Pain* distribution, the nature, severity and duration of symptoms.
- *Disability* caused by loss of function and stiffness which may result from joint problems, nerve damage or muscular weakness.
- *Deformity* resulting from congenital anatomical or developmental abnormalities, tumours, trauma or wasting.
- *Systemic features* of an underlying disease process or red flag signs (Table 9.1).

Table 9.1 The normal range of movement of the cervical spine

Direction of movement	Range of movement
Flexion/extension	120°
Axial rotation	160°
Lateral flexion	60–70°

EXAMINATION OF THE CERVICAL SPINE

The patient must be undressed appropriately, ideally in a gown that allows the whole spine and both shoulders to be examined.

GAIT PATTERN

Observe the patient walking across the examination room. Look for evidence of *pain, weakness, ataxia* and *specific gait patterns such as foot drop* (causing a high stepping gait) or a *Trendelenburg gait.*

Instruct the patient to walk heel to toe in tandem – this may elicit ataxia and suggest cervical/thoracic myelopathy or neurological diagnosis.

INSPECTION

The head should be held in a neutral position with preservation of the natural cervical lordosis. If the head is held in a different position this may be the result of muscle spasm secondary to a painful condition. If a fixed structural deformity is noted, and the patient looks at the ground, the curvature (kyphosis) may be associated with *ankylosing spondylitis*.

Look for asymmetry including shoulder height, sternocleidomastoid muscle appearance, the clavicles and the supraclavicular fossae, as well as any visible masses or scars indicating previous surgery.

PALPATION

Feel posteriorly from the occiput to the upper thoracic spine, looking for areas of tenderness or any deformity. Note that the most prominent spinous process is T1 and not C7 (vertebra prominens).

Palpate the trapezius region, the shoulders, the clavicles and then the posterior and anterior triangles of the neck, looking for tenderness and masses. Assess the thyroid, larynx and supraclavicular fossae.

RANGE OF MOVEMENT

Test actively, asking the patient to move their head, and then passively, in which you hold the head gently and move the cervical spine. Try to differentiate between active movement limited by pain and passive movement limited less by pain than by intrinsic stiffness of the cervical column.

Specific signs

Spurling's sign (Figure 9.1)

The head is extended and rotated towards the side of the patient's symptoms, and simultaneous gentle downward compression is applied to the head. The test is positive if the patient's pain is reproduced and radiates down the arm.

A positive Spurling's sign indicates cervical radiculopathy from nerve compression.

L'Hermitte's sign

On sudden flexion or hyperextension of the neck, an electric shock sensation passes down into the upper and lower limbs. This is the result of cord compression and can be caused by large disc herniation or degenerative changes.

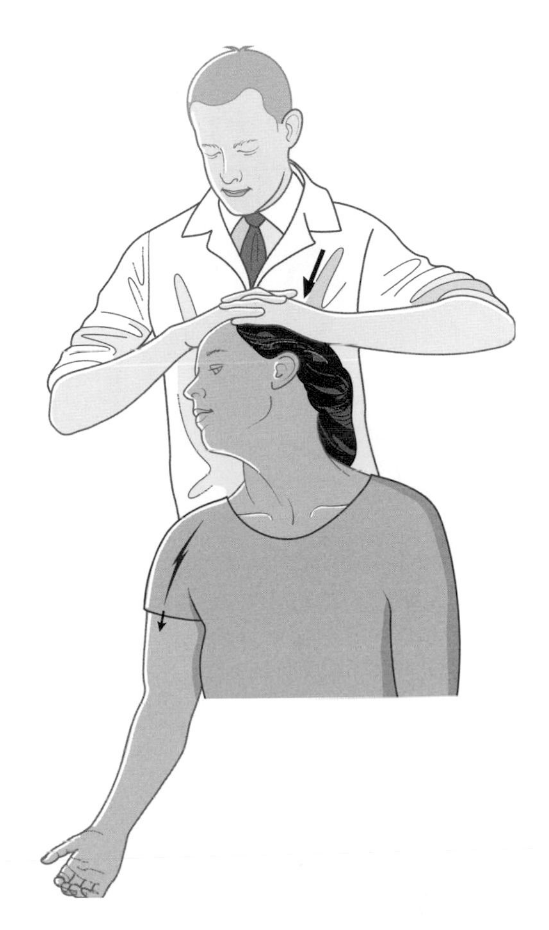

Figure 9.1 Spurling's sign.

Other systems

Where symptoms are thought to originate from the cervical spine, an examination of the shoulders and a full neurological examination of the upper and lower limbs must be carried out (see Chapter 3).

Common conditions of the cervical spine

CERVICAL AXIAL MECHANICAL TYPE NECK PAIN

This is the most common symptom arising from the cervical spine.

Age It occurs in adults, more commonly over the age of 45 years.

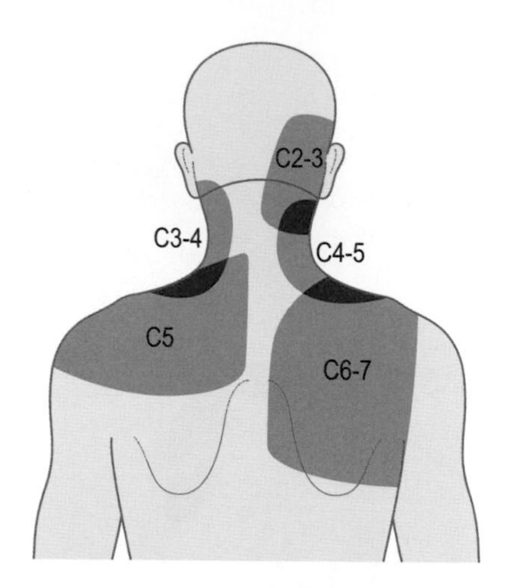

Figure 9.2 This illustrates the sites where pain is perceived from the cervical spine. The commonest origin for pain is the C5/6 and C6/7 levels with the pain felt across the shoulders and in the interscapular region, significantly below the cervical spine.

Site The pain is situated in the midline, radiating into the shoulders and down into the interscapular region of the thoracic spine, but not into the arms (Figure 9.2), unless there is also nerve compression.

Precipitating factors There may be no history of trauma.

Pain The pain is variable in intensity. There is rarely pain at night, but patients may complain of difficulty in getting to sleep.

Stiffness This is usually worse in the morning, improves on movement, but may be exacerbated by being in one position for prolonged periods of time, commonly experienced with laptop computer use.

WHIPLASH INJURY

This is a combination of a *hyperextension* and a *hyperflexion injury* of the cervical spine, usually as a consequence of being hit from behind in a motor vehicle accident.

Symptoms Patients may present immediately or 2–3 days later with neck pain, neck stiffness, occipital headaches and occasionally neurological symptoms in the upper limbs. Approximately *one quarter of patients develop chronic pain* that lasts for longer than 2 years, severe in a one-third of cases.

Examination There are no significant abnormal signs except some stiffness.

Differential diagnosis Significant injury to bones or joints needs to be excluded by appropriate investigations.

ACUTE CERVICAL INTERVERTEBRAL DISC PROLAPSE

Age and sex This is most common in the fourth decade, and slightly more common in males than females (1.4:1).

Level It most commonly occurs at the C5/6 disc level followed by C6/7 and then C4/5.

Symptoms There is *acute neck pain,* either generalized and diffuse in a mesodermal distribution, or with localized and specific pain in a nerve root distribution.

Radiculopathy and myelopathy are defined in Revision panel 9.1. There are usually no precipitating factors. Diffuse neck pain and stiffness is followed by more specific pain in a radicular pattern down one arm, sometimes into the hand. This may be severe and be associated with sensory loss and muscle weakness with decreased or absent motor reflexes. Associated myelopathy is rare but must be excluded by history and examination.

Natural history The majority of cases resolve within 3 months.

See also Chapter 3.

Revision panel 9.1

DEFINITION OF RADICULOPATHY AND MYELOPATHY

Radiculopathy: An extradural compression of a nerve resulting in a degree of pain, sensory loss, weakness and motor reflex changes, in the distribution of a spinal nerve (lower motor neuron signs).

Myelopathy: A dysfunction of the spinal cord itself caused by compression of the spinal cord producing the symptoms and signs of an upper motor neuron lesion.

CERVICAL SPONDYLOSIS AND SPONDYLITIC CERVICAL MYELOPATHY

Cervical spondylosis

Definition Cervical spondylosis is the term used to describe *degeneration of the intervertebral discs with degenerative osteoarthritis of the facet and intravertebral joints.*

Age and sex It is most common in patients aged over 50 years, although the spine begins to 'age' from the late teens, equally in males and females.

Level It is most common at the C5/6 disc level, followed by C6/7 and then C4/5.

Symptoms There is *midline neck pain* exacerbated by movement, with diffuse radiation to the shoulder, the area between the shoulder blades and the upper arms. There is associated neck stiffness, which may interfere with driving.

Night pain is not usually a major feature, although patients may complain that they find it difficult to get comfortable in order to go to sleep. They may also wake in the morning with increased neck pain and stiffness. This improves once they get up and mobilize.

Natural history The condition is usually self limiting, although some patients have episodic periods of neck pain, lasting from a few weeks to a few months, and continuing for years. A few develop significant chronic neck pain.

Spondylitic cervical radiculopathy

As the degenerative process proceeds, radiculopathy may develop caused by stenosis of the exit foramina caused by a combination of osteophytes, disc prolapse and ligamentum flavum and facet joint hypertrophy.

Spondylitic cervical myelopathy

Progressive spondylitic pathology can lead to central spinal canal stenosis and the development of a myelopathy (see Revision panel 9.1) as the spinal cord is compressed. This can be dynamic, when cord compression occurs only, or is increased, on movement. Instability of the spine may contribute to this.

Damage to the cord may lead to myelomalacia.

History

Patients complain of *clumsiness* and *dysaesthesia (abnormal sensation) of the hands,* with a loss of fine motor function. They cannot do up buttons satisfactorily, write neatly or use a keyboard. They may have associated neck pain and stiffness.

There may be a disturbance of gait, with a sense of unsteadiness. They feel a need to look at their feet on walking, with a loss of walking distance as the legs tire easily. This is caused by loss of proprioception followed by loss of motor function.

Natural history The progression of symptoms is variable, in some patients progressing very slowly, whist in others it can be rapid.

THORACIC OUTLET SYNDROME: CERVICAL RIB SYNDROME

Cause The cause may be a *cervical rib,* an associated *fibrous band* or hypertrophy of the scalenus anterior muscle compressing the subclavian artery and/or the brachial plexus, especially the T1 nerve root.

Cervical ribs occur in about 0.4% of the population (70% being bilateral), but only 60% are symptomatic (see Chapter 10).

Symptoms There is *pain* and *numbness of the arm and hand,* with *weakness of grip,* especially on prolonged carrying of heavy bags. It is made worse on abduction of the shoulder.

Vascular symptoms (axillary vein thrombosis, Raynaud's phenomenon, subclavian aneurysm) are also common (see Chapter 10). The presentation is occasionally with a lump in the neck caused by the cervical rib.

Signs There may be a palpable cervical rib in the supraclavicular fossa (see Chapter 12), decreased vascular supply to the hand, or signs of T1 nerve root compression (see Chapter 3).

Adson's test (Figure 9.3) The patient extends and turns the neck towards the affected side while abducting and extending the shoulder with the elbow in extension. This results after a few minutes in a loss of the radial pulse and an exacerbation of the patient's symptoms. Returning the neck and shoulder to the neutral position restores the pulse and relieves the symptoms.

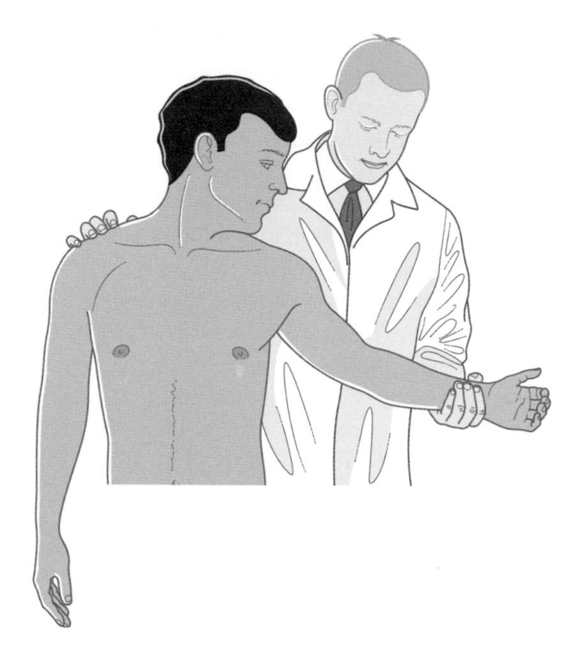

Figure 9.3 Adson's test for thoracic outlet syndrome.

Allen's test (Figure 9.4) This is similar to Adson's test, but the patient turns the neck away from the affected side while abducting and externally rotating the shoulder.

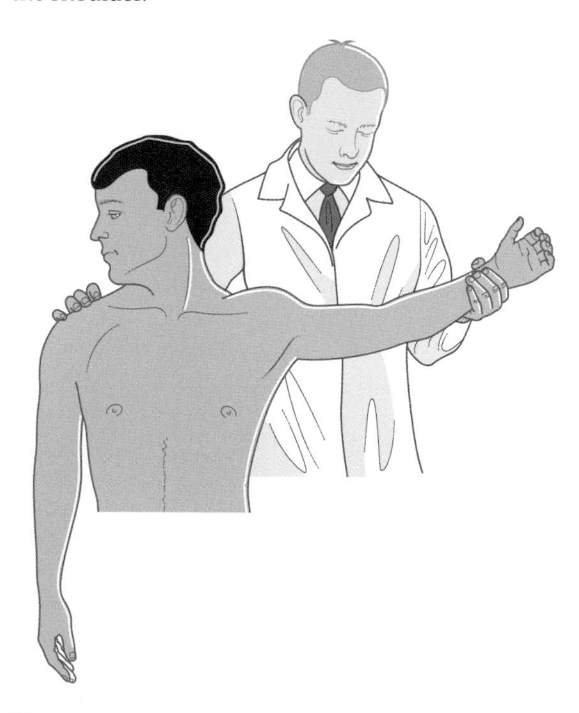

Figure 9.4 Allen's test for thoracic outlet syndrome.

Roos test. The patient is in a seated position and abducts both shoulders to 90° with the elbows flexed at 90°. The patient then open closes the hands for 3 minutes. A positive result is the reproduction of pain or paresthesia, often before the time period is complete. Symptoms are relieved by dropping the arms.

> **NOTE:** *Adson's, Allen's and Roos tests are relatively unreliable,* with both false-positive and false-negative results.

RHEUMATOID ARTHRITIS OF THE CERVICAL SPINE

Chronic, systemic autoimmune disease characterized by inflammation and destruction of the synovial joints. There may be *atlantoaxial subluxation, vertical subluxation of the second cervical vertebra* with cranial settling *(basilar invagination), or subaxial subluxation.*

Symptoms Patients present with *progressive neck pain and stiffness*. In advanced disease, cervical myelopathy (see above) may develop, but with modern treatment this is rare.

Examination of the thoracolumbar–sacral spine

The patient must be adequately undressed with exposure of the whole spine and lower limbs.

GAIT PATTERN

Look for an *antalgic gait* in which the stance phase of gait is shortened relative to the swing phase. This indicates pain on weight-bearing.

Observe any neurological deficit, such as muscle wasting or a foot drop. Heel walking may reveal a subtle weakness of tibialis anterior (L4) or extensor hallucis longus (L5), toe walking weakness of triceps surae (S1/2).

INSPECTION

View the whole spine from behind, looking for *scars*, any cutaneous stigmata of underlying spinal dysraphism such as a *hairy naevus*, a *sinus* or a *sacral dimple* indicating any underlying spinal dysraphism, for example, spina bifida. Look for any *café-au-lait spots* indicating neurofibromatosis (see Chapter 4).

Alignment

Is there a scoliosis or kyphosis (Figure 9.5)? Minor deformities are not immediately obvious. Look from the side with the patient's hips and knees in full extension to assess the sagittal plane and the presence of a kyphosis. Inspect the coronal plane from the front and back. Check the position of the shoulders. Are the scapulae and the loin creases symmetrical? Is the pelvis level?

Adam's forward bending test The patient is asked to lean forward with their arms hanging down in front of them in a relaxed and comfortable position. This will reveal more clearly any scoliosis or kyphosis (Figure 9.6).

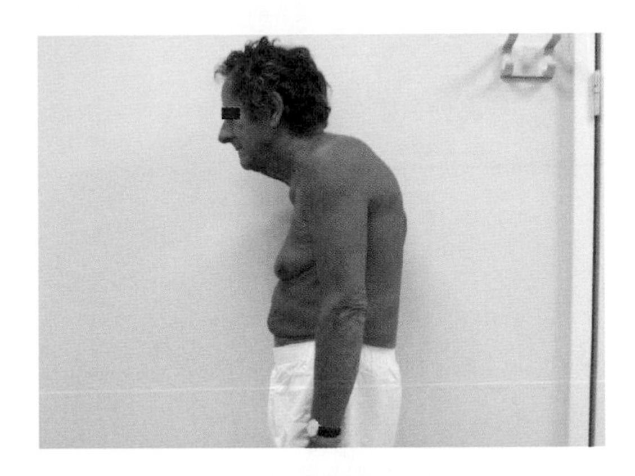

Figure 9.5 Inspection of the spine. This illustrates quite marked thoracic kyphosis in a patient with ankylosing spondylitis, with characteristic compensatory hyperextension of the neck to allow a forward horizontal gaze.

RANGE OF MOVEMENT

The bulk of forward flexion and extension on bending forwards and backwards is at the hips, so methods are needed to differentiate this from true spinal flexion and extension.

For thoracic flexion, hold a tape measure with the ends on the spines of T1 and L1, and note the increased length when the patient bends forwards from the standing into the fully flexed position. This is normally around 8 cm. A similar measurement from L1 to S1 should show an increase of 8–10 cm. Less than 3 cm indicates significant pathology.

Schober's test (Figure 9.7) Marks are made 10 cm above and 5 cm below the line that connects the two posterior superior iliac spines. On maximum forward bending, the distance should increase by 8–10 cm. Less than 3 cm indicates significant pathology.

Lateral flexion Ask the patient to run their hand down the lateral aspect of the thigh as far as they are able. The normal is approximately 30° of lateral flexion.

Rotation should be tested in the sitting position. The maximum range of thoracic and lumbar rotation

(a)

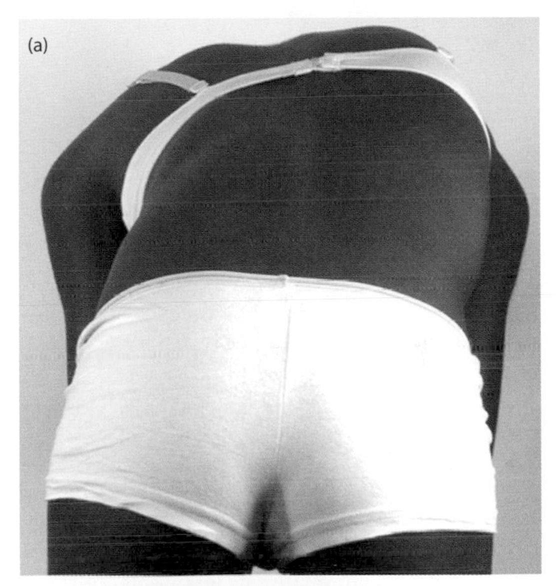

(b)

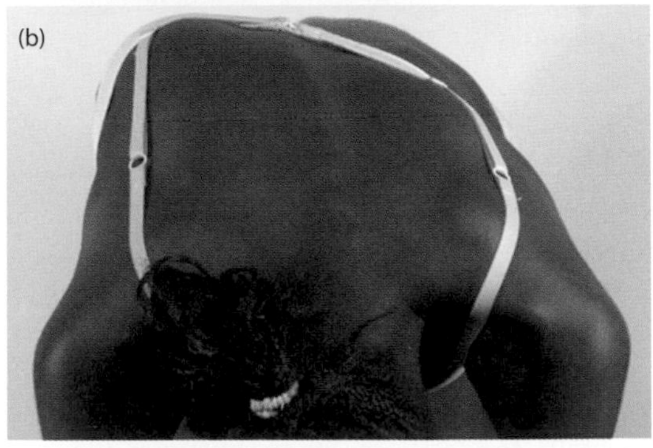

Figure 9.6 ADAM'S FORWARD BENDING TEST. (a, b) This illustrates the rib hump that is characteristic of a right thoracic scoliosis.

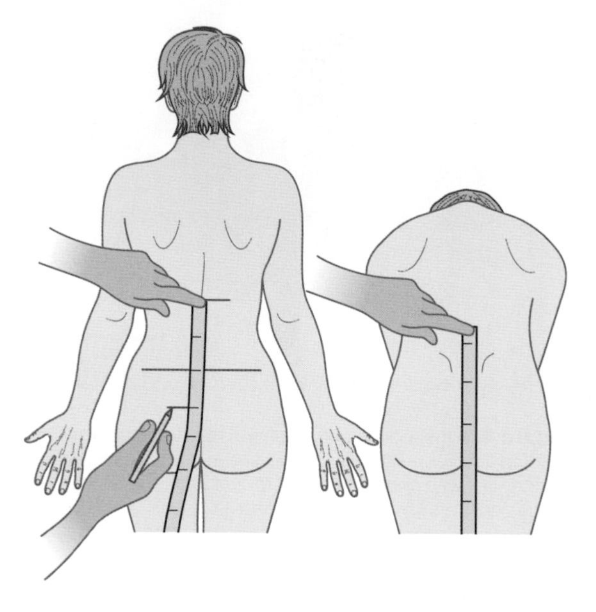

Figure 9.7 Schober's test.

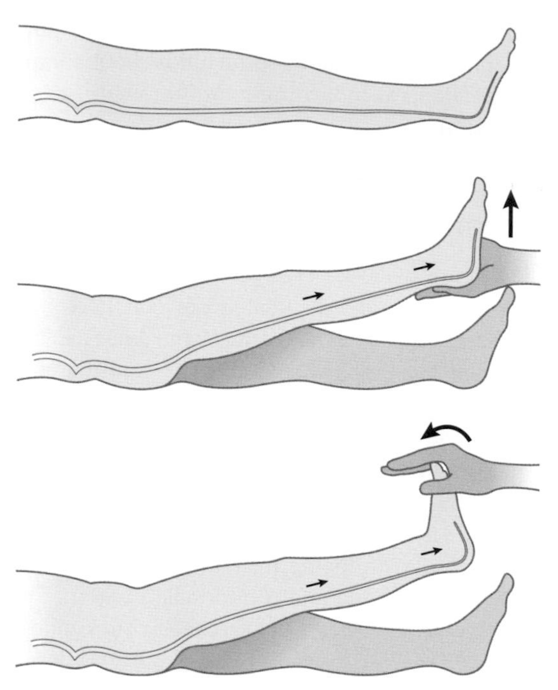

Figure 9.8 The sciatic stretch (Lasègue) test.

is approximately 40°, largely occurring in the thoracic spine, with only 5° coming from the lumbar spine.

Chest expansion Place a tape measure under the axillae. Expansion should be at least 6 cm; less than 2.5 cm is abnormal. A common cause for loss of expansion is ankylosing spondylitis.

PALPATION

Feel from T1 to the sacrum, looking for tenderness of the spine itself and the paravertebral muscles. Is there continuity of the spinous processes and the interspinous and supraspinous ligaments, or *is there a step indicating a spondylolisthesis?*

LOWER LIMB TENSION SIGNS

These are tests for radiculopathies of the lumbar and S1 nerve roots, caused by neural compression.

Sciatic stretch (Lasègue) test (Figure 9.8) With the patient lying supine, the leg is lifted until prevented by pain in a radicular distribution, that is exacerbated by dorsiflexing the ankle. If the leg can be raised above 50°, the test loses its specificity as the cause may be tight hamstring muscles.

It is known as the *bowstring sign,* if the pain is relieved by flexing the knee which suggests nerve root irritation at the L4, L5 or S1 level, caused by lower lumbar disc prolapse.

Frajersztajn's sign Raising the leg on the symptomless side reproduces the radicular pain on the affected side. This may indicate central disc prolapse, characteristically at the L4/5 level.

Femoral stretch test (Figure 9.9) The patient lies prone, and the knee is flexed and the hip extended. This tenses the femoral nerve. There is likely to be an upper lumbar radiculopathy if the radicular pain is produced down the front of the thigh in the L2-L4 distribution.

HIP AND LEG LENGTH

Leg length discrepancy is the most common cause of a functional (non-structural) scoliosis with a tilted pelvis, present only when the patient stands. It is corrected when the patient sits down and is confirmed by measuring the leg lengths (see Chapter 8).

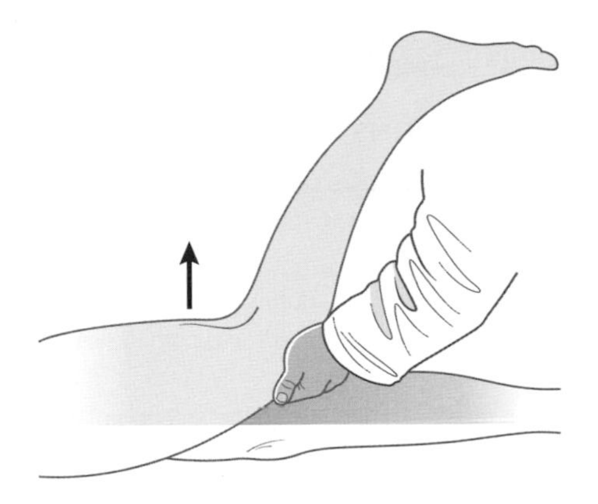

Figure 9.9 The femoral stretch test.

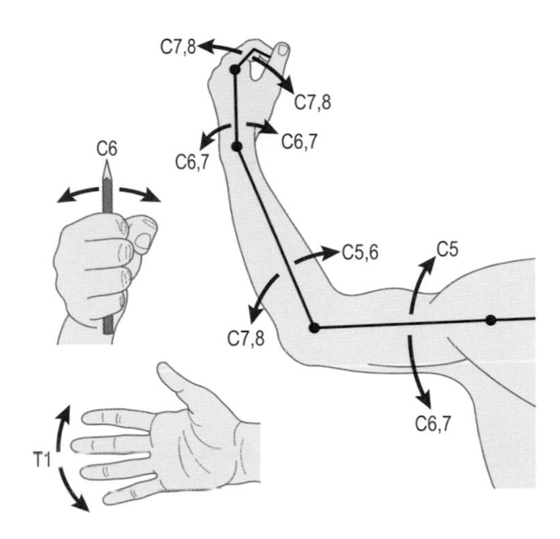

Hip examination is essential. Pain arising from the hip may mimic pain from the spine and vice versa.

NEUROLOGICAL EXAMINATION

Inspection reveals asymmetry or *muscle wasting*. *Tone* is assessed, followed by testing sensation for *light touch*, *pinprick*, *vibration* and *proprioception*, and then assessment of motor function. Finally, the reflexes are tested.

The dermatomes are shown in Figure 3.36 and the myotomes in Figure 9.10.

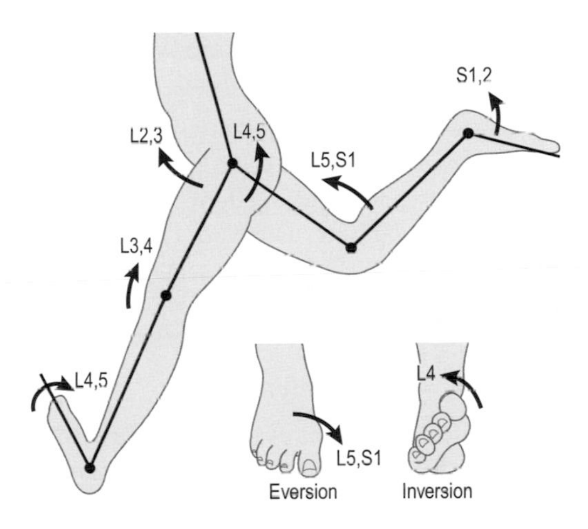

Figure 9.10 The upper and lower limb myotomes.

Rectal examination

If a cauda equina syndrome is suspected, a rectal examination is mandatory to assess the function of the S2, S3 and S4 nerve roots, which control bladder, bowel and sexual function.

There are four components:

- Assessment of *perianal light touch sensation*.
- Assessment of *perianal pinprick sensation*; may be altered in cauda equina syndrome.
- Anal sphincter digital examination to assess resting anal tone and voluntary anal contraction. In cauda equina syndrome, the *resting anal tone* is decreased or absent, with decreased or absent voluntary contraction.
- Assessment of the *bulbocavernosus reflex* (Figure 9.11). In the catheterized patient, a sharp tug on the urinary catheter produces contraction of the anal sphincter detected by an examining finger within the anus. This reflex is absent in cauda equina syndrome. It is also absent in spinal shock, and its return indicates resolution of the condition.

ABDOMINAL AND VASCULAR EXAMINATIONS

These are essential to exclude intra-abdominal pathology as a cause for back pain, and arterial ischaemia as a cause of lower limb pain (see Chapters 10 and 15).

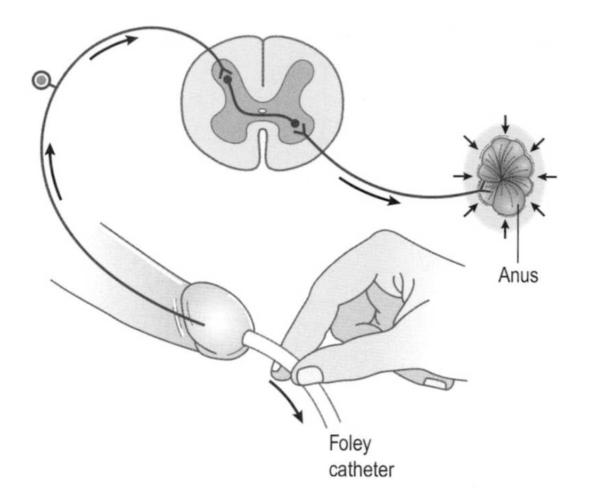

Figure 9.11 The bulbocavernosus reflex.

Revision panel 9.2

RED FLAG SIGNS FOR LOW BACK PAIN

Age – below 20 years or above 50 years
A history of significant trauma
Thoracic pain
Non-mechanical pain, namely a constant pain not related to movement and sometimes worse at night
A past medical history of cancer, steroid use, intravenous drug abuse or HIV infection
Being systemically unwell
A history of weight loss
Lumbar flexion less than 5 cm
Neurological deficit
Structural spinal deformity

Common conditions of the thoracolumbar–sacral spine

BACK PAIN

Each year, one-half of the UK population have an episode of back pain, and one-tenth of the population seek medical advice. There are three important groups:

- Simple back pain.
- Radicular pain.
- Potentially serious pathology.

The Clinical Standards Advisory Group for Back Pain has produced a set of criteria for the identification of patients presenting with low back pain who may have serious pathology. These are called the 'red flag signs' and are listed in Revision panel 9.2.

Low back pain

Definition This is pain *lasting for more than 24 hours, located between the lowest ribs and the inferior gluteal fold,* and arising from the spine. It does not radiate into the legs, and there are no neurological symptoms or signs.

Age The patient is usually between 20 and 55 years old.

Character It is mechanical in nature, namely in that it varies with activity and time. In other words, it 'comes and goes'.

Causes The causes are complex and myriad, but the most common factor is degeneration. Other causes of the pain (listed in Revision panel 9.3), must however, be excluded.

ACUTE PROLAPSED INTERVERTEBRAL DISC

Incidence Symptomatic lumbar intervertebral disc herniation affects 2% of the population at some time.

Symptoms There is back pain lasting for some weeks that lessens in severity and is replaced by leg pain radiating to below the knee. This is often described as *sciatica,* which is a radicular pain in the L4, L5 or S1 distribution, sometimes with associated neurological symptoms.

The pain *may be very severe,* exacerbated by sitting, standing and coughing, with *shooting pain down the leg.* It is relieved to a degree by changing position and walking but walking too far can further exacerbate the symptoms.

Specific enquiries Ask if there is any perineal sensory loss *(saddle anaesthesia)* or loss of normal bladder and bowel control. This may indicate cauda equina syndrome and must always be asked about.

Revision panel 9.3

CAUSES OF LOW BACK PAIN

Spondylogenic

- Degenerative:
  - Disc
  - Facet joint
  - Vertebral bodies
- Tumour:
  - Benign
  - Malignant – primary or secondary
- Sepsis:
  - Pyogenic
  - Tuberculosis
  - Fungal
  - Yeast
- Metabolic:
  - Osteoporosis
  - Paget's disease

Neurogenic

- Nerve root (radicular):
  - Disc
  - Stenosis – central, posterolateral, foraminal
- Cauda equina syndrome – often prolapsed intervertebral disc causing compression of the cauda equina but can be due to other causes, e.g. tumour or abscess

Viscogenic

- Renal
- Retroperitoneal, e.g. pancreatic
- Bowel

Vascular

- Abdominal aortic aneurysm

SYMPTOMATIC THORACIC DISC HERNIATION

This is a rare condition, affecting only one person per million per year. Symptoms include thoracic pain, burning sensations, and numbness and paraesthesia in the trunk and down the legs. There may be a full-scale myelopathy as a result of spinal cord compression (see above).

CAUDA EQUINA SYNDROME

Definition This is compression of the cauda equina leading to compromise of the nerve supply to the sphincters of the bladder and bowel.

Cause The cause is commonly *a massive central disc herniation*.

Symptoms There is usually *severe pain radiating down to the perineum*, although pain is not invariably present. This is followed by an inability to pass urine and impaired faecal continence.

Signs There is *perineal sensory loss*, a *palpable bladder* as a result of painless urinary retention, *laxity and weakness of the anal sphincter* and absence of the *bulbocavernosus reflex*.

Unless treated rapidly, the urinary and anal sphincters will not recover. *Cauda equina syndrome is therefore a surgical emergency*.

DEGENERATIVE SPINAL STENOSIS PRESENTING WITH NEUROGENIC CLAUDICATION

Degenerative changes within the lumbar spine lead to narrowing of the spinal canal, termed spinal stenosis. This may lead to *neurogenic claudication*.

Age Patients are usually over the age of 50 years.

Symptoms There is usually *low back pain* and stiffness. On walking, the pain radiates down into the legs, and may be associated with *numbness* and *paraesthesia in the feet*. Sometimes there is actual weakness of the feet, with a tendency to trip.

Neurological examination is usually normal except for the *absence of the ankle jerks*.

Relieving factors The pain may be eased to a degree by leaning forwards. The cross-sectional area of the spinal canal is increased in flexion, so the stenosis is lessened, which reduces the symptoms. Patients may say that pushing a supermarket trolley is helpful as it allows them to lean forwards with support.

Differentiation from vascular claudication The pain is relieved by resting or sitting down in both conditions. In neurogenic claudication, the symptoms recede slowly over 5–10 minutes before the patient can continue walking, and this is further improved by leaning forwards or squatting. In vascular intermittent claudication, the recovery time is much less: 1–2 minutes.

The ankle–brachial pressure index is invariably reduced in vascular claudication (see Chapter 10), but it should be remembered that the two conditions can coexist.

SPINAL DEFORMITY – SCOLIOSIS AND KYPHOSIS

Scoliosis

Scoliosis is a lateral curvature of the spine. It may be *structural* or *functional*.

A structural scoliosis is a *fixed deformity of the spine associated with a rotational deformity of the vertebral bodies*. The curvature may have some flexibility, but it cannot be corrected by a change in position (Figure 9.12).

A *functional scoliosis (Figure 9.13) is a curvature of the spine that is not associated with any rotational abnormality of the vertebral body*. It is more accurately described as a tilt or list of the spine and is corrected by sitting or lying down. The most common cause is a discrepancy in leg length.

Functional scoliosis may also occur when there is a painful lesion within the spine, such as an acute prolapsed intervertebral disc or osteoid osteoma that causes the spine to be held at an angle. The scoliosis may become fixed and structural if the source of pain is not removed.

The many causes of structural scoliosis are listed in Revision panel 9.4.

Scoliosis may be *congenital, idiopathic* or *neuromuscular*. The congenital variety may be associated with structural abnormalities of the vertebrae such as hemivertebrae or a failure of segmentation under the influence of the homeobox genes. Associated abnormalities of the genitourinary system or heart are common. Early onset idiopathic scoliosis is more common in males, while late onset (adolescent) idiopathic scoliosis is significantly more common in females.

Kyphosis

In the normal spine, there is a lordosis in the cervical and lumbar spines, and kyphosis in the thoracic

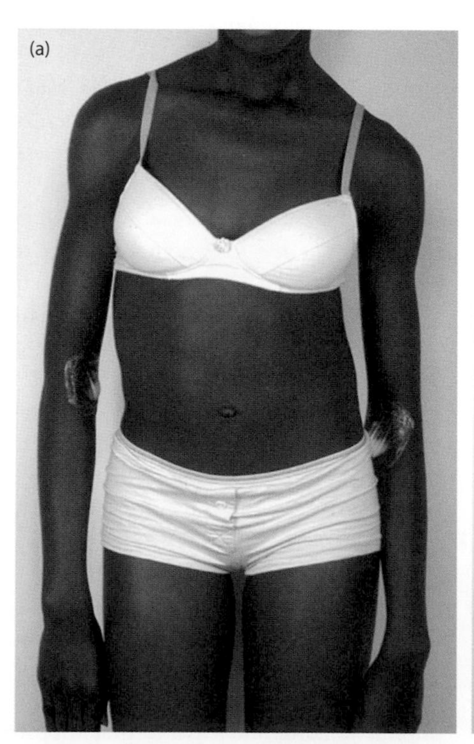

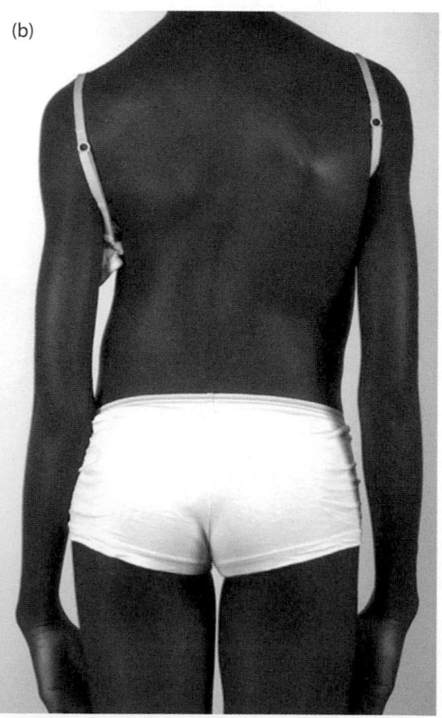

Figure 9.12 INSPECTION OF THE ALIGNMENT OF THE SPINE. (a) Showing bend to right. (b) Showing scoliosis with spine deviating in midthoracic region, to the right.

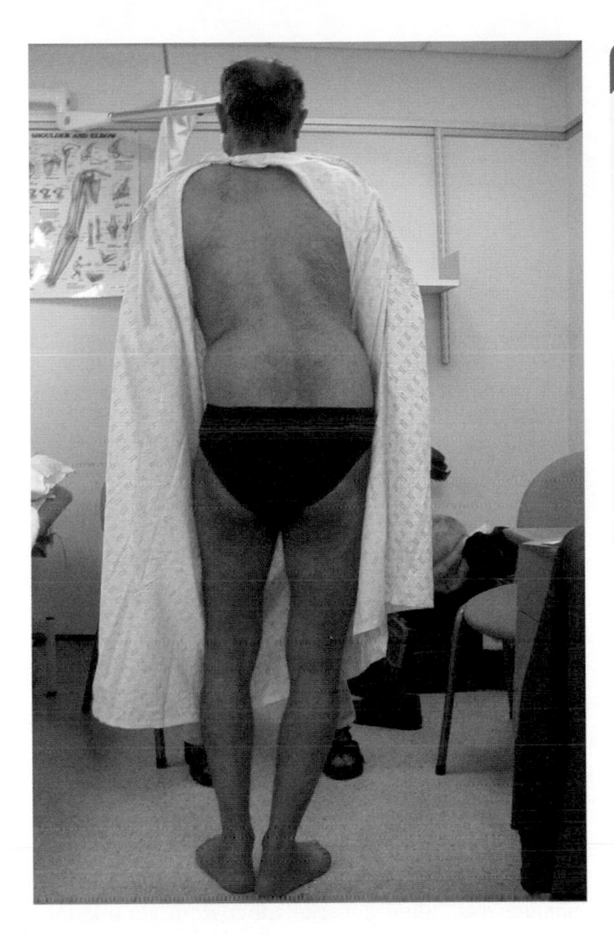

Figure 9.13 A patient with a functional scoliosis.

spine. A plumb line from the odontoid peg passes through the bodies of C7 and L1, and the posterior junction of the L5 and S1 vertebral bodies. The normal thoracic kyphosis is between 20° and 45°, and increases marginally with age to 55°, measured from T4 to T12. The lumbar lordosis is between 40° and 60°, measured from T12 to S1.

The most common sagittal plane deformity is an increase in thoracic kyphosis and a loss of lumbar lordosis. This causes increasing back pain with a positive sagittal balance (anterior position of the head in relation to the pelvis as the body tilts forwards) and fatigue on walking.

Severe kyphosis can lead to significant spinal cord compromise and the development of a progressive neurological deficit. Monitoring is essential.

Symptoms *Patients complain principally of their appearance*. Other symptoms are back pain,

Revision panel 9.4

CAUSES OF STRUCTURAL SCOLIOSIS

Idiopathic

Early onset under 5 years old
Late onset over 5 years old

Congenital

A failure of either formation or segmentation of the vertebral body, or a combination of the two

Neuromuscular

Neuropathic

Upper motor neuron:
- Cerebral palsy
- Spinal cerebellar atrophy, e.g. Friedrich's ataxia

Lower motor neuron:
- Poliomyelitis
- Spinal muscular atrophy
- Meningomyelocele – spina bifida

Myopathic

Arthrogryposis
Muscular dystrophy, e.g. Duchenne

Neurofibromatosis

Mesenchymal disorders

Marfan's syndrome
Ehlers–Danlos syndrome

Trauma

Post-traumatic deformities

Osteochondrodystrophies

Achondroplasia
Mucopolysaccharidoses, e.g. Morquio's syndrome

Spinal column sepsis

Tumours

Osteoid osteoma
Histiocytosis X

Metabolic

Rickets
Osteogenesis imperfecta
Homocystinuria

a sensation of leaning forwards, difficulty looking forwards, a sense of abdominal constriction and the need to use a stick to assist in holding themselves upright when standing or walking.

The most common causes of kyphosis in young people are *Scheuermann's disease* (osteochondritis of the spine), *ankylosing spondylitis* and *trauma*. In the older age groups, *degenerative changes* and *osteoporotic wedge compression fractures* are more common (Revision panel 9.5).

Revision panel 9.5

CAUSES OF SPINAL KYPHOSIS

Traumatic

Compression fractures

Iatrogenic

Postsurgical laminectomy
Post irradiation

Inflammatory disorders

Rheumatoid arthritis
Ankylosing spondylitis

Infectious

Pyogenic
Tuberculosis

Scheuermann's kyphosis

Degenerative conditions

Osteoarthritis
Osteoporotic wedge compression fractures
Paget's disease

Congenital

Failure of formation or segmentation, or a combination of the two

Neoplastic

Primary tumours
Metastatic tumours
Multiple myeloma

Skeletal dysplasias

Achondrodysplasia
Pseudoachondrodysplasia

A localized kyphosis with a prominent angle is termed a *kyphus*.

Scheuermann's disease

Definition This is an osteochondritis of the spine, which may cause wedging of the vertebrae and consequently a kyphosis, as a result of uneven growth of the vertebrae. It is self-limiting.

Age usually presents in teenagers.

Symptoms Patients experience pain in the lower–mid back regions, which can be severe and disabling. The pain is often worse on exercise. Patients may have a loss of height due to the kyphosis.

Natural history The cause is unknown; however, the condition is self-limiting.

SPONDYLOLISTHESIS AND SPONDYLOLYSIS

Spondylolisthesis

This is a *forward slip of one vertebra in relation to the vertebra below*. The causes are listed in Table 9.2.

Symptoms and signs *Eighty per cent of cases are symptomless*. Some patients suffer from chronic low back pain and notice tightening of the hamstring muscles. It is rare to develop radiculopathy or cauda equina syndrome.

On palpation, *a step in the spinous processes at the appropriate level may be detectable*, although this is an unreliable sign.

Spondylolysis

A spondylolysis is a *break in the pars interarticularis*, usually of the L5 vertebral body without a forward slip. The most common cause is a stress fracture of the L5 pars interarticularis.

Age There is a bimodal age presentation of symptoms.

The younger age group (8–15 years) presents with back pain made worse by exercise. There may be a *spondylolytic crisis*, namely acute severe low back pain with severe hamstring spasms and tightness. Acute gluteal muscle spasms give the appearance of

Table 9.2 Classification of spondylolisthesis

Type	Name	Cause
I	Congenital or dysplastic	Dysplasia of the lumbar/sacral posterior arch and facet joints
II	Isthmic (spondylolytic)	A defect of the pars interarticularis: Stress fracture Elongation of the pars Traumatic fracture of the pars (rare)
III	Degenerative	Degenerative changes of the facet joints and disc
IV	Traumatic	A fracture of the posterior elements, excluding the pars interarticularis
V	Pathological	Disturbance of the posterior elements and posterior tension band that allows the vertebra to slip forwards; this can be caused by tumour, sepsis or metabolic conditions such as Paget's disease
VI	Iatrogenic, after surgery	Disruption of the posterior elements due to surgical removal of the laminar, pedicles and/or facet joints

an inverted heart shape to the buttocks. There is difficulty in walking, with a semi-crouch-type gait with the hip and knees flexed. There may be neurological symptoms and signs, predominately in the L5 nerve root distribution.

Those in middle age present with back pain and L5 radicular pain from facet and disc degeneration, which causes foraminal stenosis of the L5 nerve roots.

COCCYDYNIA

This simply means pain in the coccyx.

Symptoms There is pain in the tail bone, usually with a history of slipping on a floor or stairs and landing heavily on the buttocks. The pain is worse on sitting but is only rarely felt at night. There is no disturbance of bladder or bowel function, although opening of the bowels may be uncomfortable when they need to sit on the lavatory. There are no neurological symptoms.

Natural history (see Chapter 1) The condition is self-limiting but can take up to 2 years to resolve fully.

CONDITIONS OF THE SACROILIAC JOINTS

Pain arising from the sacroiliac joints can be hard to differentiate from pain arising from the lower lumbar spine and lumbar–sacral junction. The common causes of pain are:

- Seronegative arthropathy, principally ankylosing spondylitis.
- Sepsis, including tuberculosis.
- Trauma: The sacroiliac joint is the strongest in the body, and if there is disruption, there is usually a related fracture of the pelvis.

SPINA BIFIDA AND MENINGOMYELOCELE

This condition is a consequence of *failure of fusion of the vertebral arches* with or without a defect in the neural tube, usually at a lower lumbar level.

Spina bifida occulta is a simple failure of fusion of the posterior elements and is entirely benign, occurring most commonly at the L5 or S1 level. A *meningomyelocele is when there is herniation of the neural structures through the posterior elements of the spine;* this may be associated with neurological deficits of the lower limb and of bladder and bowel function. Cutaneous appearances vary from a simple hair-filled pit to a more obvious cystic swelling with meninges bulging through the defect, or cerebrospinal fluid leaking through neural material on the surface.

A full neurological examination is essential (see Chapter 3). There is often an accompanying hydrocephalus, so look for a bulging fontanelle or excessive head circumference (see Chapter 1, Figure 1.15).

TUMOURS OF THE SPINE

These may be *benign* or *malignant*. The most common tumours are *metastatic secondary tumours*.

Symptoms Axial spinal pain that initially may be *non-specific*, progresses to be *constant pain* with non-mechanical features, and *night pain*.

Systemic features suggest a malignant process, this may include *weight loss* and *general malaise*.

Progression of the tumour may cause collapse of the vertebrae with sudden worsening of axial pain or deformity of the spine including *kyphosis*.

Neurological features may occur if the nerve roots or spinal cord are compressed. This may be caused by structural loss of the spinal column secondary to tumour destruction or to direct infiltration of the neural structures by the tumour.

Signs The gait may be painful or be affected by neurological dysfunction, including cord compression. Neurological examination is essential as well as examination of other systems as indicated by the history.

Benign tumours of the spine

- *Haemangiomas* are the most common hamartoma in the spine and consist of dilated vascular channels (see Chapters 3 and 5).
- *Osteochondromas* are benign cartilaginous tumours arising from endochondral ossification (see Chapter 6).
- *Osteoid osteomas and osteoblastomas* arise in the pedicles of vertebrae and cause night pain (see Chapter 6).
- *Aneurysmal bone cysts* are rare and produce expansile osteolytic lesions.
- *Eosinophilic granulomas* occur in children.
- *Giant cell tumours* arise in vertebral bodies and are painful. They may become malignant.

Primary malignant tumours of the spine

These are *rare*, and usually arise in the vertebral bodies:

- *Myelomas* are myeloproliferative lesions of plasma cells.
- *Chordomas* arise from notochord remnants.
- *Sarcomas* can be osteosarcomas, chondrosarcomas or Ewing's sarcomas.

Secondary malignant tumours of the spine

These are far more common than primary tumours, and are usually metastases from primary tumours of the:

- Breast.
- Bronchus.
- Kidney.
- Prostate.
- Thyroid.

Any patient with a history of cancer with back or spinal pain needs to be fully assessed and will require imaging of the spine. This is usually an MRI unless contraindicated.

SPINAL COLUMN SEPSIS

This is a rare condition but with rising incidence, which reflects an aging population but also greater ability to diagnose. There is often a significant delay in the diagnosis because of the non-specific nature of the early symptoms.

The sepsis may be

- *Pyogenic* (staphylococci, *Pseudomonas, Escherichia coli, Klebsiella, Proteus, Salmonella*).
- *Non-pyogenic* (tuberculosis and occasional fungal infection).

Ninety per cent of infections are in the thoracolumbar spine.

The infection tends to arise in disc spaces in children and end plates in adults, in both cases spreading to the adjacent discs and vertebrae. An epidural abscess may follow causing neurological compression and dysfunction.

Tuberculosis is increasing in incidence throughout the world. Airborne spread leads to lung infection, which spreads to the bones via the bloodstream. There is granuloma formation followed by caseation.

Symptoms Patients may experience *back pain* and *general malaise*. Localizing symptoms may only become apparent as the infection progresses. There may be disc and bone destruction, with secondary spinal deformity as well as neurological compression. The patient may be septic at the time of presentation, but these may not be a feature with non-specific symptoms of back pain predominating.

Revision panel 9.6

RISK FACTORS FOR SPINAL SEPSIS

Immunocompromise

Diabetes mellitus
HIV
Malnutrition
Exposure to steroids
Intravenous drug abuse
Rheumatoid arthritis
Renal failure
Liver cirrhosis

Elderly age group

Males more than females

Foreign travel

Especially for tuberculosis

History of malignancy

Sources of haematogenous spread from elsewhere

Urinary tract infection, genitourinary instrumentation
Soft tissue and respiratory infections

Spinal tuberculosis is notoriously indolent, and there is on average a delay of 6–9 months from presentation to diagnosis.

Risk factors Specific enquiry must be made about the conditions listed in Revision panel 9.6.

OSTEOPOROSIS/OSTEOMALACIA

Osteoporosis occurs with aging and is typically more common in postmenopausal women. Osteoporosis is symptomless until a pathological fracture occurs, which may occur with minimal trauma when the osteoporosis is significant. Most fractures occur in the lumbar spine but can be sustained elsewhere. Elderly patients may present with odontoid peg fractures without recalling a fall.

Patients may present with axial spine pain, spinal deformity including kyphosis, and loss of height. Vertebral body collapse or kyphosis subsequent to a fracture may lead to neural compression and symptoms related to this.

Osteomalacia affects those with a calcium and phosphate deficiency, usually caused by a vitamin D deficiency, and should be considered as a cause of kyphosis (see Chapters 6).

FRACTURES

Spine and pelvis

A *stable* spinal fracture is not displaced by normal muscle action.

Unstable fractures without immediate spinal cord damage can subsequently displace and cause cord damage leading to paresis or paralysis. Inadequate management of an unstable fracture without cord damage can therefore result in permanent and preventable cord damage.

Instability depends on the sites and extent of the damage to the vertebral bodies, the posterior arches and the stabilizing intervertebral ligaments.

Spinal fractures are usually caused by high energy mechanisms of trauma including *road traffic accidents, horse riding accidents* as well as other sports and leisure activities. These result in either *axial compression, distraction* or a combination of forces on the vertebral column, resulting in a fracture or ligament failure.

A pathological fracture should be considered and excluded if a spinal fracture occurs without a history of significant trauma. Causes include osteoporosis, spinal metastases and ankylosing spondylitis.

First aid If there is the remotest possibility of a spinal fracture, the spine must be immobilized until careful clinical and radiological assessment has shown no evidence of a fracture or displacement (see Chapter 5).

History

NOTE: Every patient with blunt injuries to the head and neck, especially if they are unconscious, should be suspected of having a spinal injury.

High-speed road traffic accidents, falls from a height and *crushing injuries* are risk factors.

Neck or back pain and the presence of neurological symptoms must also arouse suspicion of a spinal injury.

Examination

The neck must be stabilized and not moved as per the ATLS protocol. Inspect and palpate for *tenderness, bogginess, bruising, entry wounds and deformity.*

There may be a *prominent spinal process,* or an increased space between the spinous processes. All spinal movements may be limited.

The patient should then be *log-rolled* (see Chapter 5), and the *thoracolumbar spine inspected* and *palpated* as above.

Always conduct a full neurological examination including a rectal examination (see Chapter 3).

Cervical spine

These are less common than fractures of the thoracolumbar spine, but may be associated with severe, immediately fatal head injuries or severe neurological injury.

Symptoms are non-specific, and although X-rays may be useful in making the diagnosis of a fracture, often a CT scan is often required to confirm or exclude a suspected injury.

MRI may assist in assessing the cause of a neurological deficit, as well as ligament or intervertebral disc disruption, which may affect spinal stability.

C1 and C2 are 'atypical vertebrae' and the fracture patterns seen in this area are unique to the anatomy.

C3 to C7 are 'typical' cervical vertebrae and demonstrate fracture patterns related to the mechanism of injury.

With greater trauma and increased fracture displacement, the risk of associated neurological injury is increased.

FRACTURE OF C1 (JEFFERSON'S FRACTURE)

This is a *burst fracture of the ring of the atlas,* accounts for 10% of cervical fractures (Figure 9.14). and is caused by axial compression. Mechanisms include a *fall from a height*. The exact fracture pattern is determined by the degree of extension or flexion of the neck at the time of impact. There are no specific signs. Neurological problems are rare.

(a)

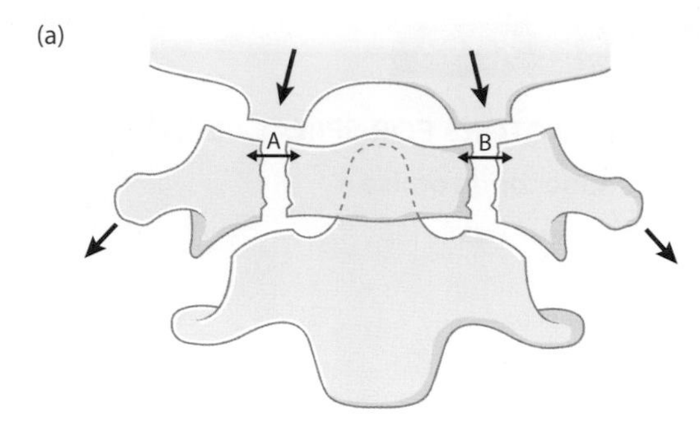

(b)

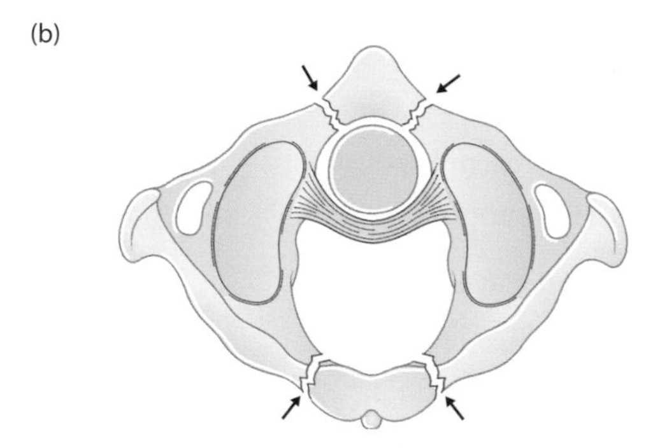

Figure 9.14 JEFFERSON'S FRACTURE. (a) AP view. If the distance A + B is >7 mm, the fracture is unstable. (b) Axial view (fractures arrowed).

FRACTURE OF THE C2 PEDICLES (HANGMAN'S FRACTURE)

Fractures of the C2 pedicles with associated disc disruption have been termed 'the hangman's fracture' and are associated with significant trauma (Figure 9.15a). The fracture may be unstable, and neurological damage may be fatal. On occasion, the fracture pattern expands the spinal canal, thus limiting trauma to the spinal cord (Figure 9.15b).

ATLANTOAXIAL DISLOCATION

This often fatal injury follows hyperextension, distraction and rotation of the craniocervical junction.

FRACTURE OF THE ODONTOID PROCESS

This is the most common fracture of the cervical spine (17%), and usually results from a direct blow on

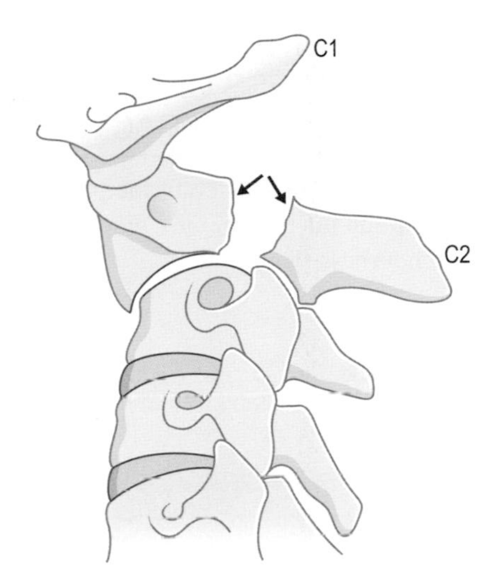

Figure 9.15 Hangman's fracture (arrows).

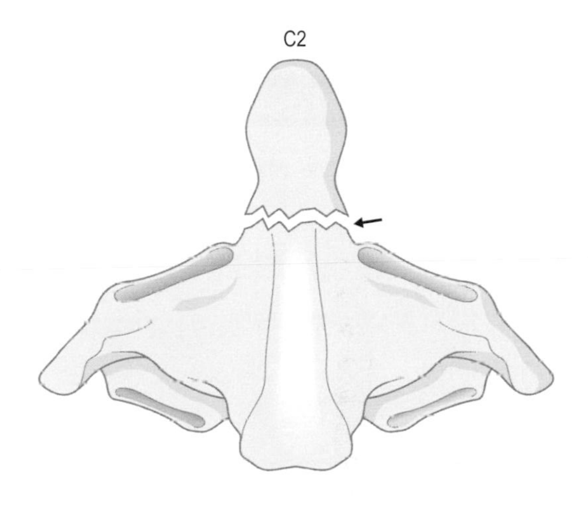

Figure 9.16 Fracture of the odontoid process (arrow)

the occiput during a fall or in a road traffic accident (Figure 9.16). There is hyperflexion in a young road traffic victim, or hyperextension in an elderly patient with osteoporosis from a fall on the face. There is cord damage in 25% of cases. There are no specific symptoms or signs.

SUBAXIAL FRACTURES (C3 TO C7)

The fracture pattern may be complex, but is determined by the mechanism of the injury, compression or distraction, and the position of the neck/head at the time of the trauma.

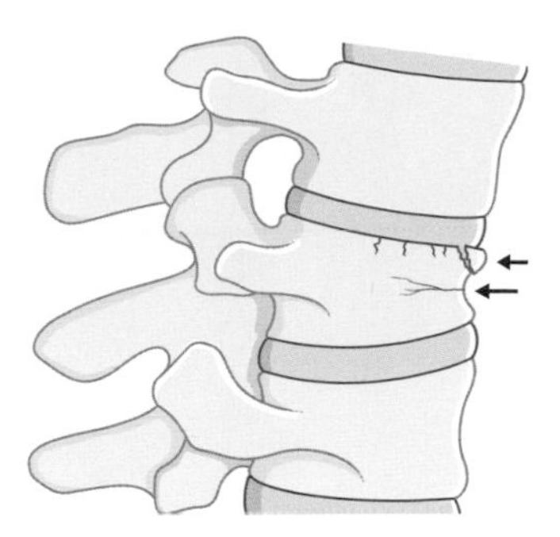

Figure 9.17 Wedge compression fractures (arrow).

WEDGE COMPRESSION FRACTURES

These follow flexion with compression. The anterior bodies of the cervical vertebra are crushed (Figure 9.17). The fracture is stable, and cord damage is rare.

BURST FRACTURES

The vertebra is crushed further than the wedge fracture and reflects a greater degree of trauma. The fracture may be comminuted and grossly disrupted. There is a greater probability of associated spinal cord injury than with a wedge compression fracture.

FLEXION DISTRACTION INJURY WITH SUBLUXATION OR DISLOCATION

There is a pure flexion or flexion–rotation injury that either tears the posterior spinal ligaments of the lower cervical spine (subluxation) or causes the articular facets to ride forwards over the facets below (Figure 9.18). There may also be associated fractures of one or both articular masses, with posterior ligamentous tears. This fracture/dislocation renders the spine unstable (Figure 9.19).

HYPEREXTENSION AVULSION FRACTURES

An avulsion fracture can occur at the anterior inferior corner of the vertebral body from a hyperextension

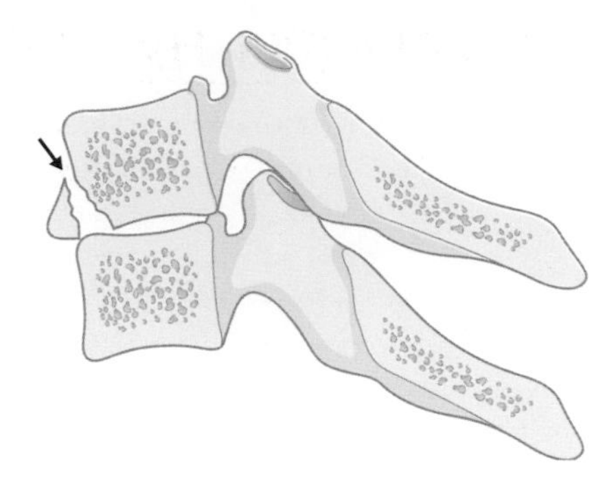

Figure 9.18 Stage IV flexion compression (arrow).

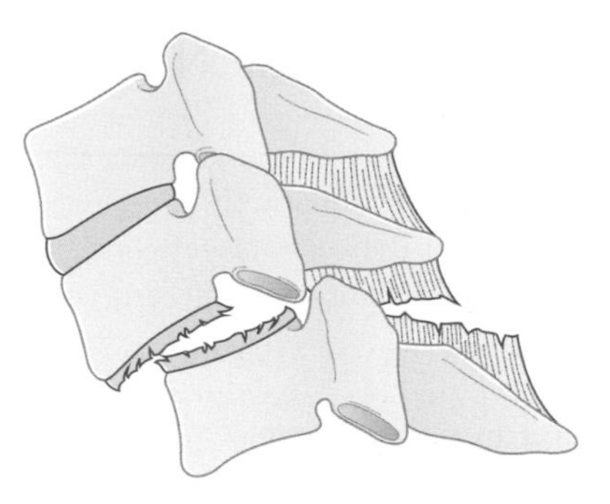

Figure 9.19 Fracture/dislocation of the cervical spine with bilateral facet dislocation. There is a high incidence of neurological injury associated with this injury pattern that may be progressive if the facets are not reduced as expeditiously as possible.

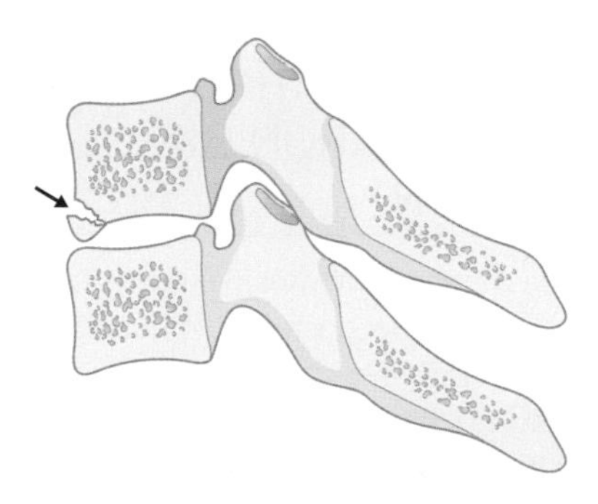

Figure 9.20 This is a stable fracture. The teardrop is the anterior portion of the vertebral body (arrow).

injury of the cervical spine (this may be referred to as a teardrop fracture) (Figure 9.20). This is rarely associated with a neurological deficit. Stability depends on the degree of disruption of the anterior longitudinal ligament and the intervertebral disc.

AVULSION INJURY OF THE SPINOUS PROCESS OF C7 (CLAY-SHOVELLER'S FRACTURE)

Severe muscular contraction of the posterior spinal muscles pulls off the spinous process. There is localized tenderness (Figure 9.21).

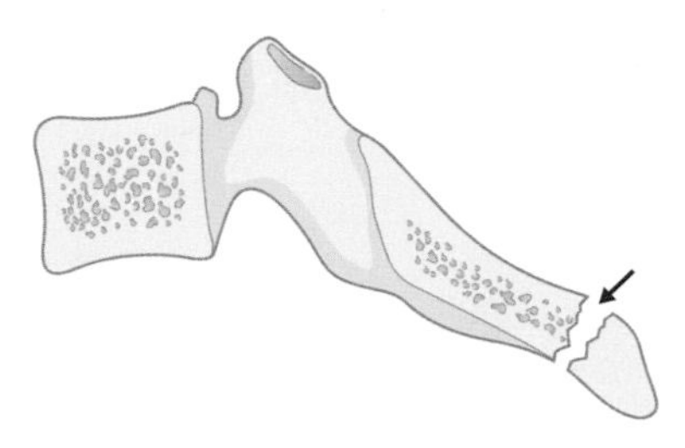

Figure 9.21 Avulsion injury of the spinous process of C7 (clay-shoveller's fracture) (arrow).

Thoracolumbar spine

Fractures of the spine can be classified by their *mechanism of injury:*

Either

- Compression.
- Burst.
- Extension.
- Fracture dislocation.

Or

- Compression.
- Extension.
- Rotational.

The stability of the fractures is based on the number of columns of the spine disrupted:

- Three column theory.
- Two column theory.

Fractures of the thoracolumbar spine usually occur after significant trauma, otherwise an underlying pathology should be considered, such as *osteoporosis*.

Fractures often occur at the cervicothoracic and the thoracolumbar junction, where a mobile area of the spine is adjacent to the more rigid thoracic spine.

In the thoracic spine, wedge compression and fracture dislocations from hyperflexion are usually stabilized by the rib cage. Where osteoporosis exists, multiple fractures may lead to kyphosis (see above).

NOTE: Fractures of the lower two thoracic and the upper lumbar vertebrae are more common, because this is the relatively mobile area between the fixed zones of the thorax and the sacrum.

The strength of the spine at this level is in three columns: anterior, middle and posterior (Figure 9.22). Fractures of the middle column and at least one other should alert to the possibility of instability.

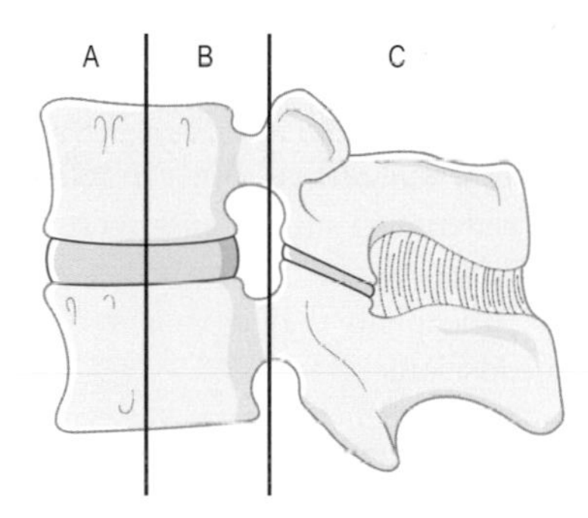

Figure 9.22 Lumbar spinal columns.

WEDGE COMPRESSION FRACTURES

These are the most common type, the result of axial compression and hyperflexion. They are stable unless a lot of vertebral height has been lost, which is indicated by *severe tenderness* and a *palpable gap between the vertebral spines.*

BURST FRACTURES

These fractures are due to axial compression that squashes the vertebral body. The pedicles are splayed, and the laminae may be fractured. Bone fragments and disc material may be pushed into the spinal canal. A significant loss of vertebral height combined with a kyphosis indicates instability.

FLEXION/DISTRACTION FRACTURES

In this type of fracture, also common in seat belt injuries, there is disruption of the posterior spinal structures, either fractures of the spinous processes (which may extend into the pedicles), ligamentous disruption or a combination of both.

Disruption of the posterior elements may be associated with fractures of the vertebral body.

They may be associated with neurological injuries or abdominal injuries, especially in children (see Chapter 5).

FRACTURE/DISLOCATIONS

These are caused by *flexion, compression, rotation and distraction, and rarely by hyperextension.* One or both facet joints are subluxed or dislocated and there are associated fractures of the vertebral body or disruption of the intervertebral disc. Associated spinal cord injury is common, especially if both facet joints are dislocated (90% complete paraplegia), and the spine is always unstable.

Minor fractures

Fractures of a transverse process are caused by muscle avulsion. They do not affect stability.

Sacrum and coccyx

These bones may be fractured by a fall or a direct blow.

Pain, local tenderness, bruising and abnormal mobility are all indicative of a fracture.

Fractures of the sacrum are often associated with fractures of the pelvis (see below).

The sacrum is divided into three zones (Figure 9.23):

- Fractures lateral to the neural foramina.
- Fractures passing through the foramina.
- Fractures medial to the foramen and involving the spinal canal.

The likelihood of neurological damage is greater in Zone 2 (30%) and Zone 3 (50%).

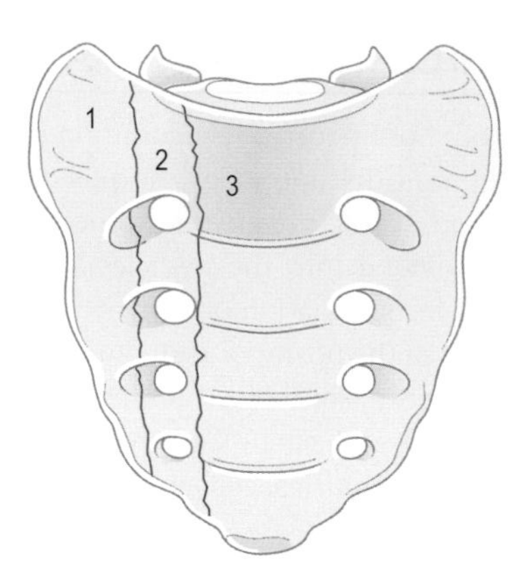

Figure 9.23 The Denis classification of sacral zones.

> **NOTE:** A full neurological examination is essential, including an assessment of anal sphincter tone and the bulbocavernosus reflex (see Chapter 3).

Pelvic fractures

Pelvic fractures are often associated with other major injuries (see Chapter 5) but may be isolated, as when for example a simple fall in an elderly patient causes a fracture of the pubis or iliac crest without any instability of the pelvic ring.

High-velocity road accidents or *falls from a height* usually cause major pelvic bone disruptions and are *often associated with other life-threatening injuries* of the head, brain, abdomen and chest.

In addition, local injuries to the *bladder* and *urethra, bowel* and *blood vessels* are also life-threatening, and effective resuscitation is essential if a successful outcome is to be achieved (see Chapter 5).

The pelvis is a strong bony ring (Figure 9.24) that carries weight from the spine to the lower limbs.

> **NOTE:** A break in one part of the ring is invariably accompanied by a break elsewhere.

They may be classified as stable where the sacroiliac complex is intact, partially unstable or completely unstable.

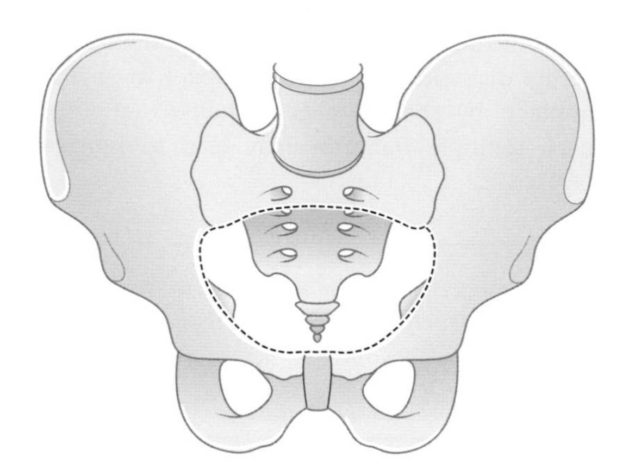

Figure 9.24 The pelvic bony ring.

Initial assessment Look for other system injuries and *hypovolaemic shock*. Then assess the degree of pelvic stability and any local organ or soft tissue damage.

History

Local pain is suggestive, but a fractured pelvis must be considered in all patients who have been subjected to high-energy trauma, especially if there are signs of unexplained hypovolaemic shock and they are unconscious.

> **NOTE:** Resuscitation precedes any assessment of the pelvic injury.

Examination

There may be no overt signs of injury, but *skin abrasions, local tenderness over the pubic symphysis, iliac crest or sacrum and the presence of crepitus* are all highly suggestive of a pelvic fracture. Leg length discrepancy and malrotation in the absence of lower limb fractures are also important signs.

A *bimanual assessment of transverse stability* should then be carried out by compressing and distracting the iliac wings (Figure 9.25). This must be done gently to avoid causing further bleeding. An experienced surgeon may be able to assess vertical and acetabular stability by pulling on the leg while palpating the pelvis.

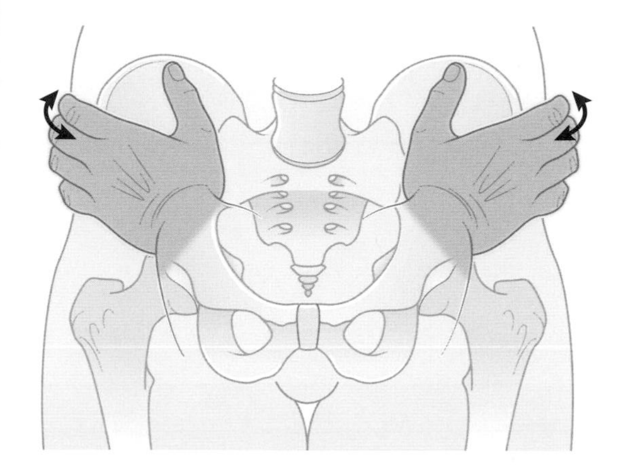

Figure 9.25 Bimanual assessment of pelvic stability.

Rectal and vaginal examinations should be performed to assess the presence of associated injuries and the presence of an occult open fracture.

Neurological examination of the lower limb (see Chapter 3) should exclude a spinal injury. The peripheral pulses should also be checked (see Chapter 10).

Urethral and bladder injuries should be looked for before catheterization in all displaced anterior ring injuries (see Chapter 17).

There may be an acetabular fracture if there is pain in the hip and lateral bruising, and the leg is in an abnormal position. Neurovascular assessment must then be carried out as sciatic, femoral and obturator nerve injuries may be associated.

Acknowledgements

The contribution of Jonathan Lucas to this chapter in the fifth edition is gratefully acknowledged.

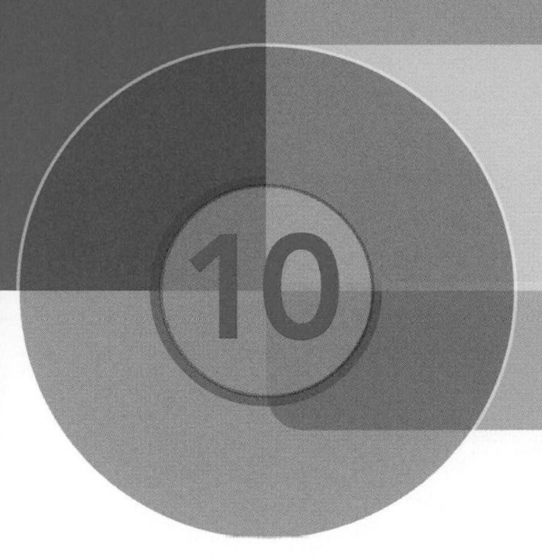

10 The arteries, veins and lymphatics

BIJAN MODARAI AND ASHISH PATEL

Techniques for examination of the arteries, veins and lymphatics are described before detailed descriptions of the history and clinical features of diseases that affect them.

THE ARTERIES

Clinical assessment of the arterial circulation of the lower limb

Always examine the patient in a warm room. A routine for assessment is listed in Revision panel 10.1.

Inspection

This is a key part of the vascular examination.

Colour

The most notable feature of an ischaemic limb is its colour. The skin may be as *white as marble* or show *varying degrees of redness or blueness,* which becomes more obvious in the lower parts of the leg and the toes (Figures 10.1–10.3). Excessive deoxygenation of the blood in the skin capillaries sometimes gives the foot a purple–blue cyanosed appearance, but the blue fades to white within a few seconds when the patient lies down. There may also be areas of blue streaks around white patches ('mottling') in the foot. When mottling becomes fixed, the area of ischaemia is usually irreversible (Figure 10.1b). Pigmented skin masks these subtle colour changes, making the diagnosis of mild and moderate arterial insufficiency more difficult. *Gangrene* turns the skin a permanent blue–black colour, which is usually first seen in the toes (see page 339).

Scars

It is important to note any scars indicating previous vascular intervention on the limb:

- Groin scars for femoral artery access.
- Medial thigh scars over the course of the long saphenous vein (indicative of vein harvesting for bypass surgery).

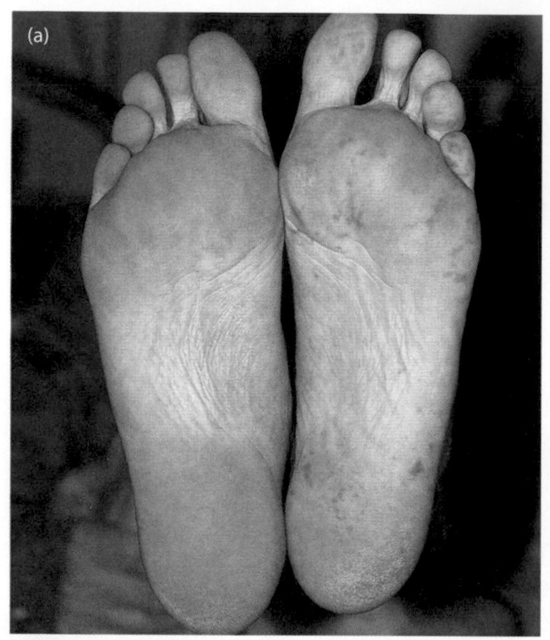

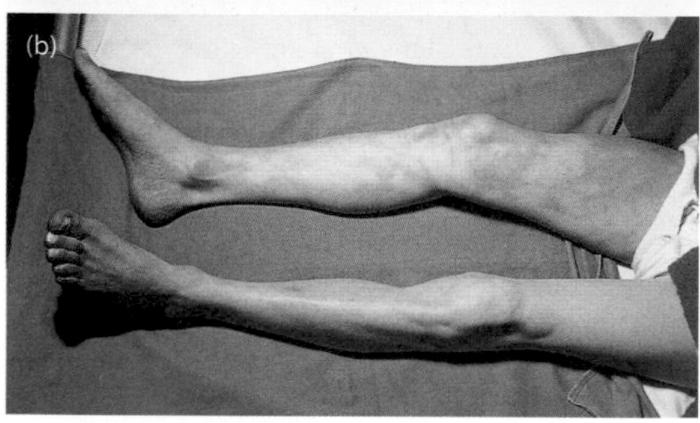

Figure 10.1 THE ISCHAEMIC LIMB. (a) The left foot becomes pallid on elevation. (b) An ischaemic right leg with fixed mottling of the skin in the thigh.

- On the medial aspect of lower leg just below the knee for popliteal access.
- On the anterolateral or medial aspect of lower leg near the calf for distal (anterior tibial, posterior tibial or peroneal) artery access.
- Behind the knee for popliteal artery access.
- Around the posterior part of the leg for short saphenous vein harvesting for bypass surgery.

Pressure areas

Very carefully inspect all areas subjected to pressure or trauma during walking or bed rest, because these are the first sites to show evidence of trophic changes, ulceration and gangrene.

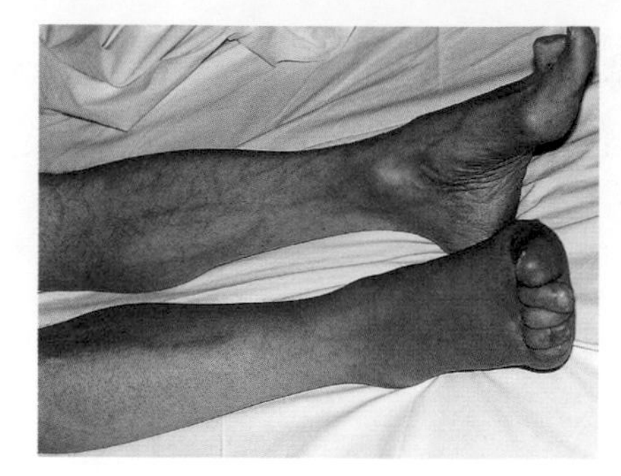

Figure 10.2 A limb showing the red/purple changes of chronic ischaemia.

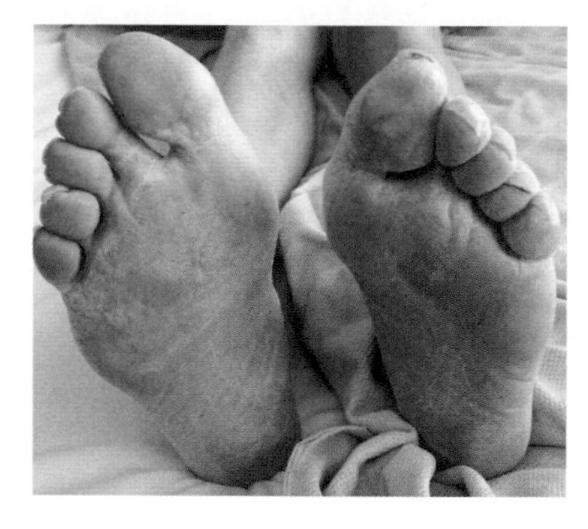

Figure 10.3 An ischaemic left great toe.

NOTE: It is important to look at the bottom, back and lateral surfaces of the heel, the ball of the foot and skin over the malleoli. The skin, especially over the head of the first and fifth metatarsals must be carefully inspected, as must the tips and in-between the toes (Figure 10.4).

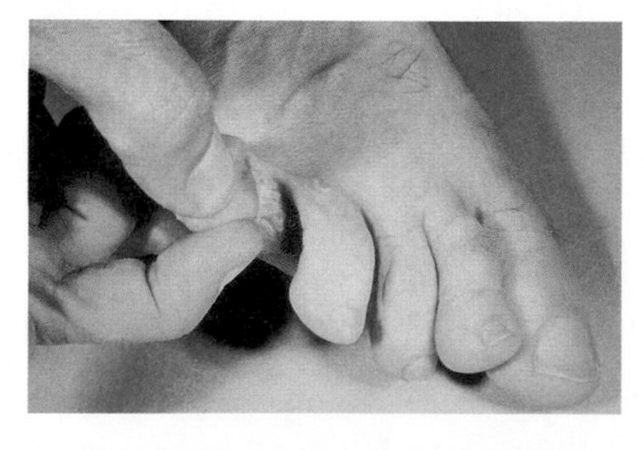

Figure 10.4 An ischaemic ulcer has developed between the toes where one toe is pressing against the other.

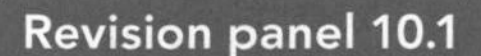

ROUTINE FOR ASSESSING THE ARTERIAL CIRCULATION

Inspection

Colour
Venous filling
Pressure areas and between the digits
Scars

Palpation

Skin temperature
Capillary refilling time
Palpate the pulses

Auscultation

Listen for bruits
Measure the ankle:brachial pressure index

Special tests

Buerger's angle

Pressure necrosis causes thickening of the skin, a purple or blue discolouration, blistering, ulceration or patches of black, dead, gangrenous skin.

> **NOTE:** Loss of hair on the skin of the lower leg is a sign of ischaemia but is unreliable and does not need to be recorded

Palpation

Temperature

The skin temperature can only be assessed reliably if both lower limbs have been exposed to the same ambient temperature for a full 5 minutes. Uncover the limbs and perform some other part of the physical examination to allow the skin temperature to adjust to the temperature of the surrounding air.

The whole limb should be assessed starting in the foot using one hand for each limb to compare which parts are warm or cold, and the level at which these changes occur. *A blue or even red foot can be very cold.*

> **NOTE:** Most clinicians prefer to use the backs of their fingers to assess temperature as the cool, dry backs of the fingers are ideal temperature sensors.

Capillary refilling

Press on the pulp of a toe or finger for 2 seconds, release pressure and then observe the time taken for the blanched area to recover. This gives a crude indication of the rate of blood flow in the capillaries and the pressure within them. This time can be compared in both limbs.

Venous filling

In a warm room, the veins of a normal foot are dilated and full of blood, even when the patient is lying horizontally. In an ischaemic foot, the veins collapse and sink below the skin surface to look like pale blue gutters. This appearance is called '*venous guttering*' (Figure 10.3) and is especially notable when performing Buerger's test (see Special tests below).

Feel all the pulses

Pulses are most easily felt where an artery is superficial and crosses a bone. In the neck, shoulder and upper limbs, the carotid, subclavian, brachial and both wrist arteries are close to the skin and easy to palpate. The pulses in the lower limb should be palpated from proximal to distal in order to determine site(s) of stenoses or occlusions.

The *femoral pulse* in the groin lies halfway between the symphysis pubis (in the midline) and the anterior superior iliac spine; this is called the mid-inguinal point (Figure 10.5a).

The *popliteal pulse* can be difficult to feel because it does not cross a prominent bone and is not superficial. There are three ways to feel it, and all three need to be tried before deciding whether the pulse is present or absent:

- The most convenient technique for feeling the popliteal pulse is to extend the patient's knee, and place both hands around the top of the calf, with the thumbs placed on the tibial tuberosity and the tips of the fingers of each

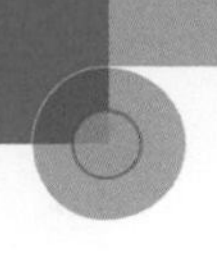

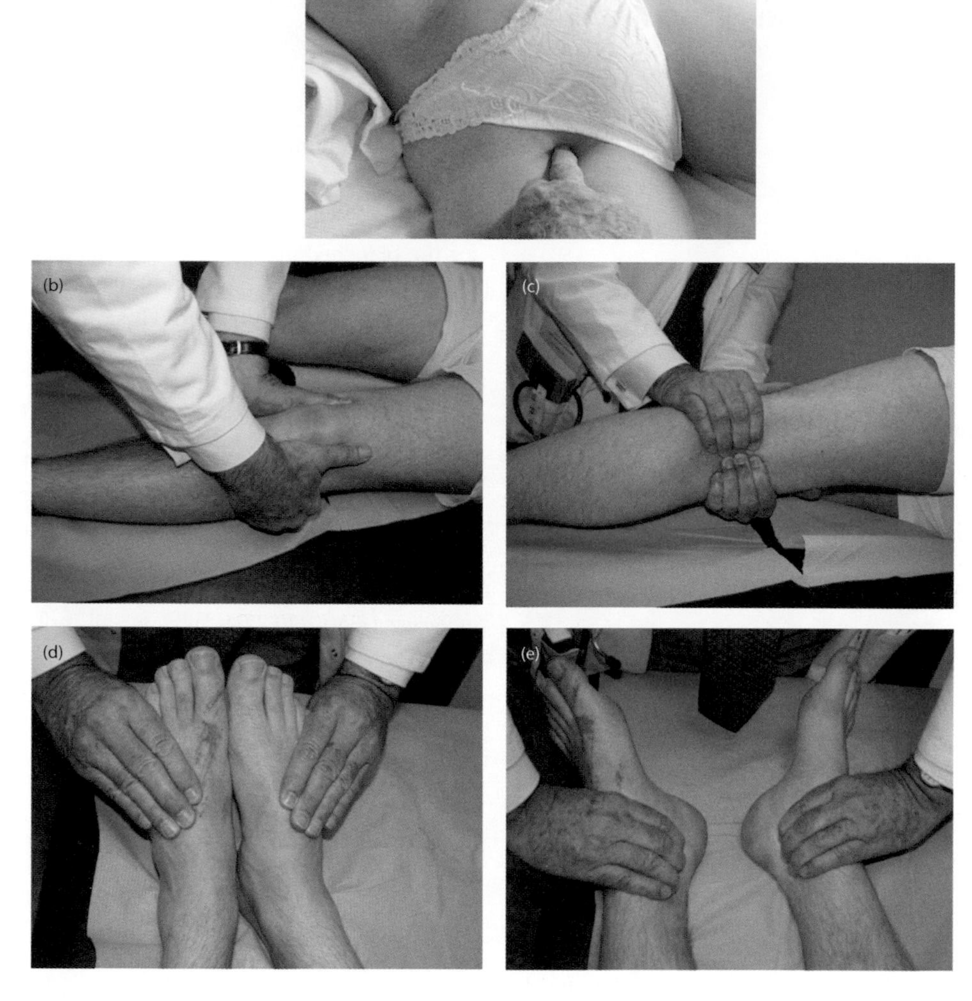

Figure 10.5 PALPATION OF THE PERIPHERAL PULSES. (a) Site of the femoral pulse at the mid-inguinal point, halfway between anterior superior iliac spine and pubic symphysis. For palpation, normally more than one finger is used for palpation of this pulse. (b) Palpating the popliteal pulse with the knee extended. (c) The position of the fingers in the midline when feeling the popliteal pulse with the knee fully extended. (d) Simultaneous palpation of the dorsalis pedis pulses using the pulps of the fingers. (e) Simultaneous palpation of the posterior tibial pulses.

hand touching behind the knee between the heads of the gastrocnemius muscle (over the lower part of the popliteal fossa). The pulps of all the fingers are then pulled forwards against the posterior part of the tibial condyle, trapping the popliteal artery between them and the posterior surface of the tibia (Figure 10.5b, c). The pulsating artery can be felt in the midline. When in doubt, count any pulse you feel against the rate detected by a second examiner feeling the radial pulse to check for synchronization.

- Flexing the knee to 135° loosens the deep fascia and may make the lower half of the artery easier to feel. The vessel is, however, moved further from the surface by bending the knee, and this may make palpation of the upper half of the artery more difficult as it sinks into the large fat pad between the femoral condyles.

- It is sometimes worth turning the patient into the prone position and feeling along the course of the artery with the fingertips of both hands.

NOTE: When the popliteal pulse is very easy to feel, it may be aneurysmal and the patient should be examined for a contralateral popliteal aneurysm as well as an abdominal aortic aneurysm.

The *dorsalis pedis* artery runs from a point on the anterior surface of the ankle joint, midway between the malleoli, towards the cleft between the first and second metatarsal bones (lateral to extensor hallucis longus) (Figure 10.5d). Ask the patient to extend their great toe towards them to identify extensor hallucis longus prior to palpating. In 10% of subjects, the anterior tibial artery is absent and replaced by a branch of the peroneal artery.

The *posterior tibial* artery lies one-third of the way along a line between the tip of the medial malleolus and the point of the heel, but is easier to feel 2.5 cm higher up, where it lies just behind the medial malleolus (Figure 10.5e).

It is important to feel the dorsalis pedis and posterior tibial pulses in both limbs simultaneously. To do this, stand at the end of the bed or couch and feel the dorsalis pedis artery of each foot simultaneously by placing the pulps of all the fingers of each hand along the line of the artery, with your thumbs beneath the arch of the foot. From this position, the hands can be rotated over the foot until the pulps of the fingers lie in the groove between the Achilles tendon and the medial malleolus. The pulps of the fingers can then be pulled up against the back of the tibia, trapping the posterior tibial artery against the bone.

Assess the muscles and nerves

Severe ischaemia causes a loss of muscle and nerve function, ultimately producing an immobile, numb limb. The sensation in the toes and dorsum of both feet should be assessed as conditions such as diabetes can have impaired sensation as a result of diabetic neuropathy rather than ischaemia.

Auscultation

It is important to use your stethoscope to listen to the arteries in the neck, the abdomen, the groin and the thigh for bruits in all patients suspected to have arterial disease (Figure 10.6).

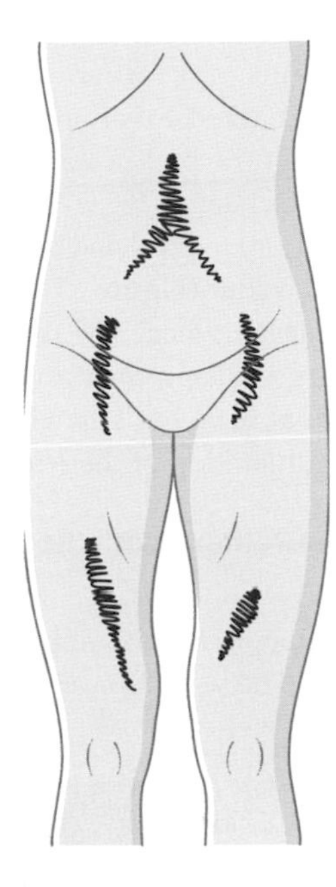

Figure 10.6 The common sites to hear bruits over the arteries of the lower limbs.

Bruits are caused by turbulent flow beyond a stenosis, or an irregularity in the artery wall. Do not press too hard over a superficial artery with the bell of your stethoscope, as pressure can distort the flow and cause a bruit. *Always remember to listen over the adductor canal.*

NOTE: Before finishing the physical examination of the lower limb, you should measure the blood pressure in both arms to exclude significant subclavian or innominate artery disease.

Special tests

Buerger's angle (the vascular angle)

Buerger's angle is the angle at which the leg becomes white when it is raised. In a normal limb the toes stay pink even when the limb is raised to 90°. In an ischaemic leg, elevation to 15° or 30° for 30–60 seconds may cause pallor (Figure 10.1a) and venous guttering. An angle of less than 20° indicates severe ischaemia. This test is often more useful as a comparator and both limbs should be raised

together; the ischaemic foot goes white, while the normal foot remains pink. After elevating the legs, patients should be asked to sit up and dangle their feet over the side of the bed. A normal foot remains pink, whereas an ischaemic leg will slowly turn from white (after elevation) to pink and then take on a suffused purple–red colour (Figure 10.2). This is a result of *reactive hyperaemia* where the re-oxygenation of the hypoxic tissue results in the washout of vasodilator metabolites that have built up whilst the leg was elevated causing dilatation of the arterioles.

Pressure measurement with the Doppler flow detector

A hand-held Doppler ultrasound should be used to detect blood flow. The sound waves generated by the device are focused into a beam and directed towards the vessel to be examined by placing the probe over the surface of the vessel, after removing any air between the probe and the skin with a coupling jelly. Moving red cells alter the frequency of the reflected ultrasound according to the Doppler principle.

The chosen vessels, usually the dorsalis pedis posterior tibial or peroneal arteries at the ankle, are located by placing the Doppler probe over their known anatomical course and listening for regular changes in the sound generated by the pulsatile flow. A sphygmomanometer cuff previously placed around the ankle is then inflated until the noise created by the flow ceases (Figure 10.7a). The pressure at which this occurs is the systolic blood pressure. This can be measured in all three ankle vessels. In addition, the

(a)

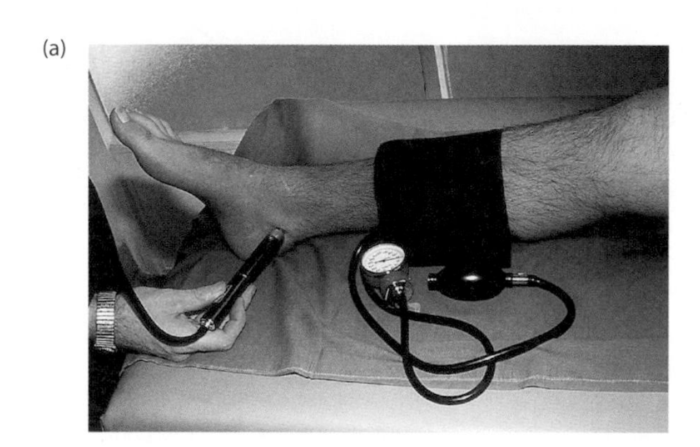

(b)

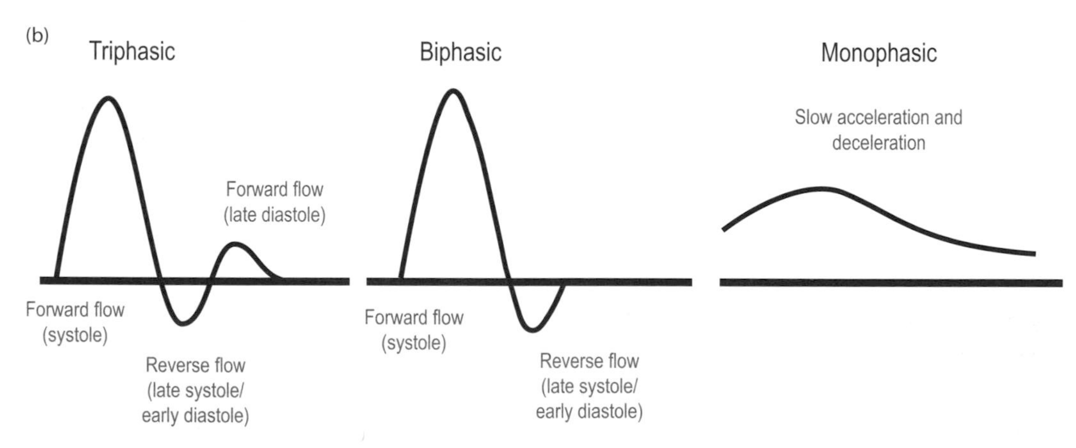

Figure 10.7 DOPPLER PRESSURE INDEX. (a) The technique for measuring the ankle pressure index, which is the pressure at which the cuff needs to be inflated to abolish the noise of the arterial flow using a Doppler. (b) Triphasic Doppler waveform shows forward flow in systole, reverse flow in late systole/early diastole and forward flow in late diastole (normal vessel). The biphasic Doppler waveform does not have forward flow in late diastole and can represent high-resistant flow (which can also be found in normal vessels). The low resistant monophasic waveform with slow acceleration and deceleration suggests arterial disease proximal to the site of the Doppler.

quality of the signal should be determined as being either *monophasic, biphasic* or *triphasic* (Figure 10.7b). A monophasic signal usually indicates compromised flow, usually from a calcified blood vessel.

The *pressure index* is the ratio between the pressure measured by this technique in an ankle vessel and the pressure in the brachial artery. It is normally 1.0, i.e. both foot and brachial artery pressures should be almost identical. Ratios above 1.1 indicate stiff, calcified limb vessels (often diabetic arteries), which cannot be compressed by the external pressure applied by the sphygmomanometer cuff. Ratios below 1 indicate occlusive disease of foot vessels upstream.

NOTE: The Doppler ultrasound flow detector is a very useful tool because it can detect pulsatile flow when the pulse is impalpable to the fingers. A more accurate assessment of the severity of the disease can be obtained by measuring the pressure before and after exercise.

Conditions of the arteries

ACUTE ARTERIAL INSUFFICIENCY OF THE LIMBS

This occurs when the arterial blood supply to a limb is suddenly interrupted, with no time for collaterals to form. It is much more common in the lower limbs. The pain comes from ischaemic muscles and nerves, which develop irreversible changes within a few hours.

Revision panel 10.2

THE SYMPTOMS AND SIGNS OF ACUTE ISCHAEMIA: THE 6 Ps

Pain
Paraesthesia and numbness
Paralysis
Pallor
Pulseless
Perishing cold

The symptoms and signs are commonly known as the 6 Ps (Revision panel 10.2). The symptoms are:

- *Pain*, usually very severe and of sudden onset.
- *Paraesthesiae* ('pins and needles') and numbness, which develop over a few hours and eventually progress to
- *Paralysis*.

The *three physical signs* are:

- *Pallor*.
- *Pulselessness*, and the limb feels
- Perishingly cold to the touch.

The limb looks white and feels cold. These findings can be compared with the appearance of the other side if the symptoms are unilateral. The capillary circulation is poor, with a prolonged refilling time. The veins are empty, and the limb may become blue and develop a blotchy, blue–white appearance.

The femoral pulse may be absent if the arterial occlusion is just above the division of the common femoral artery into the superficial and deep femoral (profunda) arteries, or present if the occlusion is situated more distally. Similarly, in the upper limb, the subclavian and axillary pulses may be palpable, whereas the distal pulses, for example, the brachial, wrist and ankle pulses, are not.

Muscle tenderness, a bad prognostic sign, especially in the muscles of the anterior and posterior calf compartments, should be sought by gently pressing the bellies of these muscles.

A full neurological examination should concentrate on power, sensation and reflexes (see Chapter 3).

The Doppler ultrasound probe should be used to confirm the absence of pulsatile blood flow in the peripheral arteries.

The leg becomes mottled and marbled if the ischaemia persists. The muscles eventually become hard, and the skin begins to blister and develop *gangrene*, which usually starts in the toes before spreading proximally. The causes of acute limb ischaemia are shown in Revision panel 10.3.

Examination

Examine the heart and general circulation with care in a patient with sudden arterial occlusion.

An *arterial embolus* is suspected if the patient is fibrillating, has had a recent heart attack or is known

Revision panel 10.3

CAUSES OF ACUTE ARTERIAL ISCHAEMIA

An arterial embolus
Thrombosis on an atheromatous plaque
Thrombosis of an aneurysm (usually popliteal)
Arterial dissection (usually aortic)
Traumatic disruption
External compression, e.g. a cervical rib or popliteal entrapment

to have heart valve disease. Patients may never have had any symptoms of chronic vascular disease such as intermittent claudication (see below) before the embolus occurs.

An *acute arterial thrombosis* (of an underlying atheromatous plaque) is usually suspected if the patient has already experienced symptoms of peripheral vascular disease, such as intermittent claudication.

A *thrombosed popliteal aneurysm* is suspected if other arteries, such as the popliteal artery of the opposite limb or the abdominal aorta, are found to be dilated.

An *aortic dissection* is suspected if the patient presents with severe chest and/or back pain. Other pulses, such as the left subclavian artery, may be absent.

A *traumatic arterial disruption* is suspected if there is a clear history of injury or vascular intervention.

A *cervical* rib is suspected if there is a palpable supraclavicular swelling (see Chapters 9 and 12). Patients with cervical ribs may have experienced neurological symptoms in the arm and hand for many years. (Special investigations are required to diagnose the other causes of subclavian artery compression.).

NOTE: Also exclude two of the major non-arterial causes of an acute limb pain of sudden onset – acute venous thrombosis (see page 356), and spinal cord compression or infarction (see Chapters 3 and 9)

Chronic arterial insufficiency of the lower limb

INTERMITTENT CLAUDICATION

Strictly speaking, intermittent claudication means *intermittent limping* (Latin claudicare, to limp, a word derived from the disability of the Emperor Claudius). This term is used to describe a *cramp-like pain in a muscle that appears during exercise.* It is caused by an inadequate blood flow to the muscles. The pain stops the patient using the muscle and, if the affected muscle is in the leg, it first causes them to limp and then to stop walking.

History

Age The majority of patients presenting with intermittent claudication are males, over the age of 50 years, with smoking-related atherosclerotic disease of the lower limb vessels. Claudication can also develop in young adults with Buerger's disease, or after an arterial embolism, thrombosis or the traumatic occlusion of a major artery.

Sex Claudication is more common in males than in females. In males, it may be associated with impotence if the occlusion disease is at the aortic bifurcation (as there is no blood flow to the internal iliac arteries). This is known as Leriche's syndrome.

Pain The pain of intermittent claudication is quite specific and must fulfil three criteria:

- The patient must experience the pain in a muscle, usually in the calf (for femoropopliteal disease) or buttock (for aortoiliac disease).
- The pain should only develop when the muscle is exercised.
- The pain ceases when the exercise stops.

Walking distance *Limitation of walking is the principal complaint.* Patients find that they can only walk a limited distance before an ache begins in the muscles of the leg, which then becomes a cramp, and eventually stops them walking any further. The distance covered by the time walking has to stop is called the *claudication distance*. This should be recorded and the patient should, if necessary, be observed walking to see when the pain develops.

They should also be asked how long they have to wait until the pain goes away and their claudication distance when walking on an incline. Some patients complain of an ache or cramp that does not stop them walking and that fades away if they force themselves to continue walking. Others find they can prevent the pain developing by walking slowly. The severity of the pain and the time taken for it to begin and cease vary from patient to patient.

Any muscle can be affected. The calf muscles are most often affected, but a claudication pain can arise in the thigh, buttock or foot muscles, and in the muscles of the upper limb and forearm.

Patients may also describe numbness and paraesthesiae in the skin of the foot at the time that the muscle pain begins. This is the result of blood being shunted from the skin to the muscle.

> **NOTE:** Pains that begin when at rest or immediately the patient stands up, and pains that occur in tissues other than muscles and that do not abate with rest, are not usually caused by vascular claudication.

Onset and progression The pain of claudication usually begins insidiously. The walking distance gradually shortens over a few months before becoming static. In one-third or more of affected patients, the walking distance then increases, with spontaneous remission of the symptoms as the collateral circulation develops.

It is always important to ask about *pain at rest in the foot,* especially when the leg is horizontal in a patient with claudication, as this symptom signifies the onset of *critical limb ischaemia* (see page 340). Patients with rest pain may have had intermittent claudication in the affected limb for many years.

Examination

General appearance

The whole cardiovascular system must be examined with care. The blood pressure must be measured in both arms and recorded, the heart examined, the major arteries auscultated and the abdominal aorta felt in case it is dilated and aneurysmal (see page 343).

An *arcus senilis* (see Chapter 1) is not diagnostic of vascular disease but is indicative.

Xanthelesmata and xanthomata, which are cholesterol deposits around the eye and in the subcutaneous tissues, are indicative of hypercholesterolaemia (see Figure 1.22). *Pallor* (see Figure 1.2) suggesting anaemia or a rubicund appearance (see Figure 1.4) suggesting *polycythaemia (rubra vera)* are worth noting, as both these conditions can predispose to claudication and rest pain.

Examination of the legs

Inspection The appearance of the limb on inspection is often remarkably normal, although if the condition is severe, there may be *some blanching on elevation of the legs* (see Figure 10.1).

Palpation The foot and leg may be cooler than the contralateral side. The pulse immediately above the affected group of muscles is likely to be weak or absent. Thus, if claudication is experienced in the calf, the popliteal pulse is usually impalpable, but the femoral pulse is likely to be present. The femoral pulse is likely to be absent if the pain is felt in the thigh muscles. Thus, the level of the symptoms and signs often indicates the level of disease. It is possible to have claudication in the calf with palpable foot pulses, but careful examination often reveals a bruit in the thigh (suggesting a significant stenosis of the superficial femoral artery), and if the pulses are re-examined after exercise, they may no longer be palpable.

The Doppler pressures are invariably reduced and fall still further with exercise.

Auscultation The common sites to find bruits in association with intermittent claudication are over the aortic bifurcation, the iliac and common femoral arteries,and the superficial femoral artery at the adductor hiatus.

Examination of the motor and skeletal systems should be normal.

Differential diagnosis

Other causes of a claudication-like pain include:

- Osteoarthritis of the hip and knee.
- Spinal stenosis.
- Prolapsed intervertebral disc.
- Venous claudication.

The hip and knee should always be carefully examined (see Chapter 8) as should the spine, especially if all the pulses are palpable.

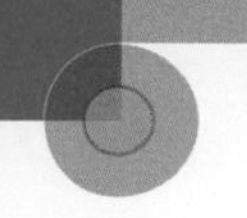

Venous claudication should be considered if the limb is swollen, or if there are skin changes of venous insufficiency such as lipodermatosclerosis of the gaiter area (see page 345).

REST PAIN

This is a term used to describe the continuous, *unremitting pain in the foot* caused by severe ischaemia. In contrast to the pain of intermittent claudication, which only appears during exercise, this pain is present at rest throughout the day and often worse at night, when the leg is horizontal.

History

Age Most patients with arterial disease severe enough to cause rest pain are 60 or more years old, but Buerger's disease and trauma can cause rest pain in young males.

Symptoms Patients complain of a continuous, severe aching pain that stops them sleeping. Rest pain is usually experienced in the most distal part of the limb, namely the toes and forefoot. The patient feels the pain at the junction of the living and dead tissues if any gangrene is present.

Rest pain is often relieved by putting the leg below the level of the heart, so patients hang their legs over the side of the bed or prefer to sleep sitting in a chair. The painful part is very sensitive. Movement or pressure exacerbates the pain. The patient can be seen siting in bed with the knee bent, holding the foot still attempting to relieve the pain. Strong analgesic drugs are the only means of providing relief. Rest pain is unremitting and gets steadily worse.

Systematic questions It is important to enquire about symptoms suggestive of pre-existing arterial disease in the affected limb, such as claudication, and any symptoms that indicate the presence of atherosclerosis elsewhere (Revision panel 10.4).

Family history Arterial disease can be familial, so it is important to ascertain the cause of death of parents and siblings, and whether they had any symptoms of vascular disease.

Risk factors These include a history of cigarette smoking, hypertension, diabetes and hypercholesterolaemia.

Revision panel 10.4

SYSTEMIC INDICATORS OF SERIOUS VASCULAR DISEASE

Chest pains
A previous myocardial infarction
Weakness or paraesthesiae in the upper limbs
Fainting
Episodes of blurred vision
Previous stroke

Examination

General appearance

Patients with rest pain usually look drawn and exhausted because of continuous pain and sleepless nights. They are often unable to lie flat on a couch with the leg horizontal for more than a short period because elevation of the leg exacerbates the pain. Again, the whole cardiovascular system must be examined with care.

Inspection

When dependent, a painful ischaemic foot is a *deep reddish–purple colour* (Figure 10.2). The tips of the toes may be grey or white if they are completely bloodless. There may be *black patches of gangrene on the toes or the heel* (Figure 10.8).

When horizontal, the foot rapidly becomes pale or marble white, and the veins empty, becoming guttered. Further elevation of the leg increases the pallor. If the foot is not white when horizontal, it will certainly become so when elevated to 20°.

It is possible to have severely ischaemic toes and a good circulation in the rest of the foot. In these circumstances, the description above applies only to the toes. The pain is unlikely to be an ischaemic pain if the whole foot is painful but stays pink above an angle of 20°. The foot may be swollen and blue if the patient has been sitting with the leg dependent to ease the pain.

The pressure areas on the heel and the skin between the toes may be gangrenous, ulcerated or infected (Figure 10.9). Ischaemic changes often develop at the site of the nail beds.

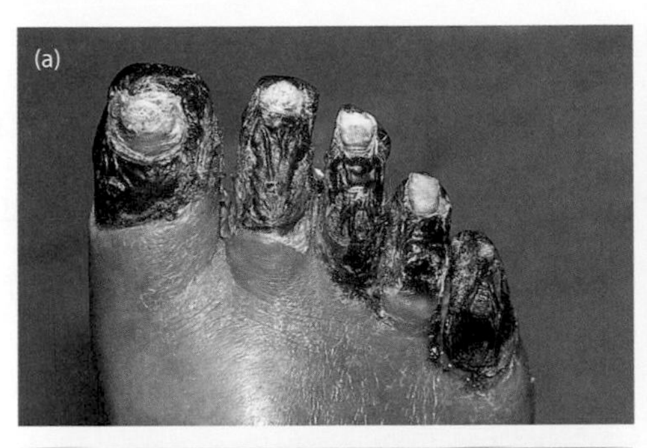

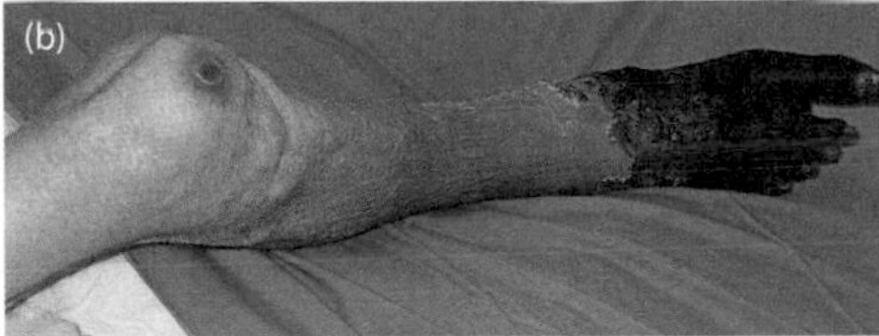

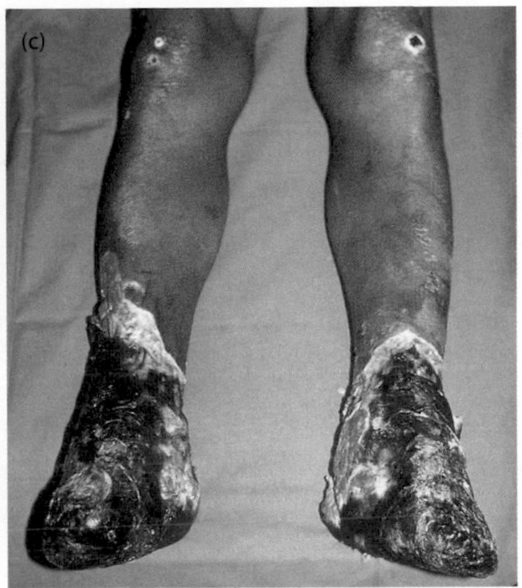

Figure 10.8 GANGRENE. (a) Black areas of clearly defined (demarcated) gangrene (dry and uninfected). (b) Gangrene caused by frostbite. (c) Gangrene caused by trenchfoot.

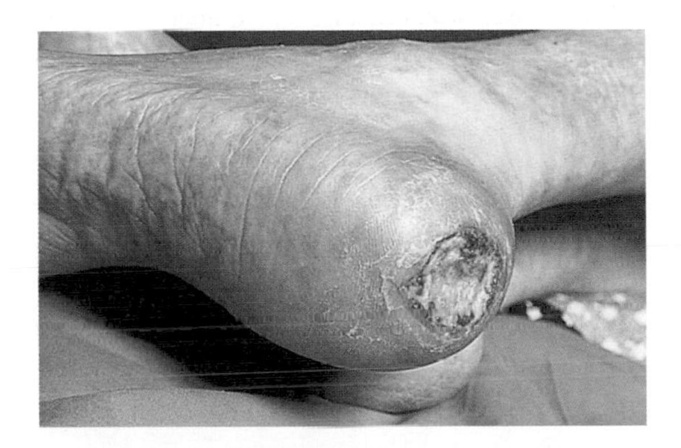

Figure 10.9 Pressure necrosis of the heel.

Palpation

The skin temperature from mid-calf downwards is usually reduced, even when the foot is dependent and congested. Capillary refilling is markedly reduced.

In general, rest pain is caused by a combination of large and small vessel disease, so it is common to find that the popliteal, foot and sometimes the femoral pulses are absent. Small vessel vasculitic disease, such as Buerger's disease should be suspected if these pulses are palpable, but the toes/forefoot are ischaemic.

Auscultation

Bruits may be heard over the iliac and femoral arteries (see Figure 10.6).

Other signs

There may be muscle wasting caused by disuse, and if the patient has been sitting holding the ischaemic foot for many weeks, there may be a fixed flexion deformity of the knee and hip joint.

Examination of the nervous system is important because a severe, constant pain in the lower limb may be caused by a neurological abnormality (see Chapter 3). The nervous system may be abnormal in individuals with diabetes, but these patients rarely have very severe rest pain as the diabetes destroys the limb's pain sensation.

Other causes of the pain include gout (which may cause severe pain in the foot, with redness and tenderness [see Chapter 8]) or an abscess or foreign body.

PREGANGRENE AND GANGRENE

This is also far more common in the lower limb, because upper limb vessels have a better collateral circulation.

Pregangrene

This term is used by clinicians to describe the changes that indicate that a tissue's blood supply is so precarious that it will soon be insufficient to keep the tissue alive.

The principal symptom of pregangrene is rest pain, which is described in detail above.

The principal signs are pallor of the tissues when elevated, congestion when dependent, guttering of the veins, thick and scaling skin and wasting of the pulps of the toes or fingers. The limb is cold and has poor capillary refilling. Ischaemic tissue is tender. Any further reduction in the blood supply will result in tissue death, or gangrene (see below). Therefore, these symptoms must be treated with the utmost urgency.

Gangrene

Gangrene is the term used to describe dead tissue. *Dead tissue is brown, dark blue or black* and gradually contracts into a crinkled, withered, hard mass. These changes can happen if a patch of skin, a toe (Figure 10.10) or the whole of the lower limb becomes ischaemic. The nerves in the dead part die, and therefore gangrenous tissues are not painful.

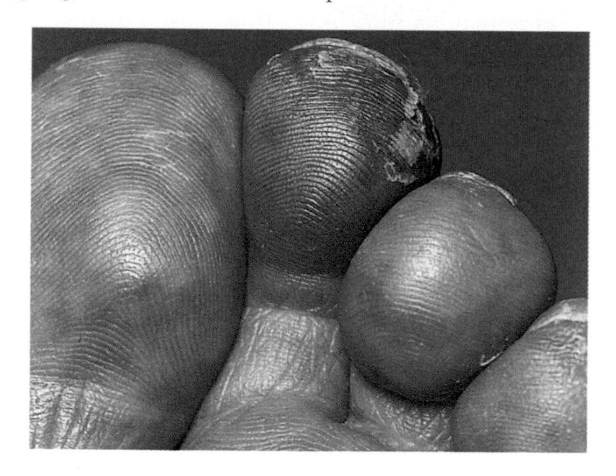

Figure 10.10 A blue ischaemic toe caused by emboli from a femoral artery stenosis.

The junction between the living and dead tissue gradually becomes distinct, provided there is adequate venous drainage and the proximal blood supply remains intact. This junction is known as the *line of demarcation*. The dead tissue may eventually separate and fall off. The living tissue on the proximal side of the line of demarcation is usually ischaemic, so is often constantly painful (rest pain) and tender. Pain is not experienced if the gangrene is the result of local trauma and the surrounding tissues are normal.

Gangrene usually develops in the extremities of the limbs – the tips of the toes and fingers – and in areas of skin subjected to pressure. The dead tissue does not become shrivelled if its venous drainage is impaired or if it becomes infected. In these circumstances, the gangrene becomes soft and boggy, and the line of demarcation is often indistinct and becomes purulent.

A hard, shrunken, non-infected patch of gangrene with a clear line of demarcation is called *dry gangrene* (Figure 10.8a). A soft, swollen, infected patch of gangrene without a clear margin is called *wet gangrene* (Figure 10.11). It is probably better to use the terms *infected* and *non-infected* rather than wet and dry. This difference is important because sometimes, as in those with diabetes, the gangrene is actually secondary to the infection and not the ischaemia. This is often associated with gas in the tissues (*tissue crepitus*) as the result of infection with gas-forming organisms that cause a foul smell.

Venous gangrene, which may complicate a massive deep vein thrombosis and phlegmasia caerulia dolens, usually affects all the toes (Figure 10.12).

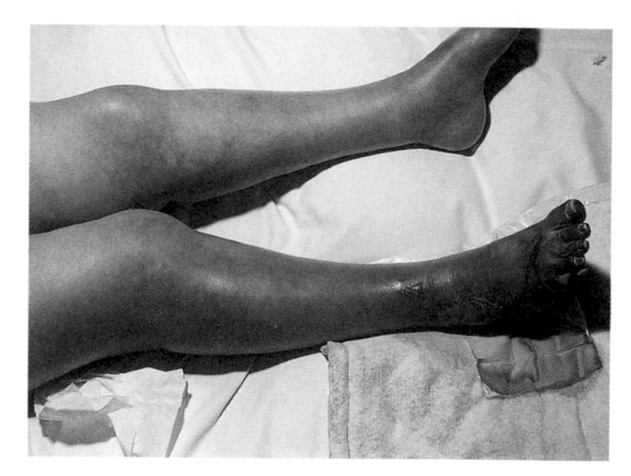

Figure 10.11 Wet gangrene with no clear line of demarcation.

ISCHAEMIC ULCERATION

An ischaemic ulcer is the aftermath of gangrene. By definition, it is caused by an inadequate blood supply.

History

Ischaemic ulcers are common in the elderly, who often also have other cardiovascular comorbidities, with symptoms of coronary or cerebral vascular

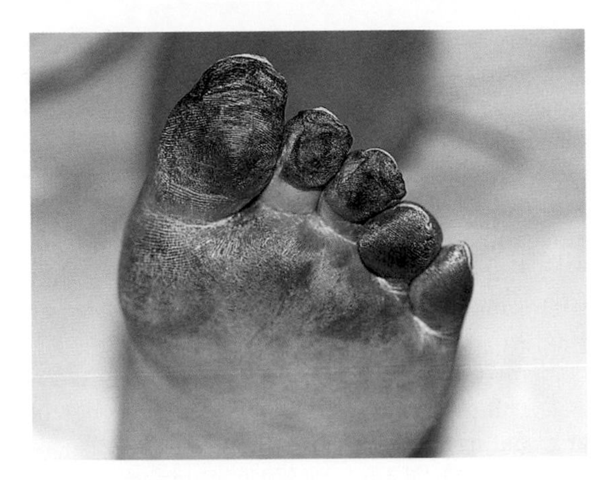

Figure 10.12 Venous gangrene in a patient with a massive venous thrombosis, which has presented with very symmetrical gangrene of all the toes combined with foot swelling.

disease. Patients sometimes remember a minor precipitating injury.

Symptoms Ischaemic ulcers, except those associated with a neurological abnormality, are very painful. They cause rest pain.

They do not bleed, but they discharge a thin serous exudate, which can become purulent. They are usually indolent, and often slowly become deeper and larger. Ischaemic ulcers may occasionally penetrate into tendons and joints, making movements very painful. The causes of ischaemic ulcers are (Revision panels 10.5, 10.6):

- Large artery obliteration: atherosclerosis and embolism.
- Small artery obliteration: Buerger's disease, atheroembolism, diabetes, scleroderma and physical agents such as prolonged local pressure, radiation, trauma and electrical burns.

Systematic questions and past history The patient may give a history of prior claudication or symptoms of generalized vascular disease such as chest pain.

Examination

Site Ischaemic ulcers are found at the tips of the toes or fingers and over the pressure points.

Size Ischaemic ulcers vary in size from small, deep defects a few millimetres across, to large, flat ulcers 10 cm or more wide on the lower leg (Figure 10.13).

Shape The ulcers are most often elliptical.

Revision panel 10.5

THE CAUSES OF ISCHAEMIC ULCERATION

Large artery obliteration

Atherosclerosis
Embolism

Small artery obliteration

Scleroderma
Buerger's disease
Embolism
Diabetes
Physical agents:
- Pressure necrosis
- Radiation
- Trauma
- Electric burns

Revision panel 10.6

THE CAUSES OF CHRONIC ULCERATION

Infection
Repeated trauma
Ischaemia
Oedema
Denervation
Localized destructive disease (tuberculosis, carcinoma)

Tenderness The ulcer and the surrounding tissues are often very tender. Removing a dressing can cause an exacerbation of the pain that lasts for several hours.

Temperature The surrounding tissues are usually cold because they are ischaemic. Adjacent, warm, healthy tissue suggests another cause for the ulceration.

Edge The edge of an ischaemic ulcer is either punched out if there is no attempt at healing by the surrounding tissues or sloping if the ulcer is beginning to heal (see Chapter 1). The skin at the edge of the ulcer is usually a blue–grey colour. There is no lipodermatosclerosis in the surrounding skin unless venous disease coexists.

Base The base of the ulcer usually contains grey–yellow slough covering flat, pale, granulation tissue.

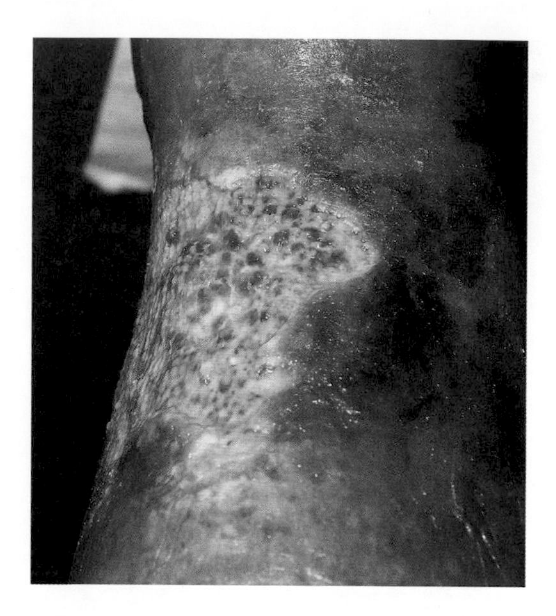

Figure 10.13 A typical ischaemic ulcer with pale granulation tissue in the base of a gently sloping ulcer edge.

Depth Ischaemic ulcers are often very deep. They may penetrate down to and through deep fascia, tendon, bone and even an underlying joint.

Discharge This may be clear fluid, serum or pus.

Relations The base may be stuck to, or be part of, any underlying structure. It is quite common to see bare bone, ligaments and tendons exposed in the base of an ischaemic ulcer.

Lymph glands Infection in an ischaemic ulcer usually remains confined to the ulcer, so the local lymph glands are not normally enlarged.

Local tissues Surrounding tissues may show signs of ischaemia – pallor, coldness and atrophy.

Distal pulses These are invariably absent.

Doppler pressures The Doppler pressure index is invariably reduced.

Neurological examination There may be a loss of superficial and deep sensation, weakness of movement and a loss of reflexes if the ulcer is caused by a neuropathy (see Chapter 3).

General examination There may be evidence of systemic cardiovascular disease elsewhere.

NEUROPATHIC ULCERATION

Pain is the mechanism by which the body appreciates that any part of the skin is becoming deprived of blood. The feet and buttocks become painful after prolonged standing or sitting, encouraging movement to remove the pressure from the painful part. When pain sensation is lost, this warning mechanism is lost, and any compressed tissue may become permanently damaged.

Neuropathic ulcers are therefore only indirectly caused by local ischaemia. The main cause is lack of sensation in the tissues, allowing unrecognized trauma to occur.

Neuropathic ulcers are deep, penetrating ulcers that occur over pressure points (Figure 10.14), but the surrounding tissues are healthy and may have a good circulation. The diagnostic features are as follows:

- The ulcers are often painless.
- The surrounding tissues have reduced sensation to painful stimuli.
- The surrounding tissues may have a normal blood supply.

These ulcers can easily be mistaken for ischaemic ulcers, which is why a neurological examination is

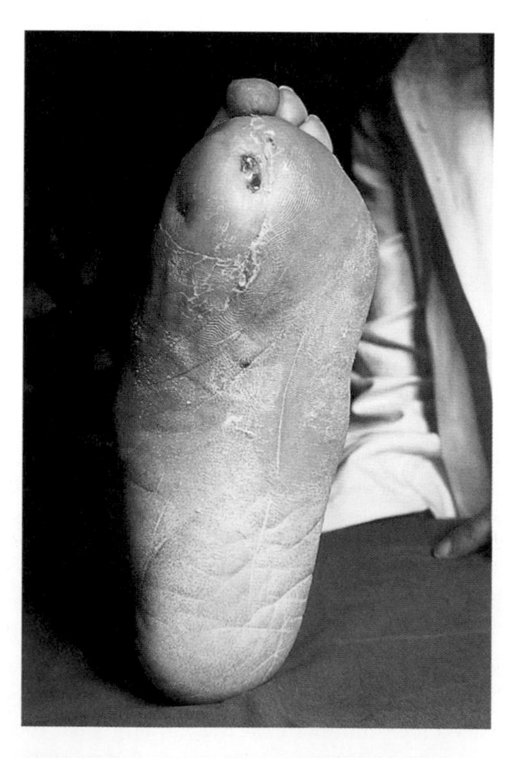

Figure 10.14 A neuropathic ulcer that is deep and painless over a pressure area in an insensate limb.

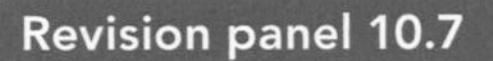

Revision panel 10.7

THE CAUSES OF NEUROPATHIC ULCERATION (ULCERS SECONDARY TO A LOSS OF SENSATION)

Peripheral nerve lesions/neuropathy

Diabetes
Vitamin B12 deficiency
Thyroid disease
Amyloidosis
Nerve injuries
Leprosy
Medications (e.g. chemotherapy, some antibiotics, phenytoin, amiodarone)

Spinal cord lesions

Spina bifida
Tabes dorsalis
Syringomyelia

Revision panel 10.8

THE CAUSES OF ANEURYSMS

Congenital/inherited

A localized weakness:
Berry aneurysm
Marfan's syndrome
Loeys-Dietz syndrome
Ehlers–Danlos syndrome
Arterial dilatation associated with a congenital arteriovenous fistula

Acquired aneurysm

Trauma
Direct injury
Infection:
Bacterial/fungal arteritis (mycotic)
Syphilis
Acquired immunodeficiency syndrome
Atherosclerotic

False (pseudo-) aneurysms

Trauma
Post-arterial surgery

always important. The causes of neuropathic ulceration (Revision panel 10.7) are:

- Peripheral nerve lesions: diabetes, nerve injuries or leprosy.
- Spinal cord lesions: spina bifida, tabes dorsalis and syringomyelia (see Chapters 3 and 9).

All these conditions may, however, occur in patients with vascular disease, so true ischaemic and neuropathic ulcers may occur together, and the combined effect of both diseases may be synergistic.

Careful examination of the arterial and neurological systems is required to identify the major cause.

Pulsatile swellings (aneurysms)

An aneurysm is a *localized dilatation of an artery.* The majority of aneurysms are caused by degeneration of the arterial wall, often with associated atherosclerosis, but some are caused by a primary weakness in the connective tissues of the arterial wall.

The causes of aneurysms are shown in Revision panel 10.8.

In a true aneurysm, all the layers of the arterial wall (intima, media and adventitia) are involved. In a false aneurysm, the arterial wall is breached, and the wall of the aneurysm consists of blood clot and compressed surrounding normal tissues.

Although an aneurysm can develop in any artery, most occur in the abdominal aorta and the femoral and popliteal arteries.

Berry aneurysms (see Chapter 3) arise in a weakened area of the circle of Willis. They are often associated with hypertension and are responsible for many subarachnoid haemorrhages at any age. It is debatable whether they are truly congenital, but the weakness responsible for their development may possibly be inherited.

Syphilitic aneurysms of the thoracic aorta were once common but are now extremely rare.

History

Age Aneurysms are rare before the age of 50 years. Thereafter, their frequency increases with age.

Sex Males are affected six times more often than females.

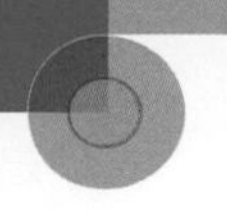

Other causative factors

- Family history.
- Cigarette smoking.
- Hypertension.

Symptoms Many aneurysms cause no symptoms during life and are discovered by chance during a routine physical examination, radiological investigation or by a screening programme.

The most common presenting symptom is *dull, aching pain*. With abdominal aneurysms, this is usually experienced over the swelling in the centre of the abdomen, *but the pain often radiates to the back*. The abdominal pain is caused by stretching of the artery, and the back pain by erosion of, or pressure on, the lumbar vertebrae (see Revision panel 9.3).

Some patients with abdominal aneurysms present with *sciatica or loin pain* as a consequence of local pressure on the nerves.

Acute pain occurs if the vessel suddenly stretches or begins to tear. This becomes a very severe pain if the aneurysm ruptures and a large haematoma forms (see Chapter 15). The patient may collapse from the accompanying hypotensive shock or suddenly die.

A few thin patients notice a *pulsatile mass*. This is a common presentation for femoral aneurysms but is rare for abdominal aneurysms.

> **NOTE:** Occasionally, patients notice their abdomen pulsating when they lie in the bath or in bed.

Severe ischaemia of the lower limb can occur if an aneurysm thromboses. This is a rare event in aortic and femoral aneurysms but is a common presentation of popliteal aneurysms.

Acute ischaemia may also be caused by emboli originating in the aneurysm. One of the best examples of this complication is the multiple small emboli that may block the digital arteries of a patient with a subclavian aneurysm. In the lower limb, emboli from an aortic or popliteal aneurysm may cause intermittent claudication or rest pain.

The aorta, femoral and popliteal arteries are closely related to the inferior vena cava and the femoral and popliteal veins, respectively. Dilatation of an artery may compress its adjacent vein by direct pressure. Patients may present with intermittent limb swelling or, if the vein thromboses off, a *massively swollen, blue, painful limb*.

Very occasionally, aneurysms rupture into an adjacent vein. The resulting acute arteriovenous fistula may cause *high output cardiac failure* with warm peripheries. The neck veins are elevated, and there is usually a loud machinery murmur over the aneurysm.

Systematic questions and past history Coronary or cerebral vascular disease can coexist.

Examination

Abdominal aneurysms

The abdominal aorta divides into the iliac arteries at about the level of the umbilicus. Consequently, most abdominal aneurysms are felt in the upper umbilical and epigastric regions (Figure 10.15). Iliac artery aneurysms present as a pulsating mass in the iliac fossa or hypogastrium.

Aneurysms produce an *expansile pulsation*. In order to feel the expansion, both hands must be placed on either side of the mass to confirm that the hands are pushed apart as well as being pushed upwards (Figure 10.15a).

Many lumps in the upper abdomen transmit aortic pulsation and may be misdiagnosed as aneurysms. Real difficulty may occasionally be encountered if the aorta is encased by pathologically enlarged lymph glands.

Aneurysms feel firm and smooth and can sometimes be moved a little from side to side. The presence of tenderness implies that there is inflammatory change, or that the wall of the aneurysm is stretching and at higher risk of rupture.

> **NOTE:** The pulses at the groins and in the legs are usually present, and the vessels often slightly dilated. All pulses must be carefully palpated and their presence or absence documented, as aneurysmal and occlusive disease may coexist in some patients (Figure 10.16).

The signs and symptoms of a ruptured aneurysm are described in Chapter 15. *When an aneurysm ruptures, it becomes very painful and tender.* The patient may collapse with signs of hypovolaemic shock – *pallor, tachycardia and hypotension*. An expanding retroperitoneal haematoma may be felt as a large mass

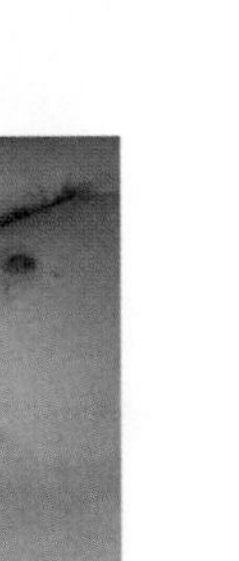

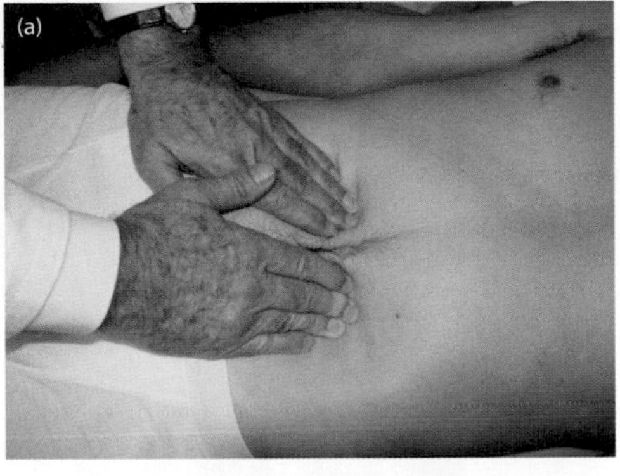

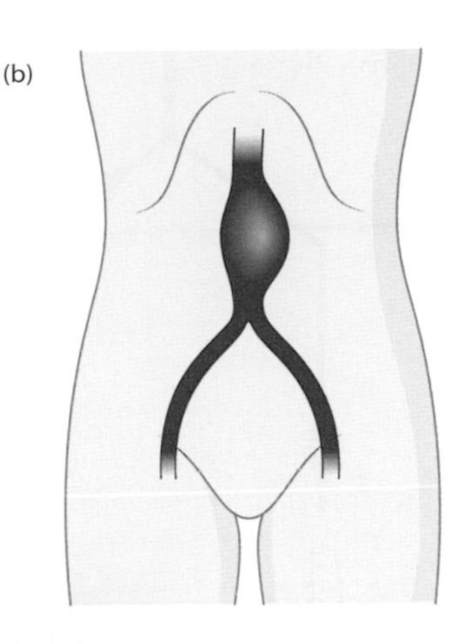

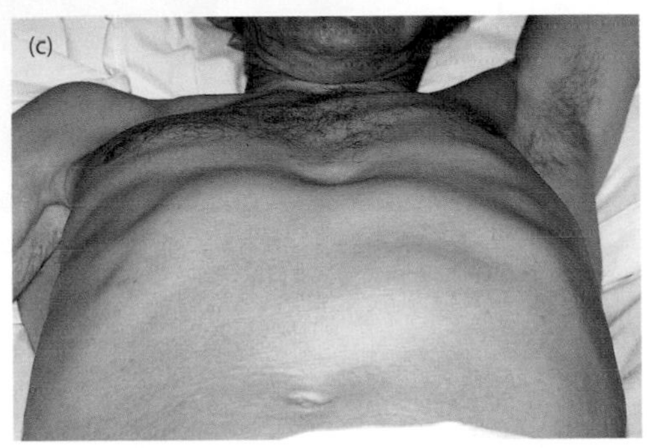

Figure 10.15 ABDOMINAL AORTIC ANEURYSM. (a) The bimanual technique used for palpating an abdominal aortic aneurysm. Assess the width of the abdominal aorta by placing your hands on either side of the pulse in the epigastrium. (b) The position of an aneurysm of the abdominal aorta. The aneurysm probably begins below the origin of the renal arteries if there is a gap between the top of the aneurysm and the costal margin. The femoral pulses are usually palpable. (c) A large central/upper abdominal expansile pulsatile mass indicative of an abdominal aortic aneurysm.

in the abdomen spreading down into the iliac fossa or posteriorly into the loins.

Femoral aneurysms

These usually arise in the common femoral artery, and produce a bulge just below the inguinal ligament (Figure 10.17). They have an *expansile pulsation*. A mass of enlarged lymph glands may transmit pulsation and can be misdiagnosed as an aneurysm (see the differential diagnosis of a groin lump, Revision panel 14.4).

NOTE: The other pulses in the leg must be documented, as there is often an associated popliteal aneurysm. Femoral and popliteal aneurysms are commonly bilateral, but do not necessarily develop or present at the same time (see page 345).

Popliteal aneurysms

Aneurysms of the popliteal artery are occasionally noticed by patients if they bulge out of the popliteal fossa. They may be found incidentally in patients presenting with *claudication*. Popliteal aneurysms should always be excluded in patients presenting with an idiopathic calf vein thrombosis. Unfortunately, popliteal aneurysms often thrombose before they are noticed, and present with *acute ischaemia of the lower limb* (see page 340).

A popliteal aneurysm should always be suspected when a popliteal pulse is easy to feel. The diagnosis is confirmed by finding an *expansile pulsation* in the popliteal fossa (Figure 10.18). The examiner's fingers are pushed apart and away by the pulse, which can often be felt on both sides of the popliteal fossa. A bruit may be present above or over an enlarged segment of the vessel.

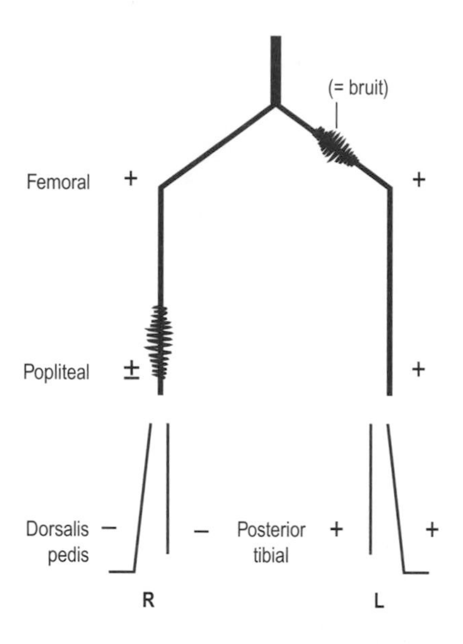

Figure 10.16 Record the pulses and bruits on a simple diagram.

A thrombosed popliteal aneurysm is smooth and solid and does not pulsate or fluctuate. It can be moved slightly from side to side, but never moves up and down. It may be confused with a Baker's cyst or semimembranosus bursa (see Chapter 8), but its size does not change when the knee is flexed, and it occupies the whole length of the midline of the popliteal fossa. The ankle pulses will not be palpable.

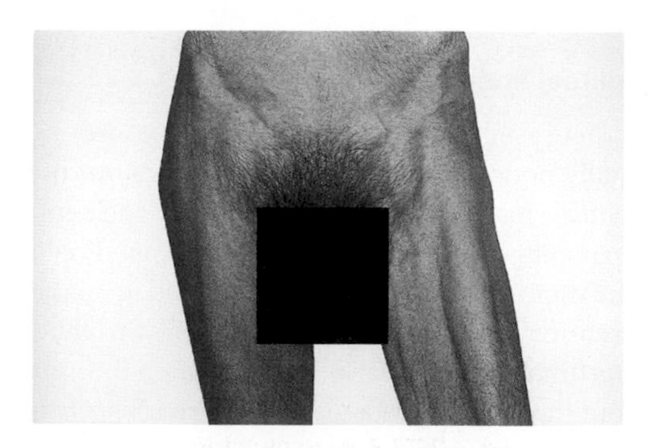

Figure 10.17 A femoral aneurysm seen as a widened vertical pulsatile mass in the left groin.

False aneurysms

A false aneurysm is a large haematoma whose centre contains fluid blood and connects with the lumen of the blood vessel. The most common causes are therapeutic or diagnostic vascular punctures; false

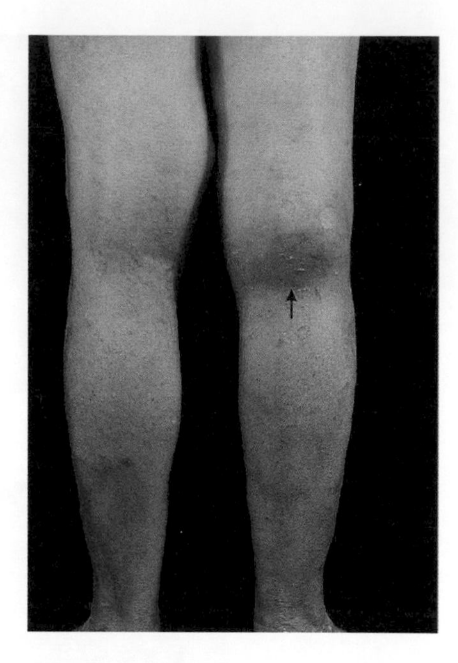

Figure 10.18 A popliteal aneurysm seen in the posterior aspect of the right leg.

aneurysms arising from a vascular anastomosis result from a suture line defect (a pulsatile mass beneath an incision in the groin at the site of a previous vascular anastomosis is most likely to be a false aneurysm) or a stab wound. Following the arterial puncture, a haematoma forms outside the artery. At first, thrombus plugs the defect, but pulsatile blood pressure gradually pushes out the haemostatic plug from the defect in the artery wall and excavates the haematoma to form a cavity connected to the vessel.

The symptoms, signs and complications of false aneurysms are exactly the same as those of a true aneurysm except for the following:

- There is a history of trauma or iatrogenic intervention (arterial puncture or vascular anastomosis), followed by
- The sudden appearance of a pulsatile swelling.
- False aneurysms tend to occur at unusual sites, for example, the wrist or ankle, although iatrogenic false aneurysms are now most common in the groin.

NOTE: False aneurysms also occur when a surgical graft separates from the native vessel.

Haemorrhage

A major vascular disruption, which may be the result of a penetrating, blunt or hyperextension injury, is likely to result in severe haemorrhage. The bleeding may be *concealed*, as when, for example, a serrated or spiculated end of a fractured long bone pierces an artery or a ruptured aneurysm bleeds into the tissues or a body cavity, or may be *revealed*, as when an aneurysm erupts through the skin or a congenital vascular malformation bleeds onto the skin surface.

Concealed haemorrhage from an arterial injury is suspected if a large swelling rapidly develops in association with signs of hypovolaemia, i.e. pallor, sweating, venoconstriction, tachycardia and eventually hypotension. The pulses distal to the injury will not be palpable if the artery has been transected, when the limb may show signs of acute ischaemia (see Revision panel 10.2).

In patients presenting with *visible revealed haemorrhage*, the diagnosis is straightforward. There is usually a jet of bright red, high pressure, pulsatile blood coming out of an obvious cutaneous defect or wound. (Venous bleeding, in contrast, is dark red and very rapidly wells up out of the wound.) The pulses distal to the injury may be absent if the artery has been transected. Direct pressure or proximal arterial compression over a bony point, or elevation and compression in the case of a venous cause, should arrest the bleeding until definitive treatment can be administered.

When the bleeding is coming from the site of a penetrating wound, it is important to assess local nerve and muscle, as other vital structures may be damaged. This may be difficult because the arrest of the haemorrhage must take precedence.

NOTE: Artery, vein, nerve and muscle injuries commonly coexist.

When haemorrhage occurs into a body cavity or is deeply seated, there may be no signs of swelling and the symptoms of hypovolaemia predominate. Haemorrhage into the peritoneum or retroperitoneum often causes pain as well as collapse and may be associated with bruising around the umbilicus (*Cullen's sign*) or flank (*Grey-Turner's sign*) (see Chapter 15).

Transient and permanent neurological weakness, paralysis and blindness

CEREBROVASCULAR ACCIDENTS

NOTE: It is important to remember that the right side of the brain controls the left side of the body, and vice versa.

The speech area (Broca's area) is invariably in the left temporoparietal area in right-handed people, although it can sometimes be in the right hemisphere in left-handed patients; nevertheless, even in left-handed patients, Broca's area is more likely to be on the left side.

Cerebrovascular accidents are more commonly caused by *infarction* than by *cerebral haemorrhage*, and are usually embolic or thrombotic, although an arterial wall dissection can occlude an artery's lumen. A sudden episode of cerebral malfunction caused by cerebral infarction or haemorrhage, both caused by vascular disease, usually takes the form of

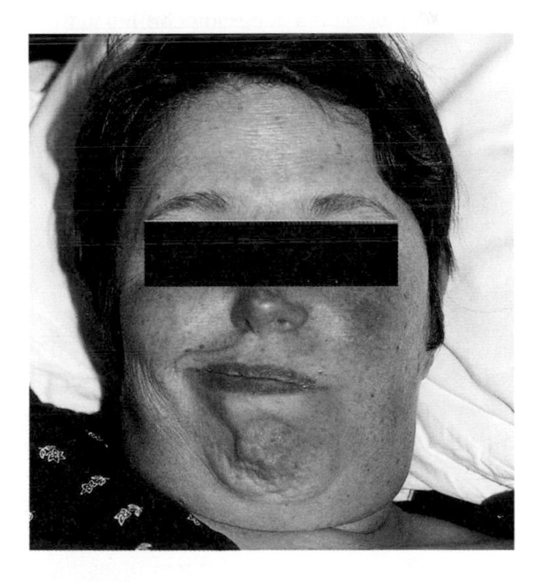

Figure 10.19 A patient who is hemiplegic with a facial weakness (upper motor; see Chapter 3) that is indicative of a cerebral infarct or bleed from a cerebral vascular accident.

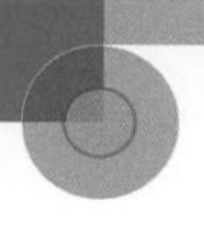

a prolonged weakness or paralysis of one half of the body (*a hemiplegia*) (Figure 10.19) and sometimes an associated sensory or speech defect, which may predominate (see Chapter 3). Ischaemia of the midbrain that damages the vital centres in this area may cause coma and cardiovascular and respiratory instability.

TRANSIENT ISCHAEMIC ATTACKS

These are defined as a brief episode of neurological or visual dysfunction (i.e. paralysis, paraesthesiae, speech or visual loss) resulting from focal temporary cerebral or retinal ischaemia not associated with permanent infarction. The classic definition stipulated that symptoms must recover completely within 24 hours (otherwise the patient is determined to have had a stroke), but this time limit has been removed as it is now considered arbitrary.

They are most commonly caused by emboli or hypoperfusion. The emboli can come from the carotid arteries, heart valves and the great vessels. Platelet clumps and cholesterol crystals originally attached to ulcerated plaques break off and are swept up into the retinal or cerebral vessels (Figure 10.20).

Retinal emboli cause transient loss of vision, known as *amaurosis fugax* (fleeting blindness), which seems to the patient like a curtain coming across the visual field or a grey veil blocking out all or part of the vision in one eye.

Other causes of transient blindness include:

- Multiple sclerosis.
- Acute glaucoma.
- Retinal tears.
- Temporal arteritis can cause transient blindness.

Multiple sclerosis can cause considerable diagnostic confusion, but multiple lesions occurring in time and space eventually indicate the likely diagnosis.

Stroke caused by cerebral haemorrhage produces identical cerebral symptoms but is more common in females and often manifests with more severe neurology that is less transient in nature. Both types of stroke usually cause upper motor neuron signs, with reduced power, spastic tone and brisk reflexes in the limbs, associated with an upgoing plantar reflex (Babinksi's sign). A cerebral haemorrhage can only be differentiated from an infarct with certainty by computed tomography (CT) scanning, and not by the history or physical signs.

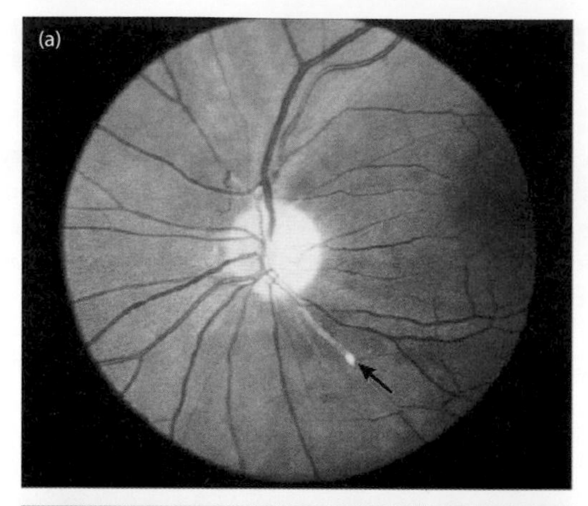

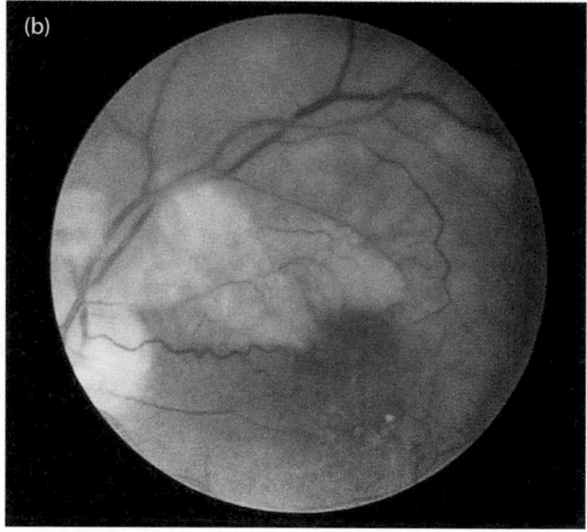

Figure 10.20 RETINAL INFARCT. (a) A retinal platelet embolus arising from a carotid plaque presenting as amaurosis fugax. (b) A retinal infarct. The pale area is the infarct.

Anyone presenting with a brief episode of weakness, paraesthesia or loss of sensation in one-half of the body that lasts a few minutes or several hours and then recovers completely must be suspected of having a transient ischaemic attack.

There are usually no physical signs by the time the patient presents, but evidence of previous ischaemic episodes – facial weakness, expressive dysphasia, upper motor neuron lesions and cholesterol emboli in the retinal vessels or areas of retinal infarction – should be sought.

The detection of a *carotid bruit* over the carotid artery just below the angle of the jaw indicates the presence of some degree of stenosis in the region of the carotid bifurcation.

> **NOTE:** A severe internal carotid artery stenosis can, however, be present without any bruit, and a loud bruit can be caused by a stenosis of the external carotid artery.

Arrhythmias and *cardiac murmurs* suggest a cardiac source for the emboli. A low pulse pressure and an ejection systolic murmur suggest the presence of aortic valve disease, while an irregularly irregular or very slow pulse suggests a possible cause of *Stokes–Adams attacks* (see Chapter 2).

Transient hypoperfusion

Whereas emboli are common, hypoperfusion is rare because autoregulation usually ensures adequate cerebral perfusion, unless there is a very severe reduction in carotid blood pressure and flow. Episodes of hypoperfusion usually occur with much greater frequency than embolic attacks, often several times a day or week, and can be brought on by exercise or vasodilatation. They may cause 'global brain ischaemia', and present with dizziness and collapse rather than motor cortical symptoms.

Differential diagnosis

The differential diagnosis of a transient ischaemic attack is shown in Revision panel 10.9.

Revision panel 10.9

THE DIFFERENTIAL DIAGNOSIS OF A TRANSIENT ISCHAEMIC ATTACK

- Embolism from carotid artery atherosclerosis
- Grand or petit mal epilepsy
- Stokes–Adams attacks from a tight aortic stenosis
- Arrhythmias
- Vasovagal attacks
- Hypoglycaemia
- Migraine
- Vertebrobasilar disease
- Subdural haematoma
- A space-occupying lesion in the brain

A history from a bystander or relative may be very helpful in making the diagnosis.

Epilepsy

Any history of aura, twitching, tongue biting or incontinence is indicative of grand mal epilepsy, whereas petit mal causes patients to lose touch temporarily with their surroundings (see Chapter 3).

Hypoglycaemic attacks

These occur during periods of food abstinence, especially at night. Patients often describe hunger, malaise and vague abdominal pain, which is accompanied by trembling, dizziness and blurred vision. They may also notice incoordination, slurred speech, diplopia and drowsiness. The blood and urinary sugar are low during an attack, the symptoms of which can be instantly relieved by glucose.

Migraine

These attacks are usually heralded by severe unilateral headache, often situated over one eye and associated with photophobia and vomiting and occasionally transient blindness. There are no physical signs, and the diagnosis relies entirely on the history. Sometimes, there is a preceding 'aura' before the migraine begins.

Vertebrobasilar insufficiency

It can sometimes be quite difficult to separate transient ischaemic attacks from vertebrobasilar insufficiency, but the symptoms of the latter from the posterior circulation (including dizziness, vertigo, vomiting, diplopia, blindness and ataxia) are often precipitated by neck movements or looking up. Neurological signs may indicate pathology in the hindbrain or cerebellum. Bruits may be heard over the origin of the vertebral artery.

Subclavian steal syndrome

This syndrome occurs when, if the subclavian artery is occluded or tightly stenosed, blood flows down the vertebral artery during arm exercise in an attempt to act as a collateral vessel to supply the arm (Figure 10.21). This steals blood away from the hindbrain, and gives rise to hindbrain and cerebellar symptoms. Patients present with transient posterior

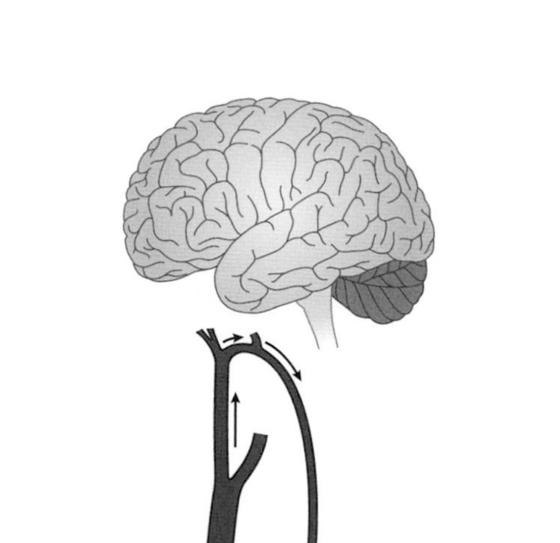

Figure 10.21 The flow of blood up the carotid artery and down the vertebral artery in a patient with subclavian steal syndrome, which results from a block in the proximal subclavian artery (shown). Use of the left arm increases the flow to the limb at the expense of flow to the hindbrain.

circulation symptoms and even loss of consciousness, after arm exercise. The presence of a weak brachial and radial pulse, reduced blood pressure in the affected arm and a bruit over the subclavian artery should suggest the diagnosis of subclavian steal syndrome.

Other intracranial disease

Patients with a *subdural haematoma* may experience fluctuations in their level of consciousness and will almost always develop some localizing neurological signs before eventually developing signs of raised intracranial pressure (see Chapter 3). This is also true of *cerebral tumours and metastases,* which can initially cause diagnostic confusion until the patient eventually develops signs of fixed and expanding defects.

COMPLETED STROKES

A full neurological examination is essential in all patients who present with a completed stroke, in order to exclude a vascular cause as well as a neurological dysfunction caused by:

- Space-occupying lesions.
- Abscesses.
- Haematomas.
- Multiple sclerosis (see Chapter 3).

The blood pressure and heart must be carefully assessed (see Chapter 2). The superficial temporal arteries should be palpated. The carotid bifurcation and lower neck should be auscultated for *bruits.* A stethoscope placed over the closed eye can occasionally detect intracerebral bruits in patients with a stenosis in the carotid siphon.

Cold, blue digits, hands and feet

Intermittent colour changes of the skin of the periphery of the limbs suggest the presence of vasospasm or recurrent minor episodes of arterial occlusion.

The supraclavicular fossa must be inspected and palpated for a fullness or occasionally a bony lump caused by a *cervical rib* or a *dilated subclavian artery.* The subclavian, axillary, brachial, radial and ulnar pulses must all be palpated and auscultated.

> **NOTE:** The blood pressure should be measured in both arms, and Doppler pressures must be measured in the radial, ulnar and brachial pulses.

Abnormalities detected by these examinations may require further imaging, including plain radiographs, dynamic Duplex scanning, magnetic resonance imaging (MRI), or CT angiography.

Patients not found to have a physical obstruction of their blood vessels are likely to be suffering from *excessive vasospasm of the small vessels* in their hands in response to cold and emotional stimuli. Some conditions can be diagnosed by the physical appearances they produce, but their aetiology is still largely conjectural, and there is a considerable overlap between each condition.

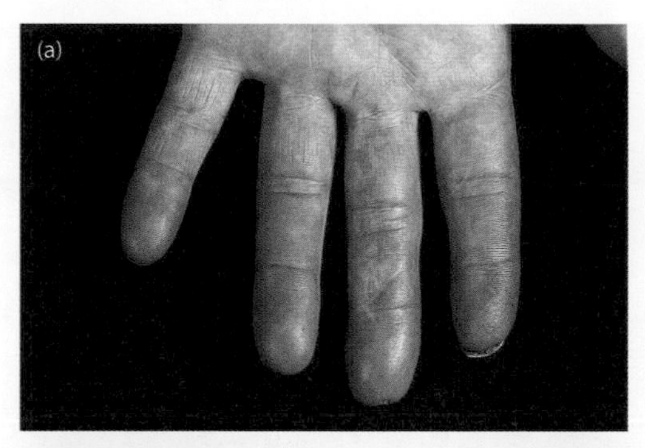

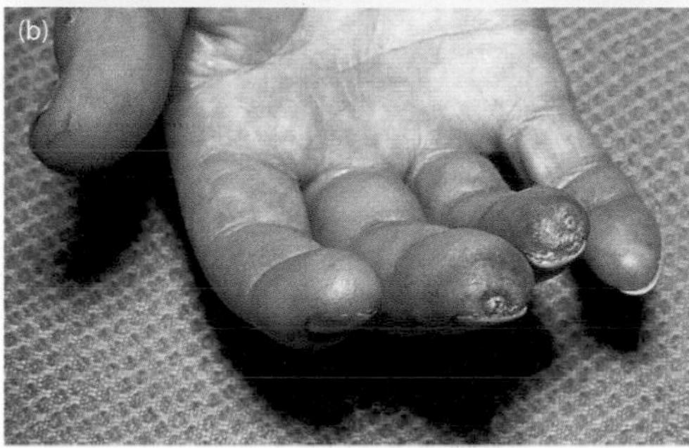

Figure 10.22 VASOSPASTIC DIGITAL CHANGES. (a) Raynaud's phenomenon. (b) Ischaemic ulceration of the fingertips. This usually indicates permanent, rather than spastic, occlusion of the digital vessels.

RAYNAUD'S PHENOMENON

This is the best-known vasospastic disorder. The term is used to describe a series of colour changes in the skin of the hands or feet following exposure to cold (Figure 10.22a). The condition can be most distressing in cold climates, especially in winter.

- The skin first turns white and becomes cold and numb.
- It next turns blue, but remains cold and numb.
- Finally, it turns red, hot and painful.

Many attacks are brought on by cold or emotion, and many do not pass through all the classic colour changes (Revision panel 10.10).

History

A clear history is essential in making an accurate differential diagnosis.

Sex Ninety per cent of those affected are female, and many are cigarette smokers. It affects 5%–20% of the population.

Revision panel 10.10

THE CAUSES OF RAYNAUD'S PHENOMENON

- Atherosclerosis and Buerger's disease
- Platelet emboli from:
  - Subclavian aneurysm (secondary to cervical rib)
  - Atherosclerotic stenosis of the subclavian artery
  - Atherosclerotic disease of the aortic arch
- Collagen disease:
  - Scleroderma
  - Systemic lupus erythematosus
  - Rheumatoid arthritis
- Vibrating tools
- Irritation of nerves:
  - Cervical spondylosis
  - Cervical rib
  - Spinal cord disease
  - Old poliomyelitis
- Repeated immersion in cold water
- Working in a cold environment
- Previous frostbite
- Blood abnormalities:
  - Cold agglutinin disease
  - Cryoglobulins
  - Polycythaemia
- Drugs:
  - Ergot
- General diseases:
  - Hypothyroidism
  - Diabetes
  - Malnutrition

Past history It is worthwhile asking patients if they have a history of frostbite, have regularly used vibrating tools or have a family history.

Joint problems, rashes and swallowing difficulty indicate the likelihood of scleroderma or another collagen vascular disease.

Examination

Those conditions which, in addition to the colour changes, cause permanent damage to the digital arteries, such as scleroderma, vibration injury and blood abnormalities, gradually cause atrophy of the pulps of the fingers, poor nail growth and ulceration of the fingertips. The fingers waste, especially the pulps, and become thin, stiff and pointed if the digital arteries become occluded. The hand is cold and the joints may be stiff. Sometimes, there are small, painful, ischaemic ulcers on the fingertips, which are slow to heal, or small scars at the site of the resolution of previous patches of ischaemia. Both are very painful and tender. The patient may eventually develop rest pain and gangrene of the fingertips. Repeated infections around the nails (paronychia) are common.

Many patients eventually develop the signs of scleroderma, evidence that the phenomenon is a secondary abnormality, not a primary disease.

When the cause of the colour changes is solely vasospasm, the hands look normal between attacks, making the diagnosis of the underlying cause far more difficult. The symptoms are often secondary to other conditions, and the diagnosis of idiopathic Raynaud's disease is only made when these have been excluded.

The common causes are:

- *Collagen vascular diseases, especially scleroderma.*
- *Excessive use of vibrating tools.*
- *Cold exposure.*

Patients with scleroderma, systemic lupus erythematosus and rheumatoid arthritis may show the characteristic changes in their skin and face (see Chapter 1, Figure 1.13).

PRIMARY RAYNAUD'S DISEASE

NOTE: When all other causes of Raynaud's phenomenon have been excluded, a diagnosis of primary Raynaud's disease is upheld.

This condition is quite common in teenage females. It is mild, familial and often associated with chilblains. It often disappears in the late twenties, but a few females have symptoms all their life, and occasionally the disease becomes very severe.

When the symptoms start in adult females, often around the menopause, they are likely to be the first sign of scleroderma.

It is always worthwhile measuring the Doppler pressures at the wrist, especially if the pulses are impalpable. The digital vessels may also be insonated with the hand-held Doppler and, in patients with collagen diseases, signals in these vessels may well be absent near the tips of the fingers.

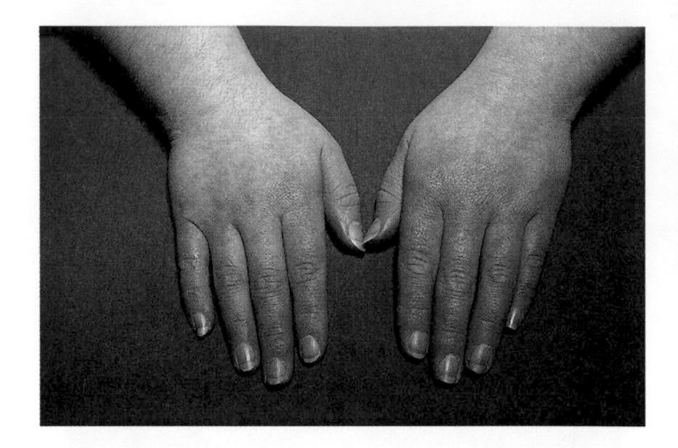

Figure 10.23 Hands demonstrating the red/blue colour changes of acrocyanosis.

Some clinicians use a cold exposure test – dipping the hands in cold water and re-mapping and re-measuring the Doppler digital pressures in the fingers – to reproduce the symptoms and confirm the existence of a cold sensitivity.

ACROCYANOSIS

This usually affects females, in which the hands and feet are persistently blue and cold (Figure 10.23). The colour of the skin does not vary with the environmental temperature as it does in Raynaud's phenomenon, but the blue discolouration may come and go. The hands may be pink and normal between attacks, or cold with sweaty palms. As the attack subsides, the hands may become warm, sweaty and painful. The fingers are susceptible to chilblains. The diagnosis is based solely on the colour, temperature and appearance of the hands.

ERYTHROCYANOSIS CRURUM PUELLARUM FRIGIDUM

This condition affects the posterior and medial aspects of the lower legs of young (15–25 years old) females in response to cold. The legs are often fat and hairless.

The affected areas become red/blue (erythrocyanotic) and swollen. *Dusky reddish–purple blotches*

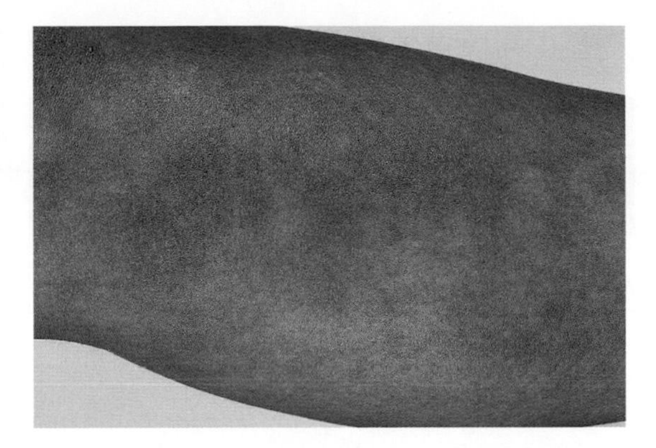

Figure 10.24 Erythrocyanosis crurum puellarum frigidum (erythrocyanosis frigida), seen as painful, red, cold areas of induration (chilblains).

appear and may feel cold to the touch. The swollen area is tender and may progress to chilblains and superficial ulceration (Figure 10.24). When the chilblains break down and ulcerate, they must be differentiated from other forms of leg ulcer.

ERYTHROMELALGIA

This is a condition in which the patient complains of burning red extremities. These symptoms may be exacerbated by the pressure of bedclothes against the skin. The condition is much more common in females. It appears to result from the release of vasodilator neurochemicals, with 5-hydroxytryptamine accumulating in the tissues. It must be differentiated from gout, Buerger's disease, systemic lupus erythematosis and rheumatoid arthritis and peripheral neuropathy.

Examination of the extremities confirms that they are red, and patients complain that dependency causes an increase in the pain.

Large limbs

Local gigantism, multiple arteriovenous fistulae and Klippel–Trenaunay syndrome all cause a limb to grow larger and thicker than the contralateral limb.

The presence of multiple arteriovenous fistulas throughout a single limb is known as *Parkes Weber syndrome* (Figure 10.25). This is a congenital abnormality. The limb, as well as being enlarged, feels hot.

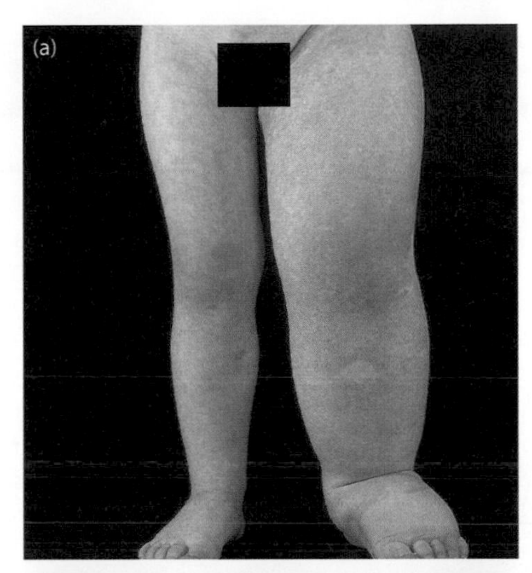

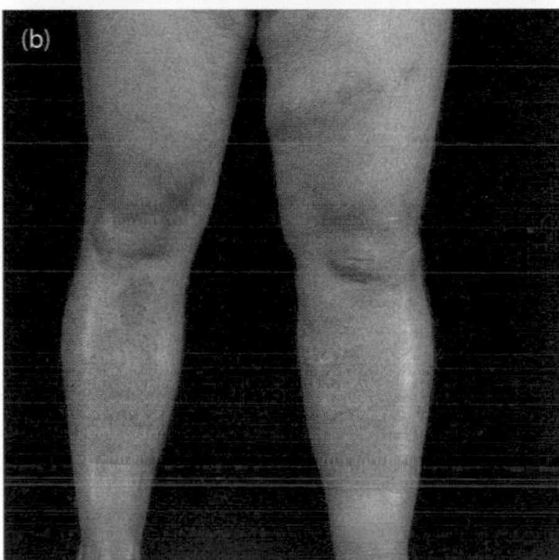

Figure 10.25 PARKES WEBER SYNDROME. (a, b) Limbs with Parkes Weber syndrome, in which the multiple arteriovenous fistulas cause limb enlargement and vascular dilatation. A machinery murmur can often be heard over the limb.

The subcutaneous veins are often dilated. There may be palpable thrills and audible machinery murmurs over the major sites of fistulation.

A tourniquet inflated around the top of the limb should cause slowing of the pulse (*the Branham–Nicoladoni sign*). This is a consequence of reducing the venous return by abolishing the shunt. The differential diagnoses are the other causes of limb hypertrophy mentioned above.

Rarely, patients with a swollen, lymphoedematous limb are misdiagnosed as having a hypertrophic limb.

Surgically correctable causes of hypertension

Renal artery stenosis, retinal haemorrhage, adrenal tumours and *coarctation of the aorta* are important, surgically correctable causes of hypertension. Renal function must be assessed, and the abdomen should be auscultated for bruits in all atherosclerotic patients who are found to be hypertensive.

A 'moon' face, abdominal striae and a 'buffalo' hump (see Chapter 1) are indicative of *Cushing's syndrome*, while the presence of neurofibromas suggests the possibility of a phaeochromocytoma (see Chapter 4).

Coarctation of the aorta is a rare but important cause of hypertension and is discussed in Chapter 2.

Intestinal ischaemia

Ischaemia of the bowel may have an acute or chronic onset.

Acute obstruction of the superior mesenteric artery by an *embolus* or by *thrombosis* causes acute, severe abdominal pain and, if untreated, can progress to peritonitis and shock (see Chapter 15).

Chronic atherosclerotic occlusion or stenosis of the coeliac or mesenteric vessels can cause intestinal angina – abdominal pain that develops 30–60 minutes after eating – causing fear of eating ('food fear') and weight loss. Because of this collateral circulation within the mesenteric vasculature, patients generally only experience symptoms when at least two of the three major mesenteric vessels are involved.

A reduced blood flow in the arteries of the colon, particularly the splenic flexure, can cause ischaemic colitis with diarrhoea and sometimes rectal bleeding (see Chapters 15 and 16).

Patients with chronic mesenteric ischaemia are often emaciated from food fear and may have other systemic features of cardiovascular disease. The only other physical sign in the chronic syndromes may be the presence of an *abdominal bruit*.

THE VEINS

Clinical assessment of the venous circulation of the lower limb

ANATOMY AND PHYSIOLOGY

The veins of the lower limb are divided into the *superficial and deep systems*, separated by the deep fascia of the leg. At certain points, veins pass through the deep fascia to provide a communication between the two systems (Figure 10.26). The valves in these *communicating* veins usually only allow blood to pass from the superficial into the deep system. The deep veins have many valves to ensure that blood only flows upwards against the force of gravity towards the heart. The deep veins accompany the arteries of the lower leg and join to form the popliteal vein, which also receives blood from the calf muscle sinusoids.

When standing, the venous return is heavily dependent on the calf muscle pump. Large venous

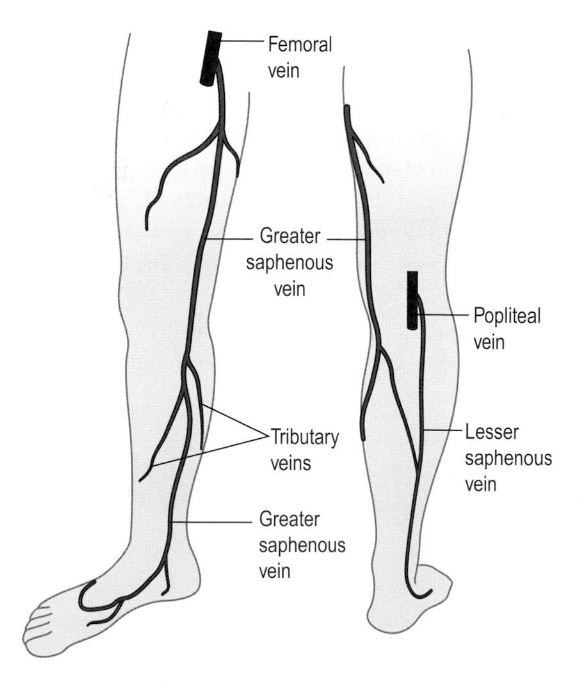

Figure 10.26 A schematic of the superficial, deep and communicating veins of the lower limb.

sinusoids within the soleus muscle are compressed during contraction of the calf muscles, for example, during walking. This forces blood out of the calf veins into the popliteal veins and on towards the heart. During calf muscle relaxation, the intramuscular veins open, but blood is prevented from refluxing back into them from the proximal deep veins by the valves in the popliteal veins. The negative pressure in the deep veins then sucks blood in from the superficial system through the communicating veins to reduce the superficial venous pressure, incrementally, with each calf muscle contraction.

The superficial veins all eventually join either the *great (long) or the lesser (short) saphenous system*. These two major subcutaneous veins end where they communicate with the femoral and popliteal veins, at the saphenofemoral and saphenopopliteal junctions respectively (Figure 10.27). The two superficial systems are also joined to the deep veins by a number of other *communicating (perforating) veins*, the most important of which are in the calf.

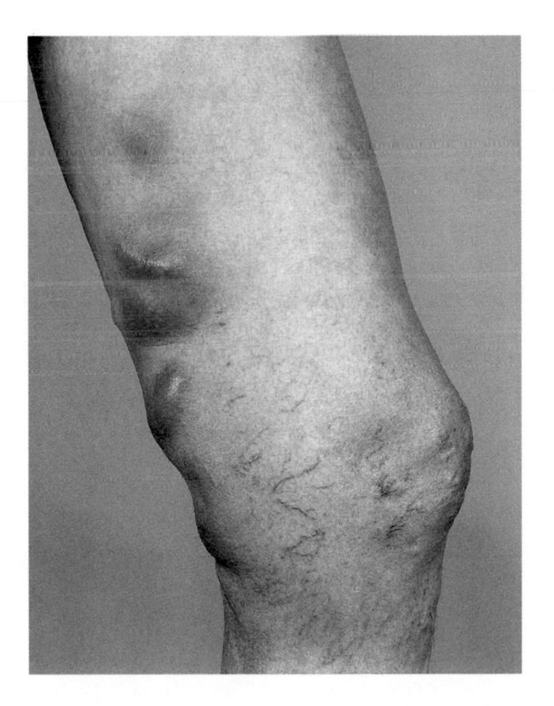

Figure 10.27 Superficial thrombophlebitis in the greater saphenous vein, shown as dark area, which is palpable as 'lumps'.

NOTE: The tributaries of the saphenous veins become varicose because they, unlike the saphenous trunks, do not contain a strong coat of smooth muscle in their wall. They lie in a more superficial position and are not bound down to the deep fascia.

A deep vein thrombosis usually starts in the soleal sinusoids and venae commitantes, before extending up into the popliteal vein, the femoral vein, the iliac veins and even into the vena cava.

SYMPTOMS OF LOWER LIMB VENOUS DISEASE

A varicose vein is a *dilated, tortuous vein* (Figure 10.28). The cause of 'primary' varicose veins is unknown, but the erect stance and abnormalities in the components and structure of the vein wall may be important factors.

'Secondary' *varicose veins* may be the result of a *proximal venous obstruction, destruction of the valves by thrombosis or an increase in flow and pressure caused by an arteriovenous fistula* (see Revision panel 10.11).

Varicosities do not cause symptoms, apart from unsightliness. Symptoms are caused by the physiological malfunction that follows the valvular incompetence and retrograde flow.

History

Age Varicose veins affect all age groups but are more common in older people. In children, they are usually caused by a congenital vascular abnormality.

Sex Ten times more females than males attend hospital with venous complaints, but surveys in the community have shown there is little difference in the incidence of varicose veins between the sexes.

Ethnic groups Varicose veins are said to be less common in Africa and the Far East than in Europe and North America.

Occupation Many patients with symptomatic varicose veins have occupations that involve standing for prolonged periods. It is doubtful whether standing, by itself, causes varicose veins, but it certainly exacerbates the leg symptoms.

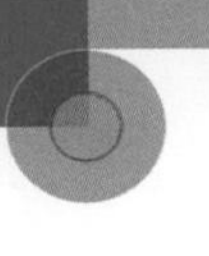

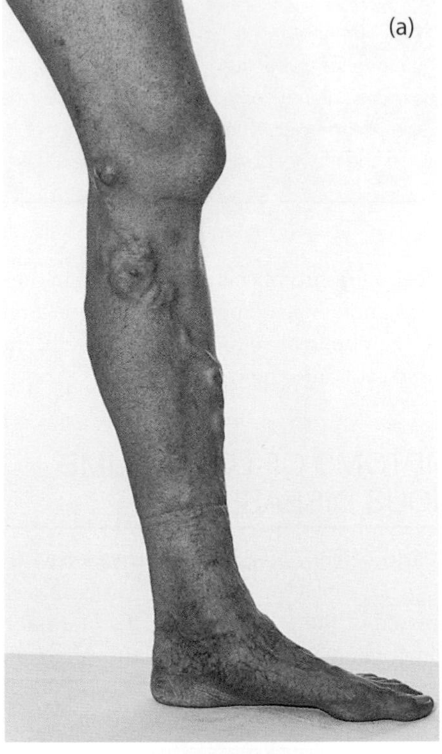

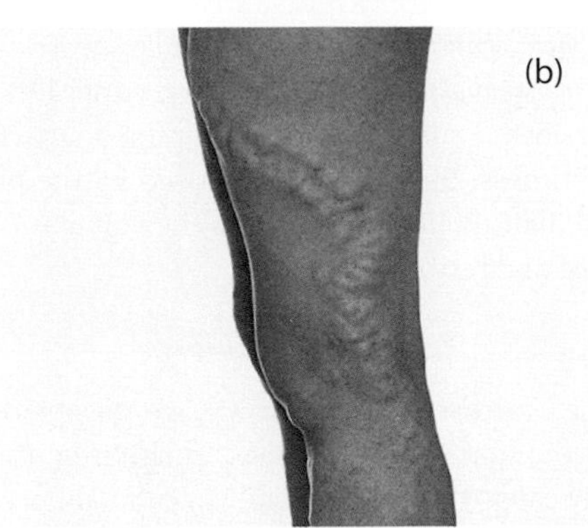

Figure 10.28 VARICOSE VEINS. Varicose veins are, by definition, dilated, tortuous and superficial veins. They occur on both the medial (a) and the lateral (b) side of the leg.

Symptoms Many patients with varicose veins have no symptoms. The disfiguring effect of the veins is often the principal complaint. The next most common complaint is pain. This is usually a dull ache felt in the calf and lower leg that gets worse throughout the day, especially when the patient is standing up for prolonged periods. *Night cramps, swelling and itching* are also common complaints.

Revision panel 10.11

THE CAUSES OF VARICOSE VEINS IN THE LOWER LIMBS

Secondary

- Obstruction to venous outflow by:
  - Pregnancy
  - Fibroids/ovarian cyst
  - Abdominal lymphadenopathy
  - Pelvic cancer (cervix, uterus, ovary, rectum)
  - Ascites
  - Iliac vein thrombosis
  - Retroperitoneal fibrosis
- Valve destruction
- Deep vein thrombosis
- High flow and pressure
- Arteriovenous fistula (especially the acquired traumatic variety)

Primary

- Cause not known; often familial
- Probably a weakness of the vein wall that permits valve ring dilatation
- Very rarely, congenital absence of the valves

Mild swelling of the ankle by the end of the day is common, but marked ankle oedema is not, and other causes of oedema should be eliminated before accepting that it is caused by the varicose veins. The symptoms are relieved by lying down for 15 or 30 minutes, or by wearing compression hosiery. The pain is often experienced in the dilated varicosities.

Some patients present with red, painful, tender lumps caused by acute *superficial thrombophlebitis* (see page 367).

NOTE: Lipodermatosclerosis, eczema and ulceration are important complications that indicate the need for treatment.

Deep vein thrombosis as a result of venous insufficiency/varicose veins presents with calf pain and leg swelling. Pleuritic chest pain, haemoptysis and dyspnea may also be present if it is complicated by a pulmonary embolism,

> **NOTE:** Always exclude conditions that may obstruct the iliac veins and cause secondary varicose veins, such as pregnancy and abdominal tumours.

Previous history

Most patients with varicose veins have had them for years, and many have had various forms of treatment such as operations and injections. *It is important to exclude a previous deep vein thrombosis* that may have accompanied previous illnesses, operations, accidents (long bone fractures) or pregnancies. All females should be asked if they had swelling of their legs or a deep vein thrombosis during pregnancy.

Family history

A definite family history is obtained in one-third to one-half of all patients who present with varicose veins.

EXAMINATION OF THE VEINS OF THE LOWER LIMB

Inspection

This is an essential part of the venous examination and ample time should be spent on this prior to palpation of the leg. The lower limbs need to be fully exposed with the patient standing in a warm, well-lit examination room. Many patients with venous disorders have visible, dilated and tortuous superficial veins, which are described as *varicose veins*.

The skin of the lower medial third of the leg, the gaiter region, must be carefully inspected. Venous hypertension caused by venous outflow obstruction or severe reflux may cause an area of skin pigmentation, tenderness and subcutaneous induration, called *lipodermatosclerosis*, and eventually *eczema and ulceration* (Figure 10.29).

The network of small dilated venules that develops beneath the lateral and/or medial malleolus of limbs with severe venous hypertension is called an *ankle flare* or *corona phlebectatica* (Figure 10.30).

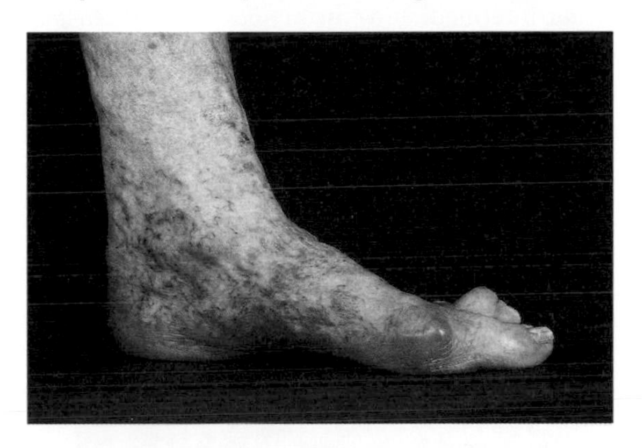

Figure 10.30 An example of an 'ankle flare' or corona phlebectatica, in which there is a considerable dilatation of the intracutaneous veins below the ankle in limbs with venous hypertension.

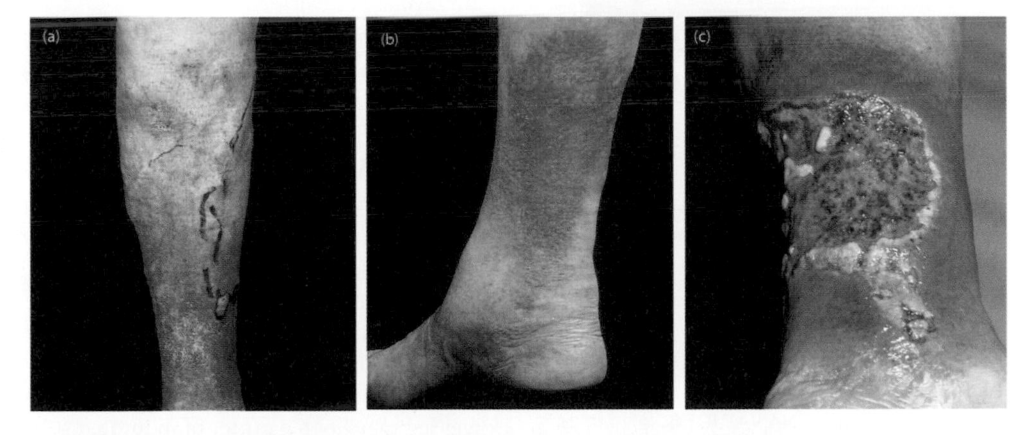

Figure 10.29 VENOUS ECZEMA, LIPODERMATOSCLEROSIS AND ULCERATION. (a) A red weepy skin rash (venous eczema) developing in a limb with venous hypertension. (b) Lipodermatosclerosis: an indurated, pigmented, inflamed plaque in the 'gaiter' area of the leg. (c) A venous ulcer. This occurs in the gaiter region of the ankle skin, surrounded by lipodermatosclerosis. The ulcer edge is sloping.

Both limbs must be examined from all aspects. The site and course of all the varicosities should be recorded on anterior and posterior outline drawings of the lower limb.

A blue-tinged bulge in the groin, which disappears on lying down, is likely to be a *saphena varix* (Figure 10.31). This is a dilation of the termination of the long saphenous vein or one of its major tributaries.

Some varicose veins are large and prominent, whereas others are minute and intradermal. The latter may cause a blue patch, which can arise from a single feeding vein. Intradermal veins are called *spider veins* or *venous stars* (Figure 10.32). Slightly larger intermediate veins are often called *reticular veins*.

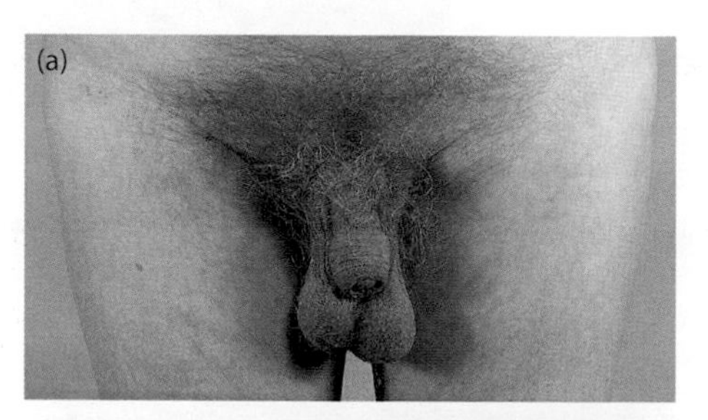

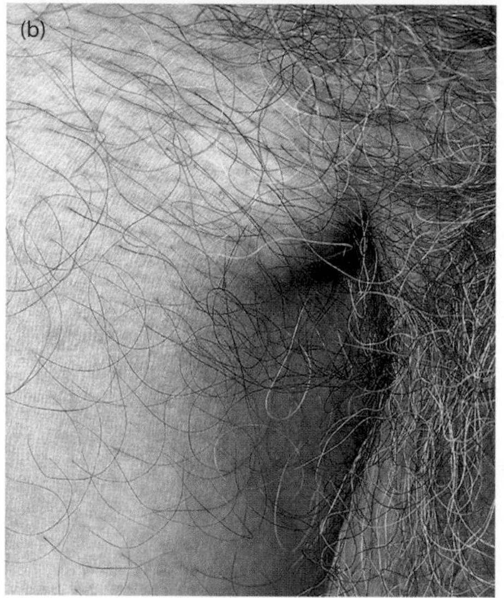

Figure 10.31 TWO SAPHENA VARICES. (a) Left, (b) right. A saphena varix is a soft bluish swelling over and below the saphenous termination, which collapses and disappears when the patient lies flat.

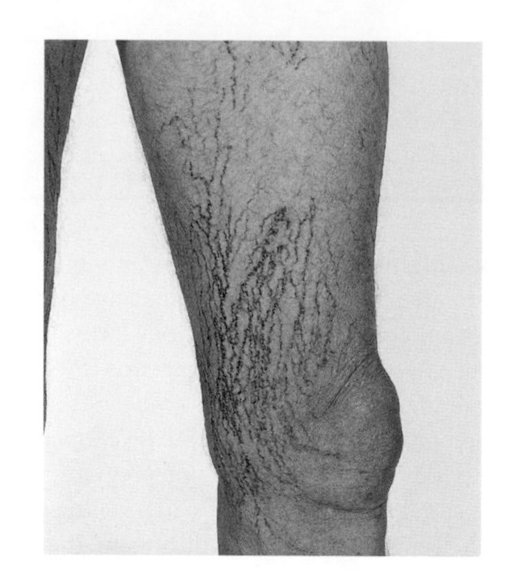

Figure 10.32 'Spider veins' are dilatations of the intracutaneous veins.

Large, prominent, distended veins on the medial side of the lower calf have been called 'ankle blowouts' if they lie in close proximity to the site of incompetent calf communicating veins (Figure 10.33).

Distended veins crossing the groins and extending up over the abdominal wall are collateral veins, and indicate the presence of a deep venous obstruction of the iliofemoral system. Cross-pubic collateral veins may be visible if one iliac system is obstructed (Figure 10.34).

Palpation

Assess the texture of the skin and subcutaneous tissue of the lower leg by palpation. There may be pitting oedema or thickening, redness and tenderness. Chronic venous hypertension results in *lipodermatosclerosis,* a term that indicates that there is a progressive replacement of the skin and subcutaneous fat by fibrous tissue, causing induration. There is often an associated inflammation caused by the fibrin deposition that precedes the fibrosis. The examiner's dominant hand should be gently run over the course of the main veins and their tributaries. Veins in the lower leg may lie in a gutter of indurated subcutaneous fat. Dilated long and short saphenous veins are usually easy to feel.

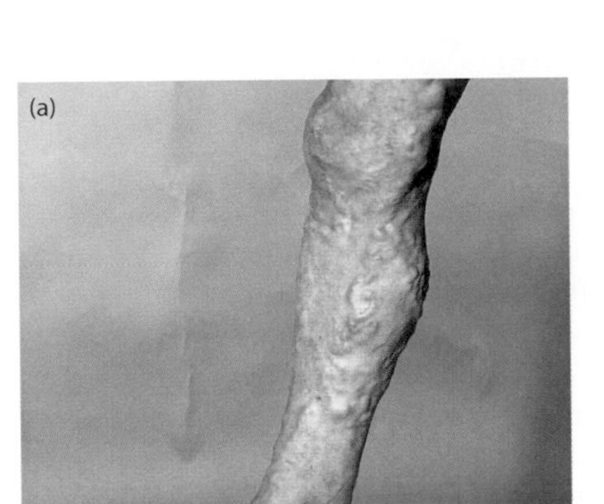

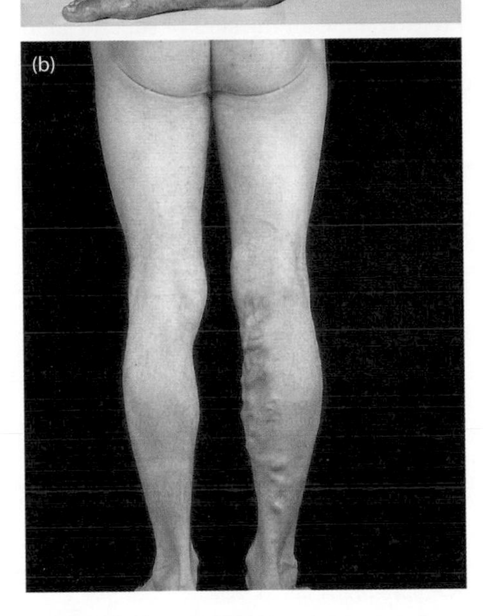

Figure 10.33 ANKLE 'BLOW-OUTS'. (a, b) Dilatations of the surface veins over or close by incompetent ankle perforating (communicating) veins.

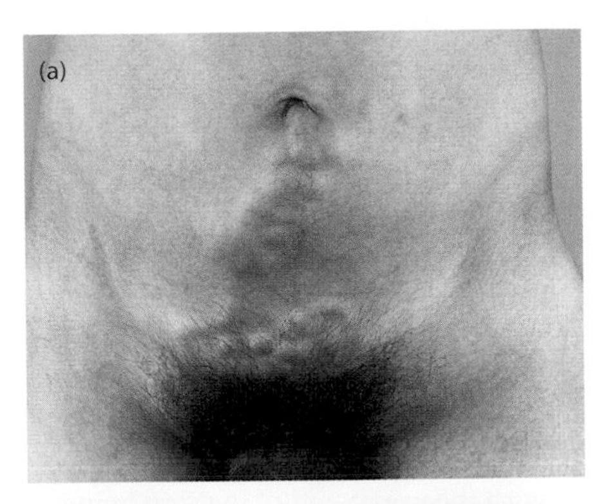

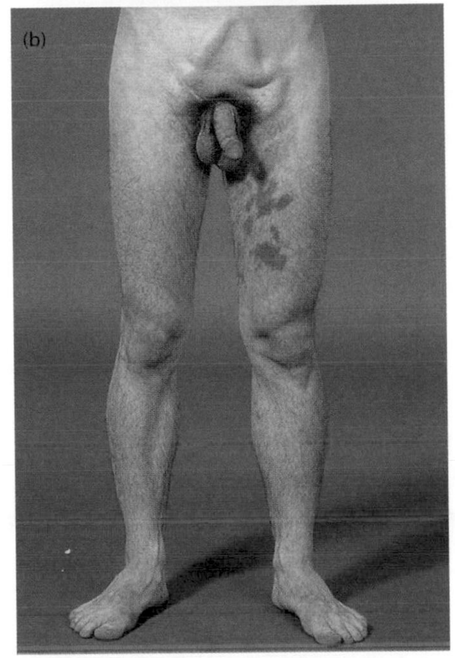

Figure 10.34 LARGE CROSS-PUBIC COLLATERAL VEINS. (a, b) These large collateral veins have formed to bypass an occlusion of the iliac veins of one limb.

> **NOTE:** The termination of a distended short saphenous vein is easier to feel if the patient is asked to bend the knees slightly to relax the deep fascia covering the popliteal fossa.

Carefully palpate the saphenofemoral junction (2.5 cm below and lateral to the pubic tubercle) and the saphenopopliteal junction, which has a variable position in the popliteal fossa (high or low). The patient should be asked to cough while the dilated veins are palpated to see if there is any *impulse or thrill (a cough impulse)*, indicating that the valves at their junctions with the deep veins are incompetent, and the back flow is turbulent.

Palpate the skin of the calf to define any areas of induration and tenderness (lipodermatosclerosis).

Percussion

The distended, dilated trunks of the long and short saphenous systems transmit a percussion wave in an orthograde direction whether or not the valves are competent. The more distended the

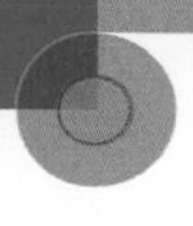

vein, the better the wave is transmitted. *The valves must be incompetent if a percussion wave is transmitted retrogradely*, i.e. downwards while the patient is standing.

Percussion can also be used to help to define the terminations of the long and short saphenous veins by placing the fingers of one hand gently over the upper end of the dilated saphenous trunk and percussing the vein below it, using the middle finger of the other hand to 'flick' distended varicosities further down the leg. The process can then be repeated in reverse, with the upper end of the vein being 'flicked' and the lower hand detecting a downward percussion wave, to check the competence of the valves.

Auscultation

Listen with your stethoscope over any large clusters of veins, especially if they remain distended when the patient lies down and the limb is elevated. A machinery murmur over such veins indicates that they are secondary to an *arteriovenous fistula*.

Special tests

Tourniquet test

NOTE: Many clinicians have abandoned tourniquet tests as a means of assessing varicose veins in favour of more sophisticated investigations such as Duplex ultrasound, but these tests are simple to perform and, if correctly carried out, can provide useful information on the major sites of communicating vein incompetence.

The patient should lie on a couch that has a small foot stool attached to it, onto which the patient can rapidly stand. The limb to be examined is then elevated – often by placing it on the examiner's shoulder – to empty the veins, a process that can be expedited by stroking the blood within the veins towards the heart. A tourniquet is then pulled tight around the upper thigh to ensure that the long saphenous vein is completely occluded (Figure 10.35).

The patient is then asked to stand up whilst the legs are observed for 10–15 seconds. If the saphenofemoral junction is the only site of superficial to deep valvular incompetence, the veins above the tourniquet will rapidly fill, but those below it will remain collapsed (Figure 10.36b). This can be confirmed by releasing the tourniquet and watching the veins below the site of the tourniquet rapidly distend from above, as blood regurgitates down the long saphenous vein. If, however, the veins below the tourniquet fill immediately the patient stands up, there must be other sites of superficial to deep incompetence below the level of the tourniquet.

This test can be repeated with the tourniquet moved progressively down the whole length of the leg to try to define all the sites of superficial to deep vein incompetence, but it is easier and simpler to apply it once below the knee to exclude short saphenous incompetence.

NOTE: Tourniquet tests are often difficult to interpret in patients with recurrent varicose veins, and the value of applying multiple tourniquets in an effort to locate the precise level of calf communicating veins has never been scientifically verified.

A modification of the tourniquet test is to empty the limb as described above and apply direct digital pressure over the upper end of the long saphenous vein while the patient stands up, to see if this prevents retrograde filling. This is called the *Trendelenburg (tourniquet) test*.

Perthes' walking test

It is important to test for deep vein obstruction or reflux when one is considering treatment of a patient's superficial veins, as they rely on the need for a competent and patent deep system for effective venous return from that limb. This can be done by asking the patient to stand up after placing a tourniquet just below the knee, to cut off long and short saphenous reflux, and then to stand repeatedly on tip toes. This exercise empties a normal superficial venous system by sucking the blood in the surface varicosities into the deep veins, through competent perforating veins. A failure to achieve superficial vein emptying, often accompanied by pain (*venous claudication*) and/or swelling indicates deep vein obstruction or reflux

Leg horizontal, superficial veins empty

Superficial vein
Muscle
Deep vein
Fascia
Tourniquet occludes the suoerficial veins

The patient stands up

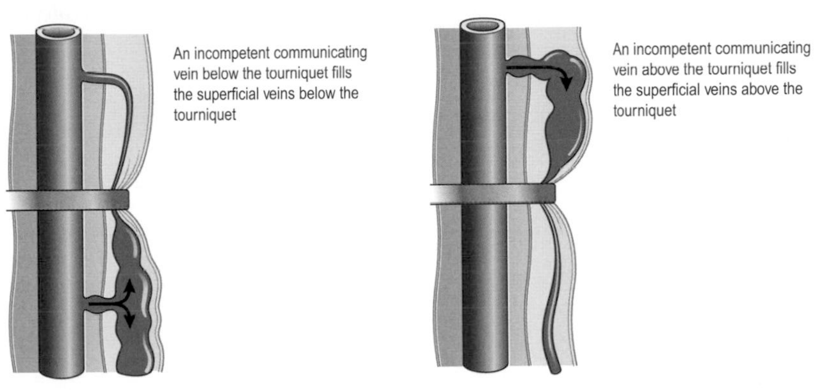

By moving the tourniquet up and down the leg it is possible to determine the level of the incompetent communicating veins.

Figure 10.35 The principles of the tourniquet test.

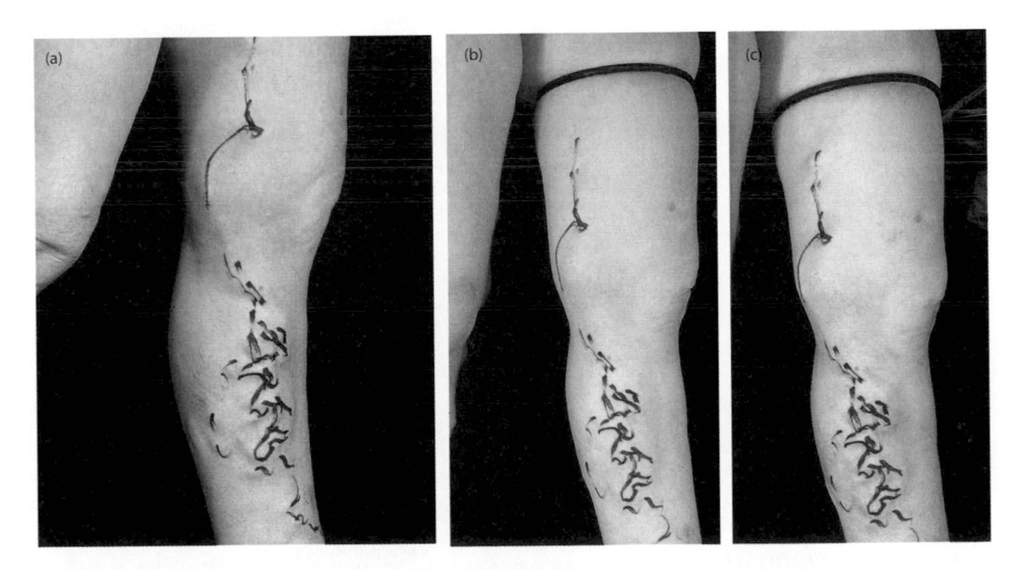

Figure 10.36 TOURNIQUET TESTS. (a) Before tourniquet applied. (b) Tourniquet controlling veins. (c) Veins distending after release of tourniquet.

through incompetent valves in the deep or communicating veins.

Venous hypertension caused by proximal vein obstruction or the presence of an arteriovenous fistula should be suspected if the varicose veins fail to collapse on elevation.

Doppler flow detector studies

The simple directional Doppler ultrasound flow probe described on page 334 can also be used to assess venous reflux. The patient is asked to stand up, and the ultrasound probe is placed over the termination of the long and then the short saphenous veins using coupling jelly. The direction of venous blood flow, augmented by rapid intermittent manual compression of the calf or any prominent varicosities in the lower limb, is then assessed.

A *uniphasic signal* on squeezing, with no sound on relaxation, indicates competent valves with forward flow (Figure 10.37a). A *biphasic signal*, with prolonged retrograde flow on releasing the compression, indicates reflux and valvular incompetence (Figure 10.37b).

Retrograde flow can also be confirmed by asking the patient to perform the *Valsalva manoeuvre*. This consists of taking a deep breath, pinching off the nose, closing the mouth and attempting a forced expiration. This causes venous flow to reverse if the valves are incompetent.

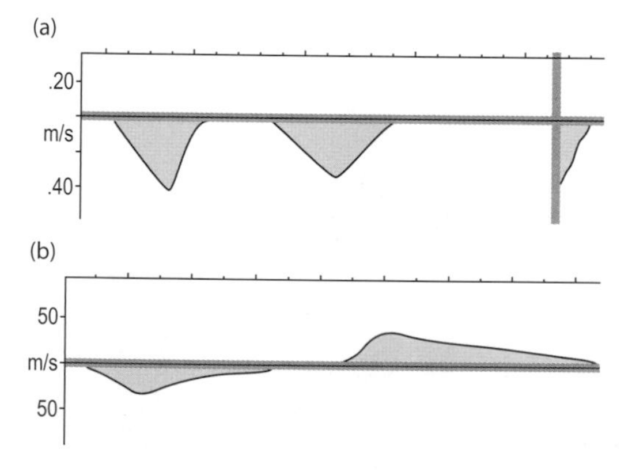

Figure 10.37 DOPPLER SIGNALS. (a) Uniphasic Doppler signal (forward flow only). (b) Biphasic Doppler signal (forward and retrograde flow).

The Doppler ultrasound flow detector can also be used in association with the tourniquet test to demonstrate retrograde flow in the saphenous trunks when the tourniquet is released.

The simple hand-held Doppler flow detector cannot detect retrograde flow in either the deep or calf perforating veins with any accuracy. The detection of deep vein flow abnormalities requires more sophisticated duplex scans.

General examination

Because varicose veins are so common, it is tempting to omit a full general examination. Never do this! *Always examine the abdomen, and make sure the patient is not pregnant.*

Revision panel 10.12

ROUTINE FOR ASSESSING THE VENOUS CIRCULATION

Ask the patient to stand up

Inspection

Site, tortuosity and size of visible veins
Ankle oedema
Skin, especially above the medial ankle, for: venous flares, atrophe blanche, spider naeviae, haemosiderin deposition, lipodermatosclerosios

Palpation

Palpate the trunks of the long and short saphenous veins
Palpate the saphenopopliteal and saphenofemoral junctions
Feel the texture of the skin and subcutaneous tissues

Percussion

Percussion wave conduction upwards or downwards

Auscultation

Listen for bruits over prominent varices

Special tests

Tourniquet tests
Doppler ultrasound

Inspection of the abdomen may reveal dilated collateral veins crossing to the other groin, or up over the abdomen and chest to join the tributaries of the superior vena cava. The direction of flow in these veins is detected by placing two fingers on the veins, sliding one finger along the vein to empty it and then releasing the other finger and watching which way the empty segment fills (Harvey's test) (Figure 10.38). This test may have to be repeated moving the fingers in either direction before the direction of blood flow can be confirmed.

A digital rectal or vaginal examination may be required to exclude a pelvic or abdominal cause for the varicose veins. In males, it is important to feel the testes. Massive enlargement of the abdominal lymph glands by metastases from small testicular tumours can cause inferior vena cava obstruction.

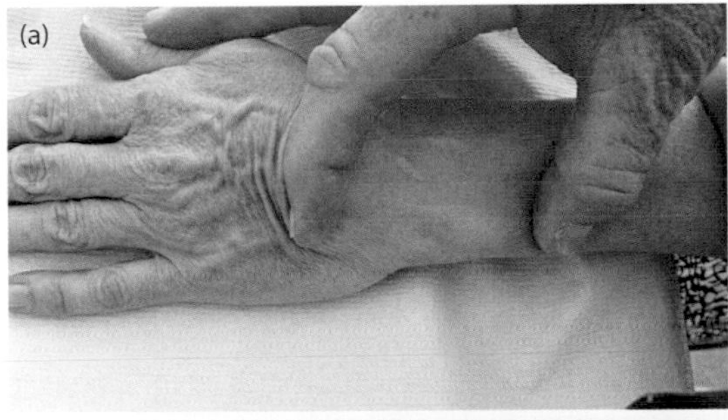

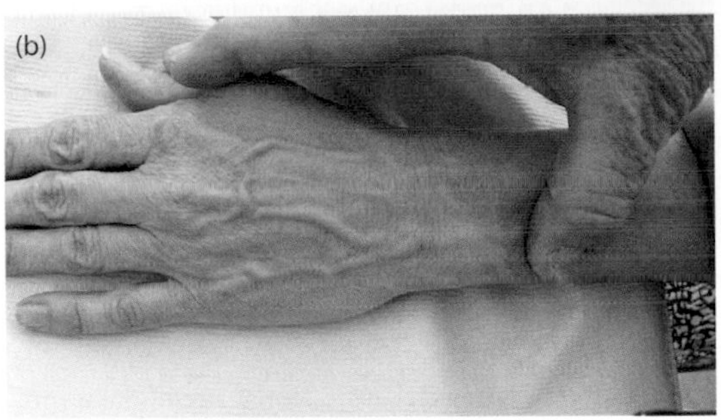

Figure 10.38 HARVEY'S TEST. (a, b) The test demonstrates that blood flows in only one direction through competent venous valves.

Lower limb venous disease

VENOUS ULCERATION

Many patients with venous ulcers do not have visible varicose veins. Approximately one-half of all venous ulcers are associated with primary varicose veins. The remainder are the result of post-thrombotic deep vein damage (see page 367).

History

Age Venous ulcers usually follow many years of venous disease, so the majority are seen in patients over the age of 40 years, many of whom have had recurrent ulceration for some years before seeking medical help. Post-thrombotic disease can cause ulceration in young adults, and ulcers can occur in children and teenagers with congenital venous malformations.

Sex Venous ulcers are more common in females than in males.

Symptoms Patients have often had aching pain, discomfort and tenderness of the skin (lipodermatosclerosis and pigmentation) for many months or years before an ulcer appears.

Some ulcers are painful, but many are not.

The discharge may be foul smelling, leading to depression and social isolation.

An episode of trauma often initiates the breakdown of the skin, but sometimes itching and scratching may start an ulcer.

Previous history Many venous ulcers are caused by deep and communicating vein damage, so there is often a history of venous thrombosis during an illness or pregnancy. The patient may have had previous episodes of ulceration.

Cause The ulcer invariably begins after the skin of the leg has been knocked and damaged. The initial incident is sometimes remembered, but often not.

Examination

Site Venous ulcers are commonly found around the 'gaiter area' of the lower leg, and usually begin on the medial aspect. Ulcers situated lower down on the foot or higher up on the fleshy part of the calf are rarely caused by venous disease.

Shape and size Venous ulcers can be of any shape and size but are most commonly oval (Figure 10.39).

Edge The edge is gently sloping and, when healing begins, pale pink as new epithelium migrates across its surface.

Base This may be covered with yellow slough but becomes covered with pink granulation tissue when the ulcer is healing. Areas of white fibrous tissue may be seen between the granulations, and there may be more white fibrous tissue than granulation tissue when the ulcer is very chronic and indolent. The base is usually fixed to the deep tissues. Tendons and the tibial periosteum may be exposed in the base of the ulcer.

Depth Venous ulcers are usually relatively shallow.

Discharge The discharge is usually seropurulent but can occasionally be bloodstained.

Surrounding tissues The surrounding tissues usually show the signs of chronic venous hypertension – induration, inflammation, pigmentation and tenderness, i.e. *lipodermatosclerosis* (see Figure 10.29b, c).

There may be old white scars (atrophie blanche) from previous ulceration, and many dilated intradermal and subcutaneous veins. Movements of the ankle joint may be limited by scar tissue, which can cause an equinus deformity of the joint. Occasionally, true cellulitis occurs.

Lymph glands Ulcers are usually colonized with bacteria rather than infected, so the inguinal lymph glands should not be enlarged or tender.

Remember that squamous cell carcinoma can arise in a chronic venous ulcer, particularly in a patient known to have a long-standing venous ulcer that has enlarged, become painful and malodorous, and especially if the edge of the ulcer is found to be raised or thickened. Malignant change is also suggested by finding enlarged inguinal lymph glands. Biopsy is indicated should any of these changes appear. Malignant change in a chronic venous ulcer is known as a *Marjolin's ulcer* (see Chapter 4) (Figure 10.39r).

The lower limbs The whole of both lower limbs must be examined for the presence of varicose veins, competent and incompetent communicating veins and skin changes, as described above. Most patients have bilateral disease, and the majority of patients with venous ulcers have incompetent communicating veins.

> **NOTE:** It is also important to assess the arterial circulation and the nerves, to exclude an ischaemic or neuropathic cause of the ulcer (see page 342).

General examination The abdomen should be examined to exclude an abdominal cause of venous insufficiency, and the other leg should be examined for signs of venous disease.

Look for any general features of the many other causes of skin ulceration, such as ischaemia, rheumatoid arthritis, skin tumours, pyoderma gangrenosum, collagen diseases, anaemia, polycythaemia, neuropathic ulcers and sickle-cell disease (Figure 10.39).

DEEP VEIN THROMBOSIS

Three-quarters of deep vein thromboses do not cause any symptoms or signs. Many occur spontaneously, but in more than one-half, there is a predisposing cause such as an operation, bed rest, thrombophilia or recent air travel.

History

Patients complain of *pain and swelling in the calf* or the whole leg. The onset of symptoms is sudden, and they are usually severe enough to make walking difficult. The first indication may be a *pulmonary embolism*, which causes symptoms such as pleuritic pain, dyspnoea, haemoptysis and collapse (See Chapter 1).

Examination

Swelling of a leg, particularly if it is unilateral, is the most significant physical sign (Figure 10.41). The ankle may be the only site of swelling if the thrombosis is confined to the calf. Swelling of both ankles needs to be differentiated from other causes of oedema. The swelling may extend up to the groin if the iliac vein is thrombosed.

The muscles that contain the thrombosed veins may become hard and tender. A change in texture of the muscle is more significant than tenderness because, although there are many conditions that make a muscle tender, there are few that make it stiff and hard.

> **NOTE:** 'Pain' on stretching the calf muscles by forced dorsiflexion is known as Homan's sign. This sign is a poor discriminator and should be abandoned.

The superficial veins may be dilated, and the leg may feel hot. A large, swollen limb that is made pale by severe oedema is called *phlegmasia alba dolens*. When

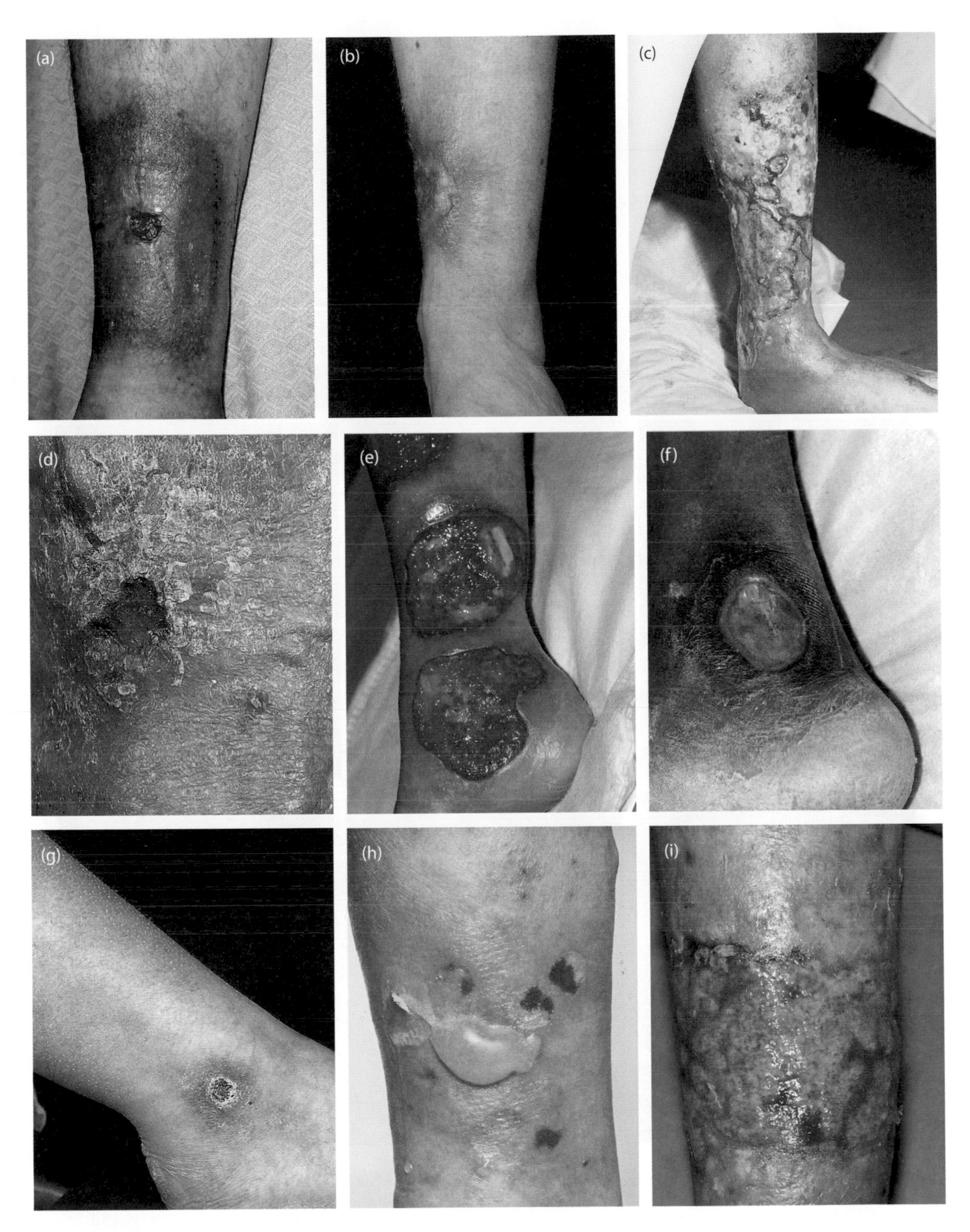

Figure 10.39 MONTAGE OF DIFFERENT TYPES OF LEG ULCER. (a) Venous. (b) Arterial. (c) Rheumatoid. (d) Neuropathic. (e) HIV (AIDS). (f) Sickle cell. (g) SLE. (h) Pemphigoid. (i) Self-induced. *(Continued)*

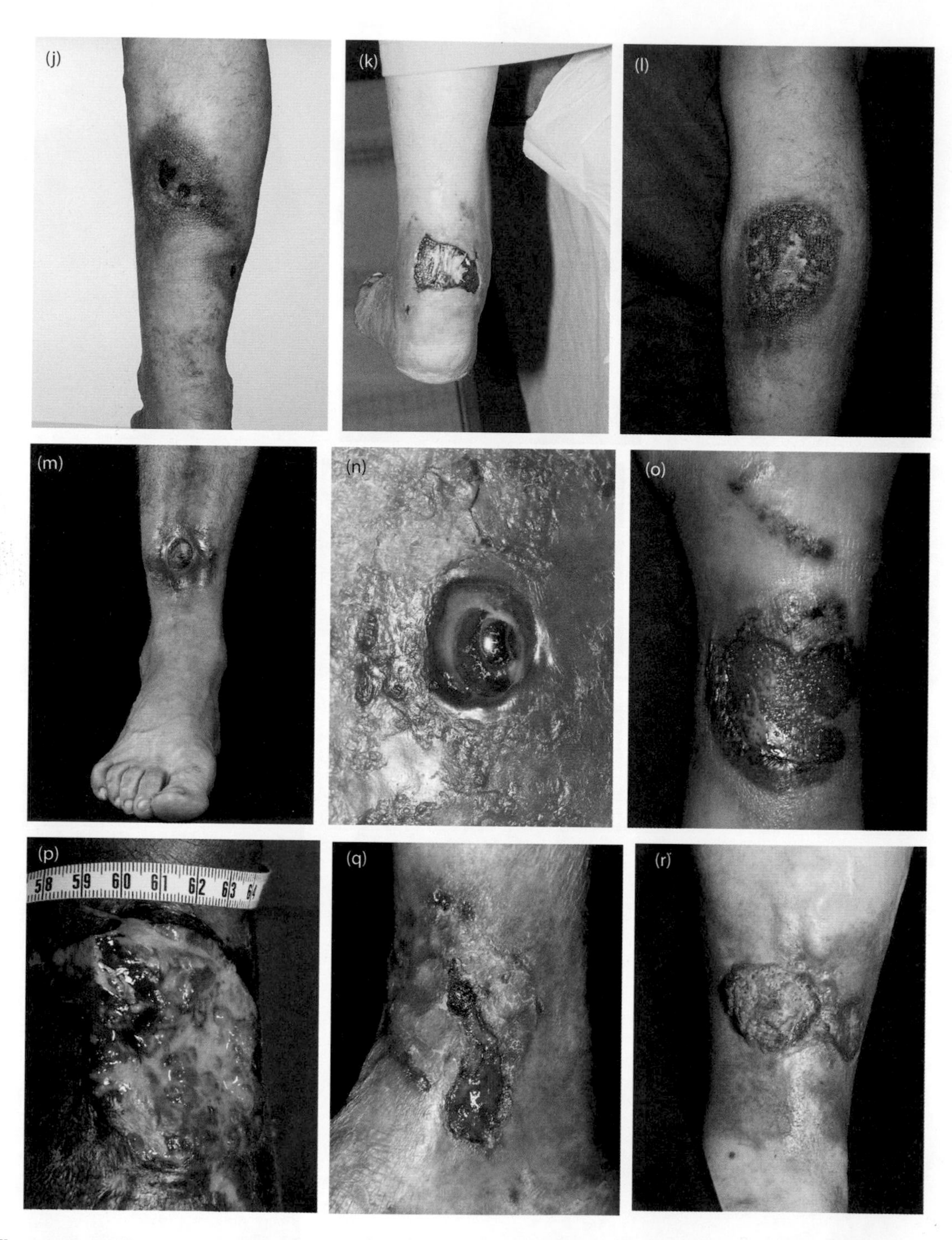

Figure 10.39 (Continued) MONTAGE OF DIFFERENT TYPES OF LEG ULCER. (j) Martorell's. (k) Gout. (l) Gumma. (m) Osteomyelitis. (n) Foreign body (orthopaedic screw). (o) Pyoderma gangrenosum. (p) Yaws. (q) Basal cell carcinoma. (r) Marjolin's.

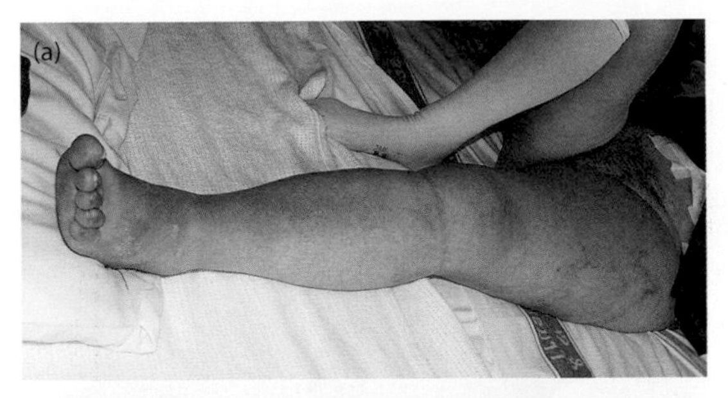

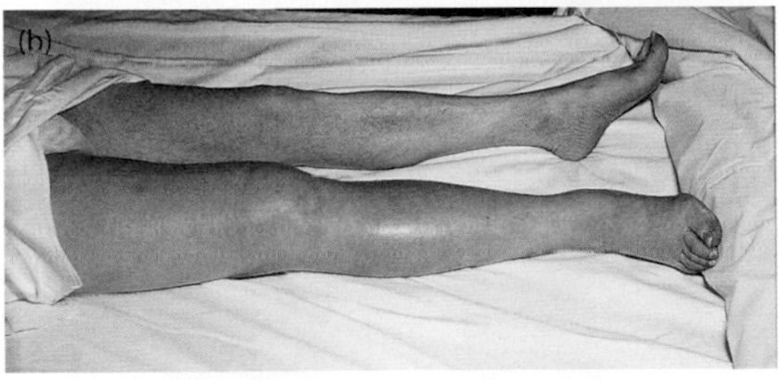

Figure 10.40 ANKLE OEDEMA/SWELLING CAUSED BY A DEEP VEIN THROMBOSIS. (a) Mild. (b) Severe.

the venous thrombosis blocks almost all the main outflow veins, the skin of the leg becomes congested and blue. This is called *phlegmasia caerulea dolens*.

Venous gangrene can develop when there is very severe venous outflow obstruction. Venous gangrene usually affects the peripheral tissues (toes or fingers, see Figure 10.12).

Chest signs The *neck veins may be dilated*, and there may be *central cyanosis* and *signs of right ventricular hypertrophy* if the patient has had a pulmonary embolus. A *fixed-split second heart sound* may be heard indicative of pulmonary hypertension, and there may be a *pleural rub* from the infarcted lung rubbing against the pleura.

The post-thrombotic limb

The symptoms and signs that follow the damage caused by a deep vein thrombosis, obstruction and valvular incompetence may appear months or years after the thrombosis. The initiating thrombosis may have passed unrecognized, but more often it has produced clinical signs and required treatment.

The earliest symptoms are usually a *slowly progressive swelling of the leg* that becomes painful as the day wears on. The skin of the gaiter area initially becomes pigmented, but eventually it can progress to *lipodermatosclerosis*. These changes may spread around the whole circumference of the gaiter area.

Varicose veins become more prominent and, if the thrombosis obstructs the venous outflow at the base of the limb, collateral veins may develop across the groins and the pubis, and the superficial veins will not empty when the patient is asked to carry out Perthe's walking test.

A proportion of patients develop true *venous claudication*. This is a severe calf and sometimes thigh pain caused by walking. It must be differentiated from intermittent claudication caused by arterial insufficiency. These patients usually have a swollen, tender limb, multiple varicose veins, collateral veins and lipodermatosclerosis, all indicating the likelihood of a previous deep vein thrombosis. The pain of venous claudication is usually accompanied by an increase of the swelling, and the pain fades very slowly.

SUPERFICIAL THROMBOPHLEBITIS

A deep vein thrombosis begins in normal veins, the vein wall becoming secondarily inflamed. In superficial thrombophlebitis, the inflammation of the vein wall is invariably the cause of the thrombosis.

The causes of superficial thrombophlebitis are given in Revision panel 10.13.

An occult carcinoma should be suspected when the episodes occur in the arms of patients over the age of

Revision panel 10.13

THE CAUSES OF SUPERFICIAL THROMBOPHLEBITIS

Varicose veins
Occult carcinoma:
Bronchus
Pancreas
Stomach
Lymphoma
Thromboangiitis obliterans (Buerger's disease)
Polycythaemia
Polyarteritis
Idiopathic
Iatrogenic
Intravenous injection and injuries

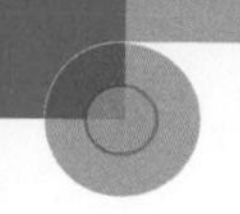

45 years, especially if they are transient and migrate. *Thrombophlebitis migrans* is, however, a rare condition.

History

Patients complain of the sudden appearance of a painful lump on their arm or leg. The pain usually subsides in 3–7 days, leaving a *tender lump* or *subcutaneous cord* that takes several weeks to disperse. There may be a preceding injury such as a venepuncture or, if the vein is varicose, a direct injury.

Examination

The swelling is in the subcutaneous tissues. It has an elongated, *cord-like shape* and may be several centimetres long, running along the long axis of the limb (see Figure 10.27). The lump is tender. *The overlying skin is at first red and inflamed,* before becoming pigmented and brown. Enlargement of the local lymph glands is rare, and other tissues in the limb are normal, unless the condition is secondary to varicose veins.

The whole patient must be examined for an occult carcinoma, even if they have varicose veins.

AXILLARY VEIN THROMBOSIS

Thrombosis of the axillary/subclavian vein may follow excessive use of the limb, especially above the head, or compression of the vein by musculoskeletal abnormalities such as a cervical rib or thoracic outlet syndrome.

History

The patient complains of a *sudden discomfort and swelling of the arm*. The arm, forearm and hand swell up, and there is discomfort on the medial side of the upper arm and in the axilla. The arm may feel hot, and if it becomes very swollen, movements may become restricted. The patient may give a history of unusual activity in the preceding 24 hours, such as painting a ceiling.

Examination

The whole arm is *swollen, congested and blue,* and the surface veins are usually distended. When the hand is raised above the level of the heart, the veins at the back of the hand do not collapse. The axillary vein may be palpable and tender. *Distended cutaneous veins develop across the anterior chest wall* and over the scapula to provide collateral drainage. The supraclavicular fossa must be carefully palpated to exclude a causative mass such as a cervical rib, a subclavian aneurysm or lymph glands enlarged by secondary malignant disease.

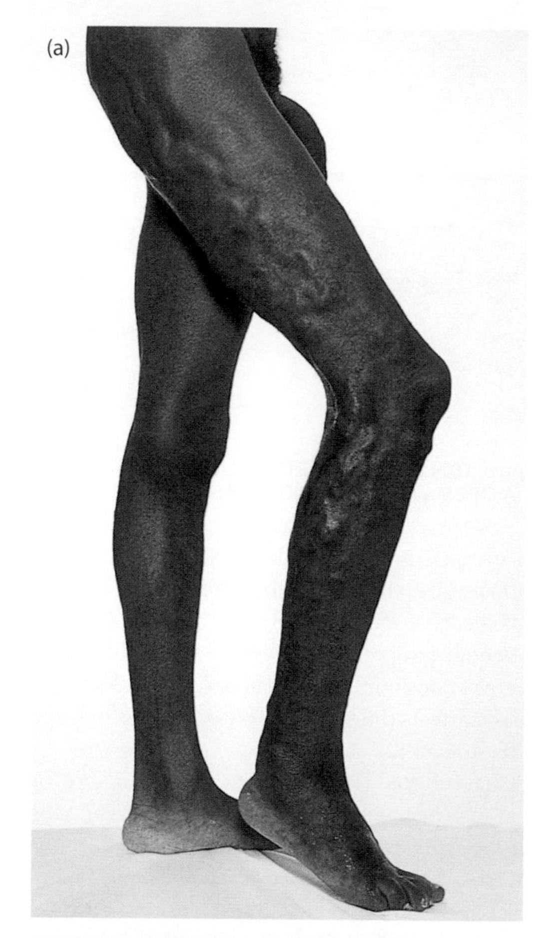

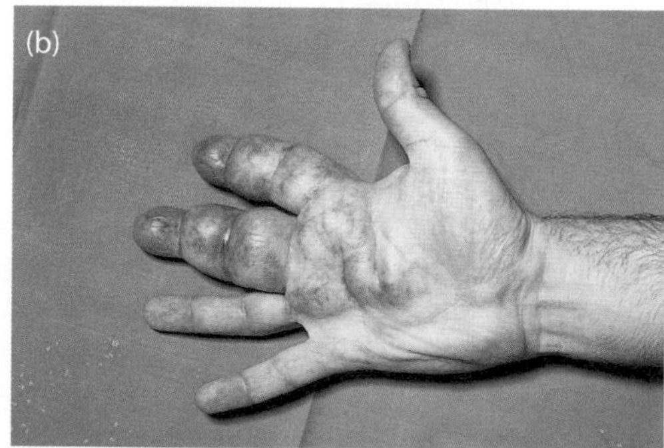

Figure 10.41 CONGENITAL VEIN ABNORMALITIES. (a) A limb with Klippel–Trenaunay syndrome that demonstrates hypertrophy, persistent vestigial veins and a capillary naevus. (b) A large venous angioma of the hand.

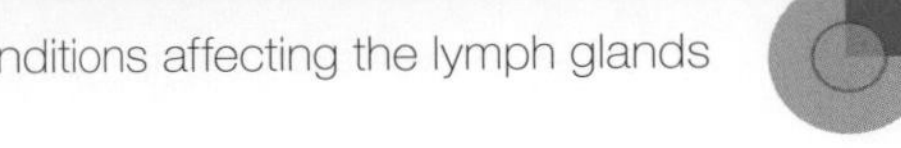

CONGENITAL VEIN ABNORMALITIES

Klippel–Trenaunay syndrome

This is a rare syndrome in which dilated veins develop early in life, often on the outer side of the leg, the leg being longer than the normal leg and covered in cutaneous angiomas (port wine stains) (Figure 10.41a).

Venous angiomas

These are localized hamartomatous overgrowths of small to middle-sized veins (Figure 10.41b). They mostly occur in the subcutaneous tissues and skin. They have a blue discolouration and become distended when dependent, collapse on elevation and are compressible.

THE LYMPHATICS

Primary abnormalities of the lymphatic vessels are rare. Disease in the lymph glands that interrupts the flow of lymph is common.

Conditions affecting the lymph glands

LYMPHANGITIS

When bacterial infection spreads through the tissues, the bacteria enter the lymphatics and pass along in the lymph to the draining lymph glands. Inflamed lymphatics close to the skin are visible as thin, tender, red streaks on the skin. Lymphangitis is most often seen as a complication of infection starting in the hands or feet. This is commonly seen in patients with diabetic foot infections.

History

The patient complains of a throbbing pain at the site of the primary infection, tenderness along the red streaks and tenderness in the groin or axilla.

Examination

Inspection of the limb reveals the *red, tender lymphatics*. The overlying skin may be slightly oedematous. The axillary or inguinal lymph glands are usually swollen and tender.

The site of the primary infection is often not obvious. It may be a small crack between the toes or alongside a fingernail.

If a lymph gland in an oedematous limb with poor lymphatic drainage becomes infected, the infection quickly spreads throughout the oedematous tissues – cellulitis.

LYMPHOEDEMA

Lymphoedema is the accumulation of lymph in the interstitial spaces as a consequence of defective lymphatic drainage. The oedema fluid is rich in protein, in contrast to the oedema of heart and kidney failure, which has a low protein content. The causes of lymphoedema are given in Revision panel 10.14.

The most common cause of lymphoedema is from disease in the lymph glands.

Revision panel 10.14

THE CAUSES OF LYMPHOEDEMA

Primary

Congenital/hereditary genetic disorders causing dilatation, incompetence, aplasia or obliteration of the lymphatics. The most common are:
- Congenital hereditary lymphoedema (Milroy disease) – shortly after birth
- Lymphoedema praecox (Meige disease) – around puberty
- Lymphoedema tarda – after the age of 35

Secondary

Neoplastic infiltration of the lymph glands:
- Secondary carcinoma
- Lymphoma (Hodgkin's, non-Hodgkin's)

Infection

- Filariasis
- Lymphogranuloma inguinale
- Tuberculosis
- Recurrent non-specific infection

Iatrogenic

- Surgical excision of the lymph glands
- Irradiation of lymph glands

> **NOTE:** Primary lymphoedema is only diagnosed when all the causes of secondary lymphoedema have been eliminated, or there is a clear family history of the condition.

History

Age Primary lymphoedema may present at birth, in young adults or, much less often, in middle age. Secondary lymphoedema presents in middle and old age and is common after treatment for cancer.

Family history Many forms of primary lymphoedema are familial and abnormal genes (such as FOXC2 and FLT4) have now been discovered in several of them.

Sex Females are affected three times more often than males. Even secondary lymphoedema is more common in females, because tumours of the uterus and ovary metastasize to the iliac lymph glands, and carcinoma of the breast spreads to the axillary lymph glands.

Geography *Filariasis*: infestation with the parasite *Wuchereria bancrofti*, which is found in tropical and subtropical countries – is a common cause of lymphoedema (elephantiasis).

Symptoms The patient notices a *slowly progressive swelling of the limb or genitalia* (Figures 10.42 and 10.43). Primary lymphoedema most often affects the lower limb, often beginning after a sprained ankle or another form of trivial injury. The swelling takes many years to develop and is often bilateral.

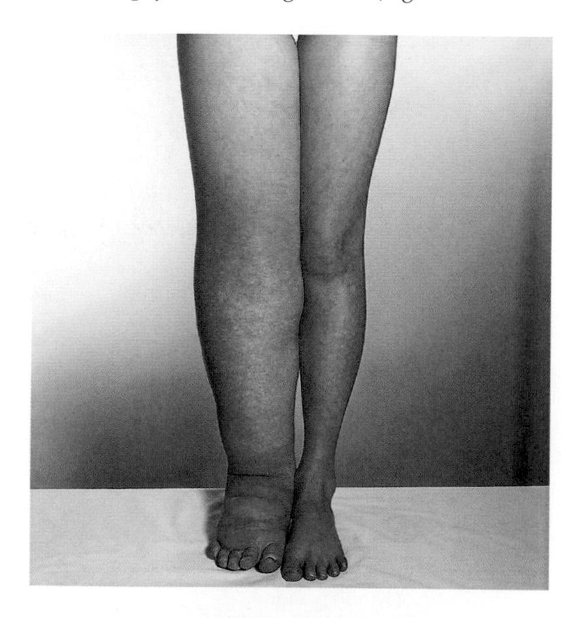

Figure 10.42 Lymphoedema of the right leg.

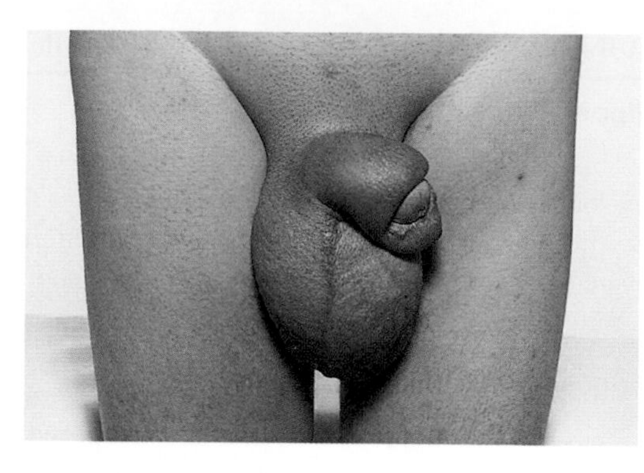

Figure 10.43 Genital oedema.

In contrast, the swelling of secondary lymphoedema (Figure 10.44) may appear in a few weeks and may progress rapidly.

The swelling is not painful. There is no discomfort in the swollen limb apart from that caused by the increased weight, which may produce a mechanical disability.

Patients with lymphoedema often develop severe episodes of acute cellulitis, which may be accompanied by

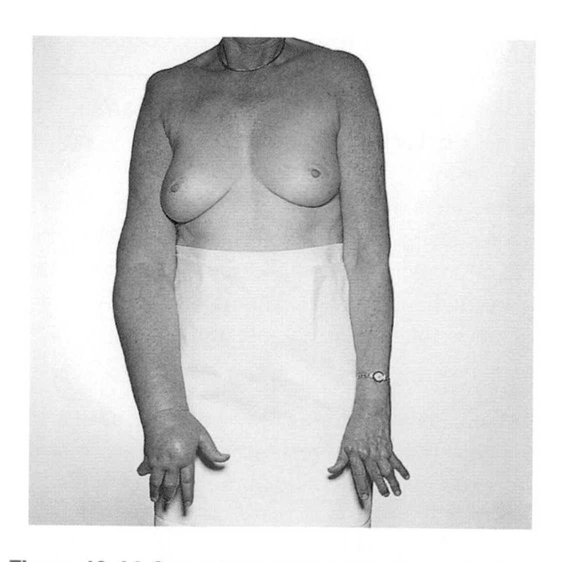

Figure 10.44 Secondary lymphoedema. The patient's right arm lymphoedema was caused by infiltration of the axillary lymph glands by metastases from a carcinoma in the right breast. Some carcinomas of the breast present in this way.

septicaemia. Acute cellulitis is often preceded by a prodromal period of sweating, rigors and malaise, which is then followed by the development of pain, tenderness, redness and swelling in the limb. The infection often gets in through cracks between the toes caused by athlete's foot (tinea pedis). Vesicles may appear on the skin and leak a clear, colourless fluid.

Examination

The swollen limb

Lymphoedema has no special characteristics.

NOTE: It is often said that lymphoedema does not pit – this is incorrect.

All oedema pits. The longer the lymphoedema has been present, the denser the accompanying fibrosis and the firmer and more 'doughy' the oedema; nevertheless, lymphoedema always pits if you press long enough.

Lymphoedema of the lower limb affects the toes much more often than other forms of oedema. If it has been present for years, the toes are squashed together and become square in cross-section. This hardly ever occurs with other types of oedema. *Stemmer's sign* is an inability to pinch the skin together on the dorsal surface of the second toe (Figure 10.45). This indicates the presence of lymphoedema and is a consequence of secondary thickening and hyperkeratosis of the skin. Skin nodules sometimes grow outwards, looking like warts.

Lymphoedema is usually diagnosed when other *general causes of oedema (cardiac, renal, hypoproteinaemia)* and other local causes (*venous obstruction, multiple arteriovenous fistulas, local gigantism and excessive fat deposition – lipodystrophy*) have been excluded. Therefore, it is essential to examine the whole patient, especially the heart, the abdomen and the veins of the limb, once the presence of oedema has been confirmed.

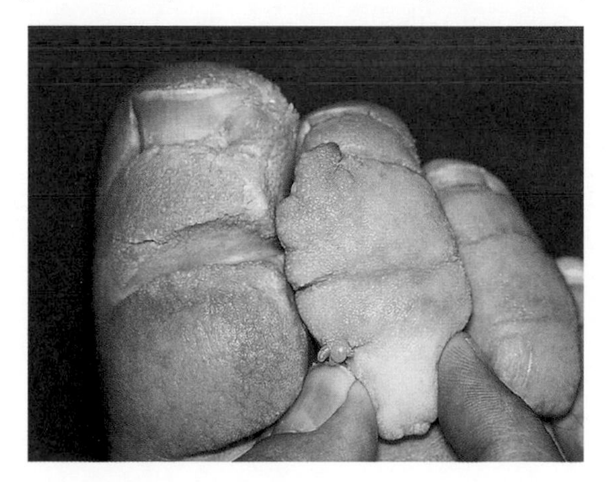

Figure 10.45 Stemmer's sign: an inability to pinch the skin together on the dorsum of the toes.

The lymph glands

The lymph glands are often slightly thickened and enlarged in patients with primary lymphoedema. They are usually enlarged and hard if they are infiltrated with primary or secondary tumour.

All the areas that drain to any palpable glands must be carefully examined.

General examination

A full examination of the patient must be carried out to look for any possible causes for secondary lymphoedema.

OEDEMA AFTER BREAST SURGERY

Swelling of the arm is a common complication of any form of axillary lymph node surgery, particularly axillary clearance, and also of axillary radiotherapy. It is not seen after simple mastectomy.

In the first days or weeks after treatment, remember the possibility of an axillary vein thrombosis.

Late swelling may be caused by recurrent carcinoma, especially if there is any enlargement of the axillary lymph glands.

LYMPHATIC REFLUX

A relatively small number of patients have dilated ectatic incompetent lymphatics that allow lymph and chyle (which is the milky lymph draining from the intestine) to reflux back into the skin, or drain into large cavities such as the peritoneum, pleura or intestine. Patients with lymphatic reflux can develop leaky vesicles on their skin, ascites and pleural effusions, and may even pass chyle in their urine (chyluria). These conditions are rare.

LYMPHANGIOMAS

These are rare malformations with distinct clinical features that are easy to recognize (see Chapter 4).

History

A patient or, in the case of a child, the parents, first notice a small soft subcutaneous swelling. There are sometimes associated small vesicles on the surface of the skin, which may weep clear fluid. These abnormalities may be present at birth or appear later in life. The subcutaneous swellings slowly enlarge, and the vesicles increase in number, but neither are usually painful.

Examination

The skin over the subcutaneous cysts usually contain many small vesicles (Figure 10.46). Lymphangiomas tend to occur at the junction of the leg, arm or neck with the trunk.

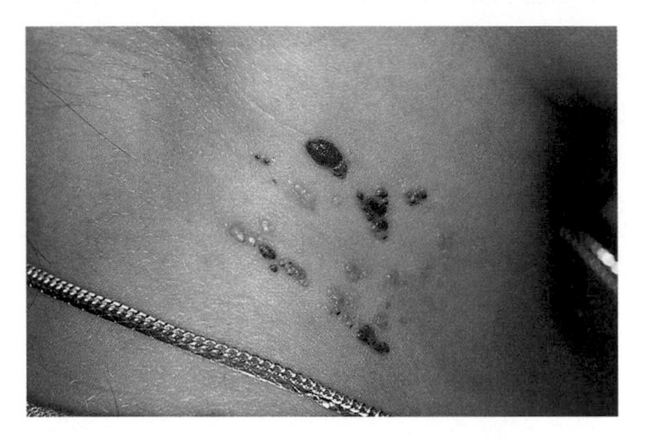

Figure 10.46 Lymphangioma circumscriptum.

The *subcutaneous swellings cannot be compressed or emptied*. They are often indistinct and multiple. They fluctuate and transilluminate if they are of a reasonable size and have the same signs as a cystic hygroma (see Chapter 12).

Regional lymphadenopathy is described in the various sections of the book, but as lymphoedema is so often secondary to lymph gland disease, you should refresh your knowledge of the causes of lymph gland enlargement by studying Revision panel 10.15.

Revision panel 10.15

THE CAUSES OF LYMPHADENOPATHY

- Infection:
  - Non-specific
  - Glandular fever
  - Tuberculosis
  - Toxoplasmosis
  - Syphilis
  - Cat-scratch fever – *Bartonella (Rochalimaea) henselae*
  - Filariasis
- Lymphogranuloma (inguinale)
- Metastatic tumour
- Primary reticuloses
- Sarcoidosis

Acknowledgements

The contribution of Matthew Waltham to this chapter in the 5th edition is gratefully acknowledged.

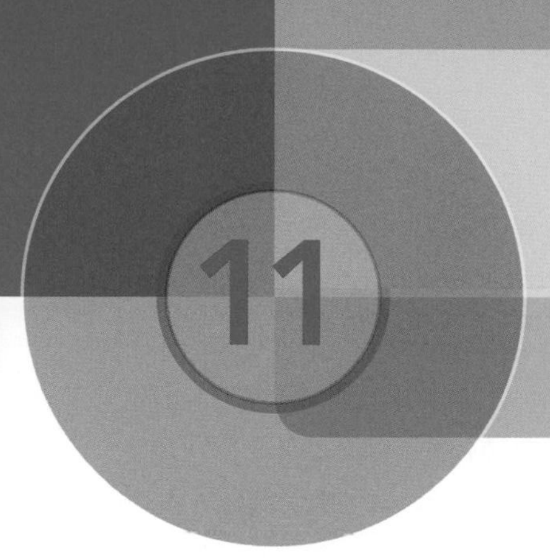

The mouth, tongue and lips

MARK MCGURK AND NAVIN VIG

Examination of the mouth, tongue and lips

It is essential to inspect the mouth with a good light and a tongue depressor or dental mirror, and to palpate the tissues. Palpation can reveal more in, or of, the soft tissues than inspection alone. A structured approach is important and should include the following steps:

- Inspect the external appearance of the lips, including the commissures.
- Retract the lips to see the labial and buccal mucosa.
- Push the cheek outwards to see the buccal side of the gum.
- Inspect the surface of the tongue.
- Ask the patient to lift their tongue to the roof of the mouth (or gently lift it away yourself) to inspect the ventral surface of the tongue, the floor of the mouth and the lingual surface of the gum.
- Ask the patient to protrude their tongue. Wrap a gauze swab around the tip and hold it firmly. This gives traction to pull the tongue forward and offers a good view of the lateral tongue back to the tonsillar fold.
- Depress the tongue to look at the fauces, tonsils and pharynx.
- Inspect the hard and soft palate.

Always wear gloves when examining. Remember to palpate the structures in the floor of the mouth bimanually and be mindful of the gag reflex when palpating in the back of the mouth.

Congenital orofacial abnormalities

CLEFT LIP AND PALATE, AND FACIAL CLEFTS

These are amongst the most common of all birth anomalies, affecting approximately 1 in 1000 births. The face, jaw and palate are formed by the fusion of the frontonasal (nose, philtrum of the upper lip, premaxilla), maxillary (cheek, upper lip, upper jaw, palate) and mandibular (lower jaw, lip) processes in the first 8 weeks of gestation. Failure of these processes to meet and fuse produces a group of congenital abnormalities: cleft lip, cleft palate and facial clefts, or a combination of these.

Failure of fusion can produce a unilateral or bilateral cleft of the lip alone, involve the bony alveolus (premaxilla, a complete cleft lip) (Figures 11.1, 11.2) and involve the hard and soft palate (secondary palate, a complete cleft lip and palate) (Figure 11.3). Total failure of fusion causes a bilateral cleft lip, a

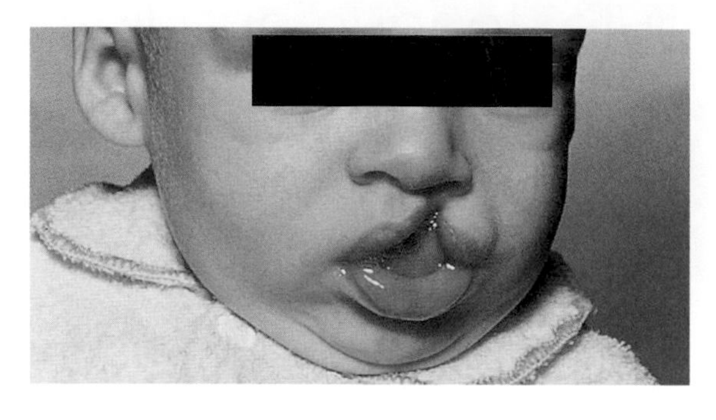

Figure 11.1 A child with a cleft lip.

cleft palate and a protuberant premaxilla (Figure 11.4). Clefts can also be limited to the palate alone and be unilateral or bilateral. It is vital that examination involves both inspection and palpation as some clefts may only become apparent on palatal palpation.

Symptoms of a cleft lip and palate include a *reduced inability to suckle and swallow, nasal regurgitation and ear infections.*

There may be interference with speech development, jaw growth and tooth position and eruption.

VASCULAR ANOMALIES (SEE CHAPTERS 4 AND 10)

These fall into major two groups, *vascular tumours* of which congenital and infantile haemangiomas are the most relevant, and *vascular malformations,* which can involve capillaries, lymphatics or veins or a combination of these structures ('low-flow' lesions). Vascular malformations also include arteriovenous malformations and fistulae ('high-flow' lesions). They can occur anywhere in the mouth including the lips, tongue and buccal mucosae and, in the presence

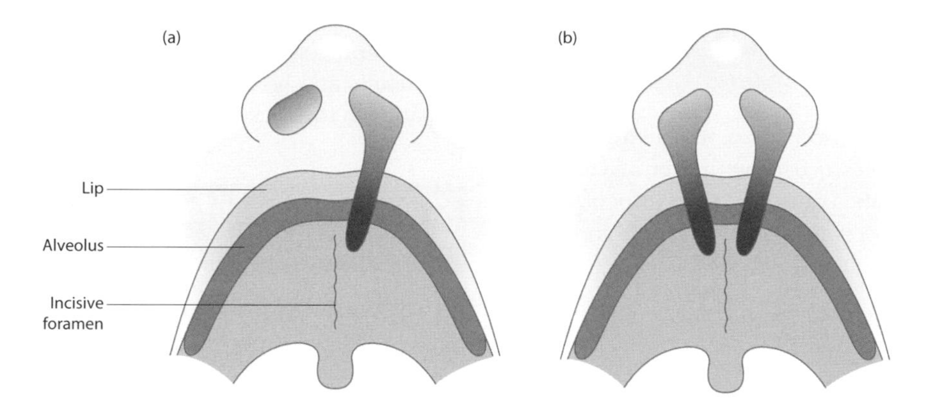

Figure 11.2 CLEFT LIP. (a) A unilateral cleft lip. A complete cleft involves the alveolus. (b) A bilateral cleft lip.

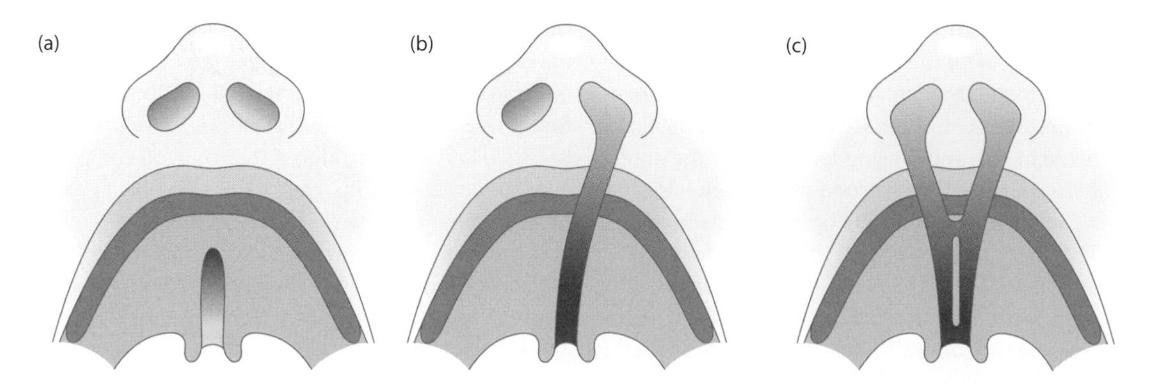

Figure 11.3 CLEFT LIP AND PALATE. (a) Cleft palate. (b) A cleft lip and palate. (c) A bilateral cleft lip and palate.

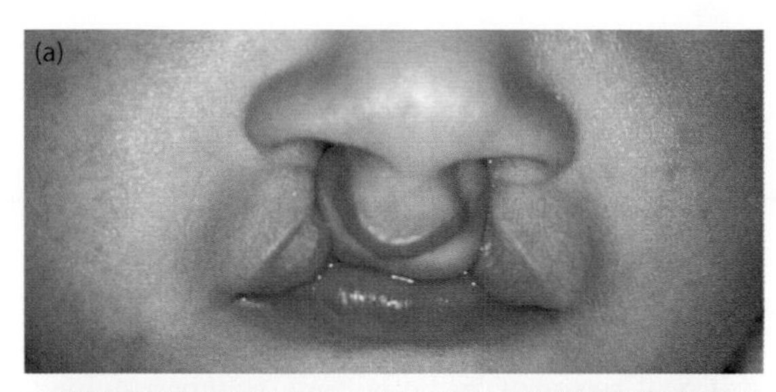

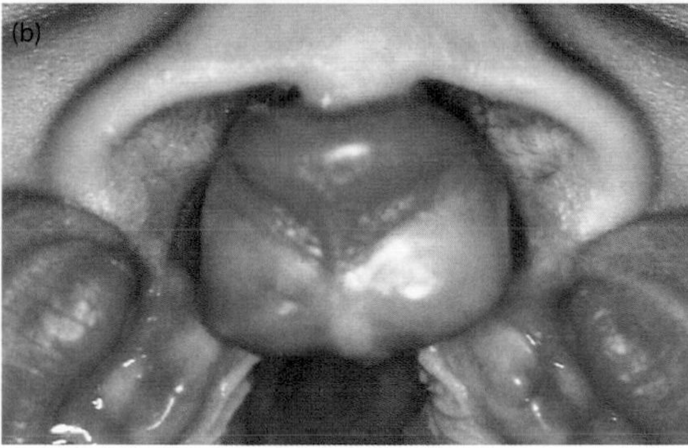

Figure 11.4 CLEFT LIP AND CLEFT PALATE. (a) Bilateral cleft lip. (b) Bilateral cleft lip and palate.

of other anomalies, may be seen as part of vascular syndromes (e.g. *Klippel–Trenaunay, Sturge–Weber or Maffucci*) (see Chapter 4).

Vascular tumours

These may be benign (congenital and *infantile haemangiomas*), locally aggressive (*Kaposi sarcoma*) or malignant (*angiosarcoma*).

Haemangiomas

Congenital haemangiomas are completely developed at birth and may completely disappear over the first 2 years (rapidly involuting congenital haemangioma). They may grow proportionally with the patient (non-involuting) or do so partially (partially involuting). They are usually red and can have an ulcerated surface with a pale halo or more grey and well circumscribed.

Infantile haemangiomas are not seen until the first few weeks after birth. They often start as small red lesions that rapidly proliferate over the first year of life and then spontaneously involute. Most will be gone by age 9 years.

Symptoms Usually only cause cosmetic problems but can ulcerate and bleed.

Size Most haemangiomas are less than 3 cm in diameter.

Colour Usually red if superficial or blue–purple if deeper.

Shape Irregular in shape.

Surface Smooth or lobulated; overlying tissue may be normal if the lesion is deep.

Composition Often firm on palpation without thrill or pulsation.

Relations Vessels usually merge with the local soft tissues.

Local tissues Normal but may be inflamed and tender if thrombosis has occurred.

Capillary malformations ('port wine stains')

Resulting from dilated capillary vessels, these are usually seen at birth as small pink spots. On the face, they affect areas supplied by the trigeminal nerve, in a dermatomal manner and can be the first sign of syndromes such as *Sturge–Weber and Klippel–Trenaunay* (Figure 11.5) (see Chapter 4).

Capillary malformations can produce significant lip and gum hypertrophy, as well as growth of the underlying jaw. The colour of the malformation deepens with age, going from red in adolescence, to purple in middle-age.

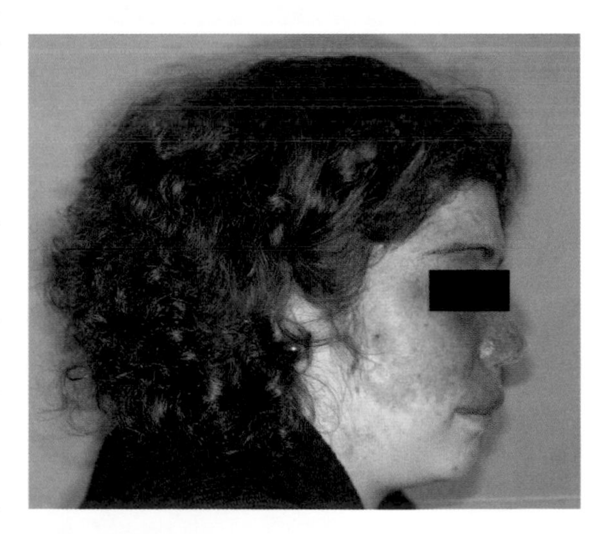

Figure 11.5 Sturge–Weber syndrome, with dermatomal involvement.

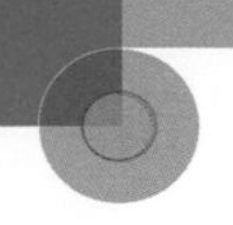

Lymphatic malformations

The majority of lymphatic malformations develop in the head and neck, with a propensity for the mouth (Figures 11.6 and 11.7). They can be very large in size (macrocystic) and cause problems with speech, swallowing and the airway. They can also present suddenly in adolescence, usually following an upper respiratory tract infection.

Age Two-thirds are present at birth, with the majority seen by age 1 year.

Symptoms Small lymphatic malformations (microcystic) are usually symptomless.

Site Mainly arise in the floor of the mouth, tongue and submandibular triangle.

Size Varies but can be very large.

Colour Same as the skin or mucous membrane under which they have developed. The cystic component in the neck transilluminates.

Shape Spherical or multilobulated.

Surface In the mouth, the small cystic lesions give a granular or 'frogspawn' appearance.

Composition Soft–spongy on palpation when small; incompressible when large.

Relations They usually merge into local structures and lie in the submucosa but may extend to the deep layers, causing obstructive problems.

Local tissues Can be normal or hypertrophied, leading to underlying bony growth.

Venous malformations (see Chapters 4 and 10)

These are the most common vascular malformation. They are *bluish lesions,* usually visible at birth and are obvious in the head and neck (Figures 11.8 and 11.9). They grow in proportion with the patient.

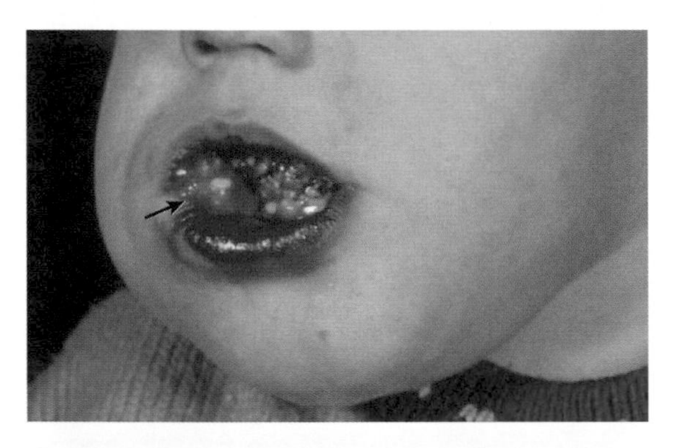

Figure 11.6 Large lymphatic malformation of the cheek and floor of mouth.

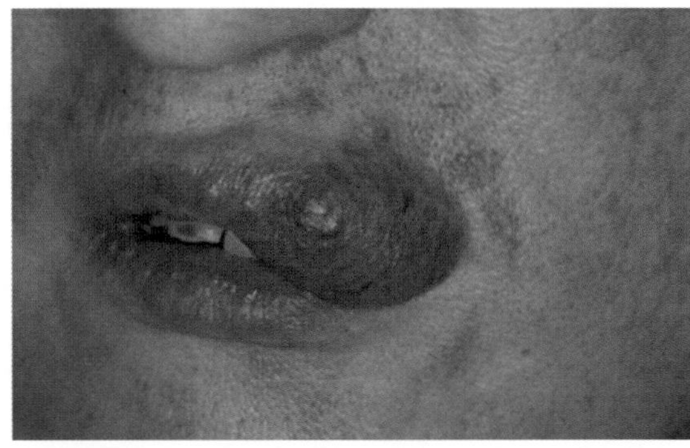

Figure 11.8 A venous malformation of the upper lip.

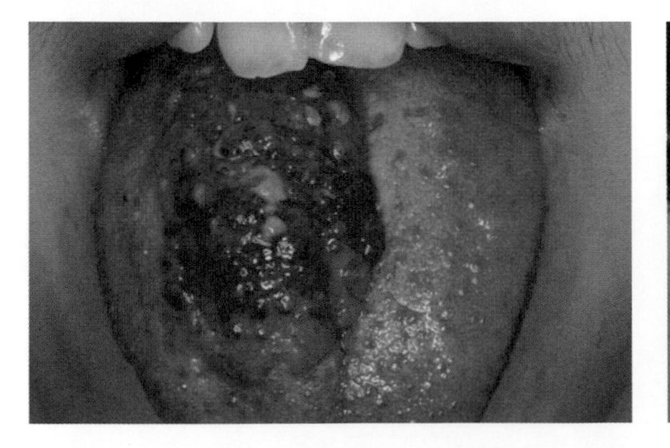

Figure 11.7 Isolated lymphatic malformation of the tongue.

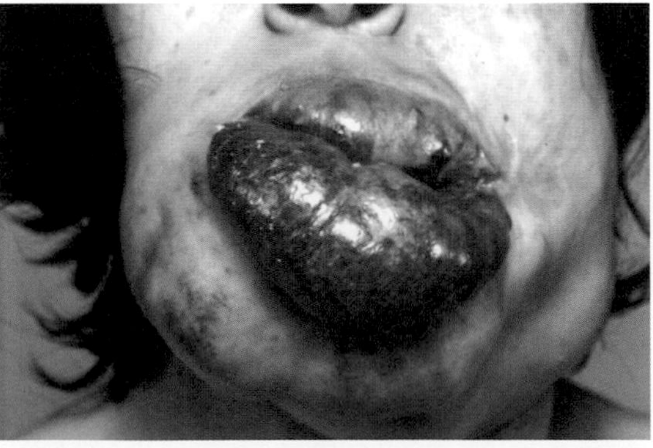

Figure 11.9 A massive venous malformation of the face.

Age Often noticed at birth as a small blue lump or bulge.

Symptoms Generally symptomless but thrombosis in larger lesions can cause pain as the lesion develops. In infants, they can become more prominent with straining, or in the head-down position.

Site Present anywhere on the head and neck, including the mouth.

Size Most tend to be small with predictable growth.

Shape Asymmetric, irregular.

Surface and colour Can be smooth or irregular. Overlying skin or mucosa is discoloured and blanches on pressure.

Composition They expand with pressure and are not pulsatile.

Local tissue Can be closely involved with local and vital structures and give rise to underlying bony growth.

Conditions of the lips, buccal mucosa and tongue

Examination of the lips may identify discolouration or pigmentation (such as that of *Addison's disease* or *Peutz–Jegher syndrome*; Figure 11.10), *telangiectasia* (hereditary haemorrhagic telangiectasia; Figure 11.11) or sun-exposure related actinic changes that can progress to lip cancer. Examination continues to identify swellings or irregularities of the lip mucosa and lining of the mouth.

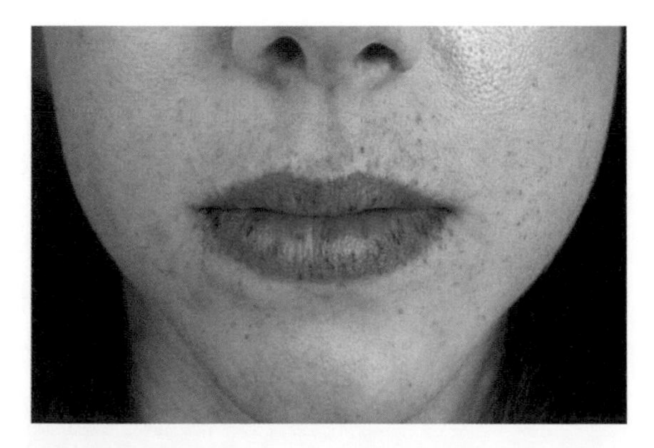

Figure 11.10 Pigmentation of lips seen in Peutz–Jegher syndrome.

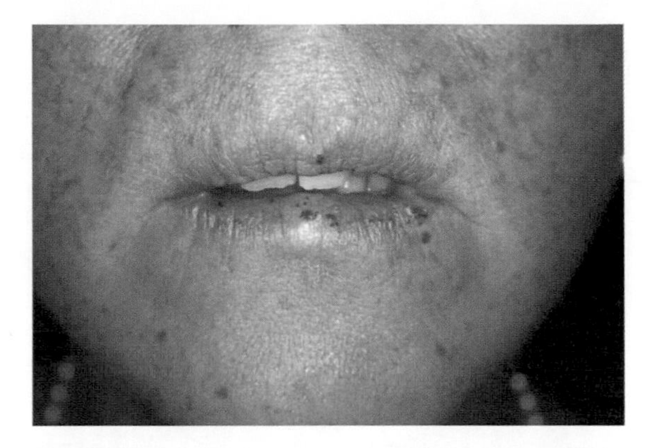

Figure 11.11 Telangiectasia in a patient with hereditary haemorrhagic telangiectasia.

MUCOCOELES (EXTRAVASATION/ RETENTION CYST)

The lining of the oral mucosa is studded with minor salivary glands whose purpose is to keep it moist. These glands continually secrete and if traumatized, saliva is secreted into adjacent tissues generating a tissue reaction. This forms a mucous extravasation cyst (Figure 11.12). Typically, they enlarge, burst and deflate and then reinflate with mucosal healing. A retention cyst is similar but saliva is retained within the gland following duct obstruction. Infection is rare.

History

Age All ages. May have a history of previous inadvertent trauma (e.g. biting) or a cheek-biting habit.

Symptoms Asymptomatic but can be caught between the teeth if large.

Examination

Site Lower lip and buccal mucosa at the level of occlusion of the teeth most commonly.

Colour Pale pink when small, but bluer as they enlarge. The epithelium may be white and the cyst partly deflated if it has been traumatized.

Shape Spherical and cystic.

Size From 0.5 to 2 cm in diameter.

Surface Smooth but may be ulcerated if the cyst has ruptured.

Composition Soft and fluctuant, to tense.

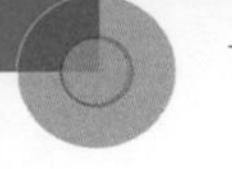

Local tissues Usually normal, but they may be inflamed if the cyst has ruptured.

Lymph glands Local lymph glands should not be enlarged.

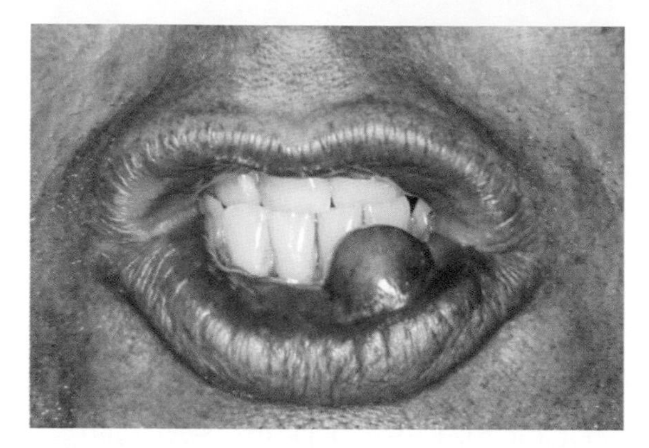

Figure 11.12 Lower lip mucocoele.

FIBROUS (FIBROEPITHELIAL) POLYP

This usually arises following local trauma that leads to connective tissue hypertrophy. This becomes an irritant to patients leading to further hypertrophy and eventually a discernible polyp.

History

Age Any age, usually in association with a history of minor repeated trauma/irritation. Denture-related in older patients.

Symptoms Polyps grow slowly and are symptomless unless caught between the teeth.

Examination

Site Commonly seen where teeth meet the cheek, tongue or lip. They may be seen under/in association with poor-fitting dentures.

Colour Normal pink mucosa, unless traumatized, in which case they can be pale and/or ulcerated.

Shape Rounded and often pedunculated (Figure 11.13). If under a denture, they can become leaf-like ('leaf fibroma').

Size Usually 0.5–2 cm in diameter.

Surface Usually smooth.

Composition Soft to firm, never fluctuant.

Relations Mobile and not fixed to the underlying tissues.

Local tissues Should be normal.

Lymph glands Should not be enlarged.

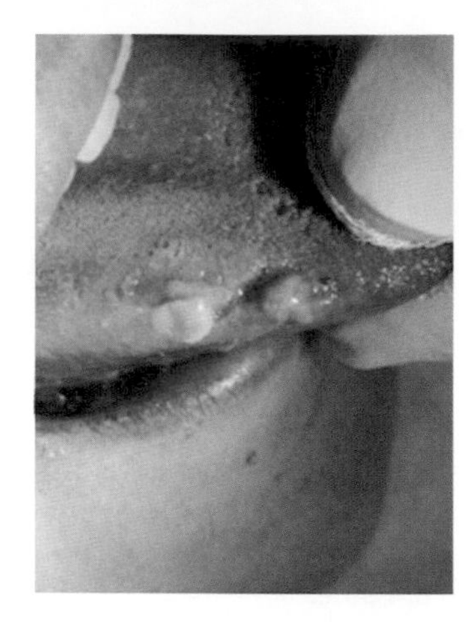

Figure 11.13 A fibroepithelial polyp on the tongue.

PAPILLOMAS

The *squamous papillomas* are small, pink, frond-like lesions that protrude from the mucosal surface (Figure 11.14). Common warts, or *verrucae vulgaris,* are discrete and sessile. The *condyloma acuminatum* subtype are uncommonly seen in the oral cavity and are often sexually transmitted warts. The human papillomavirus (HPV) is thought to give rise to most papillomas. Although HPV-16 type is firmly implicated in the pathogenesis of oropharyngeal carcinoma, there is no current evidence to suggest risk of malignant progression in oral papillomas.

History

Age Occur at any age although tend to affect adults in middle age.

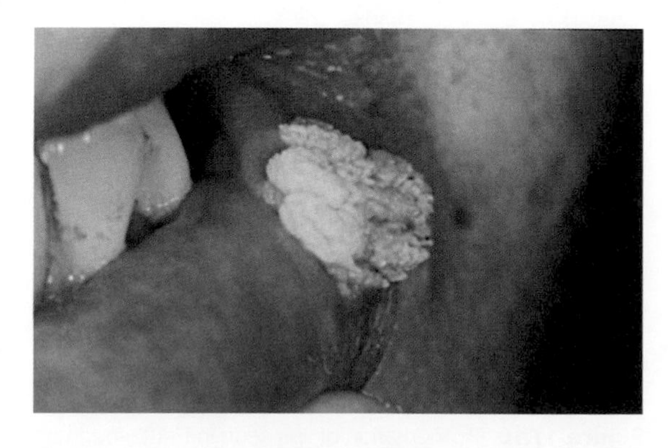

Figure 11.14 A papilloma on the lip.

Symptoms Not painful but grow slowly, causing local irritation.

Examination

Site Normally sited on the tongue, palate, mucosa of the lip.

Colour May be pink, or pale/white if keratinized.

Shape and surface: Squamous papillomas are typically spiky, exophytic, or have a cauliflower-like appearance. Verrucae vulgaris have an irregular granular surface similar to the much larger finger wart.

Size Usually less than 10 mm in diameter.

Composition Soft and fleshy lesions that are often friable.

Relations Squamous papillomas are *pedunculated* in shape, arising from a narrow, stalk-like base. Verrucae vulgaris are usually sessile.

Local tissues Normal.

Lymph glands Local lymph glands should not be enlarged.

STOMATITIS

This is a general term used to describe inflammation of the lining of the mouth. Patients complain of soreness, which may be associated with ulcers, redness and/or dryness. Pain can be severe with ulceration. In general, the mucosa is red, and the tongue may lose its papillae and become smooth. Movements of the tongue and cheeks can be uncomfortable, and eating may be difficult.

Stomatitis can be attributed to systemic causes, such as blood dyscrasias (Revision panel 11.1), when the oral manifestations are accompanied by signs and symptoms of the underlying condition. It can also arise from a local infection, trauma or be drug-induced.

A full medical history is therefore important. Painful mouths without clear clinical signs pose a diagnostic problem. They may be the result of subclinical disease, neuropathies or psychogenic causes. The key is to rule out any hidden systemic disorder.

Examination

The physical appearances vary according to the cause.

Revision panel 11.1

COMMON CAUSES OF STOMATITIS

Local causes

Dry mouth
Post-radiotherapy
Trauma: teeth, dentures

Infection and ulceration

Candidosis
Recurrent aphthae
Herpes viruses
Malignancy

Systemic disease

Blood disorders
Inflammatory bowel disease
Skin diseases
Infections

Drugs

NSAIDs
Beta-blockers
Bisphosphonates
Nicorandil
Antibiotics

Recurrent aphthous stomatitis

This is the most common oral mucosal disease. The cause is unknown but is thought to be an inappropriate and excessive immune response to minor stimuli. There may be a genetic component, and stress, hormonal disturbances and systemic disease may play a role. Most cases are mild.

There are three types; minor, major and herpetiform stomatitis:

- Minor aphthae: The most common type. Small groups of ulcers approximately 3–7 mm diameter cycle every few weeks. They last up to 10 days and heal without scarring. They do not appear on keratinized mucosa (Figure 11.15a, b).
- Major aphthae: Uncommon. Usually present as one to two ulcers as large as 1–2 cm in diameter (Figure 11.15c). They may be found on keratinized mucosa and can last for several weeks or months before they heal, often leaving a scar. They can mimic carcinoma.

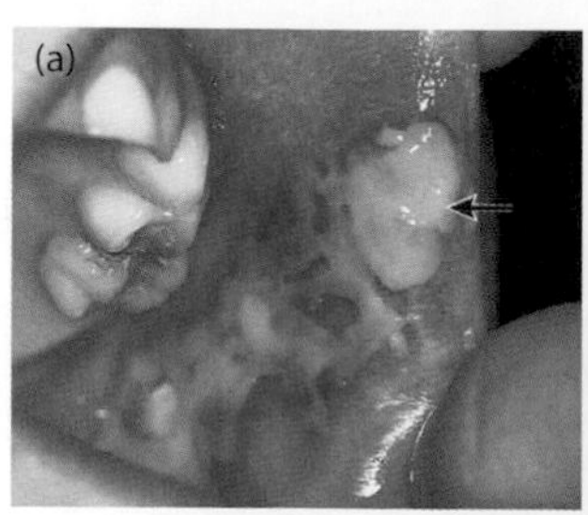

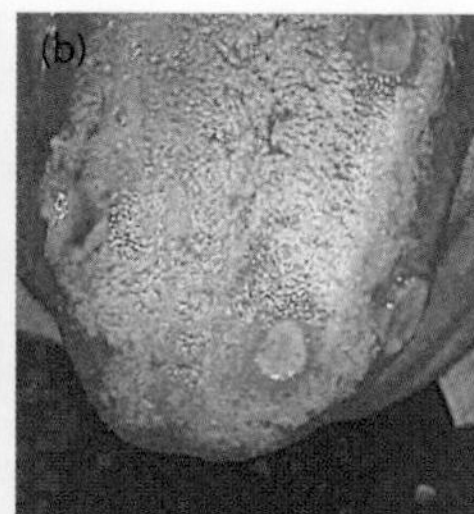

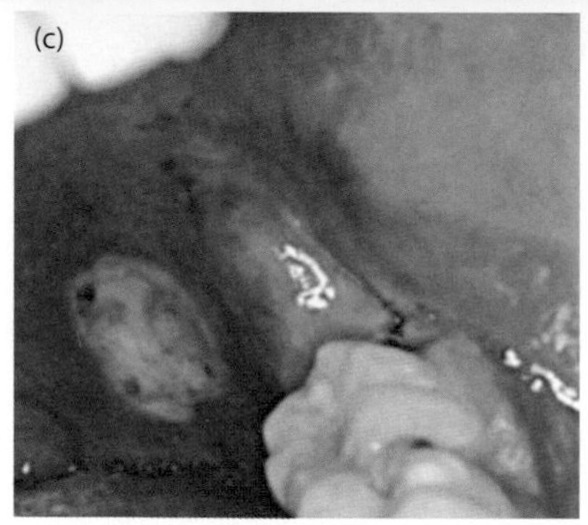

Figure 11.15 APHTHOUS ULCERS. (a) Multiple minor aphthae of the buccal mucosa. Largest ulcer is arrowed. (b) Multiple tongue. (c) Major tongue.

- Herpetiform stomatitis: Involves dozens of tiny ulcers (1–2 mm diameter) all over the mouth although not on keratinized mucosa.

Aphthous ulcers are common in otherwise healthy young people, particularly at times of stress but underlying heamatinic deficiencies need to be excluded. They tend to disappear with age.

Behçet's syndrome should be considered if the mouth ulcers are accompanied by systemic symptoms and genital ulcers.

Candidiasis

This results from the overgrowth of several species of candida fungus (usually *Candida albicans*) that are normal oral commensals. An upset to the equilibrium of the oral flora can give rise to an opportunistic infection, particularly in at-risk groups, such as the immunocompromised. The incidence has increased because of greater resistance to antifungal therapy and HIV infection.

Classifications of oral candidosis vary but is commonly divided into white or red forms, either of which can be acute or chronic.

- *White*:
  - *Pseudomembranous candidosis (thrush)*: Typically seen in neonates, the immunocompromised and in those where oral flora equilibrium has been disturbed by steroids, antibiotics or a chronically dry mouth. *Discreet creamy-white plaques* can be wiped away, leaving a red or bleeding (pseudomembranous) surface (Figure 11.16). Where infection involves the oropharynx, HIV or other immunosuppressive disease should be investigated.
  - *(Chronic) Hyperplastic candidosis* (Figure 11.17): This is a persistent plaque that does not wipe off. It may be nodular or speckled.

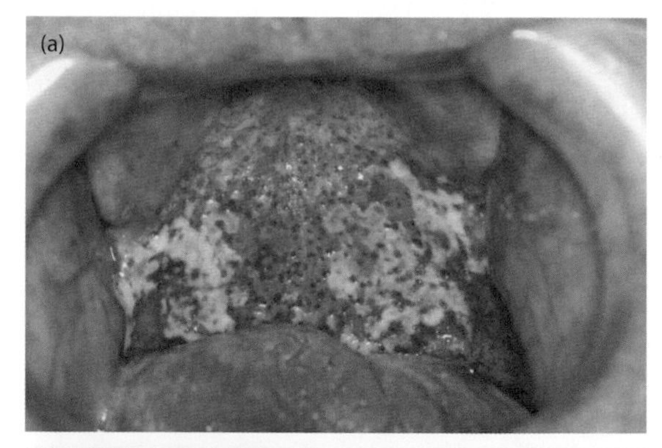

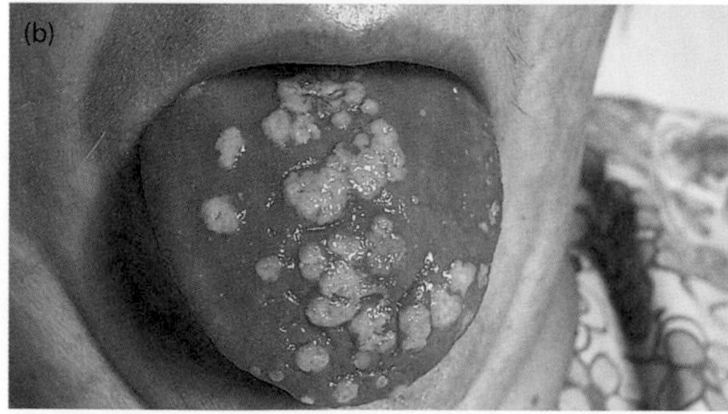

Figure 11.16 Pseudomembranous candidosis of the palate (a) and tongue (b).

The commonest site is the commissure region of the cheek, with the tongue and palate also involved. It may be associated with malignant change.

- *Red (erythematous) candidosis* accounts for two-thirds of all cases. It may be seen following:
  - Antibiotic or inhaled-steroid use.
  - Denture-induced stomatitis.
  - Angular cheilitis and median rhomboid glossitis (see below).
- *Other types include*: Chronic mucocutaneous, which is rare and associated with immunological disorders, particularly endocrine abnormalities.

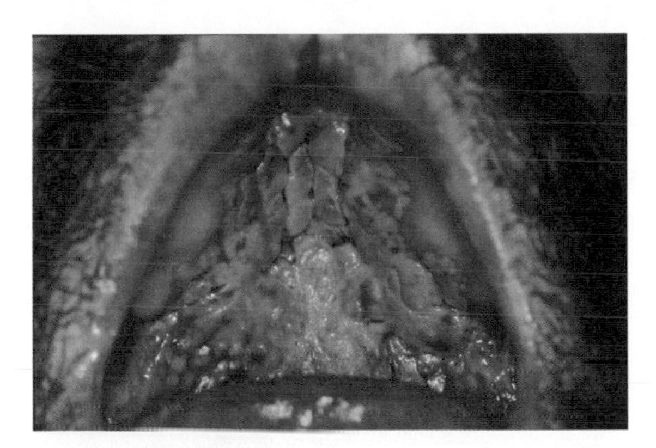

Figure 11.17 Hyperplastic candidosis of the palate.

Angular cheilitis

The corners of the mouth (angles, commissures) can become red and inflamed (Figure 11.18) more commonly seen in the elderly, particularly those using old dentures. Angle fissures become soiled with saliva, leading to maceration and subsequent superinfection with commensal organisms (staphylococci and *Candida*). Angular cheilitis may be a manifestation of iron or vitamin deficiency, especially when accompanied by glossitis and oral ulcers.

Median rhomboid glossitis

This is a symptomless area usually noticed by the patient as rhomboid-shaped red patch in the midline of the dorsum of the tongue. The mucosa may be eroded or raised, and pink-red to white-yellow (Figure 11.19) as a result of the loss of filiform papillae. Candidal infection might be intermittent. There might also be a nodular component, which can be mistaken for cancer although midline cancers of the tongue are rare.

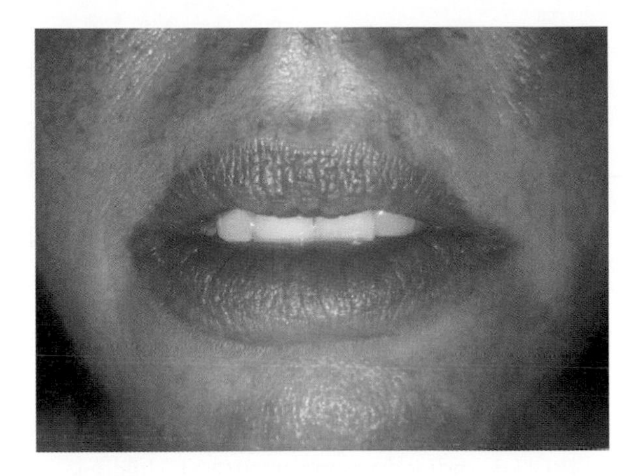

Figure 11.18 Angular cheilitis.

Acute necrotizing ulcerative gingivitis

This is a relatively uncommon infection caused by multiple spirochaete and fusiform bacteria. The appearance is dramatic, with the gums around the teeth bright red. The pathognomonic feature is

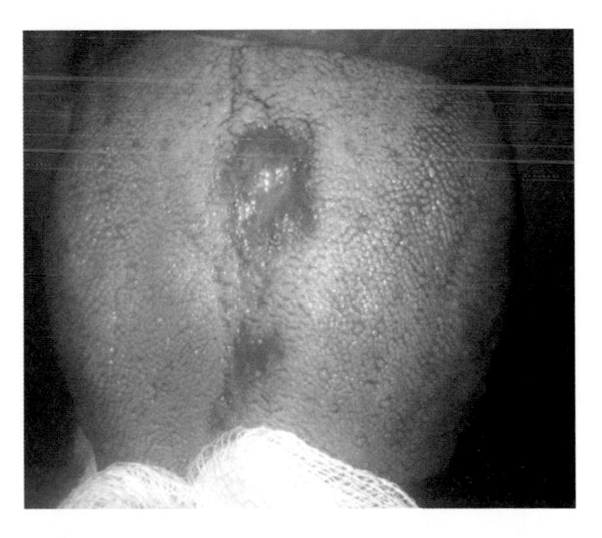

Figure 11.19 Median rhomboid glossitis.

necrosis of the papillae between the teeth. There may be bleeding, ulceration and fetor oris. It may be secondary to very poor oral hygiene, stress, local trauma or ushered in by a period of immunosuppression. The cervical lymph glands are enlarged and tender.

Noma (Cancrum Oris)

This is a serious infection that may represent a severe form of spreading acute necrotising ulcerative gingivitis. Now largely confined to parts of sub-Saharan Africa, it mostly affects young, malnourished and/or immunosuppressed children. It normally starts as a small, infected ulcerated area in the cheek or gum that spreads rapidly over 3–5 days. Necrosis follows, with tissue sloughing exposing bone and destroying the contours of the face. Mortality rates are thought to be over 80% in the absence of adequate treatment.

SYPHILIS

The prevalence of syphilis has fallen significantly in the antibiotic era, having been all but eradicated in countries with good access to healthcare. It has however shown a limited resurgence in certain high-risk populations.

- *Chancres* of primary syphilis can occur on the tongue or lips (Figure 11.20) usually as large painless ulcers or lumps.
- *Mucous patches and snail-track ulcers* are part of the skin abnormalities that develop with secondary syphilis. These patches or ulcers can be seen on the lips, tongue and tonsils most frequently.
- *Gummas* can arise in the tongue, hard palate or tonsil and present as painless masses that may ulcerate and necrose leading to perforation.

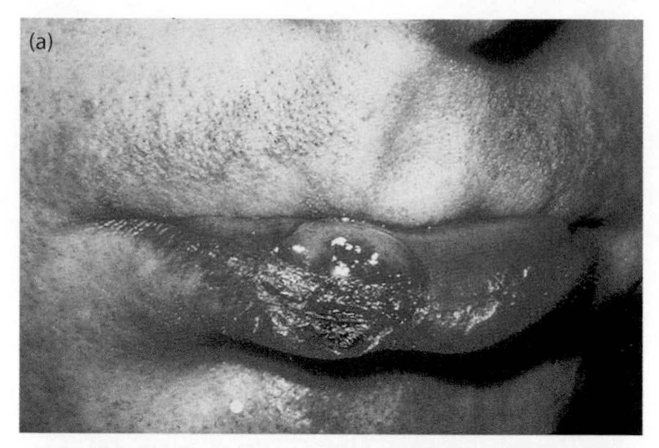

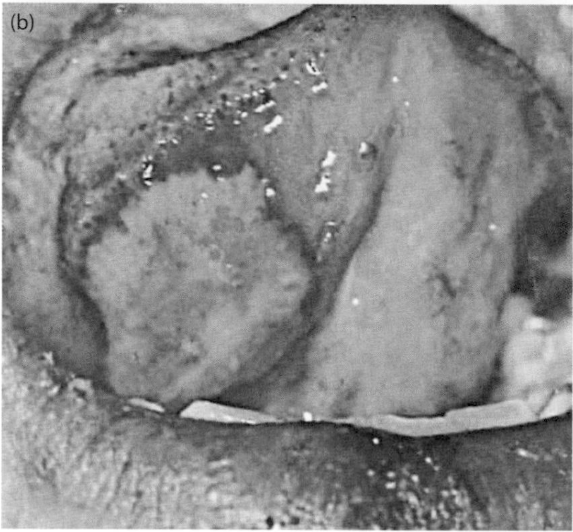

Figure 11.20 PRIMARY SYPHILIS. (a) Chancre on the lower lip. (b) Chancre on the tongue.

LEUKOPLAKIA (WHITE PATCH)

This refers specifically to 'white plaques having excluded (other) known diseases or disorders that carry no increased risk for cancer'. It is a diagnosis of exclusion and a premalignant lesion, not associated with any cause other than tobacco consumption (Figure 11.21).

Leukoplakia is usually symptomless. The malignant transformation rate depends on any underlying dysplasia, with up to 5% becoming malignant per year with severe dysplasia.

A sub-type, *verrucous leukoplakia* (Figure 11.22), is more indolent but progresses relentlessly. It may slowly migrate along the gums or oral mucosa with a 50% transformation rate to cancer in the *proliferative* form. It requires early intervention.

Site The buccal mucosa, tongue, gum and floor of mouth are the most common sites. High-risk

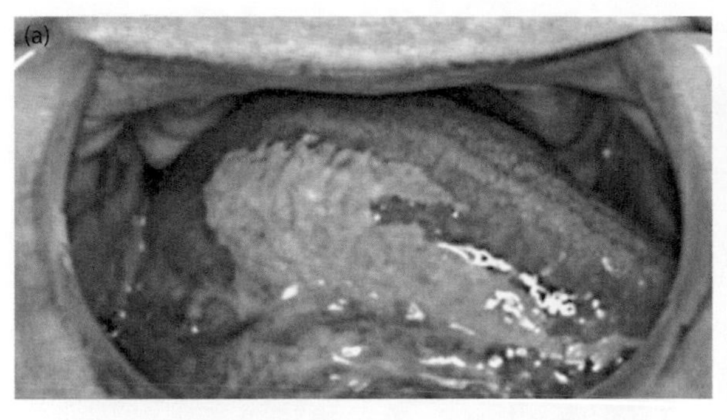

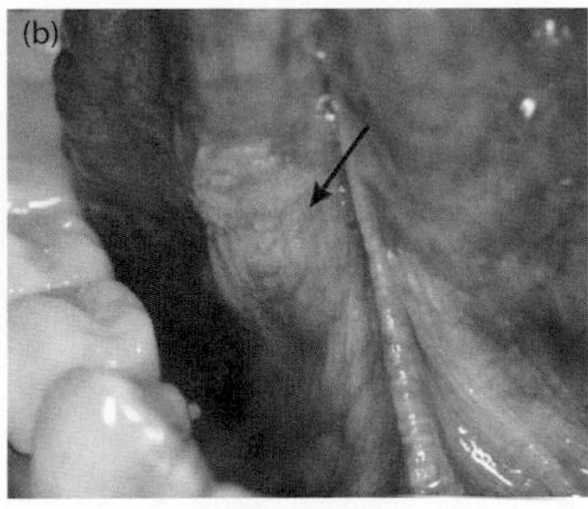

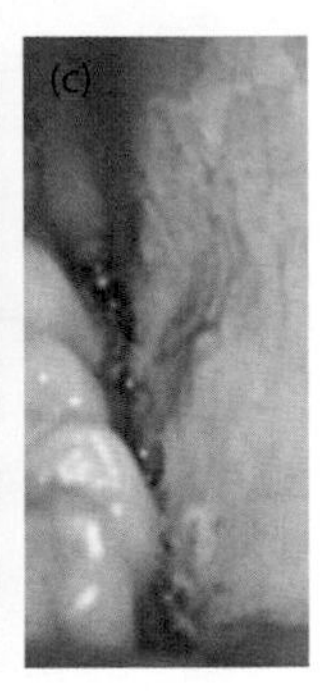

Figure 11.21 ORAL LEUKOPLAKIA. (a) Leukoplakia of the lateral tongue. (b) Leukoplakia of the ventral surface of tongue. (c) Leukoplakia of the left buccal mucosa.

regions for malignant transformation are the ventrolateral surface of the tongue and the floor of mouth.

Colour White, but there might be a red component, *erythroleukoplakia*, which has a much higher rate of malignant transformation.

Size Plaques vary in size and may occupy large areas of mucosa.

Shape and surface Can be homogenous (uniform, wrinkled, corrugated) or heterogenous (verrucous, nodular, speckled red). Heterogenous lesions have a higher rate of malignant transformation.

Local tissues Should be normal.

Lymph drainage Lymph glands should not be enlarged, and lymphadenopathy suggests a carcinoma.

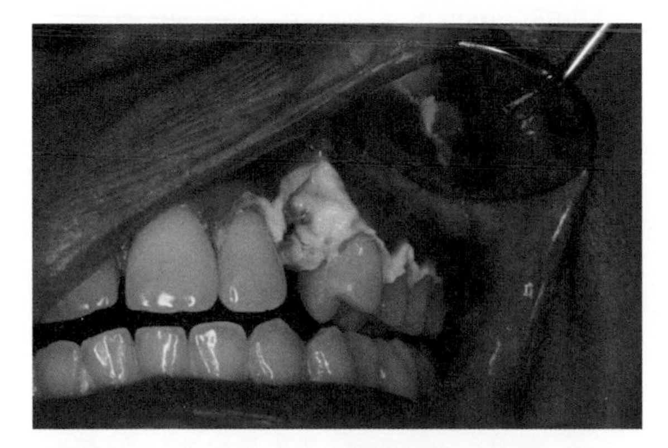

Figure 11.22 Verrucous leukoplakia of the gums, along the margins.

LICHEN PLANUS

This is an immunologically mediated condition of unknown cause affecting the mouth and skin. As the oral mucosa starts to change, it becomes white in appearance. In more aggressive forms, the tissues are friable and vulnerable to trauma. small superficial ulcers may also be seen (Figure 11.23). It affects 1–2% of the population and has a malignant transformation rate of up to 1%, mostly associated with the erosive form of the disease.

A 'lichenoid reaction' is similar to lichen planus but is caused by a known trigger, usually a dental restoration or a drug. If the former, it is an isolated patch often in contact with a large amalgam filling. Common drugs causing lichenoid reaction are beta-blockers, NSAIDs and hypoglycaemics. In contrast to lichen planus, lichenoid reactions can be distributed in multiple sites around the mouth.

Symptoms Often asymptomatic but there may be discomfort with spicy/citrus foods.

Site Predominantly buccal mucosa bilaterally but may appear on the tongue or the gums (desquamative gingivitis).

Colour Oral lesions are typically white but may have an erythematous component in erosive forms.

Size Varies widely and may occupy the whole extent of the buccal mucosa.

Shape and surface Six clinical types have been described. The two main forms of this disease that are encountered are reticular (most common) and atrophic (erosive is the extreme extension of atrophic) are the two main forms of this disease that are encountered.

Local tissues Usually normal, but there may be associated inflammation.

In the systemic form, other tissues The skin, nails, scalp and genitals may also be involved.

Lymph glands Local lymph glands should not be enlarged.

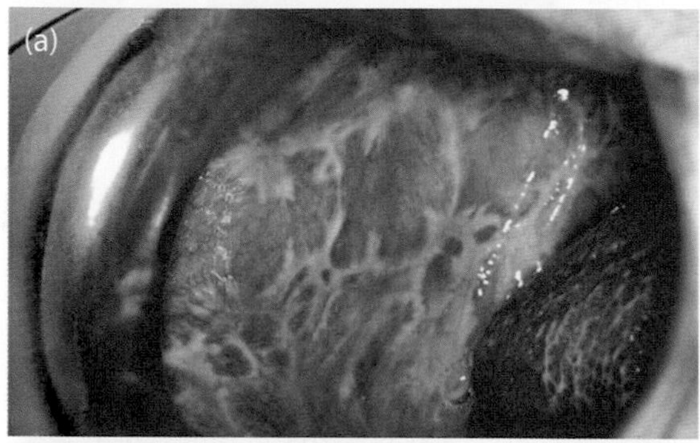

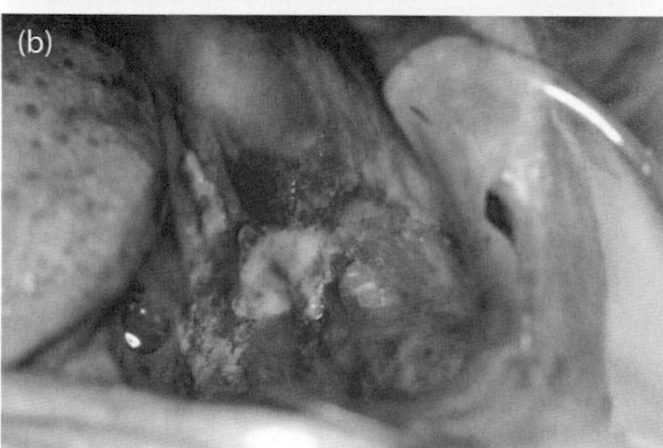

Figure 11.23 LICHEN PLANUS. (a) Reticular lichen planus of the buccal mucosa. (b) Erosive lichen planus presenting as erythroleukoplakia.

ORAL SUBMUCOUS FIBROSIS

This is a chronic, progressive fibrosis of the submucosal lining of the oral cavity. It is mediated by alkaloids released from areca nut, usually as 'paan', a betel-leaf wrap containing areca and slaked lime held against the cheek for hours at a time. This condition is most commonly found in countries of the Indian subcontinent and parts of east Asia.

It usually affects the buccal mucosa symmetrically. The diagnosis is made by palpating vertical bands of submucosal thickening. Patients may describe a burning sensation and limitation of mouth opening (trismus). Affected sites appear *shiny pale with atrophic mucosa* (Figure 11.24). It is considered to be a premalignant condition, with estimated malignant transformation rate in the UK of approximately 2%.

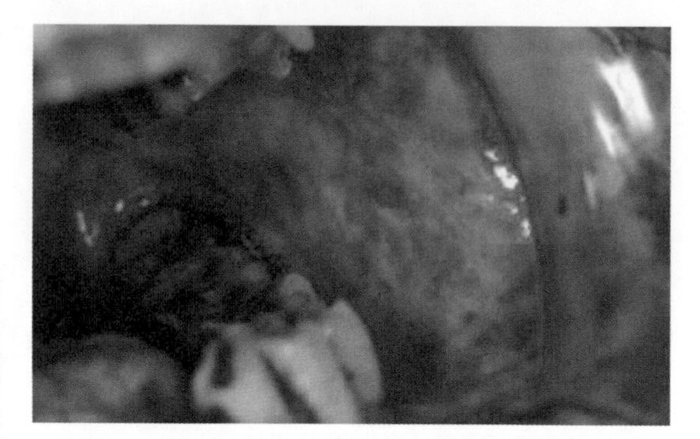

Figure 11.24 Submucous fibrosis. Note stained teeth, paler mucosa and limited mouth opening.

CARCINOMA OF THE LIP

The main cause of lip cancer is *solar radiation*. The lower lip catches the sunlight which explains why over 90% of lip cancers are found here. Actinic or solar keratosis is a pre-malignant change of the lip (Figure 11.25).

History

Age Usually over the age of 60 years with a history of chronic sun exposure.

Sex Males more than females.

Occupation More common in those with outdoor occupations such as fishermen, builders and farmers.

Ethnic group Fair-skinned people are at greatest risk particularly in sun-bleached countries, with

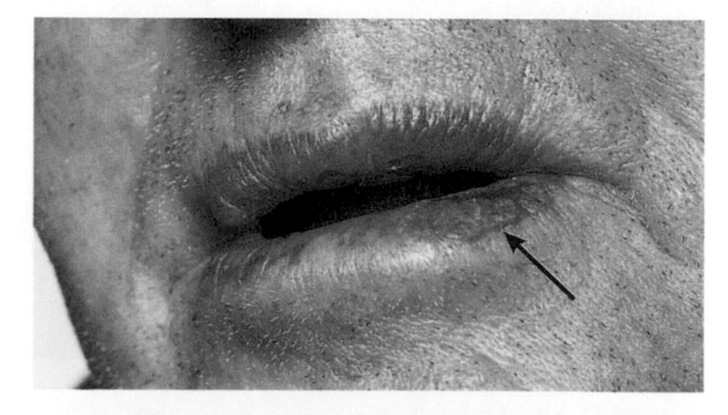

Figure 11.25 Actinic (solar) keratosis on the lower lip, a premalignant change.

greater incidence in people of European origin as one approaches the equator. Darker-skinned people are still susceptible as the vermillion does not produce melanin.

Symptoms The lesion at *first mimics a 'cold sore'* on the lip with a history of replasing ulceration, which may give false reassurance (Figure 11.26). They develop slowly and the patient may have consulted their doctor or dentist on more than one occasion. This has medicolegal implications.

Examination

Site The lower lip is involved ten times more frequently than the upper lip. Carcinoma in the angle of the lips is uncommon (Figure 11.26).

Colour There is skin or ulcer blistering, thickening and discoloration. There may be a blood-stained discharge.

Shape and size Initially a small non-healing crack in the mucosa, which crusts and ulcerates and develops into an everted-edge carcinoma. Typically less than 1 cm in diameter when the patient presents for treatment (Figures 11.27 and 11.28).

Base The base is covered with a thin, soft, friable, grey–yellow slough.

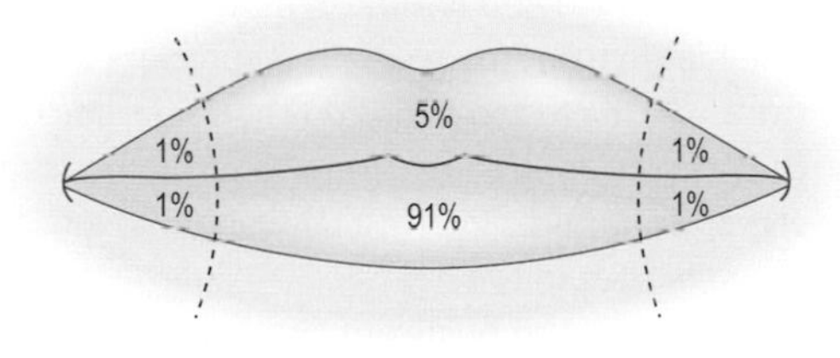

Figure 11.26 The distribution of carcinoma of the lips.

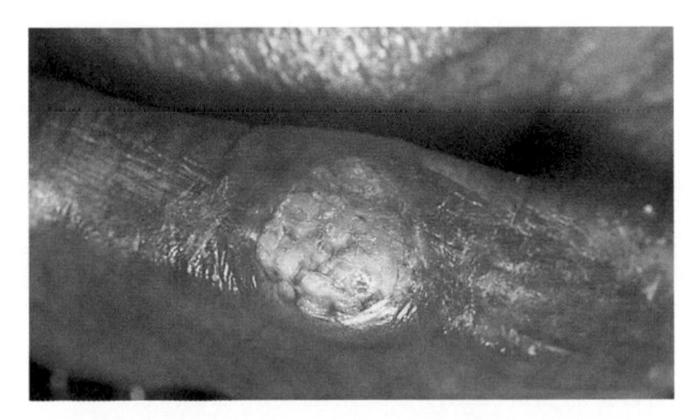

Figure 11.27 An early carcinoma that has begun to ulcerate.

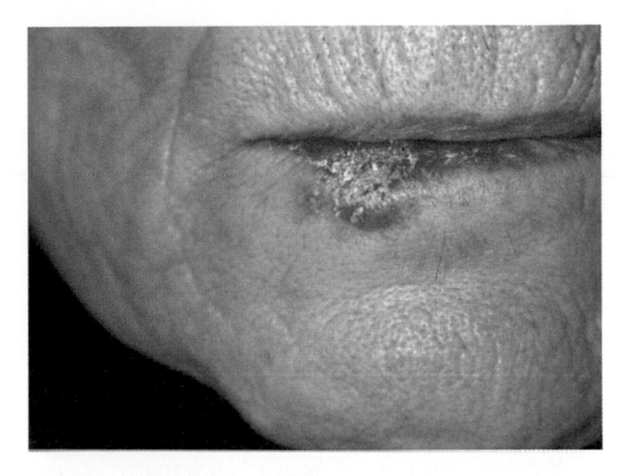

Figure 11.28 A carcinoma of the lower lip.

Depth *The ulcer is initially shallow* but can erode deep into the lip, destroying the epithelium and the underlying muscle.

Relations The lump is invariably fixed to the subcutaneous structures of the lip but can be moved, with the lip, separately from the jaw.

Lymph glands Metastasis to the cervical lymph nodes occurs only late in the disease. Lymph glands are firm and discrete if they do contain metastases.

Surrounding tissues May have actinic changes such as colour change and thinning of the mucosa.

CARCINOMA OF THE TONGUE

The tongue is the commonest site of squamous cell carcinoma in the mouth. It invades the local tissues and can spread to the regional lymph nodes in the neck. Distant blood-borne metastases are a late event of advanced disease.

Major aetiological factors include *tobacco* and *excessive alcohol consumption*, with a synergistic effect between the two.

The tongue can be divided into the anterior two-thirds and the posterior third. In a previously untreated tongue, cancers of the anterior aspect break the surface and appear as ulcers. In contrast, posterior tongue cancers can burrow into lymphoid tissue remain invisible to the eye. However, they may be palpated.

History

Age Usually over the age of 50 years, with peak incidence between 60 and 70 years.

Sex Males are more likely to be affected than females.

Symptoms Most commonly, it is a *painful ulcer* that has not settled. In one-fifth of patients, the ulcer is painless and late diagnosis tends to result. The cancer progresses inexorably. *Referred pain to the ear* is a cardinal symptom that should not be overlooked in a high-risk patient (age, alcohol and tobacco consumption) complaining of oral discomfort.

If the tumour has spread extensively, it may cause immobility of the tongue (*ankyloglossia*) leading to *difficulty with speech and swallowing*. Tumours on the base of the tongue may alter the quality of the voice, leading to 'hot-potato' speech. Alternatively, the patient may present with a lump in the neck (lymphadenopathy) before noticing any abnormality of the tongue.

Examination

Site Tongue cancer is most common on the lateral border of the tongue (Figures 11.29, 11.30) and the associated ventral surface.

Colour In the posterior third, the tongue over a deep-seated tumour may look normal, Anteriorly, the tongue may be smooth, shiny and stretched in the very early stages. The *vast majority of cancers present as ulcers* and established ones are usually covered with a transparent, yellow–grey slough.

Shape, size and composition Cancer of the tongue may present in four forms:

- An ulcer (most common).
- A nodule.
- A papilliferous or warty nodule.
- A fissure in an area of induration.

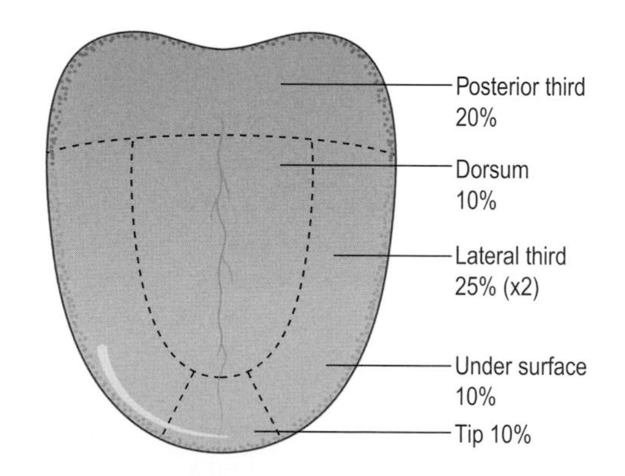

Figure 11.29 The distribution of carcinoma of the tongue.

A carcinomatous lump is *hard and indurated.* A carcinomatous ulcer of the tongue usually has the typical features of a carcinoma: a *friable, bleeding, everted edge,* a sloughing yellow–grey base, a thin serous discharge and induration.

The *papilliferous or verrucous carcinoma* is a lesion covered with an excess of proliferating filiform epithelium, usually paler than the surrounding pink epithelium, with a base broad and indurated. It may be of any size but rarely juts out far from the tongue. A *fissure* in an area of carcinomatous induration is a rare form of tongue cancer. Surrounding tissue may be inflamed or display changes associated with premalignancy.

Relations It is important to fully examine the floor of the mouth, gums, jaw, tonsils and fauces because a carcinoma can spread into any of these structures. Advanced tumour invasion may reduce the mobility of the tongue and infiltration of the gum and jaw fixes the tumour to the bone. Advanced tumours of the posterior tongue can spread into the tonsil and the pillars of the fauces.

Lymph glands

- The lymph from the tip of the tongue drains bilaterally to the submental nodes and then to the mylohyoid and jugular lymph chain.
- The lymph from the rest of the anterior two-thirds drains to the nodes on the same side of the neck, usually the mylohyoid group of deep cervical glands but metastasis can go to a wide range of sites in the neck.
- Lymph from the posterior third drains into the ring of lymph tissues around the oropharynx and into the upper deep cervical lymph glands.

NOTE: More than half of the patients who present with a cancer of the tongue have palpable cervical lymph glands.

Local tissues Involvement of the lingual nerve causes a *pain that is referred to the ear*, probably through its connections with the auriculotemporal nerve.

Differential diagnosis Causes of tongue ulcers are given in Revision panel 11.2.

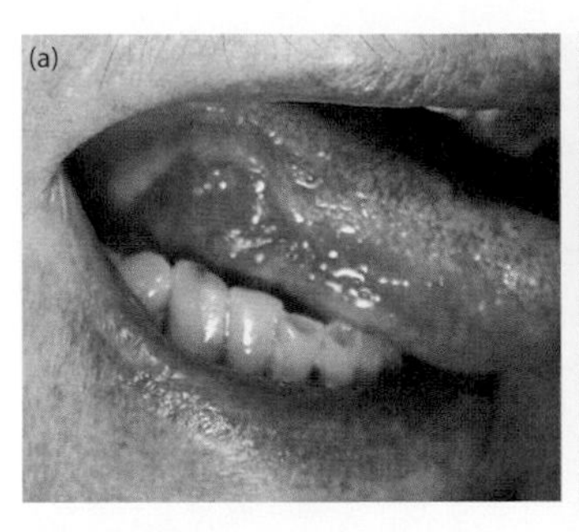

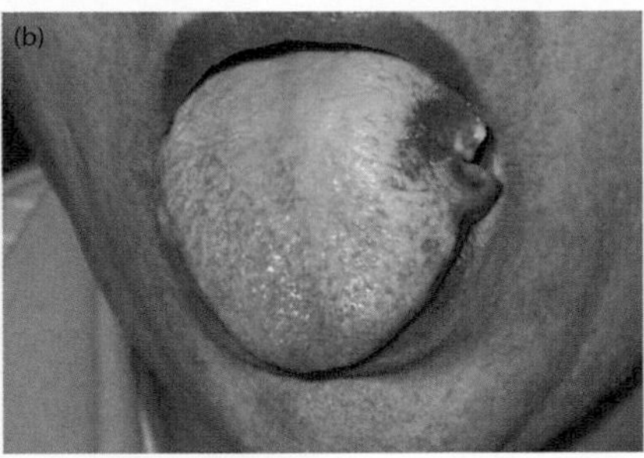

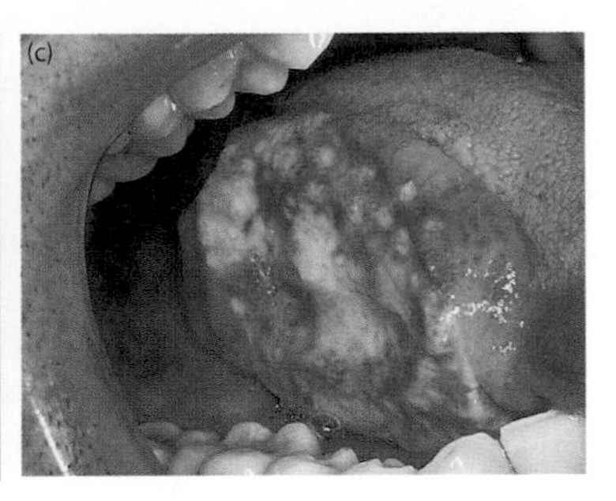

Figure 11.30 (a) An ulcer on the lateral tongue that can be disregarded by the patient in the early stages. (b) An ulcerated carcinoma on the side of the tongue. (c) A very large carcinoma with an everted edge on the side of the tongue.

Revision panel 11.2

ULCERATION OF THE TONGUE

Common causes

- Aphthous ulceration
- Drug-induced
- Trauma

Less common

- Non-specific glossitis
- Median rhomboid glossitis
- Syphilitic chancre
- Vesiculobullous disease
- Infection
- Systemic disorders

Revision panel 11.3

MACROGLOSSIA

- Acromegaly
- Amyloidosis
- Vascular malformations
- Neoplasms
- Allergy and trauma
- Down's syndrome

MACROGLOSSIA

This is an enlarged tongue. The causes of macroglossia are varied and can be either congenital or acquired (Revision panel 11.3).

TONGUE-TIE (ANKYLOGLOSSIA)

A *congenitally shortened frenulum* (Figure 11.31) can lead to a degree of tongue-tie. This does not usually interfere with feeding or cause impairment of speech development, but it can lead to parental concern.

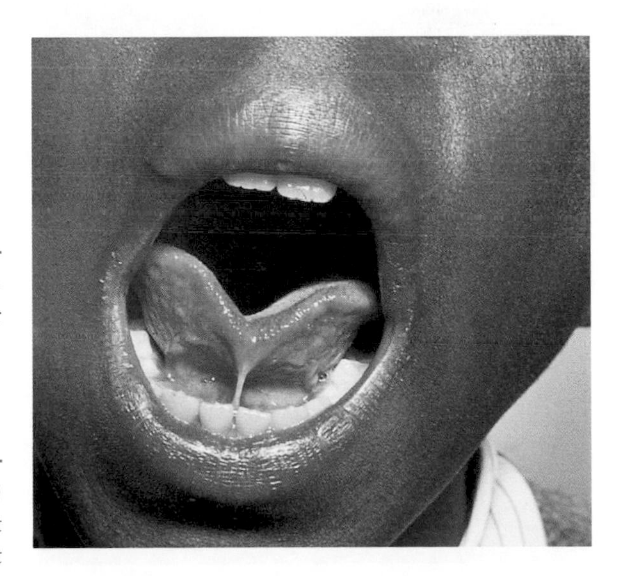

Figure 11.31 Tongue-tie rarely causes any significant impairment of speech.

WASTING OF THE TONGUE

Paralysis of the XIIth cranial nerve (the hypoglossal nerve) causes fatty degeneration and disuse atrophy of the affected side of the tongue. When patients are asked to stick out their tongue, it deviates towards the paralysed side (Figure 11.32). The cause of the hypoglossal nerve neuropathy must be elucidated (see Chapter 3).

MUCOSAL NEUROMAS

These are small, soft slow-growing lumps that are uncommon. They may be appear in conjunction with lesions elsewhere in the mouth or on the body. Their presence may be associated with the MEN2B (multiple endocrine neoplasia type 2b [see Chapter 12]) (Figure 11.33).

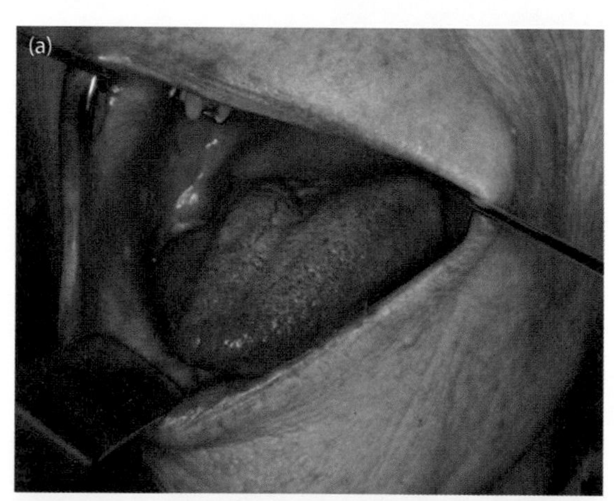

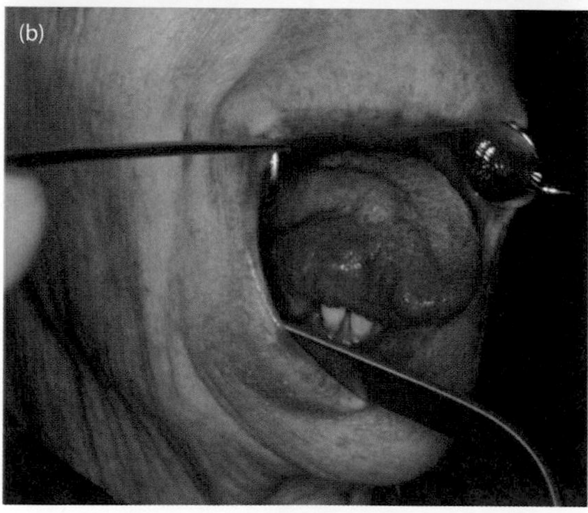

Figure 11.32 (a) When asked to protrude her tongue, it deviates to the right. (b) There is fatty degeneration and atrophy of the muscle on the right.

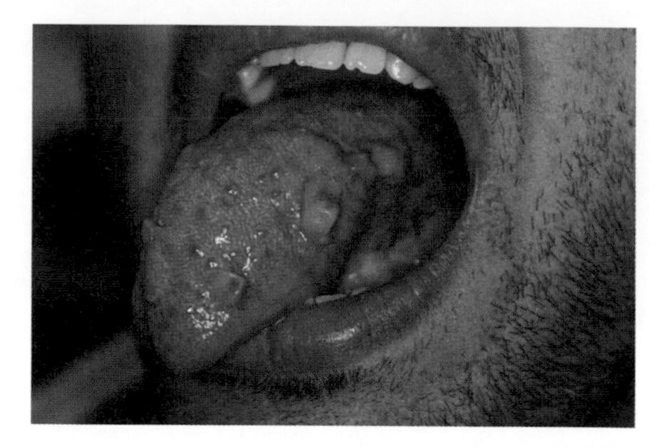

Figure 11.33 Multiple mucosal neuromas of the tongue.

Conditions of the palate

The varieties of congenital cleft palate were described earlier in the chapter.

EXOSTOSIS (PALATAL TORUS)

Bony exostoses such as those found in the palate are developmental, very common and benign. The palatal exostosis (palatal torus) is found in the midline of the hard palate. It grows slowly and is usually spherical or oval shaped (Figure 11.34). The overlying mucosa has a normal appearance, but can be traumatized easily if the exostosis is large. Tori are usually noticed in

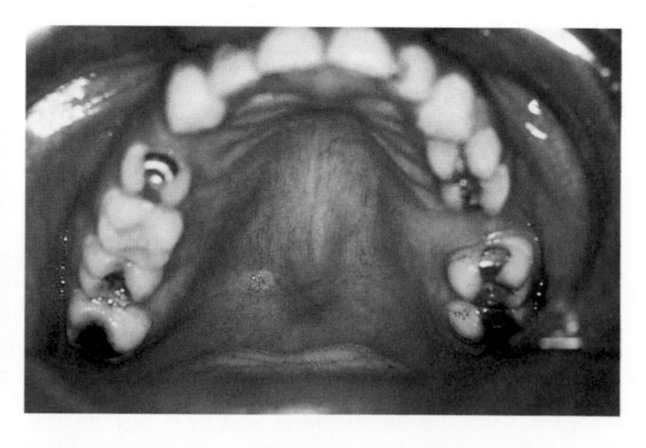

Figure 11.34 The palatal torus is rounded, usually symmetrical with a midline cleft.

middle age or later, when a new denture is required or when inadvertently traumatized resulting in osteitis. Large tori may interfere with the fitting of a denture.

PERFORATION OF THE PALATE (OROANTRAL, ORONASAL FISTULA)

A perforation in the palate can be acquired if disease or trauma destroys the bones of the palate (Figure 11.35) (Revision panel 11.4).

Revision panel 11.4

CAUSES OF PALATE PERFORATION

Extraction of an upper molar tooth.

Tumours of the maxillary antrum invading into the mouth through palate.

Granulomatosis with polyangiitis (formerly Wegener's granulomatosis): a rare vasculitis causing necrotizing granulomatous inflammation.

Gumma.

Surgery: Excision of tumours or palatal approach to the maxillary antrum.

NECROTIZING SIALOMETAPLASIA

Necrotizing sialometaplasia is a benign, tumour-like lesion that involves the minor palatal salivary glands. It usually presents as a punched out ulcerated swelling at the junction between the hard and soft palates in male smokers (Figure 11.36). It is an inflammatory condition possibly triggered by trauma and vascular infarction, but is difficult to distinguish from a neoplastic lesion without a biopsy. Although it can grow rapidly and become quite large, it is self-limiting and usually spontaneously settles within 8 weeks.

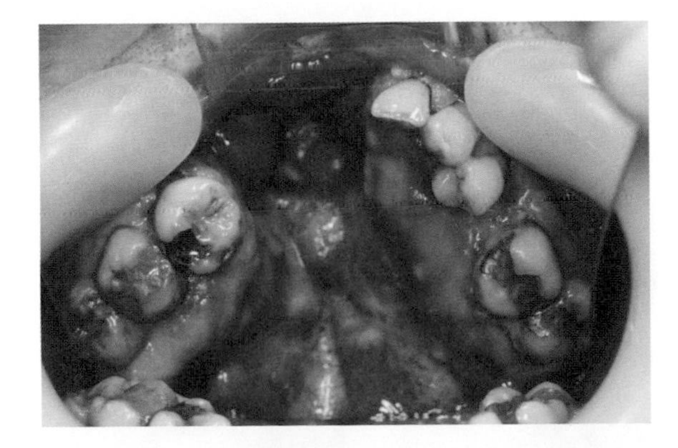

Figure 11.35 Large perforation of the anterior palate. The nasal septum and turbinates are visible.

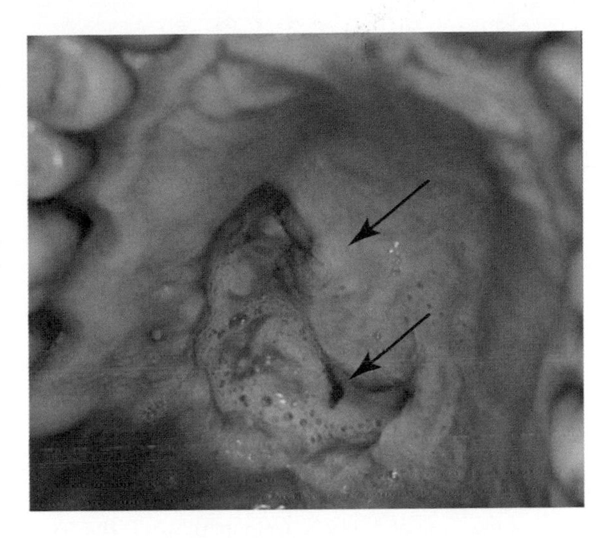

Figure 11.36 NECROTISING SIALOMETAPLASIA. Involving the hard/soft palate border and can mimic malignancy.

TUMOURS OF THE PALATE

The mucous membrane covering the hard palate is identical to that of the rest of the buccal mucosa. Cancers similar to those of the lips and buccal mucosa are not uncommon.

The posterior aspect of the hard palate contains many minor salivary glands particularly at the junction of hard and soft palate. Just over half of the tumours in the palatal minor salivary glands are benign. A *pleomorphic salivary adenoma* (mixed salivary tumour – see Chapter 12) is a benign neoplasm and is a common cause of a lump at the junction of the hard and soft palate (Figure 11.37). *Approximately 40% of minor salivary gland tumours are malignant* (adenocarcinoma, mucoepidermoid

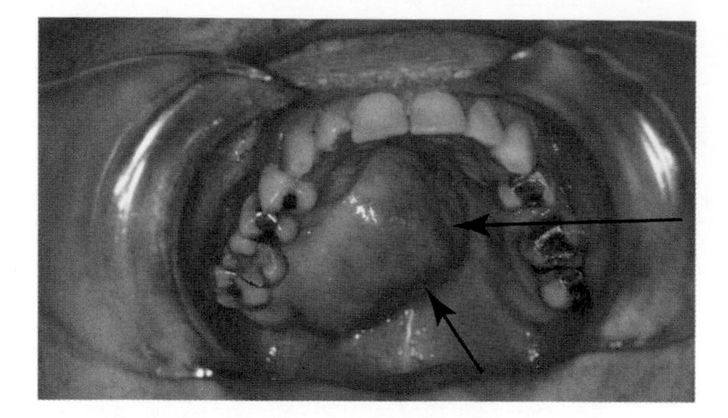

Figure 11.37 A pleomorphic adenoma of a minor salivary gland on the palate.

carcinoma, adenocystic carcinoma), and the risk increases from the soft palate down to the floor of the mouth. These lesions are best sampled by a peroral true-cut needle biopsy or a core of tissue taken from the centre of the lump so as not to violate the tumour margin.

Tumours can go unnoticed as they tend to be symptomless and only be picked up at a routine dental visit. If noticed, the patient's sole complaint is of a *slow-growing lump*. On examination, the lump feels smooth and hard. The overlying mucosa is not attached to it and, if small, the lump can be moved over the underlying palate. As it grows, it becomes less mobile and more difficult to distinguish from a tumour growing in or above the palate. Other rare tumours such as malignant melanoma can occur in the palate.

Conditions of the tonsils

TONSILLITIS

This is a very common condition that causes *a sore throat and pain on swallowing*. On examination, the tonsils are *red and enlarged*, and covered with pus. The pillars of the fauces, soft palate and oropharynx are *red and tender*, and may be covered with small yellow-based ulcers. The patient may have halitosis and be systemically unwell, with a fever and headache. Bilateral enlargement of the tonsils, together with the above signs, is diagnostic of tonsillitis.

A *tonsillar abscess* does not cause trismus, which helps to distinguish it from dental infections arising from the third molar region and which can present with similar features. Unilateral enlargement of a tonsil, even if it is red and tender, is not always caused by infection and *may be a tonsillar cancer or lymphoma*. Some of the other causes are described below.

CARCINOMA OF THE TONSIL

The tonsil is the commonest site of carcinoma in the oropharynx. Patients may complain of *difficulty with swallowing, a sore throat and then severe pain in the throat*, which is referred to the ear (otalgia). It can remain symptomless until it has spread into local structures and to the nodes of the neck.

The surface of the growth eventually ulcerates to form a *deep indolent ulcer* (Figure 11.38) that bleeds and causes *severe dysphagia*.

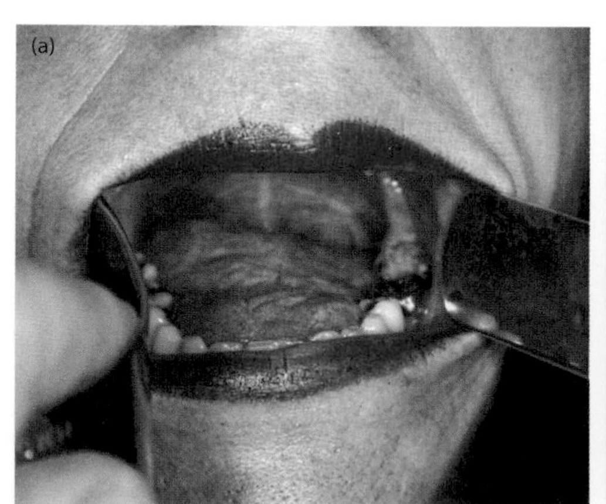

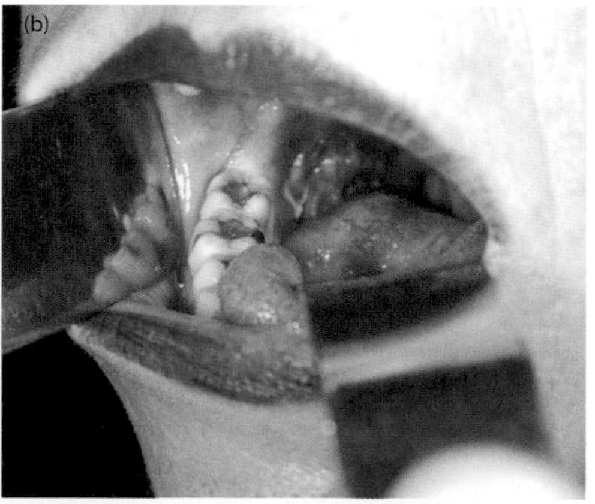

Figure 11.38 CARCINOMA OF THE RIGHT TONSIL. (a) On initial inspection, it may be difficult to see the carcinoma because of reflex retraction of the tongue. (b) The tonsillar carcinoma is evident with proper retraction of the tongue.

Tonsillar tumours are frequently contiguous with the tongue base and vice versa. They are difficult to diagnose visually and, if suspected, palpation is essential. *Cervical lymph nodes become involved* early in the disease process, and there may be palpable nodes at the time of first examination or before the primary is noticed. The clinical picture of HPV-associated oropharyngeal cancer is slightly different. These tumours tend not to ulcerate through the epithelium but burrow through the lymphoid tissues forming Waldeyer's ring.

LYMPHOMA OF THE TONSIL

This occurs in late-middle and old age. In contrast to carcinoma, it causes a painless swelling. The patient may describe a lump in the back of the mouth or throat and sometimes mild dysphagia. Gross swelling may interfere with speech. *Bilateral enlargement of the cervical lymph glands is a common feature as this is a systemic disease.* Both carcinomatous and lymphomatous tonsils can look infected, but acute tonsillitis in the elderly is not common.

PERITONSILLAR ABSCESS (QUINSY)

This is very painful and relatively common. Pus in the space around the tonsil pushes it towards the midline making the tonsil look enlarged. Over half of patients have a preceding history of tonsillitis. The diagnosis rests on observing a unilateral red bulge in the soft palate superior to the tonsil with *deviation of the uvula*, tender cervical lymph glands, fever and tachycardia. Patients describe *difficulty in swallowing and opening their mouths*, and talk with a 'hot-potato voice'.

It may be difficult to distinguish from a submasseteric abscess arising from a wisdom tooth except that the submasseteric abscess causes profound trismus.

Conditions of the floor of the mouth

MANDIBULAR EXOSTOSIS (LINGUAL OR MANDIBULAR TORUS)

As with the palatal torus, the mandibular is a benign bony lump in lingual aspect of the mandible, usually in the premolar region. Tori are typically symmetrical and grow slowly. They are spherical but may be multilobulated, with the overlying mucosa normal. They may interfere with the fitting of a denture.

RANULA

A ranula (Latin for a small frog) is a *mucus extravasation cyst* that arises from the sublingual gland. The sublingual gland has a head that is fixed to the floor of mouth by the duct of Ranvier and a tail that lies beneath the mucosa and is drained by a single duct. The head is formed by a concrescence of independent minor salivary gland units. If the duct leading from one of these units tears, saliva pours out of it into the loose spaces below the mucosa. The free saliva is an irritant and stimulates a fibrous reaction that forms a lining, which defines the ranula. This swelling can bulge up into the mouth like the pouch of a frog (Figure 11.39). An aspirate will demonstrate the presence of thick, treacly straw coloured fluid, pathognomonic of the condition.

History

Age Appear most often in children and young adults.

Sex Both sexes are equally affected.

Symptoms *A painless swelling in the floor of the mouth* that has grown gradually over a few weeks. Some ranulas can burst and discharge saliva into the mouth. Once healed they refill. Large ranulae can interfere with eating or speech.

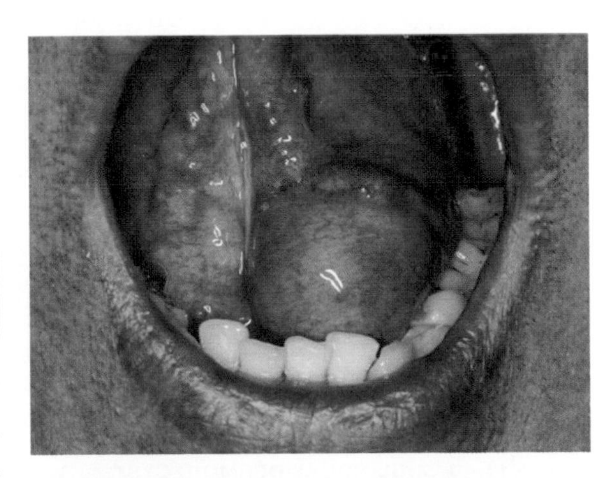

Figure 11.39 A ranula in the left floor of the mouth.

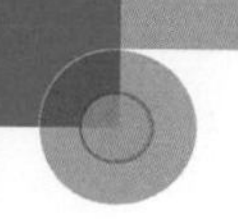

Examination

Position The swelling is often unilateral and lies in the floor of the mouth, just to one side of the midline.

Colour The lump has a characteristic *semi-transparent blue appearance*. The colour and the site are the diagnostic features.

Shape Ranulae form spherical cysts that can be larger than they first appear as they run along the floor of mouth.

Size Usually no more than 2–3 cm.

Surface Smooth, but their edge is difficult to feel because they lie deep within the arch of the mandible.

Composition *Soft, usually fluctuant* and *transilluminates*, but cannot be compressed or reduced. Saliva has bacteriocidal properties, and these cysts do not get infected.

Relations The overlying mucosa is not fixed to the wall of the cyst, and the cyst is not fixed to the tongue or the jaw. The swelling is usually closely related to the duct of the submandibular salivary gland and the lingual nerve. Ranulas can extend through the mylohyoid muscle into the neck, the *plunging ranula.*

Local tissues These should all be normal.

Lymph glands Cervical lymph glands should not be enlarged.

SUBLINGUAL DERMOID CYST

When the face and neck are formed by fusion of the facial processes, a piece of epidermis may get trapped deep in the midline just behind the jaw and later form a sublingual dermoid cyst. They may develop above or below the mylohyoid muscle (see Chapter 12). Their symptoms vary according to where they sit in relation to this muscle.

History

Age Most swellings are noticed during the second and third decades of life, with a smaller number picked up within the first year of life.

Sex Both sexes are equally affected.

Symptoms Supramylohyoid cysts can grow to quite a large size before being recognized by the patient. The patient adapts to the evolving mass and may develop slightly altered speech. Eventually, the tongue becomes elevated, which limits function. Submylohyoid cysts appear as a submental swellings just below the chin. These are generally symptomless but large ones can produce difficulty in swallowing and speech.

Examination

Position The lump is easily visible, either in the centre of the floor of the mouth between the tongue and the point of the jaw, or bulging down below the chin, looking like a double chin (Figure 11.40). They can be differentiated from other lesions by needle aspiration.

Colour Oral mucosa and skin beneath the chin overlying the lump are normal.

Tenderness Sublingual dermoid cysts are not tender.

Shape The cyst is clearly *spherical*, even although its whole surface cannot be felt.

Size By the time these cysts are noticed, they are 2–5 cm across.

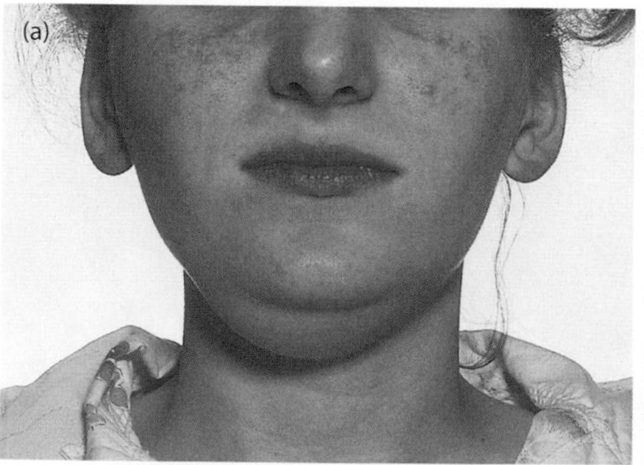

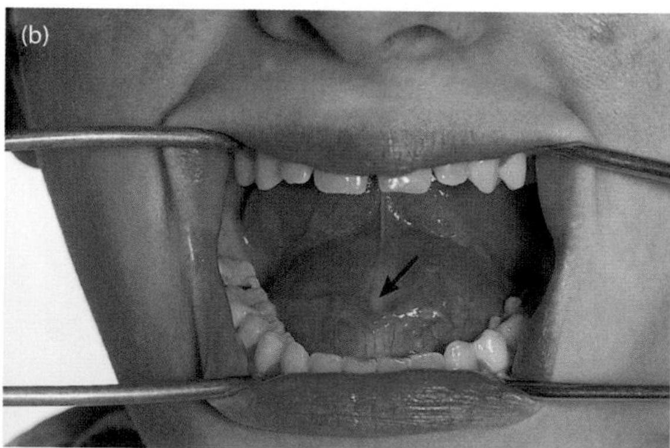

Figure 11.40 SUBLINGUAL DERMOID CYST. (a) Sublingual dermoid cyst giving the impression of a 'double chin'. (b) Bulging of the anterior floor of the mouth and displacement of the tongue posteriorly.

Surface The surface is smooth.

Edge The edge is clearly defined.

Composition The lump can feel soft and compressible, or firm. *Bimanual palpation reveals that it fluctuates.* Some describe it as 'doughy'. These cysts do not usually transilluminate as their contents are often opaque. They cannot be compressed or reduced.

Relations can be felt bimanually, with one finger in the mouth and one beneath the chin. When the tongue is lifted up, the supramylohyoid variety bulges into the mouth. The submylohyoid variety bulges out below the chin if the tongue is pushed against the roof of the mouth with the teeth clenched.

Local tissues Nearby tissues should all be normal.

Lymph glands Local lymph glands should not be enlarged.

STONE IN THE SUBMANDIBULAR DUCT

Stones (calculi, sialoliths) in the submandibular gland and duct are common (see Chapter 12). A stone may migrate to the punctum, where it becomes visible and palpable. If the stone lies in the mid-portion of the duct, it sits under the sublingual gland and may be obscured from view or palpation. *The submandibular gland is usually swollen and tender* (Figure 11.41).

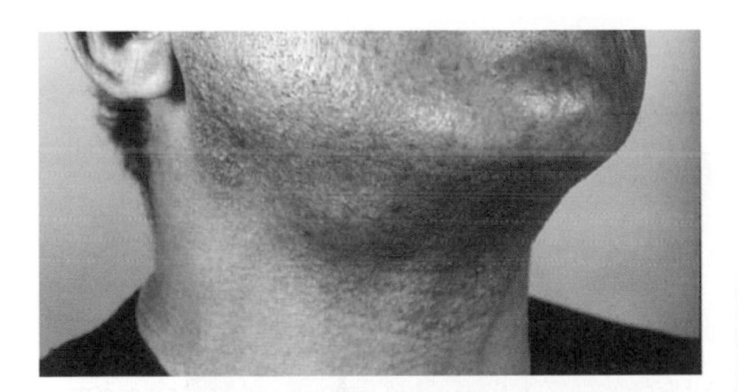

Figure 11.41 A swollen (obstructed) submandibular gland as a result of a calculus.

Conditions of the gums (gingivae)

FIBROMA (FIBROUS EPULIS)

An epulis is a benign swelling that arises from the gums. The most common variety is the fibrous epulis, which forms a firm nodule at the junction of the gum and tooth. It may be polypoid in shape (Figure 11.42).

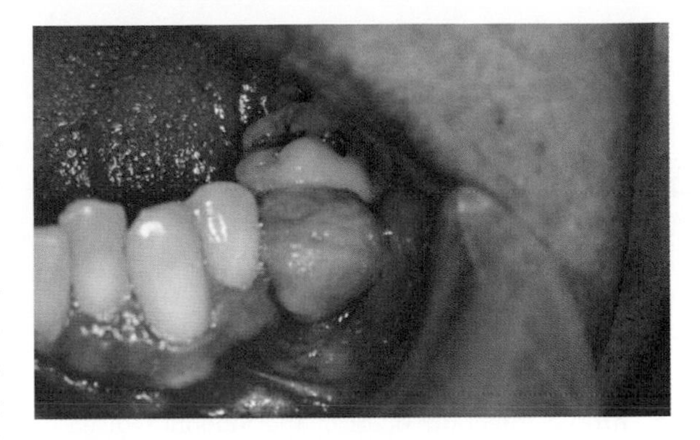

Figure 11.42 A fibrous epulis.

GRANULOMA (GRANULOMATOUS EPULIS)

This is a pyogenic granuloma arising from the mucosa of the gum (Figure 11.43). It is usually a painless and pedunculated lesion, soft and red, associated with gingivitis or local infection. It is formed of hyperplastic granulation tissue. When seen during pregnancy, it is a pregnancy epulis.

DENTAL CYST

A developmental (odontogenic) or inflammatory (radicular) cyst may cause alveolar bone and overlying gum expansion. Initially, there are few or no signs of cystic swelling on the gums and they may only identified after incidental imaging.

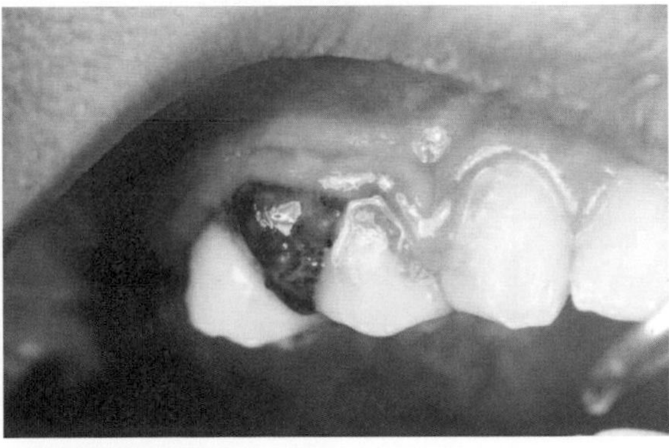

Figure 11.43 A pyogenic granuloma.

BONE TUMOUR

A variety of giant cell 'tumours' (peripheral giant cell) can extend out of the bone and have an appearance similar to that of a pyogenic granuloma (a friable gingival lump). They are distinguished by biopsy.

CARCINOMA

Carcinoma of the gum presents as a swelling that develops a *rolled edge*. In its early stages, it can mimic a chronic infection of gum (periodontal) disease. Gum disease is normally a whole mouth disorder, which can help distinguish it from a tumour. The lesion becomes painful and progresses inexorably over time (Figure 11.44). Dental extractions may be performed on suspicion of gum disease or infection, so the clinician must be alert to the 'non-healing' post-extraction socket.

Conditions of the jaw

SWELLINGS OF THE JAW

Swelling of the whole jaw may be caused by infection, a cyst or a tumour. These are classified in Revision panel 11.5.

Revision panel 11.5

CAUSES OF SWELLING OF THE JAW

Infections

- Dental (alveolar) abscess
- Acute osteomyelitis

Cysts

- Inflammatory odontogenic cysts
- Developmental odontogenic cysts
- Other non-odontogenic cysts and cystic tumours

Neoplasms:

Benign

- Ameloblastoma
- Fibro-osseous lesions
- Giant-cell lesions
- Odontogenic tumours

Malignant

- Osteosarcoma
- Secondary tumours (by direct invasion or bloodstream spread)

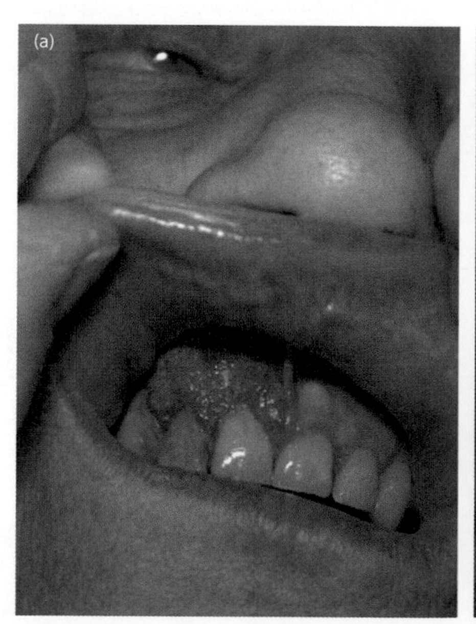

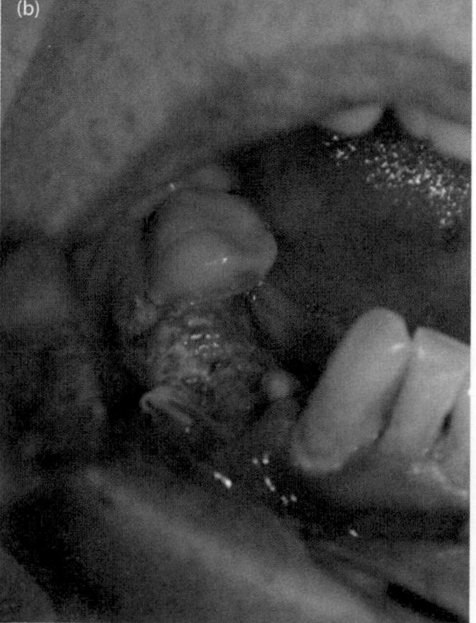

Figure 11.44 (a) Alveolar carcinoma of the anterior maxilla. (b) Alveolar carcinoma of the posterior mandible.

Alveolar (dental) abscess

The most common cause of jaw swelling is dental infection, which causes an *alveolar or gum abscess.* The abscess forms at the root base of a decaying tooth and tracks outwards, through the external surface of the mandible or maxilla. It can cause a swelling in the mouth alone or, with a spreading infection, involve the neck and/or cheek.

History

Age Can develop at any age.

Symptoms *Constant dull jaw ache,* which worsens and becomes throbbing in nature. May be associated *fever, malaise and difficulty swallowing. Toothache often precedes the abscess.* There may be a history of poor dental attendance.

Examination

Position Most alveolar abscesses point to the buccal (outer) side of the jaw. Those in the lower jaw also point downwards to the inferior margin of the mandible.

Colour Overlying skin or mucosa is reddened.

Shape Usually a flattened hemisphere, but its edges merge into the surrounding tissues, so no clear-cut shape or edge.

Surface Indistinct. The swelling is *hot and acutely tender* (Figure 11.45).

Composition Can be difficult to assess due to tenderness. Deeper aspects feel firm, but overlying tissues may be soft and boggy with oedema and pus. Large abscesses maybe fluctuant.

Relations The mass is clearly fixed to, and feels as it it is part of, underlying bone.

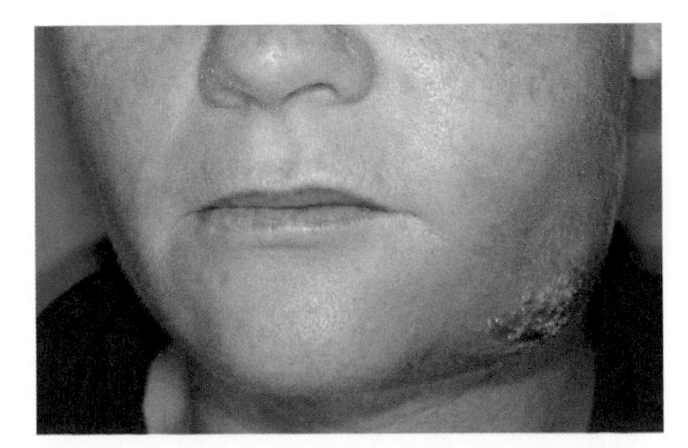

Figure 11.45 An abscess arising from a decayed lower tooth spreading to the buccal and submandibular regions.

Lymph glands Upper cervical lymph glands are usually enlarged and tender.

Local tissues Decayed teeth or roots are often seen, or there may be inflammation of gums around wisdom teeth. If the abscess is allowed to point and discharge, it may become a chronic discharging sinus.

Odontogenic cysts

These cysts arise from odontogenic epithelium left behind in the mandible as teeth develop and erupt into the mouth. These remnants can be stimulated to form a cyst (inflammatory or developmental).

An *inflammatory radicular cyst* is attached to the root of an erupted but decayed and non-vital tooth (Figure 11.46). These cysts are common and can become large. There may or may not be any swelling visible on examination. Where swelling is present, the bone may be so thin that it 'crackles' when touched, like a broken eggshell (Figure 11.47a, b).

Developmental cysts (Figure 11.48) can arise in relation to the crown of an unerupted tooth (most being third molar or canine). These are dentigerous cysts. Others include odontogenic keratocysts (Figure 11.49) which are more aggressive, tend to be larger and do not normally reside around the crown of the tooth. The distinction is made by biopsy. These cysts can enlarge, cause swelling of the jaw and produce tooth mobility.

Resorption of a root is normally associated with keratocysts, dentigerous cysts or ameloblastomas.

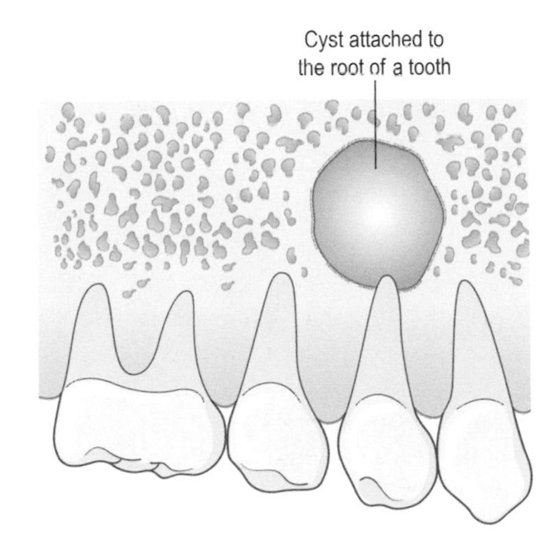

Figure 11.46 The site of origin of a dental radicular cyst (inflammatory).

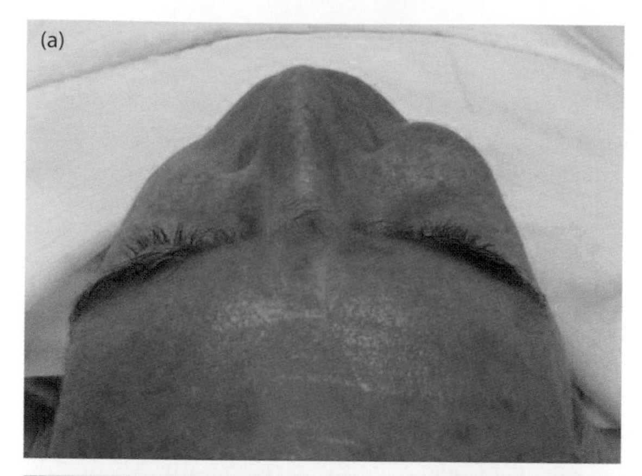

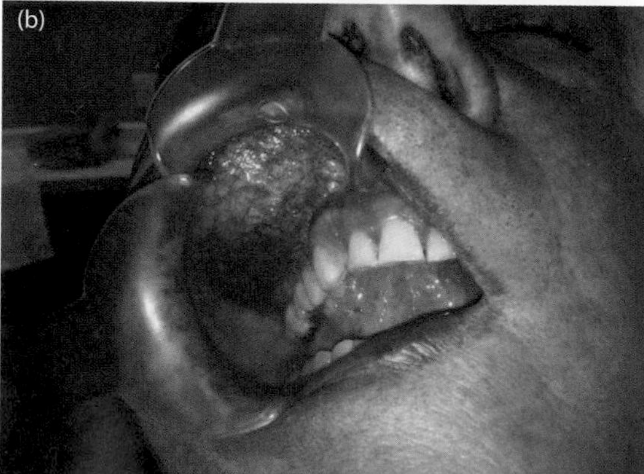

Figure 11.47 Dental radicular cyst. (a) A large radicular cyst expands the maxilla producing obvious facial asymmetry. (b) The bone thins as it grows and 'crackles' when palpated.

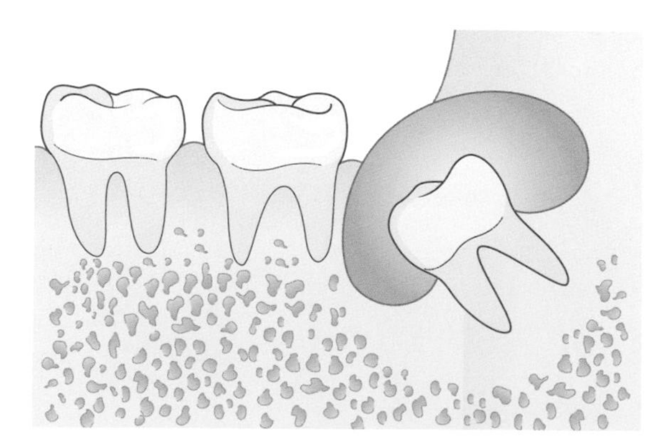

Figure 11.48 A dentigerous cyst develops around the crown of a tooth.

Biopsy will guide the treatment plan. These cysts become smaller if decompressed at the time of biopsy, by placement of a drainage tube. This encourages bone infill, covering roots and the inferior alveolar nerve which reduces chances of damage upon cyst enucleation.

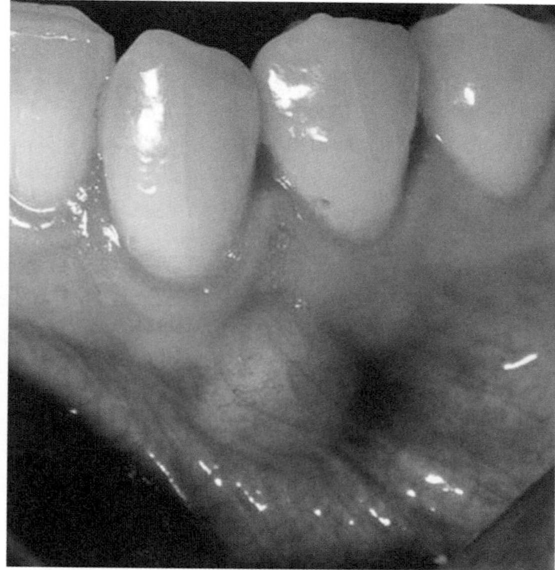

Figure 11.49 An odontogenic keratocyst (developmental) may present with a small jaw swelling.

Tumours of the jaw

Tumours of the jaw can be benign or malignant, of odontogenic origin or otherwise. Less commonly, the jaw can be the site of metastases usually from the lung, breast and kidney. Many types of benign and malignant tumours of the jaw are listed in Revision panel 11.3. Most present as a bony swelling that grows steadily, usually painlessly. Four neoplastic causes of swelling of the jaw deserve special mention.

Carcinoma of the maxillary antrum (sinus)

These are much more common than primary bone tumours. Downward invasion leads to swelling of the maxilla and palate. They are silent tumours and normally present at a late stage of development.

Ameloblastoma

This tumour arises from the epithelium associated with tooth formation and is one of the most common odontogenic tumours. Characteristically, it is a *slow-growing, painless tumour that causes progressive swelling of the jaw* (Figure 11.50). Although benign, they are locally invasive. If found to have invaded into soft tissue, there is suspicion of malignant change. The lesion requires a biopsy for definitive diagnosis.

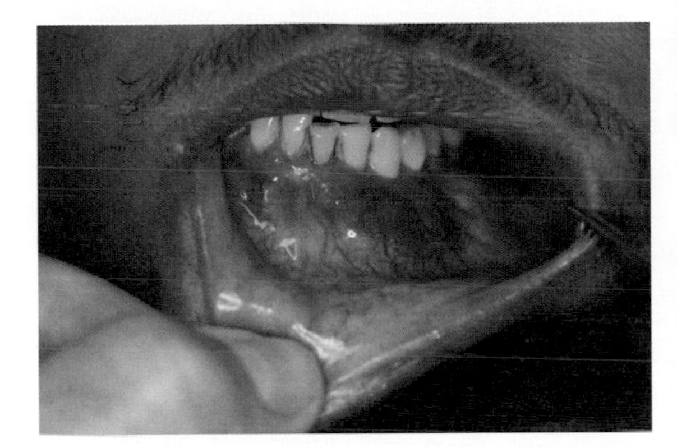

Figure 11.50 A mandibular ameloblastoma causing buccal and lingual expansion.

Osteosarcoma

These tumours can occur in both the upper and the lower jaw. Although rare, they are aggressive and seen in younger patients. Patients might complain of a dull ache, swelling, with mobile teeth and see their dentist. Osteosarcoma is diagnosed by biopsy (Figure 11.51).

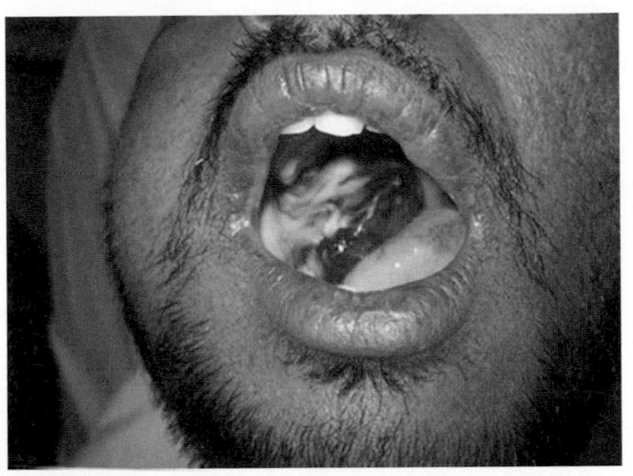

Figure 11.51 A large sarcoma of the maxilla.

Malignant Lymphoma

Burkitt's lymphoma is a *high-grade, non-Hodgkin lymphoma associated with prior Epstein–Barr virus* infection. In its endemic form, it affects children aged between 3 and 8 years of age and commonly occurs in parts of sub-Saharan Africa. Lymphoma presents with *progressive, swelling of the jaw*. It is usually painless at the outset, but pain and numbness can develop. It can distort the face, may displace the eye and partially occlude the mouth (Figure 11.52).

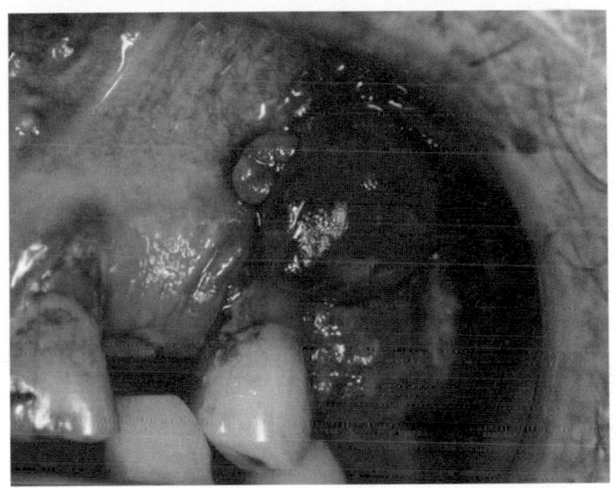

Figure 11.52 A lymphoma arising from the maxilla.

Acknowledgements

The contribution of Leandros Vassiliou to this chapter in the 5th edition is gratefully acknowledged.

The neck

JOHNATHAN G HUBBARD

History and examination of swellings in the neck

The majority of surgical conditions that arise in the neck present as a swelling. Taking the history and performing the physical examination should follow the standard pattern, but there are some important features that deserve special attention.

HISTORY OF SWELLINGS IN THE NECK

The most common cause of a swelling in the neck is an *enlarged lymph node or lymph nodes*.

Systemic illness

Symptoms such as *general malaise, fever* and *rigors* and contact with people with infectious diseases may indicate an infective cause of the swelling.

Loss of appetite, loss of weight and pulmonary, alimentary or skeletal symptoms may suggest a malignant cause.

Irritation of the skin associated with enlarged cervical lymph nodes is often seen with lymphoma.

Head and neck symptoms

The patient should be asked about pain in the mouth, discomfort on eating, sore throats or mouth ulceration, nasal discharge, blockage of the airway, pain in the throat or neck, dysphagia, odynophagia, changes in voice and difficulty with breathing.

Enquiries should be made for any lumps or ulcers on the skin of the head and face, and whether they have changed in size, shape or consistency, or have begun to bleed.

The skin, mouth, nose, larynx and pharynx are common sites for neoplasms, and although head and neck cancers commonly present with metastases in the lymph nodes, they are not usually associated with symptoms of distant metastases such as general malaise and loss of weight (see Chapter 11).

EXAMINATION OF SWELLINGS IN THE NECK

Site

It is essential to define the site of a lump in the neck.

The neck is divided into two triangles (Figure 12.1). The *anterior triangle* is bounded by the anterior border of the sternomastoid muscle, the lower edge

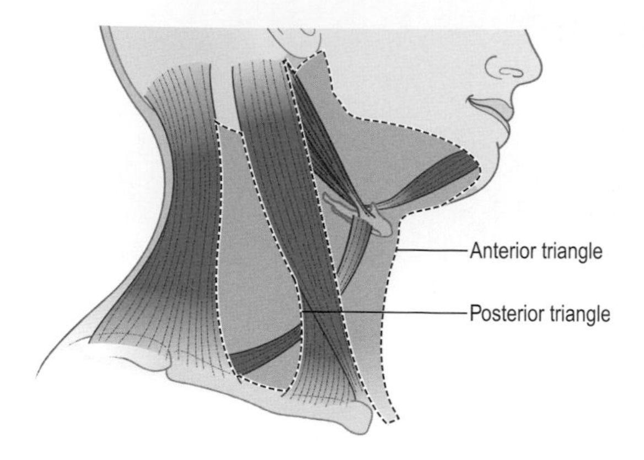

Figure 12.1 The anatomical triangles of the neck.

of the jaw and the midline. In clinical practice, the structures deep to the sternomastoid muscle are considered to be inside the anterior triangle.

The upper part of the anterior triangle, below the jaw and above the digastric muscle, is sometimes called the *digastric or submandibular triangle*.

The *posterior triangle* is bounded by the posterior border of the sternomastoid muscle, the anterior edge of the trapezius muscle and the clavicle.

The triangles are defined by getting the patient to tense their neck muscles:

- Both sternomastoid muscles are made to contract by putting your hand under the patient's chin and asking them to push their head down against the resistance of your hand.
- The trapezius muscles are made to contract by asking the patient to shrug (elevate) their shoulders against resistance.

Relation to muscles

Lumps in the neck should always be palpated with the muscles relaxed and then contracted. Lumps deep to muscle become less obvious or impalpable when the muscle contracts.

Relation to the trachea

Swellings that are attached to the trachea move when the trachea moves. The trachea is pulled upwards during *swallowing*. Assess the relationship to the trachea of every lump in the neck by observing if it moves during swallowing.

Relation to the hyoid bone

The hyoid bone moves slightly during swallowing, but ascends when the *tongue is protruded*. Ask the patient to open their mouth. Hold the jaw still and ask them to protrude their tongue. The swelling must be fixed to the hyoid bone if it moves as the tongue protrudes.

CERVICAL LYMPHADENOPATHY

Other neck swellings

The most common cause of a swelling in the neck is enlargement of the lymph nodes, as stated above (Revision panel 12.1). Even when only one lymph node is palpable, the adjacent nodes are invariably diseased.

The four main causes of cervical lymph node enlargement are:

- Infection – tonsillitis, glandular fever, toxoplasmosis, tuberculosis and cat-scratch fever.
- Metastatic tumour from a primary neoplasm in the head, neck, chest or abdomen.
- Lymphoma.
- Sarcoidosis.

Revision panel 12.1

CAUSES OF CERVICAL LYMPHADENOPATHY

Infection

Non-specific
Glandular fever
Tuberculosis
Syphilis
Toxoplasmosis
Cat-scratch fever (*Rochalimaea henselae*)

Metastatic tumour

From the head, neck, chest and abdomen

Lymphoma

Sarcoidosis

NOTE: Lymphadenopathy caused by systemic illnesses such as glandular fever, toxoplasmosis and sarcoidosis is usually associated with lymphadenopathy elsewhere.

There may be evidence of the underlying disease and special blood tests may confirm the diagnosis.

NON-SPECIFIC CERVICAL INFLAMMATORY LYMPHADENOPATHY

This can follow any inflammatory process or be associated with skin conditions, particularly of the scalp, when it is termed dermatopathic lymphadenopathy. It commonly follows recurrent bouts of tonsillitis, especially if the attacks have been treated inadequately. The upper deep cervical nodes are most often affected (Figure 12.2).

In a slim, healthy child, small normal lymph nodes are often palpable, especially in the posterior triangle.

History

Age Lymphadenopathy associated with tonsillitis, is usually found in patients younger than 10 years. Other reactive conditions can occur at any age.

Symptoms Patients, or their parents, usually discover a *painful lump just below the angle of the jaw,* often during neck washing. The pain is usually more a discomfort, which can become acute when the patient has a sore throat.

The child may snore at night or have difficulty in breathing. They often have nasal speech because of tonsillar and adenoid hyperplasia and may suffer from recurrent chest infections.

Cause The child or parents may recognize the relationship between the appearance of the lump and episodes of sore throat/tonsillitis.

Systemic effects The patient often feels ill, with a sore throat and pyrexia, and does not want to eat. Recurrent severe episodes can lead to weight loss.

Social history Recurrent sore throats and upper respiratory tract infections (URTIs) are more common in children living in poverty and poor-quality social housing.

Examination

Position Lymph from the tonsils drains to the upper deep cervical lymph nodes. The node just below and deep to the angle of the mandible is often called *the 'tonsillar' node* (Figure 12.3).

Tenderness The enlarged lymph nodes are usually tender during active infection.

Shape and size The tonsillar node is usually spherical and approximately 1–2 cm in diameter. The lymph nodes below are usually smaller.

Composition and relations Each node is rubbery in consistency and, when multiple, extend along the sternomastoid. The lymph nodes on the other side of the neck may also be enlarged and palpable.

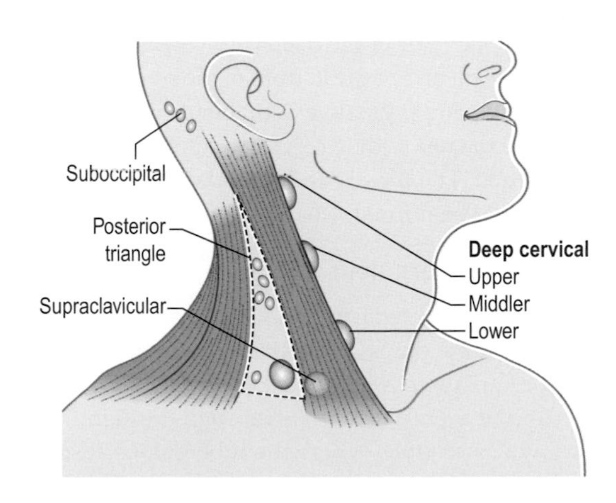

Figure 12.2 The anatomy of the cervical lymph nodes.

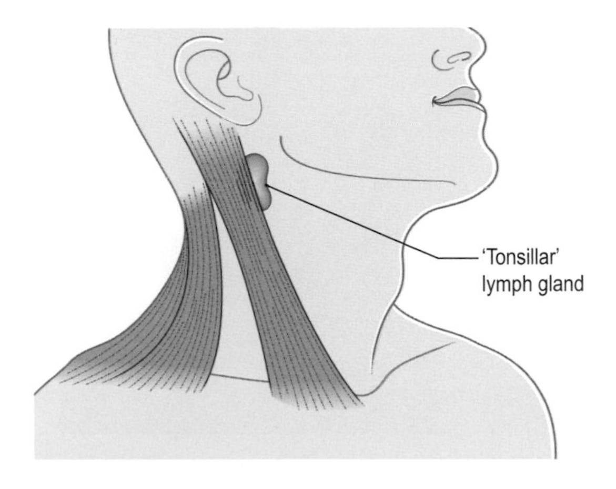

Figure 12.3 The site of the 'tonsillar' node.

Local tissues The tonsils are likely to be enlarged and hyperaemic. Pus may be seen exuding from the surface crypts.

General examination It is important to look for the presence of enlarged lymph nodes elsewhere.

Patients should be assessed for evidence of lobar collapse, bronchiectasis and lung abscess (see Chapter 2).

TUBERCULOUS CERVICAL LYMPHADENITIS AND ABSCESS

The human tubercle bacillus can enter the body via the tonsils and, from there, move to the cervical lymph nodes. The upper deep cervical nodes are frequently affected. There is no generalized infection, so there is little systemic disturbance of health. The majority of cases originated in people born outside the UK.

History

Age and ethnic groups Tuberculous lymphadenitis tends to occur in children, young adults and the elderly. In the UK, the incidence in the young diminished with the introduction of *Bacille Calmette–Guérin (BCG)* vaccination in schools, but the prevalence of cervical lymph node enlargement caused by anonymous mycobacteria is increasing. It is most commonly found in young immigrant adults (Figure 12.4).

Symptoms The patient complains of a lump in the neck. This appears gradually and is usually painless. Pain may be present if the nodes grow rapidly and necrose.

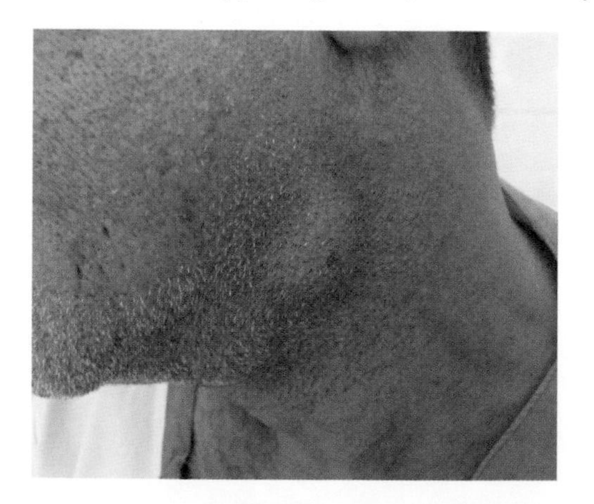

Figure 12.4 A tuberculous cervical lymph node in a young immigrant adult.

Systemic symptoms are unusual in the young, but the elderly sometimes have *anorexia and weight loss.*

The swelling increases in size if lymph nodes break down into an abscess. The patient may notice discolouration of the overlying skin, and neck movements and swallowing may be uncomfortable.

Previous history Elderly patients may have a history of swollen neck nodes when young.

Immunization Enquire for vaccination with BCG.

Family history Check for a family history of tuberculosis.

Social history The majority of UK cases currently occur in immigrant families who are often poor and socially underprivileged.

Examination

Signs of a tuberculous lymphadenitis

Position The upper and middle deep cervical nodes are frequently involved (Figure 12.5).

Temperature The mass of nodes *does not feel hot.*

Tenderness The nodes may be slightly tender, but this is not a prominent feature.

Colour The overlying skin looks normal unless an abscess has developed.

Shape, size and consistency In the early stages, the lymph nodes are firm, discrete and between 1 and 2 cm in diameter.

As caseation increases, the lymph nodes necrose, the infection spreads beyond the capsule and the nodes *enlarge and coalesce.*

An indistinct, firm mass of matted nodes that occupies the upper half of the deep cervical lymph chain, partly beneath and partly in front of the sternomastoid muscle, is highly suggestive of tuberculosis infection.

Local tissues Other cervical lymph nodes may be enlarged. The tonsils and the other tissues in the neck should be normal.

Signs of a tuberculous abscess

When an infected lymph node caseates and turns into pus, it becomes an abscess. The natural tendency of an abscess is to weaken the overlying tissues until it eventually bursts through the skin. This is known as *pointing.* Where the tuberculous abscess has burst through the deep cervical fascia into the subcutaneous tissues, it has two compartments,

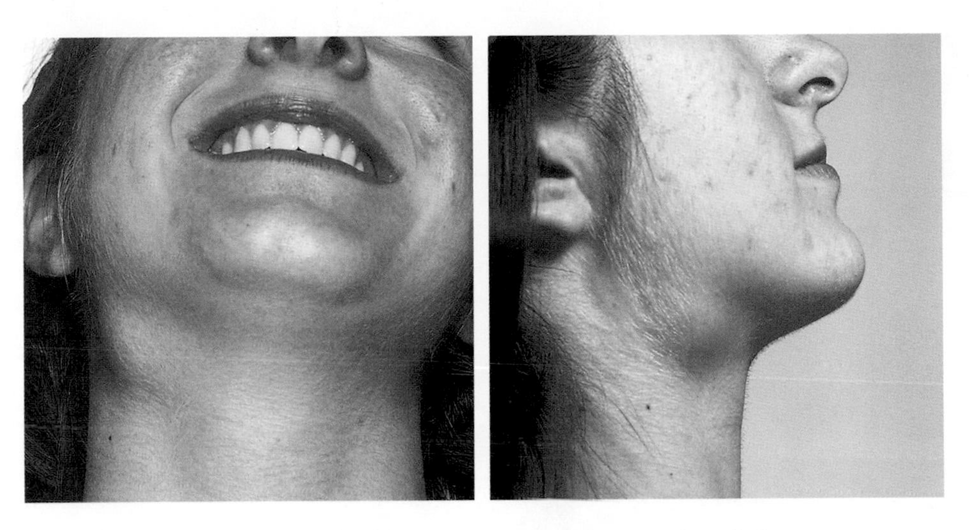

Figure 12.5 Enlargement of the upper deep cervical lymph nodes caused by tuberculosis.

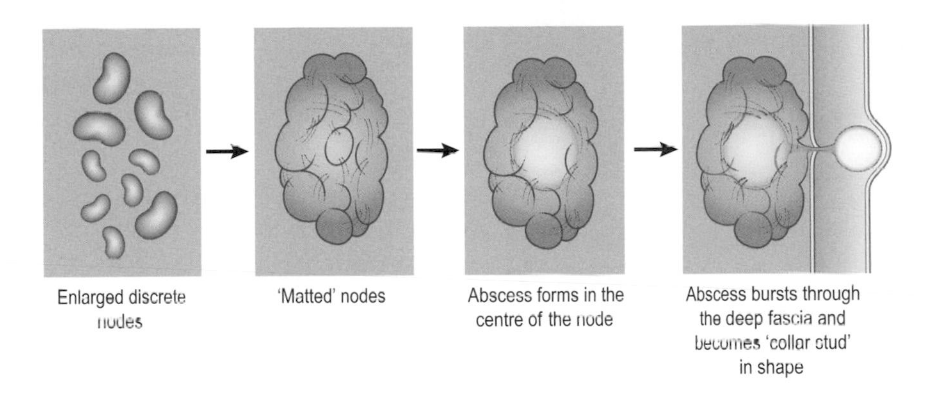

Figure 12.6 The development of a tuberculous 'collar-stud' abscess.

one on either side of the deep fascia, connected by a small central track. This is called a *'collar-stud' abscess* (Figure 12.6).

Position A tuberculous abscess is most often found in the upper half of the neck (Figure 12.7).

Colour When the pus reaches the subcutaneous tissues, the *overlying skin turns reddish–purple.*

Temperature The skin temperature is normal because the process of caseation and pus formation is slow and does not stimulate excessive hyperaemia – hence the name 'cold abscess'.

Tenderness The mass is often tender, particularly if the abscess is tense.

Shape The deep part of the abscess tends to be sausage shaped, with its long axis parallel to the front edge of the sternomastoid muscle. The superficial pocket of the abscess is usually lower than the deep part.

Size Most tuberculous abscesses are 3–5 cm across but can be larger.

Surface The surface is irregular and indistinct.

Edge The edges are often well defined unless the pocket of pus is lax.

Composition The abscess feels firm or rubbery, and *it will fluctuate if sufficient necrosis is present.* Fluctuation cannot be elicited if the abscess is small and lies deep to the sternomastoid muscle.

The subcutaneous part of a 'collar-stud' abscess is often fluctuant, but it is not usually possible to reduce the superficial pocket of pus into the deep pocket.

Relations The original abscess is deep to the deep fascia, partly under the sternomastoid muscle,

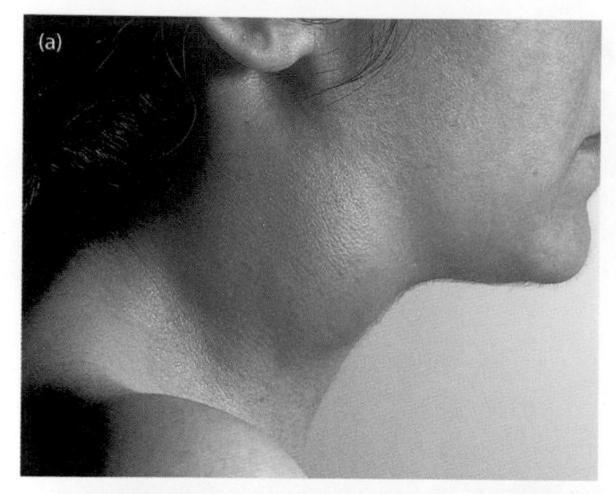

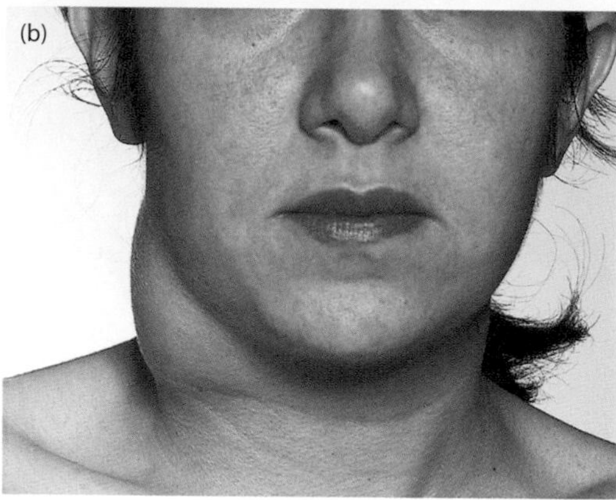

Figure 12.7 (a, b) A large tuberculous 'collar-stud' abscess.

and fixed to surrounding structures. The superficial part of a collar-stud abscess is immediately below the skin and becomes more prominent when the sterno-mastoid muscle is contracted. A chronic sinus may form if spontaneous discharge occurs. Tuberculous sinuses are painless and characterized by minimal erythema, unless secondarily infected (Figure 12.8).

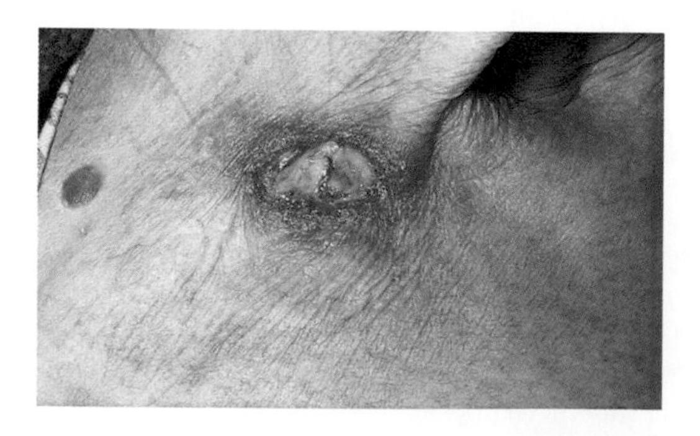

Figure 12.8 A chronic tuberculous sinus that has become secondarily infected.

The lymph nodes in the neck near the abscess may be enlarged.

General examination In tuberculous lymphadenitis, there are often no systemic abnormalities, but when a tuberculous abscess develops, there may be *tachycardia, pyrexia, anorexia and general malaise.*

NOTE: There may be signs of tuberculosis in the lungs, in other lymph nodes and in the urinary tract.

CARCINOMATOUS LYMPH NODES

Malignant metastatic deposits are the most common cause of cervical lymphadenopathy in adults.

The primary tumour is most often in the buccal cavity (tongue, lips and mucous membrane) and larynx, but every possible primary site must be examined including the skin (Figure 12.9).

History

Age Most head and neck cancers occur in patients over the age of 50 years. The exception is papillary carcinoma of the thyroid, which can occur in children and young adults.

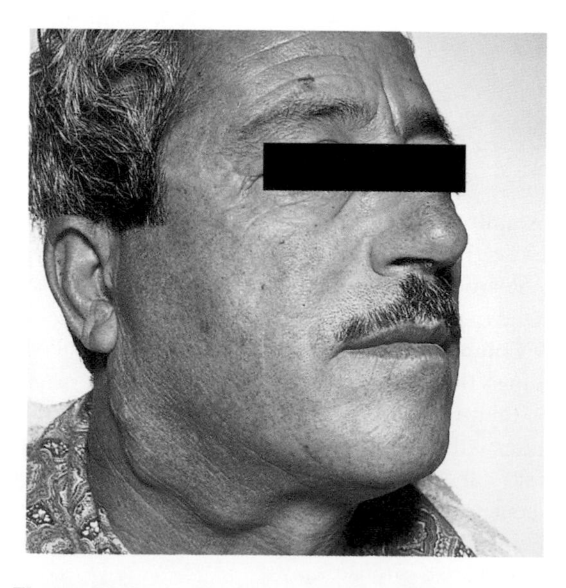

Figure 12.9 This patient presented with hard, enlarged lymph nodes in the neck. The primary lesion was the insignificant mole above his right eyebrow, a malignant melanoma.

Sex Most of the head and neck cancers, other than those of the thyroid, are more common in men.

Local symptoms The patient complains of a painless lump in the neck that tends to grow slowly. Further lumps may appear.

General symptoms The patient may have symptoms from the primary lesion in the head or neck, such as a *sore or ulcerated tongue, a hoarse voice or a separate lump in the neck such as in the thyroid or salivary glands*. They may have a cough or haemoptysis if the primary is in the chest; if it is in the abdomen, they may have dyspepsia or abdominal pain.

Head and neck cancers do not often cause anorexia and weight loss, whereas cancers in the lungs and intra-abdominal organs do.

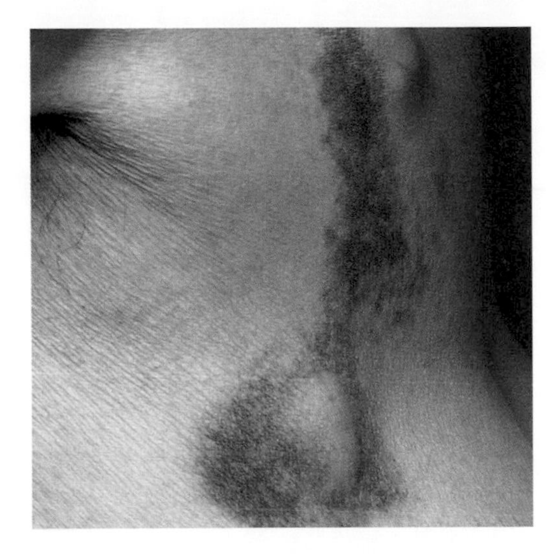

Figure 12.10 Secondary malignant deposits in the skin of the neck.

Examination

Site The site of the affected lymph nodes gives an approximate indication of the site of the primary cancer.

Lesions above the hyoid bone drain to the upper deep cervical nodes.

The larynx and thyroid drain to the middle and lower deep cervical nodes.

An enlarged supraclavicular lymph node commonly indicates intra-abdominal or thoracic disease. When enlarged by metastases, this gland is called *Virchow's node*; its presence is *Troisier's sign*.

Colour The overlying skin is a normal colour unless the mass is so large that it stretches or infiltrates the skin, which makes it pale or blotchy red (Figure 12.10).

Temperature The skin temperature is normal unless the tumour is very vascular.

Tenderness Lymph nodes containing secondary deposits are rarely tender.

Shape and size Lymph nodes containing metastases vary in size and shape depending upon the amount of tumour within them and its rate of growth. At first, the nodes are smooth, discrete and small. As they grow, they may coalesce into a large firm mass.

Composition *They are firm and may even become stony hard*. Rarely, a very vascular tumour deposit will be soft, pulsatile and compressible.

Relations Nodes can *usually be moved in a transverse direction but not vertically*. The nodes become tethered to their surrounding structures when extracapsular spread occurs. They then become fixed.

Metastatic spread is more common to the lymph nodes of the anterior triangle. These nodes lie deep to the anterior edge of the sternomastoid and may become tethered or fixed to the muscle.

Local tissues The overlying skin and muscle may be infiltrated with tumour, when it must be distinguished from secondary deposits in the skin.

Lymph nodes Other lymph nodes may be enlarged.

General examination Examine all the sites that might contain the primary lesion (Figure 12.11; Revision panel 12.2), in particular:

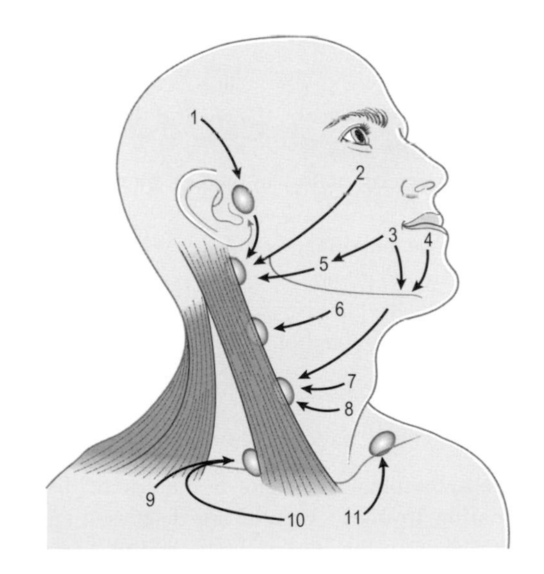

Figure 12.11 Sites of primary neoplasms that metastasize to the cervical lymph nodes.

Revision panel 12.2

SITES OF PRIMARY NEOPLASMS THAT METASTASIZE TO CERVICAL LYMPH NODES

1. Scalp:
   Parotid gland
   Upper face
   Ear
2. Maxillary antrum and other air sinuses:
   Nasal cavity and nasopharynx
3. Tongue:
   Buccal mucosa
   Floor of mouth
   Mandible
4. Lips
5. Tonsil:
   Base of tongue
   Oropharynx
6. Submandibular gland:
   Skin of neck
7. Larynx and laryngopharynx
8. Thyroid:
   Upper oesophagus
9. Upper limb and both sides of the chest wall
10. Breast
11. Lungs, stomach and all the viscera

- The skin of the scalp, the ear and the external auditory meatus.
- The lips, tongue, buccal mucous membrane and tonsils.
- The nose, maxillary antra and nasopharynx.
- The thyroid gland.
- The salivary glands.
- The skin of the upper limb.
- The breasts.
- The lungs.
- The stomach, pancreas, ovaries and testes.

The symptoms and signs of malignant disease originating in these organs are discussed in the appropriate chapters. Some aspects of this examination require special instruments, for example, a head or laryngeal mirror and light.

PRIMARY NEOPLASMS OF THE LYMPHATIC SYSTEM (LYMPHOMA)

The most common 'haematological' malignancy affecting the lymphatic system is lymphoma. It accounts for around 5% of all cancers and there are many histological subtypes. The two main categories are: *Hodgkin's* and *non-Hodgkin's lymphoma*. Subtypes of non-Hodgkin's lymphoma account for approximately 90% of cases.

History

Age Lymphoma can occur at any age but is the most common cancer in young adults (aged 15–24 years).

Sex Almost 60% of lymphomas affect males.

Symptoms Lymphoma often presents as a *painless lump in the neck*, which is noticed by chance and grows slowly.

Malaise and *weight loss* are common symptoms.

Itching of the skin (pruritus) is an unexplained but distinctive complaint.

There may be fever with rigors, occurring in a periodic fashion (*Pel–Ebstein fever*).

Lymphomatous infiltration of the skeleton may cause bone pain and some patients experience *abdominal pain after drinking alcohol*.

Superior vena cava occlusion, causing venous congestion in the neck and the development of collateral veins across the chest wall, can be the result of massive mediastinal lymph node enlargement (see Chapter 10).

Large nodal masses in the abdomen can obstruct the inferior vena cava and cause oedema of both legs.

Examination

Site *Any of the cervical lymph nodes can be enlarged* (Figure 12.12, Revision panel 12.3) even in the posterior triangle. *Other nodes in the axilla, groin and abdomen may also be enlarged.*

Tenderness The enlarged lymph nodes are not tender.

Shape, size and surface The enlarged lymph nodes in Hodgkin's disease are usually *ovoid, smooth* and *discrete* and remain separate, unlike tuberculosis where they are matted.

Consistency Lymph nodes infiltrated by lymphoma are typically *rubbery in consistency*.

Revision panel 12.3

PLAN OF EXAMINATION FOR SOURCE OF SECONDARY CERVICAL LYMPHADENOPATHY

(Start at the top and work downwards)
Examine the ***skin*** of the scalp, face, ears and neck
Look in the ***nose***
Look in the ***mouth*** at the tongue, gums, mucosa and tonsils
Palpate the parotid, submandibular and thyroid glands
Examine the arms and the chest wall – including the breast
Examine the abdomen and genitalia
Transilluminate the air sinuses
Examine the nasopharynx and larynx with mirrors

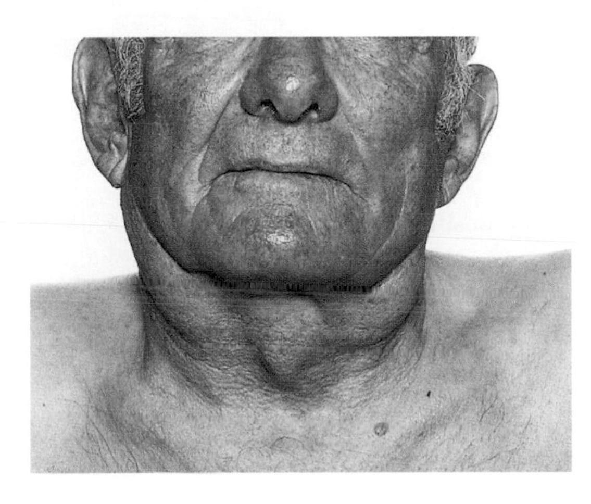

Figure 12.12 Bilateral cervical lymphadenopathy caused by Hodgkin's lymphoma.

Relations Although tethered to nearby structures, they can usually be moved from side to side and rarely become completely fixed.

Local tissues The surrounding tissues remain uninvolved.

General examination Other groups of lymph nodes may be enlarged. The *liver and spleen may be palpable*. The patient is often pale and can occasionally become jaundiced.

Spread to the skin produces elevated, reddened, scaly patches of skin known as mycosis fungoides (Figure 12.13).

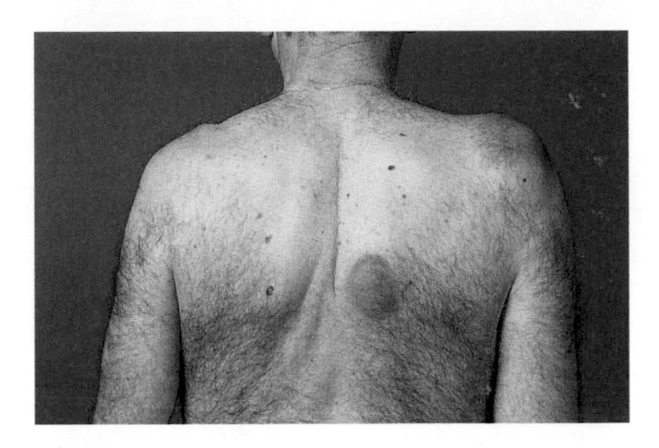

Figure 12.13 Cutaneous deposits of lymphoma.

Other causes of neck swelling

BRANCHIAL CYST

This is a *remnant of a branchial cleft* (classically the second cleft) and often appears from beneath the upper third of the sternomastoid muscle (Figure 12.14). It is lined with squamous epithelium, but there are often patches of lymphoid tissue in the wall that are connected with the other lymph tissue in the neck. It can become infected.

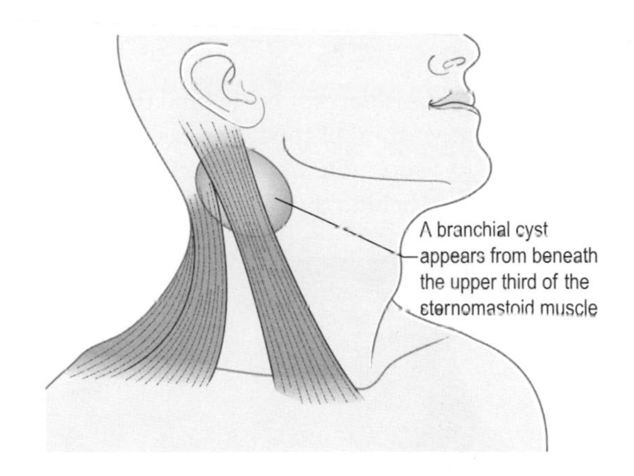

Figure 12.14 The site of a branchial cyst.

History

Age Although these cysts are present at birth, they usually do not distend and cause symptoms until adult life. The majority present between the ages of 15 and 25 years, but they can present in childhood (Figure 12.15), while a number can appear later when patients are in their 40s and 50s.

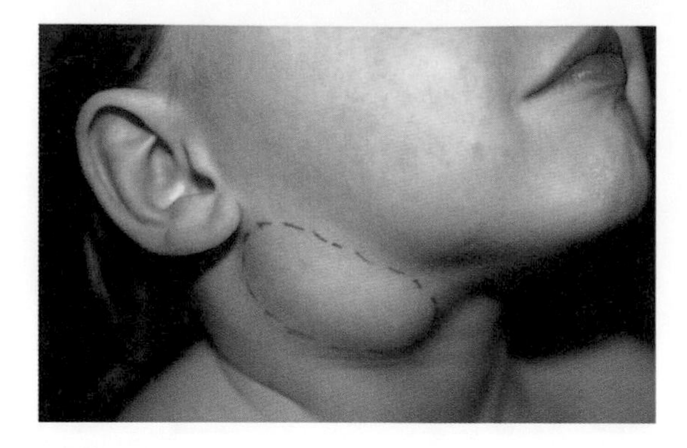

Figure 12.15 A branchial cyst presenting in childhood.

Sex Males and females are equally affected.

Symptoms Patients commonly present with a *painless swelling in the upper lateral part of the neck.*

The lump can be painful when it first appears, and later attacks of pain may be associated with an increase in size, usually caused by infection in the lymphoid tissue in the cyst wall (Figure 12.16). A severe throbbing pain, exacerbated by moving the neck and opening the mouth may then develop.

General effects These cysts have no systemic effects and are not associated with any other congenital abnormality.

Examination

Position A branchial cyst lies behind the anterior edge of the upper third of the sternomastoid muscle and bulges forwards (Figure 12.17). Rarely, it can bulge backwards behind the muscle.

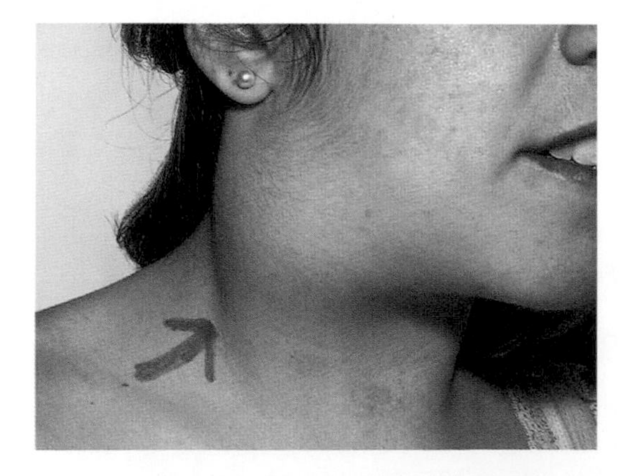

Figure 12.16 A large branchial cyst that had become painful. This commonly follows recurrent bouts of tonsillitis, especially if the infection has been inadequately treated.

Colour and tenderness The overlying skin may be reddened and the lump may be tender if the cyst is inflamed.

Shape The cyst is usually ovoid, with its long axis running forwards and downwards.

Size Most branchial cysts are between 5 and 10 cm long.

Surface Their surface is smooth and the edge distinct.

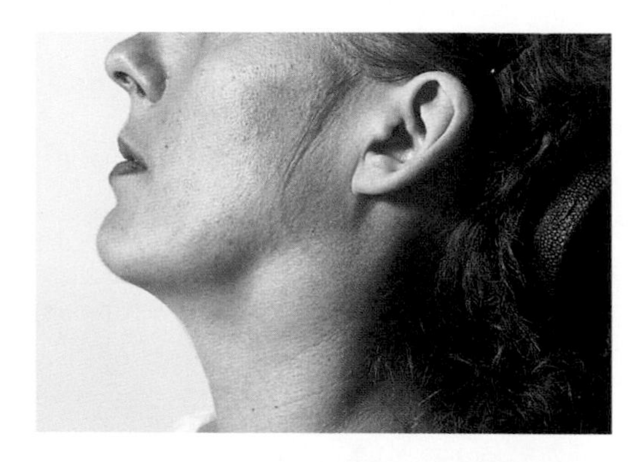

Figure 12.17 A branchial cyst that presented in adult life. The back of the swelling is clearly deep to the sternomastoid muscle.

Composition The consistency varies with the tension of the cyst. Most cysts are tense, but a lax cyst feels soft. *The lump is fluctuant, but this sign is not always easy to elicit*, especially if the cyst is small and the sternomastoid muscle thick.

The lump is usually opaque because it contains desquamated epithelial cells that make its contents thick and white. Sometimes, the fluid is golden yellow and shimmers with fat globules and cholesterol crystals secreted by the sebaceous glands in the epithelial lining. Such cysts transilluminate.

The cyst cannot be reduced or compressed.

Relations The bulk of the mass *lies deep to the upper part of the sternomastoid muscle.* It is not very mobile because it is closely tethered to the surrounding structures.

Local tissues The local tissues are normal. The surrounding tissues become oedematous and the skin hot and red if the cyst becomes infected.

Lymph nodes The local deep cervical lymph nodes should not be enlarged. If they are palpable, the diagnosis should be reconsidered in favour of an inflammatory process such as a tuberculous abscess rather than a branchial cyst. Other cystic lesions that are often presumed to be branchial cysts are secondary cystic lymph node deposits from a papillary carcinoma of the thyroid.

BRANCHIAL FISTULA (OR SINUS)

This is a rare congenital abnormality. *It is the remnant of a branchial cleft, usually the second cleft, which has not closed off.*

The patient complains of a small dimple in the skin at the junction of the middle and the lower third of the anterior edge of the sternomastoid muscle (Figure 12.18) that discharges clear mucus, and sometimes becomes swollen and painful and discharges pus.

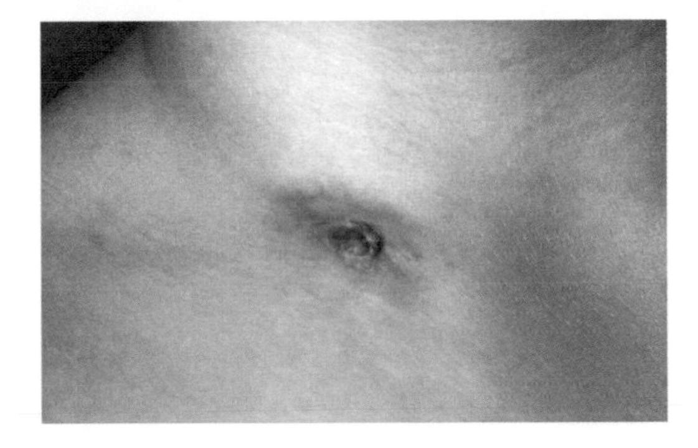

Figure 12.18 A branchial fistula opening at the lower edge of sternomastoid muscle.

When the whole branchial cleft stays patent, the fistula connects the skin with the oropharynx, just behind the tonsil. In most cases, the upper end is obliterated and the track should really be called a branchial sinus.

Swallowing accentuates the openings on the skin.

CAROTID BODY TUMOUR

This is a rare tumour of the chemoreceptor tissue in the carotid body. It is, therefore, a *chemodectoma*. It is usually benign but can become quite large and occasionally malignant.

History

Age Chemodectomas commonly appear in patients between the ages of 40 and 60 years.

Symptoms The common presentation is a painless, slowly growing lump.

Development The lump grows so slowly that many patients ignore it for many years.

Multiplicity Carotid body tumours may be bilateral.

Examination

> **NOTE:** Palpate carefully when examining a lump close to the bifurcation of the carotid artery. Heavy pressure in this area can induce a vasovagal attack.

Position The carotid bifurcation is at, or just below, the level of the hyoid bone. Therefore, carotid body tumours are found in the *upper part of the anterior triangle of the neck, level with the hyoid bone and beneath the anterior edge of the sternomastoid muscle* (Figure 12.19).

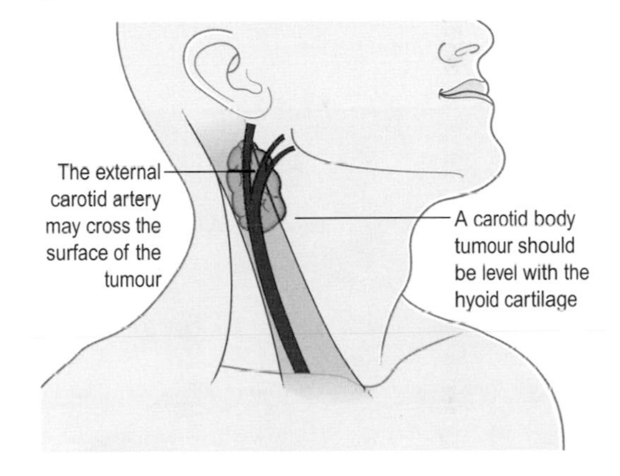

Figure 12.19 The site of a carotid body tumour.

Tenderness, colour and temperature These tumours are not tender or hot, and the overlying skin is normal.

Shape The lump is initially spherical but, as it grows, it becomes irregular in shape, often narrower at its lower end, where it is situated in the bifurcation of the common carotid artery.

Size Carotid body tumours vary from 2 cm to 10 cm in diameter.

Composition The majority of these tumours are solid, hard and do not fluctuate. They can be mistaken for an enlarged lymph node (Figure 12.20). They are often described as 'potato tumours' (Figure 12.21).

Sometimes these tumours pulsate. This is either a transmitted pulsation from the adjacent carotid artery, a palpable external carotid artery running over

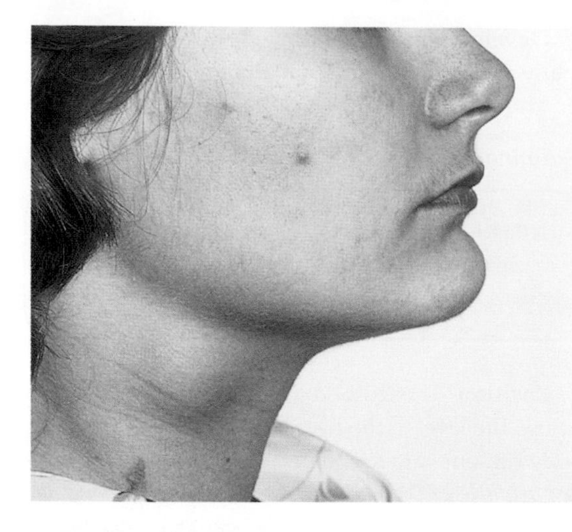

Figure 12.20 A carotid body tumour. Note that the visible mass is lower than that of a branchial cyst (see Figure 12.17) but indistinguishable on inspection from enlarged cervical lymph nodes.

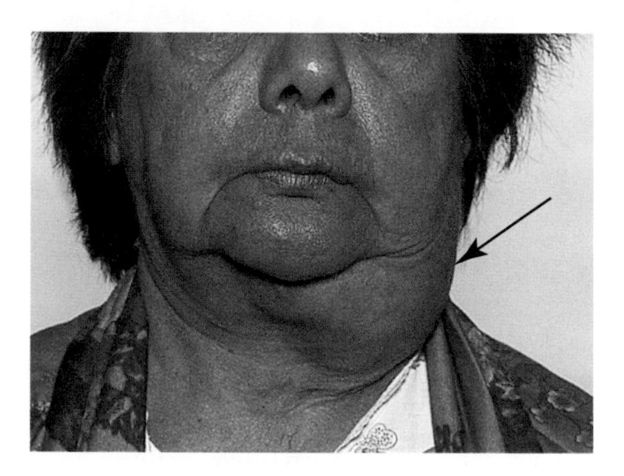

Figure 12.21 A very large, firm, bosselated carotid body tumour – hence the name 'potato tumour'.

the superficial aspect of the lump or a true expansile pulsation from a soft or very vascular tumour or an aneurysm (Figure 12.22).

It is surprising that, in spite of their vascularity, most of these tumours are hard. Those that are soft and very vascular not only have an expansile pulsation, but can also be compressed and may exhibit a bruit.

Relations The lump is deep to the cervical fascia and beneath the anterior edge of the sternomastoid muscle.

The common carotid artery can be felt below the mass, and the external carotid artery may pass over its superficial surface. Without this close relationship to the arteries, this tumour is indistinguishable from an enlarged lymph node.

NOTE: Because of their intimate relationship with the carotid arteries, these tumours can be moved from side-to-side but not up and down.

CYSTIC HYGROMA

A cystic hygroma is a congenital collection of lymphatic sacs that contain clear, colourless lymph. They are usually found in the neck but can be located anywhere in the body (e.g. junction of the body with arm and the leg). They are probably derived from clusters of lymph channels that failed, during intrauterine development, to connect with and become normal lymphatic pathways. Cystic hygroma occurs on its own or as part of a genetic syndrome, e.g. Turner syndrome or Down syndrome.

History

Age The *majority of cystic hygromas present at birth* or within the first few years of life (Figure 12.23a and b), but they occasionally stay empty until infection or trauma in adult life causes them to fill up and become visible. Occasionally, large lymphoceles can be seen in elderly patients (Figure 12.23c).

Symptoms The only symptom is the complaint about the lump, but the parents of an affected child are usually more concerned about the disfigurement caused by the cyst.

Family history This condition is not familial.

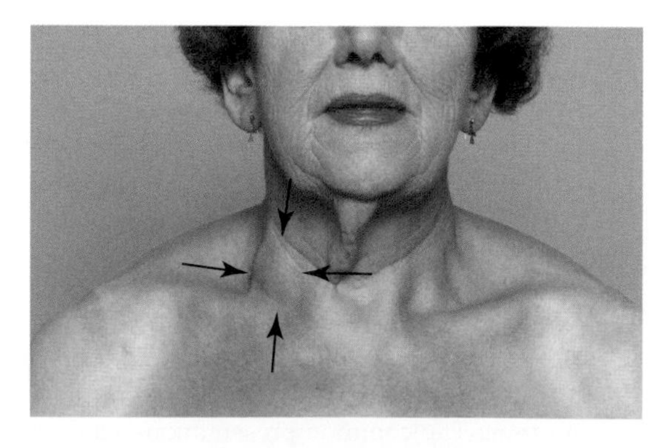

Figure 12.22 A carotid artery aneurysm.

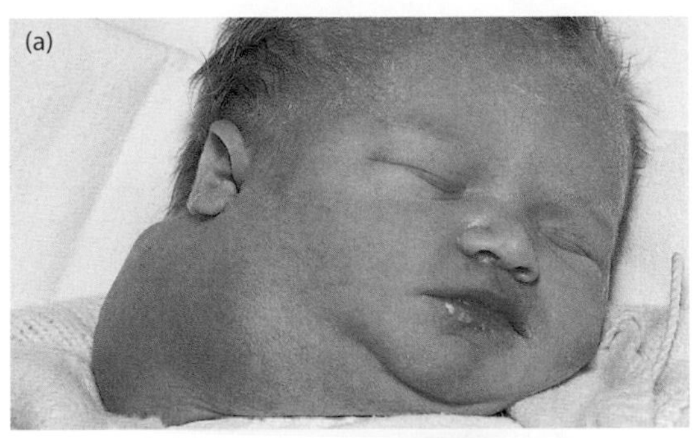

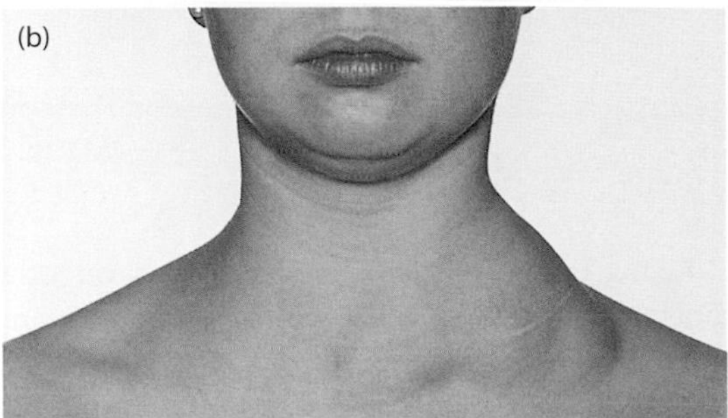

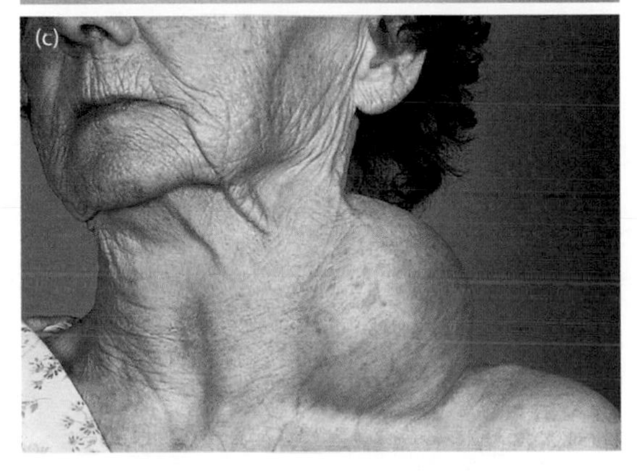

Figure 12.23 CYSTIC HYGROMA. Two examples of cystic hygroma: (a) in a very young child – the common age of presentation; (b) in a young adult; (c) an elderly woman.

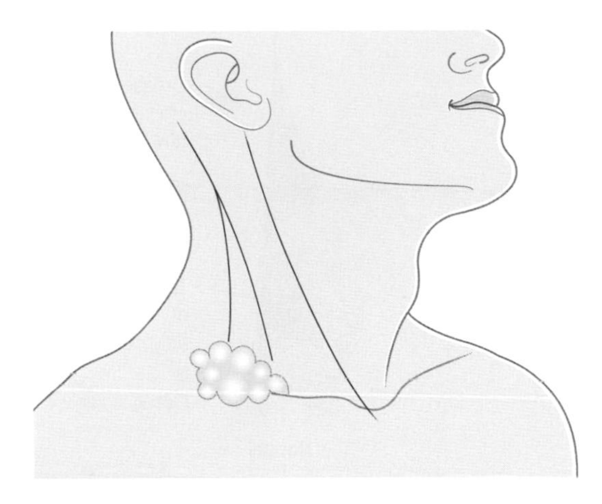

Figure 12.24 The cystic hygroma is commonly found in the subcutaneous tissue at the base of the posterior triangle. It is brilliantly translucent.

Examination

Position Cystic hygromas are commonly found around the base of the neck (Figure 12.24), usually in the posterior triangle, but they can be very big and occupy the whole of the subcutaneous tissue of one side of the neck.

Temperature and tenderness They are not hot or tender and the overlying skin is normal.

Shape A cystic hygroma is a mixture of soft unilocular and multilocular cysts, so the whole mass looks *lobulated* and *flattened*.

Size Small cysts are a few centimetres across. Large cysts can extend over the whole of one side of the neck.

Surface If the cysts are close to the skin, it may be possible to feel a distinct surface. Deep cysts feel smooth, but because they are lax, their edges are often indistinct.

Composition Cystic hygromas are soft and dull to percussion. They *fluctuate easily, but their distinctive physical sign is a brilliant translucence.*

Large cysts will conduct a fluid thrill and, in some multilocular swellings, the fluid in one loculus can be compressed into another.

They cannot be reduced.

Relations Cystic hygromas develop in the subcutaneous tissues. Thus, they are superficial to the neck muscles and close to the skin but are rarely fixed to the skin. A cyst in the posterior triangle may extend deeply beneath the sternomastoid muscle into the retropharyngeal space.

Local tissues The local tissues are normal.

Lymph nodes The local lymph nodes should not be enlarged and, as the lymph drainage of the tissues around the cyst is normal, there is no lymphoedema. If there is associated lymphadenopathy, the diagnosis should be reconsidered, as cystic nodal metastases of papillary thyroid carcinoma can present as large, painless cystic swellings in the neck.

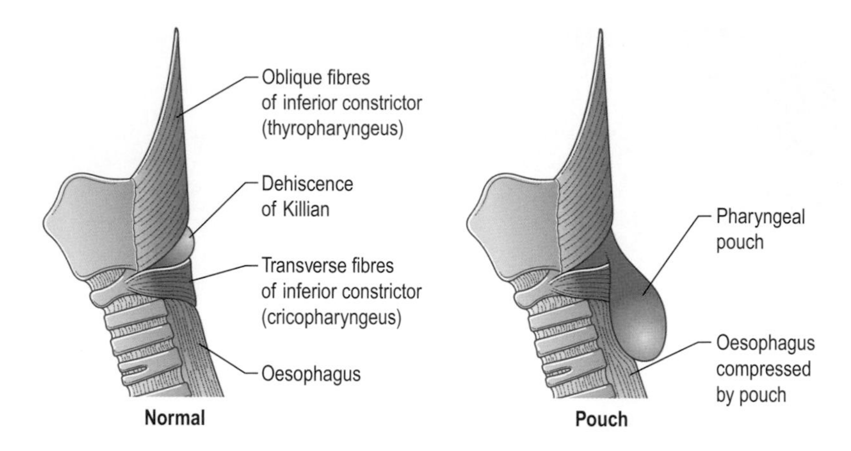

Figure 12.25 The anatomy of a pharyngeal pouch.

PHARYNGEAL POUCH

This is a 'pulsion' diverticulum of the pharynx through the gap between the horizontal fibres of the cricopharyngeus muscle below and the lowermost oblique fibres of the inferior constrictor muscle above. If swallowing is uncoordinated so that the cricopharyngeus does not relax, the weak unsupported area just above these fibres (known as *Killian's dehiscence*) bulges out (Figure 12.25). The bulge eventually grows into a sac, which hangs down and presses against the side of the oesophagus.

History

Age Pharyngeal pouches appear in middle and old age.

Sex They are more common in males than in females.

Symptoms Patients often have a long history of *halitosis and recurrent sore throats* before noticing the common presenting symptom of *regurgitation of froth and food*. The regurgitated food is undigested and comes up into the mouth at any time. There is no bile or acid taste to it.

> **NOTE:** Regurgitation at night causes bouts of coughing and choking and, if pieces of food are inhaled, a lung abscess may develop.

As the pouch grows, it presses on the oesophagus and causes *dysphagia*. Patients can sometimes swallow their first few mouthfuls of food (until the pouch is full), but thereafter have difficulty in swallowing.

By the time these symptoms become severe, the patient may have *noticed a swelling in the neck* and find that *pressure on the swelling causes gurgling sounds and regurgitation*. The *swelling changes in size and often disappears*.

The patient may become malnourished and lose weight if the dysphagia continues.

Examination

Position In most patients, there is no palpable swelling, but when a swelling caused by a pharyngeal pouch is apparent, it appears behind the sternomastoid muscle, below the level of the thyroid cartilage (Figure 12.26).

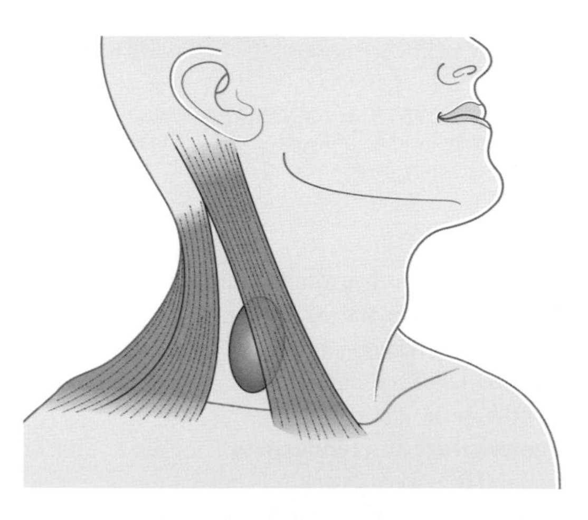

Figure 12.26 A pharyngeal pouch rarely causes a detectable swelling. If it does, the swelling is behind the sternomastoid muscle.

Shape Its shape is indistinct because only part of its surface is palpable. It feels like a bulging deep structure.

Size Most pouches cause a swelling of only 5–10 cm diameter. The pouch is not palpable when it is smaller, so *many patients have symptoms but no abnormal physical signs.*

Surface and edge When palpable, the surface is smooth, but the edge is not definable.

Composition The lump is soft and sometimes indentable. It is dull to percussion and does not fluctuate or transilluminate.

It can be compressed and sometimes emptied. Compression may cause a gurgling sound and be associated with regurgitation. Although the mass may disappear with compression, not to return until the patient eats again, it cannot be said to have been 'reduced' according to the usual meaning of the word.

Relations A pharyngeal pouch lies deep to the deep fascia, behind the sternomastoid muscle, and is fixed deeply. Its origin from a structure behind the trachea can be appreciated during palpation, but the neck of the pouch and its attachment to the oesophagus cannot be felt.

It cannot be moved about in the neck.

Local tissues The surrounding tissues feel normal. Indeed, when the pouch is empty, the neck feels normal.

Lymph nodes The cervical lymph nodes should not be enlarged.

General examination Pay special attention to the chest, as there may be an aspiration pneumonia, collapse of a lobe or a lung abscess.

STERNOMASTOID 'TUMOUR'

This is a swelling of the middle third of the sternomastoid muscle and is also known as ischaemic contracture of a segment of the sternomastoid muscle (Figure 12.27). In neonates, it consists of oedema around an infarcted segment of the muscle, caused by the trauma of birth. As the patient grows, the lump disappears and the abnormal segment of muscle becomes fibrotic and contracted.

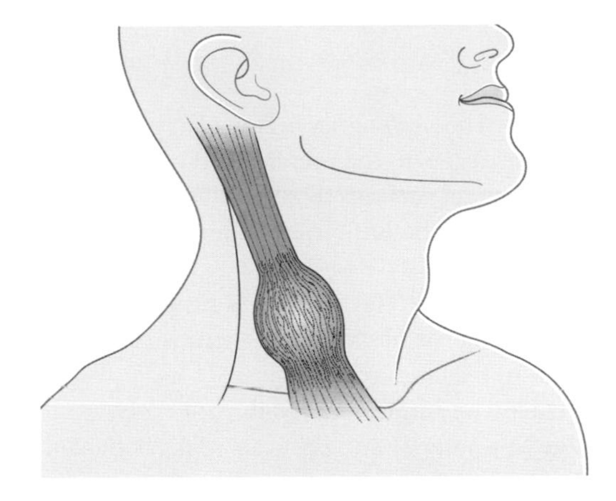

Figure 12.27 A sternomastoid 'tumour' is an area of oedema and necrosis in the lower third of the sternomastoid muscle.

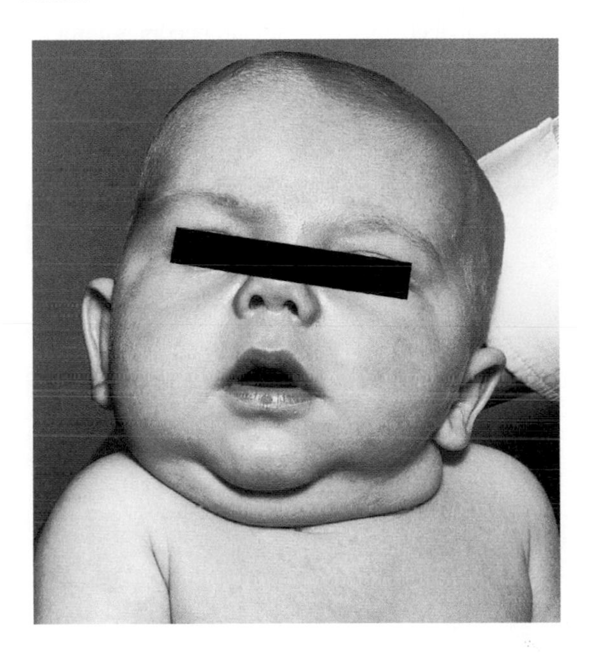

Figure 12.28 An infantile torticollis caused by ischaemia of the sternomastoid muscle.

History

Age The lump is noticed at birth or in the first few weeks of life.

Symptoms The mother may notice the lump or that the child keeps their head turned to one side – torticollis (Figure 12.28). Attempts to turn the head straight may cause pain or distress.

If the muscle is not extensively damaged, the swelling slowly subsides, the muscle spasm relaxes and the torticollis disappears. If the muscle damage becomes an area of permanent fibrosis, the twist and tilt of the head to one side becomes more noticeable as the child grows.

Examination

The lump

Position The *swelling lies in the middle of the sternomastoid muscle* (i.e. in the middle third of the neck on the anterolateral surface) (Figure 12.29).

Tenderness The lump may be tender in the first few weeks of life.

Shape and size The swelling is *fusiform*, with its long axis along the line of the sternomastoid muscle. It is usually 1–2 cm across.

Surface The surface is smooth.

Edge The anterior and posterior edges of the lump are distinct, but the superior and inferior edges, where the lump becomes continuous with normal muscle, are indistinct.

Composition At first, the lump is firm and solid and easy to feel, but as it gradually becomes harder, it begins to shrink and may become impalpable.

Local tissues and lymph nodes These should be normal.

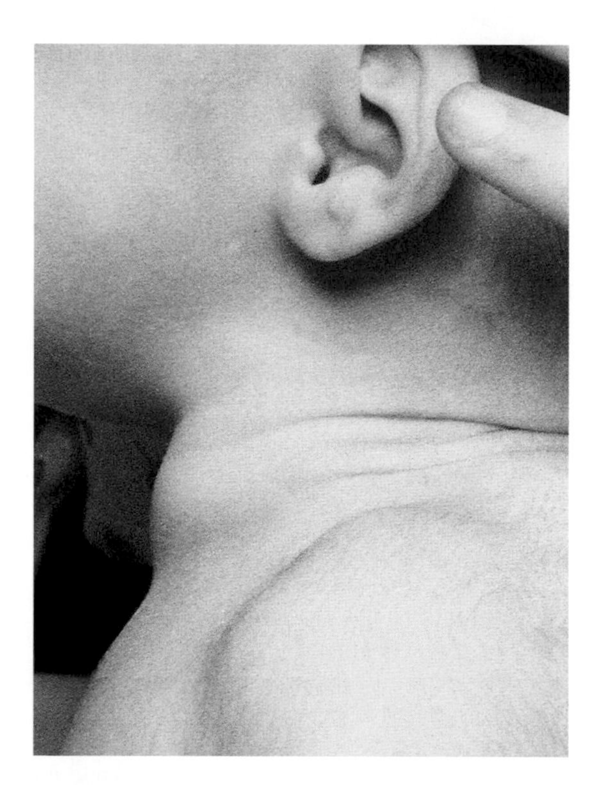

Figure 12.29 A localized swollen segment of sternomastoid with a slight torticollis in an older child, caused by ischaemia and fibrosis of the muscle after birth; this is a typical sternomastoid 'tumour'.

The neck

Examine the movements of the neck. As the child is too young to obey commands, watch how they move their head when lying in their cot, and then manipulate the head and neck very gently.

The sternomastoid muscles rotate and tilt the head. Contraction of the left sternomastoid turns the head towards the right but tilts the head to the left. Both these deformities may be present. Forced movement to correct the deformity may cause pain and be resisted by the child.

Apart from the restriction of movement caused by spasm of the sternomastoid muscle, the neck movements should be normal.

The eyes

Look at the eyes and watch their movements to detect any squint. Torticollis can be a means of correcting a squint. Move the head into a vertical and central position and watch the eyes. If the torticollis is secondary to a squint and not a sternomastoid tumour, the squint will appear as the head is straightened.

The head

An uncorrected torticollis may affect the growth of the facial bones and cause facial asymmetry.

In adults, recent-onset torticollis usually just represents muscle spasm (Figure 12.30).

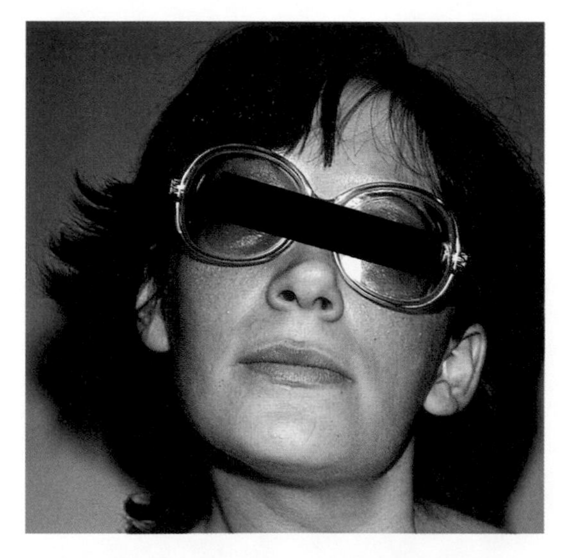

Figure 12.30 An adult form of torticollis caused by muscular spasm.

CERVICAL RIB

Although a cervical rib can cause serious neurological and vascular symptoms in the upper arm, clinical examination of the neck does not usually reveal any abnormalities (see Chapters 7 and 9). The abnormal rib is usually detected with an X-ray (Figure 12.31). Sometimes, there is a fullness at the root of the neck, but it is rarely distinct enough to justify a firm clinical diagnosis of cervical rib (Figure 12.32). It can occasionally be associated with aneurysmal change in the subclavian artery.

The common neurological symptoms caused by a cervical rib are *pain in the C8 and T1 dermatomes and wasting and weakness of the small muscles in the hand.*

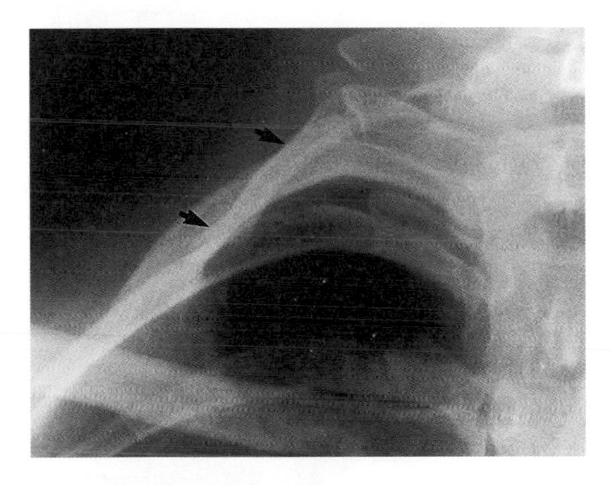

Figure 12.31 An X-ray demonstrating a cervical rib.

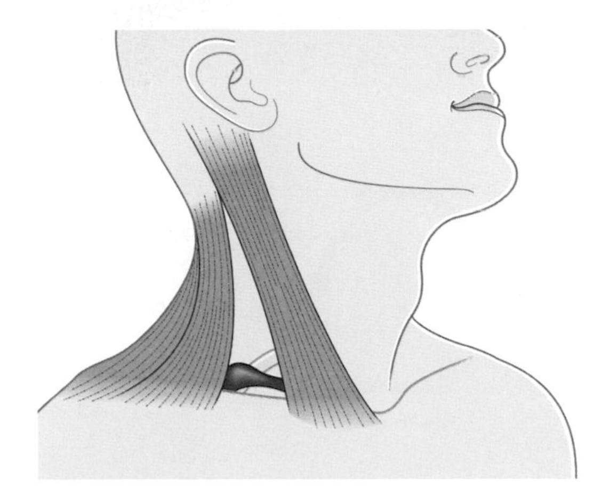

Figure 12.32 A cervical rib rarely causes a visible swelling. It may cause a subclavian artery aneurysm.

Vascular symptoms such as Raynaud's phenomenon, trophic changes and even rest pain and gangrene may occur but are uncommon.

THE SALIVARY GLANDS

Saliva is produced by the paired parotid, submandibular and sublingual glands and many other small, unnamed glands scattered beneath the buccal mucous membrane.

The most common surgical conditions affecting the salivary glands are:

- Infection and calculus formation in the submandibular gland.
- Tumours of the parotid gland.

Sialolithiasis accounts for about 50% of disease affecting the salivary glands.

Most tumours of the salivary glands are benign and around 80% occur in the parotid. Malignant tumours most frequently affect the parotid, while less frequent tumours of the other salivary glands are more likely to be malignant (40% submandibular and 70%–90% sublingual, 50% minor salivary glands).

Mumps is the most common medical disease; all other diseases of the salivary glands are uncommon (Revision panel 12.4).

Revision panel 12.4

CAUSES OF SWELLING OF A SALIVARY GLAND

Acute infection

Viral (e.g. mumps)
Bacterial (e.g. *Staphylococcus*)

Duct obstruction

Sialectasis (chronic infection)

Tumour

Benign
Malignant

Sarcoidosis (Mikulicz's syndrome)

Sjögren's syndrome

Conditions of the submandibular salivary gland

SUBMANDIBULAR CALCULI

Submandibular calculi are common because the submandibular gland lies below the opening of its duct on the floor of the mouth, and because the secretion of the submandibular gland contains a considerable quantity of mucus, two factors that encourage stasis in the duct. *Calculi in the parotid gland are less common.*

A salivary gland calculus is composed of cellular debris, bacteria, mucus and calcium and magnesium phosphates – a mixture similar to the 'scale' (tartar) on the teeth.

History

Age Most submandibular salivary calculi occur in young to middle-aged adults.

Sex Males and females are equally afflicted.

Symptoms The main symptoms are *pain and swelling beneath the jaw,* caused by obstruction of Wharton's duct.

Swelling is usually the principal complaint because it appears before, and persists after, the pain. The pain is a dull ache, which occasionally radiates to the ear or into the tongue.

Both *symptoms appear, or worsen, before and during eating.* The swelling begins just before eating, and the pain develops as the gland enlarges. Both symptoms last through the meal, but afterwards the pain goes away before the swelling. If the gland becomes irreparably damaged, the swelling persists between meals and the dull aching pain may also become constant.

Very rarely, the patient may notice discomfort and a swelling in the floor of the mouth caused by distension of the duct and/or the stone.

Patients may be able to relieve their symptoms by pressing on the gland, and they may notice that this action produces a foul-tasting fluid in their mouth (purulent saliva).

Development The symptoms may recur and remit for periods of a few days or weeks if the stone moves in the duct, causing intermittent obstruction.

The symptoms disappear if the stone passes through the orifice of the duct.

Persistent obstruction damages the gland, making it harder and tender.

Previous history The patient may have had similar symptoms on the other side of the face. Simultaneous bilateral calculi are uncommon.

Examination

The lump

Position The submandibular gland lies beneath the horizontal ramus of the mandible on the mylohyoid muscle (Figure 12.33). *It is 2–3 cm in front of the anterior border of the sternomastoid muscle* and should not be confused with enlarged upper deep cervical lymph glands, which are deep to the sternomastoid muscle.

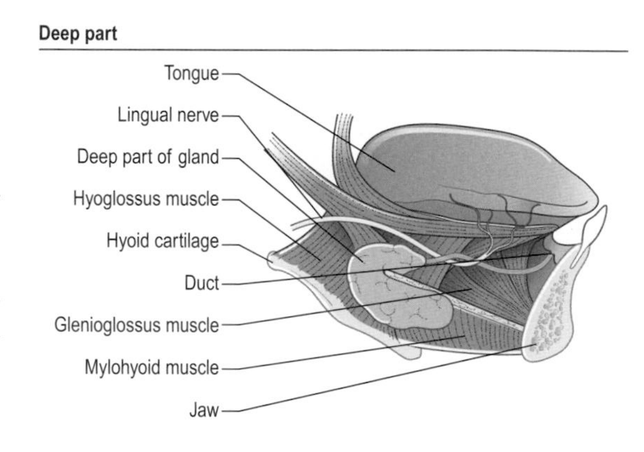

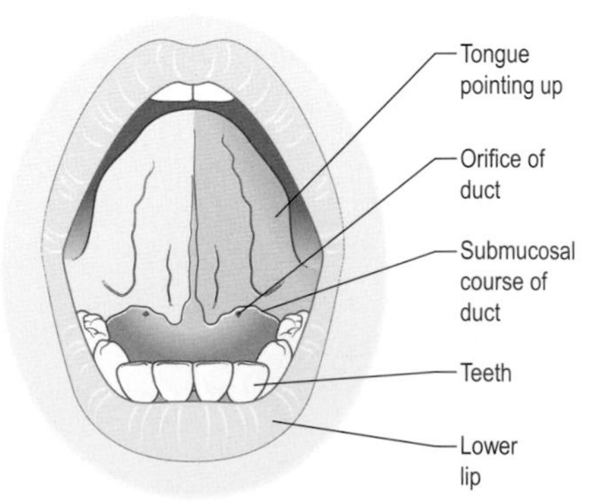

Figure 12.33 The anatomy of the submandibular gland.

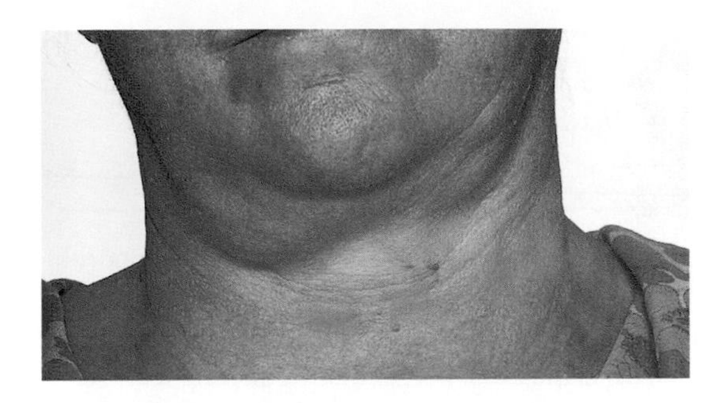

Figure 12.34 A swollen right submandibular gland. Although some of the swelling seems to spread over the jaw, the upper part of the gland is actually deep to the mandible.

Colour and temperature If the gland is not infected, the overlying skin will have a normal colour and temperature (Figure 12.34). If the gland is infected, the skin becomes red, oedematous and hot.

Tenderness The gland is tender when it is tense (before and during eating) but resolves between meals unless it is infected.

Shape The shape of the superficial part of the submandibular gland is a flattened ovoid (almond shaped).

Size If the gland is enlarged solely by obstruction of its duct, it rarely becomes more than 3–5 cm across. If it becomes infected, it may get much larger.

Surface Its surface is smooth but the lobules of the gland may make it bosselated.

Edge The anterior, posterior and inferior edges of the gland are distinct and easy to define, but the upper edge is wedged between the mandible and the mylohyoid muscle and is impalpable.

Composition A distended submandibular gland has a *rubbery, hard consistency* and will not fluctuate, transilluminate or reduce. It is dull to percussion and has no bruit.

Prolonged pressure on the gland may make it a little smaller and produce a jet of saliva from the orifice of the submandibular duct.

Relations The skin is freely mobile over the swollen gland, while the gland can be moved a little from side-to-side, but movements are restricted by the tethering to the underlying muscles. When the muscles of the floor of the mouth are tensed by asking the patient to push their tongue against the roof of the mouth, the gland becomes less mobile.

It is important to ascertain the relations of the lump to the floor of the mouth and the tongue by *bimanual palpation*. Feel the lump between the gloved index finger of one hand inside the mouth and the fingers of the other hand on the outer surface of the lump.

It should be possible to appreciate that the lump is outside the structures that form the floor of the mouth. It should not be fixed to the mucosa of the floor of the mouth or to the tongue.

Local tissues The nearby tissues, except the submandibular duct in the floor of the mouth, should be normal.

Lymph nodes Lymph from the submandibular gland drains to the middle deep cervical lymph nodes, but there is also some lymphoid tissue within the gland that can contribute to its enlargement.

The local lymph nodes are usually not enlarged unless the gland is infected.

The floor of the mouth

Inspection Ask the patient to open their mouth and lift their tongue up to the roof of the mouth. This displays the orifices of the submandibular ducts on their small papillae on either side of the frenulum of the tongue.

> **NOTE:** If a stone is impacted at the end of the duct, its grey–yellow colour may be visible in the open orifice of the duct.

The presence of a stone in the duct makes that side of the floor of the mouth bulge upwards, look asymmetrical and a little reddened (see Figure 12.35).

Press the gland gently and watch for any discharge from the orifice of the duct.

Palpation Feel along the course of the duct in the floor of the mouth for lumps and tenderness.

A *stone in the duct will not feel stony hard* if it is small and surrounded by inflammatory oedema. The lump caused by such a stone will feel soft with a hard centre.

General examination Examine all the salivary glands in case the symptoms are the result of systemic disease such as Sjögren's syndrome (see page 425) and not just a stone.

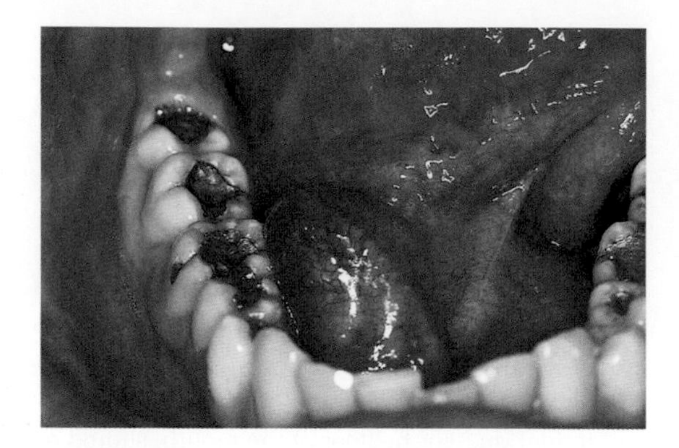

Figure 12.35 Stone in the submandibular duct. When a stone impacts at the end of the submandibular duct, the floor of the mouth looks asymmetrical. In this patient, there is a bulge over the right submandibular duct due to an impacted stone.

Submandibular sialadenitis

Infection of a submandibular gland invariably occurs secondary to the presence of a stone in its duct or damage done by a stone that has passed through the duct. The infecting organism is usually *Staphylococcus*.

The symptoms are identical to those caused by a stone except that when the gland is infected the pain is severe, throbbing and continuous.

The physical signs of the lump in the neck are similar to those of the obstructed gland, with the addition of heat and tenderness. An infected gland may become large (5 × 10 cm). If the duct system becomes dilated (*sialectasis*), pus may pool in the gland and the whole structure turn into a multilocular abscess, which may then point onto the skin.

Submandibular salivary gland tumours

The tumours that often occur in the parotid gland may occur in the submandibular gland, but they are rare. Tumours are more likely to be malignant.

The physical features of tumours in the submandibular gland are the same as tumours arising in the parotid gland, apart from the site.

A *pleomorphic adenoma* forms a painless, slow-growing, non-tender, hard, well-defined, spherical mass within the gland.

Carcinoma causes an indistinct, warm, slightly tender, rapidly growing, painful mass.

NOTE: Numbness of the anterior two-thirds of the tongue indicates infiltration of the lingual nerve and is diagnostic of carcinoma.

It may be difficult to distinguish a pleomorphic adenoma from enlargement of the lymph tissue within the gland. A long history of slow, gradual growth is the most useful distinguishing feature.

Conditions of the parotid gland

ACUTE INFECTIVE PAROTITIS

The most common infection of the parotid gland is *mumps* (Figure 12.36). This is an epidemic viral parotitis that typically causes *bilateral painful, swollen glands* and excessive oedema that spreads down into the neck giving the child a double chin; it is relatively straightforward to diagnose. When there is unilateral gland enlargement (Figure 12.37), little pain and no oedema, and there are no obvious contacts with the infection, it can be much more difficult to diagnose.

Non-specific parotitis, usually a staphylococcal infection, is caused by:

- Poor oral hygiene.
- Dehydration.
- Obstruction of Stensen's duct by a stone or scar tissue.

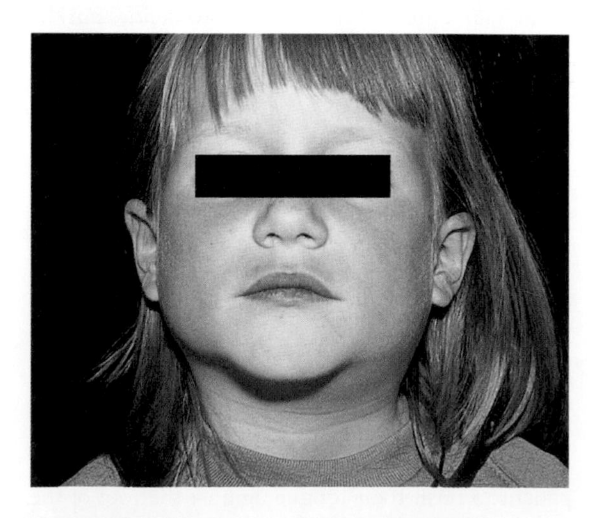

Figure 12.36 Bilateral mumps in a young female.

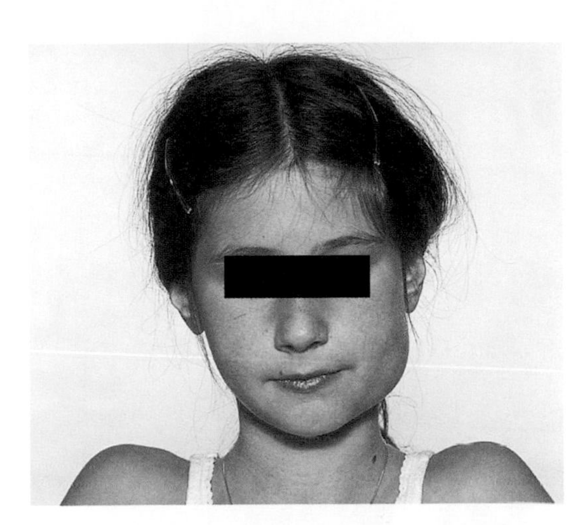

Figure 12.37 Unilateral mumps. A young female with diffuse swelling of the left parotid gland caused by mumps. Much of the swelling is caused by oedema.

> **NOTE:** In the days before the fluid balance of sick or postoperative patients was properly controlled and administered, fulminating parotitis, with subsequent septicaemia, was a common cause of death.

History

Age Acute parotitis is more common in the elderly and the debilitated.

Symptoms The patient complains of a sudden onset of *pain and swelling in the side of the face.*

The pain is continuous and throbbing and radiates to the ear and over the side of the head.

Speaking and eating cause pain because movement of the temporomandibular joint is painful.

The patient feels hot, sweaty and ill and may complain of shivering attacks (rigors).

Systematic questions Systematic questioning may reveal symptoms of another illness, such as a bronchial carcinoma, which has caused the debility and dehydration.

Previous history The patient may have recently undergone a major operation or suffered a severe medical illness.

Examination

The lump

Position The parotid gland lies in front of and below the lower half of the ear. It is wrapped around the vertical ramus of the mandible, with its deep portion in between this bone and the mastoid process (Figure 12.38).

In acute parotitis, the whole gland is swollen, so the whole of the face in front of the lower half of the ear bulges outwards.

Colour and temperature The skin over the swelling is discoloured a reddish–brown, feels hot and is smooth and shiny.

Tenderness The swelling is very tender.

Shape The *mass has the shape of the normal parotid gland*: a semi-circular anterior edge, a vertical edge just in front of the ear and a bulge running into the gap between the mandible and the mastoid process.

Size The swollen parotid may be three to four times larger than normal.

Surface Its surface is smooth but difficult to define because of oedema, inflammation and tenderness.

Composition The texture of the swelling is often described as 'brawny'. This means that it has a firm consistency but is indentable. It is dull to percussion, not fluctuant and not compressible.

Relations If the overlying skin is red and oedematous, it will be tethered to the swelling. The swelling cannot be moved over the deep structures and becomes more prominent when the patient contracts the masseter muscles by clenching their teeth.

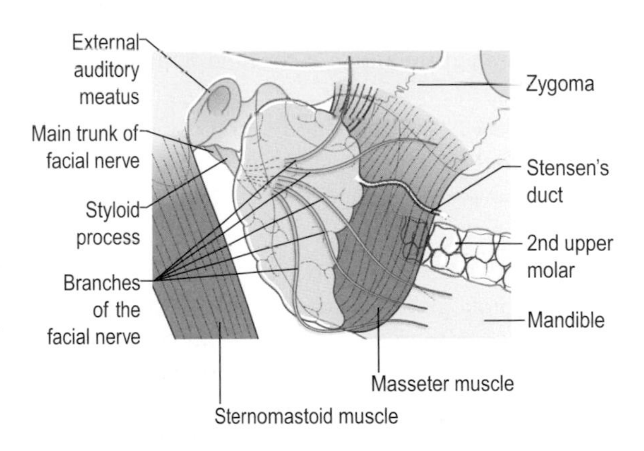

Figure 12.38 The anatomy of the parotid gland. Note that the parotid gland extends below and behind the angle of the mandible. Lumps in this part of the gland are easily mistaken for enlarged upper deep cervical lymph nodes.

Local tissues Apart from the changes in the skin and the restricted movements of the temporomandibular joint, the surrounding tissues are normal. The function of the facial nerve is **not** impaired.

Lymph nodes The upper deep cervical lymph nodes are usually enlarged and tender.

The mouth

Inspection *The orifice of Stensen's duct is opposite the second upper molar tooth.* The mouth of the duct may be patulous and the buccal mucosa over the course of the duct slightly oedematous.

Palpation Feel the mouth of the duct for any thickening or swelling.

The parotid gland cannot be palpated bimanually because it lies behind the anterior edge of the masseter muscle and the vertical ramus of the mandible.

Gentle pressure on the gland may produce a purulent discharge from the orifice of the duct.

Chronic parotitis

This is usually caused by a small calculus or a fibrous stenosis blocking the drainage of Stensen's duct.

History

The patient complains of *recurrent swelling of the parotid gland*. The swelling is particularly noticeable before eating and is associated with an aching pain.

In severe cases, the gland becomes permanently swollen, but the pain is usually not constant.

Chronic parotitis maybe bilateral.

Examination

The whole gland is easy to feel because it is bigger and firmer than a normal gland and its edges are distinct (Figure 12.39). It is also tender and feels rubbery hard.

Pressure on the gland may produce a copious squirt of fluid through the orifice of the duct if there is partial obstruction to the flow of saliva.

Examine all the other salivary glands to exclude a general abnormality.

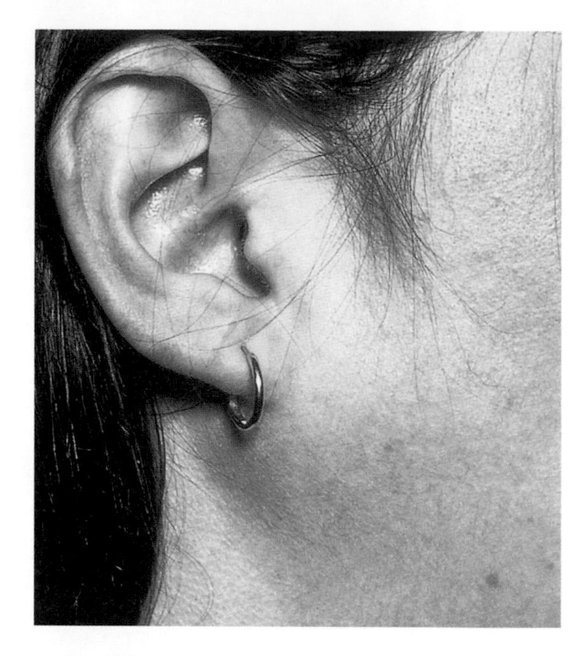

Figure 12.39 Chronic parotitis. A firm, slightly tender enlargement of the whole of the parotid gland caused by recurrent infection secondary to a stone in Stensen's duct.

PAROTID TUMOURS

The 2005 WHO classification of salivary gland tumours includes 10 benign and 23 malignant tumours of epithelial origin. There are also rare non-epithelial tumours that are frequently of squamous cell origin; 80% of SGT affect the parotid.

Common benign tumours include:

- Pleomorphic adenoma (>50%).
- Warthin tumour.

Common malignant tumours include:

- Mucoepidermoid carcinoma (35%).
- Polymorphous low-grade adenocarcinoma.
- Adenoid cystic carcinoma.
- Acinic cell carcinoma – a type of adenocarcinoma, of which there are many others.

Pleomorphic adenoma

This is the commonest tumour, accounting for more than half of tumours. It has a mixed histological appearance of *epithelial* and *myoepithelial cells* that are variably arranged on a variable background (of *mucin, chondroid or myxoid*). The epithelial cell types are also variable (e.g. cuboidal, clear, spindle).

NOTE: The tumours old name was *mixed parotid tumour.*

It is a slow-growing adenoma with an incomplete capsule. The small pieces of tumour that protrude through the defects in its capsule limit its treatment by enucleation and allow rapid extension if it undergoes malignant transformation which affects <10% of long-standing lesions.

History

Age Peak incidence is in the 3rd to 4th decades.

Sex They occur more often in males.

Symptoms The patient complains of a painless swelling on the side of their face that has been present for months or years and is slowly growing.

The lump may be more prominent when the mouth is open or when eating. The latter symptom can cause confusion, so it is important to find out whether the lump just becomes more prominent because of contraction of the masseter muscle or actually increases in size.

Examination

Position The majority of adenomas begin in the portion of the gland that lies over the junction of the vertical and horizontal rami of the mandible, just anterior and superior to the angle of the jaw.

Colour and temperature The temperature and colour of the overlying skin are normal.

Tenderness The lump is not tender.

Shape Adenomas are spherical when they are small, but as they grow, they become flat on their deep surface and slightly pointed superficially. They may become lobulated when very large (Figure 12.40).

Size Can vary from pea-sized nodules to large, almost pendulous, masses 20 cm across (Figure 12.41).

Surface Their surface is smooth, sometimes bosselated, and occasionally crossed by deep furrows.

The surface of any deep extension between the mandible and the mastoid process is impalpable.

Edge The edge is quite distinct and easy to feel.

Composition The tumour mass has a *rubbery, hard consistency*, is dull to percussion, not fluctuant or translucent, and not compressible.

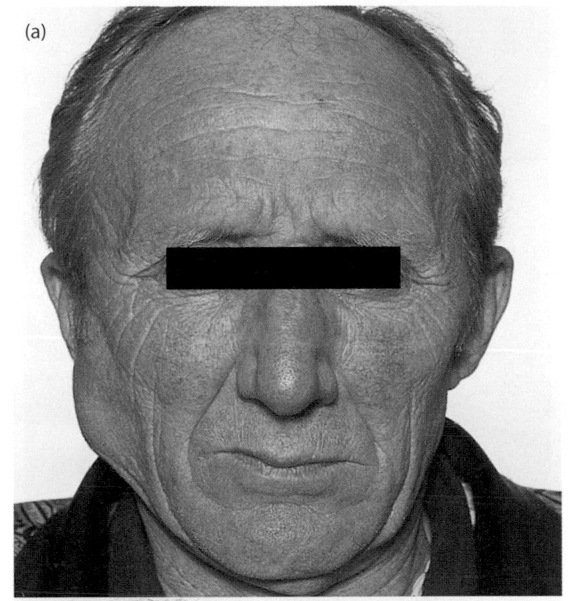

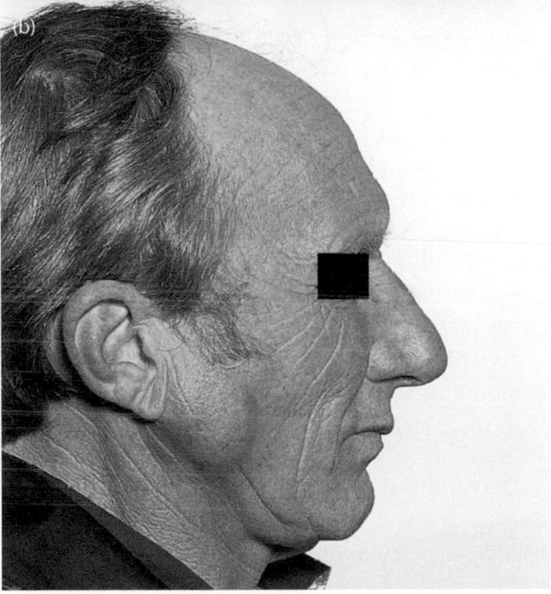

Figure 12.40 PLEOMORPHIC ADENOMA. (a, b) These photographs show the typical site, the healthy overlying skin, the absence of facial nerve involvement and the lobulation that develops as the tumour grows.

Relations The overlying skin and the ear are not attached to the lump.

Small tumours can be moved about over the deep structures, but large tumours are less mobile.

Lymph nodes The cervical lymph nodes should not be enlarged.

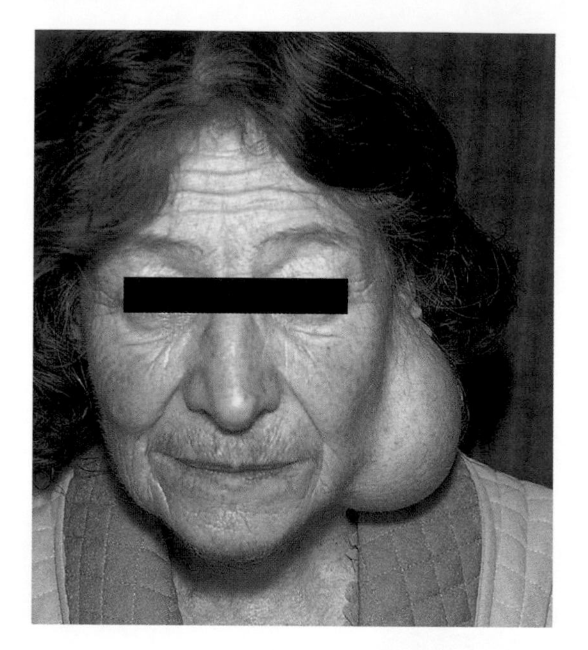

Figure 12.41 A very large, almost pendulous, pleomorphic adenoma of the parotid gland.

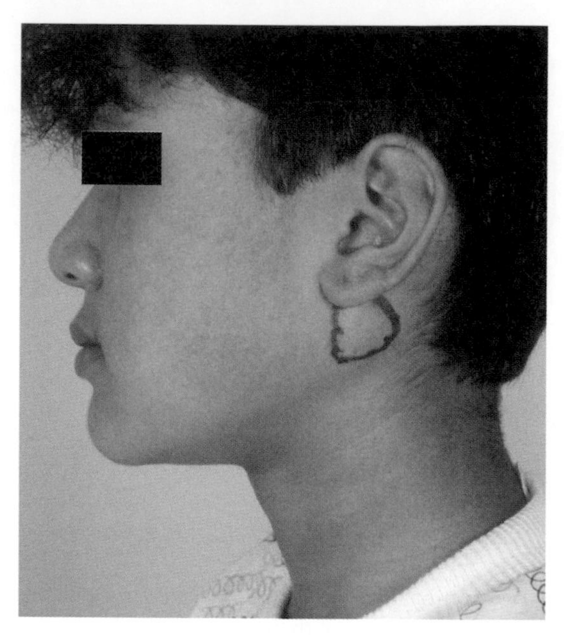

Figure 12.42 An acinic cell tumour of the parotid gland, which is difficult to differentiate from a pleomorphic adenoma on simple clinical examination.

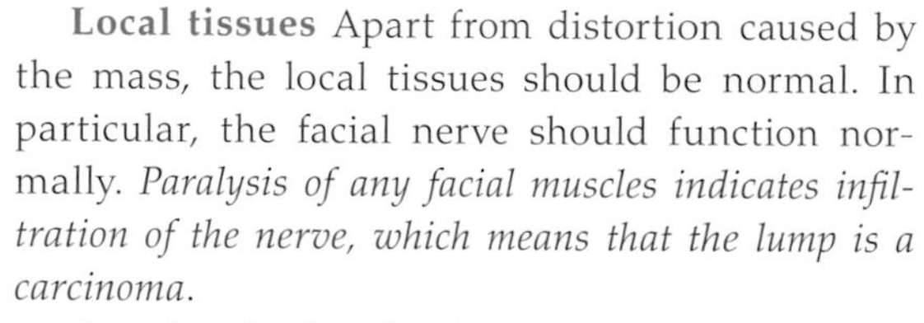

Local tissues Apart from distortion caused by the mass, the local tissues should be normal. In particular, the facial nerve should function normally. *Paralysis of any facial muscles indicates infiltration of the nerve, which means that the lump is a carcinoma.*

Examine the inside of the mouth A pleomorphic adenoma in the deep part of the parotid gland will push the tonsil and the pillar of the fauces towards the midline.

Differential diagnosis *Other parotid tumours,* such as acinic cell tumours (Figure 12.42), can be difficult to differentiate simply on examination. *A preauricular lymph node,* enlarged by secondary infection or metastases, can also present as a firm, smooth swelling just in front of the tragus and be indistinguishable from a pleomorphic adenoma if it is not tender. The most distinctive physical sign of an enlarged preauricular lymph node is its mobility. Most tumours in the parotid gland can only be moved a short distance because they are tethered to the gland; the preauricular lymph node lies outside the capsule of the parotid gland and is usually very mobile.

Warthin tumour

This is the second most common benign tumour, although much less common than pleomorphic adenoma. It is composed of *glandular and cystic structures and contains epithelial and lymphoid tissue.* It has a thin capsule. The epithelial element is believed to originate from embryonic parotid ducts that have become separated from the main duct system of the gland. The lymphoid element comes from normal lymph tissue associated with the developing gland.

History

Age These tumours usually occur in patients over 60 years age.

Sex They are more common in males.

Ethnic group They do not occur in black people.

Symptoms The patient complains of a slow-growing, painless swelling over the angle of the jaw. They are multicentric in up to 20% and, less frequently, bilateral.

Examination

Position The *tumour arises in the lower pole of the parotid, near the lower border of the mandible*

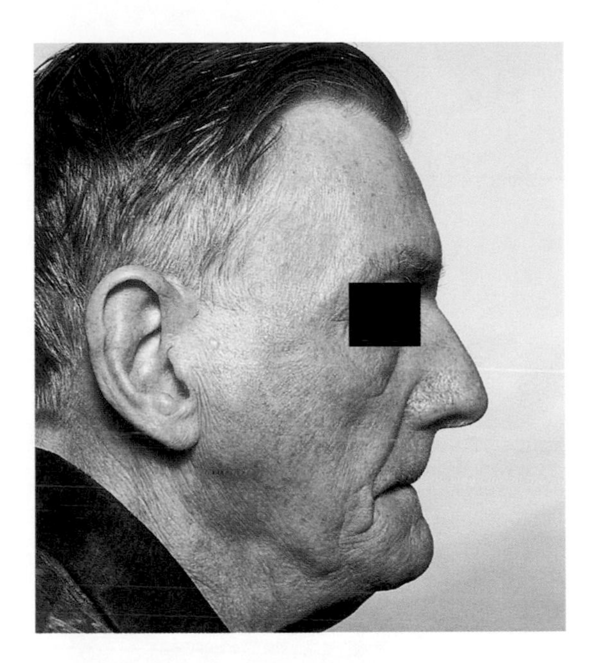

Figure 12.43 Warthin tumour of the parotid gland demonstrating the typical site, just over the angle of the jaw. Although it looks similar to the pleomorphic adenoma shown in Figure 12.41, it had a soft consistency.

(Figure 12.43). This is slightly lower than the common site of the pleomorphic adenoma.

Temperature and colour The overlying skin is normal.

Tenderness The lump is not tender.

Shape Warthin tumours are spherical or hemispherical.

Size They are usually 1–3 cm in diameter.

Surface The surface is smooth and well defined.

Edge Its edge is distinct and sometimes makes the lump seem separate from the parotid gland.

Composition *Tumours are soft and fluctuate.* They do not transilluminate.

Relations The lump can usually be moved a little in all directions and is not attached to the skin.

Local tissues The adjacent tissues are normal.

Lymph nodes The cervical lymph nodes should not be enlarged.

Carcinoma of the parotid gland

Salivary gland carcinomas are uncommon and represent approximately 6% of head and neck cancers and less than 1% of all cancers.

NOTE: Carcinoma of the parotid gland can arise *de novo* or in a long-standing pleomorphic adenoma.

History

Age The patient is usually over the age of 50 years.

Sex Males and females are equally affected.

Symptoms The common complaint is of a solitary, rapidly enlarging swelling on the side of the face. *There may be pain* especially during movements of the jaw. The pain may *radiate to the ear and over the side of the face* (Figure 12.44). The patient may give a history of a preceding painless lump that has been present for many years.

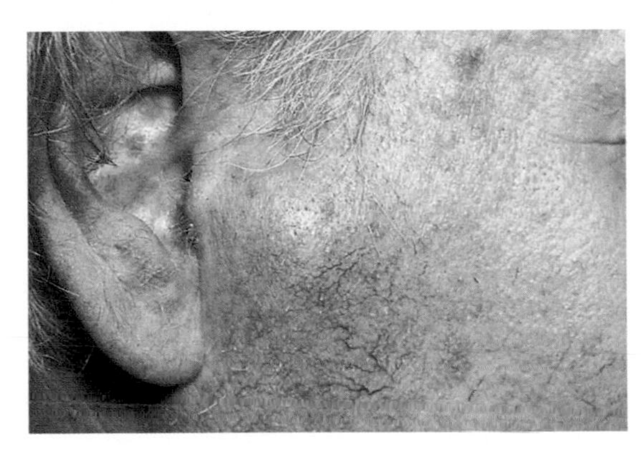

Figure 12.44 Carcinoma of the parotid gland. This patient complained of a painful swelling in front of his ear. The swelling was hot and the overlying skin reddened. Although the swelling was not very large, there was some weakness of the muscles of facial expression.

The patient may also complain of asymmetry of the mouth (Figure 12.45) and difficulty in closing the eyes from facial nerve involvement.

Examination

Position The swelling is in the site of the parotid gland.

Colour If the overlying skin is infiltrated by the tumour, it may be reddish–blue.

Temperature The skin and the mass are hyperaemic and hot.

Tenderness The mass is not very tender, an important difference from acute parotitis, which also presents as a hot swelling.

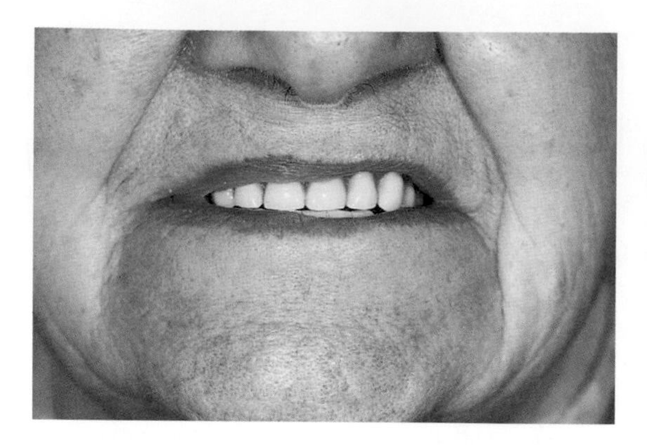

Figure 12.45 Asymmetry of the mouth due to facial nerve palsy.

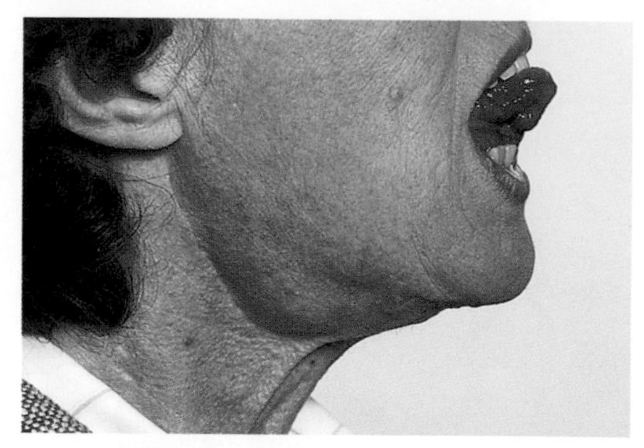

Figure 12.46 The submandibular swelling in this woman was a lymph gland enlarged by secondary deposits from a carcinoma of the tongue, and not a lesion of the submandibular gland.

Shape The tumour may be of any shape. It is basically a flattened hemisphere, but as it spreads in different directions, its shape becomes irregular.

Size Its size increases inexorably.

Surface The surface is smooth but irregular.

Edge The edge is often indistinct.

Composition The mass has a firm, *sometimes hard consistency*, is dull to percussion but is not fluctuant or translucent. Although it may be very vascular, it does not have an audible bruit.

Relations Carcinoma of the parotid becomes *fixed to the deep structures* early in its growth and may also become fixed to, and *infiltrate, the skin*.

The thickening of the tissues around the temporomandibular joint may restrict jaw movements.

Local tissues The patient will be unable to use the muscles of facial expression if the facial nerve is infiltrated by tumour. The signs may vary from mild weakness of the lower lip when baring the teeth to a *complete VIIth cranial nerve palsy*.

The jaw will be swollen and tender if the tumour has infiltrated into the mandible.

Lymph nodes The cervical lymph nodes are likely to be enlarged and hard.

General examination There may be evidence of disseminated blood-borne metastases.

Differential diagnosis Not all swellings in the parotid or submandibular region are caused by salivary gland pathology. Lymph nodes in these areas can mimic salivary gland enlargement (Figures 12.46, 12.47) while primary skin lesions in these areas may potentially be misdiagnosed (Figure 12.48).

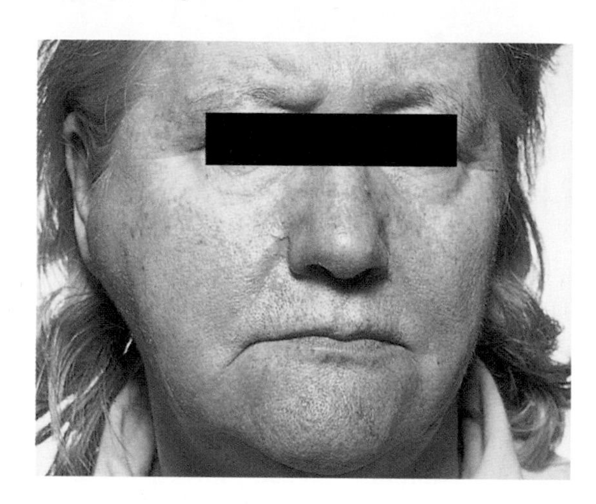

Figure 12.47 Preauricular lymphadenopathy. Preauricular lymphadenopathy is a condition that is commonly mistaken for parotid gland enlargement. However, this woman's preauricular swelling was caused by a secondary deposit of carcinoma in the ascending ramus of the mandible.

AUTOIMMUNE DISEASE

There are two syndromes of slow, progressive, but relatively painless enlargement of the salivary glands in which biopsy reveals that the swelling is caused by replacement of the glandular tissue by lymphoid tissue.

Mikulicz's syndrome

This is a rare chronic condition. Its cause is unknown but it may be an IgG4-related disease. It

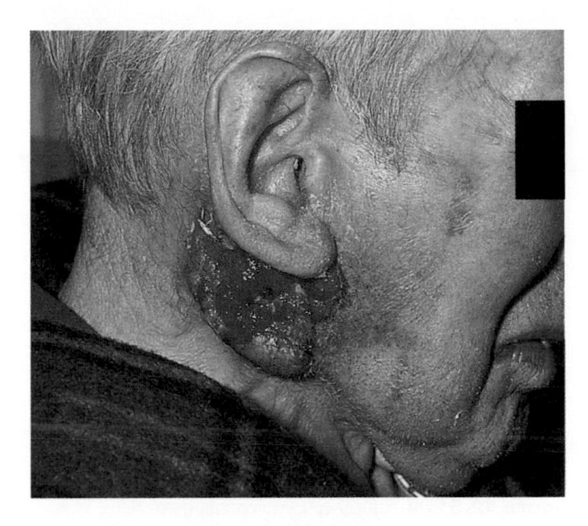

Figure 12.48 This ulcerating lesion over the parotid gland was initially diagnosed as a parotid carcinoma. However, there was no facial weakness and the lesion was actually in the skin. A biopsy revealed that it was a squamous cell carcinoma of the skin.

usually occurs in association with an underlying disorder including TB, Hodgkin's lymphoma, leukaemia and sarcoid. It is frequently associated with *Sjögren's syndrome* and has previously been considered a form of Sjögren's. It presents with:

- Benign enlargement of the salivary glands: usually both the parotid and both submandibular glands enlarge, but the syndrome can begin and remain in one gland for quite a long time.
- Enlargement of the lachrymal glands: this causes a bulge at the outer end of the upper eyelids and narrowing of the palpebral fissures.
- A dry mouth, which may be the presenting symptom: the patient is not thirsty.

Sjögren's syndrome

Sjögren's syndrome is an autoimmune condition that exhibits all the above characteristics, although the degree of salivary gland enlargement is often not so gross, plus:

- Dry eyes.
- Generalized arthritis.

THYROGLOSSAL CYST

The thyroid gland develops from the lower portion of the thyroglossal duct, which begins at the foramen caecum at the base of the tongue and passes down to the pyramidal lobe of the isthmus of the thyroid gland. If a portion of this duct remains patent, it can form a thyroglossal cyst.

> **NOTE:** Thyroglossal cysts are commonly found between the isthmus of the thyroid gland and the hyoid bone; and just above the hyoid bone (Figure 12.49).

History

Age Thyroglossal cysts can appear at any age, but most are seen in young adults.

Sex They are more common in females.

Symptoms They present as a painless lump in a prominent part of the neck (Figure 12.50). Pain, tenderness and an increase in size occur if the cyst becomes infected.

Duration of symptoms The lump may be noticed acutely or have been present for many years before an increase in its size causes the patient to complain.

Systemic symptoms There are no systemic symptoms.

Examination

Position Thyroglossal cysts lie close to the midline, between the chin and the second tracheal ring. In the fetus, the thyroglossal duct is in the midline but, in

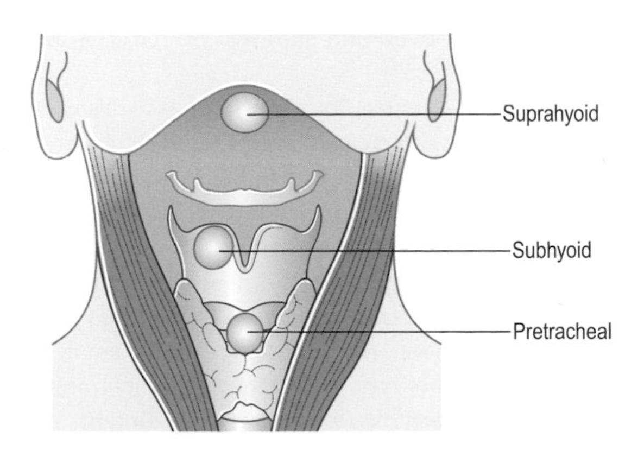

Figure 12.49 The sites of a thyroglossal cyst.

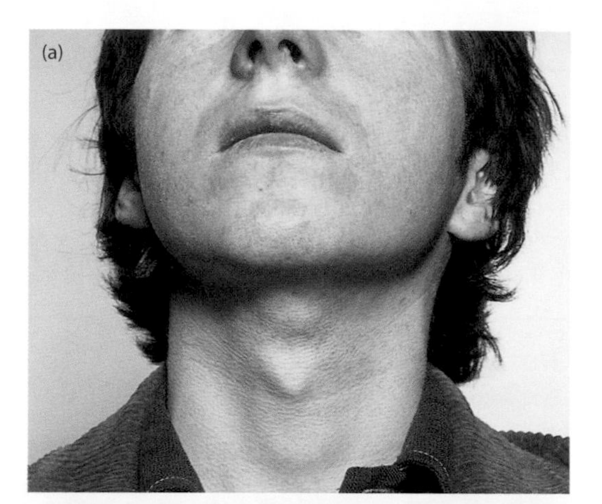

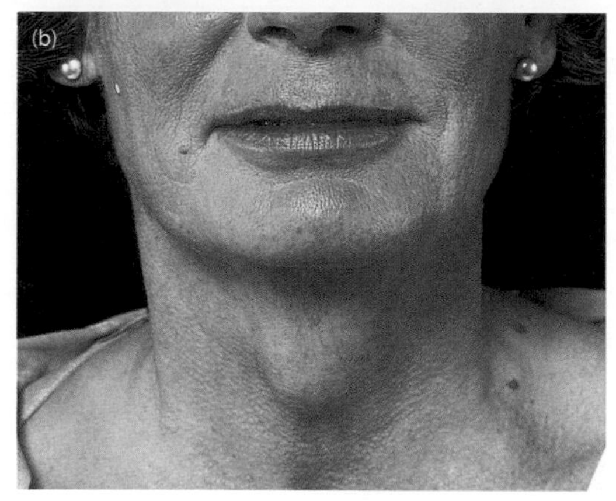

Figure 12.50 TWO THYROGLOSSAL CYSTS. (a) Subhyoid cyst. (b) Pretracheal cyst.

adult life, the cyst often slips to one side of the midline, especially if it develops in front of the thyroid cartilage.

Colour, temperature and tenderness If the cyst is infected, the overlying skin will be red, hot and tender (Figure 12.51).

Shape and surface Thyroglossal cysts are *spherical and smooth*, with a clearly defined edge.

Size They vary from 0.5 to 5 cm in diameter. Because a lump in the front of the neck is so noticeable, patients may present when cysts are small.

Composition Consistency depends upon the tension within the cyst and varies from *soft to hard*. Some cysts are too tense and others too small to fluctuate, but the *majority fluctuate*. Some transilluminate but many do not because the contents are thickened by desquamated epithelial cells or debris of past infection.

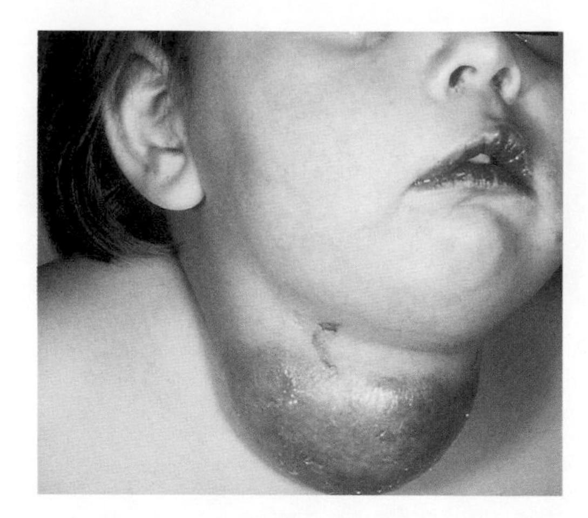

Figure 12.51 An infected thyroglossal cyst.

Relations Thyroglossal cysts are tethered by the remnant of the thyroglossal duct. This means that *they can be moved sideways but not up and down.*

The thyroglossal duct is always closely related to the hyoid bone. When the hyoid bone moves, the cyst moves. The hyoid bone moves upwards when the tongue is protruded. First, ask the patient to open their mouth and keep the lower jaw still; next, hold the cyst with your thumb and forefinger, and then ask the patient to *protrude their tongue*. If the cyst is fixed to the hyoid bone, you will feel it tugged upwards as the tongue goes out. This is a difficult sign to elicit so it is easier to feel the tugging sensation than actually to see movement. *Although this test is diagnostic, the absence of movement does not exclude the diagnosis.*

Local tissues Remember to examine the base of the tongue for ectopic (lingual) thyroid tissue. A lingual thyroid looks like a flattened strawberry sitting on the base of the tongue.

Lymph nodes should not be enlarged unless there is secondary infection, or rarely a thyroid cancer can present within a thyroglossal cyst.

THE THYROID

Symptoms of thyroid disease

The thyroid gland can causes symptoms and signs related to:

- Neck swelling.
- Endocrine dysfunction.

In order to appreciate fully the symptoms and signs that may be produced by diseases of the thyroid, a clear understanding of the physiology of the thyroid is essential. The history and examination should be directed towards detecting both the local and general symptoms and signs that may be produced.

NECK SYMPTOMS

A lump in the neck

The majority of thyroid swellings grow slowly and painlessly. Frequently, the patient will notice a swelling coincidentally when washing, or it will be pointed out to them by someone. Swellings may have been present for years before the patient seeks medical advice. Lumps can appear suddenly or a long-standing lump may change or enlarge. Examples include haemorrhage into a necrotic nodule, a fast-growing carcinoma or subacute thyroiditis (Revision panel 12.5).

Slow-growing thyroid cancers can be present as a static lump for several years before metastasis or local growth occurs. The length of time that a lump has been present is not a clear indication of its underlying nature.

Revision panel 12.5

SCHEME FOR THE DIAGNOSIS OF SWELLINGS IN THE NECK (DEEP TO THE DEEP FASCIA)

1. Is there one or more than one lump?
2. Where is the lump?
3. Is it solid or cystic?
4. Does it move with swallowing?

Multiple lumps are invariably lymph glands

A single lump

In the anterior triangle that does not move with swallowing

Solid:
- Lymph node
- Carotid body tumour

Cystic:
- Cold abscess
- Branchial cyst

In the posterior triangle that does not move with swallowing

Solid:
- Lymph node

Cystic:
- Cystic hygroma
- Pharyngeal pouch
- Occasionally, a secondary deposit of a papillary thyroid carcinoma

Pulsatile:
- Subclavian aneurysm

In the anterior triangle that moves with swallowing

Solid:
- Thyroid gland
- Thyroid isthmus lymph gland

Cystic:
- Thyroglossal cyst

Discomfort during swallowing

Large thyroid swellings may cause a tugging sensation in the neck with swallowing. This is not true dysphagia. Thyroid swellings are less likely to obstruct the oesophagus because it is a muscular tube that is easily stretched and pushed aside. However, because the thyroid has to be pulled upwards with the trachea in the first stage of deglutition, an enlarged gland can make swallowing uncomfortable.

Dyspnoea

An early symptom of tracheal impingement by a thyroid mass is a cough, frequently at night. Deviation or compression of the trachea may cause difficulty in breathing. This symptom is often worse when the neck is flexed or when the patient lies down. The whistling sound of air rushing through a narrowed trachea is called stridor.

Pain

Pain is not a common feature of thyroid swellings. Acute and subacute *thyroiditis* can present with a painful gland, and Hashimoto's disease often causes an uncomfortable ache in the neck.

Thyroid carcinoma can rarely cause local pain and pain referred to the ear if it infiltrates surrounding structures.

Hoarseness

A change in the quality of the voice of a patient with a lump in the neck is a very significant symptom because it may be the result of a paralysis of one of the recurrent laryngeal nerves, which means that the lump is likely to be malignant and infiltrating the nerve.

SYMPTOMS OF ENDOCRINE DYSFUNCTION

Patients with a thyroid disorder should be carefully questioned and examined for symptoms of endocrine dysfunction (Figure 12.52, Revision panel 12.6).

Symptoms of hyperthyroidism/thyrotoxicosis

Nervous system Symptoms include:

- nervousness
- irritability
- insomnia
- nervous instability
- a thyrotoxic psychosis may be present
- proximal muscle myopathies may occur with muscle wasting and weakness.

Cardiovascular system Symptoms include:

- palpitations
- breathlessness on exertion
- swelling of the ankles
- chest pain (may manifest as tachycardia, atrial fibrillation, dyspnoea and peripheral swelling).

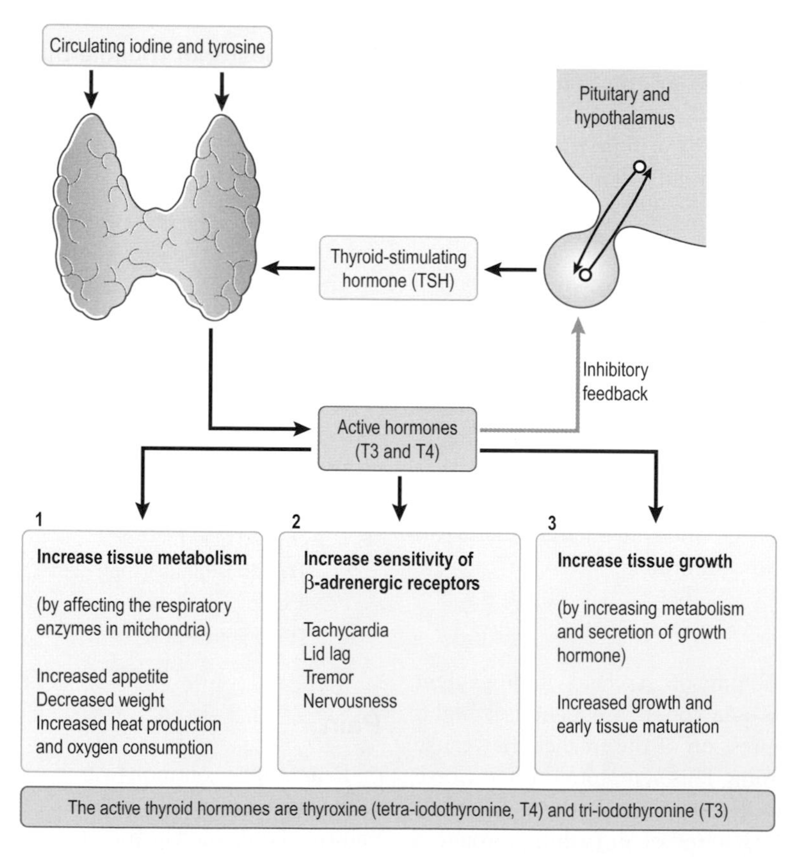

Figure 12.52 The physiology of the thyroid gland.

Revision panel 12.6

PHYSIOLOGY OF THE THYROID GLAND

Changes in hormone activity can be assessed by:

Clinical examination
Measuring thyroid stimulating hormone (TSH) and free tri-iodothyronine (FT3) and thyroxine (T4) levels
Measuring the rate and quantity and pattern of uptake of radio-labelled technetium or iodine

Hormone secretion can be suppressed by:

High-dose iodine transiently inhibits hormone release (Wolf Chaikoff effect)
Potassium perchlorate, which interferes with iodine trapping
Carbimazole and propylthiouracil, which inhibit the iodination of tyrosine and the coupling of tyrosines to make thyronines
Destroying the gland surgically or with radioiodine

Metabolic and alimentary systems There is:

- an increase in appetite but weight loss or absence of weight gain
- possible change of bowel habit, usually diarrhoea
- a preference for cold weather
- intolerance of hot weather
- excessive sweating
- some women have a change of menstruation, usually amenorrhoea.

Symptoms of hypothyroidism/ myxoedema

Symptoms include:

- increase in weight, with deposition of fat across the back of the neck and shoulders
- slow though, speech and action
- intolerance of cold weather
- loss of hair, especially the outer third of the eyebrow
- muscle fatigue
- a dry skin
- constipation.

Conditions of the thyroid gland

Concentrate on both the nature of any thyroid enlargement and changes in endocrine activity. It is best to assess both aspects together.

NOTE: Confirm that the swelling in the neck is in the thyroid gland by watching to see if it moves when the patient swallows.

All thyroid swellings ascend during swallowing. The patient may need a sip of water to help deglutition. Observe the general contours and surface of the swelling. The *skin can be tethered* and pulled up by swallowing in an advanced thyroid carcinoma that has infiltrated skin, although this is very uncommon.

Ask the patient to open their mouth and then to put out their tongue. If the lump moves up as the tongue comes out, it must be attached to the hyoid bone, and is likely to be a *thyroglossal cyst*.

The *neck veins will be distended* if there is a mass obstructing the thoracic inlet. Raising both arms above the head may cause venous compression at the inlet inducing facial redness (*Pemberton's sign*).

Look at the position of the thyroid cartilage. Is it in the centre of the neck or deviated to one side?

Then look at the whole patient.

NOTE: Are they sitting still and composed, or fidgeting about, and looking nervous and agitated, or are they slow and ponderous in their movements?

Are they thin or overweight? What is the distribution of any wasting or excess weight? Patients with thyrotoxicosis have a generalized loss of weight, especially about the face, but may also have *localized wasting of their hands, face and shoulder muscles.*

Are they *under-clothed and sweaty*, or wrapped up in a large number of jumpers but still cold?

LOOK AT THE HANDS

Feel the pulse. *Tachycardia* suggests thyrotoxicosis (hyperthyroidism); *bradycardia* suggests hypothyroidism. Thyrotoxicosis may cause atrial fibrillation – it may be the only sign in elderly patients.

Are the palms moist and sweaty?

Is there a tremor? Test for a tremor by asking the patient to hold their arms out in front of them, with the elbows and wrists straight, and fingers straight and separated. Thyrotoxicosis causes a *fine, fast tremor*. If in doubt, hold out your own hand beside the patient's for comparison. A fine tremor may be accentuated by placing a sheet of paper over the fingers.

EXAMINE THE EYES

Patients who suffer from thyrotoxicosis may complain of *staring* or *protruding eyes* and difficulty closing their eyelids (*exophthalmos*), double vision caused by muscle weakness (*ophthalmoplegia*) and swelling of the conjunctiva (*chemosis*). Very rarely, they get pain in the eye if the cornea ulcerates (see Revision panel 12.7). These are symptoms and signs that are pathognomonic for *Graves' disease*. They can be unilateral or bilateral. They are discussed in the section on Thyrotoxicosis (see page 437) (see Figures 12.53, 12.54). Lid retraction and lag can occur in any cause of thyrotoxicosis,

Revision panel 12.7

EYE SIGNS OF THYROTOXICOSIS

- Lid retraction and lid lag
- Exophthalmos, which also causes difficulty with convergence and absent forehead wrinkling when looking upwards
- Ophthalmoplegia, particularly of the superior rectus and inferior oblique muscles (cannot look 'up and out')
- Chemosis

Lid retraction and lid lag

Sensitization of sympathetic nerves carried via the IIIrd cranial nerve causes overactivity of the involuntary (smooth muscle) part of the levator palpabrae superioris muscle, resulting in lid lag and retraction. The patient has *lid retraction* if the upper eyelid is

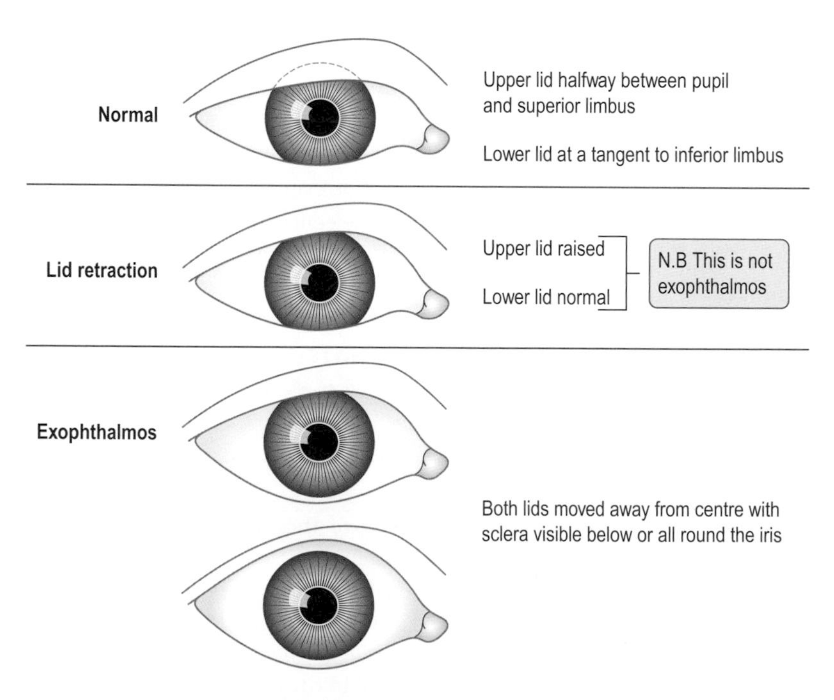

Figure 12.53 The relations of the eyelids to the iris.

higher than normal (midway between the pupil and the superior limbus of the iris) and the lower lid is in its correct position. Do not be deceived into thinking this abnormality is caused by exophthalmos. When the upper lid does not keep pace with the eyeball as it follows a finger moving from above downwards, the patient has *lid lag*.

Exophthalmos

The normal relationship of the eyelids to the iris is changed if the eyeball is pushed forwards by an increase in retro-orbital fat, oedema and cellular infiltration. The sclera becomes visible below the lower edge of the iris (the inferior limbus).

Ophthalmoplegia

The cause of the weakness of the ocular muscles (ophthalmoplegia) associated with severe exophthalmos is oedema and cellular infiltration affecting the muscles. The muscles most often affected are the superior rectus and inferior oblique muscles.

> **NOTE:** Weakness and tethering of these muscles prevents the patient looking upwards and outwards.

Chemosis

Chemosis is *oedema of the conjunctiva*. The normal conjunctiva is smooth and invisible. A thickened, crinkled, oedematous and slightly opaque conjunctiva is easy to recognize.

Chemosis is caused by the obstruction of normal venous and lymphatic drainage of the conjunctiva by increased retro-orbital pressure.

EXAMINE THE NECK

Palpate the neck from the front

> **NOTE:** The most important part of palpation is done from behind.

It is worthwhile placing your hand on any visible swelling while standing in front of the patient, to confirm your visual impression of its size, shape and surface, and to find out if it is tender.

Check the position of the trachea. This is best done by feeling with the tip of two fingers in the suprasternal notch. The trachea should be exactly central

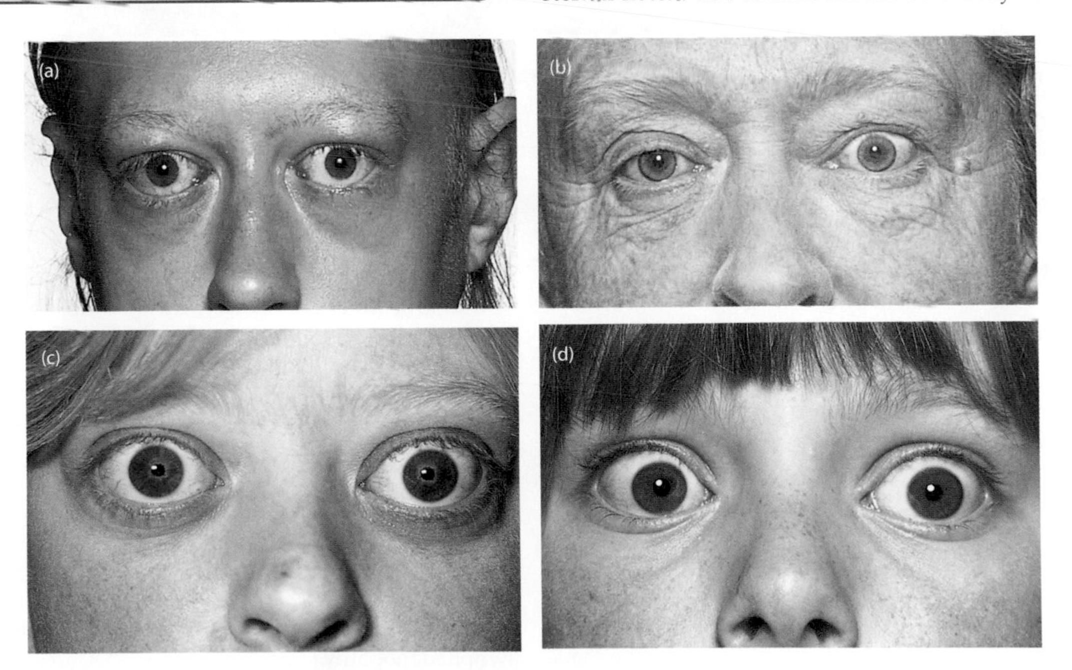

Figure 12.54 SOME EYE SIGNS ASSOCIATED WITH THYROTOXICOSIS. (a) Exophthalmos. (b) Unilateral lid retraction. (c) Exophthalmos and lid retraction. (d) Severe lid retraction but no exophthalmos. *(Continued)*

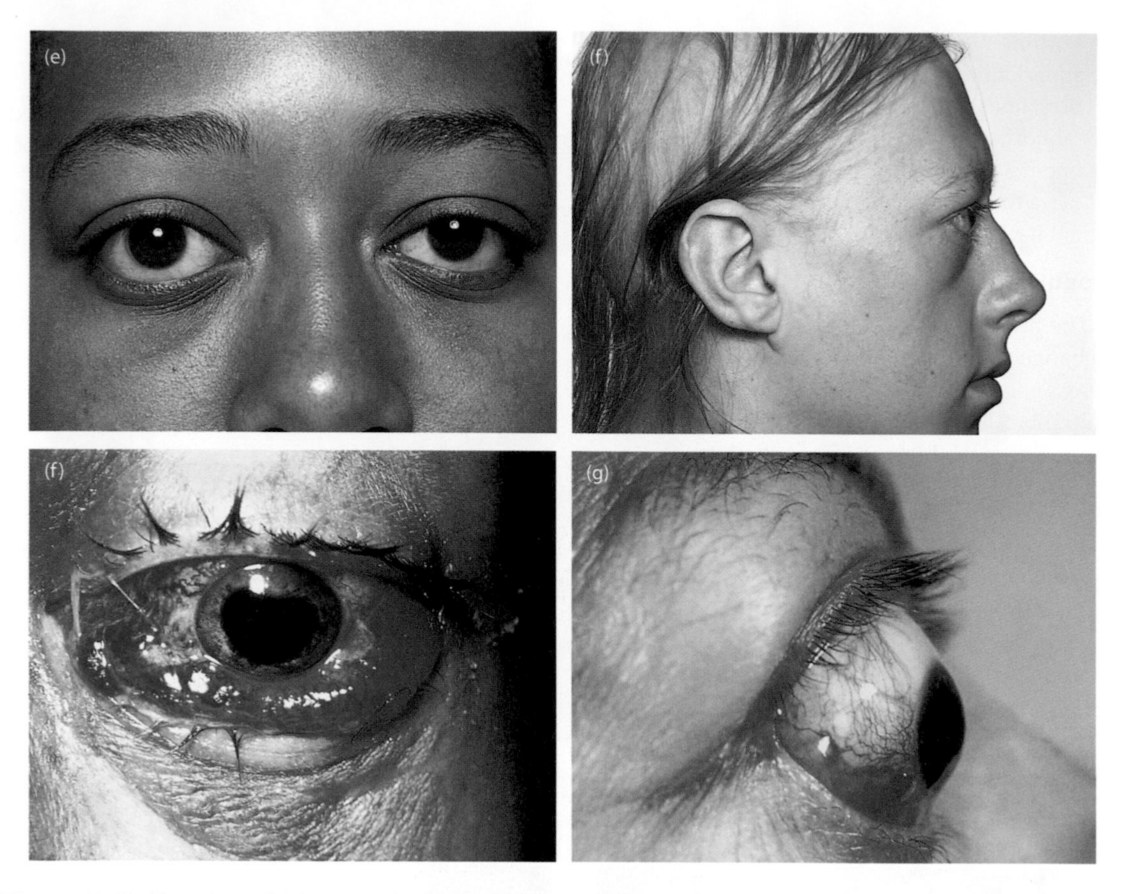

Figure 12.54 (Continued) SOME EYE SIGNS ASSOCIATED WITH THYROTOXICOSIS. (e) Exophthalmos but no lid retraction. (f) Wasting and loss of hair (and exophthalmos). (g) Chemosis. The conjunctiva is hyperaemic and bulging over the eyelid. There is exophthalmos, lid retraction and periorbital oedema. (h) This patient had gross chemosis and exophthalmos but the eye was pulsating. The cause of these abnormalities was a carotid artery–cavernous sinus fistula.

at this point. When a thyroid mass extends below the suprasternal notch and obscures the trachea, you must examine the thyroid cartilage. A mass that is displacing the trachea will tilt the thyroid cartilage laterally.

Palpate the neck from behind the patient (Figure 12.55)

Stand behind the patient. Place your thumbs on the ligamentum nuchae and tilt the patient's head slightly forwards to relax the anterior neck muscles. Let the palmar surface of your fingers rest on each side of the neck; they will be resting on the lateral lobes of the thyroid gland. A small lobe can be made prominent and easier to feel by pressing firmly on the opposite side of the neck.

Ask the patient to swallow while you are palpating the gland to confirm that the swelling moves and is part of the thyroid, again the patient may need a sip of water. This manoeuvre also lifts up lumps that are lying behind the sternum into the reach of your fingers.

NOTE: It is important to assess whether you can feel the lower border of the thyroid on swallowing or whether significant retrosternal extension remains.

Palpate the neck for cervical and supraclavicular lymphadenopathy.

Following palpation, you should be able to describe the thyroid/lump and any cervical

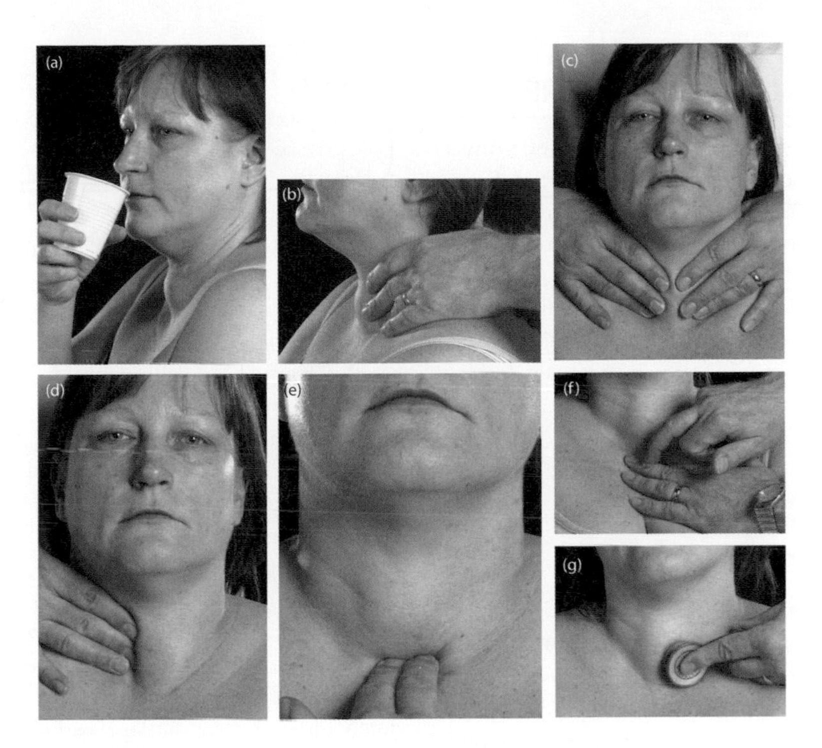

Figure 12.55 EXAMINATION OF THE THYROID GLAND. (a) Look at the eyes and the neck and ask the patient to swallow. (b) Palpate the neck from behind, with the thumbs pushing the head forwards to flex the neck slightly. (c) Palpate both lobes and the isthmus with the fingers flat. (d) If one lobe is difficult to feel, make it more prominent by pressing firmly on the opposite side. (e) Feel the trachea. (f) Percuss the lower limit of the gland. (g) Listen over the gland for a systolic bruit.

lymphadenopathy: location (diffuse, solitary or multiple); tenderness, shape; size; surface; consistency.

PERCUSSION

Percussion is used to define the lower extent of a swelling that extends below the suprasternal notch by percussing along the clavicles and over the sternum and upper chest wall (Figure 12.55). This can be done when standing in front of or behind the patient. Percussion is not an overly reliable assessment of the extent of a retrosternal goitre. Inability to get below the thyroid by palpation during swallow is a better clinical indicator of significant retrosternal extension. Percussion of the lump in the neck itself is rarely helpful.

AUSCULTATION

Listen over the swelling. Thyrotoxic and vascular glands and lumps may have a systolic bruit (Figure 12.55).

GENERAL EXAMINATION

Pay particular attention to the cardiovascular and nervous systems for evidence of hyperthyroidism or hypothyroidism, the signs and symptoms of which are described above.

Revision panel 12.8

PLAN FOR THE EXAMINATION OF A PATIENT WITH A GOITRE

- Inspect the **neck** to check for goitre
- Look at the **whole patient** for agitation, nervousness or lethargy
- Examine the **hands** for sweating, tremor and tachycardia
- Examine the **eyes** for exophthalmos, lid lag, ophthalmoplegia and chemosis
- Examine the **neck**: always check that the lump moves with swallowing
- Palpate the **cervical lymph nodes**

SIMPLE HYPERPLASTIC GOITRE AND MULTINODULAR GOITRE

Simple enlargement of the thyroid gland is invariably caused by excess stimulation with TSH. Several causes are recognized that produce a relative deficiency in iodine for increased TSH hormone production. *Frequently, the underlying cause in a given patient is unknown.* An initial diffuse thyroid hyperplasia (*hyperplastic goitre*) may progress through areas of focal hyperplasia, combined with necrosis, haemorrhage and scarring to the development of nodules (*multinodular goitre*).

Causes of hyperplastic and multinodular goitre

1. *Iodine deficiency*: dietary deficiency still occurs in certain geographic areas, e.g. central Africa, central Asia. Iodination of salt has reduced the incidence in many countries.
2. *Physiological demand*: usually diffuse hyperplasia transiently during puberty and pregnancy.
3. *Goitrogens:*
   Dietary, e.g. found in cassava and cabbage (especially when combined with iodine deficiency).
   Medication, e.g. amiodarone, lithium.
4. *Defects in thyroid hormone synthesis pathway.* Defects in many steps of the pathway have been identified, e.g. impaired transport of iodine.
5. *Genetic mutations*, e.g. PDS gene; Pendred's syndrome (goitre associated with deafness).

Hyperplastic goitre

History

Age In areas where goitre is endemic, hyperplastic goitres appear in childhood.

Sporadic physiological hyperplastic goitres appear at puberty, during pregnancy and during severe illnesses and emotional disturbances.

Sex Hyperplastic goitres are five times more common in females.

Local symptoms The principal complaint is of a *swelling in the neck*. This appears slowly and without pain.

NOTE: A large goitre can cause pressure symptoms such as dyspnoea, venous engorgement and mild discomfort during swallowing.

General symptoms Patients are usually euthyroid.

Examination

Position The swelling occupies the anatomical site of the thyroid gland.

Tenderness It is not tender.

Shape The swelling usually follows the configuration of the gland and can be seen to have two lobes and an isthmus.

Size Physiological goitres are only two or three times larger than a normal gland, but iodine-deficiency goitres can become very large.

Surface The surface of a hyperplastic goitre is smooth (Figure 12.56a). Its surface becomes bosselated and, in time, nodular. The late stage of a hyperplastic goitre can be termed 'colloid goitre' but, in clinical practice, the terms colloid and multinodulatr goitre are interchangeable.

Composition The gland feels firm. Hyperaemic physiological goitres may have a very soft systolic bruit.

Relations The gland moves upon swallowing. The other tissues in the neck should be normal.

Lymph nodes The deep cervical lymph nodes should not be palpable.

The eyes The eyes should be normal.

General examination The patient is usually euthyroid.

Multinodular goitre

Multinodular goitres may develop from a hyperplastic picture and can, therefore, be *endemic* (in iodine-deficient areas) or *sporadic*. Genetic defects may be responsible for goitre formation e.g. Pendred's syndrome. Mutations in the PDS gene cause deafness in childhood and a high frequency (75%) of subsequent multinodular goitre.

A nodular goitre results from a disorganized response of the gland to stimulation, and contains areas of both hyperplasia and hypoplasia. Nodules coalesce, rupture and fibrosis occurs, making the

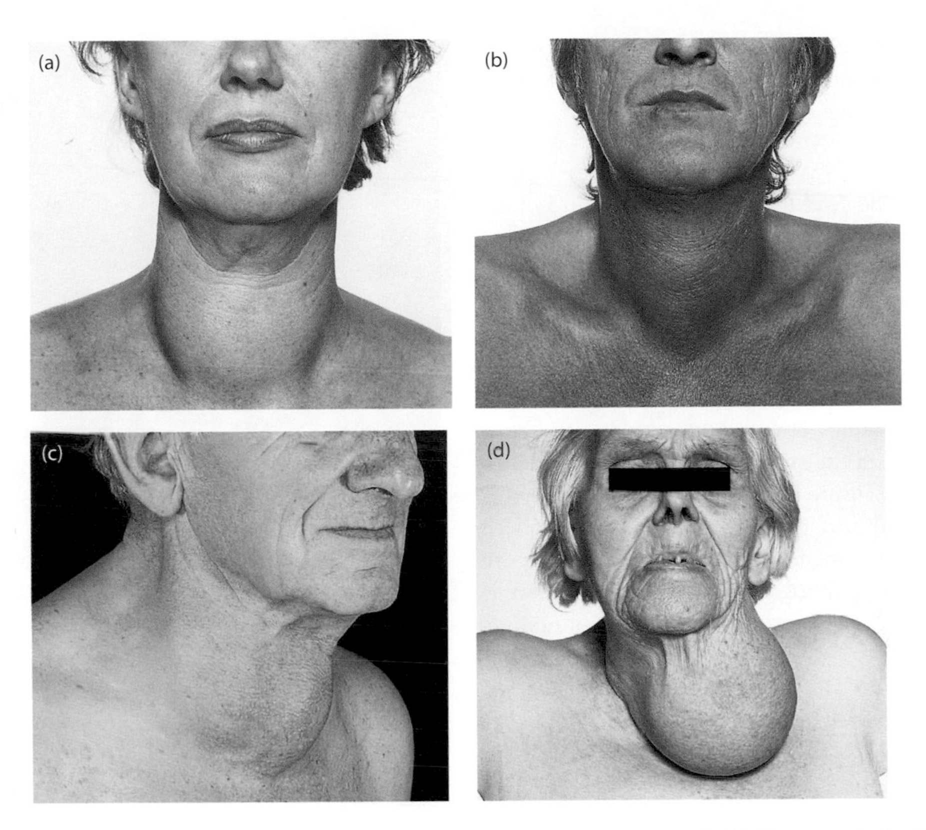

Figure 12.56 VARIOUS GOITRES. (a) A large colloid goitre. The patient was euthyroid. (b) A large central solitary nodule. (c) A nodular goitre extending below the sternum and causing venous obstruction. Distended veins are visible above the right clavicle. The patient was euthyroid. (d) Beware! Not all lumps in the neck are thyroid swellings. This mass was soft and did not move with swallowing. It was a lipoma. Never make a spot diagnosis; examine every lump carefully and thoroughly.

process irreversible. The cut surface of a nodular goitre reveals nodules with haemorrhagic necrotic centres separated by normal tissue.

> **NOTE:** Multinodular goitres tend to gradually enlarge over time in the path of least resistance.

Growth can be anterior, superior, posterior or inferior extending to the superior mediastinum, or a combination growth pattens can be seen. A large goitre may, therefore, be clinically obvious or 'hidden'.

History

Age In endemic areas, nodular goitres appear in early adult life (15–30 years). Sporadic nodular goitres appear later, between the ages of 25 and 40 years.

Sex Nodular goitres are six times more common in females.

Geography Goitres are common in areas where the drinking water is deficient in iodine.

Symptoms The most common presenting symptom is an *enlarging, painless swelling in the neck*, which may cause dyspnoea, discomfort when swallowing, stridor and engorged neck veins.

> **NOTE:** Sudden enlargement and pain can occur if there is haemorrhage into a necrotic nodule.

The majority of patients with multinodular goitre are euthyroid. Long-standing goitres can occasionally develop secondary thyrotoxicosis (*Plummer's syndrome*). Typically, this occurs in the elderly and may be triggered by the administration of iodine-containing contrast in medical imaging. Toxic multinodular goitre is the commonest cause of thyrotoxicosis in those over 60 years of age.

Examination

Position The swelling is in the lower third of the neck in the anatomical site of the thyroid gland and is usually asymmetrical.

Tenderness A nodular goitre is only tender when there has been a recent haemorrhage into a nodule.

Shape and size *The nodules are asymmetrical and the gland can become any shape.* Nodules in the isthmus are prominent. The nodules may extend below the clavicles and the sternal notch, into the superior mediastinum (Figure 12.56c).

Surface The surface of a nodular goitre is smooth but nodular. Frequently, only one nodule may be palpable, even although the rest of the gland is grossly diseased. This is termed a 'dominant nodule' (Figure 12.56b).

Composition The consistency of nodules varies: some feel hard, others feel soft.

> **Note:** There is an old saying that 'solid lumps in the thyroid feel cystic, whereas cystic lumps feel solid'.

Thyroid tissue is soft, whereas a nodule full of blood and liquefied necrotic tissue is tense and feels hard.

The nodules do not fluctuate or transilluminate.

There should be no bruit over the gland.

Relations As with all thyroid swellings, the lump will move up during swallowing, indicating that it is fixed to the trachea. It should not be fixed to any other nearby structures.

Local tissues *The trachea may be compressed and/or deviated.* Bilateral nodules may compress the trachea into a narrow slit, causing dyspnoea and stridor, exacerbated by neck flexion. Large unilateral nodules push the trachea laterally.

When the trachea is pushed to one side, the 'keel' of the larynx is tilted away from the midline.

If the gland is jammed in the thoracic inlet, it may obstruct and distend the jugular veins.

Rarely, the goitre is so large that it starts to cause pressure on the overlying skin and may even start to ulcerate through (Figure 12.57).

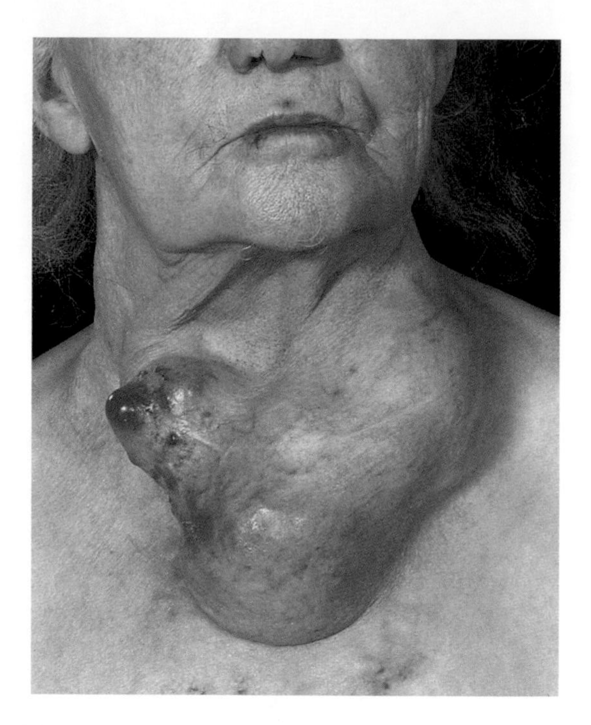

Figure 12.57 A large goitre causing skin changes and imminent ulceration.

Lymph nodes The cervical lymph nodes should not be palpable.

Eyes The eyes should be normal. Lid lag and lid retraction may occur with marked thyrotoxicosis.

General examination The majority are euthyroid. There may be signs of thyrotoxicosis, particularly cardiovascular signs in the elderly with a toxic goitre.

The nature of a multinodular goitre is evaluated as per the solitary thyroid nodule (below). Clinical suspicion of tracheal compression or retrosternal extent is further evaluated with CT scans.

THE SOLITARY NODULE (Figure 12.56b)

> **NOTE:** Although only one nodule may be palpable, many patients presenting with a solitary nodule actually have a multinodular goitre, i.e. a clinically dominant nodule in a macroscopical multinodular goitre (Revision panel 12.9).

Revision panel 12.9

CAUSES OF A 'SOLITARY' MODULE IN THE THYROID GLAND

A dominant nodule in a multinodular goitre
Haemorrhage into a nodule
A cyst
Adenoma
Carcinoma (papillary, follicular or medullary)
Enlargement of the whole of one lobe (usually Hashimoto's disease)

It is not possible to confirm the pathological nature of a solitary nodule by clinical examination. *Although the majority of solitary nodules are benign, they must all be investigated.* Within a multinodular thyroid, the clinically dominant nodule may not be the 'suspicious' nodule on further evaluation.

Ultrasound scan is the key investigation of palpable and non-palpable thyroid nodules, remaining thyroid tissue and lymph nodes. Thyroid nodules are risk stratified using ultrasound criteria. Nodules at increased risk of malignancy are further assessed with ultrasound-guided fine needle aspiration for cytology.

THYROTOXICOSIS

This is the clinical syndrome that results from exposure to elevated circulating levels of thyroid hormones. Hyperthyroidism refers to thyrotoxicosis from overproduction of thyroid hormones by thyroid follicular cells. 95% are the result of three causes (Table 12.1):

- Graves' disease – 70%.
- Toxic multinodular goitre – 20%.
- Toxic solitary adenoma – 5%.

Graves' disease is an autoimmune condition that occurs in all age groups. Stimulatory antibodies to the TSH receptor (TRAb) are present in the sera of 90% of patients and cause unregulated overproduction of thyroid hormone. Extrathyroidal manifestations include:

1. Eye manifestations (*ophthalmopathy*).
2. Skin (*dermopathy*): pretibial myxoedema.
3. *Acropachy*: clubbing.
4. *Lymphoid hyperplasia.*

Table 12.1 Causes of thyrotoxicosis

Cause	%
Thyrotoxicosis (overproduction)	
Graves' disease	70%
Toxic multinodular goitre	20%
Toxic nodule	5%
Iodine induced	<1%
TSH secreting pituitary adenoma	<1%
Associated with thyroid destruction	
Subacute thyroiditis	3%
Silent thyroiditis	3%
Amiodarone induced (Type 2)	<1%
Non-thyroidal origin – all very rare	
Factitious	
Struma ovarii	
Metastatic thyroid cancer	

The thyroid hormones T3 and T4 have three effects:

- They increase the metabolic rate of all cells.
- They increase the sensitivity of ß-adrenergic receptors.
- They stimulate all cells to grow, but the effect on growth is only significant before natural growth has finished.

The increased tissue metabolism causes an *increased appetite, a decrease in weight and an increase in heat production.*

The increased adrenergic receptor sensitivity causes *tachycardia, extrasystoles, atrial fibrillation, tremor, nervousness, lid retraction and lid lag.*

Stimulation of growth during childhood produces early maturation and a slight increase in the rate of growth.

In hypothyroidism, all of these symptoms are reversed. The lack of growth stimulation in a child causes short stature and impacts mental development (IQ).

History

Age Graves' disease typically affects women, with peak incidence aged 20–40 years.

Toxic autonomous nodules can occur at any age.

Toxic multinodular goitre typically occurs in those over 45 years of age and is the commonest cause of hyperthyroidism in patients over 60 years age.

Sex Graves' disease is ten times more common in females.

Metabolic symptoms An *increased appetite* is common, but, despite this, patients either lose weight or do not gain weight.

Patients *may feel hot and prefer cold weather* and dislike warm weather.

There may be *excessive sweating.*

Cardiovascular symptoms The patient may have *palpitations, shortness of breath* during exertion, and *tiredness.*

Neurological symptoms Symptoms such as *nervousness, irritability, insomnia,* depression and excitement, may be noticed by family long before the patient is aware of them.

There may be *hyperaesthesia, headaches, vertigo* and *tremors of the hands and tongue.*

The patient may complain that their eyes have become more protuberant and that some eye movements are difficult.

Alimentary symptoms There may be *increased bowel frequency and mild diarrhoea.*

Genital tract symptoms *Oligomenorrhea* or *amenorrhoea* are common.

Musculoskeletal symptoms In addition to generalized weight loss, there may be specific wasting and weakness of the small muscles of the hand, shoulder and face.

Examination

Signs in the neck

The *thyroid gland is usually enlarged,* but hyperthyroidism can be present without significant enlargement of the gland.

The enlargement may be diffuse, nodular or tender, depending on the pathology (Figure 12.58).

A diffusely enlarged hyperaemic gland usually has a *systolic bruit audible over its lateral lobes.*

Signs in the eye

Thyrotoxicosis is associated with four groups of physical signs in the eyes (see Figures 12.53, 12.54)

Specific Graves' disease ophthalmopathy is thought to be the result of an immune response to retro-orbital antigens similar to the thyroid, or cross reactivity of TRAb to TSH receptors present on fibroblasts and adipocytes within the retro-ocular tissues. Resulting inflammation, oedema and fibrosis affects the retro-orbital tissue and ocular muscles. There is an association with smoking (frequency and severity of symptoms).

Exophthalmos, ophthalmoplegia and chemosis are specific eye signs of Graves' disease; 30% of patients with Graves' disease have eye signs that are pathognomonic for Graves' disease. Signs can be unilateral.

Lid retraction and lid lag These are common signs (see page 432). Ask the patient to follow your finger as you move it slowly from above, downwards. If the upper eyelid does not keep pace with the eye, the patient has *lid lag.* The patient may also blink less frequently than normal.

Exophthalmos/proptosis Oedema of the retro-orbital tissues pushes the eye forwards. The first abnormality is the appearance of sclera below the inferior limbus but, when the condition is extreme, the eye appears to be popping out and the eyelids cannot be completely closed.

Exophthalmos makes convergence difficult and allows the patient to look up without raising their eyebrows or wrinkling their forehead. Corneal ulceration may complicate severe exophthalmos.

Ophthalmoplegia Infiltration of the ocular muscles weakens the eye muscles and diminishes the eye movements. The muscles most often affected are the superior rectus and inferior oblique muscles. As these muscles normally turn the eye upwards and outwards, this is the first movement to become weak.

Chemosis Obstruction of normal venous and lymphatic drainage of the conjunctiva by increased retro-orbital pressure causes the conjunctiva to become oedematous, thick, boggy and crinkled and may bulge over the eyelids. The eyes water excessively.

General signs

These are best described in systems.

Metabolic signs The patient looks thin and their face and hands may be particularly wasted. They may look hot and be sweating, even in a cold room.

Cardiovascular signs There is usually a tachycardia > 90 beats per minute.

The pulse will be irregular if there are extrasystoles or atrial fibrillation.

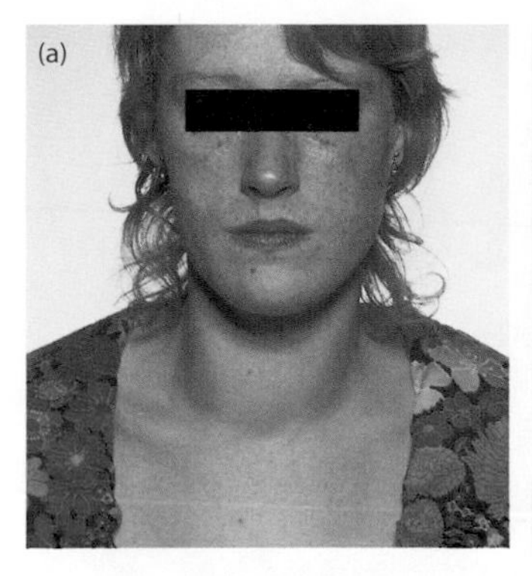

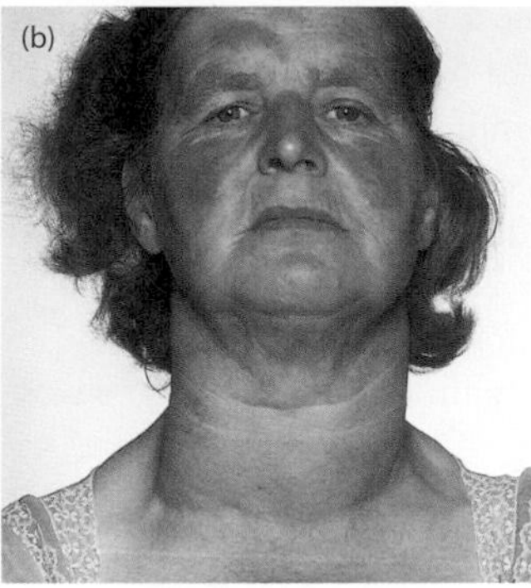

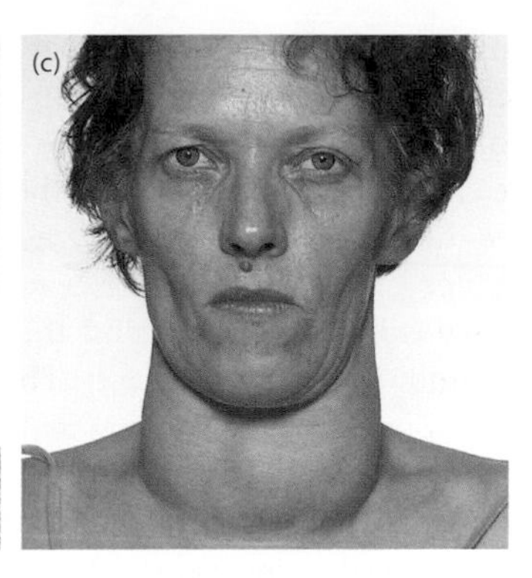

Figure 12.58 THE VARIED APPEARANCES OF THYROTOXICOSIS. (a) A small goitre, nervousness and agitation, with the start of weight loss. (b) A nodular goitre. No eye or nervous system signs, but palpitations, breathlessness and atrial fibrillation. (c) A large goitre, increasing appetite but weight loss – particularly of the face and shoulder girdle – with no eye signs.

If there is mild heart failure, there may be râles at the bases of the lungs and oedema of the ankles.

Neurological signs The patient looks worried and nervous and moves in an agitated, jerky way.

A *fine tremor* may be demonstrated when they stretch out their hands with their fingers spread. A similar tremor may be present in the protruded tongue.

Musculoskeletal signs The muscles of the hands, shoulders and face may be wasted and weak and the fingertips enlarged.

Skin Pretibial myxoedema This is is a *violaceous, non-pitting induration of pretibial skin* that occurs in 1–5% of patients with Graves' disease. Skin biopsy reveals mucin in the lower dermis with overlying epidermal thickening (hyperkeratosis) (Figure 12.59).

HYPOTHYROIDISM AND MYXOEDEMA

History

Hypothyroidism is the term used to describe the deficiency of thyroid hormone and is common in clinical practice. The prevalence of hypothyroidism in the UK is around 2% and is 10 times more common in women. A further 6–8% have subclinical hypothyroidsim (raised TSH but normal T3 and T4). Severe *hypothyroidism/myxoedema is the clinical state* that follows a chronic severe lack of thyroid hormone, which today is uncommon. The term myxoedema means 'mucous swelling' and was first described as it was believed that the increase in weight and body swelling was caused by a new form of oedema. Hypothyroidism can be a result of:

- a primary thyroid disorder
- autoimmune thyroid disease
- following treatment for hyperthyroidism (surgery and radioiodine)
- thyroidectomy for benign and malignant thyroid disease.

Congenital hypothyroidism affects 1 in 1500 births Secondary causes include pituitary disease with low production of TSH.

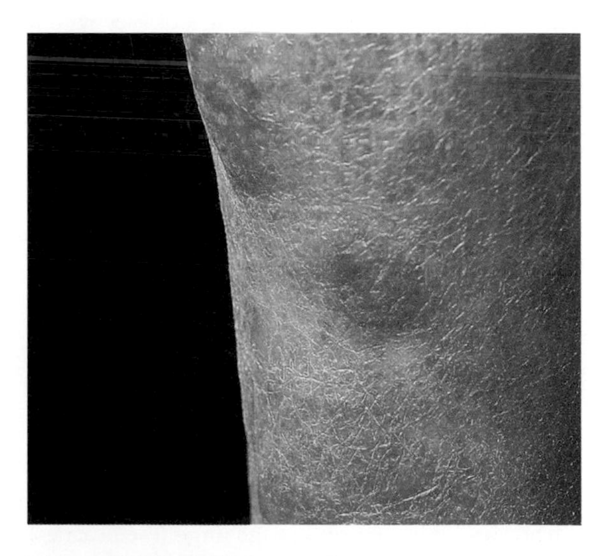

Figure 12.59 Pretibial myxoedema.

Metabolic symptoms The patient complains of *tiredness and weakness*, which can lead to intense physical and mental lethargy. These symptoms may come on insidiously and, therefore the patient simply ascribes their symptoms to their age or the everyday pace of life.

The *patient may feel cold*, and therefore like hot weather and dislike cold weather. They gain weight but have a poor appetite.

Cardiovascular symptoms *Breathlessness* and *ankle swelling* indicate the onset of cardiac failure.

Neurological symptoms The patient finds it difficult to think and to speak quickly and clearly. *Hallucinations, dementia* ('myxoedema madness') and, in severe cases, 'myxoedema coma' can occur.

Alimentary symptoms Constipation is common.

Genital tract symptoms Menorrhagia is common

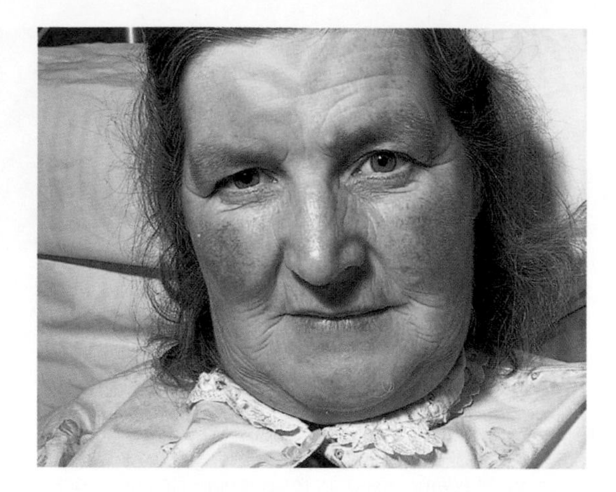

Figure 12.60 The facies of myxoedema. Thinning of the hair, loss of the outer third of the eyebrows, a 'peaches and cream' complexion and thickening and heaviness of the eyelids.

Examination

Signs in the neck

The thyroid gland may be enlarged by long-standing disease such as a nodular goitre but, in many cases, the neck is normal. The thyroid may be small, firm and atrophic in long-standing Hashimoto's thyroiditis, consistent with a 'burnt out' gland. There may be a scar suggesting previous thyroid surgery.

Signs in the eyes

The eyes are normal but the *eyelids become swollen and heavy*, making the patient look sleepy and lethargic.

The *hair of the outer third of the eyebrows falls out*.

General signs

Hypothyroidism may be detected on biochemical testing before the physical signs of hypothyroidism occur. Today, most patients seek medical advice at an early stage. Chronic severe hypothyroidism/myxoedema produces a *puffy face*, a generalized, non-pitting increase in the subcutaneous tissues of the trunk and limbs and a *dulling of thought, speech and action*. In a white-skinned patient with myxoedema, the *complexion is said to resemble 'peaches and cream'*. The skin is smooth and has a pale-yellow (the cream) colour. The cheeks are often slightly flushed and have a pink-orange tinge (the peaches) (Figure 12.60).

The skin is dry and inelastic and does not sweat. Although it may look oedematous, it does not pit after prolonged pressure.

The patient is *overweight*, with excess connective tissue and fat in the supraclavicular fossae, across the back of the neck and over the shoulders.

The *hair is thin and falls out*.

The *hands are puffy and spade-like*.

The *tongue enlarges* and seems to fill the mouth during speech and interferes with the articulation of words. The voice becomes deep and hoarse.

All the signs of myxoedema may develop insidiously and may not always be obvious; therefore, they must be looked for carefully if a hypothyroid state is suspected (Figure 12.61).

Cardiovascular signs The *pulse rate is slow* (40–60 beats per minute) and the *blood pressure is low*. Both these changes may be reversed if heart failure develops.

The hands are usually cold and the *fingertips blue*.

Neurological signs Mental alertness and the ability to respond to questions and solve problems are noticeably retarded. Conversation is hampered by the difficulty in articulation caused by enlargement of the tongue.

All movements are slow and deliberate.

The *reflexes are sluggish and their relaxation period prolonged*.

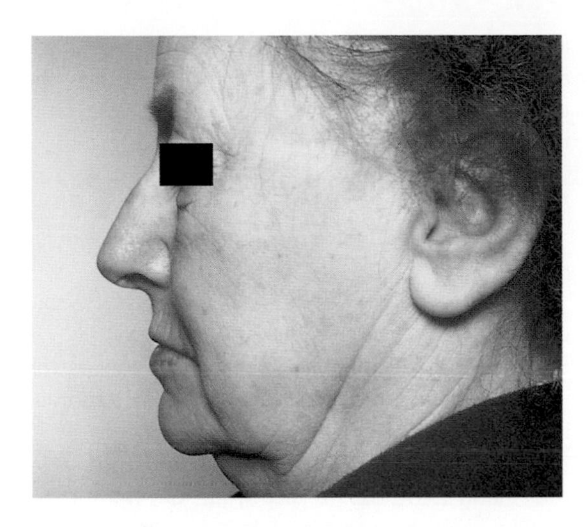

Figure 12.61 This woman has myxoedema. There is some loss of hair, especially the outer third of the eyebrows, and heaviness of the face and creamy skin, but none of these features is diagnostic. This emphasizes that early myxoedema is difficult to recognize.

CONGENITAL IODINE DEFICIENCY SYNDROME (FORMERLY *CRETINISM*)

Untreated neonatal and childhood hypothyroidism causes *stunting of mental and physical development*. Today, this condition is very rare because the hormone deficiency can be replaced. There is routine screening for hypothyroidism in women antenatally, and for the newborn.

Congenital iodine deficiency syndrome can still occur in those places where goitre remains endemic. The child may have a goitre.

NOTE: The child has an underdeveloped skeleton and a large protruding tongue, the eyes are wide apart, and the skull is also wide. The limbs and neck are short and the hands spade-like.

The skin is dry and there are supraclavicular pads of fat.

The abdomen is *distended and protruberant*, and there is often an *umbilical hernia*.

The child has a *reduced IQ*.

There has been a worldwide increase in thyroid cancer, primarily because of the increased detection of small subclinical nodules on high-quality ultrasound. The best treatment for some of these tiny lesions is under debate.

The thyroid gland is a very vascular organ, and secondary tumour deposits from primary lesions such as the kidney, melanoma, breast, colon and lung can be found at autopsy. These secondary deposits rarely become large and noticeable and rarely present as a thyroid swelling.

Increasingly, secondary deposits and small subclinical primary cancers are incidentally detected on PET scanning during oncology follow up.

NOTE: The majority of the neoplasms in the thyroid gland that present as a lump in the neck are primary thyroid tumours.

There are three varieties of carcinoma of the thyroid follicular cells:

- Papillary carcinoma.
- Follicular carcinoma.
- Anaplastic carcinoma.

The first two are 'well differentiated' thyroid cancers. This means that the majority maintain thyroid function and take up iodine. Anaplastic cancer is an undifferentiated malignancy and does not take up iodine or function like usual thyroid cells.

The parafollicular (C) cells can undergo malignant change, leading to *medullary thyroid carcinoma*.

Lymphoid tissue within the thyroid can undergo malignant change to become a *lymphoma*.

This is more common in patients with Hashimoto's disease.

PAPILLARY CARCINOMA

This is the *commonest thyroid cancer* and two-thirds are confined to the thyroid at presentation.

It spreads to local *lymph nodes*. The cervical lymph glands may be palpable long before the primary lesion in the thyroid gland becomes palpable. *30–50% of tumours are multifocal.*

A preoperative diagnosis can be made for classical papillary thyroid carcinoma on fine needle aspiration cytology (Thy5) due to distinctive cytological features: nuclear inclusions and grooves, papillary formations, absence of colloid.

Histology: Growth pattern is typically finger-like papillary structures with nuclear characteristics similar to cytology. Psammoma bodies are present in 50%.

FOLLICULAR CARCINOMA

This spreads via the haematogenous route. Ultrasound scan show a suspicious nodule and fine needle aspiration is reported as indeterminate follicular lesion (Thy3F).

A definitive cytological diagnosis is not possible in local disease because distinguishing between a benign follicular adenoma and a follicular cancer requires histological detail of capsular and vascular invasion.

History

Age Papillary thyroid carcinoma occurs in children and young adults. The mean age of presentation is 35–45 years.

Follicular thyroid carcinoma has an older mean age at presentation of 40–60 years.

Sex Females are affected more than males for both types; 70–75% of all cases.

Symptoms The common presenting symptom is a *lump in the neck*. The lump may be in the region of the thyroid gland or there may be *secondary deposits* in the *cervical lymph glands*. Lymph node metastases are common in papillary thyroid carcinoma but rare in follicular thryoid carcinoma, affecting less than 10% of patients.

The patient may complain of breathlessness, or pain or swelling in a bone, caused by lung and bone metastases.

Duration of symptoms This is variable. Typically, patients have just become aware of a lump or have a lump that has been growing over some months. Palpable nodules that the patient was unaware of are now often detected on health screening ultrasound. Patients with metastatic follicular carcinoma may present with a pathological fracture.

Cause There is a greater incidence of papillary carcinoma *in children who have had their neck or chest irradiated* intentionally for conditions such as asthma, TB, enlargement of the thymus, tonsillitis and acne (a treatment no longer practised), or unintentionally following a nuclear reactor accident. It is important to ask about this.

Examination

The principal abnormality is a *lump or lumps in the neck*.

Position The lump is in the region of the thyroid gland or deep to the sternomastoid muscle.

Temperature and tenderness The skin of the neck should be normal, provided there is no tumour infiltration. The lumps are usually not tender.

Shape and size The primary nodule in the thyroid gland may vary in size from less than 1 cm, impalpable nodule to a nodule >5 cm in diameter. When palpable, it is usually *spherical, smooth* and *clearly defined*, but its surface may be bosselated. The lump may present as a *dominant nodule* in a multinodular goitre.

Composition The consistency of both the primary nodule and the secondary lymph nodes is firm or hard.

Relations The primary nodule in the thyroid gland moves upon swallowing and is not usually fixed to superficial structures unless there is local invasion.

Enlarged lymph nodes move more easily in a transverse than in a vertical plane and do not move with swallowing.

Lymph nodes All the lymph nodes in the neck must be examined with care if a nodule is felt in the thyroid gland.

Lymph nodes containing thyroid carcinoma metastases are ovoid or nodular, and usually smooth and clearly defined. Occasionally they may be cystic. The thyroid gland lymph drains to the pretracheal and paratracheal lymph nodes and then to the *lower deep cervical lymph nodes*, which lie beneath the anterior edge of the lower third of the sternomastoid muscle.

General examination The patient usually appears well, without systemic signs to suggest a disseminated neoplasm or thyroid dysfunction.

Examine the chest carefully for any evidence of consolidation or collapse. Pulmonary secondary deposits are quite common but may not cause abnormal physical signs.

Metastases in the skeleton may be painful and tender, and rarely may be visibly deformed, swollen and hot. Some thyroid cancer metastases are so vascular that they are soft and pulsatile and have an audible bruit.

ANAPLASTIC CARCINOMA

This is the most aggressive variety of thyroid cancer, rapidly infiltrating local structures and obstructing the trachea. Most patients with this cancer die within months of diagnosis. Its cells do not synthesize thyroid hormone, and it is frequently inoperable and non-responsive to radioiodine treatment.

History

Age Anaplastic carcinoma typically affects the elderly, between *60–80 years of age*.

Sex Females are affected more often than males.

Symptoms The common complaint is of a *rapidly enlarging neck swelling* rather than 'a lump', because the tumour is diffuse and infiltrating.

A dull *aching pain* in the neck is quite common.

Dyspnoea occur when the tumour compresses the trachea and may also be the result of multiple pulmonary metastases.

Dysphagia occurs when the oesophagus is compressed or locally invaded.

Hoarseness or a change in the quality of the voice implies infiltration of the recurrent laryngeal nerve.

Pain in the ear, caused by infiltration of the vagus nerve, is not uncommon.

There may be *bone pain* and pathological fractures may occur.

General malaise and weight loss occur with disseminated disease.

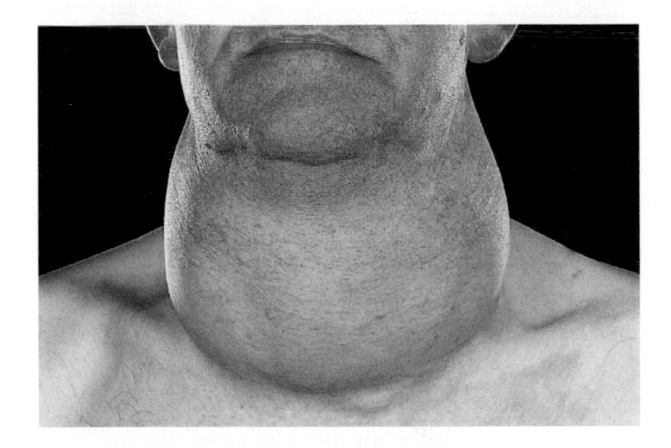

Figure 12.62 A poorly differentiated follicular carcinoma arising in a long-standing multinodular goitre.

Duration of symptoms The symptoms of an anaplastic carcinoma often *develop rapidly*. Local invasion and compression of the trachea can lead to death from asphyxia or precipitate a fatal pneumonia.

Examination

Position and shape The neck swelling is in the region of the thyroid gland. It may be localized at first to one lobe but, in advanced cases, the entire thyroid may be enlarged (Figure 12.63).

Colour The overlying skin often has a red–blue tinge because the underlying infiltration interferes with venous drainage.

Temperature The skin temperature is normal or slightly raised.

Tenderness The mass often becomes tender as the tumour infiltrates beyond the thyroid.

Size A large mass may interfere with neck movements.

Surface and edge The *surface is irregular* and the *margin may be indistinct* and difficult to define if there is invasion beyond the thyroid.

Composition The mass is *hard and solid*.

Relations Provided the mass is not infiltrating the whole neck, it will move during swallowing.

When it becomes fixed to one or both sternomastoid muscles, the lump no longer moves during swallowing.

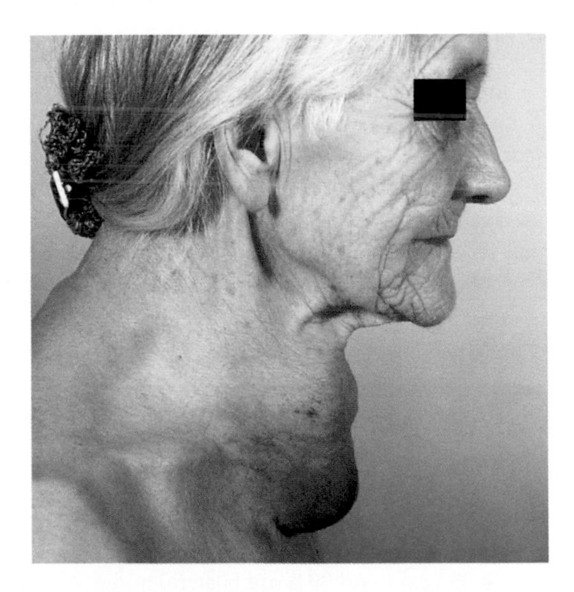

Figure 12.63 Anaplastic carcinoma of the thyroid.

Local tissues The skin *may be tethered or fixed to the lump* or infiltrated with tumour, making it thick, nodular and a reddish–brown colour.

The *trachea is often compressed and deviated, causing stridor.*

One vocal cord may be paralyzed by infiltration of the recurrent laryngeal nerve. This may be suspected if the patient has a *hoarse voice* but must be confirmed by laryngoscopy.

Lymph nodes The deep cervical lymph nodes are invariably involved, their enlargement may be obscured by the primary thyroid mass.

> **NOTE:** When the local lymph nodes are palpable, they are typically hard and fixed because of extra capsular spread.

General examination There is often wasting and anaemia.

Basal pneumonia or collapse as a consequence of pulmonary metastases or the narrowed trachea may occur.

There may be evidence of skeletal metastases and pathological fractures.

In advanced cases, the liver may be enlarged and there may be other skin metastases

MEDULLARY CARCINOMA

This accounts for 5–10% of thyroid cancers. It is a *neuroendocrine tumour of the parafollicular C-cells, which are derived from the neural crest.* They may present with a thyroid nodule. All the family must be investigated if any one member is affected. The common presentation is a firm, smooth and distinct lump in the neck, indistinguishable from any other form of solitary thyroid nodule. *There is a high frequency of cervical lymph node metastases.*

Calcitonin is produced by the C cells and used as a tumour marker. Serum levels are elevated on blood tests preoperatively.

- Seventy-five percent of cases are *sporadic* with a mean age 40–60 years and 20% are multifocal.
- Twenty-five percent are *familial* with a mean age 35 years and 90% are bilateral and multifocal, and associated with diffuse C-cell hyperplasia that precedes the development of cancer. It is caused by germ-line RET protooncogene mutations on chromosome 10 and is associated with other endocrine conditions:
  - Multiple endocrine neoplasia (MEN) type 2A and 2B.
  - Familial medullary thyroid cancer.

Common features of MEN type 2A include:

- Phaeochromocytoma.
- Primary hyperparathyroidism.

Common features of MEN type 2B include:

- Phaeochromocytoma.
- Mucosal neuromas of the tongue, lips and conjuctivae (Figure 12.64).
- Pale-brown birthmarks (see Chapter 1).
- Gastrointestinal complaints, e.g. constipation.
- A marfanoid habitus.

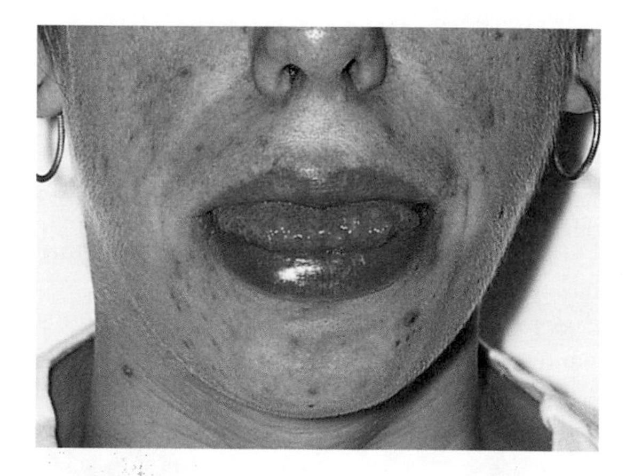

Figure 12.64 Tongue neuromas in a patient with multiple endocrine neoplasia type 2b and medullary carcinoma of the thyroid.

It is important to exclude the presence of a pheochromocytoma once a diagnosis of medullary carcinoma has been made.

Patients with a medullary carcinoma are offered genetic screening.

This is a mixed group of disorders that result in inflammation of the thyroid (Table 12.2).

Table 12.2 Classification of thyroiditis

Classification
Infections: Bacterial, fungal, parasitic
Subacute thyroiditis
Autoimmune thyroiditis: Hashimoto's thyroiditis Lymphocytic thyroiditis Postpartum thyroiditis
Thyroiditis associated with other disorders: Graves' disease
Radiation thyroiditis
Miscellaneous: Sarcoidosis Drug associated (amiodarone, lithium) Amyloidosis Reidlel's De Quervain's

INFECTIOUS THYROIDITIS

Infection affecting the thyroid is rare. It presents with pain and tenderness over the thyroid. There may be systemic features with fever and tachycardia. Inflammatory markers such as white cell count and C-reactive protein are elevated. Gram-positive *Staphylococcus* or *Streptococcus* species are the likely cause and spread to the thyroid via the blood. Blood cultures and ultrasound with fine needle aspiration cytology are considered. Antibiotics are usually curative.

HASHIMOTO'S DISEASE

This is an autoimmune thyroiditis with associated lymphocytic infiltration of the thyroid leading to the destruction of thyroid cells and function. Initially, the thyroid cells respond by becoming hyperplastic, potentially causing a degree of transient thyrotoxicosis (hashitoxicosis), but the gradual destruction of the thyroid cells may ultimately lead to hypothyroidism for many patients. The precise nature and aetiology has not been fully elucidated. Elevated levels of thyroid antibodies (anti-thyroid peroxidase and anti-thyroglobulin) are usually identified.

History

Age and sex Hashimoto's disease is most common in middle-aged females but can occur in both sexes and at all ages.

Symptoms in the neck The clinical presentation is variable. *Some are symptomless. Some have a neck lump.* Pressure symptoms with discomfort out of proportion to goitre size are fairly common.

The voice should not alter.

Systemic effects Most patients are euthyroid although hypothyroidism is a common finding and may develop over time and requires monitoring.

Family history Other members of the family may have suffered from the same or other forms of autoimmune disease, such as pernicious anaemia and autoimmune gastritis.

Examination

The main complaint is usually a *lump in the neck*, which may be associated with *local discomfort*.

Shape The swelling may be any shape – a solitary nodule, the whole of one lobe or the whole gland. When one lobe or more is involved, the swelling is usually lobulated.

Size Hashimoto's disease usually causes a moderate swelling of the entire thyroid, easily visible but rarely gross. In later stages, the gland becomes impalpable as a consequence of atrophy.

Surface and composition The thyroid may have a *smooth surface through to a small firm, rubbery nodular texture* as inflammation and fibrosis progresses. The composition and mild tenderness are the features that may alert you to the possibility of the diagnosis.

Relations The swelling moves with swallowing but is not fixed to any other structures.

Local tissues All the local tissues should be normal.

Lymph nodes The nearby lymph nodes should not be enlarged.

General examination The majority of patients are euthyroid, but some will have the signs of hypothyroidism. Rarely, there may be features of mild thyrotoxicosis.

DE QUERVAIN'S THYROIDITIS

This is a true subacute inflammation of the thyroid gland, often associated with a transient mild hyperthyroidism typically resolving over 3 months. It may be caused by a *virus infection* and sometimes occurs in epidemics. Thyroid inflammation causes sudden release of stored thyroid hormone. The thyroid itself is not 'overactive'.

History

De Quervain's thyroiditis occurs in adults. The main complaint is of the *sudden appearance of a painful swelling in the neck*. The patient feels ill, may have a sore throat and may notice that they are anxious, sweaty and hungry and have palpitations.

Examination

Examination reveals a *diffuse, firm, tender swelling of the whole of the thyroid gland*. There may be signs of mild thyrotoxicosis.

RIEDEL'S THYROIDITIS

This is a very rare condition where the *thyroid is gradually replaced by dense fibrous tissue*, which may infiltrate beyond the gland into surrounding structures. It can be part of a systemic disorder of multifocal fibrosclerosis, which features retroperitoneal and mediastinal fibrosis and sclerosis cholangitis.

The patient complains of a *lump in the neck* and rarely, increasing dyspnoea caused by compression of the trachea and hoarse voice from recurrent laryngeal nerve involvement.

Dysphagia may feature when the oesophagus is compressed.

Examination reveals a *stony hard swelling of the thyroid gland*, which may initially be unilateral, but eventually the entire thyroid is affected. The lump moves with swallowing but may be fixed to the surrounding tissues.

It is important to exclude malignancy, typically with needle core biopsy for histology. As fibrosis progresses, hypothyroidism may develop.

NOTE: A scheme for diagnosing thyroid swellings is shown in Figure 12.65.

PARATHYROID DISEASE AND SYMPTOMS

Parathyroid conditions are rarely accompanied by clear physical signs. It is extremely uncommon to be able to palpate an abnormal parathyroid gland in the neck. A palpable neck lump is more likely to be of thyroid origin. The only physical signs that may be noted in parathyroid disease relate to the functional abnormalities of the parathyroid glands.

HYPOPARATHYROIDISM

The most common cause of hypoparathyroidism with consequent hypocalcaemia is *damage or removal of the parathyroids at the time of thyroidectomy*.

Early symptoms are tingling and numbness in the fingertips, feet and peri oral. *Facial nerve irritability with a positive Chvostek's sign* may be demonstrated, which is contraction and twitching of facial muscles when the skin over the facial nerve is tapped at the angle of the jaw where the nerve leaves the parotid gland. With a very low calcium, the patient may also suffer from *spontaneous carpopedal spasm*. Latent tetany can be produced by inflating a sphygmomanometer cuff on the arm above systolic blood pressure, when carpal spasm can occur (Figure 12.66). This is known as Trousseau's sign.

Revision panel 12.9

SUMMARY OF THYROID PATHOLOGY

Once you have examined the patient, you should be able to draw conclusions on the nature and texture of the gland and on its endocrine activity.

The gland

1. Solitary palpable nodule.
2. Multinodular goitre.
3. Diffusely enlarged gland.

Activity of the gland

1. Normal (euthyroid).
2. Hypersecretion (hyperthyroidism).
3. Hyposecretion (hypothyroidism).

Having established the configuration of the gland and its endocrine activity, a table of possible differential diagnoses can be drawn up (Table 12.3). This allows a degree of clarity in interpreting the presenting clinical features and in arriving at a working diagnosis.

If only one lump is palpable it may be:

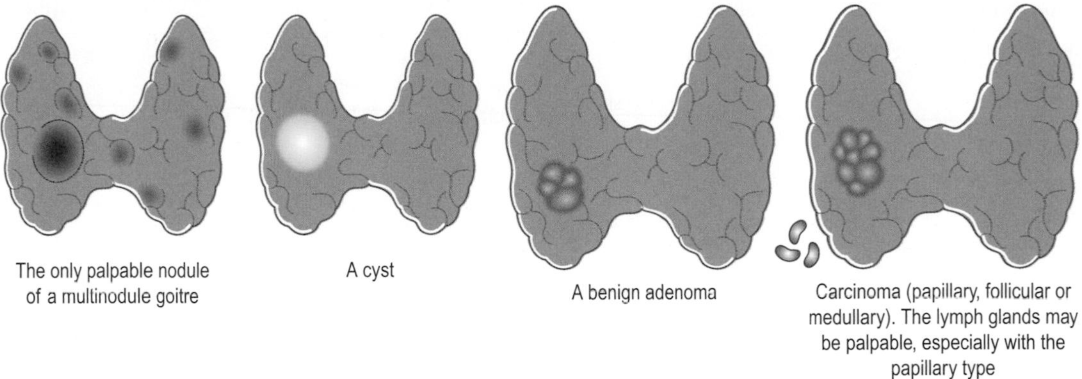

If more than one lump is palpable the swelling may be:

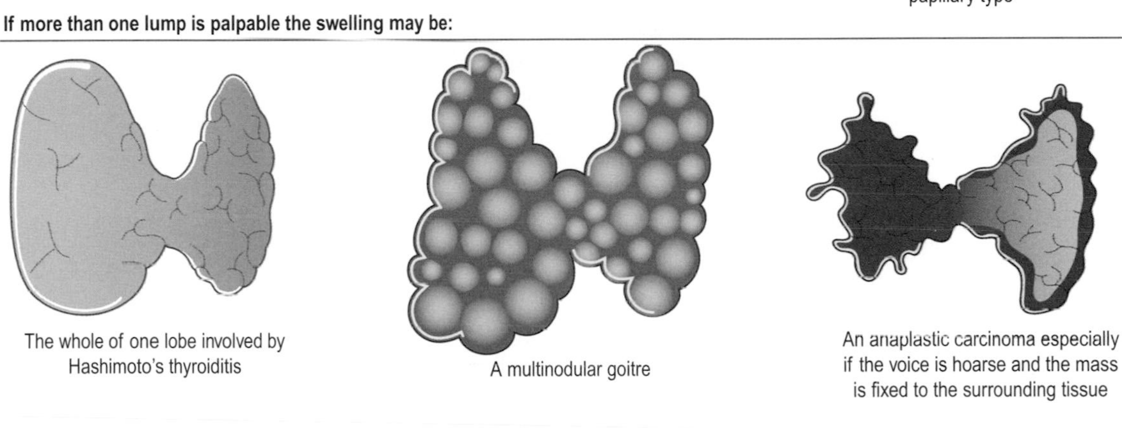

If diffusely enlarged it may be:

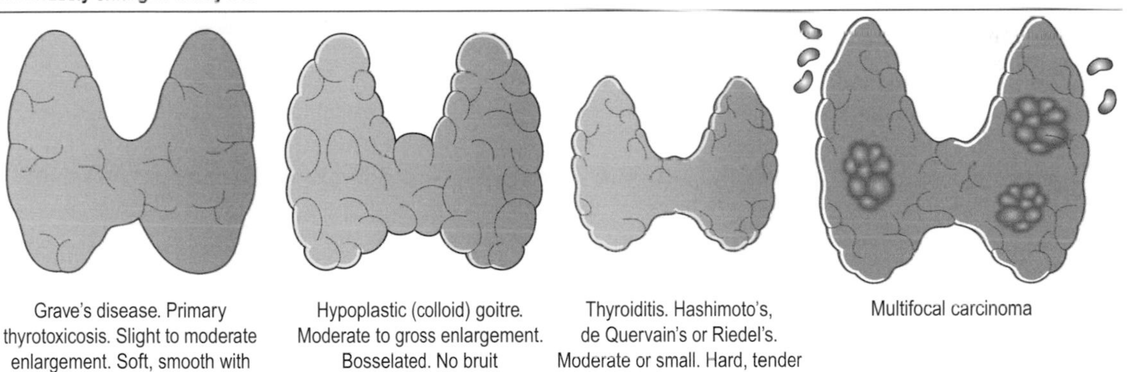

Figure 12.65 Scheme for the diagnosis of thyroid swellings.

Table 12.3 Correlation between clinical state of the thyroid gland, endocrine function and pathological diagnosis

Clinical state	Hypothyroid	Euthyroid	Hyperthyroid
Diffuse enlargement	Thyroiditis	Iodine deficiency Enzyme defects Thyroiditis Amyloid Physiological (pregnancy, puberty)	Graves' disease
Multinodular enlargement	Multinodular goitre with gross degeneration	Multinodular goitre Lymphoma Anaplastic carcinoma Medullary carcinoma	Toxic multinodular goitre (Plummer's syndrome)
Solitary nodule	Coincidental nodule with hypothyroidism	Cyst Dominant nodule Adenoma Follicular or papillary carcinoma	Autonomous toxic nodule
No palpable goitre	Thyroiditis Primary hypothyroidism Post-thyroidectomy or postradioactive iodine	Normal gland	Graves' disease Thyroxine overdose

HYPERCALCAEMIA AND HYPERPARATHYROIDISM

Primary hyperparathyroidism and cancer are the most frequent causes of hypercalcaemia (Table 12.4). Distinguishing between primary hyperparathyroidism and other sources is relatively straightforward with modern assays for intact parathyroid hormone and corrected or ionized calcium levels.

The normal physiological response of raised calcium is a low parathyroid hormone. Parathyroid hormone remains inappropriately raised in hyperparathyroidism, while in other causes of hypercalcaemia, Parathyroid hormone is low.

PRIMARY HYPERPARATHYROIDISM

Symptoms are classically described as *'stones* (renal calculi), *bones* (osteitis fibrosa cystica), *abdominal* groans (constipation, ileus, pancreatitis) and psychic moans (depression, confusion, dementia-type symptoms). Severe bone disease of osteitis fibrosa cystica (bone resorption of terminal phalanges, brown tumours, salt and pepper appearance on skull X-ray), are rarely seen today with earlier diagnosis. Bone pain and evidence of osteopenia and osteoporosis on DEXA scan are relatively common. Symptoms are attributable to both the direct effects of parathyroid hormone on the organs such as the kidneys and bones and to the effects of the resultant hypercalcaemia. A small number of patients are truly symptomless.

Direct questioning may reveal symptoms that are attributable to hyperparathyroidism; however, many such symptoms are common in the population at large. Non-specific symptoms can include tiredness, emotional lability, lack of concentration, thirst, polyuria, anorexia and muscle weakness. Many patients have marked improvement of symptoms following surgery, confirming their relationship to the underlying diagnosis.

There are generally no physical signs of primary hyperparathyroidism. Neck examination may reveal a lump in the thyroid region. This could represent an enlarged parathyroid (adenoma or rarely a cancer) but it is far more likely to be a coincidental thyroid nodule.

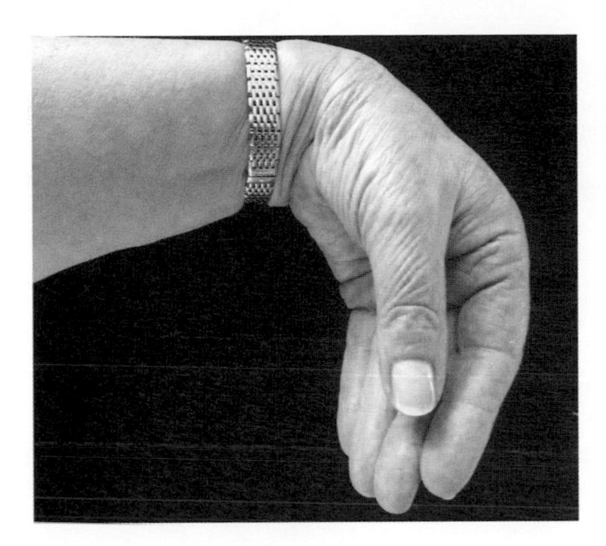

Figure 12.66 Trousseau's sign of hypocalcaemia.

MEN1

HPT can be part of MEN1 (Multiple Endocrine Neoplasia Type 1). It may be a presenting feature before other conditions become evident. MEN1 includes:

- Pituitary adenomas.
- Growth hormone.
- Prolactinoma.
- Gastro-entero-pancreatic neuroendocrine tumours.
- Insulinoma.
- Gastrinoma.
- Glucagonoma.
- Pancreatic polypeptide.
- VIPoma.
- Adrenocortical adenoma.

Table 12.4 Common causes of hypercalcaemia

Common causes of hypercalcaemia
Endocrine:
Primary hyperparathyroidism
Tertiary hyperparathyroidism
Thyrotoxicosis
Malignancy:
Secondary spread – bronchus, breast, thyroid, prostate, kidney
Rare tumours, e.g. bronchus-secreting PTH-related peptide
Multiple myeloma
Lymphoma
Infection:
Tuberculosis
Other:
Sarcoid
Drugs:
Vitamin D/calcium tablets
Lithium
Thiazide diuretic

Acknowledgements

The contribution of William Thomas to this chapter in the 5th edition is gratefully acknowledged.

The breast

JENNA MORGAN AND LYNDA WYLD

The majority of women attending breast clinics require simple reassurance but approximately *10% will have symptoms denoting breast cancer.* Identification of this latter group requires skill and knowledge.

Breast cancer has the best prognosis of the common solid-organ malignancies, with an up to 80% 10 year survival rate. Nevertheless, public perception and media attention fuel high rates of anxiety about breast symptoms.

DEVELOPMENT AND PHYSIOLOGY OF THE BREAST

Female breast development commences shortly before the menarche, initially triggered by androgens and, as puberty commences, by oestrogens and a range of other growth factors. It has five stages, as described by Tanner (Figure 13.1) and may be asymmetrical and uncomfortable, resulting in concern. Some degree of breast asymmetry is common and reassurance is all that is required if this is less than half to 1 cup size, but more than this may cause embarrassment. Rarely, a breast may fail to develop, sometimes in conjunction with failure of development of pectoral girdle muscles and upper limb deformities (*Poland's anomaly*).

Some children are born with *multiple nipples* along the embryonal milk line that runs from the axilla to the groin (Figure 13.2). Usually, these accessory nipples are small and non-functional but may occasionally lactate.

In the postpubertal female, the breasts increase in size in the second half of each menstrual cycle, following ovulation. Mild pain, increased nodularity and tenderness are common during this phase.

In pregnancy and lactation, the size and texture of the breasts change profoundly, making clinical assessment more difficult.

History and examination of breast disease

History

The following factors should be explored in taking a history:

Age The age of the patient is a good pointer to the diagnosis (see Table 13.1). Young females rarely have cancer, but over the age of 70 years, up to 50% of all breast lumps turn out to be malignant. It is however worth noting that 5% of all breast cancers occur in women under 40, with a small number of cases reported in women in their early 20s every year.

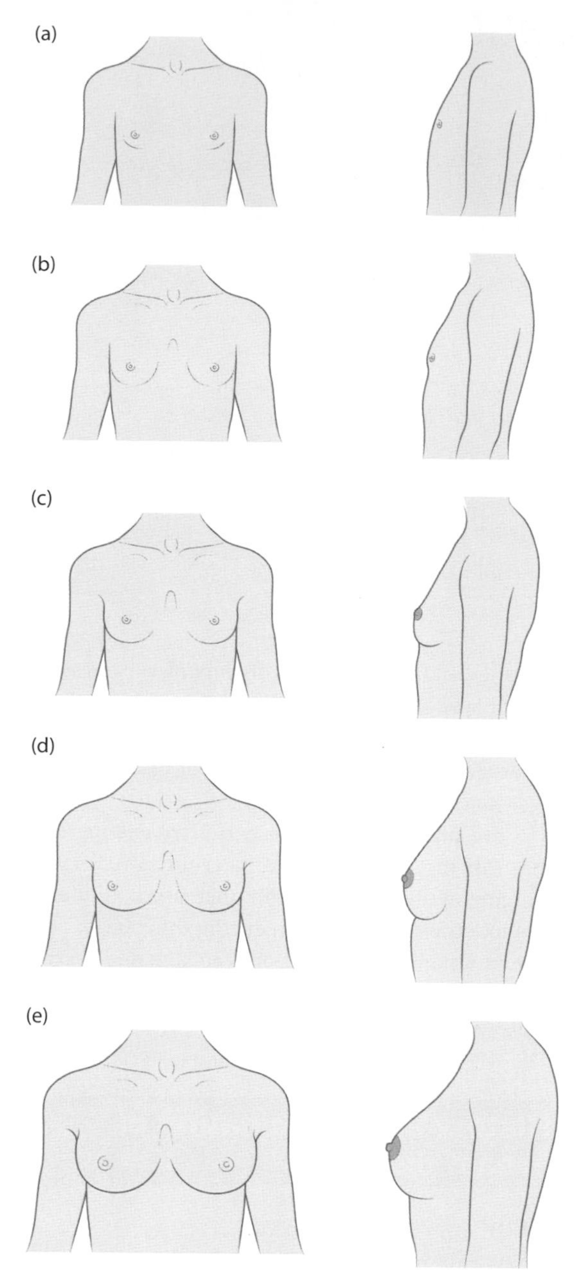

Figure 13.1 FIVE STAGES OF FEMALE BREAST DEVELOPMENT. (a) Preadolescent. (b) Breast budding. (c) Continued enlargement. (d) Areola and papilla form secondary mound. (e) Mature female breasts.

Family history Are there any first- or second-degree relatives who have been diagnosed with breast or ovarian cancer and at what age? If so, a detailed family tree should be drawn including relatives on both maternal and paternal sides of the family.

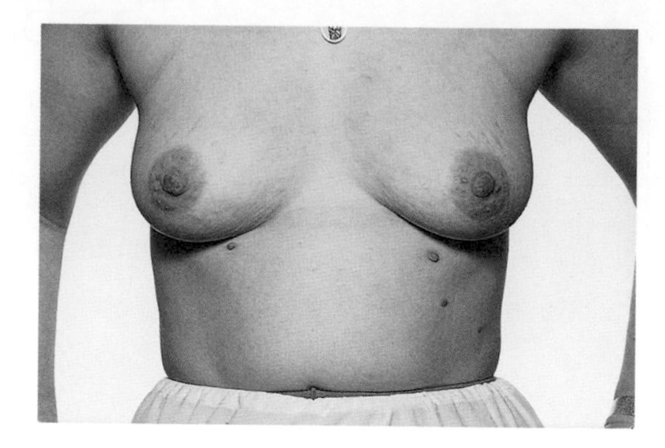

Figure 13.2 Accessory nipples.

Pregnancy and history of previous pregnancy. How many children has the patient had? Were the children breastfed and, if so, for how long? Parity before the age of 30 and breastfeeding reduce the incidence of breast cancer slightly. It is important to establish if a women is currently pregnant or breast-feeding as both are linked to increasing breast nodularity and an increased risk of breast sepsis.

Relation of symptoms to menstruation Breast symptoms that alter with the menstrual cycle are more likely to be caused by benign disease.

Medication Is the patient taking drugs containing female sex hormones? *Oral contraceptive pills* reduce the severity of cyclical change in the breasts. *Hormone replacement therapy* taken by menopausal and postmenopausal patients extends the age at which they are likely to suffer from benign conditions such as breast cysts. Both oestrogen-containing oral contraceptive use and use of hormone replacement treatment increase the risk of breast cancer slightly.

Lifestyle factors Some lifestyle factors have an association with the development of breast cancer, such as alcohol consumption, lack of exercise and postmenopausal obesity. A summary of breast cancer risk factors is shown in Table 13.2.

History of previous breast surgery In the western world there is increasing use of *cosmetic breast implants* and many women attend with implant-related symptoms such as lumps, leakage of silicone, swelling and distortion related to *capsule formation* around the implant. The type of implant and when inserted should be ascertained if possible.

Table 13.1 A comparison of the clinical features of four common breast lumps

Type of lump	Age (years)	Pain	Surface	Consistency	Axilla
Fibroadenoma	15–35	No	Smooth and bosselated	Rubbery	Normal
Benign nodularity	20–55	Often	Indistinct	Mixed	Normal
Solitary cyst	40–55	Occasional	Smooth	Soft to hard	Normal
Carcinoma	35+	Uncommon	Irregular	Hard	Nodes may be palpable

A *history of previous breast cancer* may be a cause for breast symptoms (scar, pain, nodules of recurrence in the breast, lymphoedema of the arm, metastatic recurrence).

Examination (Figure 13.3 and Revision panel 13.1)

Breast examination is a sensitive examination and must always be performed gently, with full permission and explanation and in the presence of a chaperone (Revision panel 13.1).

The woman should be asked to undress to the waist and wear a front-opening gown.

The examination starts with the women seated and facing the clinician (Figure 13.3a).

Inspection Examine for asymmetry, indentation and tethering, which may be accentuated by *asking the women to lift her hands above her head* (Figure 13.3b) and *contract her pectoral muscles* (Figure 13.3c).

The patient should then be asked to rest on the examination couch with her upper body raised at 45°. When a patient says that the lump can only be felt in a certain position they should also be examined in this position.

Table 13.2 Relative risks for breast cancer

Factor	Relative risk
Hormone replacement therapy use for >5 years	2.00
OCP use	1.25
Postmenopausal obesity	1.25
Alcohol (2 units per day)	1.20
Moderate exercise (30 mins per day)	0.82
BRCA 1 gene carrier	8.00
First-degree relative with breast cancer	1.80

Palpation The patient should be asked if the breasts are painful or tender in a particular area before palpating the breasts with the *flat of your fingers* (Figure 13.3d), pressing the tissue against the chest wall in all areas, including behind the nipple.

The normal breast should be examined first. If a lump is found, categorize its size, consistency, surface contour, fixity to the underlying ribs and pectoralis muscle (by assessing mobility with the muscle tense and relaxed by asking the patient to tense her pectoral muscle by pushing her hands on her hips).

Examine the axilla for lymphadenopathy, which is present in 10% of women with breast cancer. The patient's arm should be lifted out at an angle of 45° supported along your own ipsilateral forearm (Figure 13.3e). This allows the anterior and posterior axillary fold muscles to relax allowing easy palpation of the axillary contents. *Lastly, palpate for infra- and supraclavicular lymphadenopathy* (Figure 13.3f).

Size There is great variation, with individual sensitivity at each extreme.

Ptosis (droopiness) This is highly variable from no ptosis where the nipple is above the inframammary fold to marked ptosis where the nipple points vertically downwards well below this fold. In markedly ptotic breasts remember to examine the inframammary fold.

Symmetry It is quite normal for there to be a difference between sides. Any size difference of recent onset, outside of puberty or pregnancy, may be caused by significant pathology.

Skin The skin may be *pulled in or puckered* by an underlying cancer. There may be oedema caused by obstruction of skin lymphatics by cancer cells, which is commonly referred to as *peau d'orange*. Other skin changes include *visible tumour nodules* or a *malignant ulcer* caused by direct invasion of the skin by a cancer.

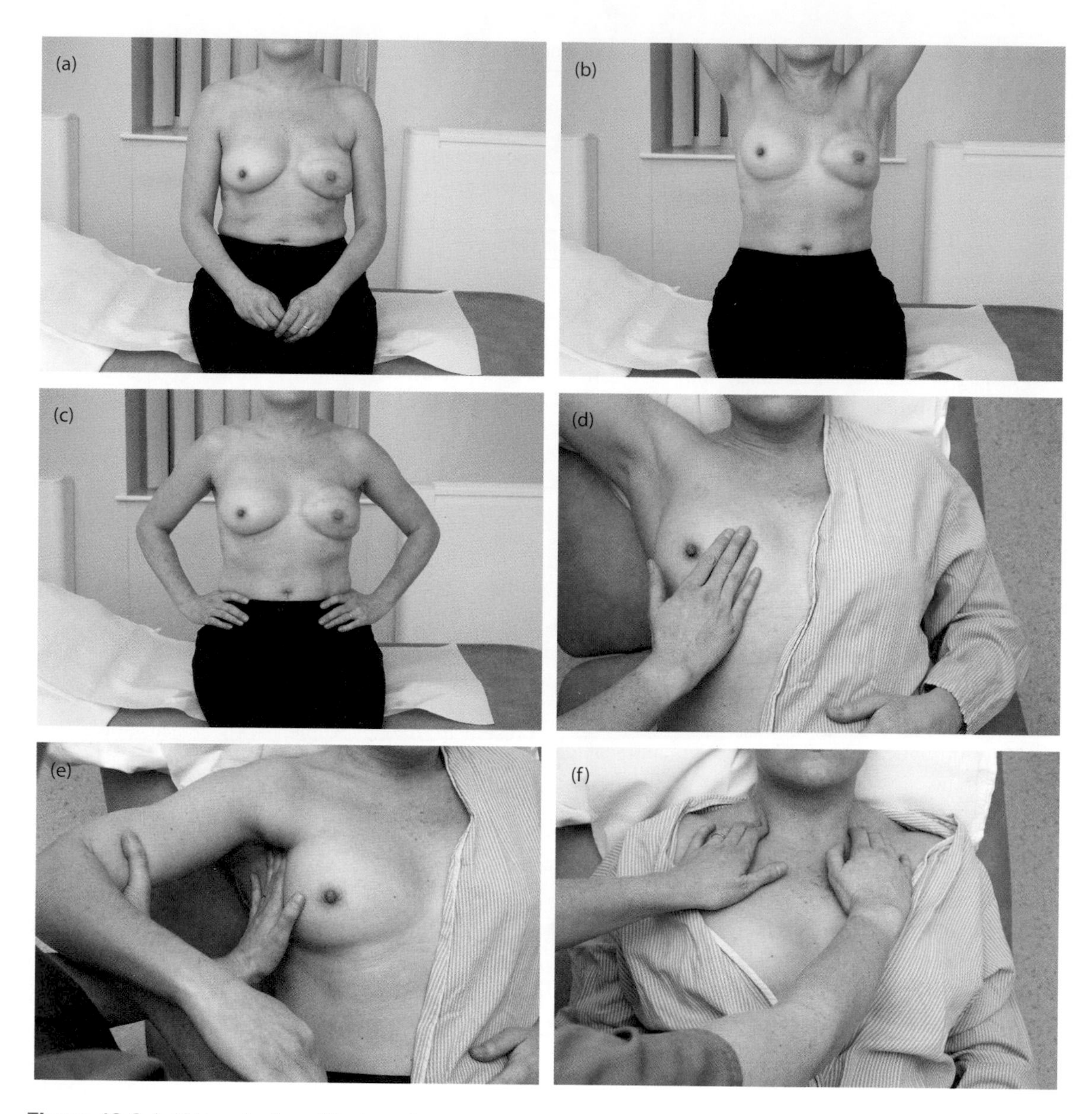

Figure 13.3 (a-h) Examination of the breast.

The colour of the nipples and areolae changes with age, and there is darkening during pregnancy. The areolar skin is naturally corrugated with small nodules known as *Montgomery's tubercles,* which secrete a natural moisturiser to keep the areolar skin healthy.

The *nipple may be inverted,* which may be normal for some women. However, if it is unilateral and of recent origin it may denote underlying malignancy.

Duplication There may be *accessory nipples* along the milk line from axilla to groin (Figure 13.2), or visible *accessory breast* tissue in the anterior axillary fold (Figure 13.4).

There is a difference between *skin fixation* and *skin tethering* (Figure 13.5):

- When *a lump is fixed to the skin,* it has spread into the skin and cannot be moved or separated from it.

- A *tethered lesion* is one which is more deeply situated and distorts the fibrous septa (*Cooper's ligaments*) that separate the lobules of breast tissue. This puckers the skin, but the lesion remains separate from it and can be moved independently.

Most lumps can be moved anywhere within the arc depicted, without moving the skin.

It is *tethered* when a lump is pulled outside the arc, the skin indents.

If a lump cannot be moved without moving the skin, it is *fixed*.

Revision panel 13.1

POINTS TO REMEMBER WHEN EXAMINING THE BREAST

History

Menarche, menopause, changes during the menstrual cycle, pregnancies, lactation, family and drug history

Examination

Expose the trunk above the waist

Inspect the breasts at rest and ask the patient to raise her arms above her head

Look at:

- Size
- Symmetry
- Skin:
  - Puckering
  - Peau d'orange
  - Nodules
  - Discolouration
  - Ulceration
- Nipples and areolae
- Axillae, arms and neck

Feel the normal side first

Examine the axillae

Carry out a focused examination for metastatic disese if locally advanced breast cancer or history indicates. This should include checking for spinal tenderness, pleural effusions and hepatomegaly.

Examine the supraclavicular fossae

Carry out a general examination

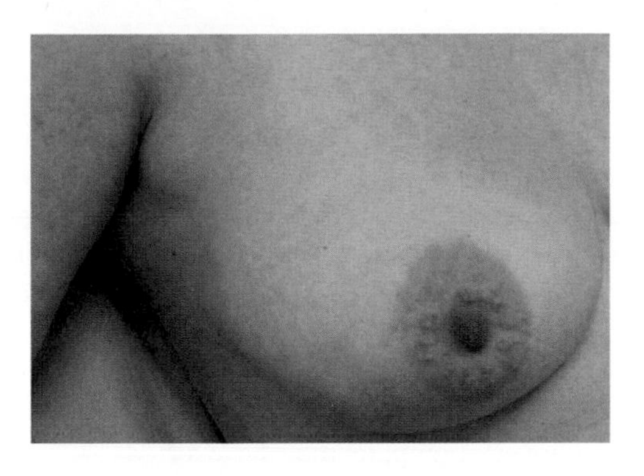

Figure 13.4 Accessory breast tissue in the axillary tail. This is easily mistaken for a pathological abnormality.

Most lumps can be moved anywhere within the arc depicted, without moving the skin

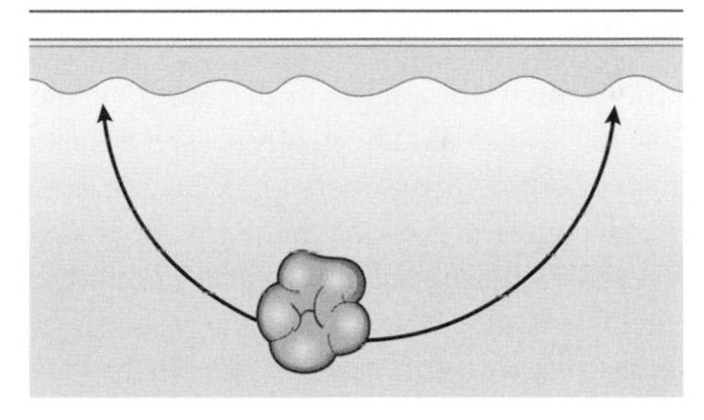

If when a lump is pulled outside the arc the skin indents, it is **tethered**

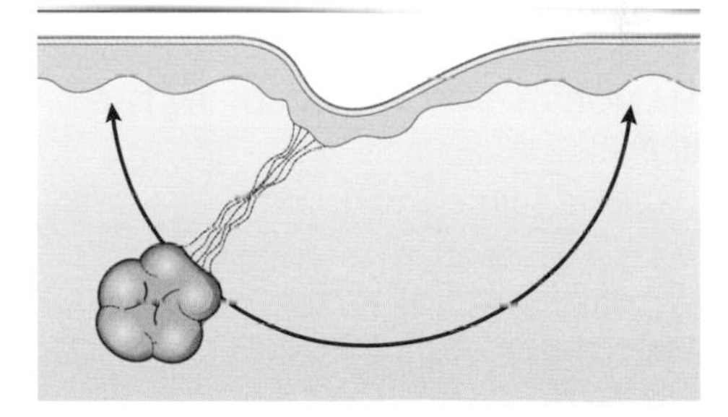

If a lump cannot be moved without moving the skin, it is **fixed**

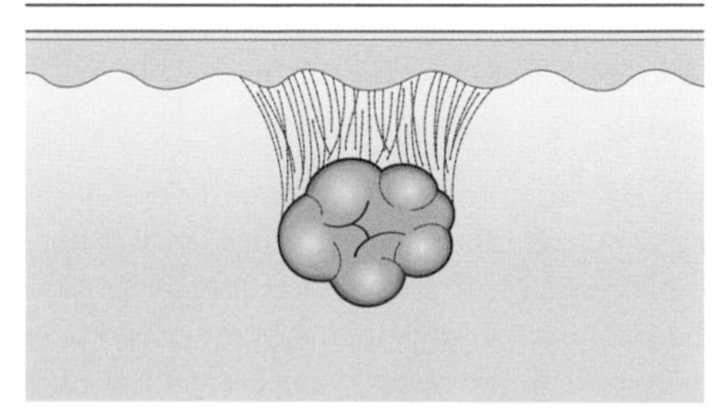

Figure 13.5 Tethering and fixation.

Relations to the structures beneath the breast

The difference between fixation and tethering to deep structures is less obvious because the muscles beneath the breast are invisible when relaxed. If there is a deep-seated lump, ask the patient to press her hand against her hip, which tenses the pectoral muscles. If the lesion is then less mobile, it is either fixed or tethered.

The nipple (Figure 13.8 and Revision panel 13.2)

An inverted nipple may be everted by gentle squeezing the areolar edge or by asking the patient do it for you.

Nipple inversion that is easily everted is normal.

If the nipple will not evert, there may be underlying disease.

Unilateral inversion of recent onset is more significant than bilateral inversion.

If the patient complains of discharge, it may be possible to express fluid by gently pressing the areola (or the patient will again help). Observe whether any fluid comes from one or many duct orifices. Physiological discharge is creamy white/yellow. Duct ectasia may cause creamy or greenish brown discharge. Bloody discharge or single duct spontaneous discharge requires investigation.

Revision panel 13.2

CHANGES THAT CAN OCCUR IN THE NIPPLE

Destruction
Depression (retraction or inversion)
Discolouration
Displacement
Deviation
Discharge
Duplication

The axilla

Small, firm, glands can commonly be felt in thin patients, but usually on both sides. In the obese, it may be impossible to feel even enlarged glands.

The axillary contents form a three-sided pyramid whose apex is in the narrow gap between the first rib and the axillary vessels.

Stand on the patient's right side. Take hold of her right elbow with your right hand and let her forearm rest on your right forearm. Persuade her to allow you to take the weight of her arm. Place your left hand flat against the chest wall and sweep the tips of your fingers from the top of the axilla and from side-to-side to feel the nodes against the chest wall.

To reach the apex of the axilla, you will have to push the tips of your fingers upwards and inwards.

Next, move your left hand anteriorly over the anterior axillary fold and downwards into the axillary tail and behind the edge of the pectoralis major muscle.

To palpate the left axilla, lean across the patient, hold her left elbow with your left hand and use your right hand to feel the axilla.

Finally, feel the supraclavicular fossae and the neck. Whilst examining the axillae, check the arms for lymphoedema.

TRIPLE ASSESSMENT

The diagnostic mainstay is *triple assessment*, comprising:

1. History and examination.
2. Imaging by mammography and/or ultrasound scanning.
3. Biopsy (Revision panel 13.3).

Revision panel 13.3

TRIPLE ASSESSMENT OF A BREAST LUMP

History and examination
Imaging by mammography and/or ultrasound scanning
Ideally histology by core biopsy

Followed by discussion at the MDT meeting to ensure concordance

Imaging

For women over the age of 40 years, mammography is usually performed. Mammography is usually of low sensitivity in younger women as they have dense breasts.

Women of all ages should have an ultrasound to investigate new breast symptoms.

Histology

Ultrasound-guided core biopsy is the histological examination of choice. Fine needle aspiration cytology (FNAC) is less reliable, less accurate and less often performed.

Presentation of breast disease

Breast disease presents in three main ways:

- *A lump,* which may or may not be painful.
- *Pain,* which may or may not be cyclical.
- *Nipple discharge* or a change in appearance.

The most likely diagnoses when the patient presents with one or more of the above are listed below (Table 13.3).

Remember that carcinoma may present in almost any way, to which must be added the findings on screening mammography in asymptomatic females.

Carcinoma of the female breast

Breast cancer is the most common cancer in females and the second most common cause of cancer death.

There are many macroscopic varieties and histological types and this can affect the clinical presentation; for example, *ductal carcinomas tend to present as hard lumps,* lobular carcinomas tend to be softer, triple-negative cancers tend to grow rapidly and so have pushing borders and can be difficult to distinguish from benign pathologies like fibroadenomas.

In a proportion of cases, the malignant cells arising from the duct are confined to the ducts and do not invade through the basement membrane. This is termed *ductal carcinoma-in-situ.* It may present with nipple discharge, as a lump in a manner similar to invasive cancer or be asymptomatic and diagnosed via the screening programme as microcalcification on mammography (Figure 13.6).

Should carcinoma cells migrate along the ducts to the nipple, they produce the skin changes known as *Paget's disease.*

In a small percentage of cases, a patient with breast cancer may present with locally advanced (<5%) or metastatic (<5%) disease.

History

Age Carcinoma of the breast is extremely rare in teenagers and in the 20s. Fewer than 5% of cases occur in women less than the age of 40 years. Peak incidence is in the 60s and the condition remains common into old age.

Symptoms Classically, the patient notices a *painless lump in the breast;* however, the first symptom

Table 13.3 Most likely diagnoses according to presentation

Painless lump	Painful lump	Pain and tenderness, but no lump	Nipple discharge	Changes in the nipple/areola	Changes in breast size or shape
Carcinoma	Area of fibroadenosis	Cyclical breast pain	Duct ectasia	Duct ectasia	Pregnancy
Cyst	Cyst	Non-cyclical breast pain	Intraductal papilloma	Carcinoma	Carcinoma
Fibroadenoma	Periductal mastitis	Rarely, a carcinoma	Ductal carcinoma-in-situ	Paget's disease	Benign hypertrophy
Area of fibroadenosis	Abscess		Associated with a cyst	Eczema	Rare large tumours
	Occasionally a carcinoma				

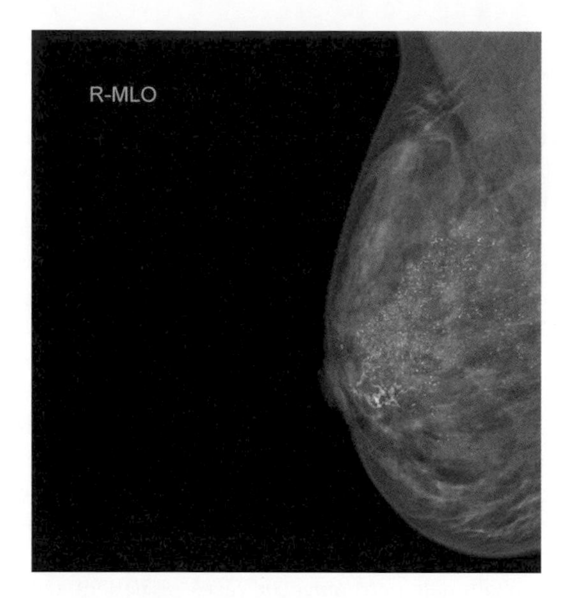

Figure 13.6 Microcalcifications of the breast. (Reproduced with kind permission from Dr Emma Craig MB ChB, FRCR, Consultant Radiologist, Doncaster and Bassetlaw Teaching Hospitals NHS Foundation Trust.)

may be an *axillary lump*, with the primary lesion in the breast being less obvious or even impalpable.

The patient may notice *skin dimpling*.

The *nipple may become retracted or destroyed* (Figure 13.7) and Revision panel 13.2. The breast may have changed shape or feel hard.

Backache caused by bony metastases is a common symptom of advanced disseminated disease, but an uncommon mode of presentation. Occasionally, a *pathological fracture or hypercalcaemia* (see Chapters 6 and 12) may be the first sign of the disease, as may symptoms from cerebral, lung or abdominal deposits – such as fits or breathlessness.

Systemic symptoms commonly associated with cancer, such as *malaise* and *weight loss*, are rarely found in patients with breast cancer.

Family history Most cases of breast cancer (75%) are sporadic, with no genetic predisposition. Breast cancer is a common disease, so finding several sufferers in one family is not unusual.

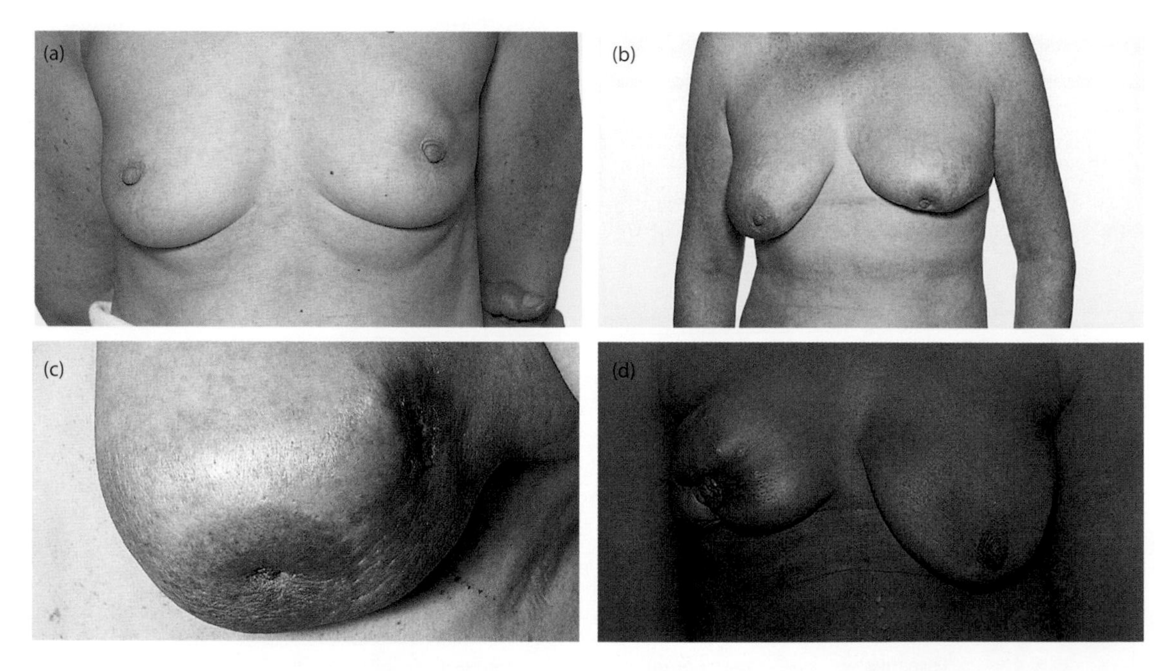

Figure 13.7 CHANGES IN THE NIPPLE CAUSED BY AN UNDERLYING CARCINOMA. (a) *Displacement* and *deviation*. The left nipple is elevated (displaced) and pointing downwards and inwards, not downwards and outwards (deviation). The tumour can be seen just above the areola. (b) *Retraction and displacement*. The left nipple has been pulled into the breast (retraction) and pulled upwards (displacement) by the underlying carcinoma. (c) *Retraction and peau d'orange*. This carcinoma has invaded the skin and ulcerated. The skin of the lower part of the breast is oedematous and looks like the skin of an orange. (d) *Destruction*. The right nipple and areola have been invaded and destroyed by the underlying carcinoma.

NOTE: Approximately 5–8% of women with breast cancer carry highly penetrant, usually autosomal dominant gene mutations.

These give the individual up to an 80% life-time risk of developing breast cancer (i.e. BRCA1, BRCA2, Li Fraumeni syndrome/TP53, TPEN, CDH1 [hereditary gastric cancer], STKII [Peutz Jeghers] mutations and PALB2). A further 20% of breast cancer cases have some genetic contribution from moderate-risk genes that only increase the woman's risk to a small or moderate degree.

Parity Carcinoma of the breast is more common in nulliparous females, and less common with increasing numbers of children and with breastfeeding.

Examination

A technique for examining the breast has been described.

Site *Half of all breast cancers occur in the upper outer quadrant,* including the axillary tail. Remember to examine the entire breast.

Tenderness Most tumours are not tender, but palpation may produce discomfort.

Temperature Only the very rare 'inflammatory' type of breast cancer feels warm.

Shape A carcinoma of the breast may grow into any shape. Multiple tumours in the breast are seen in 10% of cases (Figure 13.8).

Surface The surface is usually *indistinct,* which makes it difficult to define the shape except when the lesion is small. A few cancers (especially triple-negative type) feel smooth, mimicking cysts and fibroadenomas.

Composition Carcinomas are solid, so they usually feel *firm to hard*. Some tumours (especially lobular type) are however soft thickenings so do not attribute too much significance to consistency.

Relations to surrounding structures The terms 'fixation' and 'tethering' are defined above. Figure 13.8 shows how the nipple may be affected by an underlying cancer.

Fixation of a lump to the skin is almost diagnostic of a carcinoma. The only other condition producing skin fixation is traumatic fat necrosis (or, of course, a pointing abscess, which should be obvious).

A cancer may also attach to or infiltrate the chest wall muscle. Such a lesion will be *fixed*. If neglected, the tumour will invade and consume the whole breast, leaving only a large malignant ulcer on the chest wall. Such advanced lesions are still seen (Figure 13.9).

When a tumour spreads alongside the fibrous septae of the breast, it blocks the associated lymphatics. This produces oedema of the overlying skin between the many small pits that mark the openings of the hair follicles and sweat glands. The result is the *orange-peel appearance known as peau d'orange*.

Local tissues Extensive (but not always palpable) *involvement of the axillary lymph glands* may cause *lymphoedema of the arm or venous thrombosis and oedema* (Figure 13.8).

NOTE: The other breast may contain a lump that the patient has not noticed. A second primary lesion is far more likely than a metastasis.

Lymph glands The axillary lymph glands are often palpable, depending on the build of the patient, but this may not be pathological, especially when bilateral. Involved nodes may even be visible, but conversely impalpable glands are quite commonly found on investigation to contain tumour.

Palpable lymph glands containing metastases are usually firm and discrete. As they enlarge, they may mat together.

General examination A full general examination is essential to detect the presence of metastases, which occur commonly at the following sites:

- *The skeleton* (see Chapter 5): especially the lumbar spine, causing back pain and reduced spinal movements and pathological fractures in the long bones. There may even be paraplegia from cord compression (see Chapter 8).
- *The lungs*: causing pleural effusions or nodules. Lung parenchymal involvement, in the form of diffuse lymphatic involvement known as *lymphangitis carcinomatosa,* may cause severe dyspnoea (see Chapter 2).
- *The liver*: making it palpable and causing jaundice and ascites (see Chapter 15).

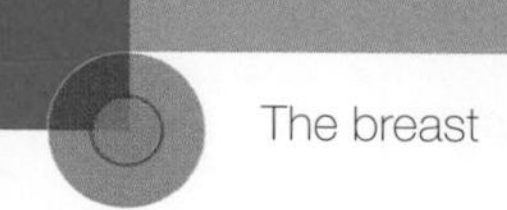

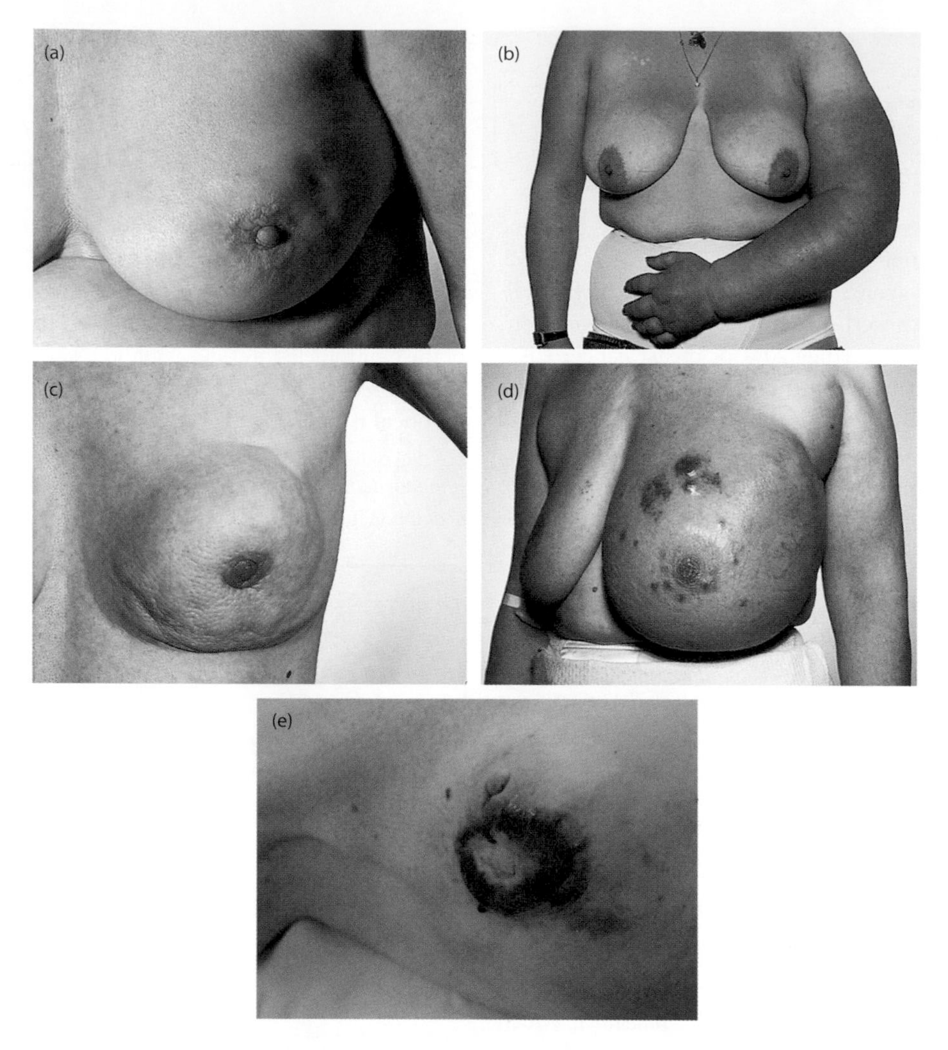

Figure 13.8 SOME DIAGNOSTIC FEATURES IN ADVANCED CARCINOMA OF THE BREAST. (a) Retraction, deviation and displacement of the nipple. Puckering and tethering of the skin. Visible axillary lymphadenopathy. (b) Secondary lymphoedema of the left arm caused by metastases in the lymph glands. (c) Fixation to the skin and the underlying muscle. (d) Massive enlargement of the breast with secondary nodules of tumour in the skin. (e) A fungating carcinoma with local secondary tumour nodules in the surrounding skin. The axillary lymphadenopathy is again visible as well as palpable.

- *The skin*: producing multiple hard nodules within the skin. These are usually in the skin of the breast containing the cancer, but may be seen in the neck, trunk and further away (see Chapter 4).
- *The brain*: producing any variety of neurological symptoms and signs (see Chapter 3).

STAGING OF BREAST CANCER

Breast cancer is staged using the TNM system – see Table 13.4 for a simplified version.

CONDITIONS MIMICKING BREAST CANCER

Fat necrosis

Fat necrosis occurs after an injury, not necessarily noticed by the patient. There is focal necrosis of fatty tissue with local scarring and possibly skin tethering. There may be a history of trauma or of bruising. The condition resolves spontaneously, although some cases may leave a permanent scar within the breast.

Table 13.4 Simplified TNM staging system for breast cancer

	Primary tumour (T)		Lymph node status (N)		Metastases (M)
Tx	Primary tumour cannot be assessed	Nx	Unable to assess lymph node status	Mx	Unable to assess for metastases
T0	No evidence of primary tumour	N0	No evidence of lymph node spread	M0	No evidence of metastasis
Tis	Carcinoma in situ DCIS: ductal LCIS: lobular Paget's disease with no invasive component	N1	Metastasis in moveable axillary lymph nodes	M1	Metastatic spread
T1	Tumour ≤2 cm in greatest dimension	N2	Metastasis in fixed axillary lymph nodes +/– internal mammary nodes		
T2 T3 T4	Tumour ≥2 cm, <5 cm Tumour is >5 cm Tumour of any size with direct invasion into chest wall or skin; inflammatory type	N3	Metastasis in supraclavicular lymph nodes +/– axillary/ internal mammary nodes		

Mondor's disease

Mondor's disease is *thrombophlebitis* of the lateral thoracic vein, which produces a cord like, linear skin puckering. It is usually idiopathic but may be triggered by trauma, inflammation or very rarely linked to a malignancy elsewhere. It resolves spontaneously but may benefit from topical NSAIDs.

Benign breast tumours

FIBROADENOMA

A fibroadenoma is a benign neoplasm of the breast with a dominant fibrous element, common in young women.

Examination

A mobile, discrete lump.

Position It may be anywhere in the breast.

Shape and size Fibroadenomas are usually *spherical or ovoid but sometimes lobulated*, and may be any size.

Surface The *surface is smooth*, the edge definite and the consistency like firm rubber.

Mobility A fibroadenoma is the most mobile of all breast lesions and fully merits the description 'breast mouse'.

PHYLLODES TUMOUR

This is a rare condition, that may be benign, borderline or malignant. The malignant ones may metastasize and all types may recur locally after simple excision and require excision with a margin.

It presents in middle-aged individuals as a *slow-growing, smooth swelling*, rather like a large fibroadenoma, from which it can only be distinguished on histology.

Most fibroadenomas present in the teens and 20s, occasionally later, but not in the elderly. They enlarge slowly and, if left, can become sizeable.

History

A painless lump in the breast. Occasionally, there is more than one lesion.

INTRADUCT PAPILLOMA

This uncommon condition is a *benign papillary neoplasm* arising from the duct epithelium and enlarging into the duct system. It usually presents with a *bloodstained discharge* from the nipple, although there may be a soft swelling near the areola. The majority are just a few mm in size and impalpable.

LIPOMA OF THE BREAST

Lipomas may occur anywhere in the body (see Chapter 4).

Subcutaneous lipomas on the breast are just like lipomas elsewhere, and there may be others on the trunk or limbs. If more deeply seated, they may have clinical features similar to those of cysts and fibroadenomas.

Benign breast disease

The various symptom complexes seen in benign breast 'disease' are termed *fibroadenosis* or *fibrocystic disease*. Use of the term disease is a misnomer as these changes are essentially a spectrum of normal. These names are derived from the histological features of breast biopsies, such as:

- fibrosis
- adenosis
- microcyst formation
- epithelial hyperplasia
- lymphocytic infiltration.

Studies of normal breasts have shown that all these changes are non-specific and are commonly present in females without breast complaints. They are the histological manifestations of the dynamic changes that occur throughout normal reproductive life during breast development, cyclical menstrual change, pregnancy and menopausal involution.

Most patients' symptoms fall, with considerable overlap, into three categories:

- Lumps and nodularity.
- Pain.
- Cysts.

LUMPS AND NODULARITY

History

The symptoms of lumps and nodularity occur between menarche and menopause, beginning in the early 20s and reaching a peak in the 30s. Most patients present with one or more tender lumps in the breast, the tenderness frequently drawing the patient's attention to the lump. The swelling is variable and clearly related to the menstrual cycle, usually being more obvious in the premenstrual phase and resolving when menses begin.

Examination

Benign breast swelling can vary from a *diffuse nodularity* to quite *discrete lesions* that mimic a fibroadenoma, a cyst or cancer (Table 13.3; Revision panel 13.4).

Benign nodules tend to be rubbery and mobile.

> **NOTE:** Experience is needed to differentiate discrete lesions that might be malignant from diffuse swellings that require only reassurance and perhaps reassessment at a different phase of the menstrual cycle. Any woman with persistent asymmetry after a menstrual cycle should be investigated.

Revision panel 13.4

A SIMPLIFIED PLAN FOR THE DIAGNOSIS OF COMMON BREAST LUMPS

Define the surface and shape and then define the consistency

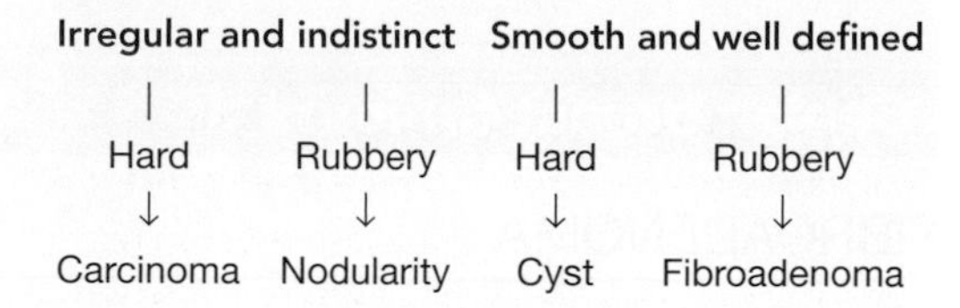

BREAST PAIN

Breast pain may be cyclical or non-cyclical.

For premenopausal women or those on hormone replacement therapy, the patient should be encouraged to keep a breast pain diary to identify cyclical pain.

In postmenopausal women, the pain cannot be hormonal and so is usually musculoskeletal in origin or due to underlying pathology, such as cysts.

Cyclical breast pain

Cyclical breast pain is very common. Almost all females experience it to some degree during reproductive life. It comes on during the second half of the cycle and is relieved, when menstruation commences.

It is often unilateral. It may be felt throughout the breast, or more in the upper outer quadrants. There may be associated tenderness, sometimes to the extent that the sufferer cannot bear any pressure on the breasts. The pain is usually reduced by the use of oral contraceptives.

On examination, there may be tenderness but no discrete lump. Diffuse nodularity is common, particularly in the upper outer quadrants.

Cyclical breast pain is not a symptom of cancer. Several studies have shown that females with breast pain are no more likely to have an impalpable carcinoma than females without pain.

Non-cyclical breast pain

Non-cyclical breast pain is less common than cyclical breast pain and has many causes.

Females at the menarche sometimes experience discomfort during early breast development.

Females in their 20s may present with a persistently painful, tender area in one breast, but this usually resolves spontaneously.

Non-cyclical breast pain without any physical signs is also seen around the menopause and again resolves on its own.

> **NOTE:** Older females sometimes complain of unilateral breast pain, many years after hormonal activity has ceased. Careful examination is essential, as there is very occasionally an underlying cancer.

Breast pain in the elderly is often musculoskeletal in origin, e.g. from a pectoralis muscle strain.

COSTOCHONDRITIS (TIETZE'S SYNDROME)

This is an uncommon condition in which pain and tenderness arise from a costochondral junction. The patient complains of pain that may be exacerbated by movement and finds what she thinks is a breast lump. Examination will demonstrate that the lump is behind the breast and is part of the chest wall.

BREAST CYST

This is probably the most common discrete breast swelling.

A fluid-filled cyst appears in the breast, without a demonstrable epithelial lining or a capsule. The condition is age related and occurs during menopause. Cysts may be multiple and recurrent.

History

Age Breast cysts are unusual before age 40, peaking between 40 and 55. Hormone replacement therapy has extended the age range.

Presentation Cysts often appear quite suddenly and there may be associated discomfort and tenderness.

Past history Many patients have multiple cysts and whilst most cysts resolve, there is a small increased risk of cancer in women with cysts, so affected women should be encouraged to attend clinic with each new 'cyst'.

Examination

Shape and surface A solitary cyst is *smooth, spherical and of variable consistency, from soft and cystic* to quite hard. The clinical diagnosis usually rests upon the smooth, spherical shape, but the swelling may be more diffuse.

Size Large breast cysts may even be visible and appear blue or green through the skin, but there will not be tethering or fixation to the skin or muscles.

Consistency It is rarely possible to elicit fluctuation or a fluid thrill or to transilluminate the lesion.

Comment Patients with breast cysts should be sent for imaging assessment. The cyst is usually aspirated under ultrasound (Figure 13.9). The fluid obtained is variable in colour and clarity, varying from very dark green or almost black, to clear yellow. Bloodstaining is unusual and may indicate more sinister pathology. Such fluid should be sent for cytology and the cyst wall biopsied.

Occasionally, a breast cyst communicates with the duct system and there is concomitant nipple discharge. This resolves when the cyst is aspirated.

A *galactocele* is a milk-containing cyst and occurs during lactation. It presents as above and the physical

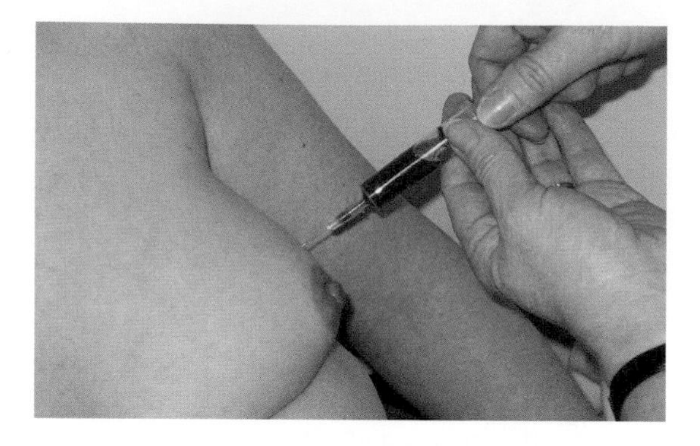

Figure 13.9 Aspiration of a breast cyst, although this would normally be performed under ultrasound guidance. The aspirate has the typical brownish–green colour seen with a benign cyst.

signs are similar. Aspiration produces milk, but the cyst rapidly refills and resolution must await cessation of breastfeeding.

Conditions of the nipple

The symptoms associated with the nipple are discharge, inversion and skin changes.

NIPPLE DISCHARGE

Nipple discharge is a common symptom and, if bilateral and from multiple ducts, is usually either physiological or the result of *duct ectasia*.

It occurs in any age group, but is most common during reproductive life. Most females who have breastfed can express fluid for some time afterwards.

The fluid may be thick or thin, cloudy or clear, or bloodstained. The discharge may be unilateral or bilateral.

The most common cause of nipple discharge is duct ectasia. Other causes include duct papilloma and DCIS, which are more likely if the discharge is single duct, spontaneous and bloodstained.

NOTE: Nipple discharge is rarely associated with invasive cancer and endocrine causes (such as hyperprolactinaemia) are very rare.

NIPPLE INVERSION

Unlike nipple discharge, this condition may be associated with significant disease and always merits full assessment. The most common cause is *duct ectasia*, but nipple inversion is a regular presentation of breast cancer.

NIPPLE SKIN CHANGES

Eczema of the nipple is sometimes seen and usually responds to a short course of topical steroids. This may represent *Paget's disease of the nipple* if it persists.

PAGET'S DISEASE OF THE NIPPLE (FIGURE 13.10)

This is caused by cancer cells migrating along the duct system from an invasive carcinoma or DCIS situated more deeply in the breast.

The presence of carcinoma cells in the skin of the nipple appears similar to eczema (Table 13.5). Patches of skin first become *red and then encrusted* and oozy. The *edges of these lesions are distinct*, unlike eczema, and they do not itch, although the patient may complain of abnormal sensations and prickling. *In time, the nipple is destroyed and ulcerates.*

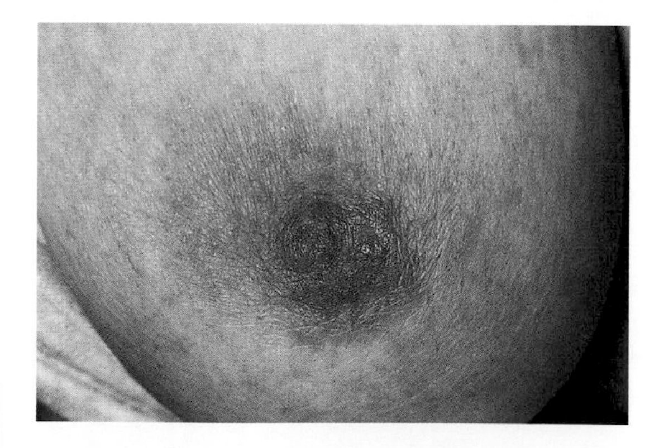

Figure 13.10 Paget's disease of the left nipple. The skin of the outer lower quadrant of the areola is red and slightly thickened.

Table 13.5 The differences between eczema and Paget's disease of the nipple

Eczema	Paget's disease
Unilateral or bilateral	Unilateral
Any age	Older females
Itches	Does not itch
Vesicles	No vesicles
Nipple intact	Nipple may be destroyed in later stages
No lumps	May be an underlying lump
May affect just the areolar	Always arises from the nipple but may spread into the areolar

DUCT ECTASIA AND PERIDUCTAL MASTITIS

This is a common condition of unknown aetiology. The characteristic pathological feature is *dilatation* of the *larger mammary ducts,* which are full of inspissated material containing macrophages and chronic inflammatory debris. The inflammatory complications are closely related to smoking.

There are several presenting features:

- *Nipple inversion,* which is at first readily everted. There is a highly characteristic transverse slit appearance (Figure 13.11).
- *Purulent nipple discharge* from the dilated ducts.
- Chronic low-grade infection of the periareolar area, with tender thickening around the nipple known as *periductal mastitis,* which may progress to abscess formation and even fistula formation after the abscess discharges. Typically, this results in a small scabbed area at the areolar margin which intermittently discharges pus (Figure 13.12).

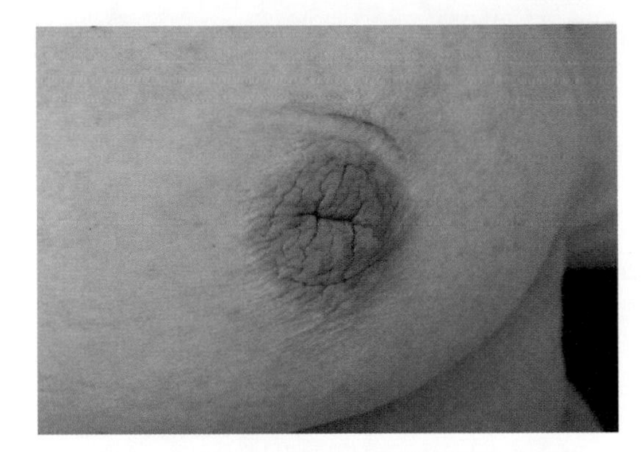

Figure 13.11 The typical appearance of the nipple in duct ectasia. Note the transverse slit. The scar above the areola is the aftermath of an incision made to drain an abscess caused by periductal mastitis.

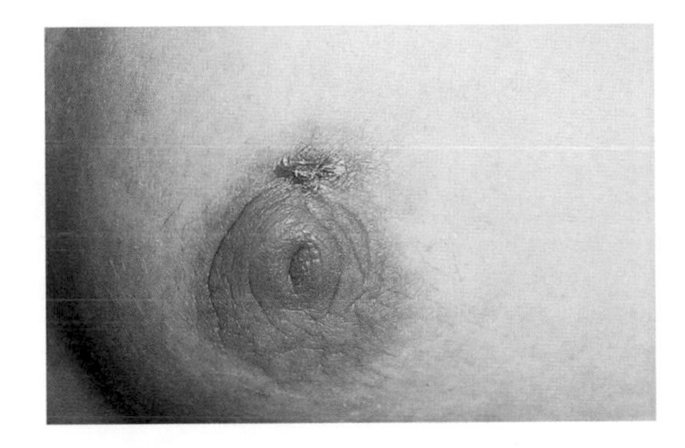

Figure 13.12 A mammary duct fistula. This tract connects with a duct. Recurrent infection causes recurrent acute breast abscesses.

Breast abscess

ACUTE BREAST ABSCESS

History

Acute breast abscess is usually associated with either lactation or periductal mastitis as above.

During breastfeeding, bacteria may gain access to the engorged breast lobules via the nipple and duct system or via the circulation.

The patient develops *malaise* and *fever* accompanied by a *painful lump in the breast.*

Examination

The infected breast will be *red, warm, painful* and *swollen*. Eventually, the abscess will point and discharge through the skin. There may be very obvious tender lymphadenopathy in the ipsilateral axilla.

NOTE: It is safe for the infant to continue breast feeding even from the breast containing an abscess, providing the mother can tolerate the process.

RECURRENT AND CHRONIC BREAST ABSCESS

Recurrent and chronic breast abscess is usually associated with *duct ectasia*, described above.

Tuberculosis of the breast remains common in some parts of the world and is occasionally seen in the UK.

Both forms of infection present with a painless mass and may mimic carcinoma.

Pregnancy

Pregnancy is always associated with changes in the breast (Revision panel 13.5). Within a few weeks of the ovum being fertilized, the breasts become tense, heavy and slightly uncomfortable.

Revision panel 13.5

BREAST CHANGES OF PREGNANCY

Fullness and prickling sensations
Enlargement
Distended subcutaneous veins
Increased nipple and areolar pigmentation
Circumareolar pigmentation
Hypertrophy of the subareolar sebaceous glands (Montgomery's tubercles)
A clear, expressible secretion (colostrum)

By 2 months, the breasts are enlarged and feel granular – even 'lumpy' – in texture. The subcutaneous veins dilate and become prominent, and the skin of the breasts is warm. The nipples enlarge and the areolae darken permanently. The sebaceous glands of the areola, *Montgomery's tubercles*, become larger.

The male breast

There are two causes of enlargement of the male breast: gynaecomastia, which is benign and common, and carcinoma, which is malignant and rare.

GYNAECOMASTIA (FIGURE 13.13)

All males have nipples and rudimentary breasts with very little development of the branching duct and lobule structures as seen in the female. The rudimentary ducts are close to the nipple. Gynaecomastia is an abnormal development of both the ductal and/or stromal elements, with the following patterns of presentation:

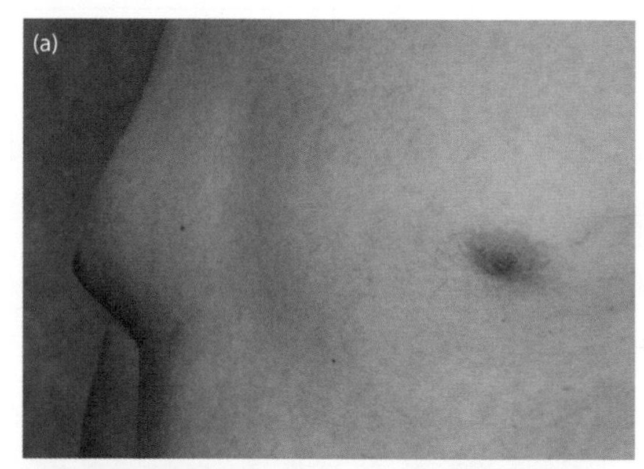

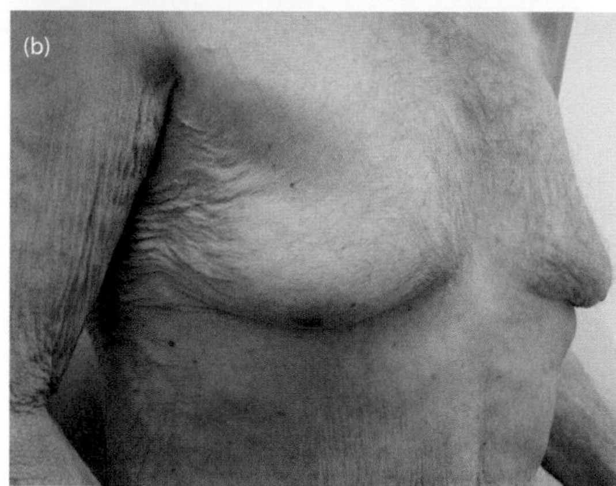

Figure 13.13 GYNAECOMASTIA. (a) Unilateral gynaecomastia in a young male. (b) Bilateral gynaecomastia in an elderly male.

Physiological

This may occur in three age groups:

- Transient breast enlargement in male infants due to maternal oestrogens crossing the placenta.
- Breast development in adolescents, caused by a temporary imbalance of adrenal and testicular steroid hormones during puberty and maturation. All males have a rise in oestrogen

levels during puberty which is important for bone maturation and may stimulate transient breast enlargement and tenderness.
- Middle-aged and older males: this may be predominantly fatty and linked to obesity or more glandular when it reflects subtle changes in male to female hormone ratios with aging.

All males see a slight age-related decline in testosterone levels and as they age, usually gain weight. Adipose tissue metabolizes adrenal androgens to oestrogens and this may be enough to trigger a mild degree of glandular breast enlargement.

Pathological

- Drug-induced, typically associated with drugs used for prostate cancer which have an anti-androgenic effect, digoxin, proton pump inhibitors (PPIs) to name but a few.
- In younger males recreational drug use is an important cause: *anabolic steroids* and cannabis may both cause gynaecomastia. Some body builders even use *tamoxifen* to prevent breast enlargement during anabolic steroid use.

NOTE: A very few cases are caused by inappropriate hormone secretion, as may occur in testicular carcinoma and bronchial carcinoma.

Liver disease

Impaired liver function, of whatever cause, reduces the ability of the liver to metabolize oestrogen, resulting in breast stimulation and gynaecomastia.

History

The patient complains of painless, or slightly tender, enlargement of one or both breasts.

There may be a history of a recent illness. Taking a drug history is essential.

Examination

Sometimes, there is a *clearly palpable disc of firm breast tissue behind the areola*. This is the usual form of gynaecomastia seen in younger males. In older males, enlargement tends to be more diffuse, usually with a fatty element. Tenderness may occur. There is no associated axillary lymphadenopathy.

A general examination, especially of the abdomen (liver) and scrotum (testes), may yield information that indicates the likely cause.

CARCINOMA OF THE MALE BREAST

This is an uncommon condition, usually of middle-aged and elderly males, occurring 10 years later, on average, than in the female. Its symptoms and physical signs are identical to those of carcinoma of the female breast, although the cancer is almost always centrally located as this is where almost all of the glandular elements of the male breast are found. (Figure 13.14).

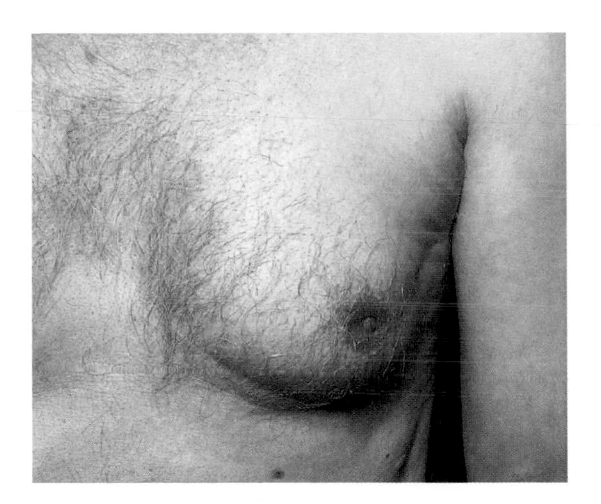

Figure 13.14 Carcinoma of the male breast. Although the mass of tumour is relatively small, it has already caused retraction of the nipple and is fixed to, and dimpling, the skin.

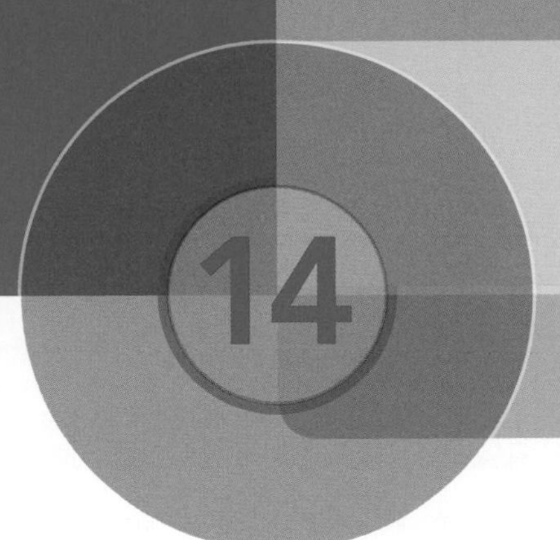

The abdominal wall, hernias and the umbilicus

JAMES A GOSSAGE AND KATHERINE M BURNAND

EXAMINATION OF THE ABDOMINAL WALL

The abdominal wall has a complex structure, and many of the surgical conditions affecting it are embryological in origin. It develops laterally from the vertebral column, envelops the intestinal tract and finally fuses around the umbilical cord in the midline to form a seam-like fibrous cord, the *linea alba*. The umbilical cord forms by the fifth week of gestation, developing from and containing the remnants of the yolk sac and allantois. It carries nutrients to the embryo. The testes develop in the peritoneum of the posterior abdominal wall and migrate into the scrotum through the muscles just above the inguinal ligament. These are both weak spots in the abdominal wall.

NOTE: To decide whether an abdominal swelling is deep to, or part of, the abdominal wall, palpate the lump with the abdominal wall relaxed and then with it tense. A deep lump becomes impalpable when the abdominal muscles contract. A lump superficial to the muscles becomes more prominent.

All the lesions of skin, subcutaneous tissue, fascia and muscle described elsewhere can develop within the abdominal wall.

CONTRACTING THE ABDOMINAL MUSCLES

If you ask a patient to lift their head and shoulders off the couch, the abdominal muscles contract – provided they do not lever themselves up with their elbows. Alternatively, lift the patient's heels and then ask the patient to hold them in that position. This tenses the muscles so any mass deep to them will become impalpable unless it is huge.

SWELLINGS IN THE RECTUS SHEATH

Acute haematoma

The inferior and superior epigastric arteries lie deep to, or within, the rectus abdominis muscles. If these muscles contract suddenly and violently, the epigastric arteries or muscle fibres can tear. The subsequent haematoma within the muscle produces pain and swelling.

Rupture of the *inferior epigastric artery* occurs during severe exercise, but also during coughing in elderly patients, especially if they are taking steroid medication. The blood is contained within the rectus sheath superiorly, but below the arcuate line (the lower edge of the posterior rectus sheath, midway between the pubis and the umbilicus) there is no posterior layer so the blood collects in the extraperitoneal space in the iliac fossa.

The patient complains of iliac fossa pain and tenderness of sudden origin, which is made worse by contracting the abdominal muscles. Examination reveals a diffuse, tender mass in the iliac fossa, deep to the abdominal wall. Skin discolouration may appear a few hours later.

Rupture of the *superior epigastric artery* follows a bout of violent coughing and causes pain and tenderness in the upper abdomen, made worse by tensing the abdominal muscles and by deep breathing. On the right-hand side, it might be confused with cholecystitis.

Tumours

Lipoma (see Chapter 4)

The most common swelling in the anterior abdominal wall superficial to the rectus sheath is the subcutaneous lipoma. This is clearly in the subcutaneous layer and displays the characteristic smooth surface, rounded edge and pseudo-fluctuant consistency. Solitary lipomas may be sizeable as they cause no trouble.

Dercum's syndrome (see Chapter 4) is familial, and there are multiple, sometimes tender, lipomas in the abdominal and chest walls and limbs. The lesions are rarely bigger than 2–3 cm.

Sarcoma (see Chapter 4)

Sarcomas are a rare desmoid tumour, which can arise in the rectus sheath and be associated with the gene causing familial adenomatous polyposis.

Abdominal hernia

A hernia is the protrusion of an organ, or part of an organ, through its containing wall (Revision panel 14.1). For an organ or tissue to herniate, there must be a weakness in the retaining wall. This may be caused by a congenital abnormality, may be related to the normal anatomy, such as a place where a vessel or viscus enters or leaves the abdomen, or may be acquired as a result of trauma or disease (Revision panel 14.2).

Revision panel 14.1

BASIC FEATURES OF ALL HERNIAS

They occur at a weak spot
They reduce on lying down, or with manipulation
They have an expansile cough impulse

This chapter deals with abdominal hernias, excluding those at the oesophageal hiatus (Figure 14.1).

Common abdominal hernias in order of frequency in adult life are:

- Inguinal.
- Umbilical/paraumbilical.
- Incisional.

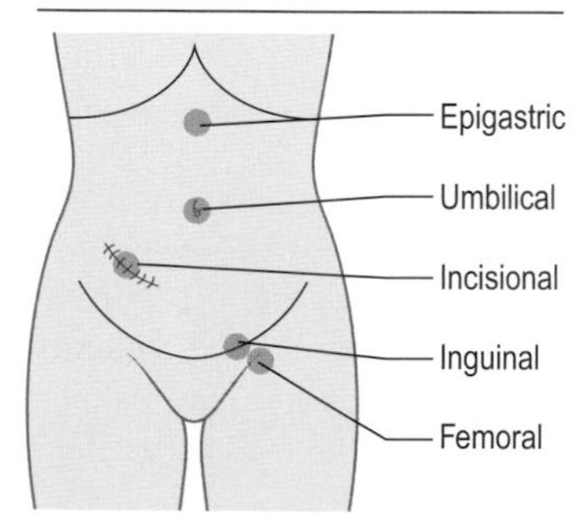

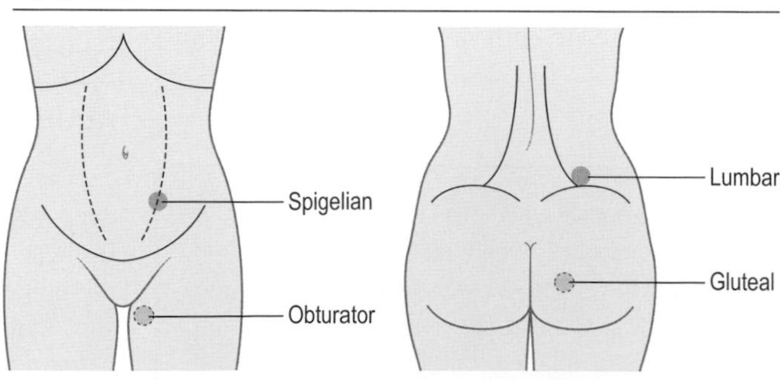

Figure 14.1 The sites of hernias.

- Femoral.
- Epigastric.

Rarer hernias include:

- Spigelian.
- Obturator.
- Lumbar.
- Gluteal.

Revision panel 14.2

CAUSES OF ABDOMINAL HERNIAS

Congenital anatomical defect
Alongside structures penetrating the abdominal wall
Acquired weakness from trauma, previous surgery or disease
Associated with raised intra-abdominal pressure

You may not have a detailed knowledge of all the rare conditions, but you should be aware that hernias occur in strange places and can incarcerate, obstruct or strangulate, even culminating in the death of a patient. They should always be assessed promptly if irreducible.

Hernias are more common in men than women: Nine percent of males and 1% of females develop an inguinal hernia at some time in their lives.

Although a femoral hernia is found more often in females than in males, the most common hernia in females is still inguinal.

Certain physical signs are common to all hernias but are not always present.

- They occur at congenital or acquired weak spots in the abdominal wall.
- Most hernias can be reduced.
- Most hernias have an expansile cough impulse.

The last two signs may be absent if the hernia has a narrow neck or the contents do not include bowel.

The diagnosis of a hernia is suggested by the site of the swelling and confirmed by the presence of *reducibility and an expansile cough impulse*. If these signs are absent, then the hernia maybe incarcerated/strangulated or other causes of a lump must be considered.

Inguinal hernia

To understand inguinal hernias, it is necessary to understand the anatomy of the inguinal canal (Figure 14.2).

SURFACE ANATOMY

The inguinal ligament runs between the anterior superior iliac spine, which is easy to see and feel, and the pubic tubercle, which is not. Follow the inguinal ligament downwards and medially, and you will find the tubercle 2–3 cm from the midline.

MUSCLES

Beneath the skin and subcutaneous tissue lies the *aponeurosis* (a flat tendon) of the external oblique muscle. The lower inwardly folded edge of this aponeurosis, which runs between the anterior superior iliac spine and pubic tubercle, is the inguinal ligament. The fibres of the aponeurosis run parallel to the inguinal ligament in the direction taken by a hand when placed in a trouser pocket, and separate above the crest of the pubis to form the external or superficial inguinal ring.

Deep to the external oblique aponeurosis are the lowermost fibres of the internal oblique muscle, arising from the lateral half of the *inguinal ligament*. They run medially in an arch, convex upwards, to the edge of the rectus abdominis muscle, where they join the aponeurosis of the transverse abdominal muscle to form the anterior rectus sheath. At this point, the fused aponeuroses are known as the *conjoint tendon*.

THE INGUINAL CANAL

The half-moon-shaped gap beneath the arch of the internal oblique muscle is the weak spot of the inguinal region. The weak, attenuated tissue filling the gap is called the *transversalis fascia*. This area is crossed by the *inferior epigastric artery* as it runs upwards from the femoral artery, curving medially towards the rectus sheath.

The point where the vas deferens and testicular artery pierce the transversalis fascia is *lateral* to the inferior epigastric artery and known as the internal or deep inguinal ring. Indirect inguinal hernial

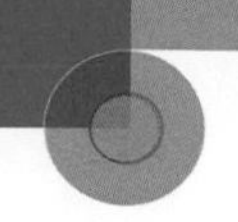

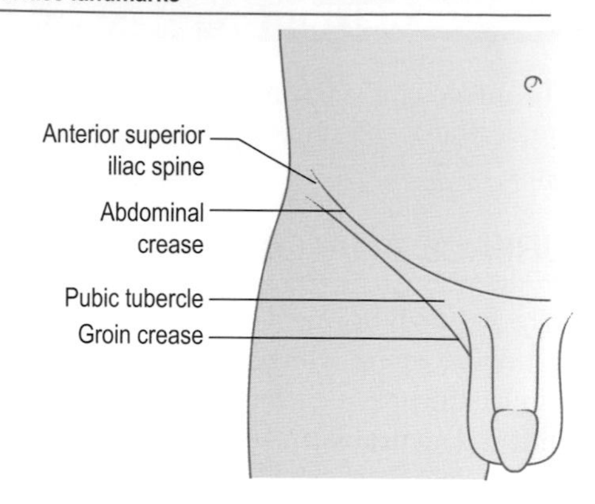

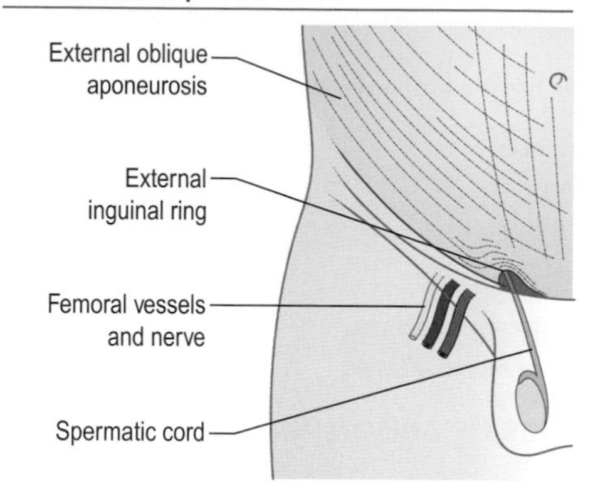

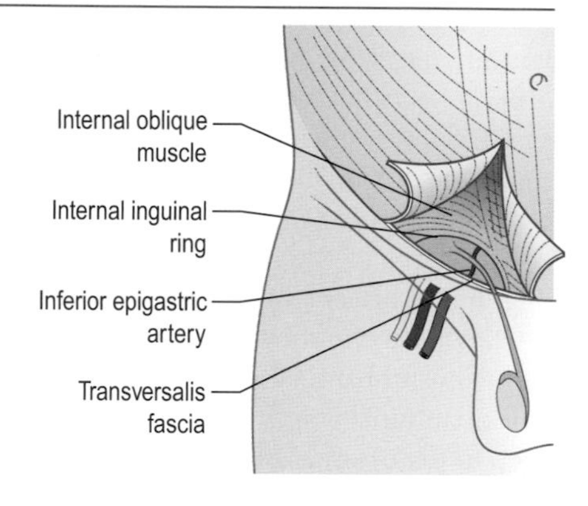

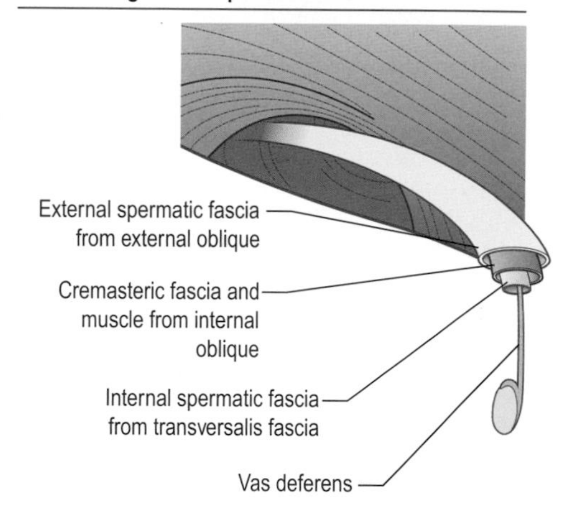

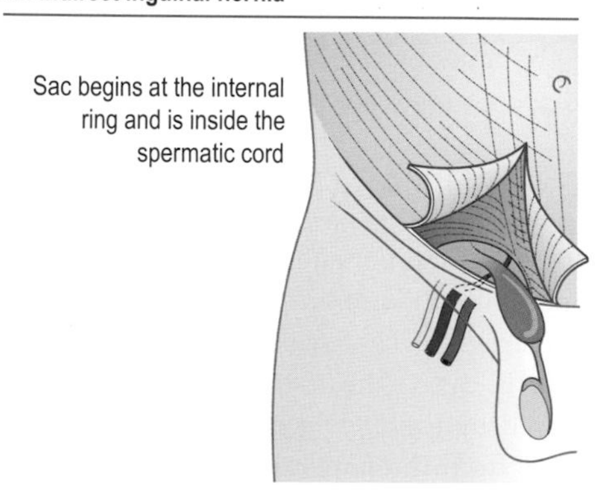

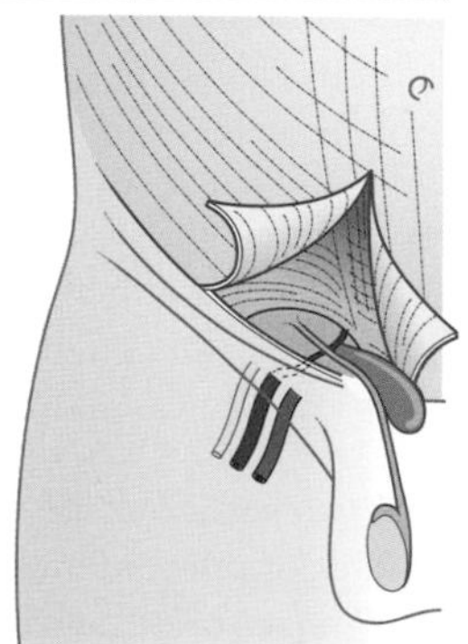

Figure 14.2 The anatomy of the inguinal region.

sacs leave the abdomen at this point. Direct inguinal hernias push through the weak area of the posterior wall *medial* to the inferior epigastric artery. You cannot palpate the inferior epigastric artery, but the femoral pulse, which can be felt at the mid-inguinal point (half way between the anterior superior iliac spine and the midline), will tell you where it begins. The important clinical point is that the exit point of an indirect hernia is lateral to that of a direct hernia (Revision panel 14.3).

As the vas deferens enters the inguinal canal, it takes with it a thin layer of fascia derived from the transversalis fascia, called the *internal spermatic fascia*. Further down the canal, it collects a covering of muscle fibres and fascia from the internal oblique muscle. These coverings are called the *cremaster muscle and cremasteric fascia*. Finally, as the vas passes through the external ring, it acquires another thin layer of fascia derived from the external oblique aponeurosis and called the *external spermatic fascia*.

Because the sac of an indirect inguinal hernia comes down obliquely alongside the vas deferens inside the spermatic cord, it has an easy path of little resistance down into the scrotum. The three fascial layers of the cord funnel the peritoneal sac towards the scrotum. By contrast, the sac of a direct inguinal hernia begins medial to the epigastric artery, outside the spermatic cord, so has no easy path to the scrotum, which as a consequence it rarely enters.

Revision panel 14.3

INDIRECT OR DIRECT INGUINAL HERNIA?

Indirect inguinal hernia

- Can (and often does) descend into the scrotum
- Reduces upwards, then laterally and backwards
- Controlled, after reduction, by pressure over the internal inguinal ring
- After reduction, the bulge reappears in the middle of the inguinal region and flows medially and obliquely towards the scrotum
- Found in all age groups including children

Direct inguinal hernia

- Does not go down into the scrotum
- Reduces upwards and then straight backwards (hence the name 'direct')
- Not controlled after reduction by pressure over the internal inguinal ring
- After reduction, the bulge comes directly forwards
- Rare in children and young adults

TECHNIQUE FOR THE EXAMINATION OF AN INGUINAL HERNIA

Ask the patient to stand up

It is not possible to examine or even detect an uncomplicated inguinal hernia when the patient is lying down. If you suspect the diagnosis from the history, *start the examination with the patient standing*. As part of any routine supine abdominal examination, conclude by asking the patient to stand up to look for hernias (Figure 14.3).

NOTE: Always examine both inguinal regions.

Look at the lump from in front

Determine the exact site and shape of the lump. With practice, you may be able to distinguish an inguinal from a femoral hernia on sight.

Inspection will also reveal whether the lump extends down into the scrotum, whether there are any other scrotal swellings and whether there are any swellings on the symptomless side.

Feel from the front

Examine the scrotum and its contents. It is not unusual to find an epididymal cyst or a hydrocele as well as a hernia because they are all common conditions.

In males, first decide whether the lump is a hernia or a true scrotal lump by seeing if you can 'get above it', namely feel its upper edge with a normal spermatic cord above. If you can, it is a scrotal swelling and not a hernia. If the lump has no upper edge because it passes into the inguinal canal, it is a hernia.

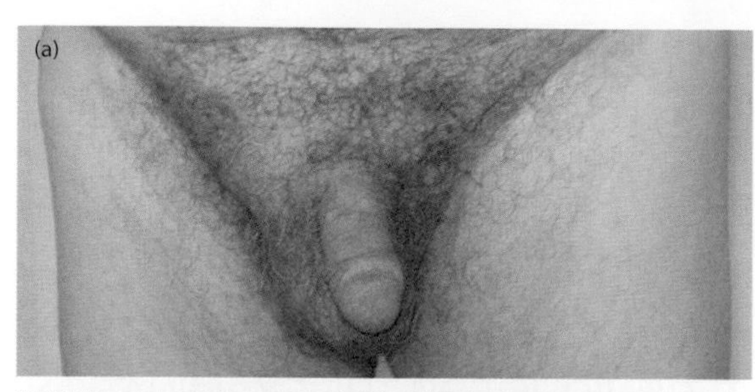

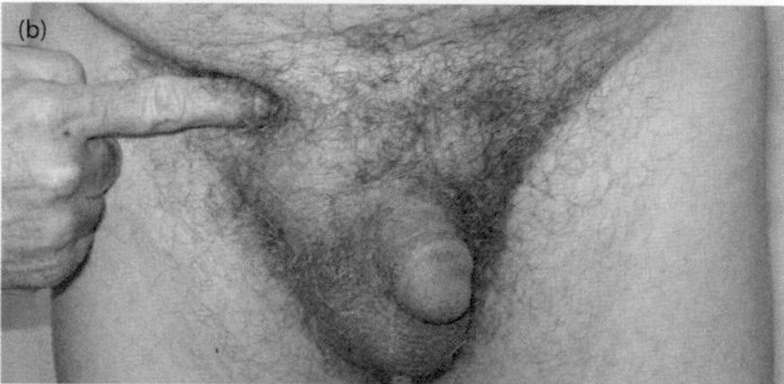

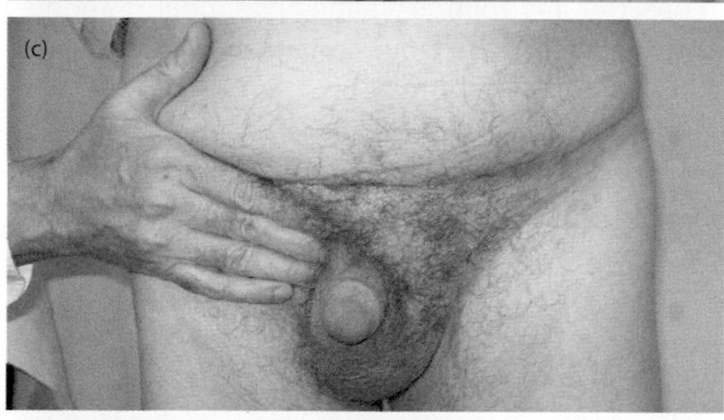

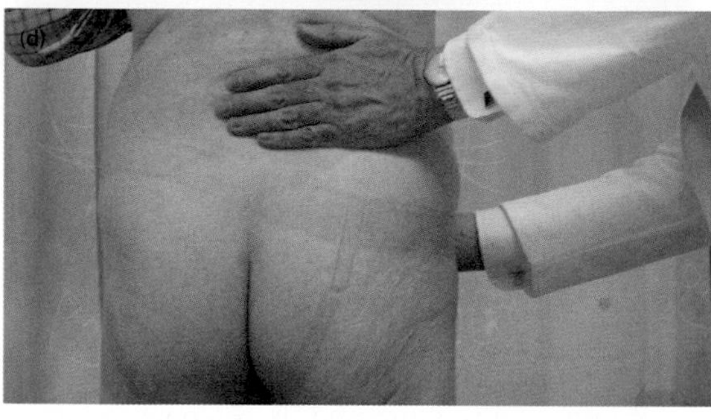

Figure 14.3 TECHNIQUES FOR THE EXAMINATION OF AN INGUINAL HERNIA. (a) Ask the patient to stand up. When palpating the groin, stand at the patient's side. (b) The pubic tubercle. Note that it is not low down in the crease of the groin. (c, d) Place your examining hand flat on the groin parallel to the inguinal ligament, and your other hand on the patient's back to stop you pushing him over. You will then be able to manipulate and probably reduce the hernia.

Feel from the side

Having examined the scrotal contents and decided that you cannot get above the lump, you can make a provisional diagnosis of inguinal hernia and proceed to examine the lump itself.

Stand by the side of the patient with one hand in the small of the patient's back to support him, and your examining hand on the lump with your fingers and arm roughly parallel to the inguinal ligament.

Assess the following features of the lump (discussed in detail below):

- Position.
- Temperature.
- Tenderness.
- Shape.
- Size.
- Tension.
- Composition (solid, fluid, or gaseous).
- Reducibility.

Expansile cough impulse

Compress the lump gently with your fingers; then ask the patient to turn away from you and cough. If the swelling becomes tense and expands with coughing, it has a *cough impulse*.

Movement in one direction of the swelling is not a cough impulse – it has to expand or become more tense. The presence of an expansile cough impulse is diagnostic of a hernia, but its absence does not exclude the diagnosis because the neck of the sac may be blocked or the contents may be something other than intestine.

Is the swelling reducible?

The main reason for standing at the side of the patient is to be able to place your hand in exactly the same position as the patient places his own hand when he is reducing or supporting the hernia. He puts his hand on the lump and lifts it upwards and backwards. You must do the same. You can only do this if your arm comes from a position above and behind the hernia.

First, gently compress the lower part of the swelling. As the lump gets softer, lift it up towards the external ring. It is important not to hurt the patient during this procedure as the muscles will become tense and make further efforts at reduction impossible. Once it has all passed in through this point, slide your fingers upwards and laterally towards the internal ring to see if the hernia can be controlled (kept inside) by pressure at this point.

NOTE: If the hernia can be held in the reduced position by pressure over the internal ring, it is an indirect inguinal hernia. If it is above the inguinal ligament and cannot be controlled by pressure over the internal ring, it is a direct hernia.

With large hernias, it is often difficult and inappropriate to try and reduce the hernia with the patient standing up. In this case, ask the patient to lie down. In most cases, the hernia will reduce.

Finally, be very gentle with hernias that appear incarcerated. It is possible to *reduce the hernia* 'en masse', which means reducing the bowel together with the peritoneal sac. The hernia contents may still be incarcerated or even strangulated within the peritoneal sac.

Remove your hand and watch the hernia reappear

A reappearing indirect hernia slides obliquely downwards along the line of the inguinal canal, whereas a direct hernia will project directly forwards (Figure 14.4).

Feel the other side

Move to the other side of the patient and examine that inguinal region. *Inguinal hernias are quite often bilateral*, particularly when they are direct. Even when you cannot see or feel a lump, ask the patient to cough while you are palpating the inguinal canal. There may be a small hernia that is palpable with coughing but is not visible.

Examine the abdomen

Look particularly for anything that may be raising the intra-abdominal pressure, such as a *large bladder, ascites, abdominal distension or pregnancy*.

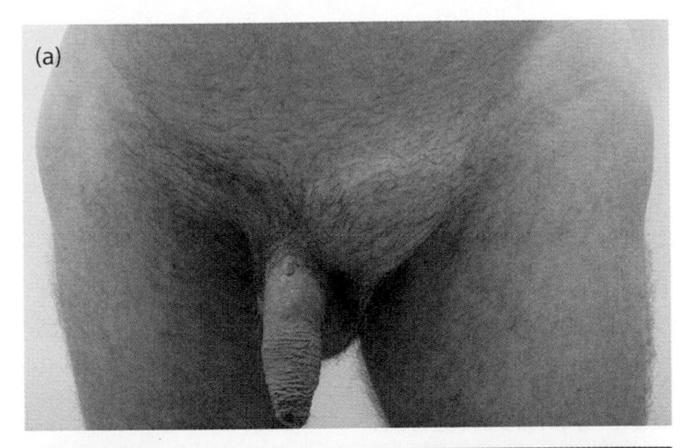

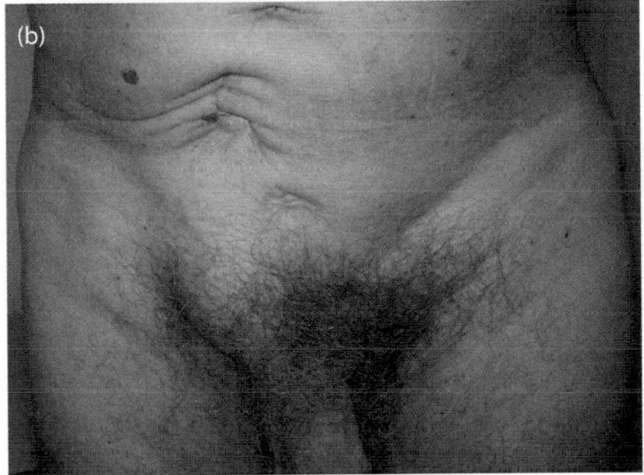

Figure 14.4 INGUINAL HERNIAS. (a) A left indirect inguinal hernia, moving obliquely down towards the scrotum. (b) This is a right direct recurrent inguinal hernia. The original inguinal hernia probably developed because of the disruption and distortion of the abdominal wall caused by the previous abdominal operation. Always look for a scar in the groin. The bulge is coming out directly towards you.

With the patient lying flat, ask the patient to cough as you observe the groin. Particularly in a slim adult, you may see the contents entering the sac, which will help you to decide if the hernia is direct or indirect, as described above in the standing position. With a direct hernia, the swelling will advance directly upwards towards you. With an indirect hernia, you may be able to see oblique motion from the internal ring to the neck of the scrotum. Indirect hernias have sometimes been referred to as *oblique hernias*.

With the patient in this position, it is easier to decide whether a hernia is femoral.

NOTE: Femoral hernias only rarely reduce, lie below the inguinal ligament and are rather more lateral than an indirect inguinal sac extending through the external inguinal ring downwards to the same level.

Cardiovascular and respiratory assessment

Assess the cardiovascular and respiratory systems with the patient's fitness for operation in mind.

Inguinal hernia

History
Elective presentation

Age Inguinal hernias may appear at any age from birth to old age.

Occupation If there is an underlying weakness, the appearance of a hernia may coincide with strenuous physical effort, or it may be first noticed at such a time. Despite the fact that hernias are no more common in manual workers than in office workers, compensation law in many countries accepts that a hernia may be an industrial injury.

Local symptoms The usual symptom is the patient finding a *painless swelling*. Some patients notice a dragging, aching sensation in the groin, which gets worse as the day goes on. A few present with *groin pain*, and the hernia is only detected by the doctor.

Other abdominal symptoms Large hernias may interfere with bowel activity and cause a change in bowel habit.

It is important to consider other conditions causing an increase in abdominal pressure. Patients with a carcinoma of the left colon, or diverticular disease, may experience progressive constipation and hence increased straining during defaecation. This increase in abdominal pressure may make a coincidental hernia more prominent and lead the patient to attribute their symptoms to the hernia. You must always enquire about changes in bowel habit in patients presenting with a hernia. Other diseases that may cause an increase in abdominal pressure, such as chronic bronchitis with persistent coughing, and difficulty with micturition should also be excluded.

History
Emergency presentation

Hernias, pre-existing or just discovered, may present as a surgical emergency. The patient notices that the *groin swelling will not reduce or that it is painful and tender*. This may be associated with the cardinal symptoms of intestinal obstruction – *colicky abdominal pain, vomiting, distension and absolute constipation*. The griping pain is felt not in the groin but in the midline of the abdomen, at a level that depends on which part of the intestine is involved.

> **NOTE:** The hernial orifices of any patient with intestinal obstruction must always be carefully examined, as the patient may not have noticed a small lump in their groin. This is particularly so with femoral hernias.

The terms 'irreducible', 'incarcerated', 'obstructed' and 'strangulated' are used freely in the description of hernias. They must be defined carefully (Figure 14.5).

Irreducible means simply what it states, that the contents of the hernia sac cannot be replaced into the abdomen. An irreducible hernia may be associated with three other categories of complication – incarceration, obstruction and strangulation.

Incarcerated means that contents are literally imprisoned in the sac of the hernia (usually by adhesions) but are alive and functioning normally. An incarcerated hernia is not tender.

Obstructed means that a loop of bowel is kinked or trapped within the sac of the hernia in such a way that its lumen, but not its blood supply, is obstructed. Therefore, the bowel is alive, and the patient has the signs and symptoms of intestinal obstruction but not of strangulation. The hernia will not be unduly tender.

Strangulation means that compression or twisting has compromised the blood supply to the contents of the sac, which are ischaemic or infarcted. The patient will be obviously unwell, and the swelling will be acutely tender. An entrapment that interferes with the blood supply to the bowel wall will commonly obstruct the lumen as well, so most strangulated hernias containing bowel have intestinal obstruction.

There is a variety of strangulated hernia in which only a segment of the bowel wall is trapped and the lumen remains patent. The strangulation makes the hernia very tender, but there are no symptoms or signs of intestinal obstruction. This is called *Richter's hernia*. It occurs when the hernia has a narrow neck, so is more commonly seen with femoral than inguinal hernias.

Neck of sac

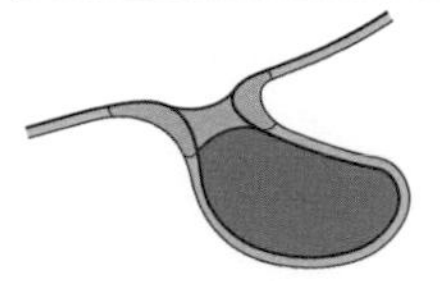

This tight ring of peritoneum is usually the site of any strangulation

A strangulated hernia

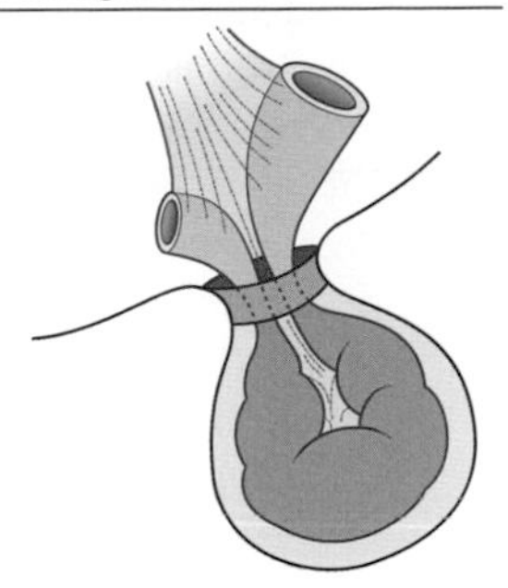

The blood supply of the contents of the hernia is cut off. When a loop of the gut is strangulated there will also be intestinal obstruction

A strangulated hernia

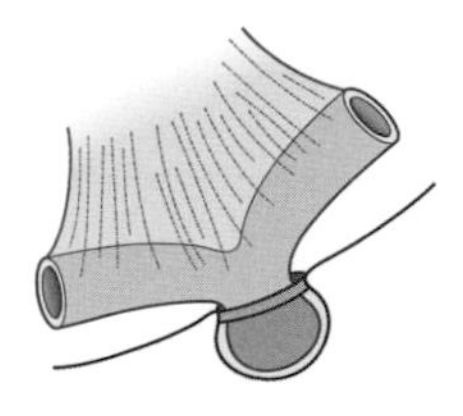

If the sac is small, a knuckle of bowel can be caught in the sac and strangled without causing intestinal obstruction. This is called a *Richter's hernia*

Maydl's hernia

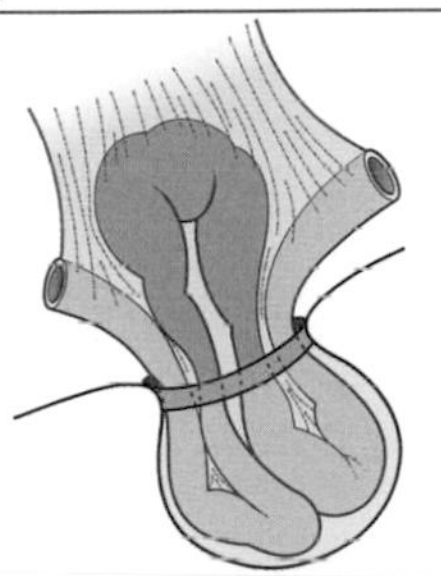

When two adjacent loops of bowel are in the sac, the intervening portion in the abdomen is the first to suffer if the neck of the sac is tight, because it is the centre of the whole loop involved. Thus the strangulation piece is intra-abdominal. This is a rare variety of strangulation

Sliding hernia

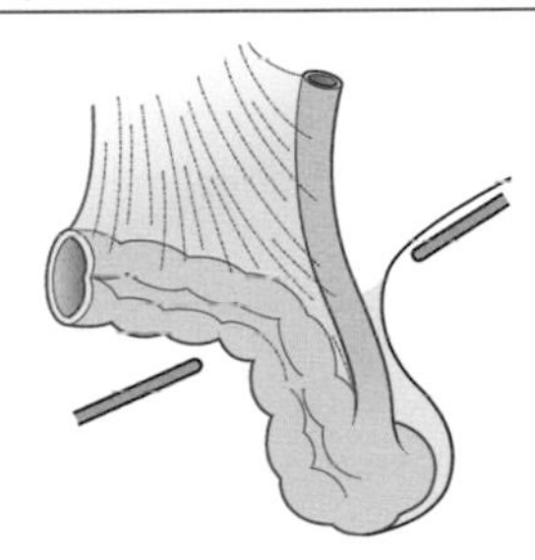

If bowel which is normally extraperitoneal forms one side of the sac, it is thought to have slid down the canal pulling peritoneum with it, hence the name *hernia-en-glissade*. The sac can contain other loops of bowel, and the gut forming the wall of the sac can be strangled by the external wall ring

Incarceration

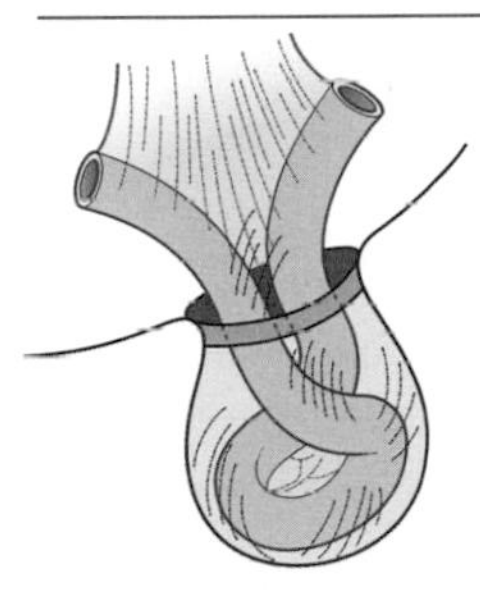

The contents are fixed in the sac because of their size and adhesions. The hernia is irreducible but the bowel is not strangulated or obstructed

Reduction-en-masse

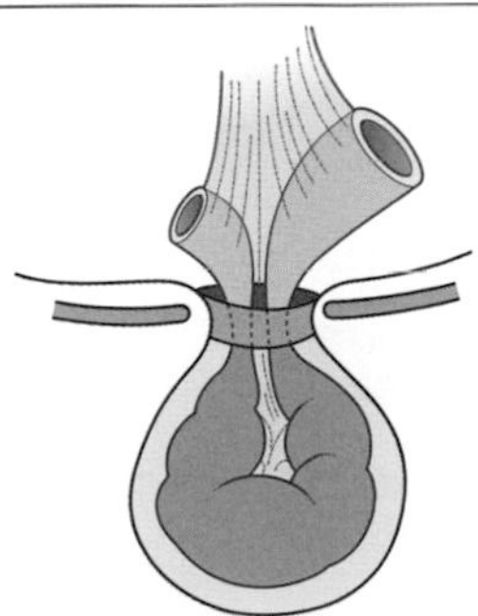

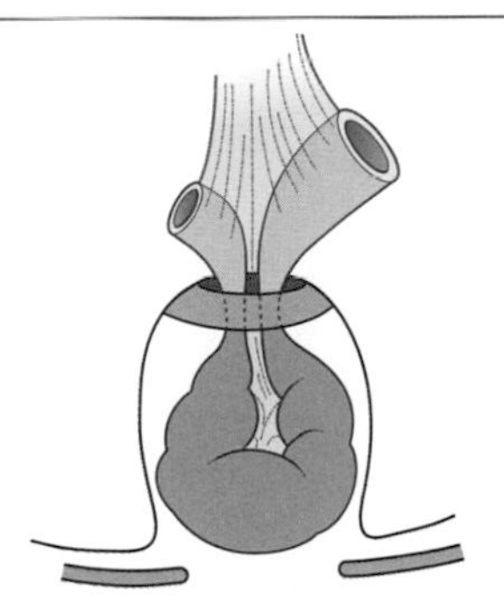

It is possible to push a hernia back through the abdominal wall, so apparently reducing it, without actually pushing the contents out of the sac. If they were strangulated in the first position they will still be strangulated in the second. Never push hard when trying to reduce a hernia

Figure 14.5 Some definitions.

Examination

This is the same as for a non-emergency hernias but particular attention should be paid to:

- **Colour** The skin may be erythematous with strangulation.
- **Temperature** The overlying skin may be warm if strangulated but not incarcerated.
- **Tenderness** A strangulated hernia is very tender. An irreducible, non-strangulated hernia is not tender to light pressure, but any attempt at reduction by excessive pressing and squeezing can cause considerable pain.
- **Reducibility** This means that it is possible to return the contents of the hernia to their normal anatomical site – the abdomen.

NOTE: Look carefully for any scars near the hernia. It may have been repaired in the past.

There is an increased incidence of direct right inguinal hernia in patients who have had an appendicectomy through a right iliac fossa incision, because this incision weakens the adjacent muscles and occasionally divides the iliohypogastric or ilioinguinal nerves.

SPECIAL VARIETIES OF INGUINAL HERNIA

The differences between a direct and an indirect inguinal hernia are listed in Revision panel 14.3. The distinction between the two is not totally irrelevant, as well as being an excellent exercise in clinical anatomy (see Figure 14.4). When an inguinal hernia strangulates, the usual site of constriction is the internal ring. Hence a direct hernia, which does not pass through this ring, is much less likely to place the patient's life at risk by becoming strangulated. This may influence management in a poor-risk patient. Bilateral hernias are more likely to be direct than indirect.

It is not uncommon to find both a direct and an indirect hernia in the same groin. When this occurs, the two sacs are straddled by the inferior epigastric artery and the hernia is sometimes called a *pantaloon hernia*. This is usually detected only at operation.

A *sliding hernia* occurs when a partly extraperitoneal segment of bowel (the caecum or terminal ileum on the right, sigmoid colon on the left, or fallopian tube in women) slides down into the inguinal canal, pulling a sac of peritoneum with it. The viscus involved is part of the wall of the sac. Clinical differentiation of this variety is never certain, but it is far more common on the left, and involvement of the sigmoid colon may produce disproportionate pain and even symptoms of bowel dysfunction. *Maydl's hernia* (hernia-en-W; Figure 14.5) is a rare condition in which there are two loops of bowel in the sac, with strangulation of a loop of bowel between them in the abdomen. Diagnosis is made at operation.

RECURRENT HERNIAS

This is a common condition as not all of the many surgical repairs that are performed are successful.

Recurrent hernias are more likely to present with local pain. They tend to be direct and, because of the scarring from the previous surgery, are unlikely to be large. They are very rarely scrotal. The hernia may consist of extraperitoneal fat without a peritoneal sac, infiltrating itself into the defects that have arisen in the previous repair. Recognition is important because strangulation is more likely than with an untreated hernia.

DIFFERENTIAL DIAGNOSIS

There are very few conditions that can be mistaken for an inguinal hernia provided you remember to check the scrotum, feel for a cough impulse and test reducibility (Revision panel 14.4).

Confusion may occasionally be caused by swellings that occur in the line of the spermatic cord that can pop in and out of the external ring, such as an undescended testis and a hydrocele of the cord in children. With the first, routine examination of the scrotum should reveal an absent testis. Neither has an expansile cough impulse.

Revision panel 14.4

DIFFERENTIAL DIAGNOSIS OF AN INGUINAL HERNIA

Femoral hernia
Hydrocele of the cord or the canal of Nuck
Undescended testis
Lipoma of the cord

INGUINAL HERNIA IN FEMALES

In females, the equivalent of the spermatic cord is the round ligament, which joins the uterus just as the vas deferens joins the prostate. Hernias in females nearly always follow the round ligament and are therefore indirect. The sac passes obliquely towards the labium in the same way as it would pass towards the scrotum in the male.

There are two conditions of the groin unique to females:

- *Hydrocele of the canal of Nuck* is a fluid-filled distal sac of an indirect hernia. The proximal part of the sac is too narrow to admit bowel or other abdominal contents. It is analogous to the encysted hydrocele of the cord seen in boys. It presents with a *smooth, fluctuant swelling without a cough impulse,* that will transilluminate.
- *Haematocele of the round ligament* is a curious condition in which the round ligament becomes distended with multiple small sacs containing bloodstained fluid. It presents in pregnancy with a soft, sausage-like swelling in the groin extending into the labium. This may have a weak cough impulse and when gently squeezed feels spongy and reduces in size. It is commonly confused with a hernia, but it resolves when the pregnancy is over, which hernias certainly do not.

INGUINAL HERNIAS IN CHILDREN

Groin hernias in male children are almost always indirect and are caused by *failure of the processus vaginalis to obliterate* after the testicle enters the scrotum. There are three clinical manifestations of this abnormality, but it is important to appreciate that the pathological process in all three is identical, namely a patent processus vaginalis.

The three clinical manifestations are:

- Infantile hydrocele.
- Encysted hydrocele of the cord.
- Inguinal hernia.

An infantile hydrocele is a fully patent processus vaginalis (i.e. one extending right down to the scrotum) that is too narrow to admit bowel but allows fluid from the peritoneal cavity to accumulate within it. The condition may present at birth or shortly afterwards as a scrotal swelling that is usually large, tense, *brilliantly translucent* and often bilateral. It should be possible to get above the swelling, i.e. to feel or see that its upper limit is at or below the external inguinal ring. It is rarely possible to squeeze the fluid back into the abdomen as the narrow neck of the processus acts as a non-return valve. It does not have an expansile cough impulse.

When the child cries, intra-abdominal pressure is raised and the scrotal swelling may become harder. It is important to reassure the parents that the child is not crying because the hydrocele is tense, but that the swelling is tense because the child is crying.

The usual natural history is spontaneous resolution during the first year of life as the processus slowly obliterates but, once the child begins to walk, this is less likely. In ambulant children, the swelling often increases in size during the day.

An *encysted hydrocele of the cord* is the least common variety of patent processus vaginalis; in this, a narrow-necked patent processus that does not reach the testis becomes dilated distally and filled with fluid. It presents as a discrete swelling in the spermatic cord below the external inguinal ring and above the testicle (Figure 14.6). It *transilluminates brilliantly* and has no cough impulse.

An inguinal hernia in a child (Figures 14.7, 14.8) displays the physical signs listed above for an indirect inguinal hernia. The contents reduce easily, and the swelling does not transilluminate.

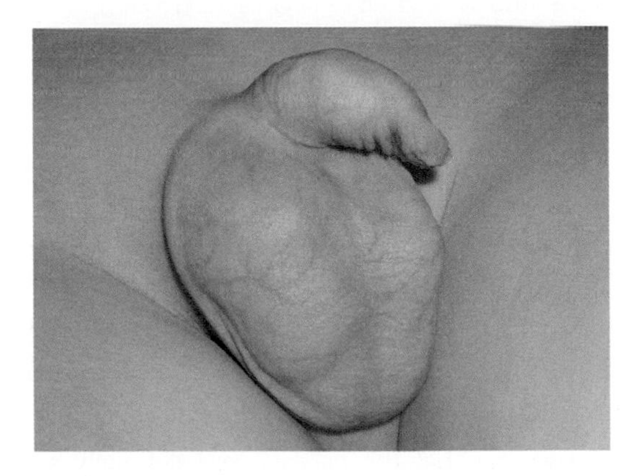

Figure 14.6 A right encysted hydrocele of the cord. It is clearly separate from the testicle. You can get above it, and there is no cough impulse in the swelling or in the groin above it.

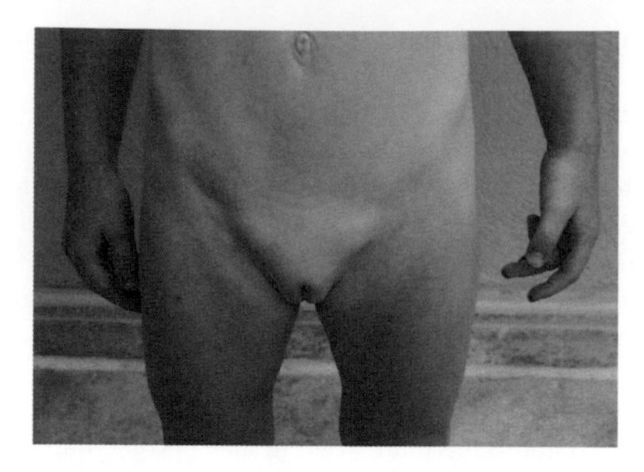

Figure 14.7 This young girl's parents gave a history of an intermittent left groin swelling and pointed to the inguinal canal, but nothing was visible when she came to the clinic. Nevertheless, the history was good enough for an operation to be planned. But, later a lump appeared in the other groin, and the parents took this photograph confirming the presence of bilateral inguinal hernias.

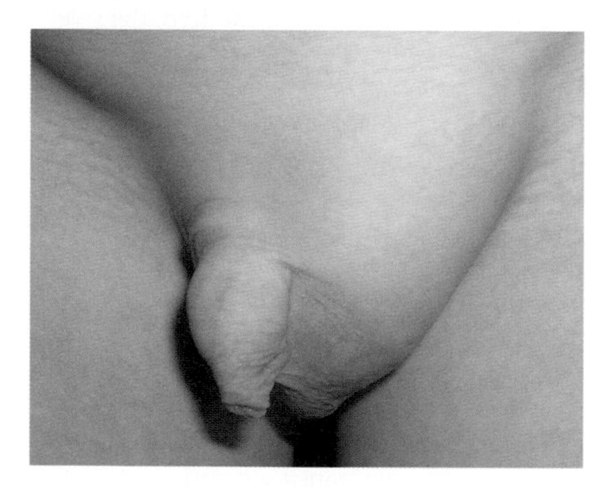

Figure 14.8 A large left inguinal hernia in a child.

Children's groin hernias occasionally become irreducible, but strangulation is rare. If strangulation does occur, the gonadal vessels are more likely to be damaged than the vessels of the bowel, so testicular infarction is more common than bowel infarction.

NOTE: Direct hernias do occur in children but are very rare.

Children's hernias may only appear intermittently. The swelling that the parents have definitely seen often obstinately refuses to appear in the presence of the examining doctor (Figure 14.7). If the site of the swelling indicated by the parents is the inguinal canal, exploration is justified on the history or camera phone evidence, and an indirect sac is invariably found.

In females, the wall of the sac may include the ovary and fallopian tube. In these cases, when the contents are reduced, there may remain a small mass, which is tender to touch. The child may also complain of pain in the area.

NOTE: Do not confuse the infantile with the adult hydrocele.

In children, the condition is a fluid-filled congenital inguinal hernia with a narrow sac that communicates with the peritoneal cavity on every occasion.

The adult hydrocele is an acquired condition in which fluid accumulates around the testicle, within the tunica vaginalis, in response to a local abnormality. It has no communication with the peritoneum.

Femoral hernia

ANATOMY

A femoral hernia is a protrusion of extraperitoneal fat, a peritoneal sac and sometimes abdominal contents through the femoral canal (Figure 14.9). The anatomical margins of this canal are the inguinal ligament anteriorly, the pubic ramus and pectineus muscle posteriorly, the lacunar ligament and pubic bone medially, and the femoral vein laterally.

The femoral canal provides a space into which the femoral vein can expand. It normally contains loose areolar tissue and a lymph gland known as the *gland of Cloquet*. With bone or ligament on three sides and a major vessel on the fourth, the femoral canal cannot distend easily. A peritoneal sac coming through it therefore has a stiff, narrow neck, and any contents are at risk of strangulation.

A characteristic but not invariable feature of the sac of a femoral hernia is that it is thick walled with layers of fat and connective tissue, which when cut across look like an onion. This means that the sac remains palpable even when empty, so seems to be irreducible.

History

Age Femoral hernias are rare in children and do not become common until over the age of 50 years, with no upper age limit.

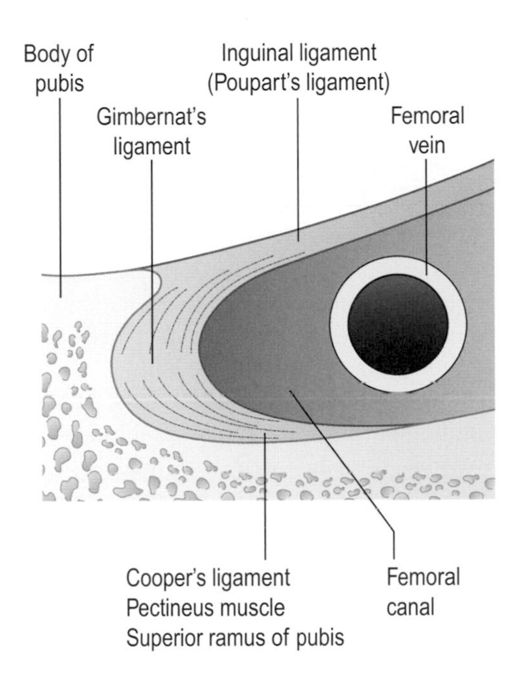

Figure 14.9 The boundaries of the left femoral canal.

Sex *Femoral hernias are much more common in females than in males.* Nevertheless, do not forget that, even in females, the most common hernia in the groin region is the inguinal hernia, and that a male can have a femoral hernia.

Symptoms Usually, the patient discovers the swelling. The other main presentation is in the elderly, with *obstruction or strangulation* of a previously unnoticed hernia. Partial strangulation of the bowel wall (*Richter's hernia*) is likely, because of the narrow neck.

Femoral hernias are occasionally bilateral.

Examination (Figure 14.10)

Because of the thick-walled sac, a femoral hernia can be seen and felt when the patient is lying flat. It is easier in that position to find the pubic tubercle and other related anatomical landmarks.

Position The neck of a femoral hernia, or the point at which it disappears into the abdomen, is below the inguinal ligament and lateral to the pubic tubercle (Figure 14.11). The *bulge usually appears to be directly behind the skin crease of the groin,* whereas the inguinal hernia bulges out above the groin crease. With experience, this feature allows spot diagnosis.

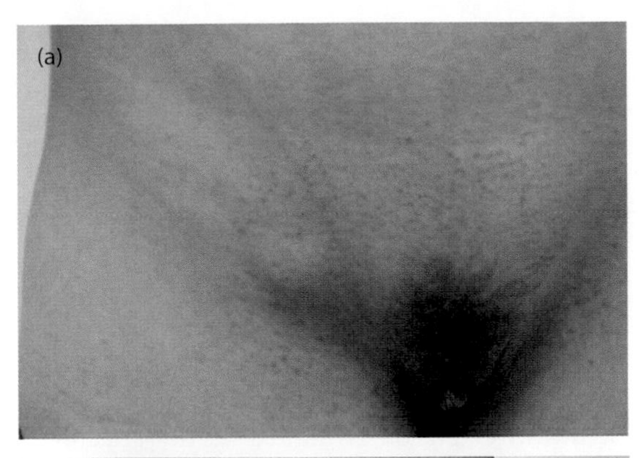

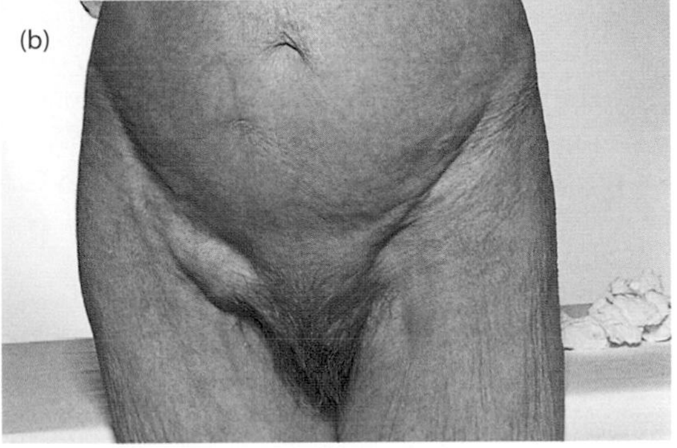

Figure 14.10 FEMORAL HERNIAS. (a) A right femoral hernia. Note that the femoral hernia bulges into the crease of the groin. (b) A larger femoral hernia, in an elderly female, with a wide neck stretching laterally over the femoral vein.

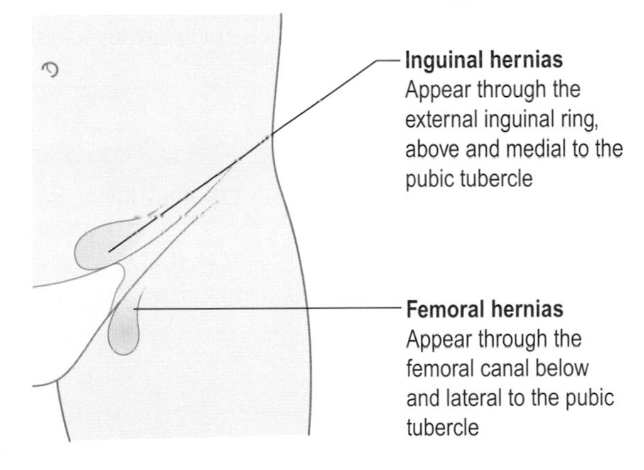

Figure 14.11 The sites of appearance of inguinal and femoral hernia.

A small hernia in a fat person is very difficult to feel, so take great care when examining this region in a patient with intestinal obstruction.

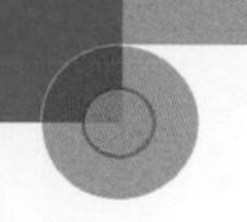

Colour The overlying skin will be of normal colour. Even if the hernia is strangulated, the sac and superficial fascia provide good camouflage.

Temperature The skin temperature is normal for the same reasons.

Tenderness Femoral hernias are not usually tender unless strangulated.

Shape and size The lump is *almost spherical,* and the neck cannot be defined clearly. Most femoral hernias are small. Should they enlarge, they extend or spread upwards towards the fold of the groin because downward extension is limited by the attachment of the membranous layer of the superficial fascia (Scarpa's fascia) to the deep fascia of the upper thigh.

Surface The surface of the sac is usually smooth.

Composition The majority of femoral hernias feel firm because they consist of a thick-walled fatty sac. The peritoneal sac is small and is either empty or contains omentum.

Reducibility The majority of femoral hernias cannot be reduced, as most of the swelling is the sac itself.

Cough impulse Femoral hernias do not usually have a cough impulse.

Relations Diagnosis depends upon the site of the lump, hence the importance of clearly defining its relations to the surrounding structures (Revision panel 14.5).

Local tissues Femoral hernias develop through a natural defect but are sometimes seen after the repair of an inguinal hernia. Look out for groin scars.

Revision panel 14.5

DIFFERENTIAL DIAGNOSIS OF A LUMP IN THE GROIN

- Inguinal hernia
- Femoral hernia
- Enlarged lymph glands
- Saphena varix
- Ectopic testis
- Femoral aneurysm
- Hydrocele of the cord or hydrocele of the canal of Nuck
- Lipoma of the cord
- Psoas bursa
- Psoas abscess (Figure 14.13)

General examination As ever, this should be routine.

Prevascular hernia

This is a rare variety of femoral hernia (Figure 14.12). The femoral canal expands laterally under the inguinal ligament in front of the femoral artery and vein. It has a wide neck and a flattened wide sac, which bulges downwards and laterally.

Prevascular hernias usually reduce, and have a cough impulse. They rarely strangulate. They are difficult to repair by open techniques because the femoral vessels form the posterior wall of the defect.

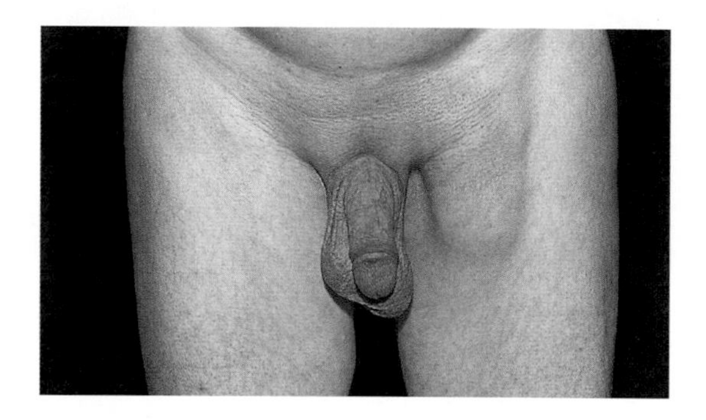

Figure 14.12 A prevascular femoral hernia.

Figure 14.13 Psoas abscess.

Umbilical hernia

All hernias related to the umbilicus may be called umbilical hernias. They may be congenital or acquired. All congenital umbilical hernias come through the umbilical defect itself. In adults, most umbilical hernias are acquired and come through a defect adjacent to the umbilical cicatrix, rather than through the umbilical scar itself, and should be termed *paraumbilical* (Figure 14.14). In practice, the simple expression 'umbilical hernia' is used commonly for both varieties.

Skin dimple

The normal umbilicus

Rectus abdominis muscle

Scar in linea alba tethered to the skin

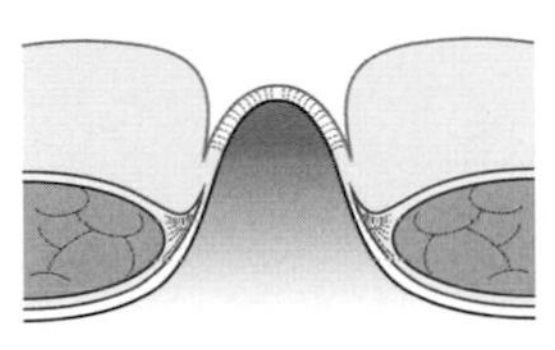

A congenital umbilical hernia

The umbilical scar fails to form or is weak. The abdominal contents bulge through the weak spot and evert the umbilicus

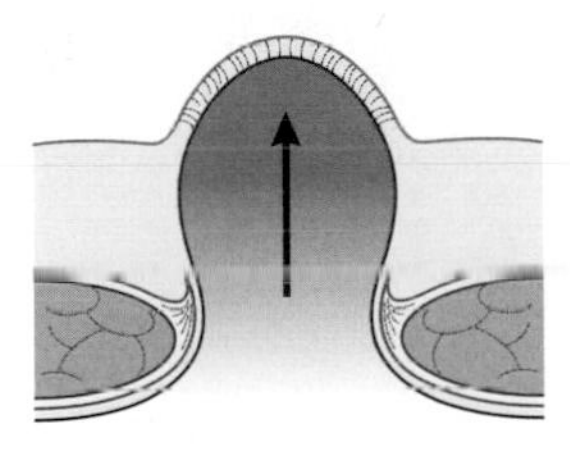

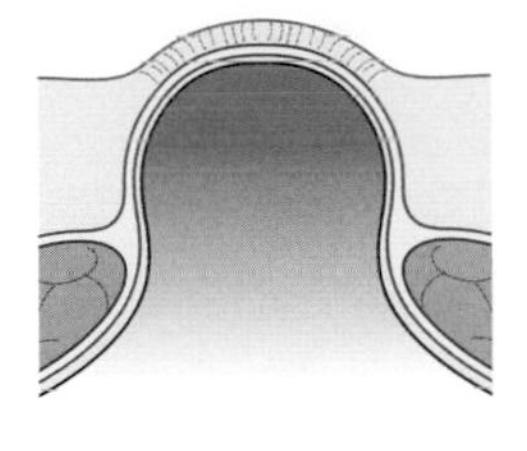

An acquired true umbilical hernia

The umbilical scar is stretched by a raised intra-abdominal pressure and the umbilicus everts

A paraumbilical hernia

The hernial orifice is at the side of the umbilical scar so the sac bulges out the umbilicus, turning it into a crescent-shaped slit

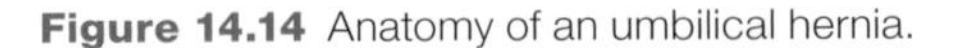

Figure 14.14 Anatomy of an umbilical hernia.

CONGENITAL UMBILICAL HERNIA

In early fetal life, the whole of the mid-gut protrudes through the umbilicus. As it returns into the abdomen, the gap in the abdominal wall gradually closes, leaving a small central defect through which the umbilical vessels connect the fetus with the placenta. Should the process to obliterate the peritoneal sac fail and the defect persists, there will be a congenital umbilical hernia (Figure 14.15).

NOTE: A congenital persisting protrusion of bowel through the umbilical defect without a covering of skin is called an *exomphalos*. This is a failure of development of the abdominal wall and not a true hernia.

History

Age Although the weakness is present at birth, the hernia may be very small and not immediately noticed.

Ethnicity Congenital umbilical hernias are more common in Afro-Caribbean people.

Symptoms The swelling rarely causes any symptoms for the patient, but parental anxiety is common. Intestinal obstruction or irreducibility is extremely rare. A visible hernia may be embarrassing to a child when noticed by others. 'Tummy ache' in children may be attributed to the hernia, but it is unlikely that there is ever a genuine association.

Natural history The vast majority of congenital umbilical hernias resolve spontaneously during the first few years of life. It is difficult to explain how a large defect in an active child will close, but this is usual. The hernia becomes gradually smaller and then disappears. However, if there is still a defect by the age of 4 years, it is unlikely to close and operation is advised.

Examination

Shape and size Congenital umbilical hernias are usually hemispherical and overlie a palpable defect in the abdominal wall. The size of the lump is variable. Very small hernias can only be found by gently palpating the umbilicus with the tip of a finger. Although the hernia may be sizeable, the palpable defect is often small.

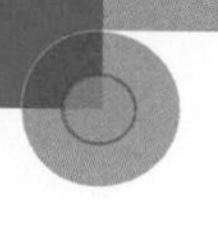

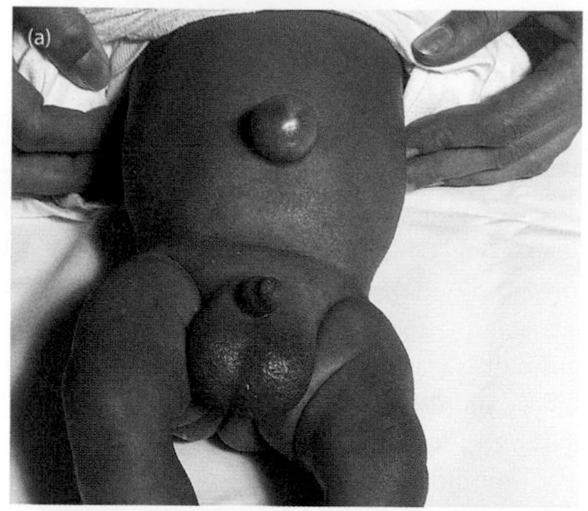

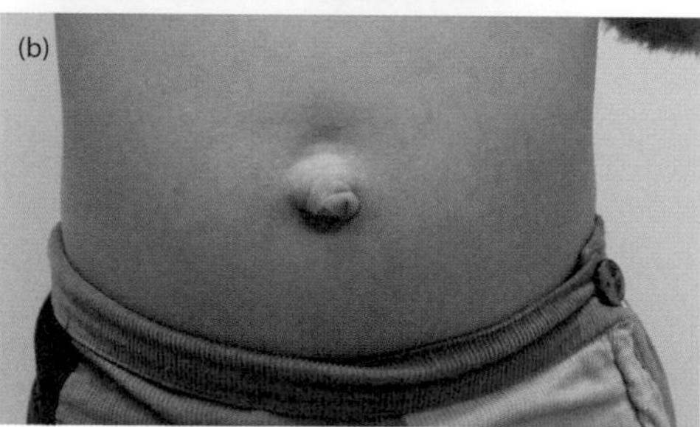

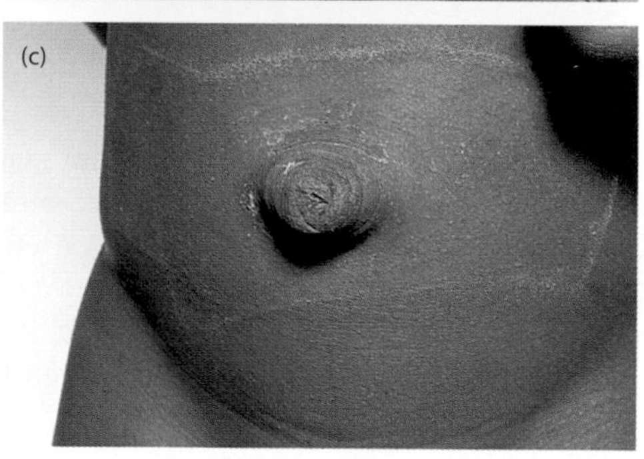

Figure 14.15 CONGENITAL UMBILICAL HERNIAS. (a) This baby also has a left inguinal hernia and a right hydrocele. (b) An umbilical hernia in a 3-year-old female. (c) A regressing congenital umbilical hernia. The defect has almost closed, and the overlying skin is collapsing inwards to become a normal umbilicus.

In neonates, the remnants of the umbilical cord may be visible.

Composition Congenital umbilical hernias are *soft, compressible and easy to reduce*. They usually contain bowel so would be resonant to percussion, which is difficult to elicit in a small child. They reduce spontaneously when the child lies down and become tense when the child cries.

Cough impulse An expansile cough impulse is invariable.

UMBILICAL HERNIA IN ADULTS

A true umbilical hernia comes through the umbilical scar and has the umbilical skin tethered to it. It is not common in adults and is usually secondary to raised intra-abdominal pressure. The causes of an acquired umbilical hernia include pregnancy and ascites.

Paraumbilical hernia

This is the common acquired umbilical hernia. It appears through a defect adjacent to the umbilical scar (Figure 14.16). It does not bulge into the centre of the umbilicus, and the umbilical skin is not attached to the centre of the sac.

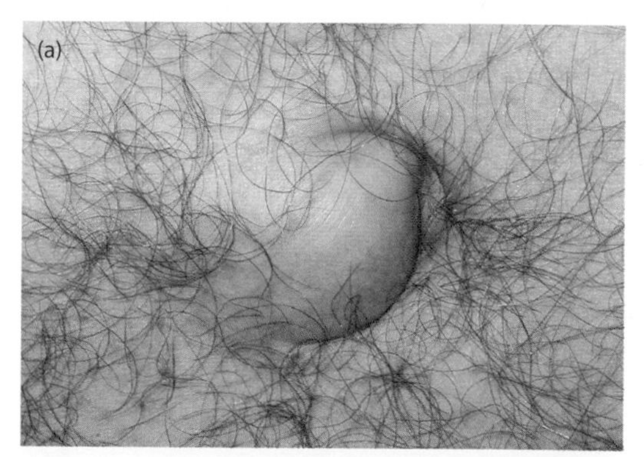

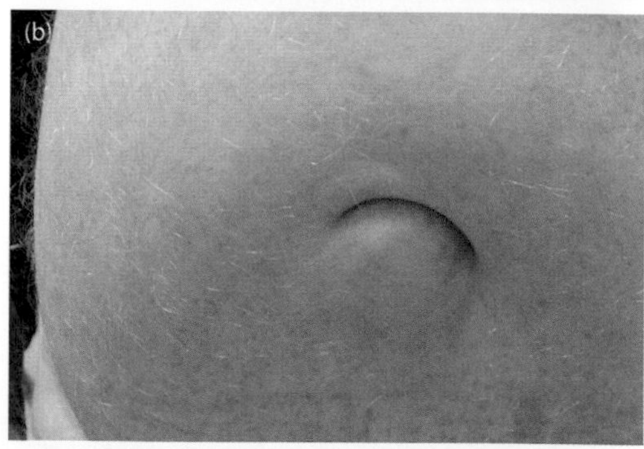

Figure 14.16 PARAUMBILICAL HERNIAS. (a) Note that the hernia is clearly coming out alongside the true umbilical scar. (b) A large paraumbilical hernia, partially obscured by a very fat abdominal wall. Note the classical crescent shape of the umbilicus.

History

Age Paraumbilical hernias usually develop in middle and old age. They are more common in females than in males, and are associated with parity and obesity.

Symptoms The symptoms are *swelling and discomfort*. Sometimes, the only symptom is pain and tenderness around the umbilicus, made worse by prolonged standing or strenuous exercise, and the doctor finds the hernia.

Strangulation of an umbilical hernia, whether or not it has been previously noticed by the patient, regularly occurs. The usual contents are extraperitoneal fat or omentum, so even although the hernial contents may be strangulated, bowel is not obstructed or damaged.

Examination

Position The main bulge of the hernia is beside the umbilicus, which is pushed to one side and stretched into a crescent shape. With a large hernia in a fat patient, there may be a crescent-shaped pit, with attachment of the skin to the umbilicus at the bottom. This pit may be too deep to clean and, in consequence, there may be a foul-smelling discharge and even a collection of dried-up sebaceous secretions, an *ompholith* (see page 489).

Surface and edge The surface is smooth and the edge easy to define, except when the patient's abdominal wall is very fat.

Composition The lump is firm as it usually contains omentum. If it contains bowel, it is soft and resonant to percussion. It will be reducible unless the contents are adherent to the sac or the defect is very narrow.

Cough impulse Most of these hernias have an expansile cough impulse.

Relations The skin at the centre of the umbilicus is not attached to the centre of the sac as in the true umbilical hernia, but the umbilical skin is usually firmly applied to the side of the sac and may be fixed to it.

If the hernia can be reduced, the firm fibrous edge of the defect in the linea alba is easy to feel.

General examination Although abdominal distension usually causes a true umbilical hernia, it can exacerbate a paraumbilical hernia, so look for underlying causes of distension.

Epigastric hernia

This is a protrusion of extraperitoneal fat, and sometimes a small peritoneal sac, through a defect in the linea alba somewhere between the xiphisternum and the umbilicus (Figure 14.17).

The patient complains of epigastric pain, which is localized exactly to the site of the hernia, but often does not notice the underlying lump.

The pain is sometimes associated with eating, so the patient calls it 'indigestion' and makes a self-diagnosis of peptic ulceration. A likely explanation for this is that the fatty hernia is 'nipped' by the linea alba on leaning forward in the sitting position adopted at the dining table. Thus, when a patient complains of epigastric discomfort, palpate the

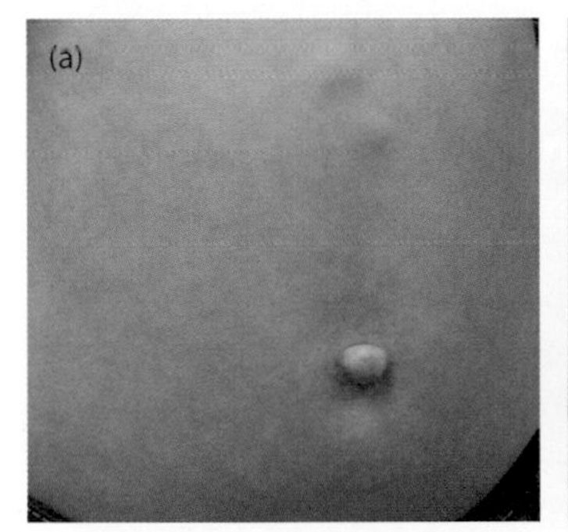

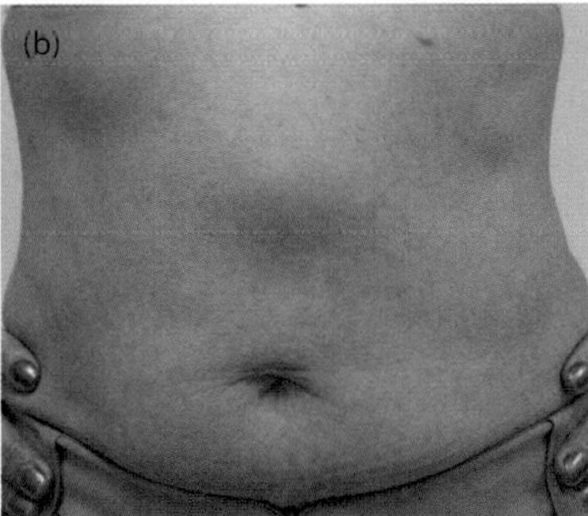

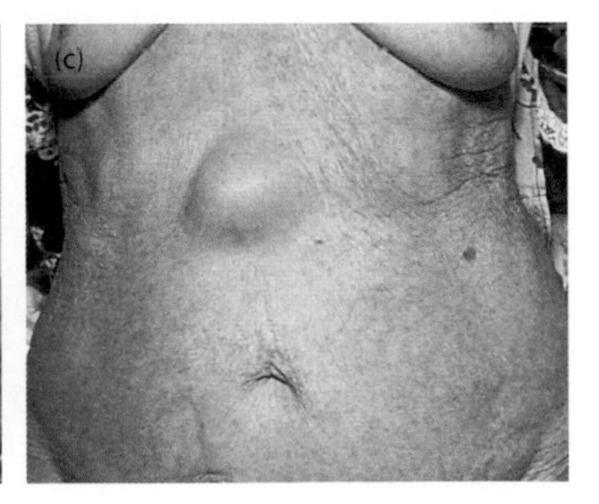

Figure 14.17 THREE PATIENTS WITH EPIGASTRIC HERNIAS. (a) A 3-year-old male with two epigastric hernias and an umbilical hernia. These small hernias can be the source of epigastric pain. (b) A female with a large epigastric hernia, which was misdiagnosed as a lipoma and ignored for 5 years. (c) An elderly female with an epigastric hernia. This reduced easily and caused no symptoms.

abdominal wall very carefully before concentrating on deep palpation, because all the symptoms may be caused by a small, fatty epigastric hernia.

On examination, these hernias feel firm, *do not usually have a cough impulse and cannot be reduced*. It is sometimes impossible to distinguish them from lipomas, only the typical position suggesting the correct diagnosis. The defect is always exactly in the midline, but the sac and hence the palpable swelling may lie to one side.

EPIGASTRIC HERNIA IN CHILDREN

This condition is reasonably common in childhood, sometimes associated with divarication of the rectus abdominis muscles (Figure 14.17). A small hernia may only be visible intermittently, leading to diagnostic uncertainty. As strangulation of such a sac in a child rarely occurs, it is safe to wait until the hernia is seen before discussing surgery, unlike inguinal hernia in children, for which an operation may be indicated on the history alone.

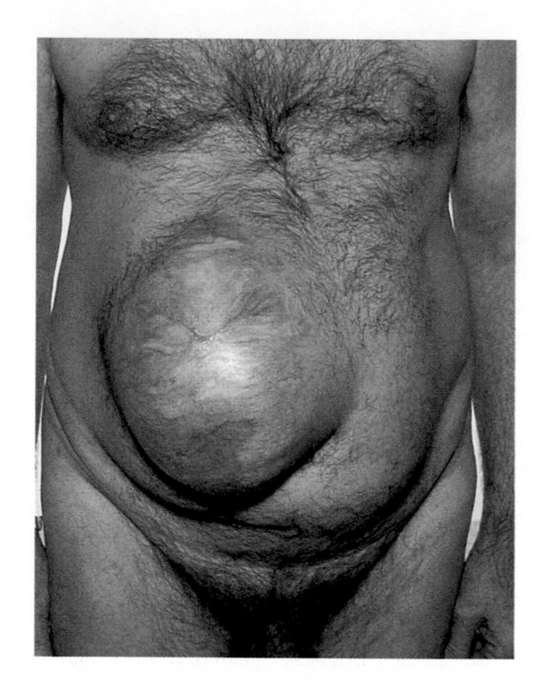

Figure 14.18 A large incisional hernia.

Incisional hernia

An abdominal incisional hernia is a hernia through a scar in the abdominal wall, caused by a previous surgical operation or injury. Scar tissue is inelastic and stretches progressively if subjected to constant stress.

History

Patients usually remember the operation or wound that caused the scar, but may not recall any complications in the original wound such as a haematoma or infection, which weakened it and made it more susceptible to the development of a hernia. There may be a history of factors likely to weaken the abdominal musculature, such as chronic cough, obesity or steroid therapy.

Age Incisional hernias occur at all ages but are more common in the elderly.

Symptoms The most common symptoms are a *lump and pain*. Intestinal obstruction and strangulation can occur.

Examination (Figure 14.18)

Commonly, there is a *lump with an expansile cough impulse, beneath an old scar*. The defect in the abdominal wall may be palpable. Incisional hernias are not infrequently irreducible, the defect being plugged with adherent omentum.

If the lump does not reduce and does not have a cough impulse, it may not be a hernia, but rather a deposit of tumour, a chronic abscess or haematoma or a foreign-body granuloma. All these conditions, except recurrent tumour, appear shortly after the initial surgery.

The first signs of incisional hernia usually appear in the first year after surgery but sometimes many years later.

Divarication of the recti

This is separation of the rectus abdominis muscles with extenuation of the linea alba, from the xiphisternum to umbilicus and occasionally below.

It may be seen in children in the first few years of life. It is only noticeable when the abdominal wall is tensed. Children have a relatively larger abdominal cavity than adults; even the slimmest appear somewhat 'pot-bellied'.

The condition usually improves and eventually disappears as the child grows, but occasionally it persists into adult life. There may be a coincidental umbilical hernia or an epigastric hernia.

The only clinical concern is the appearance, as strangulation is impossible with such a wide-necked bulge.

Divarication of the recti is also seen in adults, in females during and immediately after childbirth. There may be a wide separation of the muscles, with stretched overlying abdominal skin. The examiner may be able to put a hand into the abdominal cavity. (Ask permission to do this!)

As abdominal tone recovers, the defect closes, although it may become permanent after multiple pregnancies.

Divarication is best observed with the patient lying supine and raising their head and legs together, the recti are fully tensed and the abdominal pressure rises. The thinned-out linea alba then bulges, producing a visible swelling. Patients of all ages learn the best way to produce the swelling.

Rare abdominal hernias

Spigelian hernias *occur* at the edge of the rectus sheath, below the umbilicus and above the inguinal area. They are seen in obese patients and may be difficult to diagnose.

Obturator hernias come through the obturator foramen, and the small sac is concealed amongst the adductor muscles of the thigh. Only on very rare occasions will there be a palpable mass. The usual presentation is small bowel obstruction of unknown cause. The sac may compress the obturator nerve and cause pain in the medial side of the thigh.

Lumbar and gluteal hernias are rare. They are commonly associated with previous surgery near to the defect, such as a loin incision or an excision of the rectum. Diagnosis is difficult and often requires imaging by magnetic resonance imaging.

Conditions of the umbilicus

The most common abnormality of the umbilicus is an umbilical hernia, described above.

Other important congenital abnormalities of the umbilicus are exomphalos and persistent fistulas. The acquired conditions are inflammation and invasion by tumour.

EXOMPHALOS

NOTE: This condition, present at birth, represents an intrauterine failure of the intestines to return to the abdomen, combined with a failure of the two sides of the laterally developing abdominal wall to unite to cover the embryonic defect.

All layers of the abdominal wall are deficient over the protruding intestines except for a translucent sac consisting of peritoneum, Wharton's jelly and amnion (Figure 14.19). Once it is exposed to air it quickly opacifies. Surgical management will depend on the size of the defect, visceroabdominal disproportion and respiratory status.

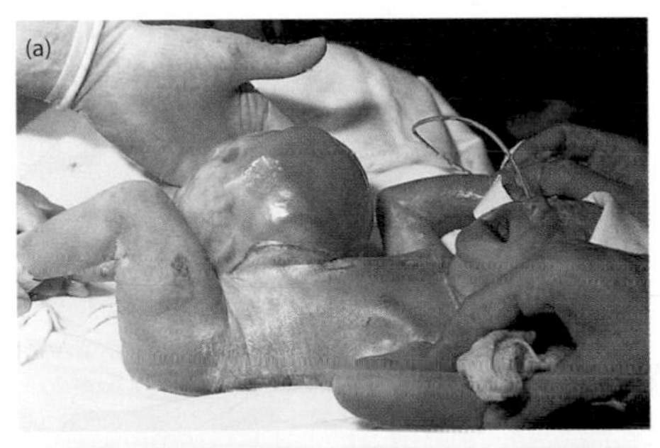

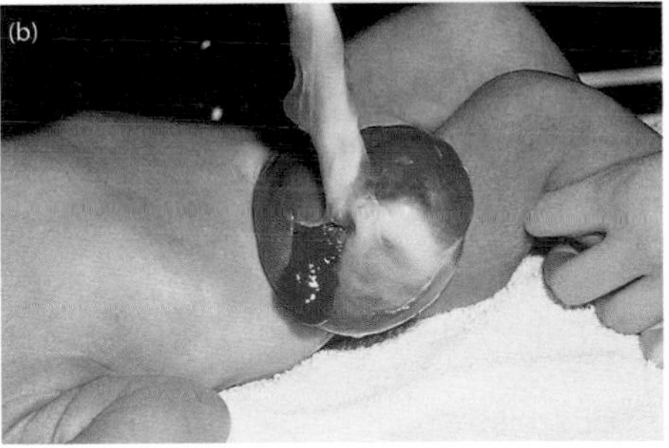

Figure 14.19 TWO EXAMPLES OF EXOMPHALOS. (a) The bowel can be seen through the thin membrane. (b) The thin membrane is covered with fibrin but has, nevertheless, ruptured. The umbilical cord is still present.

UMBILICAL FISTULAS

Four structures pass through the umbilicus during fetal development: the umbilical vein, the umbilical

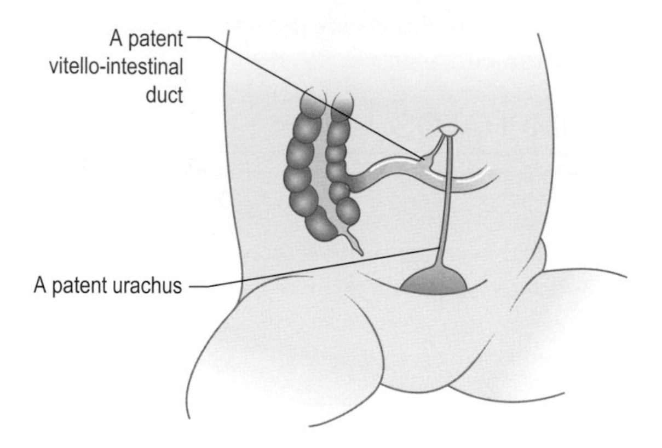

Figure 14.20 A patent vitellointestinal duct or patent urachus can become an intestinal or urinary fistula, respectively.

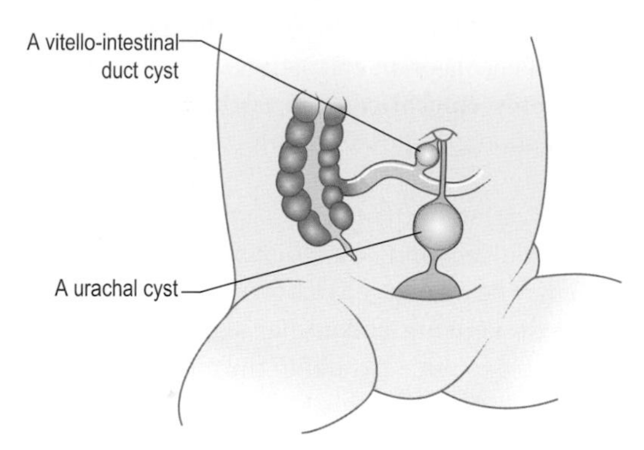

Figure 14.21 If the vitellointestinal duct or urachus are not completely obliterated, they may turn into cysts.

arteries, the vitellointestinal duct and the urachus. If either of the last two tubes fails to close properly, there will be an *intestinal or a urinary fistula, sinus or cyst.*

A *patent vitellointestinal duct* (Figure 14.20) in the neonate produces an intermittent discharge of *mucus and sometimes faeces from the umbilicus.* It is a rare abnormality. Sometimes, there is visible small intestinal mucosa lining an obvious fistula but, on other occasions, there may only be a small fluid leak and the condition mimics an umbilical granuloma. The duct connects to the ileum at the site of a Meckel's diverticulum.

A *vitellointestinal duct cyst* is a small, spherical, mobile swelling deep to the umbilicus that is tethered to the umbilicus and to the small bowel by a fibrous cord (Figure 14.21). Very occasionally, when the duct closes late there can be persistent intestinal columnar epithelium presenting as an umbilical adenoma. This will not resolve with time unlike an umbilical granuloma.

A *patent urachus* can become a track through which *urine can leak* onto the external surface of the abdomen through the umbilicus. This rare condition occasionally presents in childhood, but more commonly in adult life, in association with bladder dysfunction most commonly due to chronic retention of urine caused by disease of the prostate.

The patient complains of a watery discharge from the umbilicus.

An *urachal cyst* is an immobile swelling below the umbilicus deep to the abdominal muscles. It may become large enough to fluctuate and have a fluid thrill. If it is still connected to the bladder, it may vary in size and be difficult to distinguish from a chronically distended bladder.

UMBILICAL GRANULOMA

This is a very common condition affecting newborns. After the umbilical cord has been severed and tied, the proximal remnant shrivels and separates spontaneously. This leaves an area of chronic inflammation at the line of demarcation, which is quickly covered by epithelium. If the inflammatory process becomes florid, with associated infection, excess granulation tissue is formed that prevents the raw area becoming epithelialized.

The baby presents with a pouting umbilicus surmounted by a *bright red, moist, friable, sometimes hemispherical mass of bleeding granulation tissue* (Figure 14.22). This condition is similar to the pyogenic granuloma seen in other parts of the skin. It usually regresses spontaneously in the first month or so of life. If the condition persists longer than this, the possibility of a patent vitellointestinal duct or an umbilical adenoma should be considered.

OMPHALITIS

Infection within the umbilicus is not uncommon in adults (Figure 14.23). It is usually associated with inadequate hygiene and a sunken umbilicus caused by obesity, made worse by any coexisting paraumbilical hernia. The condition is similar to the intertrigo

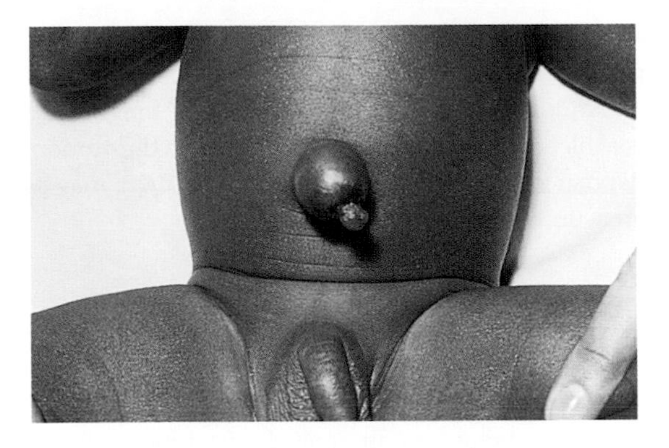

Figure 14.22 An umbilical granuloma. This is an excessive amount of granulation tissue at the point where the umbilical cord separated. These granulomas are often associated with an umbilical hernia.

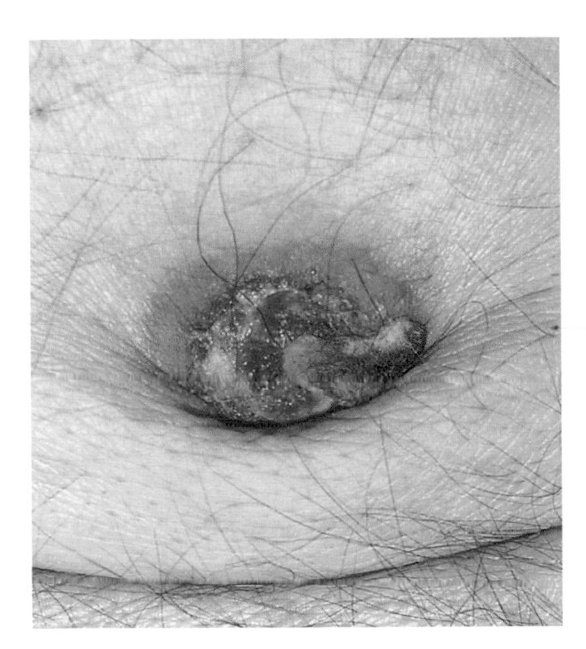

Figure 14.23 Omphalitis. A protruding mass of infected granulation tissue caused by a large ompholith, the brown tip of which is just visible.

that occurs between folds of skin elsewhere associated with obesity and sweating, which become secondarily infected with skin organisms that produce an unpleasant smell.

The patient complains of umbilical discharge, pain and soreness.

On examination, the skin within and around the umbilicus is red and tender, and exuding a seropurulent discharge with a characteristic *foul smell*. The whole umbilicus may feel indurated, especially if there is an ompholith or a tumour deposit.

Although simple dermatitis or skin infection is by far the most common cause of a discharge from the umbilicus, it is essential to exclude the other causes of an umbilical discharge, which are listed in Revision panel 14.6.

True omphalitis is infection of the stump of the umbilical cord following inadequate postnatal care and cleanliness.

Revision panel 14.6

CAUSES OF DISCHARGE FROM THE UMBILICUS

Congenital

Vitellointestinal remant (fistula/sinus)/patent urachus

Acquired

Umbilical granuloma
Dermatitis (intertrigo)
Ompholith (umbilical concretion)
Fistula (intestinal)
Secondary carcinoma
Endometriosis

OMPHOLITH

When the sebaceous secretions that accumulate in the umbilicus are mixed with the broken hairs and fluff from clothing that become sucked into the umbilicus, the mixture can form a firm lump, worthy of the name umbilical stone or ompholith. The outside tip of the concretions dries out and may protrude like a sebaceous horn.

Routine personal hygiene will usually prevent the formation of an ompholith, but this can be challenging in obese patients.

Small concretions are common and uncomplicated. An abscess will occasionally develop in a narrownecked umbilicus containing an ompholith. The patient feels unwell and has a very painful,

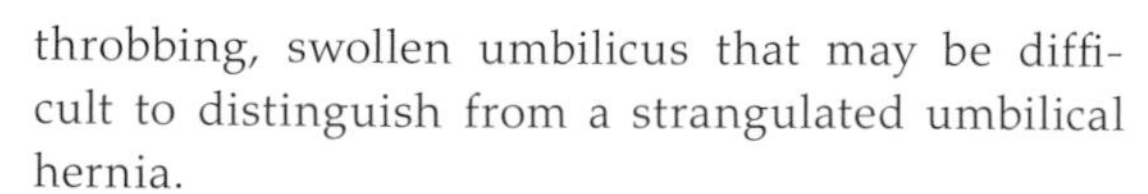

throbbing, swollen umbilicus that may be difficult to distinguish from a strangulated umbilical hernia.

Pus tracking from an intra-abdominal abscess may occasionally point at the umbilicus, the most common cause being diverticular disease.

SECONDARY CARCINOMA (SISTER JOSEPH'S NODULE)

A firm or hard nodule bulging into the umbilicus, underneath the skin or eroding through it, in a patient who is losing weight and looks unwell is likely to be a nodule of metastatic cancer (Figure 14.24). This presentation always indicates advanced, widespread intra-abdominal disease, and the primary tumour is usually in the abdomen.

The tumour cells reach the umbilicus via lymphatics that run in the edge of the falciform ligament alongside the obliterated umbilical vein, or by transperitoneal spread.

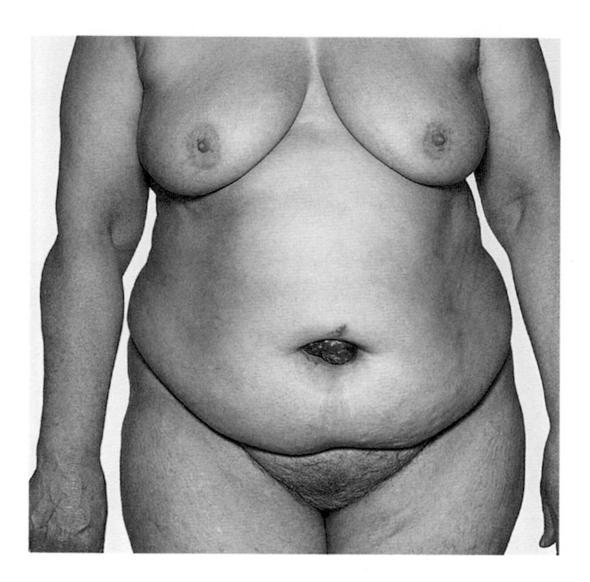

Figure 14.24 A nodule of metastatic carcinoma bulging through the umbilicus causing a serosanguinous discharge. This is known as a Sister Joseph's nodule.

Nodules of secondary carcinoma may ulcerate, bleed and become infected. Rarely, the tumour deposit is in continuity with bowel and there may be an acquired intestinal fistula.

ENDOMETRIOMA

If, in a female patient, the umbilicus enlarges, becomes painful and discharges blood during menstruation, it may contain a patch of ectopic endometrial tissue.

DISCOLOURATION OF THE UMBILICUS

The following physical signs are rare, but the diseases that cause them are common and serious.

A blue tinge around the umbilicus, caused by dilated, tortuous, sometimes visible, veins, is called a *caput medusae*, after Medusa, the mythical Gorgon who had small snakes on her scalp instead of hair. The dilated veins are collateral vessels that have developed to circumvent portal vein obstruction. There will be other signs of portal hypertension and liver failure.

Yellow-blue bruising around the umbilicus (*Cullen's sign*) and in the flank (Grey Turner's sign; see Chapter 15) may be caused by pancreatic enzymes that have tracked along the falciform ligament to the umbilicus or across the retroperitoneal space to the loin and digested the subcutaneous tissues following an attack of severe acute pancreatitis. Both appear a few days after the beginning of the acute symptoms.

Bruising at the umbilicus can also be associated with *intra-abdominal bleeding*, particularly when it is extraperitoneal. Causes include ruptured aortic aneurysms, ruptured ectopic pregnancy and accidental periuterine bleeding in pregnancy.

The abdomen

JAMES A GOSSAGE AND KATHERINE M BURNAND

Examination of the abdomen

The abdomen contains the stomach, duodenum, small and large bowel, liver, gallbladder, spleen, pancreas, kidneys, uterus, bladder, aorta and vena cava and, in females, the uterus, ovaries and Fallopian tubes. Therefore, this relatively small cavity contains a number of vital organs, all of which are susceptible to disease or malfunction. Many are inaccessible to palpation, being hidden behind the lower ribs or inside the bony pelvis (Figure 15.1).

The close proximity of the abdominal organs to each other can make the brain incapable of distinguishing which organ is the source of a pain. Symptoms and signs will help to distinguish the likely organ and the pathology responsible for the pain.

PREPARATION

The environment

The examination room must be warm and private if the patient is to lie undressed and relaxed. A cold couch placed in a draught or in the view of other patients makes proper examination impossible. A good light is essential, ideally with daylight as artificial light can obliterate the soft shadows that may provide the first indication of asymmetry.

The examination couch or bed

A hard, flat couch makes the patient lie absolutely flat and opens the gap between the pubis and the xiphisternum but, unfortunately, stretches and

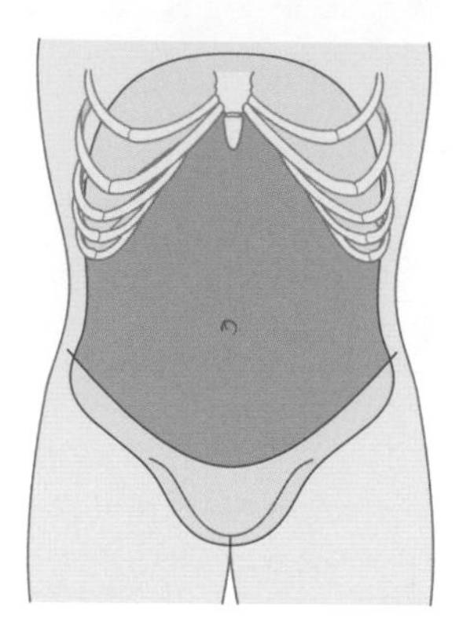
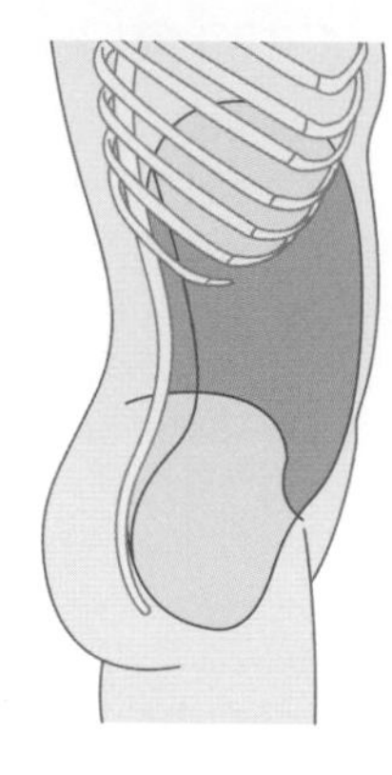

Figure 15.1 These drawings show the extent of the abdominal cavity. The paler areas indicate the parts of the abdomen shielded from palpation by the ribs and the pelvis.

tightens the abdominal muscles. Conversely, a soft bed lets the lumbar spine sink into a deep curve closing the gap between the pubis and the ribs. The best compromise is a hard couch with a backrest that can be raised by 15–20°. The hard couch ensures that patients retain their lumbar lordosis, opening access to the abdomen and pushing the central contents anteriorly. The elevation of the thoracic cage relaxes the anterior abdominal wall muscles.

Exposure

The full extent of the abdomen should be visible and, ideally, patients should be uncovered from nipples to knees. To maintain patient dignity, a compromise is to cover the lower abdomen with a sheet or blanket while the abdomen is being palpated. At the end of the examination, you must never forget to examine the genitalia and the hernial orifices.

Getting the patient to relax

It is not possible to feel anything within the abdomen if the patient is tense. There are several ways in which relaxation can be achieved:

- Ask the patient to rest their head on the couch or a pillow to avoid tensing the rectus abdominis muscles.
- Ask the patient to place their arms by their sides, not behind their head.
- Encourage the patient to sink their back into the couch and breathe regularly and slowly.
- Only press your hands into the abdomen during expiration as the abdominal muscles relax.

If the above manoeuvres do not work, ask the patient to flex their hips to 45° and their knees to 90° and place an extra pillow behind their head. These procedures tilt up the pelvis and reduce the access to the abdomen, but they usually relax the abdominal muscles.

The position of the examiner

The examiner's hands should be clean and warm with short nails. The whole hand should rest on the abdomen by keeping the hand and forearm horizontal, in the same plane as the front of the abdomen. To achieve this, the examiner must sit or kneel beside the bed. Do not examine the patient from a standing position by leaning forwards and dorsiflexing your wrist.

Sitting or kneeling beside the patient with your forearm level with the front of the abdomen puts your eyes about 50 cm above your hand, an ideal level for seeing any soft shadows caused by lumps and bumps (Figure 15.2).

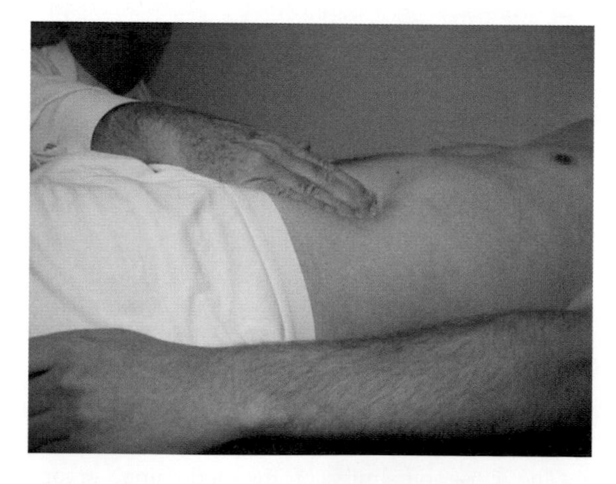

Figure 15.2 When you palpate the abdomen, sit or kneel so that your forearm is horizontal and level with the anterior abdominal wall, and your eyes are 50 cm above this level. If you are higher, your wrist will be extended and you will not be able to palpate comfortably and firmly. In this illustration, the abdomen is inadequately exposed.

EXAMINATION

This should follow the standard routine of inspection, palpation, percussion and auscultation.

Inspection

Look at the whole patient (see Chapter 1). Look for any general abnormality indicative of intra-abdominal pathology such as *cachexia, pallor or jaundice*.

Inspection of the abdomen from the end of the bed reveals whether there is any *asymmetry* or *distension*.

Note the position, shape and size of *any bulge*, any changes in its shape and whether it moves with respiration or increases with coughing.

Observe the reaction of the patient to coughing or moving. Patients with peritonitis find movement extremely painful and, consequently, tend to lie very still, while patients with colic roll around with each bout of pain.

Record the presence of any *scars, sinuses* or *fistulas*.

Dilated surface veins may indicate the possibility of portal hypertension or inferior vena caval occlusion.

Palpation

Palpate gently but deliberately, firmly and with purpose. Rapid, jerky or circular movements reminiscent of kneading dough are distressing for patients and cause them to lose confidence. Keeping your hands still and feeling the intra-abdominal structures moving beneath them gives more information than rapid and thoughtless palpation.

Finish by feeling the areas that might otherwise be forgotten (see Revision panel 15.1):

Revision panel 15.1

NEVER FORGET TO EXAMINE

Supraclavicular lymph glands
Hernia orifices
Femoral pulses
Genitalia
Anal canal and rectum

- Feel the supraclavicular fossae and neck for lymph glands.
- Feel the hernial orifices at rest and when the patient coughs.
- Feel the femoral pulses.
- Examine the external genitalia.
- Look at the hands, nails and facies.

General light palpation for tenderness

This should be done by gently *resting a hand on the patient's abdomen and pressing lightly*. The hand should be systematically moved over the whole of the abdomen. If you are right-handed, start in the left iliac fossa and move round in an anticlockwise direction to finish in the right iliac fossa.

When a patient complains of pain, ask them to indicate its site before you begin your palpation, so that you can *start over a non-tender area* and move towards the tender spot. Carefully define the area of tenderness so that you can depict it as a hatched area on a drawing of the abdomen.

Assess the degree of tenderness. Palpation over an area of mild tenderness just causes pain. **Guarding**, the tightening of the patient's abdominal muscles in response to pressure, indicates severe tenderness.

The sudden withdrawal of manual pressure may cause a sharp exacerbation of the pain, which is known as **rebound** or **release tenderness**. This test may be distressing for the patient, and it is preferable to assess rebound tenderness by the patient's response to light percussion.

> **NOTE:** The release of pressure in a distant non-tender part of the abdomen sometimes causes pain in the tender area.

General palpation for tenderness

When no pain is elicited by systematic light palpation over the whole abdomen, repeat the process, pressing more firmly and deeply to see if there is any deep tenderness.

Palpation for masses

The whole abdomen must be carefully palpated for the presence, position, shape, size, surface, edge, consistency, fluid thrill, resonance and pulsatility of any masses.

Tender masses in the abdomen are very difficult to feel because of the protective guarding of the abdominal wall muscles. The surface and size of a tender mass may be obtained by resting your hand gently on the tender area and pressing a little deeper during expiration and feeling the mass as it moves beneath your hand.

Rapid, hard pressure achieves nothing because the patient tightens their abdominal muscles and it is inappropriate.

Palpation of the normal solid viscera

The liver To feel the liver, place your right hand transversely and flat on the right side of the abdomen at the level of the umbilicus, parallel with the right costal margin (Figure 15.3a). Then ask the patient to take a deep breath. If the liver is grossly enlarged, its lower edge will move downwards and bump against the radial side of your index finger. If nothing abnormal is felt, repeat the process after moving your hand upwards, inch by inch, until the costal margin is reached.

The liver edge may be straight or irregular, thin and sharp, or thick and rounded. The surface may be smooth or knobbly. Palpation beginning just below the costal margin can easily miss a large liver. Gross hepatomegaly may fill the whole abdomen so, if in doubt, begin your palpation in the right iliac fossa. An enlarged liver is *dull to percussion*, and its upper margin should be percussed out to assess its full dimension.

The spleen An enlarged spleen appears below the tip of the tenth rib along a line heading towards the umbilicus and, if really large, may extend into the right iliac fossa. A normal spleen is not palpable.

To feel the spleen, place the fingertips of your right hand on the right iliac fossa just below the umbilicus (Figure 15.3b). Ask the patient to take a deep breath. If nothing abnormal is felt, move your hand in stages towards the tip of the left tenth rib. When the costal margin is reached, place your left hand around the lower left rib cage, and lift the lower ribs and the spleen forwards as the patient inspires. Occasionally, this manoeuvre lifts a slightly enlarged spleen far enough forward to make it palpable.

It is *dull to percussion* as it lies immediately beneath the abdominal wall with no bowel in front of it, unlike a renal mass (see page 533).

NOTE: The spleen is recognized by its shape and site and, when present, the notch on its superomedial edge.

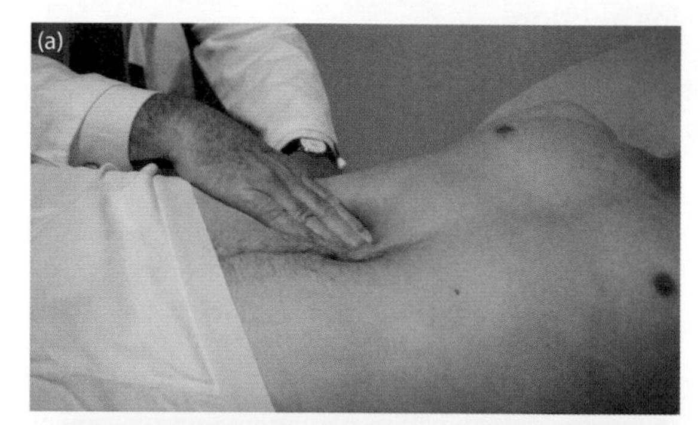

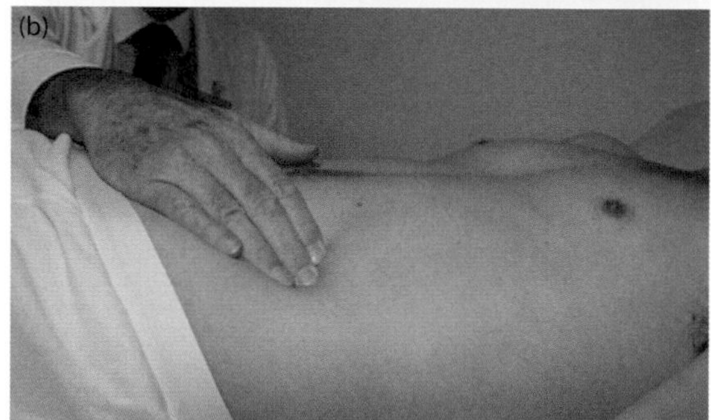

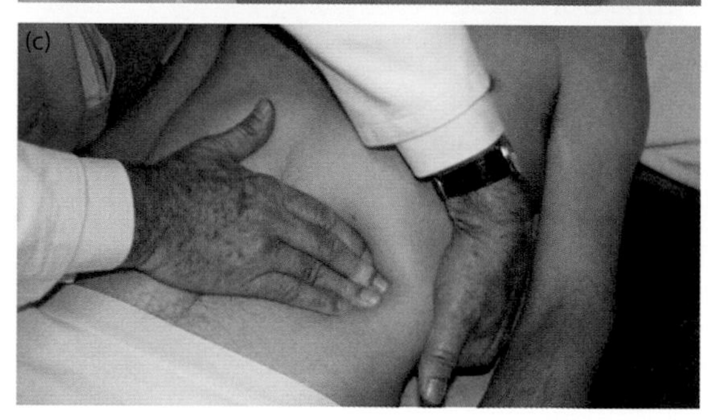

Figure 15.3 PALPATING THE ABDOMEN. (a) Palpate the liver by resting your fingers on the abdomen almost parallel to the right costal margin, and ask the patient to breathe in. The liver edge can be made more prominent by putting your left hand under the lower ribs and lifting them forwards. (b) Palpate the spleen with your fingers lying transversely across the abdomen so that the tip of the spleen will hit the tips of your index and middle fingers when the patient breathes in. You can make the spleen more prominent by lifting the lower ribs forwards with your left hand, as you do when palpating the left kidney. (c) Palpate the kidneys by pressing firmly into the lumbar region during inspiration while lifting the kidney forwards with your other hand in the loin.

The kidneys Normal kidneys are usually impalpable, except in very thin people, but both lumbar regions should always be carefully examined.

To feel the patient's right kidney, place your left hand behind the patient's right loin between the 12th rib and the iliac crest, so that you can lift the loin and kidney forwards (Figure 15.3c). Then place your right hand on the right side of the abdomen just below the right costal margin. As the patient breathes in and out, palpate the loin between both hands. The lower pole of a normal kidney may be felt at the height of inspiration in a very thin person. When a kidney is very easy to feel, it is either enlarged or abnormally low.

To feel the left kidney, lean across the patient, place your left hand around the flank into the left loin to lift it forwards, then place your right hand on the abdomen and feel any masses between the two hands.

An enlarged kidney can be pushed back and forth between the anterior and posterior hands. This is called *balloting*. It feels like patting a ball back and forth in a pool of water. Balloting is also used to palpate a fetus in a pregnant uterus.

Percussion

The whole abdomen must be percussed, particularly over any masses. A dull area may draw your attention to a mass that was missed on palpation and indicate a more detailed and careful palpation of the area of dullness. When there is a circumscribed mass, a tap on one side while feeling the opposite side with the other hand may reveal that it conducts a *fluid thrill*. Any area of dullness should be outlined by percussion with the abdomen in two positions to see if it moves or changes shape. Free fluid (*ascites*) changes shape and moves (*shifting dullness*; see page 545).

Percussion causes pain if peritonitis is present and is a useful method for mapping out a tender area (see above).

When a part or the whole of the abdomen appears distended, the patient should be held at the hips and the abdomen shaken from side-to-side. Splashing sounds – *a succussion splash* – indicate that there is an intra-abdominal viscus, usually the stomach, distended with a mixture of fluid and gas.

Auscultation

Listen to the bowel sounds. Peristalsis produces gurgling noises because the bowel contains a mixture of fluid and gas. The pitch of the noise depends upon the distension of the bowel and the proportions of gas and fluid. *Normal bowel sounds are low-pitched* gurgles that occur every few seconds.

The absence of bowel sounds indicates that peristalsis has ceased. This may either be a primary or a secondary phenomenon. If you can hear the heart and breath sounds but no bowel sounds over a 30-second period, the patient probably has a *paralytic ileus*.

Increased peristalsis increases the volume and frequency of the bowel sounds. Distension of the bowel caused by a *mechanical intestinal obstruction* is associated not only with *increased bowel sounds,* but also with *a change in the character of the sounds*. They become *amphoric* in nature with runs of high-frequency gurgles, sounding like sea water entering a large cave through a narrow entrance, often described as 'tinkling'.

Having assessed the quality of the bowel sounds, it is important to listen for any *systolic vascular bruits,* which indicate arterial stenosis or increased blood flow through, for example, a fistula.

Revision panel 15.2

FEATURES OF PAIN THAT MUST BE ELICITED

- Time and nature of onset
- Site
- Character (burning, throbbing, stabbing, constricting, colicky, aching)
- Severity
- Progression
- Duration
- End
- Radiation
- Relieving factors
- Exacerbating factors
- Associated symptoms, e.g. vomiting, diarrhoea, painful micturition, missed or absent periods

Abdominal pain

Time spent taking a careful history is never wasted, as abdominal pain is the only symptom of many intra-abdominal diseases. The two most significant properties of an abdominal pain are its *site* and its *character* (Revision panel 15.2).

THE SIGNIFICANCE OF THE SITE OF ABDOMINAL PAIN

The abdomen can be divided into three horizontal zones – upper, central and lower – by two horizontal lines. These are the *transpyloric plane* (a line circling the body midway between the suprasternal notch and the symphysis pubis) and the *transtubercular plane* (a line circling the body that passes through the two tubercles of the iliac crest) as shown in Figure 15.4. Each of these three zones can be further vertically subdivided into three regions – central, right and left – by the two mid-clavicular lines.

The anatomical names of these nine regions are:

- The epigastrium.
- The right hypochondrium.
- The left hypochondrium.
- The umbilical region.
- The right lumbar region.
- The left lumbar region.
- The hypogastrium or suprapubic region.
- The right iliac fossa.
- The left iliac fossa.

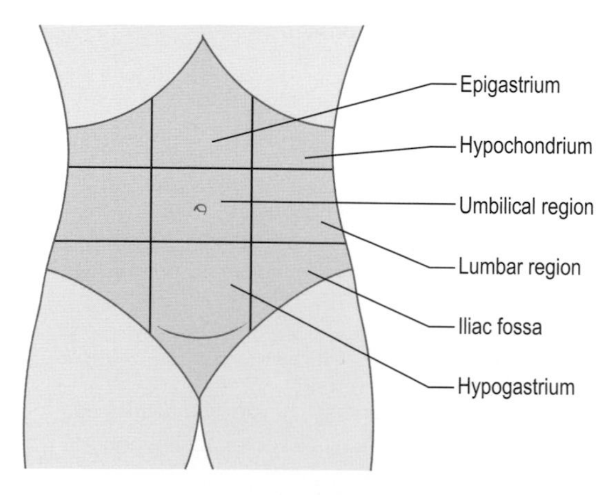

Figure 15.4 The names of the regions of the abdomen.

> **NOTE:** Sometimes, patients are only capable of localizing pain to the upper or lower half of the abdomen and/or to the left or right side.

Colicky pain is referred to the *centre of the abdomen* whatever its source, as it is a *visceral sensation*, whereas the pain from the parietal peritoneum is felt over the inflamed area (a *somatic sensation*).

Pain in the upper abdomen is most likely to arise from the biliary tree, stomach, duodenum or pancreas (Figure 15.5). These structures produce right-sided, central and left-sided pain, respectively. The pain from these three organs radiates in different directions:

- Gallbladder pain may radiate through to the back and to the right, to reach the tip of the scapula. When felt in this area, it often seems to the patient to be a separate, independent pain.
- Ulcers in the posterior wall of the stomach or duodenum cause a pain that radiates through to the back.
- Pancreatic pain also tends to go through to the back and sometimes to the left.

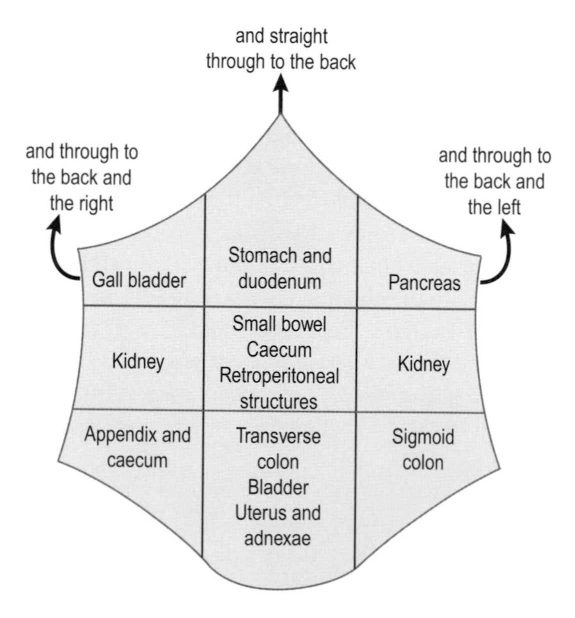

Figure 15.5 The structures that commonly cause pain in the nine anatomical regions of the abdomen, with the pain often radiating through to the back.

Pain in the centre of the abdomen is most likely to arise from the small bowel, caecum and midline retroperitoneal structures such as the aorta.

Pain from retroperitoneal structures often radiates through to the back. Pain in the lateral zones of the central region is most likely to come from the kidneys.

Pain from the kidney is also felt in the loin, and may radiate down to the groin. All visceral pain may move and become localized if the inflammatory process in the viscus involves the parietal peritoneum.

Pain in the lower abdomen is most likely to come from the appendix, caecum, colon, bladder, uterus, ovaries and Fallopian tubes. Pain in the hypogastric region usually arises from the bladder, rectum, uterus and its adnexae. Pain in the right iliac fossa usually comes from the caecum and the appendix. Pain in the left iliac fossa usually comes from the sigmoid colon.

Lower abdominal pains rarely radiate, but pain from pelvic structures may be referred to the lower back or perineum.

THE SIGNIFICANCE OF THE CHARACTER OF ABDOMINAL PAIN

It is possible to subdivide the character of the pain of the majority of the painful conditions that occur within the abdomen into two large categories: a *constant pain* associated with inflammation, ischaemia, infarction and neoplastic infiltration, and a *colicky pain* associated with obstruction of a muscular conducting tube such as the bowel or the ureter (colic).

The constant pain caused by:

- Inflammation.
- Infiltration.
- Ischaemia.
- Infarction.

whether it is the mild inflammatory response around a chronic peptic ulcer or the acute response to a perforated appendix, is made worse by any local or general movement and persists until the underlying cause subsides. Inflammation within the abdomen does not throb or burn in the same way that inflammatory pains do elsewhere.

The colic caused by obstruction to a muscular conducting viscus is a pain that fluctuates in severity at frequent intervals and feels griping in nature. The source of bowel colic can be suspected from *the time interval between the peaks of the pain* – short in the jejunum, longer in the ileum, and longer still in the colon.

In biliary and renal colic, the peaks of pain are short, and the pain seldom goes away completely between exacerbations. Prolonged obstruction to the outflow of any hollow viscus ultimately causes it to distend. This produces a constant 'stretching' pain, which is different from the ache of inflammation but not colicky in nature. A similar pain can come from conditions that stretch the retroperitoneal tissues.

Colic can also be caused by muscular dysfunction, i.e. disorders of gastrointestinal motility such as irritable bowel syndrome.

THE SIGNIFICANCE OF RADIATION

Radiation of a pain signifies that other structures are becoming involved. For example, when the pain from a duodenal ulcer radiates through to the back, it indicates that the inflammation has spread beyond the duodenum into adjacent structures in the posterior abdominal wall, such as the pancreas. Radiation, therefore, not only indicates the source of the pain, but may also hint at the extent of the disease.

THE SIGNIFICANCE OF THE RATE OF ONSET AND SEVERITY

Patients with severe abdominal pain of *acute onset* are usually collectively grouped as having an 'acute abdomen'. These patients usually consult their GP or seek emergency medical help once their pain has persisted for more than an hour or so. Many, however, will have had chronic symptoms over the preceding months or years caused by the condition currently causing their acute symptoms, i.e. the same condition can present acutely or chronically.

Therefore, although the rate and severity of presentation may indicate the urgency of the problem, they do not always indicate the nature of the underlying pathology.

Whatever the urgency and underlying pathology, a full history and clinical examination (as described above) must be carried out so that a working diagnosis or differential diagnosis can be made and the patient assigned to one of the following management categories:

- An acute abdomen, e.g. peritonitis, with a known or unknown underlying cause requiring urgent treatment.
- An abdominal pain of known or unknown cause requiring pain palliation pending further investigation and treatment.
- An abdominal pain with no evidence of any clinically detectable intra-abdominal pathology that can be observed and investigated later if necessary, i.e. time to wait and see.

In almost every case, additional investigations are likely to be required to refine the diagnosis and plan treatment, but when the diagnosis is 'uncertain', careful monitoring and repeated re-examination are essential to detect any progression or resolution of the problem and ensure that important new physical signs are not missed. Acute physical signs often develop over several hours and become clear cut, often diagnostic, by the time of a later examination. In contrast, the signs of chronic conditions may take months to develop.

PATHOLOGY OF THE ACUTE ABDOMEN

The principal causes of acute abdominal pain are:

- Inflammation of a viscus.
- Perforation of a viscus.
- Obstruction of a viscus.
- Infarction of a viscus.
- Intra-abdominal or retroperitoneal haemorrhage.
- Extra-abdominal or medical causes of acute abdominal pain.

Inflammation of a viscus

Inflammation of a viscus results in localized pain and a condition known as *peritonitis*. The clinical features of peritonitis are as follows.

Tenderness and guarding

The tenderness is initially localized to the site of the inflammation, but can become more generalized as the condition worsens. Guarding is an excellent indication of the severity of the tenderness. If the whole abdomen is tense, there is likely to be general peritonitis.

Rebound tenderness or tenderness on percussion

This is just another way of detecting that the abdomen is very tender. It can be a valuable sign because the patient is not expecting pain when you suddenly remove your hand, so the apprehension, which can cause guarding during direct palpation, is absent. It can however cause considerable discomfort so should be used sparingly.

Localized pain during distant palpation

The structures in the painful area are likely to be very inflamed. When you press on a distant non-tender part of the abdomen pain can often be felt in the actual inflamed area (e.g. *Rovsing's sign* in appendicitis).

Absence of bowel sounds

The absence of bowel sounds *per se* does not indicate peritonitis, but their absence in a tender, rigid abdomen makes it highly likely that there is generalized peritonitis.

An increasing tachycardia

There is likely to be serious disease within the abdomen if the pulse rate increases gradually during 1–2 hours of observation.

Pyrexia

The temperature rises only when the peritoneal cavity becomes heavily infected.

NOTE: Remember that steroids damp down the inflammatory response. Patients on corticosteroids with a severe peritonitis may have a normal temperature.

When a peptic ulcer erodes through the wall of the stomach or duodenum at a point where it is covered only by visceral peritoneum, acid gastric juice enters the peritoneal cavity. This causes a chemical peritonitis, which later becomes infected with bacteria.

Perforation of a viscus

A perforation in the wall of a hollow viscus allows its contents – acid, bacteria, small bowel contents, faeces, bile or urine – to enter the peritoneal cavity, where they rapidly cause a *chemical or infected peritonitis*. The history and physical signs may indicate the site and cause of the perforation, but whether they do or do not, it is usually necessary to perform a laparotomy to confirm the diagnosis and close the perforation. It is essential, therefore, to recognize the signs of peritonitis (see above). The pain usually begins near the site of the perforation but rapidly spreads across the whole abdomen (Revision panel 15.3).

Revision panel 15.3

CONDITIONS LIKELY TO CAUSE PERFORATION OF A VISCUS

Peptic ulceration
Acute diverticulitis
Ischaemia
Gangrenous appendicitis
Trauma
Ulcerative colitis (toxic megacolon)
A perforated gallbladder
Small bowel disease (Crohn's disease, strangulation, a foreign body, typhoid)
Carcinoma of the colon
Boerhaave's syndrome
Radiation necrosis

Obstruction of a viscus/intestinal obstruction

There are many causes of intestinal obstruction (Revision panel 15.4).

Revision panel 15.4

COMMON CAUSES OF ALIMENTARY TRACT OBSTRUCTION BY AGE

Neonates

Atresia (duodenum, ileum, anorectal)
Meconium obstruction
Malrotation with volvulus
Hirschsprung's disease (functional obstruction)

3 weeks

Congenital hypertrophic pyloric stenosis

6–9 months

Intussusception

Teenage

Inflammatory masses (appendicitis, Crohn's disease)
Intussusception of Meckel's diverticulum or polyp

Young adult

Hernia
Adhesions
Inflammation (appendicitis, Crohn's disease)

Adult

Hernia
Adhesions
Inflammation (appendicitis, Crohn's disease)
Carcinoma

Elderly

Carcinoma
Inflammation (diverticulitis)
Sigmoid volvulus

Although it is normally possible to tell whether the site of the obstruction is in the small bowel or large bowel on the basis of the history aided by physical signs and plain abdominal X-rays, the clinician must always attempt to answer these three questions:

1. Is there intestinal obstruction?
2. Is the bowel strangulated?
3. Is the site of the obstruction in the small bowel or large bowel?

Revision panel 15.5

CARDINAL SYMPTOMS OF INTESTINAL OBSTRUCTION

Pain
Vomiting
Distension
Absolute constipation

The *signs of strangulation* are the same as the signs of local peritoneal inflammation, which have been described above, namely, pain, tenderness, guarding and rebound tenderness.

The cardinal symptoms of intestinal obstruction are pain, vomiting, distension and absolute constipation (Revision panel 15.5), but the severity and time of onset of each of these symptoms depend on the level of obstruction.

PAIN

The pain of intestinal obstruction is *true colic*. It occurs as a severe central griping pain interspersed with periods of little or no pain. Colic is uncommon with obstructions above the pylorus. Small bowel colic is felt in the centre of the abdomen, and large bowel colic usually in the lower third of the abdomen. Small bowel colic occurs every 2–20 minutes, depending on the level of obstruction in the small bowel. Large bowel colic occurs about every 30 minutes or more.

VOMITING

Intestinal obstruction causes frequent vomiting. The nature of the vomitus depends on the level of the obstruction. With pyloric obstruction, the vomitus is watery and acid with no bile staining. High small bowel obstruction produces a greenish–blue, bile-stained vomit. Obstruction in the lower part of the small bowel is associated with a brown vomit that becomes increasingly foul-smelling as the obstruction persists. It becomes so thick, brown and foul that it is often called *faeculent vomit*. Vomiting is unusual and is usually a late symptom in patients with large bowel obstruction.

DISTENSION

The lower the site of the obstruction, the more bowel there is available to distend. High obstructions are not associated with distension, particularly if the patient is vomiting frequently.

Obstruction of the colon causes the colon to distend around the periphery of the abdomen. The distension then extends into the small bowel if the ileocaecal valve is incompetent. If this valve remains competent, the *right side of the colon, especially the caecum, can become grossly distended*, causing a visible bulge in the right iliac fossa that is hyper-resonant. This is known as a *closed-loop obstruction* and is a surgical emergency, a perforation or ischaemia can occur particularly of the caecum (law of LaPlace).

Small bowel obstruction tends to cause distension in the centre of the abdomen and occasionally in a very thin patient *visible peristalsis* may be visible in which loops of small bowel become visible with peristaltic waves running across them during episodes of colic (Figure 15.6).

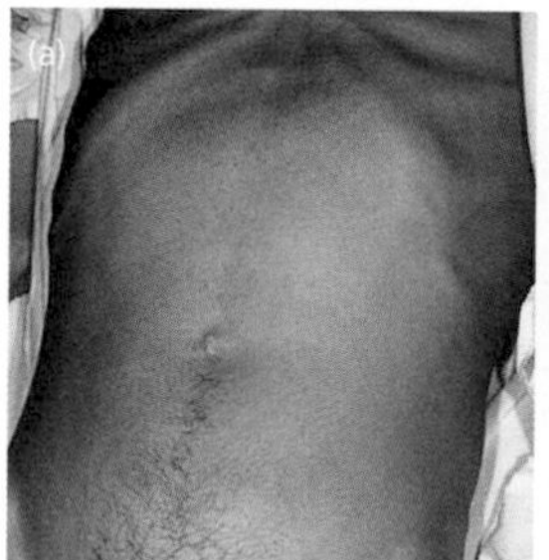

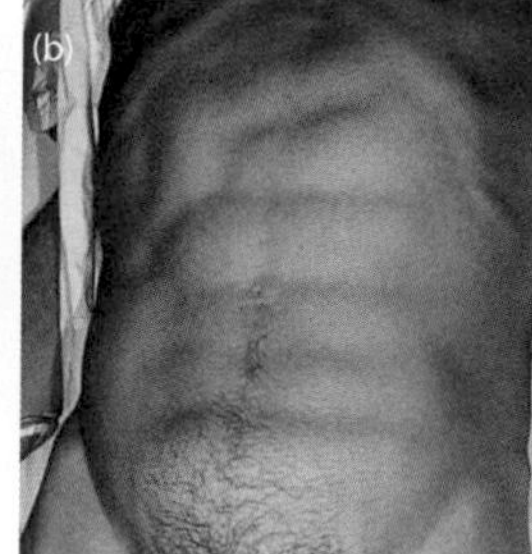

Figure 15.6 DISTENSION. (a) Mild distension of the abdomen. (b) Visible peristalsis in the same patient.

ABSOLUTE CONSTIPATION

Once an obstruction is complete and the bowel below is empty, absolute constipation develops. This means that *neither faeces nor flatus is passed*. This occurs early in lower large bowel obstructions and late in high small bowel obstructions.

TO SUMMARIZE

A high small bowel obstruction causes frequent colic and vomiting. The distension is slight and central, and absolute constipation is rare.

A low large bowel obstruction causes infrequent colic, absolute constipation and peripheral abdominal distension. Vomiting is absent or occurs very late on.

The bowel sounds in a patient with mechanical obstruction are at first loud, frequent and obstructive in nature. As the bowel distends, the sounds become more resonant and high-pitched, before eventually becoming amphoteric.

Strangulated hernias and adhesions are the most common causes of small bowel obstruction, therefore, *all the hernial orifices* must be carefully examined (see Chapter 14).

Abdominal scars suggest adhesions.

Carcinoma, diverticulitis and volvulus are the most common causes of large bowel obstruction.

Rectal examination and sigmoidoscopy are essential before more detailed investigations are carried out. It is important to remember that some patients with large bowel obstruction have a *pseudo-obstruction (Ogilvie's syndrome)* in which large bowel peristalsis ceases as a consequence of retroperitoneal pathology.

Infarction of a viscus

Table 15.1 lists the abdominal organs that may infarct and present with acute abdominal pain, together with the common pathological processes responsible for infarction.

Table 15.1 The intra-abdominal organs that may infarct

Organ	Mechanism
Small and large bowel	Volvulus Arterial thrombosis Arterial embolism Dissecting aneurysm Venous thrombosis
Ovary	Torsion of pedicle
Omentum/mesentery	Strangulation of appendix epiploica
Stomach	Volvulus
Spleen/kidney/liver	Arterial occlusion

Acute pain develops when the blood supply of an organ is obstructed. When the obstructing mechanism is an external constriction or a torsion of a vascular pedicle (e.g. a volvulus), the process is gradual but the end result is the same – severe abdominal pain – as the nerve endings are damaged and die. Pain is also experienced through the somatic nerve endings of the peritoneal cavity if they are directly stimulated by the proximity of the dead organ.

History

The pain of infarction is usually severe and continuous and quickly develops all the hallmarks of peritonitis. The patient often finds it difficult to locate the site of the pain, which becomes progressively worse if left untreated and which is aggravated by any movement and is only relieved by strong analgesics. Vomiting may accompany the pain, and most patients are severely nauseated.

Vomiting and complete dysphagia occur in the few patients who develop the rare condition of infarction of the stomach caused by a *gastric volvulus.*

Some patients may describe a 'classical colic' in which the pain becomes continuous and much more severe as the blood supply of an obstructed loop is compromised by the *process of strangulation.* Patients may know they have a hernia that has become irreducible and painful, or they may provide a history of *previous abdominal surgery,* indicating the possibility of adhesions as a cause of strangulation.

A history of *angina, heart attacks, strokes* or *intermittent claudication* indicates coexisting atherosclerotic disease and increases the likelihood of a mesenteric thrombosis (see Chapter 10).

Splenic infarction is common in patients with *sickle-cell disease,* who may also develop bowel ischaemia, as may patients with autoimmune vasculitis.

Severe chest pain preceding the abdominal pain indicates the possibility that an *aortic dissection* has compromised the mesenteric vessels and led to infarction.

Examination

General features Patients with abdominal infarction lie still and are often pale and sweating from the associated hypovolaemic shock. There is a tachycardia, which increases during the period of observation. An *irregularly irregular pulse* (atrial fibrillation) should suggest the possibility of a mesenteric embolus.

Pyrexia The temperature may be mildly elevated at first, but a high temperature only develops if treatment is delayed and bowel wall necrosis or perforation occurs.

Tenderness and guarding These signs may be mild at first but become more pronounced as the condition of the bowel wall deteriorates. The abdomen also becomes more distended, and rebound or percussion tenderness can be elicited.

Bowel sounds These may be present while the infarction is beginning, but a major intra-abdominal infarct always eventually causes a paralytic ileus.

The presence of an *intra-abdominal bruit* (see Chapter 10) indicates the presence of atherosclerotic disease in the intra-abdominal vessels.

The hernial orifices These must be carefully examined (see Chapter 14), together with all visible incisions, and palpated for the presence of tender and irreducible lumps.

Rectal examination and sigmoidoscopy The presence of a *sigmoid volvulus* is usually suspected from typical appearances on plain abdominal X-rays, but sigmoidoscopy may be both diagnostic and therapeutic in this condition. Gentle pressure of the sigmoidoscope against a blind end of bowel, or the passage of a flatus tube through the sigmoidoscope, usually leads to the passage of a massive flatus with abdominal decompression and relief of pain, provided infarction has not developed.

Peripheral pulses Absence of the brachial or femoral pulses indicates the possibility of a dissecting aneurysm, especially in a patient whose pain began in the chest.

NOTE: Infarction of the bowel must always be considered in a patient with severe abdominal pain and few signs. The most likely differential diagnoses are a perforated viscus causing peritonitis, severe acute pancreatitis and a ruptured abdominal aortic aneurysm.

Abdominal pain caused by haemorrhage

The common conditions that cause intraperitoneal or retroperitoneal haemorrhage are:

- Ruptured aortic aneurysm.
- Ectopic pregnancy.
- Blunt or penetrating trauma (liver, spleen, retroperitoneum).

COMMON FEATURES OF INTRAABDOMINAL HAEMORRHAGE

History

The onset of pain is always rapid, but the signs of shock and collapse may precede the pain and be the predominating symptoms.

Although patients may die from untreated hypovolaemia, the accompanying hypotension sometimes reduces the bleeding, giving a false impression of recovery, but this fortunately allows time to transfer the patient to hospital.

Examination

General appearance The patient often looks very pale and may be sweating, restless and breathless, a condition known as *air hunger*. A *tachycardia* is invariably present, and this is often marked if the patient is hypovolaemic. The blood pressure is maintained at first, especially in fit young adults, but eventually may fall suddenly and disastrously. The peripheral circulation is shut down so that the extremities of the limbs are pale and cold. The pupils may be dilated. The *jugular venous pressure* is very low and may not be visible even when the patient is lying flat.

RUPTURED ABDOMINAL AORTIC ANEURYSM

History

Patients with abdominal aortic aneurysms invariably are, or have been, smokers and may have a family history of atherosclerotic aneurysms.

A previous history of angina, myocardial infarction, intermittent claudication, transient ischaemic attacks or strokes indicates the presence of generalized atherosclerosis.

Symptoms The *pain* from a ruptured abdominal aortic aneurysm *begins in the centre of the abdomen but commonly radiates to the back* and may radiate to the groin along the course of the genitofemoral nerve.

Examination

Abdomen inspection The abdomen is often distended. If the patient is thin, a large central pulsating mass may be visible in the epigastrium or umbilical region.

Cullen's sign and *Grey Turner's sign* – bruising around the umbilicus and in the flank, respectively – are late indicators (3–4 days) of a longstanding rupture.

Palpation The presence of an expansile pulsatile mass may be confirmed (Figure 15.7). It is usually tender and consists of the aneurysm and the surrounding haematoma. The upper and lower limits of the aneurysm should be defined. A clear separation between the upper end of the aneurysm and the costal margin indicates that the aneurysm is likely to begin below the renal arteries. The finding of additional pulsatile masses in the iliac fossae suggests associated iliac aneurysms (usually in the common iliac arteries). The femoral, iliac and foot pulses must all be palpated. The presence of *dilated popliteal arteries* strengthens the possibility that the patient has an abdominal aneurysm. The peripheral pulses may be absent.

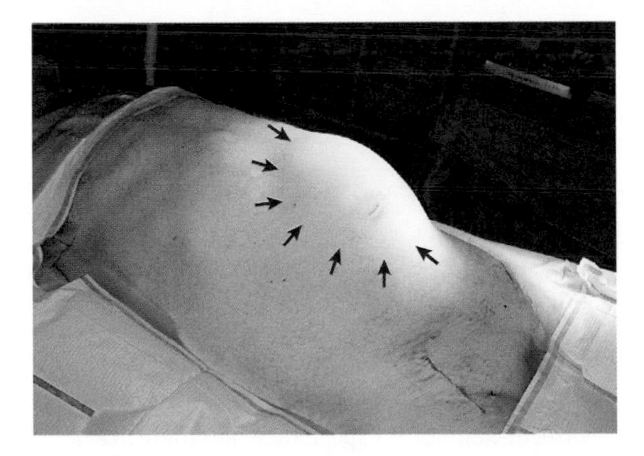

Figure 15.7 Large pulsatile abdominal mass present in the centre and upper abdomen.

Large amounts of free blood in the abdomen, obesity, marked guarding and hypotension may all conspire to render a leaking aneurysm impalpable.

Severe abdominal pain and collapse (see Chapter 10) with clear evidence of hypovolaemia are strongly suggestive of a leaking aneurysm in an elderly male who is known to be hypertensive and a smoker, but special investigations may be needed to confirm the diagnosis.

Auscultation The bowel sounds may be diminished as a consequence of the irritation caused by intraperitoneal blood. Vascular bruits may be heard.

Rectal and vaginal examination Rectal examination is usually unhelpful, but occasionally an internal iliac artery aneurysm can be palpated.

SPECIAL FEATURES OF OTHER ABDOMINAL ANEURYSMS

Aneurysms can arise in all the visceral arteries, but they are rare. Splenic artery aneurysms are the most common.

RUPTURE OF THE SPLEEN

The spleen may be ruptured by blunt or penetrating injuries. When the spleen is ruptured by an external injury, the left lower ribs are often fractured.

Splenic haemorrhage usually causes pain in the left hypochondrium and upper abdomen. It may be associated with *left shoulder tip pain* if blood or a haematoma is irritating the left hemidiaphragm. Shifting dullness and flank dullness may be detected.

There will be local pain and tenderness and sharp pain on inspiration if the ribs are broken.

Very occasionally, a ruptured pathologically enlarged spleen is palpable in the right hypochondrium.

ABDOMINAL TRAUMA

Blunt and penetrating injuries can damage any of the intra-abdominal viscera. The *spleen and liver* are the most *susceptible organs,* and both may bleed profusely.

A history of blunt or sharp injury to the abdomen, even if trivial, provides an important clue to the diagnosis.

There may be signs of the external injury, such as cutaneous bruising or marks along the line of a seat belt, if the patient has had blunt trauma to the abdomen (see Chapter 5).

ECTOPIC PREGNANCY

When an ectopic pregnancy is the source of haemorrhage, the *patient may know she is pregnant* (morning sickness, amenorrhoea, breast swelling or a positive pregnancy test) and is likely to have experienced some intermittent lower abdominal pain before the *sudden onset of severe pain* in this area. This is usually *associated with faintness and collapse*, although less acute presentations are common. The lower abdominal pain becomes generalized if left untreated.

A history of any abnormality in the menstrual cycle in a female of child-bearing age, coupled with the sudden onset of severe abdominal pain, should suggest the possibility of an ectopic pregnancy. A previous history of *pelvic inflammatory disease* (see below) or *fertility problems* also raises suspicions of the diagnosis. If available, a rapid pregnancy test can be very helpful.

PHYSIOLOGICAL RUPTURE OF OVARIAN LUTEAL CYSTS

These can cause minor episodes of bleeding and lower abdominal pain when they rupture at the middle of the menstrual cycle. This is called *mittleschmerz*.

RUPTURE OF PATHOLOGICAL OVARIAN CYSTS

Large pathological ovarian cysts can sometimes rupture and bleed profusely. Patients may collapse from the associated hypovolaemic shock or present with lower abdominal pain and then develop the signs of internal bleeding.

RUPTURE OF LIVER ADENOMAS

Liver adenomas can develop in young females taking the contraceptive pill and may rupture spontaneously. The pain is usually felt in the upper abdomen, and hypovolaemic collapse is common.

SUMMARY

All the conditions described above present with a combination of *abdominal pain* and *haemorrhagic shock* in varying proportions (Revision panel 15.6). Their presentation needs to be distinguished from the symptoms of intra-abdominal infarction and peritonitis caused by a perforated viscus and acute pancreatitis, all of which can produce a similar clinical picture.

Revision panel 15.6

SOURCES OF INTRA-ABDOMINAL HAEMORRHAGE

- Ruptured abdominal aortic aneurysm
- Blunt or penetrating abdominal trauma (liver, spleen, retroperitoneum)
- Ruptured ectopic pregnancy (tubal rupture)
- Ruptured ovarian cyst
- Haemorrhage from a liver adenoma
- Ruptured visceral aneurysms:
  - Splenic
  - Hepatic
  - Mesenteric
- Torn mesentery
- Retroperitoneal haemorrhage (over-anticoagulation)

EXTRA-ABDOMINAL AND MEDICAL CONDITIONS CAUSING ACUTE ABDOMINAL PAIN

The conditions described in Revision panel 15.7 are not unusual causes of abdominal pain, which emphasizes the need to conduct a full clinical examination on every patient however obvious it may seem that their problem is in the abdomen.

The chest and heart must be examined and special tests must be performed, such as chest X-ray and electrocardiography, especially when there are no or minimal signs in the abdomen.

Revision panel 15.7

EXTRA-ABDOMINAL AND MEDICAL CONDITIONS CAUSING ACUTE ABDOMINAL PAIN

- Pneumonia/pleurisy
- Pulmonary embolus
- Myocardial infarction
- Spinal disorders, e.g. prolapsed disc
- Epigastric artery haematoma
- Testicular torsion
- Acute porphyria
- Infectious hepatitis
- Curtis–Fitz-Hugh syndrome
- Herpes zoster
- Diabetic ketoacidosis
- Syphilis (lightening pains)
- Henoch–Schönlein purpura
- Post-transplant lymphoproliferative disorder (PTLD)/immunodeficiency
- Collagen disease
- Sickle-cell disease
- Retroperitoneal fibrosis
- Mesenteric adenitis
- Non-specific abdominal pain
- Factitious disorder

The pain of spinal abnormalities can radiate to the abdomen, so the back should be examined carefully, especially if the pain is felt in the lumbar region.

Acute porphyria

This is associated with severe intestinal colic that is particularly precipitated by barbiturates and alcohol. The urine is often dark and turns red–purple on standing (Figure 15.8).

Mesenteric adenitis

This is associated with an upper respiratory tract infection (URTI) and cervical lymphadenopathy. It can cause pain in the right iliac fossa, which may be mistaken for appendicitis. The pain is caused by swollen glands in the mesentery, so the area of tenderness may move when the patient moves from side-to-side.

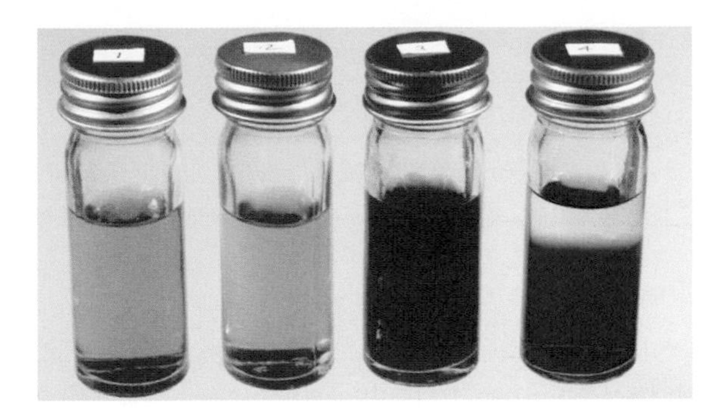

Figure 15.8 Acute porphyria. These are a series of urine samples taken from a patient with acute porphyria showing the characteristic development left to right of the red–purple pigment over time.

Epigastric artery haematoma

Both superior and inferior epigastric arteries may rupture causing swelling and subsequent haematoma (Figure 15.9).

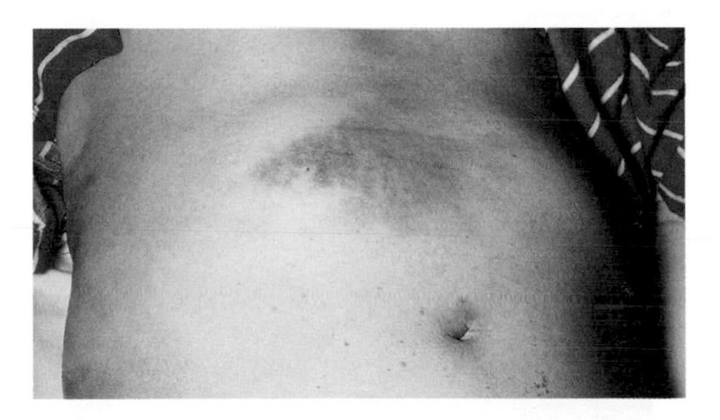

Figure 15.9 Swelling and haematoma caused by rupture of a superior epigastric artery.

Infectious hepatitis and glandular fever

These conditions cause pain in the right hypochondrium. The pain is caused by swelling of the liver stretching the liver capsule. Jaundice usually develops within a few days.

Curtis–Fitz-Hugh syndrome

The pain of this syndrome is caused by a pericapsulitis around the liver that is related to pelvic inflammation with *Chlamydia*. A preceding vaginal discharge suggests the diagnosis, which has to be differentiated from acute cholecystitis.

Herpes zoster

This causes pain in the abdomen if an appropriate dermatome is involved (see Chapter 4). The diagnosis is only confirmed when the characteristic rash develops (see Figure 4.38).

Diabetic ketoacidosis

This can cause marked abdominal pain. The diagnosis is confirmed by finding glycosuria and elevated blood glucose levels. Patients are often very thirsty and drowsy.

Syphilis

Syphilis can cause abdominal pain during a tabetic crisis, but tertiary syphilis is uncommon nowadays. Argyll Robertson pupils and evidence of destruction of the dorsal columns of the spinal cord causing loss of deep pain and proprioception indicate the diagnosis.

Henoch–Schönlein purpura

Purpura can present with intestinal colic (Figure 15.10) The diagnosis should be suspected in children who have a purpuric rash over their thighs and buttocks.

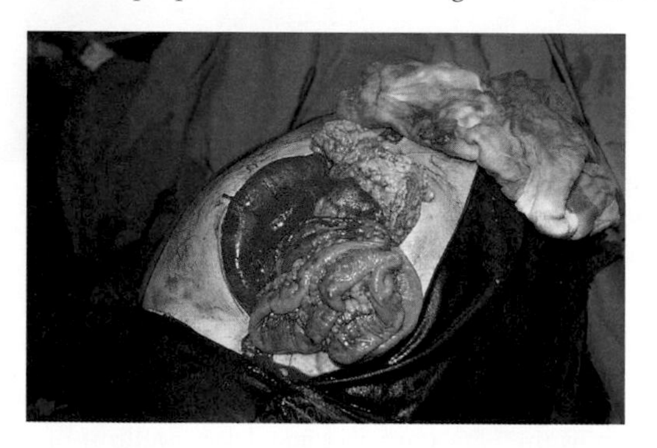

Figure 15.10 Haemorrhage under the serosa and in the mesentery of the upper segment of bowel wall caused by the Henoch–Schönlein purpura. The lower loops are normal. Apart from tenderness, this produces no physical signs in the abdomen.

Post-transplant lymphoproliferative disorder/immunodeficiency

This is a serious complication following transplantation causing lymphoma (most commonly abdominal). It is related to an interaction of Epstein–Barr virus infection and immune suppression. It is most common after intestinal transplantation. Any compromised state of a patient's immune system can lead to appendicitis or other intra-abdominal infections having a fulminating course.

Collagen diseases

A number of collagen diseases, especially systemic lupus erythematosus, are associated with abdominal pain with an increased risk of intestinal infarction secondary to small vessel obstruction.

Sickle-cell crisis

This can cause abdominal pain, usually from intestinal and splenic infarction.

Non-specific abdominal pain

In some patients, no cause for acute abdominal pain can be found, despite hospital admission, re-examination and special investigations. These patients are categorized as having non-specific abdominal pain, and account for nearly one-third of the many patients admitted as acute surgical emergencies with abdominal pain. In the great majority, the pain disappears spontaneously and does not recur. In some, however, the cause eventually becomes apparent.

Factitious disorder

A very small group of patients with factitious disorder can invent or exaggerate symptoms of abdominal pain.The cause of this disorder is often unknown; however, it is a serious psychiatric illness. The physical signs are often minimal, but some of these patients are very good at mimicking guarding and rebound tenderness.

NOTE: Beware the patient who has come from many miles away, or even a different country, whose abdomen bears the scars of many incisions (Figure 15.11), especially if the pain is difficult to control and requires increasing quantities of analgesic drugs.

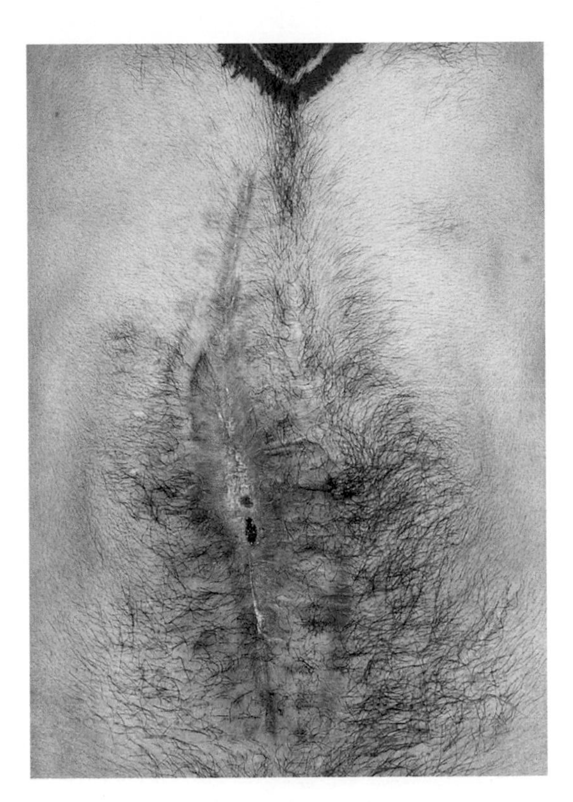

Figure 15.11 Factitious disorder. This is an abdomen showing many relatively recent laparotomy scars, which, in a newly presenting patient at a different hospital, should arouse suspicion.

CAUSES OF ACUTE UPPER ABDOMINAL PAIN

The common sites of inflammation and malignant disease in the upper abdomen causing upper abdominal pain are in the stomach and duodenum, gallbladder and pancreas.

The conditions causing acute upper abdominal pain are summarized in Revision panel 15.8.

OESOPHAGITIS

This occurs when acid pepsin refluxes up out of the stomach into the oesophagus through the lower oesophageal sphincter onto the squamous epithelium lining the oesophagus, which is not able to resist these powerful chemicals. In many instances, the reflux occurs because of incompetence of the gastro-oesophageal junction caused by a hiatus hernia.

Revision panel 15.8

COMMON CONDITIONS THAT PRESENT WITH ACUTE UPPER ABDOMINAL PAIN

Gallstones/biliary colic
Acute cholecystitis
Acute pancreatitis
Acute gastritis/duodenitis
Peptic ulcer
Perforated peptic ulcer
Oesophagitis
Gastric volvulus
Boerhaave's syndrome
Haemorrhage/infarction
Extra-abdominal causes

History

Patients complain of *heartburn*, which is a severe burning discomfort felt in the centre of the chest behind the heart, often experienced at night. The frequency and severity of the heartburn is made worse by lying flat, so patients sleep propped up on pillows to try to reduce its occurrence. Heartburn is often initiated by bending, stooping or heavy lifting. When reflux occurs, patients may experience a *bitter taste developing in the mouth*, which is often accompanied by *flatulence and coughing* if any of the refluxing acid spills over into the lungs. Sometimes, the burning pain may only be experienced in the epigastrium.

After many years, patients may complain of difficulty with swallowing and of food sticking in their gullet. Although the presence of dysphagia suggests the development of a stricture caused by the acid reflux, achalasia or a carcinoma of the oesophagus or cardia must be excluded.

Examination

This rarely reveals any diagnostic signs. The diagnosis relies on endoscopy and other investigations.

ACUTE GASTRITIS/DUODENITIS/ PEPTIC ULCERATION

Benign gastric and duodenal ulcers are classified together as *peptic ulceration*. Mucosal infection with *Helicobacter pylori* is a major factor in their development.

Gastric ulcers are now rare in the UK, so any patient presenting with indigestion, non-specific upper abdominal pain and a recent onset of weight loss should be *suspected of having a gastric cancer.*

Duodenal ulcers are still common throughout the world and affect both sexes in equal numbers. They can occur at any age, but most often arise in middle-aged patients.

History

Symptoms Patients with acute peptic ulceration present with *acute pain of short duration,* but may have had previous similar episodes *interspersed with periods of relief lasting for many months or even years.*

The main symptom of acute peptic ulceration is an *epigastric discomfort or pain,* which is related to meals and described as *indigestion* or *dyspepsia.* It can vary from a mild discomfort to a very severe pain that forces the patient to lie down. The severity and tenderness may equal those of a perforated peptic ulcer.

Patients with *gastric ulcers* are typically afraid to eat because the pain is induced by food. Vomiting often relieves the pain.

Patients with *duodenal ulcers* typically have a good appetite and rarely lose weight because they eat frequently to relieve their pain. *Acid brash, water brash* and *heartburn* are rare symptoms. *Haematemesis and melaena* may complicate all forms of peptic ulceration.

Drugs Many drugs, but especially *aspirin* and the *non-steroidal anti-inflammatory drugs* (NSAIDs) that are used to treat arthritis, irritate the gastric mucosa and cause ulceration, so it is essential to ascertain the precise details of any drug ingestion.

Social history Cigarette smoking and periods of stress may be important risk factors.

Examination

Abdominal examination often reveals *epigastric tenderness,* with guarding if the pain is severe. The patient may be anaemic if there has been chronic silent bleeding before the acute episode.

PERFORATED PEPTIC ULCER

Acid gastric juice enters the peritoneal cavity if a peptic ulcer erodes the wall of the stomach or duodenum at a point where it is covered only by visceral peritoneum. This causes a chemical peritonitis, which later becomes infected with bacteria.

History

Age and sex Perforated peptic ulcers are most common between the ages of 40 and 60 years, but also occur in the very old because many old people are given *NSAIDs* for joint disease. Males and females are equally affected.

Symptoms A perforation causes *sudden severe and constant pain.* This usually *begins in the epigastrium,* reaches its maximum intensity quickly and remains severe for many hours. It gradually extends to involve the whole of the abdomen. All movement, including respiration, makes the pain worse, causing the patient to lie immobile on the bed.

NOTE: Many patients give no history of previous dyspepsia, but it is important to ask if they have ever suffered from indigestion in the past.

Drug history It is important to enquire whether the patient has taken steroids, NSAIDs or salicylates, because these dispose to perforation.

Examination

General appearance The patient looks ill and is *obviously in pain, lying completely still.* A tachycardia is common and respiration is shallow, but the temperature is usually normal.

Abdomen inspection The abdomen is flat and does not rise and fall with respiration. *The abdominal muscles can be seen to be tightly contracted.*

Palpation In the early stages, *tenderness* and *guarding may be confined to the epigastrium and right side,* but eventually, when the entire peritoneal cavity is contaminated, the *whole abdomen* becomes very tender, with intense guarding, often described as *board-like rigidity.* No intra-abdominal viscus or masses can be felt because the abdominal musculature is permanently contracted.

Percussion This is usually painful. The liver dullness may be diminished or completely absent if a large quantity of air has escaped into the peritoneal cavity.

Auscultation The bowel sounds disappear once generalized peritonitis is established.

> **NOTE:** After 4–6 hours, the acid in the peritoneal cavity becomes diluted and the pain and guarding can decrease. Patients think they are improving, but they are in fact getting worse. The peritonitis is progressing and hypovolaemia is developing. An increasing tachycardia and absent bowel sounds associated with increasing abdominal distension and sunken eyes indicate that the patient is becoming extremely ill.

GALLSTONE COLIC/BILIARY COLIC

There is an overlap between gallstone colic and acute cholecystitis. Gallstone colic is a severe pain caused by spasm of the gallbladder as it tries to force a gallstone down the cystic duct, which is why 'gallstone colic' is a preferable term to 'biliary colic'. About one-fifth of patients who present in this way become jaundiced. *Many cases of gallstone colic progress to acute cholecystitis.*

History

Symptoms Gallstone colic begins suddenly across the upper abdomen. Patients are often unable to indicate which side is more affected. *The pain is severe and constant with excruciating exacerbations.* It is not a true colic because it does not remit between exacerbations. The severe pain seldom lasts longer than a few hours unless acute cholecystitis develops. It is usually accompanied by nausea and vomiting and is relieved only by strong analgesia.

> **NOTE:** Many patients give a history of flatulent dyspepsia and previous episodes of upper abdominal pain.

Examination

General appearance The patient is frightened and becomes restless as a consequence of the intensity of the pain. A mild tachycardia is often present in the early stages, but the temperature is usually normal. Jaundice may be present.

Abdomen The abdomen is often *extremely tender,* with *intense guarding* in the upper abdomen.

ACUTE CHOLECYSTITIS

Acute inflammation of the gallbladder is commonly caused by obstruction of the cystic duct by a small stone causing gallbladder distension, chemical inflammation of its wall and, eventually, secondary infection.

History

Age Patients are commonly 30–60 years of age and female. Younger patients with disorders of haemolysis such as sickle-cell disease or hereditary spherocytosis often form pigment stones, which may precipitate an attack of acute cholecystitis.

Sex Acute cholecystitis is more common in females than in males.

Symptoms The main symptom is a *sudden pain,* often without any previous symptoms of chronic indigestion. *It is felt in the right hypochondrium and often radiates through to the back close to the tip of the right scapula.* The pain is continuous, lasting more than 6 hours, and is exacerbated by moving and breathing. Nothing except analgesic drugs brings relief. Some patients recognize the pain as a severe version of their chronic indigestion pain but, as stated above, it often occurs *de novo.* Patients nearly always feel *nauseated* and often vomit.

> **NOTE:** The urine may be dark, the stools pale and the skin itchy, if there is an associated obstructive jaundice.

Previous history There may be a history of flatulent dyspepsia or previous attacks of gallstone colic.

Examination

General appearance The patient is distressed by the pain and *lies still, breathing shallowly.* There is usually a *tachycardia and pyrexia,* although in the early stages of the attack the temperature is often normal. *Jaundice may be present* and the patient may be sweating.

Abdomen inspection Rarely, there may be a fullness in the right hypochondrium in the early stages of the inflammation.

Palpation There is almost always *tenderness and guarding in the right hypochondrium.*

Palpate the abdomen just below the tip of the ninth costal cartilage and ask the patient to take a deep breath. When the liver and the attached gallbladder descend and strike the palpating hand, the patient will experience a sharp pain that prevents further inspiration. This is called *Murphy's sign*.

At an early stage, before there is any guarding, *an enlarged gallbladder may be palpable*. At a later stage, when the inflammation has been present for several days and the tenderness is beginning to subside, an inflammatory mass may become palpable (*Zackary Cope's sign*). This will still be very tender and moves little with respiration. It usually indicates that there is pus in the gallbladder (an *empyema*).

Occasionally, the contents of an obstructed gallbladder do not become infected, and a large *mucocele* may develop. This may reach down to the level of the umbilicus.

Because gallbladder pain often radiates through to the tip of the scapula, the affected dermatome may be hyperaesthetic, a change detected by lightly drawing a pin down the back of the patient's chest. This is called *Boas' sign*.

Percussion A dull area just beneath the costal margin indicates the presence of an inflammatory mass.

Auscultation The bowel sounds are normally present unless the gallbladder has infarcted or ruptured and caused biliary peritonitis. This complication is rare.

ACUTE PANCREATITIS

Acute pancreatitis is a condition in which activated pancreatic enzymes autodigest the pancreatic gland. It may be caused by obstruction of the pancreatic duct, usually by a small gallstone obstructing the ampulla of Vater. It is also commonly secondary to alcohol abuse.

Viral infections, trauma, periampullary carcinoma and a number of rarer conditions may also cause acute pancreatitis. In about one-third of cases, a cause is never discovered (Revision panel 15.9).

Revision panel 15.9

CAUSES OF ACUTE PANCREATITIS

- Gallstones
- Alcohol
- Metabolic (hypercalcaemia, hyperlipidaemia)
- Endoscopic retrograde cholangiopancreatography
- Trauma
- Idiopathic
- Autoimmune
- Medication (thiazides, steroids)
- Infections (mumps, Coxsackie virus)
- Structural abnormalities (pancreatic divisum, choledochocele)
- Periampullary carcinoma

Pancreatitis can vary from a very mild inflammation to an acute haemorrhagic destruction of the whole gland – a condition with a high mortality.

History

Age and sex Pancreatitis is equally common in males and females. The peak incidence is in the fourth and fifth decades of life, but it can occur at any age.

Symptoms The common presenting symptom is *pain that begins suddenly, high in the epigastrium,* and steadily increases in severity until it is very severe, causing the patient to lie still and breathe shallowly. *It usually radiates through to the back.* Nothing relieves the pain, which is exacerbated by movement. Frequent *vomiting* and *retching* are very common, and are an important pointer to the correct diagnosis. There is persistent nausea between the bouts of vomiting.

> **NOTE:** In the UK, nearly half of patients who present with acute pancreatitis have biliary tract disease. Therefore, many patients have a previous history of indigestion.

Social history A careful history of the patient's alcohol intake is important. Mumps is a very rare cause of pancreatitis, but ask about any recent contacts with children or the disease.

Examination

General appearance *Patients lie still* because the pain is severe, and, if they are *pale and sweating*, it is likely that they have become hypovolaemic. When respiration is impaired, they become grey, apprehensive, dyspnoeic and cyanosed. The sclerae may reveal a *slight tinge of jaundice* if the pancreatitis has been caused by a stone lodged in the lower end of the bile duct. Mild jaundice may also appear on the second or third day of the illness if oedema in the head of the pancreas causes compression of the bile duct. There is usually a *tachycardia* and, if the patient has become hypovolaemic, the jugular venous pressure and blood pressure may be low. Pyrexia is usually mild.

Abdomen inspection There is always *tenderness* and *guarding in the upper abdomen* but the signs may be mild. Any patient with severe pain but minimal abdominal signs may have acute pancreatitis.

If the pain is severe and the tone of the abdominal muscles is increased, the abdomen will not move with respiration. A paralytic ileus may develop, causing mild abdominal distension.

Bruising and discolouration in the left flank (*Grey Turner's sign*) and around the umbilicus (*Cullen's sign*) only develop in patients with very severe haemorrhagic pancreatitis. These are rare and late signs, and indicate extensive destruction of the gland.

> **NOTE:** Remember that they may also occur after a large intraperitoneal or retroperitoneal haemorrhage from another cause, such as a leaking abdominal aortic aneurysm.

A number of patients develop a collection of inflammatory exudate in the lesser sac. This is initially suggested by fullness in the epigastrium, which may become a more prominent mass if a *pseudocyst or abscess develops*.

Percussion Percussion may cause pain if there is peritonitis and be dull over any pseudocysts that are developing.

Auscultation Bowel sounds are usually present in the first 12–24 hours but fade away if a paralytic ileus develops.

> **NOTE:** Acute pancreatitis can be extremely difficult to diagnose and, as it has no distinctive features, is often forgotten and missed. Whenever you examine an acute abdomen and cannot find a obvious cause, think 'Could this be acute pancreatitis?' 'Or a mesenteric vascular infarction?' 'Or possibly a leaking abdominal aortic aneurysm?'

GASTRIC VOLVULUS

History

This is a rare condition and usually occurs in association with a giant hiatus hernia.

Age and sex It is equally common in males and females. The peak incidence is in elderly patients.

Symptoms Patients report a *sudden onset of severe upper abdominal/chest pain* in association with retching.

Previous history The pre-existing hiatus hernia may have caused a *history of reflux, regurgitation*, breathlessness, early satiety and upper abdominal discomfort.

Examination

General appearance The patient appears *distressed* with an increased respiratory rate and *tachycardia*. Cardiovascular collapse develops if the stomach becomes ischaemic.

Abdomen inspection There may be tenderness and guarding in the upper abdomen but often the abdominal signs are minimal.

Percussion Percussion may cause pain if there is peritonitis from ischaemia or perforation.

Auscultation Bowel sounds are usually present.

The lack of abdominal signs can often be misleading.

> **NOTE:** A gastric volvulus should be suspected if a patient has sudden onset epigastric pain and intractable retching, and passing a nasogastric tube is difficult (*Borchardt's triad*).

BOERHAAVE'S SYNDROME

This syndrome is caused by a full-thickness tear at the oesophagogastric junction, perhaps as a consequence of *attempting to suppress a vomit*.

The patient complains of the *sudden onset of a severe pain in the upper abdomen or lower chest after a bout of vomiting*. The condition should be suspected if, in addition to tenderness, guarding and rigidity in the upper abdomen, there is *supraclavicular subcutaneous emphysema*.

Subcutaneous bubbles of air – emphysema – feel like the little plastic air pockets in 'bubble wrap', which compress, crackle and pop beneath the fingers during gentle palpation.

NOTE: The triad of pain, vomiting and subcutaneous emphysema is known as *Mackler's triad*.

HAEMORRHAGE/INFARCTION

As previously mentioned, intra-abdominal or retroperitoneal haemorrhage can result in acute upper abdominal pain. Rupture of the spleen or a liver adenoma will result in upper abdominal pain. Pain from a ruptured aneurysm can be felt in any part of the abdomen or the back depending on the site of the rupture.

EXTRA-ABDOMINAL CAUSES

Extra-abdominal causes such as pneumonia are often perceived to be arising in the upper abdomen and can mimic conditions such as acute cholecystitis. Splenic infarction is seen in patients with sickle-cell disease. This can cause acute left upper quadrant pain, which may radiate to the tip of the left shoulder.

Acute central abdominal pain

Causes are listed in Revision panel 15.10.

Revision panel 15.10

CAUSES OF ACUTE CENTRAL ABDOMINAL PAIN

- Small bowel obstruction
- Small bowel perforation
- Mesenteric infarction
- Intussusception
- Spontaneous bacterial peritonitis
- Meckel's diverticulitis
- Acute gastroenteritis
- Inflammatory bowel disease
- *Yersinia* ileitis
- Typhoid
- Tuberculosis
- UTI
- Ruptured aortic aneurysm

SMALL BOWEL OBSTRUCTION

Intestinal obstruction produces a *severe central griping pain interspersed with periods of little or no pain*. Small bowel colic is felt in the *centre of the abdomen* and is associated with *vomiting* (see page 500). The pain becomes more severe, is constant and will become more generalized if the bowel becomes ischaemic or perforates.

SMALL BOWEL PERFORATION

Small bowel perforation causes *sudden onset central abdominal pain* progressing to generalized peritonitis. It is usually the result of ischaemia from small bowel volvulus or a closed loop obstruction.

MESENTERIC ISCHAEMIA

Infarction of the bowel caused by a sudden mesenteric artery occlusion causes *acute abdominal pain*. The patient is usually a middle-aged male smoker with other signs of arterial disease such as:

- Atrial fibrillation.
- Intermittent claudication.
- Angina.
- Previous myocardial infarction.

It can also be the result of a twist in the intestinal mesentery – *volvulus*. Venous occlusion can be seen in some prothrombotic conditions and presents in a similar manner.

The *vasculitides such as systemic lupus erythematosis* and conditions such as *sickle-cell disease* can also cause acute and chronic abdominal pain, which is thought to be related to mesenteric ischaemia.

INTUSSUSCEPTION

Intussusception occurs as a segment of bowel invaginates and enters the bowel beyond it, and is driven on by peristalsis (Figure 15.12). The apex of the intussusception can be:

- Lymphoid tissue (Peyer's patches).
- An appendix.
- A Meckel's diverticulum.
- A polyp.
- Submucosal haemorrhage.
- Tumour.

Initially, the pain may be similar to that of intestinal obstruction. The most common site is an *ileocolic intussusception* leading to small bowel obstruction. As the condition progresses, the bowel may become ischaemic and perforate. This will cause generalized peritonitis, and the abdominal signs will change accordingly. The intussusception can sometimes be felt as a *sausage-shaped mass* in the right hypochondrium with a emptiness in the right lower quadrant. Patients occasionally pass *'redcurrant jelly' stools.*

Rarely, the intussusception can be felt on rectal examination.

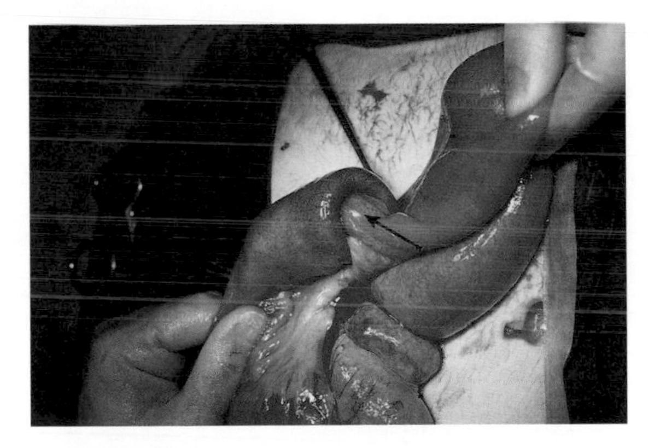

Figure 15.12 An intussucepted loop of small bowel (arrowed). It may be palpable as a sausage-shaped mass.

SPONTANEOUS BACTERIAL PERITONITIS

This condition is seen in patients on peritoneal dialysis or with ascites (Figure 15.13). Patients may have minimal tenderness until the later stages, but equally can present with generalized peritonitis. The dialysate or ascitic fluid is usually altered in appearance and can be tested for bacterial contamination and the presence of white cells.

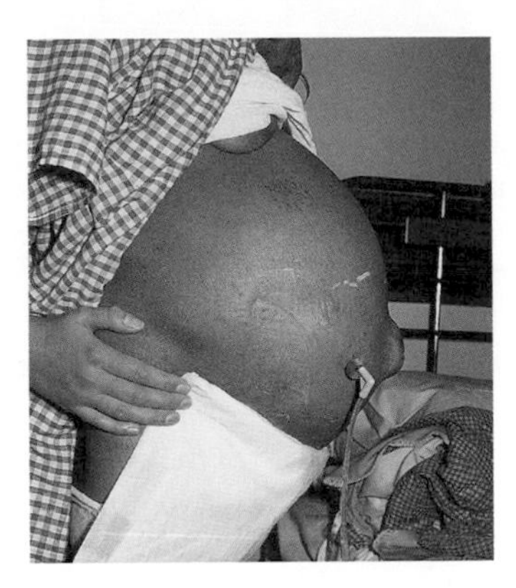

Figure 15.13 Patient on peritoneal dialysis with ascites.

ACUTE MECKEL'S DIVERTICULITIS

This is the *remnant of the vittelointestinal duct.* It contains all layers of the bowel wall and can contain ectopic gastric or pancreatic mucosa, it occurs in about 2% of the population and causes abdominal pain if it becomes inflamed.

Inflammation of a Meckel's diverticulum produces symptoms and signs that are *indistinguishable from those of acute appendicitis,* although the pain and tenderness are generally felt more towards the centre of the abdomen than in the right iliac fossa.

It may also cause colicky abdominal pain if it acts as the head of an intussusception or if a congenital band arising from its apex causes small bowel obstruction or a volvulus.

ACUTE GASTROENTERITIS

Gastroenteritis is usually caused by a *Campylobacter* or a viral infection, but must be differentiated from food poisoning. The symptoms of vomiting and diarrhoea usually predominate over the abdominal pain, which may be non-existent or very mild.

Occasionally, it causes severe colicky, cramping pains that must be differentiated from the colic of small bowel obstruction caused by diseases such as Crohn's disease, *Yersinia* infections (see page 514) or acute appendicitis.

There are usually few signs on abdominal examination.

The stool should be cultured to exclude *Campylobacter, Giardia,* ova and parasites, particularly if the patient has recently travelled to a foreign country.

INFLAMMATORY BOWEL DISEASE

Crohn's disease and *ulcerative colitis* may present with acute or chronic central abdominal pain together with a variety of other gastrointestinal symptoms.

Acute Crohn's disease may present with *central or right iliac fossa discomfort and signs similar to those of appendicitis.* A thick and tender terminal ileum may be palpable in the right iliac fossa, and thickened ileum and jejunum may also be palpable in the umbilical region.

Acute fulminating ulcerative colitis may present with acute abdominal pain, especially when complicated by acute toxic dilatation or perforation of the colon. The abdominal pain is invariably preceded by *severe incessant diarrhoea accompanied by the passage of blood, mucus and pus.*

ACUTE *YERSINIA* ILEITIS

This condition is indistinguishable from acute Crohn's disease and appendicitis on the history and physical signs. A mass is rarely palpable. It is usually incorrectly diagnosed as acute appendicitis.

TYPHOID

Typhoid normally presents with toxaemia and diarrhoea. Severe abdominal pain and all the signs of peritonitis can be present if a typhoid ulcer perforates the small bowel.

URINARY TRACT INFECTION (CYSTITIS AND PYELONEPHRITIS)

The symptoms and signs of urinary tract infections are discussed in Chapter 17. Pain from pyelonephritis is felt mainly in the *lumbar region,* but may spread to the centre of the abdomen. When patients are asked to describe the site of their renal pain, they usually put their hands on their waist with their thumbs pointing forwards and their fingers spread backwards between the 12th rib and the iliac crest. It is easier to detect tenderness in the renal angle if the patient is sitting up and leaning slightly forwards.

Deep abdominal palpation must be carried out to ensure that there is not an enlarged kidney caused by another pathology responsible for the infection, such as a hydronephrosis. The bladder may be enlarged and should be palpated and percussed. Examination of the external genitalia and a rectal examination are essential (see Chapters 16 and 18). The *urine should be examined for red and white cells and organisms.* The presence of red cells in the urine suggests that the pain is more likely to be coming from a calculus or a tumour than an infection.

INTRA-ABDOMINAL OR RETROPERITONEAL HAEMORRHAGE

As previously mentioned, intra-abdominal or retroperitoneal haemorrhage, for example, with a ruptured abdominal aortic aneurysm, can result in acute central abdominal pain.

Acute lower abdominal pain

Causes are listed in Revision panel 15.11.

Revision panel 15.11

CAUSES OF ACUTE LOWER ABDOMINAL PAIN

Acute appendicitis
Meckel's diverticulitis
Mesenteric adenitis
Crohn's disease
Diverticulitis
Salpingitis/pelvic inflammatory disease (PID)
Ectopic pregnancy
Twisting or degenerating fibroid
Acute urinary retention
Cystitis/pyelonephritis/renal colic
Colonic carcinoma/diverticulitis/perforation

ACUTE APPENDICITIS

This is the most common cause of acute abdominal pain in the Western world. The cause remains unknown, but obstruction of the lumen by a faecolith, swollen Peyer's patches, a stricture or a carcinoid tumour at its base all can play a part. Threadworms, which are often found in the appendix, may be an aetiological factor, as may diet and childhood infections.

History

Age and sex Appendicitis can and does occur at any age, but *most often affects young adults or teenagers of* either sex.

Symptoms The condition most often presents with a vague often 'colicky' pain that begins in the *centre of the abdomen*. At first, this is often thought to be indigestion and ignored, but after a varying period, usually a few hours but sometimes 2–3 days, *the pain shifts* to the *right iliac fossa* and becomes more severe.

> **NOTE:** This 'typical' history is almost diagnostic of appendicitis but only occurs in about half the patients.

The remainder present with a variety of patterns of pain. It may begin and remain in the right iliac fossa, or only be felt in the centre of the abdomen. The central pain is a referred pain. The normal visceral innervation of the appendix comes from the tenth thoracic spinal segment. The corresponding somatic dermatome encircles the abdomen at the level of the umbilicus (T10). The midline pain is higher if the spinal segment visceral innervation is higher. Some patients have retrosternal pain that shifts to the right iliac fossa. Therefore, the important feature of the initial pain is its central location and not its precise level.

The inflamed appendix most commonly lies behind the caecum (*retrocaecal*) so causes pain in the lateral part of the right iliac fossa and the flank, but it may hang down into the pelvis and lie against the bladder or a loop of large bowel (Figure 15.14). In these circumstances, the *patient may present with misleading bladder or large bowel symptoms.*

Acute appendicitis may also present with intestinal obstruction – colic and abdominal distension – if the appendix lies too close to and inflames the terminal ileum (preileal or postileal).

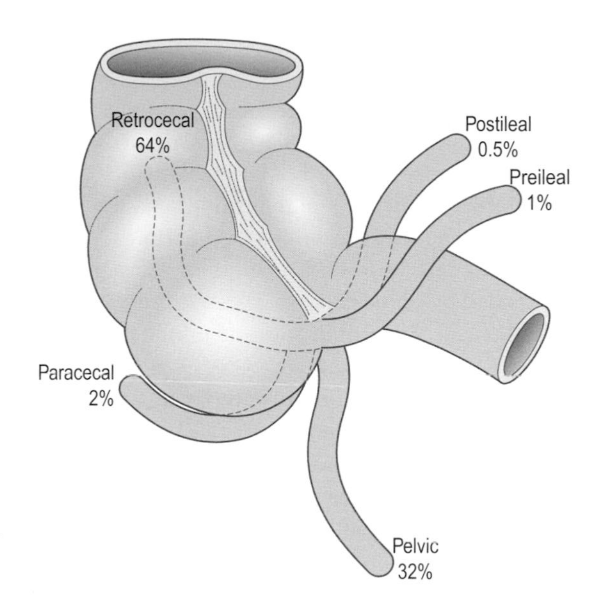

Figure 15.14 The different positions that the appendix may lie in relation to the caecum and terminal ileum.

A *loss of appetite* usually precedes the onset of pain by a few hours, and most patients feel slightly nauseated. *Many patients vomit once or twice.* Most patients with appendicitis state that they had been constipated for a few days before the pain started, but a few complain of diarrhoea, which may lead to a mistaken diagnosis of gastroenteritis, especially in children.

Some patients present with *symptoms of generalized peritonitis* – generalized abdominal pain, nausea and vomiting, sweating and sometimes rigors – especially if the initial stages of the disease go unoticed.

> **NOTE:** Atypical presentations are common in the very young, in pregnant females and in the very old, when the appendicitis may be related to obstruction of its ostium by a carcinoma of the caecum.

Examination

General appearance Patients often look unwell with flushed cheeks. A *low-grade pyrexia* is usually present, while a high temperature should suggest another cause for the pain, or general peritonitis associated with a ruptured appendix. The *pulse rate is usually elevated* and rises as the infection spreads.

Head and neck The *tongue is usually furred*, and most patients have a distinctive *fetor oris*. Palpable lymph glands in the neck and enlarged tonsils indicate that the patient may have mesenteric adenitis rather than appendicitis, but beware – acute appendicitis often follows a viral infection.

Chest The lung examination findings should be normal. It is important to exclude any signs of a right-sided basal pneumonia, because this can occasionally cause abdominal pain and mimic appendicitis, especially in children.

Abdomen inspection The abdomen, although it may be slightly distended, usually looks normal. The right hip may be kept slightly flexed if the appendix is lying against the psoas major muscle. Coughing and sudden movements cause pain if peritonitis has developed.

Palpation *The right iliac fossa is tender, and the overlying muscles show guarding.* The maximum site of tenderness must be carefully assessed by gentle palpation.

It is classically maximal over *McBurney's point*, one-third of the way along a line joining the anterior superior iliac spine to the umbilicus. High or low tenderness may indicate that the appendix is lying in an unusual position.

There may be *release or rebound tenderness in the right iliac fossa*. Pressure on the left iliac fossa may cause pain in the right iliac fossa (*Rovsing's sign*). Release of pressure on the left iliac fossa may cause pain on the right. All these manoeuvres cause pain because they move the inflamed appendix as it lies in the right iliac fossa against the overlying peritoneum, which contains many somatic pain fibres.

When the appendix is behind the caecum, the tenderness may be experienced in the lateral part of the lumbar region – the flank.

When a subhepatic appendix produces pain and tenderness below the right costal margin, it must be differentiated from acute cholecystitis.

A *tender, indistinct mass* may be felt in the right iliac fossa. It is usually impossible to feel below it because it is fixed posteriorly. It is dull to percussion. An appendix mass *usually takes a few days to develop*. An appendix abscess should be suspected if the temperature is high and the mass is very tender. The features of an appendix mass and abscess are described on pages 528, 529.

Percussion This causes pain if peritonitis is present. Dullness on percussion may suggest the presence of an underlying mass that is obscured by tenderness and guarding.

Auscultation Bowel sounds are present unless perforation and general peritonitis have caused a paralytic ileus.

Rectal examination There is considerable debate about the usefulness of this examination, especially in young children, but the presence of tenderness high in the pelvis usually indicates an inflamed pelvic appendix.

Hip movement Extension of the right hip joint exacerbates the pain if the appendix is in a retrocaecal position lying against the psoas muscle. Pain on external and internal rotation of the hip indicates that the appendix is lying against the obturator internis muscle.

MECKEL'S DIVERTICULITIS

Inflammation of a Meckel's diverticulum produces symptoms and signs that are *indistinguishable from those of acute appendicitis*, although the pain and tenderness are generally felt more towards the centre of the abdomen.

MESENTERIC ADENITIS

This condition is usually seen in children and is associated with a preceding upper respiratory tract infection and *cervical lymphadenopathy*. It often causes a more *central abdominal pain* but can cause pain in the right iliac fossa, mimicking appendicitis. The *pain can sometimes be shown to move* when the patient is placed in the lateral decubitus position as the glands move over with the mesentery.

CROHN'S DISEASE

Acute Crohn's disease affecting the terminal ileum can present with symptoms and signs similar to those of appendicitis. *Occasionally, a mass will be palpable* and has to be differentiated from an intussusception or a tumour.

ACUTE DIVERTICULITIS OF THE COLON

Acquired diverticula develop in the colon, especially the sigmoid colon, probably as a result of changes in bowel motility and the consistency of the faeces. The condition may be related to the low-roughage diet popular in the USA and Europe. Diverticula often cause no symptoms, but they may become obstructed and *acutely inflamed – acute diverticulitis*. This may progress to a pericolic abscess situated on the outside of the colon, which may then *perforate, causing generalized peritonitis* (see below).

When a *solitary diverticulum of the caecum* becomes inflamed, the signs are indistinguishable from those of acute appendicitis or a carcinoma of the colon.

History

Age, sex and ethnic group Patients with diverticulitis are commonly between the ages of 50 and 70 years. The condition is slightly more common in females than in males. Native Africans and Asians are rarely affected.

Symptoms The first symptom is often a *mild intermittent lower abdominal pain* that then shifts to the *left iliac fossa* (for the same reasons as appendicitis moves to the right), where it becomes a more constant ache. The pain begins gradually before becoming more severe and constant. It may become colicky if the large bowel becomes obstructed. The pain is often associated with *nausea* and a *loss of appetite*, but rarely vomiting. Most patients are constipated, but a few develop diarrhoea. If the colon lies against the vault of the bladder and the bladder wall becomes inflamed, there may be painful and increased frequency of micturition. Some patients can relate their attacks to the type of food they have eaten.

Previous history Some patients give a history of chronic diverticular disease, flatulence, distension and left iliac fossa pain.

Examination

General appearance Patients lie still because of the pain and often look flushed. They are usually pyrexial and have a tachycardia.

Abdomen inspection If there is a generalized peritonitis or intestinal obstruction, the abdomen moves with respiration and may be distended.

Palpation There is *tenderness* and *guarding* in the left iliac fossa, where there may be a *palpable, tender, sausage-shaped mass*. Pressure on the right side of the abdomen may induce pain on the left (*reversed Rovsing's sign*). Rebound tenderness will be present if generalized peritonitis has developed. In the latter stages of peritonitis or obstruction, there may be considerable abdominal distension.

Percussion Any palpable mass in the left iliac fossa should be dull to percussion.

Auscultation The bowel sounds may be normal, amphoric if there is intestinal obstruction or absent if a generalized peritonitis develops causing a paralytic ileus.

Rectal examination Pain may be experienced when the finger is pushed high into the left side of the pelvis. Rectal examination is important to exclude a carcinoma of the rectosigmoid junction, which can perforate and cause similar symptoms. Sigmoidoscopy is indicated to exclude a carcinoma but often causes pain when attempting to negotiate the rectosigmoid junction. The findings are rarely diagnostic unless a carcinoma is seen.

Differential diagnoses Acute diverticulitis must be differentiated from:

- Carcinoma of the colon.
- Pericolic abscess.
- Ischaemic colitis.
- Acute appendicitis.
- Crohn's disease.

ACUTE SALPINGITIS/PELVIC INFLAMMATORY DISEASE

Acute salpingitis is an infection in one or both fallopian tubes, and is often associated with infection within the surrounding supporting tissues around the adnexae – hence the term 'pelvic inflammatory disease'. The common infecting organisms are *Gonococcus* and *Streptococcus*. These organisms usually reach the Fallopian tubes by direct spread through the vagina and uterus, and rarely from the bloodstream. Salpingitis is a well-recognized complication of the puerperium and following abortion.

History

Age and sex Salpingitis usually occurs in sexually active females between the ages of 15 and 50 years.

Symptoms A *purulent, yellow–white vaginal discharge* usually precedes, by a few days, the *gradual onset of lower abdominal pain*. The pain is constant and can become severe. It may radiate to the lower part of the back. Sometimes, the abdominal pain is preceded by a low backache. Menstruation may have been irregular over the previous months, and patients often give a history of dysmenorrhoea and dyspareunia (painful sexual intercourse). *Sweating and rigors are common*, but there is usually no nausea, vomiting or change in bowel habit. By contrast, urinary tract symptoms, such as painful and frequent micturition, are common as the urinary tract is often also infected.

Previous history Patients may have had previous attacks of infection or know that they have had or have been exposed to gonorrhoea.

Examination

General appearance The patient looks flushed and feverish. There is no distinctive fetor oris, and *the oral temperature is often higher than in appendicitis*, being between 38°C and 39.5°C.

Abdomen inspection The abdomen moves normally and looks normal.

Palpation Tenderness and some guarding are present across the lower abdomen. *The tenderness is often bilateral* as both Fallopian tubes may be infected, but can be asymmetrical if one tube is more inflamed than the other. It is usually lower and nearer to the midline than the tenderness of acute appendicitis. A *huge pyosalpinx is occasionally palpable*, but even large swollen tubes can often only be felt by manual examination (see below).

Percussion This seldom causes pain, but may do so if there is associated peritonitis.

Auscultation The bowel sounds are usually normal.

Vaginal examination Examination of the vaginal introitus may reveal a *yellow–white discharge*, a specimen of which should be sent for culture. The cervix and uterus should be of normal size, but bimanual palpation of the adnexae will cause pain. *Moving the cervix (cervical excitation) is also painful*. Speculum examination may demonstrate pus coming from the cervical canal. If a pyosalpinx or tubo-ovarian abscess is present, a mass may be felt to one side of the uterus.

ECTOPIC PREGNANCY

A sudden onset of lower abdominal pain in a female of child-bearing age should be immediately treated as a suspected ectopic pregnancy. The patient usually gives a history of *delayed menstruation followed by a few days history of mild abdominal pain or cramps*. If it is associated with a major intra-abdominal bleed, the patient will be showing *signs of haemorrhagic shock and will require immediate resuscitation*. The pain initially arises in the lower abdomen on the side of the ectopic pregnancy. The pain becomes more generalized if there is significant bleeding, with shoulder tip pain if blood collects beneath the diaphragm.

TWISTED/DEGENERATING FIBROIDS

Pedunculated fibroids can twist and infarct, leading to severe lower abdominal pain. Degeneration occurs when the fibroid reaches a size at which it can no longer maintain an adequate blood supply. This can result in acute lower abdominal pain, which can last for several weeks.

UROLOGICAL CAUSES

Acute urinary retention, cystitis, bladder colic, ureteric colic and pyelonephritis can all cause acute lower abdominal symptoms and are discussed in Chapter 17.

UTERINE COLIC

This is always associated with pregnancy. The presence of a large pelvic mass should confirm the presence of a pregnant uterus.

CARCINOMA OF THE COLON

A carcinoma of the caecum may cause appendicitis. The physical signs are indistinguishable from those of simple acute appendicitis. Even when a mass is palpable, it is rarely possible to be certain that this is not an inflammatory mass, and even if the mass is very hard, discrete, knobbly and not very tender, it may simply be the result of inflammation.

> **NOTE:** The possibility of a cancer of the caecum must always be considered in a patient over 40 years old who presents with acute appendicitis.

Other possible diagnoses include an inflamed solitary caecal diverticulum, Crohn's disease and ileocaecal tuberculosis. Localized perforation of the caecum can also occur, leading to initially localized and then generalized peritonitis.

Tumours in the left side of the colon can present with generalized peritonitis. In such cases, severe generalized abdominal pain develops, accompanied by signs of shock with tachycardia, hypotension, distension, tenderness, loss of liver dullness and absent bowel sounds. *In many cases, the peritonitis is caused by a rupture of a distended caecum caused by an obstructing left-sided tumour.*

CHRONIC ABDOMINAL PAIN

Causes of chronic upper abdominal pain are listed in Revision panel 15.12.

Revision panel 15.12

COMMON CONDITIONS PRESENTING WITH CHRONIC UPPER ABDOMINAL PAIN

- Chronic peptic ulceration
- Carcinoma of the stomach
- Chronic pancreatitis
- Chronic cholecystitis
- Carcinoma of the pancreas
- Liver metastases
- Splenomegaly

CHRONIC PEPTIC ULCERATION, GASTRITIS AND DUODENITIS

History

Age Peptic ulceration tends to occur between the ages of 20 and 60 years.

Sex Both gastric and duodenal ulcers are more common in males than females.

Occupation There is a higher incidence amongst those in the professions and those with executive appointments!

Symptoms Although a few patients present to hospital with an acute, sometimes very severe upper abdominal pain of short duration as described above.

> **NOTE:** The great majority of patients with chronic peptic ulceration present with a chronic, less severe and more intermittent pain, which they usually call 'indigestion' or dyspepsia because it is directly related to the ingestion of food.

Nevertheless, some patients experience continuous pain over many hours or days that is unaffected by food.

Night pain, which wakes the patient and seems to be unrelated to food, is a *common symptom of duodenal ulceration.* This is thought to be caused by the drop in pH in the stomach at night, when the acid secretions are no longer buffered by the presence of food. The pain is usually experienced in the *epigastrium and may radiate into either the back or the right hypochondrium* if the ulcer is situated in the posterior part of the stomach or the second part of the duodenum. The pain is usually described as a continuous gnawing or boring ache and is rarely very severe.

It is usually episodic, occurring for 2 or 3 weeks at a time before resolving spontaneously, only to recur a few months later – a feature known as *periodicity.*

The rapid onset of pain after food, causing *food fear and loss of weight,* suggests the presence of a gastric ulcer. Pain that is *relieved by eating indicates the probability of a duodenal ulcer.*

The pain is usually relieved by commercially available antacids, H2 receptor blockers and PPIs.

Peptic ulcers commonly arise in middle-aged smokers, but are also common in middle-aged and elderly patients on long-term NSAIDs.

Vomiting is rare unless a pyloric stenosis has developed.

Excessive salivation (water brash) and *acid brash* are highly suggestive of duodenal ulceration. Some patients develop heartburn.

Haematemesis and *melaena* are important complications that occur in a small proportion of patients with chronic, and acute, peptic ulceration. Chronic blood loss may cause an iron deficiency anaemia, which presents with *tiredness* and *shortness of breath*.

Chronic peptic ulceration must be differentiated from other causes of chronic abdominal pain. A clear history of weight loss suggests a gastric carcinoma, whereas acid heartburn and reflux suggest oesophagitis. Gallstones and chronic cholecystitis may coexist and are important differential diagnoses.

Examination

General Anaemia and cervical lymphadenopathy with obvious cachexia should suggest the possibility of carcinoma of the stomach rather than peptic ulceration.

Abdomen inspection Epigastric distension and visible peristalsis may be present if a *pyloric stenosis* has developed.

Palpation Minor tenderness in the epigastrium is often the only abnormality. The presence of a *succussion splash indicates the presence of pyloric stenosis.*

Percussion and auscultation These should be normal.

> **NOTE:** The diagnosis of chronic peptic ulcer is now almost exclusively made on flexible endoscopy and biopsy. The importance of *Helicobacter pylori* as a cause has already been described, and a breath test is available to confirm its involvement.

CARCINOMA OF THE STOMACH

This is a common cause of death in males. Pernicious anaemia, gastric polyps and chronic gastric ulcers are known to be premalignant conditions, but the majority of gastric cancers arise spontaneously. *Helicobacter pylori* is an important predisposing factor.

History

Age The incidence of gastric carcinoma reaches its peak between 50 and 70 years, but it can arise at an earlier age.

Sex Gastric cancer is two to three times more common in males than in females.

Geography There are unexplained variations in the incidence of this disease. It is very common in Japan, closely followed by Chile, Austria and Finland. In the UK, it affects approximately 20–30 per 100,000 of the population. Genetic and dietary factors may be important, as may be the ingestion of nitrites.

Symptoms The onset of *indigestion* or *epigastric pain,* however vague, in a patient over 40 years of age should be treated very seriously. The pain may be mild and related to food, but, unlike the indigestion associated with peptic ulcer, the pain of a gastric ulcer is constant and not solely brought on by eating. When patients have had symptoms of a peptic ulcer for many years, they are usually aware that the nature of the pain has changed. Often their periodic pain becomes constant.

Patients with stomach cancer do not want to eat, and *loss of appetite is a cardinal symptom*. The inevitable consequence of a loss of appetite is *loss of weight*. The patient may lose 10–20 kg in 1 or 2 months. The loss of appetite and weight often occur long before any other symptoms.

Tumours near the cardia may cause obstruction of the oesophagogastric junction and cause the patient to complain of difficulty swallowing (*dysphagia*). As the dysphagia increases, undigested food may be regurgitated from the oesophagus.

Cancers in the pyloric region often obstruct the outflow of food from the stomach. If so, the patient may vomit large quantities of undigested food – *projectile vomiting* – (undigested because of the low acid production associated with the accompanying atrophic gastritis) and notice epigastric discomfort and distension.

> **NOTE:** Some cancers grow to a considerable size without producing symptoms, apart from mild weight loss.

Systematic questions A systematic review of the other systems may reveal symptoms that suggest that the tumour has metastasized, such as weakness, tiredness or dyspnoea.

Previous history The patient may have a long history of peptic ulceration or have had an ulcer some years previously that was cured with medication. Pernicious anaemia and atrophic gastritis predispose to gastric cancers. The patient may have been taking vitamin B12 supplements for their anaemia.

Examination

General appearance The most noticeable features are *wasting* and *pallor.* The wasting is often most apparent in the face and hands. The pallor is usually caused by an iron deficiency anaemia that is the result of chronic bleeding and lack of iron in the diet. Many patients present at an advanced stage with multiple hepatic metastases or metastases in the lymph glands around the porta hepatis. Mild jaundice suggests the latter.

Neck *The supraclavicular fossa must be carefully examined,* as secondary deposits in the supraclavicular lymph glands are common. A palpable supraclavicular gland in a patient with a carcinoma of the stomach is called *Virchow's gland,* and its presence is referred to as *Troisier's sign.*

Lungs The presence of a pleural effusion suggests pulmonary metastases.

Abdomen inspection The abdomen is often scaphoid as a consequence of weight loss but, paradoxically, there may be generalized abdominal distension if ascites is present. Pyloric obstruction causes *epigastric distension and visible peristalsis.* These physical signs can only be seen in thin patients. In the majority, the primary tumour is too small, too high or too deep to be seen.

Palpation In the majority of patients, the only physical sign is epigastric tenderness. Deep palpation on full inspiration may reveal an *epigastric mass.* In a thin patient with advanced disease, there may be a hard, irregular, dull epigastric mass that moves with respiration. The liver may be palpable and its edge and surface knobbly and irregular. The epigastrium may be distended, and there may be a *succussion splash* if there is pyloric obstruction.

Percussion Shifting dullness may be present if there is an associated ascites.

Auscultation The bowel sounds should be normal.

Rectal examination Metastatic nodules may be felt in the pelvis and in the ovaries (*Krukenberg's tumours*).

Often physical signs are minimal, and endoscopy is required for diagnosis.

LYMPHOMA OF THE STOMACH

This presents with symptoms and signs similar to those of a carcinoma of the stomach – vague epigastric pain and weight loss. It may arise in middle-aged patients. Endoscopic deep biopsy is required for diagnosis.

CHRONIC PANCREATITIS

This progressively destroys the exocrine and endocrine tissues of the pancreatic gland.

History

Age and sex Many patients are middle-aged, and 80% are males. It is a rare condition, affecting between three and ten patients per million in Western countries.

Symptoms Patients complain of *severe, recurrent episodes of upper abdominal pain* that usually radiates through to the back. The pain is a gnawing, dull, persistent ache. The pattern and periodicity of the attacks vary greatly, but they are often related to episodes of excessive alcohol drinking. The condition can develop after multiple attacks of acute pancreatitis (acute relapsing pancreatitis) but more often develops *de novo* in patients who subject themselves to chronic alcohol abuse.

Weight loss and *nausea* are common.

Diabetes, *steatorrhoea* and *jaundice* develop in about 10% of affected patients.

Drug addiction is common, as long-term opiate analgesics are often required to relieve the persistent, intolerably severe pain.

Examination

There are often few physical signs. Patients often look distraught and dishevelled. *Weight loss* and *jaundice* may be apparent. A *mass* (a pseudocyst) may be palpable in the epigastrium. The diagnosis ultimately relies on special tests.

Chronic pancreatitis can cause thrombosis of the portal vein, in which case, the signs of portal hypertension will be present.

NOTE: Carcinoma of the pancreas is the important differential diagnosis (see below).

CHRONIC CHOLECYSTITIS

Chronic or recurrent infection in the gallbladder is *almost always associated with gallstones*. The combination of stones and infection may present various clinical pictures: indigestion, flatulent dyspepsia (chronic cholecystitis), acute pain (acute cholecystitis), gallstone colic, obstructive jaundice and, less commonly, ascending cholangitis, acute pancreatitis and intestinal obstruction. Most of these complications are associated with abdominal pain.

History

Age Gallstones can form at any age. The majority of patients with symptoms are between 30 and 60 years old, but a number of females between the ages of 15 and 25 years develop gallstones. Younger patients with sickle-cell disease develop pigment stones.

Sex Gallstones are far more common in females than in males.

Ethnic group Native north Americans are particularly liable to develop gallstones.

Symptoms The common complaint is of an *upper abdominal indigestion-like pain after eating*. The pain normally begins gradually, 15–30 minutes after a meal, and lasts for 30–90 minutes. When it becomes severe, it tends to move over into the *right hypochondrium and may radiate through to the back*. It is not relieved by anything except analgesic drugs. *Patients often notice that the pain is worse after eating a fatty meal,* such as bacon and eggs or fish and chips. The *attacks of pain are irregular,* lasting for weeks or months, with pain-free intervals of varying length. There is often postprandial belching, hence the description *flatulent dyspepsia*. The patient's appetite remains good, and their weight stays steady or increases. *Nausea* and *vomiting* can occur during acute exacerbations.

Previous history Apart from previous episodes of dyspepsia, the patient may have been jaundiced or noticed their stools were pale, offensive and floated on the water in the lavatory pan.

Examination

General appearance *Medical students believe that almost every patient with gallstones is female, fair, fat, fertile and forty*. Many are, but enough are male, thin, dark and of any age to make one pay scant attention to the 'five Fs' as an aid to diagnosis. The skin or sclerae may show signs of *jaundice*, indicating that there may be stones in the common bile duct (*choledocholiathiasis*).

Abdomen inspection The abdomen usually looks normal.

Palpation The patient is *tender in the right hypochondrium just below the tip of the ninth rib*, the point where the edge of the rectus abdominis muscle crosses the costal margin. It may be necessary to palpate deeply behind the costal margin as the patient takes a deep breath to detect mild tenderness or a small mass.

A *mass present in the right hypochondrium* suggests that a stone is obstructing the cystic duct and that a *mucocele* or *empyema* is developing.

Percussion, auscultation and rectal examination These should be normal.

CARCINOMA OF THE PANCREAS

Eighty-five per cent of pancreatic cancers arise in the head of the pancreas. Although many present with *jaundice and weight loss, abdominal pain* is the presenting symptom in more than half, and occurs at some stage in over 90%.

The pain is usually a *continuous, dull, boring pain, felt in the epigastrium and radiating through to the back*. It is often worse at night and may be relieved by sitting forward.

Radiation of the pain to the right hypochondrium is common with tumours of the head of the pancreas, while radiation to the left hypochondrium indicates an infiltrating tumour of the tail of the gland.

Jaundice develops in almost 90% of patients at some stage of the disease, and is characteristically progressive but rarely painless. *Pale stools, dark urine and skin itching* indicate obstructive jaundice. Weight loss is almost universal.

Steatorrhoea, epigastric bloating, flatulence, diarrhoea, vomiting and constipation may all occur in between 20 and 30% of patients.

Ten per cent of patients present with *thrombophlebitis migrans* (see Chapter 10).

Examination

Obstructive jaundice, a palpable gallbladder and an enlarged liver indicate a carcinoma of the head of the pancreas, but in the early stages, physical signs are rarely present. Carcinomas of the tail or body of the pancreas often present late with the symptoms and signs of distant metastases.

LIVER METASTASES/TUMOURS

Distension of the liver capsule stimulates pain fibres. Liver metastases are a common complication of all intra-abdominal malignancies. A *constant dull ache in the right hypochondrium, general malaise, weight loss* and sometimes *mild jaundice* may be the first indication of their presence.

> **NOTE:** Patients with liver cirrhosis who develop a hepatocellular carcinoma often complain of epigastric or right hypochondrial pain. This should be suspected when severe pain and weight loss develop in a patient who is known to have cirrhosis.

SPLENOMEGALY

The causes of splenomegaly are listed in Revision panel 15.19. A large spleen can cause dull, persistent left hypochondrial pain. Splenic infarction, which is often associated with sickle-cell disease, causes a more severe pain that may be exacerbated by deep respiration.

Chronic central abdominal pain

See Revision panel 15.13.

IRRITABLE BOWEL SYNDROME

This is a functional disorder of the bowel of unknown aetiology, which causes *chronic intermittent abdominal pain* that may be associated with changes in bowel habit and abdominal distension. Combinations of these symptoms occur in at least 10% of the population, suggesting the possibility that the syndrome is simply a variant of normality.

Many aetiological factors have been proposed, including the quantity of fibre in the diet, food allergies, disorders of bowel motility, abnormalities of visceral autonomic nerve perception, psychological disorders and social and behavioural problems.

The *diagnosis is based solely on the history*, as there are no physical signs except for an indefinite, ill-localized abdominal sensitivity on palpation.

> **NOTE:** *It is important to exclude all other causes* of abdominal pain, so enquire about any symptoms or signs that might indicate the presence of organic disease, such as anaemia, bleeding, weight loss, fever or a change in bowel habit.

Revision panel 15.13

CAUSES OF CHRONIC CENTRAL ABDOMINAL PAIN

Irritable bowel syndrome
Inflammatory bowel disease
Recurrent adhesive obstruction
Small bowel tumours
Mesenteric ischaemia
Radiation damage
Carcinomatosis
Retroperitoneal fibrosis/tumours
Tuberculosis
Lumbar spine pain
Chronic constipation
Psychosomatic

The following symptoms suggest the diagnosis:

- Continuous or recurrent abdominal pain or discomfort for at least 3 months that is relieved by defaecation; and/or
- A change in the frequency of defaecation; and/or
- A change in the consistency of the stool.

These symptoms are diagnostic when presenting together with two or more of the following complaints:

- An altered frequency of defaecation.
- An altered stool consistency.
- Problems with defaecation (straining/incomplete evacuation).
- Bloated feelings of abdominal distension.
- The passage of mucus.

CROHN'S DISEASE

This disease usually runs a chronic course. It generally presents with a *long history of colicky central or lower abdominal pain* coming on every 15–30 minutes, *associated with diarrhoea*. Thickened segments of small bowel may be palpable, but some patients have no detectable abdominal physical signs.

The patient may show other stigmas of a chronic inflammatory disease (Revision panel 15.14).

Revision panel 15.14

EXTRA-ABDOMINAL MANIFESTATIONS OF CROHN'S DISEASE

Finger clubbing
Erythema nodosum
Arthritis – sacroiliitis
Aphthous ulceration
Episcleritis/uveitis
Pyoderma gangrenosum
Anal sepsis/fistulation
Sclerosing cholangitis
Gallstones
Renal stones
Anaemia
Osteoporosis
Hypoproteinaemia

RECURRENT ADHESIVE OBSTRUCTION

Adhesive obstruction is suggested when the signs and symptoms of small bowel obstruction develop in a patient with an abdominal scar. Congenital bands and internal hernias may also cause recurrent episodes of small bowel obstruction.

NOTE: Adhesive obstruction is a difficult diagnosis to make and is often applied incorrectly to any patient who experiences pain after abdominal surgery. The diagnosis can only be made with certainty when the obstruction becomes acute and laparotomy confirms the presence of adhesions obstructing the bowel.

TUMOURS OF THE SMALL BOWEL

These are rare and often found incidentally at autopsy. They present late with unexplained small bowel obstruction. Adenomas that occur in association with *familial polyposis* and *Gardner's syndrome* may cause intussusception and acute small bowel obstruction. *Lipomas* and *hamartomas* can also arise in the small bowel. The latter are known to occur in the *Peutz–Jeghers syndrome*, together with *circumoral pigmentation* (see Figure 11.10).

Carcinoid tumours are common in the appendix, where they are usually benign, but they can also arise in the small bowel, where they are more likely to be malignant.

Lymphomas can occur anywhere in the intestine but, quite commonly, arise in the small intestine.

Adenocarcinomas of the small bowel are extremely rare.

All these rare tumours can present with chronic subacute small bowel obstruction causing a *central colicky abdominal pain, weight loss and a change in bowel habit*. Acute obstruction may develop, and a mass may be palpable.

MESENTERIC ISCHAEMIA

Less acute occlusions of the mesenteric vessels may cause *chronic central or general abdominal pain*. This pain is often brought on by eating and is called *intestinal angina*. It begins insidiously with umbilical epigastric cramping pains, vomiting and diarrhoea, which lead to *'food fear', anorexia and weight loss*.

An *abdominal bruit* from a stenosed mesenteric artery may be the only detectable physical sign, but is often not present. Chronic mesenteric ischaemia should be considered in all patients with unexplained abdominal pain associated with severe weight loss.

Mesenteric venous thrombosis can complicate abdominal trauma, portal vein thrombosis, splenectomy and other causes of a hypercoagulable state.

RADIATION DAMAGE

Both the small and large bowel can be damaged by the external beam radiation used to treat pelvic malignancies such as cancer of the uterus, cervix and bladder.

Most patients develop transient diarrhoea at the time of the radiation, but some present months or years later, when fibrosis and strictures form, with colicky or continuous pain, vomiting, weight loss, constipation or diarrhoea.

Eventually, the endarteritis in the small mesenteric vessels, caused by the irradiation, may lead to ischaemia, necrosis and perforation of the bowel.

Radiation bowel injury must be differentiated from a recurrence of the primary tumour and/or widespread metastatic spread throughout the abdominal cavity (see below).

CARCINOMATOSIS

Patients with extensive 'seeding' of metastases throughout the peritoneal cavity may develop a *non-specific aching abdominal pain* that they find difficult to describe and that may be associated with few physical signs.

Eventually, *clinical ascites, abdominal masses*, evidence of tumour at other sites and *generalized weight loss and cachexia* make the diagnosis obvious. In the early stages, the nebulous nature of the pain and the lack of physical signs can lead the physician to give, mistakenly, calming reassurance or make an incorrect diagnosis of irritable bowel syndrome.

RETROPERITONEAL FIBROSIS

This not only obstructs the ureters, but may also involve the abdominal aorta and inferior vena cava. It often causes a *vague central, persistent abdominal* pain. The kidneys may be enlarged by a hydronephrosis, or there may be a tender abdominal aneurysm. The patient may present with the symptoms of an acute deep vein thrombosis or oedema of the lower limbs if the fibrosis obstructs the vena cava. (see Chapter 10).

TUBERCULOSIS

Intra-abdominal tuberculosis is relatively rare in Western countries but is still quite common in India and Africa, where it may be associated with the increasing incidence of AIDS.

Ileocaecal tuberculosis may cause colicky or *continuous central abdominal pain, often associated with abdominal distension* and weight loss.

There may be a *mass of matted glands* in the right iliac fossa, a dough-like feeling to the abdomen, ascites or signs of chronic intestinal obstruction, together with evidence of tuberculous infection at other sites such as the lungs or cervical lymph glands.

LUMBAR SPINE DISORDERS

Pain caused by abnormalities in the spine may radiate from the back to the front of the abdomen and cause diagnostic difficulties. Any suggestion that an abdominal pain is affected by movement and position should indicate the possibility that the pain is arising in the back. This can sometimes be confirmed by careful examination of the spine.

CONSTIPATION

This may cause a rather indeterminate abdominal pain and general abdominal distension. In these cases, there are hard faeces in the rectum and palpable, *indentable masses* in the abdomen.

PSYCHOSOMATIC PAIN

This is a dangerous diagnosis to make, especially knowing how difficult it is to recognize the pain of widespread intra-abdominal malignancy. There are, however, some patients with profound psychological disturbances, severe anxiety or 'cancer phobia' who persistently present with abdominal pain for which no cause can be found.

Beware of adopting the 'cry wolf' attitude. Each new episode of pain requires an open-minded new history and examination.

Chronic lower abdominal pain

See Revision panel 15.15.

Revision panel 15.15

CAUSES OF CHRONIC LOWER ABDOMINAL PAIN

- Diverticular disease
- Crohn's disease
- Carcinoma of the colon
- Gynaecological malignancy
- Chronic infections
- Chronic appendicitis
- Chronic pelvic sepsis
- Endometriosis
- Degenerating fibroid
- Urological causes
- Uterine colic

CHRONIC DIVERTICULAR DISEASE

Although diverticular disease may present with acute abdominal pain or large bowel obstruction as described above, it most commonly presents in middle-aged or elderly patients with *episodes of central or lower left-sided abdominal pain, often associated with or preceded by constipation*. The pain is dull or colicky and there may be weeks, months or years between attacks. The condition needs to be differentiated from carcinoma of the colon, irritable bowel syndrome and other causes of inflammatory bowel disease.

Examination of the abdomen may reveal some tenderness in the left iliac fossa and, very *occasionally, a palpable mass*. Rectal examination and sigmoidoscopy are rarely helpful and the diagnosis is made by special investigations.

CROHN'S DISEASE

Crohn's disease usually presents with a long history of colicky central or lower abdominal pain associated with an altered bowel habit. Patients may also report the systemic manifestations of Crohn's disease (see Revision panel 15.14).

CARCINOMA OF THE CAECUM AND RIGHT COLON

Cancer of the caecum is often silent until it has grown to a considerable size.

History

Most right-sided colonic and caecal tumours present with symptoms of *anaemia* (tiredness and shortness of breath), *weight loss and a mass*. They can also present with a dull pain in the right iliac fossa or with the colicky pains of small bowel obstruction. *Sometimes, the symptoms closely mimic acute appendicitis.*

Examination

General appearance Patients usually appear pale and thin.

Abdomen inspection The abdomen may be generally distended or full in the right iliac fossa. *A mass may be visible in a thin patient.*

Palpation The right iliac fossa is often tender, with some guarding of the overlying muscles. A *firm, irregular mass* may be felt in the right iliac fossa or right lumbar region, which may be fixed or freely mobile (Figure 15.15). The liver may be palpable, enlarged and irregular.

Percussion The mass is usually dull to percussion.

Auscultation Bowel sounds are normal unless obstruction or peritonitis is present.

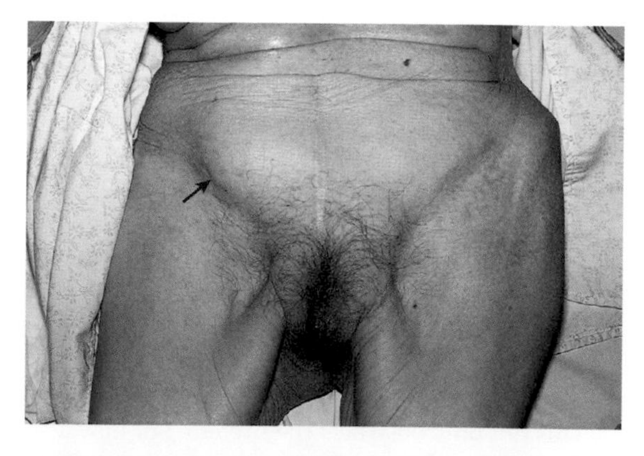

Figure 15.15 A mass clearly visible in the right iliac fossa (arrowed).

Rectal examination This is usually normal, as is sigmoidoscopy, although the latter may show the presence of rectal polyps. Occult blood may be detected in the faeces with the appropriate test.

CANCER OF THE LEFT COLON

The symptoms of cancer of the left colon differ according to the part of the colon involved. The majority of colon cancers are found in the sigmoid colon and at the rectosigmoid junction, where they are usually small, annular and ulcerated. They usually present with a *change in bowel habit*, often with variable periods of constipation interspersed with episodes of explosive diarrhoea and the passage of a number of loose stools.

History

Age The majority of patients are over 50 years old, but colon cancer can occur in young adults with ulcerative colitis or familial polyposis.

Sex Both sexes are equally affected.

Symptoms Pain is a rare symptom and, when it is present, it is usually a *mild lower abdominal colic* or ache. After some weeks or months, it usually becomes a persistent pain in the left lower abdomen. *Alternating constipation and diarrhoea* is typical of the annular variety of carcinoma of the left colon. The constipation is caused by the intestinal obstruction, and the diarrhoea by liquefaction of faeces above the obstruction. The diarrhoea may be increased by inflammation of the colonic mucosa and an excessive secretion of mucus.

The episodes of colicky abdominal pain are accompanied by distension, but early *loss of weight and appetite* is uncommon. The weight loss often precedes the anorexia.

Thin patients may feel a lump in their abdomen.

Rectal bleeding is not a common symptom of a tumour of the sigmoid or descending colon but, when it occurs, the *blood is dark and plum-coloured*, sometimes with clots of blood interspersed amongst the faeces. When the tumour is at the rectosigmoid junction or within the rectum, it is more likely to cause bleeding and it may prolapse, causing tenesmus.

Rectal tumours usually present with bleeding rather than abdominal pain or large bowel obstruction (see Chapter 16). Painful frequent micturition indicates involvement of the bladder.

Examination

General appearance Weight loss may be apparent.

Abdomen inspection In thin patients, there may be swelling in the left iliac fossa. The colon, especially the caecum, may be visibly distended with faeces.

Palpation A *large tumour may be palpable*, often in the left lumbar region or iliac fossa. Part of the mass may be hard faeces above the tumour rather than the tumour itself, in which case, the mass is indentable. The mass is tender if there is any surrounding inflammation or a pericolic abscess associated with a perforation.

The *liver may be palpable* with an irregular knobbly surface and edge.

Percussion A mass in the left iliac fossa will be dull to percussion.

Auscultation Loud, high-pitched continuous gurglings can be heard during the attacks of colic, but if the colon perforates, the abdomen becomes silent and, of course, tender.

Rectal examination A tumour in the apex of a loop of the sigmoid colon hanging down into the pelvis may be palpable on *bimanual examination*. Secondary nodules may be felt within the pelvis, and blood may be visible on the fingerstall. Rectal and rectosigmoid tumours should be visible on rigid sigmoidoscopy (see Chapter 16).

Tumours in the left side of the colon can present with generalized peritonitis. In such cases, severe generalized abdominal pain develops accompanied by signs of shock with tachycardia, hypotension, distension, tenderness, loss of liver dullness and absent bowel sounds.

> **NOTE:** In many cases, the peritonitis is caused by a rupture of a distended caecum, not a rupture at the site of the cancer (LaPlace's law).

GYNAECOLOGICAL MALIGNANCY

Signs and symptoms of gynaecological malignancy are insidious and often absent early in the disease.

Patients can report abdominal pain, bloating, weight loss, urinary urgency and fatigue. Ovarian malignancy should be suspected and investigated before a diagnosis of irritable bowel syndrome is given.

CHRONIC INFECTIONS

- **Tuberculosis** Ileocaecal tuberculosis can lead to chronic lower abdominal pain. Fistulation of the small bowel can lead to chronic abdominal pain, but may present acutely if associated with abscess formation or cellulitis.
- **Actinomycosis** Abscesses form in the gastrointestinal tract. They are painful and enlarge before discharging, commonly in the right iliac fossa.
- ***Yersinia* pseudotuberculosis** This causes a short-lived terminal ileitis similar to Crohn's disease.
- ***Enterobius* vermicularis** These are small threadworms, often found in the appendix, and may cause right lower abdominal pain.
- ***Ascaris* lumbricoides** These worms can form a tangled mass resulting in intestinal obstruction.

'CHRONIC' APPENDICITIS

Two forms of chronic inflammation may develop in the appendix: the *mucocele* and the *empyema*. Both follow an attack of acute inflammation, and both may cause recurrent pain in the right iliac fossa that is sometimes colicky in nature. Worms and faecoliths may produce similar symptoms.

NOTE: Recurrent episodes of mild acute infection, commonly classified as a 'grumbling' appendix, are extremely rare. Do not make that diagnosis; look for another cause for the patient's pain.

CHRONIC PELVIC SEPSIS

A number of patients with acute pelvic inflammatory disease develop lower abdominal pain, which is often related to the menstrual cycle. Adnexal tenderness on bimanual examination in association with a low-grade fever and a continuing *vaginal discharge* indicates the diagnosis. There may be associated urinary frequency and dysuria. Gonococcus and other pathogens found on a high vaginal swab confirm the diagnosis.

ENDOMETRIOSIS

This is a condition in which ectopic endometrial tissue is present in sites in the abdomen other than the uterus, such as the large and small bowel and the lining of the abdominal cavity. It causes abdominal pain at the time of menstruation.

DEGENERATING FIBROIDS

The pain is initially acute, but can last up to a number of weeks.

UROLOGICAL CAUSES

Urinary retention, cystitis, bladder colic, ureteric colic and pyelonephritis can all cause chronic lower abdominal symptoms and are discussed in Chapter 17.

UTERINE COLIC

Abdominal pain during pregnancy is always concerning. It is important to exclude other causes as they can be difficult to differentiate.

CONDITIONS PRESENTING WITH DYSPHAGIA

Some serious alimentary diseases do not cause abdominal pain, but do affect swallowing and may cause retrosternal pain.

FOREIGN BODY

A swallowed foreign body can become impacted in the oesophagus, leading to obstruction and complete dysphagia. An underlying stricture or malignancy should be ruled out by endoscopic examination.

MOTILITY DISORDERS

The common forms of dysmotility are *diffuse oesophageal spasm, non-specific motility disorder and achalasia*. All of these can present with dysphagia with or without pain.

The connective tissue disorder *systemic sclerosis* also causes poor oesophageal motility. This can lead to a failure of acid clearance from the oesophagus, resulting in stricture formation.

NEUROLOGICAL DISEASES

Conditions such as myasthenia gravis, multiple sclerosis (MS) and cerebrovascular disease can lead to oropharyngeal dysmotility.

REFLUX OESOPHAGITIS

This causes a retrosternal burning sensation, described by the patient as *heartburn*. Patients may also develop dysphagia. Apart from the nature of the pain, the clue to the diagnosis of reflux oesophagitis is its relationship to posture. Bending, stooping, heavy lifting and tight clothes all force acid up into the oesophagus and cause heartburn. It is often worse at night if the patient slips off their pillow. This is often the only symptom of a hiatus hernia. Recurrent or persistent reflux can result in a peptic stricture or a Schatzki ring, causing dysphagia. Strictures can also be the result of ingestion of a corrosive substance.

OESOPHAGEAL WEBS

A postcricoid web is found in patients with *Plummer–Vinson syndrome*, which is associated with iron deficiency anaemia. Other causes include bullous diseases such as pemphigus.

PHARYNGEAL POUCH

This condition leads to regurgitation, aspiration and dysphagia as the pouch enlarges (see Chapter 12).

OESOPHAGEAL CARCINOMA

The diagnosis is suspected when the patient complains of dysphagia and weight loss. Palpable supraclavicular lymph glands often develop. At first, large pieces of food stick, but ultimately fluids cannot be swallowed. Benign neoplasms of the oesophagus can occur, but are rare.

CONDITIONS PRESENTING WITH VOMITING

Acute gastroenteritis

Symptoms usually begin 12–72 hours after infection. Patients may present predominantly with either *diarrhoea or vomiting*. Bacterial infections are associated with severe abdominal cramps and blood in the stool.

Pyloric stenosis or obstruction

This occurs in *neonates with congenital hypertrophic pyloric stenosis*, and in adults with either a cicatrizing peptic ulceration of their pylorus or duodenum, or a carcinoma of the antrum of the stomach.

Neonates, with congenital *hypertrophic pyloric stenosis*, usually present between 2 and 6 weeks after birth. After feeding, they vomit large quantities of curdled and unpleasant-smelling milk. The vomit is forcefully ejected, justifying the adjective '*projectile*'. The child becomes thin and dehydrated, but retains its appetite. Careful abdominal examination shortly after a feed may reveal a *smooth ovoid mass just below the right costal margin and to the right of the rectus muscle*, sometimes called a pyloric 'tumour'. This is most easily achieved when standing to the *left* of the patient with the right hand. This is the hypertrophied pylorus, and is a diagnostic physical sign.

Adults with pyloric stenosis present with vomiting. The *vomit is usually large in volume, not bile stained* and, when the condition is long-standing, not acidic because the chronic gastric retention causes achlorhydria. The stomach contents are, therefore, not digested, and the patient may notice that their vomit contains food that was eaten 24 or 48 hours previously. *Epigastric distension, visible gastric peristalsis* and a *succussion splash* may be present.

Small bowel obstruction

As previously described in this chapter, small bowel obstruction presents with vomiting as one of the main symptoms.

Gastric volvulus

Patients report severe epigastric or retrosternal pain. They are unable to tolerate liquids and suffer from continuous retching.

Acute gastric dilatation

This condition can occur after surgery or in association with metabolic disturbances such as hyperglycaemia. The abdomen is distended and tender. There may be a succussion splash. Vomiting places the patient at risk of aspiration pneumonia.

Delayed passage of meconium

Delayed passage of meconium is often the presenting symptom in children with either cystic fibrosis, Hirschsprung's disease, intestinal atresias or anorectal malformations.

Vomiting and abdominal distension occur at or soon after birth. Cystic fibrosis can lead to meconium ileus as a result of thickened meconium inspissated within the small bowel lumen causing bowel obstruction secondary to pancreatic insufficiency. Hirschsprung's disease typically affects just the large intestine (colon) (>95% cases) and causes failure/difficult passing stool due to missing nerve cells (ganglion cells) in the colon.

Duodenal atresia

This presents with vomiting that occurs soon after birth. In 85% of patients, the level of obstruction is distal to the ampulla of Vater so the vomiting is bilious. The diagnosis may have been detected during antenatal checks and is often associated with other congenital abnormalities (25% have trisomy 21).

Medical causes

Medical causes of vomiting are listed in Revision panel 15.16.

Revision panel 15.16

MEDICAL CAUSES OF VOMITING

Medications, e.g. opioids
Alcohol
Chemotherapy
Pregnancy
Uraemia
Hyper/hypoglycaemia
Cerebrovascular accident
Migraine
Brain neoplasm
Concussion
Adrenal insufficiency
Ménière's disease

CONDITIONS PRESENTING WITH HAEMATEMESIS OR MELAENA

Haematemesis is the *vomiting of blood*. This must be differentiated from haemoptysis, when the blood is coughed up and originates from the respiratory tract. Patients describe vomit that resembles coffee grounds. This is the result of the blood becoming altered by the acid present within the stomach.

Melaena refers to the *black, tarry stool* produced in the presence of upper gastrointestinal haemorrhage. The black appearance of the stool is caused by oxidation of iron in the haemoglobin as it passes through the ileum and colon. The causes are listed in Revision panel 15.17.

CONDITIONS PRESENTING WITH JAUNDICE

The term 'jaundice' is derived from the French word jaune, meaning yellow. The yellow discolouration of the skin is caused by an excess of bile pigments in the plasma. This is initially visible against the white background of the sclerae, and then becomes more obvious as the skin turns yellow with elevation of the serum levels. The conditions that cause jaundice can be subdivided as below:

Revision panel 15.17

CAUSES OF HAEMATEMESIS AND MELAENA

- Peptic ulceration:
  - Spontaneous
  - Steroid ingestion
- Acute gastric erosions:
  - Aspirin
  - NSAIDs
  - Steroids
  - Trauma
  - Burns
- Carcinoma:
  - Stomach
  - Oesophagus
- Oesophageal varices

- *Haemolytic jaundice* (prehepatic) is associated with increased red-cell fragility and high levels of *unconjugated bilirubin* in the bloodstream, which does not enter the urine (acholuric). Causes include:
  - Sickle-cell anaemia.
  - Spherocytosis.
  - Thalassaemia.
  - 6-phosphate dehydrogenase deficiency.
- *Hepatocellular jaundice* is the result of parenchymal liver abnormalities, leading to a mixed picture of *elevated unconjugated and conjugated bilirubin*. Causes include:
  - Chronic active hepatitis.
  - Cirrhosis.
  - Drug-induced hepatitis.
  - Alcohol-induced liver disease.
- *Obstructive jaundice* (posthepatic) is associated with *pruritis, pale stools and dark urine*. This is as a result of obstruction of the biliary tree, leading to a systemic absorption and *elevation of conjugated bilirubin*. In extrahepatic cholestasis.

> **NOTE:** Courvoisier's law holds that the presence of a palpable gallbladder that is non-tender and accompanied by jaundice is unlikely to be due to gallstones and malignancy is likely.

Posthepatic causes include choledocholithiasis, cholangitis, pancreatic malignancy, Mirizzi's syndrome (see below), bile-duct strictures (benign and malignant), choledochal cyst and biliary atresia.

CAUSES OF OBSTRUCTIVE JAUNDICE

Choledocholithiasis

Gallstones can pass from the gallbladder into the common bile duct. Obstructive jaundice occurs when the stone becomes impacted within the duct. This often occurs at the ampulla, where the stone can also cause acute pancreatitis by obstructing the pancreatic duct. The jaundice is often fluctuating and the gallbladder is not palpable.

Cholangitis

This is an ascending infection as a result of a poorly draining or obstructed biliary tree. This is most commonly caused by bile-duct stones, but is also caused by malignancy of the pancreas, bile duct, ampulla or bile-duct strictures.

> **NOTE:** The classic Charcot's triad of symptoms include pain, obstructive jaundice and fever (often with rigors).

Pancreatic malignancy

The jaundice is usually *painless and progressive*. It is often associated with weight loss and pruritis. The gallbladder maybe palpable.

Mirizzi's syndrome

Obstruction of the common hepatic duct can be caused by a stone impacted in the cystic duct leading to oedema and direct compression of the extrahepatic biliary tree.

Bile-duct strictures

Benign causes include *primary sclerosing cholangitis, iatrogenic injury from previous biliary surgery and fibrosis secondary to choledocholithiasis*. Malignant causes include *cholangiocarcinoma*, adenocarcinoma of the pancreas and ampullary tumours.

Choledochal cyst

This condition usually presents in childhood and can manifest as one or all of the following: *jaundice, pain* and an *upper abdominal mass*. It is most commonly the result of a fusiform dilatation of the common bile duct. The condition carries an increased risk of cholangiocarcinoma.

Biliary atresia

Presentation is usually in the early neonatal period with persistent neonatal jaundice. It occurs in approximately 1 per 15,000 live births, and the cause is unknown.

CONDITIONS PRESENTING WITH DIARRHOEA

This is defined as the frequent passage of loose or liquid stool exceeding three or more bowel actions per day. Some diseases of the large bowel cause diarrhoea without any other symptoms. The nature of the diarrhoea may suggest the diagnosis, but it often relies on the results of investigations such as flexible sigmoidoscopy, biopsy, colonoscopy, barium enema or stool cultures.

INFECTIONS OF THE GI TRACT

Infections from food, such as *Salmonella* and *staphylococcal toxins, are called food poisoning*. The stools are watery, brown and passed with great frequency. Abdominal colic is common and may be associated with nausea, vomiting and thirst.

In tropical countries, the most common causes of diarrhoea are *bacillary dysentery* and *amoebic dysentery*. The diagnosis is confirmed on stool culture.

Cholera presents with vomiting, cramps and severe diarrhoea. The diarrhoea lasts for up to three or four days. The patient passes colourless, watery stools (known as *rice-water stools*), which consist of an inflammatory exudate, mucus, flakes of epithelium, the casts of villi and the infecting organism. *Salmonella, Giardia* and *Campylobacter* are also common infections causing abdominal pain and diarrhoea, and will be differentiated by stool culture.

Norovirus is a common viral cause in institutions and rotavirus is commonly seen in children.

Clostridium difficile is an important infection that can occur in patients on broad-spectrum antibiotics. The toxins produced can lead to a condition known as *pseudomembranous colitis*. White plaques can be seen over the mucosa when performing sigmoidoscopy. Severe infections can result in a life-threatening condition known as *toxic megacolon*.

SMALL BOWEL AND PANCREATIC DISORDERS

Pancreatic damage as a consequence of cystic fibrosis or chronic pancreatitis leads to a loss of pancreatic digestive enzyme production (i.e. lipases and amylases) and this, in turn, causes *pale frothy and offensive stools, known as steatorrhoea*.

Small bowel infiltration, infestation or fistulation can also cause diarrhoea. *Tropical sprue* and *coeliac disease* can also present with loose or frequent stools.

Patients who have had extensive previous bowel resections may have *short bowel syndrome*, leading to a rapid bowel transit time resulting in malnutrition, dehydration and weight loss.

INFLAMMATORY BOWEL DISEASE

Patients with *ulcerative colitis* and less commonly *Crohn's disease* can develop chronic frequent diarrhoea often associated with diffuse intermittent abdominal pain. They sometimes pass a watery brown fluid, while at other times they pass just mucus containing red flecks of blood or dark, altered blood. Patients may have 20–30 bowel actions a day.

NOTE: Worsening pain may be the result of acute toxic megacolon, which can be complicated by bowel perforation. The patient is dehydrated, thin, ill and feverish, with signs of abdominal distension and acute peritonitis, i.e. tenderness and guarding with a loss of liver dullness and an absence of bowel sounds.

CARCINOMA OF THE COLON AND RECTUM

Most *cancers of the left-hand side of the colon* cause a change in bowel habit, which may be associated with pain and bleeding. Persistent copious diarrhoea is not usually a prominent feature.

A *villous papilloma* is a benign or malignant rectal tumour that causes excessive mucus secretion. Patients frequently pass stools of pure mucus. This may cause dehydration and the loss of large quantities of sodium and potassium.

Spurious *(overflow) diarrhoea* occurs when a very constipated patient passes loose, watery stools around a mass of faeces impacted in the rectum. Diagnosis is by rectal examination.

Cancers of the rectum can present with diarrhoea, especially if they are locally advanced, when a frequent and sometimes painful urge to defaecate (*tenesmus*) may develop.

DRUGS

Medications are a common cause of diarrhoea, and a complete drug history including non-prescribed medications should be established. Drugs such as orlistat (which inhibits the absorption of fat), chemotherapy agents, antibiotics and overuse of laxatives can all lead to increased bowel frequency.

ENDOCRINE CAUSES

Hormone-secreting tumours (VIPomas, glucagonomas, Zollinger–Ellison syndrome) and conditions such as hyperthyroidism and Addison's disease can also cause increased bowel frequency.

ABDOMINAL MASSES

The techniques for palpating the liver, spleen and kidneys are described on pages 483, 484.

HEPATOMEGALY

The causes of enlargement of the liver (Figure 15.16, Revision panel 15.18) are listed and classified according to their clinical presentation.

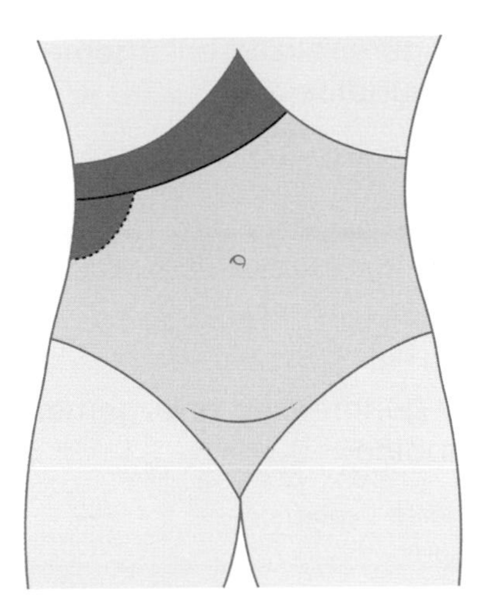

Figure 15.16 Hepatomegaly.

Revision panel 15.18

CAUSES OF HEPATOMEGALY

Infection
Congestion
Bile duct obstruction
Cellular infiltration
Cellular proliferation
Space-occupying lesions

Smooth generalized enlargement, without jaundice

- Congestion from heart failure.
- Cirrhosis.
- Lymphoma.
- Hepatic vein obstruction (Budd–Chiari syndrome).
- Amyloid disease.
- Kala-azar (leishmaniasis).
- Gaucher's disease.

Smooth generalized enlargement, with jaundice

- Infective hepatitis.
- Biliary tract obstruction (gallstones, carcinoma of pancreas, atresia).
- Cholangitis.
- Chronic active hepatitis.

Knobbly generalized enlargement, without jaundice

- Metastatic deposits.
- Cirrhosis.
- Polycystic disease.
- Primary liver carcinoma (hepatocellular and cholangiocarcinoma).

Knobbly generalized enlargement, with jaundice

- Metastatic deposits.
- Cirrhosis.

Localized swellings

- Riedel's lobe.
- Secondary carcinoma.
- Hydatid cyst.
- Liver abscess.
- Primary liver carcinoma.
- Cholangiocarcinoma.
- Benign liver adenoma.

The physical signs of an enlarged liver are as follows:

- It descends below the right costal margin.
- You cannot feel its upper limit.
- It moves with respiration.
- It is dull to percussion up to the level of the 8th rib in the mid-axillary line.
- It may have a sharp or rounded edge with a smooth or irregular surface.

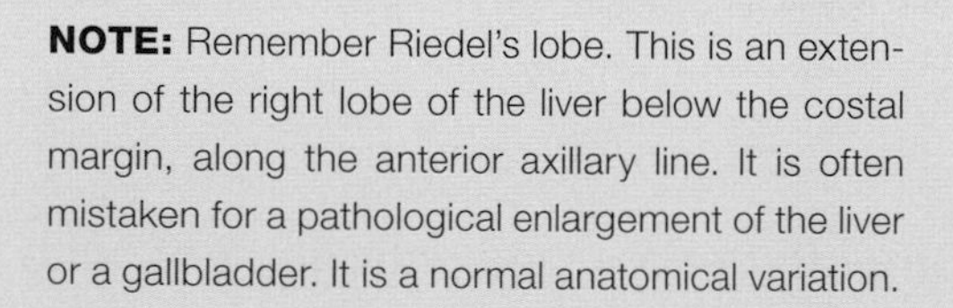

NOTE: Remember Riedel's lobe. This is an extension of the right lobe of the liver below the costal margin, along the anterior axillary line. It is often mistaken for a pathological enlargement of the liver or a gallbladder. It is a normal anatomical variation.

SPLENOMEGALY

The spleen is almost always uniformly enlarged (Figures 15.17–15.19). The causes of splenomegaly

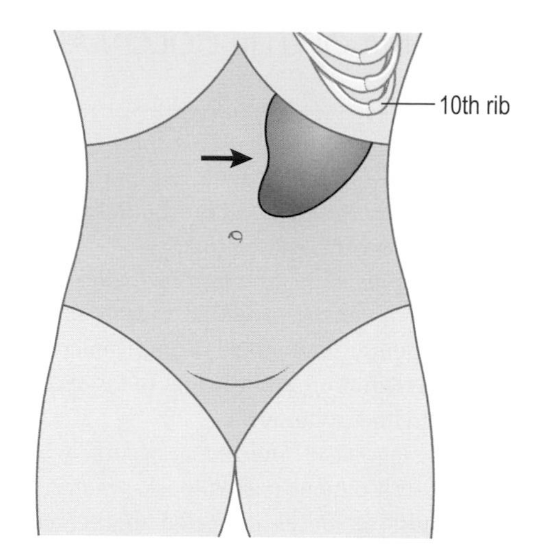

Figure 15.17 Splenomegaly. The notch is not always palpable.

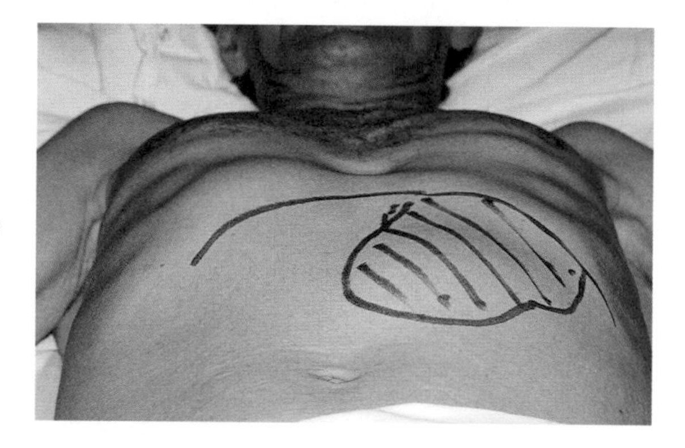

Figure 15.18 Patient with splenomegaly; swelling outlined on the surface with a marker pen.

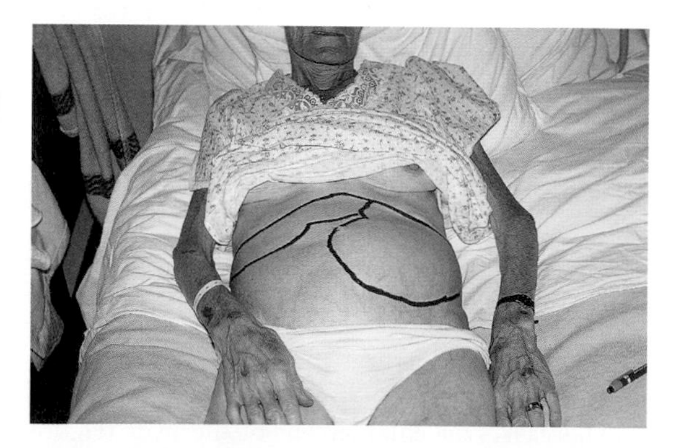

Figure 15.19 Massive hepatosplenomegaly in a patient with lymphoma.

are classified according to the underlying disease (Revision panel 15.19).

Infection

Bacterial

- Typhoid.
- Typhus.
- Tuberculosis.
- Brucellosis.
- General septicaemia.

Viral

- Glandular fever.
- Epstein–Barr virus.

Spirochaetal

- Syphilis.
- Leptospirosis (Weil's disease).

Protozoal

- Malaria.
- Kala-azar (leishmaniasis).
- Schistosomiasis.

Cellular proliferation

- Myeloid and lymphatic leukaemia.
- Lymphomas.
- Pernicious anaemia.
- Polycythaemia rubra vera.
- Spherocytosis and other haemolytic anaemias, for example elliptocytosis, autoimmune haemolytic anaemia and thalassaemia.
- Thrombocytopenic purpura.
- Myelofibrosis.
- Sarcoidosis.

Congestion

- Portal hypertension (cirrhosis, portal vein thrombosis).
- Hepatic vein obstruction.
- Congestive heart failure.

Infarction and injury

- Emboli from bacterial endocarditis.
- Splenic artery or vein thrombosis caused by polycythaemia or sickle-cell disease.
- Haematoma.

Cellular infiltration

- Amyloidosis.
- Gaucher's disease.

Collagen diseases

- Felty's syndrome.
- Still's disease.

Space-occupying lesions

- True solitary cysts.
- Polycystic disease.
- Hydatid cysts.
- Angioma.
- Lymphomas.
- Secondary tumours (very rare).

The physical signs of an enlarged spleen are:

- It appears from below the tip of the left 10th rib and enlarges along the line of the rib towards the umbilicus.
- It is firm, smooth and usually spleen shaped; it often has a definite notch on its upper edge.
- You cannot get above it.
- It moves with respiration.
- It is dull to percussion.
- Although it may be possible to bring it forwards by lifting the left lower ribs forwards, it cannot be felt bimanually or be balloted.

Revision panel 15.19

CAUSES OF SPLENOMEGALY

Infection
Cellular proliferation
Congestion
Infarction
Cellular infiltration
Collagen diseases
Space-occupying lesions

ENLARGEMENT OF THE KIDNEY

One or both kidneys may be enlarged (Figure 15.20, Revision panel 15.20). The common causes of renal enlargement are:

- Hydronephrosis.
- Pyonephrosis.
- Malignant disease: carcinoma of the kidney and nephroblastoma.
- Solitary cysts.
- Polycystic disease.
- Perinephric abscess.

A mobile or low-lying kidney may be easily palpable and seem to be enlarged, especially if the patient is thin.

Hydronephrosis may be bilateral if the obstructing lesion is in or distal to the neck of the bladder.

Nephroblastoma is occasionally bilateral. Polycystic disease is very likely to affect both kidneys.

The physical signs of an enlarged kidney are as follows:

- It lies in the paracolic gutter or can be pushed back into this gutter – that is to say, it can be reduced into the loin.
- It is usually only possible to feel the lower pole, which is smooth and hemiovoid.
- It moves with respiration.
- It is not dull to percussion because it is covered by the colon; even when a large kidney reaches the anterior abdominal wall, it has a band of resonance across it.
- It can be felt bimanually.
- It can be balloted (see page 495).

Revision panel 15.20

CAUSES OF ENLARGEMENT OF THE KIDNEY

Distension of the pelvicalyceal system
Space-occupying lesions:
- Single:
  - Cyst
  - Abscess
  - Tumour
- Multiple:
  - Polycystic disease

Compensatory hypertrophy

PANCREATIC PSEUDOCYSTS

This is a non-epithelialized collection of walled-off pancreatic juice, almost exclusively following pancreatitis (see page 510). They form on the surface of the pancreas and may bulge compressing the stomach.. Patients may develop epigastric fullness, pain, nausea and vomiting. If the cysts become infected, the patient develops severe pain, sweating and rigors.

With pancreatic pseudocysts *the epigastrium contains a firm, sometimes tender, mass with an indistinct lower edge*; the upper limit is rarely palpable (Figure 15.21). These swellings can be very difficult to feel

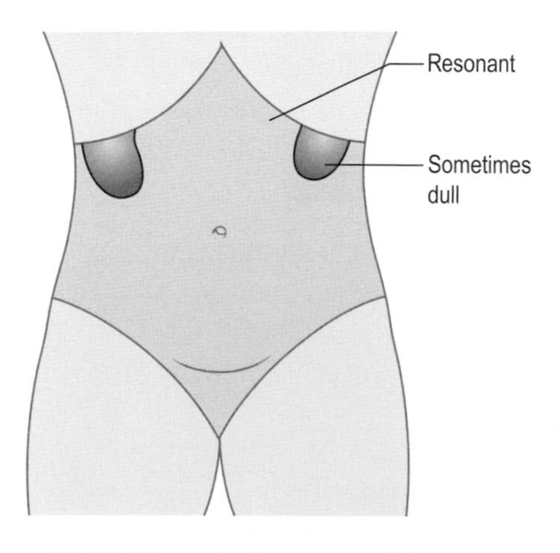

Figure 15.20 Bilateral enlargement of the kidneys.

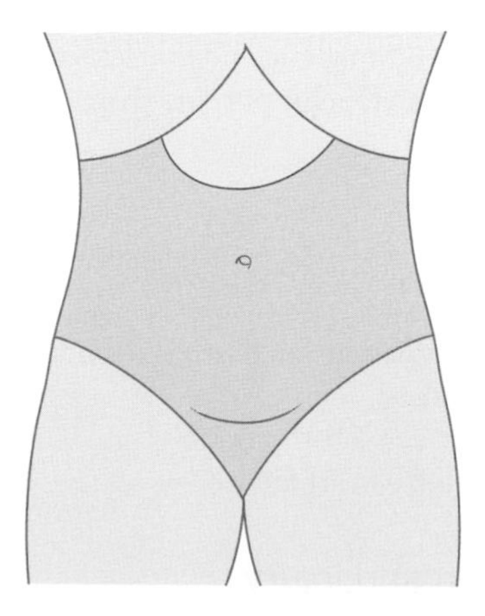

Figure 15.21 A pancreatic, lesser sac, pseudocyst.

as most of their bulk is in the retroperitoneum and beneath the costal margin. They can be complicated by rupture or bleed.

MESENTERIC CYSTS

These are cysts containing clear fluid that develop in the mesentery. They arise from the vestigial remnants of reduplicated bowel and are usually found by chance. They can, rarely, cause abdominal distension or recurrent colicky pain. Like all cysts, they can twist, rupture or bleed.

The physical characteristics of a mesenteric cyst are as follows:

- It forms a smooth, mobile, spherical swelling in the centre of the abdomen (Figure 15.22).
- It moves freely at right angles to the line of the root of the mesentery, but only slightly along a line parallel to the root of the mesentery.
- It is dull to percussion.
- Large cysts may be felt to fluctuate and have a fluid thrill.

NOTE: It can be difficult to discriminate between a very large cyst and tense ascites.

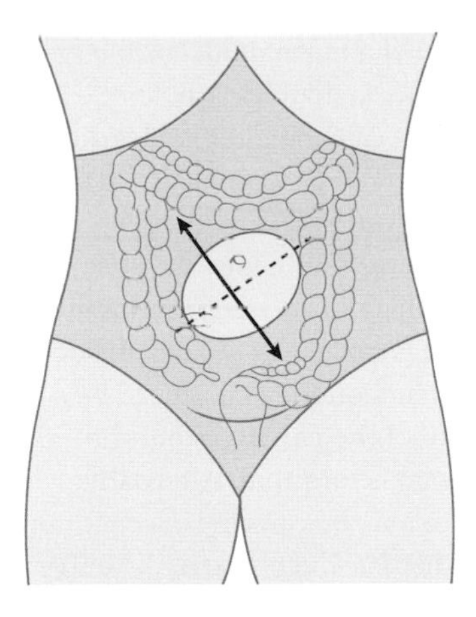

Figure 15.22 A mesenteric cyst.

RETROPERITONEAL TUMOURS

Apart from primary and secondary tumours of the lymph glands, retroperitoneal tumours are rare. The most common variety is the *liposarcoma*. They grow slowly and silently and usually become quite large before they are noticed by the patient or become palpable. The patient complains of distension, a vague abdominal pain and sometimes anorexia and weight loss.

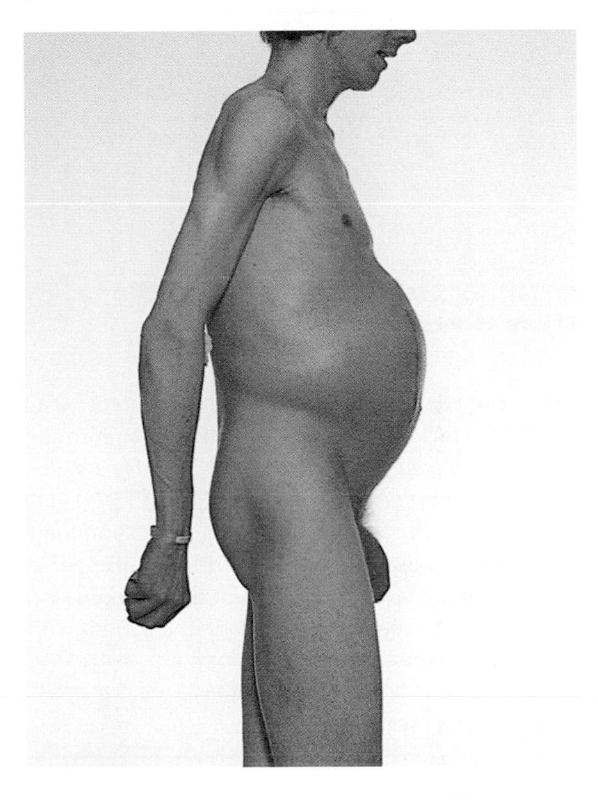

Figure 15.23 Abdominal distension caused by a retroperitoneal liposarcoma in a young male.

They produce the following physical signs:

- Abdominal distension.
- A smooth or bosselated mass with an indistinct edge and a soft to firm consistency.
- Resonance while they are covered with bowel, but when they reach the anterior abdominal wall and push the bowel out to the flanks, they become dull to percussion (Figure 15.23).
- Very little movement with respiration.

CARCINOMA OF THE STOMACH

The symptoms of carcinoma of the stomach are described on page 520. Although stomach cancers

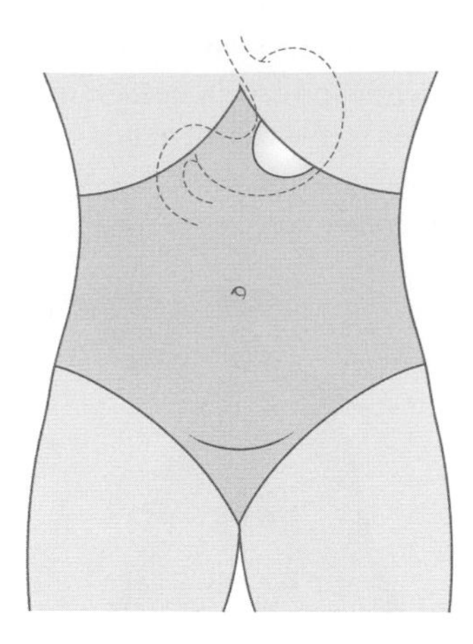

Figure 15.24 Stomach mass.

can become large, hard masses, they are notoriously difficult to feel because they are situated high in the abdomen. A *palpable tumour is hard and irregular, disappearing beneath the costal margin* (Figure 15.24). It is rarely possible to feel its upper edge. The symptoms of abdominal pain or indigestion with loss of appetite and weight are far more significant than the physical signs. Do not expect to feel a mass in a patient with carcinoma of the stomach.

GALLBLADDER

An enlarged gallbladder is usually easy to recognize from its shape and position (Figure 15.25).

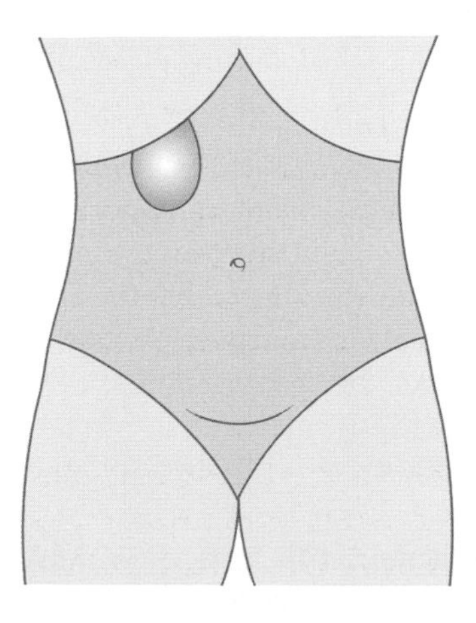

Figure 15.25 An enlarged gallbladder.

The causes of enlargement of the gallbladder are:

- *Obstruction of the cystic duct,* usually by a gallstone, and rarely by an intrinsic or extrinsic carcinoma – the patient is not jaundiced and the gallbladder often contains bile, mucus (a mucocele) or pus (an empyema). Patients are often overweight so a gallbladder can be difficult to palpate.
- *Obstruction of the common bile duct,* usually by a stone or a carcinoma of the head of the pancreas – the patient will be jaundiced.

NOTE: *Courvoisier's law* states that when the gallbladder is palpable but non-tender and the patient is jaundiced, the cause is unlikely to be gallstones because previous attacks of inflammation result in a thick-walled, fibrotic and non-distensible gallbladder.

This is a useful clinical rule but there are a number of exceptions:

- Stones that form in the bile duct rather than in the gallbladder may obstruct the duct in the presence of a normal distensible gallbladder.
- There may be double pathology – a stone in the cystic duct causing gallbladder distension, and a carcinoma or a stone blocking the lower end of the bile duct.
- The converse of the law, jaundice without a palpable gallbladder, does not mean that jaundice is caused by stones. In such cases, the obstruction may be caused by a cancer of the head of the pancreas, but the gallbladder distension is minimal. Alternatively, the jaundice may be caused by a carcinoma of the bile or hepatic ducts above the entry of the cystic duct into the bile duct.
- *Mirizzi's syndrome*: when the cystic duct is closely applied to the common hepatic duct or is very short, a stone impacted in it can inflame and obstruct the bile duct and cause jaundice. The gallbladder is often distended.

The physical features of an enlarged gallbladder are as follows:

- It appears from beneath the tip of the right 9th rib.
- It is smooth and hemiovoid.
- It moves with respiration.
- There is no space between the lump and the edge of the liver.
- It is dull to percussion.

When an acutely inflamed gallbladder becomes surrounded by adherent omentum and bowel, it loses some of its characteristics. A gallbladder mass is diffuse and tender, lies in the right hypochondrium and does not move much with respiration. As the infection subsides, it becomes more discrete and mobile, and less tender.

FAECES

The colon can become grossly distended with faeces as a result of a mechanical obstruction or chronic constipation. The patient may complain of diarrhoea, but this is actually mucus and a little watery faeces leaking out around the main mass of faeces (spurious diarrhoea).

The physical characteristics of faeces are as follows:

- The masses lie in that part of the abdomen occupied by the colon – the flanks and across the lower part of the epigastrium (Figure 15.26).
- They feel firm or hard but are *indentable*. This means that they can be dented by firm pressure with the fingers, and this dent persists after releasing the pressure.
- There may be multiple separate masses in the line of the colon, but in gross cases the faeces coalesce to form one vast mass that is easy to mistake for a tumour.
- When there is no mechanical obstruction, *rectal examination confirms a rectum full of very hard faeces*, but if there is a blockage in the lower colon, the rectum will be empty.

NOTE: Do not forget that faecal masses can form above an annular stenosing carcinoma of the colon.

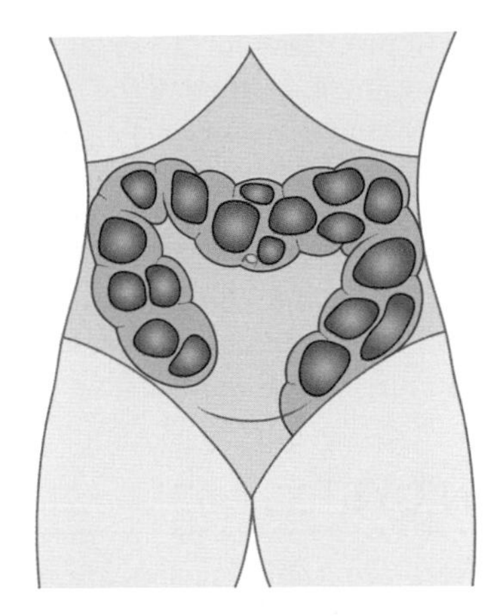

Figure 15.26 A colon distended with faeces. The masses are indentable. Faecal impaction of this degree is likely to be caused by Hirschsprung's disease or gross constipation.

URINARY BLADDER

The causes of retention of urine are listed in Revision panel 17.4, page 582. The bladder may be tense and painful (acute retention) or enlarged and painless (chronic retention) (see Figure 17.3).

The physical features of an enlarged bladder are the following:

- It arises out of the pelvis so has no lower edge (Figure 15.27).
- It is hemiovoid in shape, usually deviated a little to one side.
- It may vary in size: a very large bladder can extend up to and above the umbilicus.
- It is not mobile.

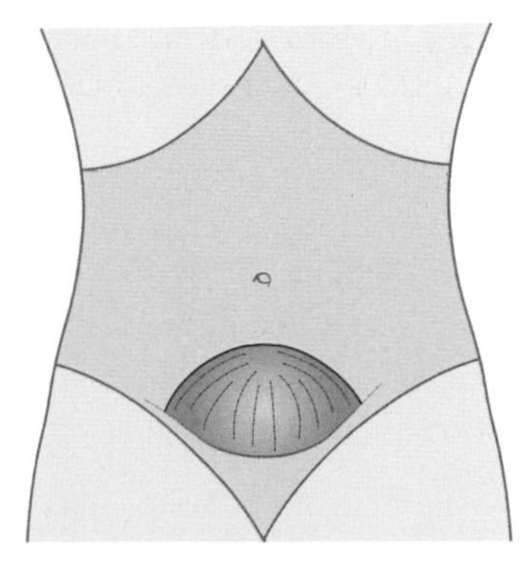

Figure 15.27 A distended urinary bladder.

- It is dull to percussion.
- If it is large enough to permit the necessary simultaneous percussion and palpation, it will have a fluid thrill.
- Direct pressure on the swelling often produces a desire to micturate.
- It does not bulge into the pelvis and can only be felt indistinctly on bimanual (combined rectal and abdominal) examination.

OVARIAN CYST

Small cysts are common and are impalpable. When they enlarge, they rise up out of the pelvis into the lower abdomen and become palpable.

The physical features of a large ovarian cyst are as follows:

- It is smooth and spherical with a distinct outline.
- It arises from the pelvis, so its lower limit is not palpable; i.e. you cannot 'get below it' (Figure 15.28).
- It may be mobile from side-to-side but cannot be moved up and down.
- It is dull to percussion.
- It has a fluid thrill.

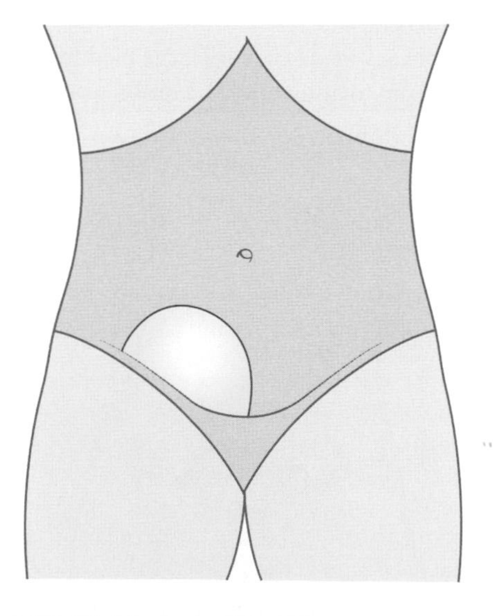

Figure 15.28 A large ovarian cyst.

- Its lower extremity may be palpable in the pelvis during rectal or vaginal examination, and movement of the cyst may produce some movement of the uterus.

PREGNANT UTERUS

Never forget that pregnancy is the most common cause of enlargement of the uterus, and of abdominal distension.

The diagnosis of pregnancy is more difficult in the first 20 weeks, when the uterus is still relatively small and there are no fetal movements.

A pregnant uterus is a smooth, firm, dull swelling arising out of the pelvis. The uterus enlarges to the xiphisternum by the 36th week of pregnancy. At this stage, the fetus is palpable (ballotable) and moves.

The diagnosis of pregnancy is confirmed if bimanual examination reveals that the mass cannot be moved independently of the cervix and that the cervix is soft and patulous.

> **NOTE:** An enlarged uterus must not be squeezed during a bimanual examination, as this can theoretically cause the patient to go into labour and abort the fetus.

FIBROIDS

These are benign fibromyomatous uterine tumours that can grow to an enormous size and fill the whole abdomen. They are usually multiple. They can cause irregular and heavy periods, disturbed micturition, lower abdominal pain and backache.

The physical signs of a fibroid uterus are the following:

- It arises out of the pelvis, so its lower edge is not palpable (Figure 15.29).
- It is firm or hard, bosselated or distinctly knobbly, each knob corresponding to a fibroid.
- It moves slightly in a transverse direction, and any movement of the abdominal mass moves the cervix.
- It is dull to percussion.
- It is palpable bimanually: a moderately enlarged uterus can be pushed down into the pelvis.

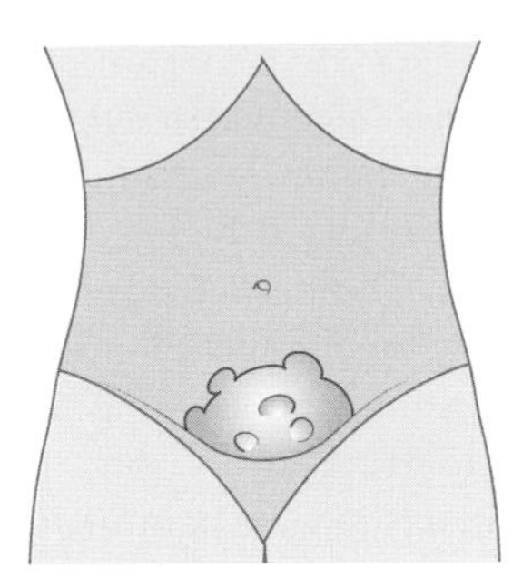

Figure 15.29 A large fibroid uterus.

A MASS IN THE RIGHT ILIAC FOSSA

A mass in the right iliac fossa is a common physical finding (Figures 15.30 and 15.15, Revision panel 15.21). There are a number of conditions that may be responsible. This section describes the important features in the history and examination of each cause.

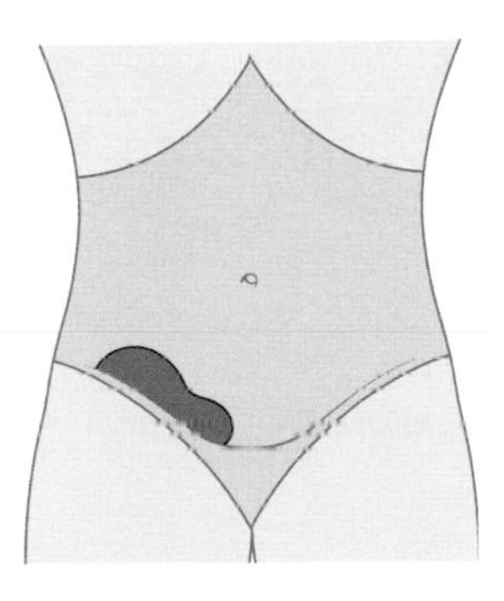

Figure 15.30 A common diagnostic problem: a mass in the right iliac fossa.

Revision panel 15.21

CAUSES OF A MASS IN THE RIGHT ILIAC FOSSA

- Appendix mass
- Appendix abscess
- Carcinoma of the caecum
- Crohn's disease (terminal ileitis)
- Iliac lymphadenopathy
- Iliac artery aneurysm
- Psoas abscess
- Chondrosarcoma or osteosarcoma of the ileum
- Tuberculosis
- Actinomycosis
- Spigelian hernia
- Ruptured epigastric artery
- Kidney transplant
- Ovarian cyst/tumour
- Fibroid
- Malignant change in an undescended testis

APPENDIX MASS

History

The patient usually complains of *a period of central abdominal pain followed by a pain in the right iliac fossa*. The pain often persists for several days, and is usually accompanied by malaise, loss of appetite and pyrexia.

Examination

There is a *tender, indistinct mass,* which is dull to percussion, *fixed to the iliac fossa posteriorly* and accompanied by a persistent low fever and tachycardia. An appendix mass must be differentiated from carcinoma of the caecum.

APPENDIX ABSCESS

History

This is the same as for an appendix mass, with the additional symptoms of an abscess, namely, *fever, rigors, sweating and increased local pain.*

Examination

There is a *tender mass* that, in its late stages, may be associated with oedema and reddening of the overlying skin. The patient will have a swinging, intermittent fever and an increasing tachycardia.

CARCINOMA OF THE CAECUM

History

Often there is no acute pain, just a dull discomfort in the right iliac fossa. Some patients present with anaemia, diarrhoea or intestinal obstruction.

Examination

The *mass is firm, distinct and hard*. It is usually fixed to the posterior abdominal wall, but is sometimes mobile. It is not tender and does not resolve with observation. The patient's temperature and pulse are normal unless there is an associated pericolic abscess.

CROHN'S DISEASE (TERMINAL ILEITIS)

History

The patient will have experienced recurrent episodes of pain in the right iliac fossa, general malaise, weight loss and episodes of diarrhoea.

Examination

The swollen terminal ileum forms an *elongated sausage-shaped mass* that usually lies transversely in the right iliac fossa and feels rubbery and tender.

ILIAC LYMPH GLANDS

History

The symptoms depend on the cause of the lymphadenopathy. There may be a generalized disease, or local disease in the limb, perineum or genitalia.

Examination

Enlarged iliac lymph glands form an *indistinct mass with no clear contours*. The mass follows the line of the iliac vessels and may bulge forwards just above the inguinal ligament. It can be easy to feel, or be no more than a fullness in the depths of the iliac fossa.

All the other lymph glands must be examined, as must the lower limb, to try to find the cause of the lymphadenopathy.

ILIAC ARTERY ANEURYSM

History

The patient may have noticed a pulsating mass or felt an aching pain in the right iliac fossa.

Examination

The common iliac artery dilates more often than the external iliac artery, so the smooth, distinct mass with an *expansile pulsation* is usually in the upper medial corner of the iliac fossa.

PSOAS ABSCESS

History

The patient is likely to have felt ill for some months, with night sweats and loss of weight. Back pain and abdominal pain can also occur.

Examination

The iliac fossa is filled with a *soft, tender, dull, compressible mass*. There may be a fullness in the lumbar region that is accentuated by pressing on the mass in the iliac fossa. The *swelling may extend below the groin*, and it may be possible to empty the swelling below the groin into the swelling above, and vice versa (Figures 15.31).

Back movements may be painful and limited.

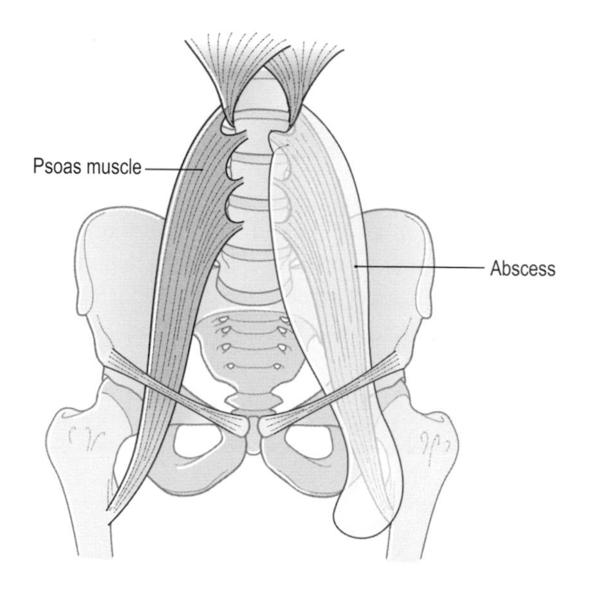

Figure 15.31 Psoas abscess.

CHONDROMA AND SARCOMA OF THE ILIUM

Rarely, chondromas and chondrosarcomas arise in the iliac bones. They grow slowly and may bulge into the iliac fossa. They are *large, hard, non-tender* and *clearly fixed to the skeleton*. They usually lie in the lateral part of the iliac fossa. Osteomas and osteosarcomas of the ilium are rare.

TUBERCULOSIS

In many parts of the world, tuberculosis is more often the cause of an inflammatory mass in the right iliac fossa than is appendicitis. The mass consists of the *inflamed ileocaecal lymph glands* and parts of the caecum and terminal ileum that are also inflamed.

History

The patient has often had a vague central pain for months, with general ill-health, loss of weight and changes in bowel habit. The pain then becomes intense and settles in the iliac fossa. An acute episode of central abdominal pain moving to the right iliac fossa, similar to appendicitis, is uncommon.

Examination

The mass is *firm, tender and very indistinct.* The surface and the edge are difficult to define. If there is a tuberculous peritonitis, the abdomen will be swollen and less pliable – often described as a 'doughy' abdomen.

ACTINOMYCOSIS

This invariably develops as a complication of appendicitis, but may present *de novo* as a mass in the iliac fossa with a *number of discharging sinuses* that produce characteristic 'sulphur granules'. It is a rare condition.

SPIGELIAN HERNIA

These hernias appear at the outer edge of the rectus abdominis muscle along the linea semilunaris. *The lump is still palpable when the abdominal wall muscles are contracted,* and it is felt to lie above them (see Chapter 14).

RUPTURED INFERIOR EPIGASTRIC ARTERY

This occurs as a result of straining or coughing. The haematoma tracks beneath the abdominal wall, extraperitoneally, to produce a mass in the iliac fossa. It is diffuse, and there may be *discolouration* of the skin. It is attached to the anterior abdominal wall but, as it is on its deep surface, it becomes impalpable when the muscles contract. Contraction of the abdominal muscles is usually painful (see Chapter 14).

TRANSPLANTED KIDNEY

The mass is situated beneath the transplant scar and a history of transplantation makes the diagnosis easy. The lump is smooth, kidney shaped and rubbery.

OVARIAN CYSTS AND FIBROIDS

These can fall to the right into the right iliac fossa. They will be felt to be *connected to the uterus on bimanual examination*. A huge pyosalpinx may occasionally be palpable in the right iliac fossa.

MALIGNANT CHANGE IN AN UNDESCENDED TESTIS

NOTE: This is a rarity but is easily suspected provided you remember always to examine the scrotum as part of the abdominal examination (see Chapter 18, page 611).

A MASS IN THE LEFT ILIAC FOSSA

Diverticulitis and carcinoma of the colon are the common causes of a mass in the left iliac fossa. It must be remembered that the normal sigmoid colon is palpable in one out of three patients. An appendix mass on the left side only occurs if the patient has situs inversus.

Tuberculosis and Crohn's disease only cause masses in the right iliac fossa. All the other causes of a mass in the right iliac fossa mentioned above can also cause a mass in the left iliac fossa (Revision panel 15.22).

DIVERTICULITIS

When sigmoid diverticula become inflamed, the swollen colon and surrounding pericolic abscess may be palpable.

History

The patient may have suffered from *recurrent lower abdominal pains* and chronic constipation for years. The acute episode starts suddenly with a severe left iliac fossa pain, nausea, loss of appetite and constipation.

Examination

The left iliac fossa contains a *tender, indistinct mass* whose long axis lies parallel to the inguinal ligament. There may be signs of general or local peritonitis and intestinal obstruction. The diagnosis depends upon the site of the tenderness. There are very few other

Revision panel 15.22

CAUSES OF A MASS IN THE LEFT ILIAC FOSSA

- Diverticulitis
- Carcinoma of the left or sigmoid colon
- Crohn's disease
- Iliac lymphadenopathy
- Iliac artery aneurysm
- Psoas abscess
- Chondrosarcoma or osteosarcoma of the ileum
- Actinomycosis
- Ruptured epigastric artery
- Spigelian hernia
- Kidney transplant
- Ovarian cyst/tumour
- Fibroid
- Malignant change in an undescended testis

acute inflammatory conditions that present with a mass in the left iliac fossa.

CARCINOMA OF THE SIGMOID COLON

History

The patient may present with:

- Lower abdominal pain.
- Abdominal colic.
- Intestinal obstruction.
- Change in bowel habit.
- Rectal bleeding.
- General cachexia.

Examination

The mass is hard, *easily palpable and not tender*. It may be mobile or fixed. The colon above the mass may be distended with indentable faeces. The tumour can perforate locally and cause a 'pericolic' abscess similar to that of diverticular disease.

A LUMP IN THE GROIN

The inguinal region is part of the iliac fossa and swellings within it and just below it in the groin can be confused with iliac fossa masses (see Revision panels 15.22, 15.23). The diagnosis is made from the site and shape of the lump and, if present, its reducibility and an expansile cough impulse.

Revision panel 15.23

CAUSES OF A MASS IN THE GROIN

Hernia (inguinal or femoral)
Lymph glands
Saphena varix (see Figure 10.31, page 358)
Psoas abscess
Psoas bursa
Femoral aneurysm
Hydrocele of a femoral hernial sac
Hydrocele of the cord or canal of Nuck
 (see pages 478–479)
Ectopic testis (see page 602)

ABDOMINAL DISTENSION

The causes of abdominal distension can be remembered by repeating the letter 'F' six times: fetus, flatus, faeces, fat, fluid (free and encysted) and fibroids; and other solid tumours (Revision panel 15.24).

Revision panel 15.24

CAUSES OF ABDOMINAL DISTENSION

Fetus
Flatus
Faeces
Fat
Fluid:
 Free (ascites)
 Encysted
Large solid tumours such as:
 Fibroids
 Enlarged liver
 Enlarged spleen
 Polycystic kidneys
 Retroperitoneal sarcomas

FETUS

Pregnancy is the most common cause of abdominal distension. The features of a pregnant uterus have already been described on page 540.

FLATUS (TYMPANITES)

Gas in the intestine can cause considerable abdominal distension.

In the early stages, the distension may be localized to that part of the abdomen containing the distended bowel, such as the epigastrium when the stomach is distended, or the right iliac fossa when the caecum is distended, but as the distension affects the whole bowel, the whole abdomen swells.

The distension remains localized if the bowel twists into a *volvulus*. This is a common complication of a long sigmoid colon combined with a narrow base of the mesocolon.

Distended bowel has no palpable surface or edge. The only diagnostic features are hyper-resonance and, when there is obstruction, visible peristalsis. The bowel sounds may be hyperactive. Shaking the patient causes a splashing sound as the thin layer of fluid in the distended bowel splashes about. This is known as a *succussion splash* and is particularly common when there is gastric distension caused by pyloric stenosis.

Acute dilatation of the stomach, mechanical intestinal obstruction, paralytic ileus, aerophagy (air swallowing) and massive amounts of free gas from a perforation all cause hyper-resonance on abdominal percussion.

FAECES

Faecal impaction may present as abdominal distension or an abdominal mass. The physical features of faecal masses in the abdomen are described on page 539. The diagnosis can usually be suspected from a history of the patient's bowel habits. The common causes are Hirschsprung's disease, chronic intestinal obstruction, chronic constipation and antidepressant drugs.

FAT

Fat rarely causes distension, but frequently makes the patient pot-bellied. A large fat abdomen may be caused by a thick layer of subcutaneous fat or by excess fat in the omentum and mesentery. These two sites of fat deposition do not necessarily enlarge together. A protuberant, round abdomen often has a thin layer of subcutaneous fat but contains a heavy, thick omentum.

FLUID: ASCITES

Free fluid in the peritoneal cavity is called ascites. It is caused by a variety of conditions, but they all fall into one of four groups: those that raise the portal venous pressure, those that lower the plasma proteins, those that cause peritonitis and those that allow a direct leak of lymph into the peritoneal cavity (Revision panel 15.25).

Revision panel 15.25

AETIOLOGY OF ASCITES

Raised portal venous pressure

Prehepatic, intrahepatic and posthepatic
Cardiac
Pulmonary

Hypoproteinaemia

Renal
Hepatic
General

Peritonitis

Acute and chronic
Traumatic, chemical, infective, neoplastic

Lymphatic obstruction (chylous ascites)

Causes of an increased portal venous pressure

Prehepatic

- Portal vein thrombosis.
- Compression of the portal vein by lymph glands.

Hepatic

- Cirrhosis.

Posthepatic

- Budd–Chiari syndrome.

Cardiac

- Constrictive pericarditis.
- Right heart failure caused by mitral stenosis, tricuspid incompetence and pulmonary hypertension.

Pulmonary

- Pulmonary hypertension and right heart failure.

Causes of hypoproteinaemia

- Kidney disease associated with albuminuria.
- Cirrhosis of the liver.
- The cachexia of wasting diseases, malignancy and starvation.
- Protein-losing enteropathies.
- Malnutrition.

Causes of chronic peritonitis

Physical

- Postirradiation
- Starch granuloma.

Infection

- Tuberculous peritonitis.

Neoplasms

- Secondary peritoneal deposits of carcinoma.
- 'Mucus'-forming tumours (pseudomyxoma peritonei).

Causes of chylous ascites

This is caused by the leakage of lymph from the lacteals or the cisterna chyli as a result of congenital abnormalities, trauma and primary or secondary lymph gland disease.

Physical signs of ascites

- A fluid thrill.
- Shifting dullness.

A *fluid thrill* is elicited by flicking one side of the abdomen with the index or middle finger, and feeling the vibrations when they reach the other side of the abdomen with your other hand. Before doing this, you must place the edge of the patient's (or an assistant's) hand on the abdomen at the umbilicus to prevent the percussion wave being transmitted through the fat in the abdominal wall. A fluid thrill is present in any fluid-filled cavity, so that the difference between free and encysted fluid depends on the recognition of shifting dullness.

Shifting dullness is a dull area that moves or changes shape when the patient changes position. The dullness of ascites is found in the flanks and across the lower abdomen. Percuss the medial limits of the flank dullness carefully, and place vertical marks on the abdomen with a marker pen. Then ask the patient to turn onto one side to an angle of approximately 45°. Wait a few seconds and percuss again. If there is free fluid moving under the influence of gravity, the medial limits of dullness will have moved towards the midline on the lower side of the abdomen and away from it on the upper side.

FLUID: ENCYSTED

Fluid trapped in a cyst, in the renal pelvis or between adhesions has a fluid thrill, is dull to percussion, but does not shift.

The position and features of a cyst depend on its anatomical origin. The following cysts or fluid-filled swellings may become large enough to present as abdominal distension:

- Ovarian cysts.
- Hydronephrosis.
- Urinary bladder.
- Pancreatic pseudocysts.
- Mesenteric cysts.
- Hydatid cysts.

A large aortic aneurysm can also distend the abdomen. It is distinguished by the presence of an expansile pulsation.

FIBROIDS AND OTHER SOLID TUMOURS

Solid tumours that can become very large and cause abdominal distension are, in approximate order of frequency:

- Hepatomegaly (Budd–Chiari syndrome or metastatic liver tumours).
- Fibroids.
- Splenomegaly (myelofibrosis).
- Large cancers of the colon.
- Polycystic kidneys.
- Primary carcinoma of the liver.
- Retroperitoneal sarcoma and lymphadenopathy.
- Neuroblastoma/ganglioneuroblastoma/ganglioneuroma (in children).
- Nephroblastoma (in children).
- Neurofibroma/schwannoma.

The physical signs of most of these tumours are described in the preceding parts of this chapter.

16 The rectum and anal canal

MARK GEORGE

Applied anatomy

The rectum has a continuous layer of longitudinal muscle outside the inner circular muscle, unlike the sigmoid colon where the longitudinal muscle is in three bands, the taeniae. The anorectal junction forms a right angle, held in this position by the *puborectalis muscle*.

At the anus, the gut joins the skin. The anus is lined by squamous epithelium, while the rectum is lined by columnar epithelium. The location where the epithelium changes is known as the *mucocutaneous junction* and is visible as a wavy white line in the lower third of the anal canal (sometimes called *Hilton's white line or dentate line*); above this junction is the rectum. The rectum has the following features:

- It has autonomic sensation and is sensitive only to stretching.
- It receives its arterial blood supply from the mesenteric vessels.
- It drains venous blood into the portal circulation.
- It drains lymph into the mesocolic and eventually into the preaortic lymph nodes.

Below the mucocutaneous junction is anal skin, which has the following features:

- It has somatic sensation and is as sensitive as skin.
- It receives its arterial blood supply from the iliac vessels.
- It drains venous blood into the iliac veins.
- It drains lymph into the inguinal lymph glands.

This differentiation explains the way in which cancers spread and the genesis of many symptoms.

Symptoms of anorectal disease

Embarrassment often inhibits patients from describing their 'anorectal' symptoms in precise detail although, as ever, the history is often crucial in making the correct diagnosis. The principal symptoms include bleeding, pain, pruritus, incontinence, prolapse, tenesmus and a change of bowel habit, mentioned in Chapter 1, but now discussed in detail.

BLEEDING

Blood passed per rectum may be *fresh* or *altered*. When blood is degraded by intestinal enzymes and bacteria, it becomes black and acquires a characteristic smell. Such a black, tarry stool is called *melaena* (see Chapter 15). To have time to turn black before it reaches the rectum, the blood has usually come from the stomach or duodenum.

Recognizable blood may appear in four ways:

- Mixed in with the faeces.
- On the surface of the faeces.
- Separate from the faeces, either after or unrelated to defaecation.
- On the toilet paper after wiping.

Blood mixed with the faeces or on the surface of the faeces

These are difficult to differentiate. Blood 'mixed in' with the faeces should theoretically have come from above the sigmoid colon to give sufficient time for mixing, while blood 'on' the faeces has usually come from the rectum or anal canal.

Blood separate from the faeces

An anal condition such as haemorrhoids is usually responsible for bleeding following defaecation.

When blood is passed by itself, it has accumulated rapidly, causing a strong desire to defaecate. Causes include *diverticular disease* and *angiodysplasia*.

NOTE: Bleeding from the upper gastrointestinal tract is occasionally sufficiently rapid to be passed as recognizable blood and not melaena, but usually the brighter red the blood is, the lower down is its source.

Blood on the toilet paper

This is usually the result of minor bleeding from conditions *close to the anal margin,* such as haemorrhoids or a fissure.

PAIN

Pain from the anal canal is felt principally on defaecation and is often protracted, cramp-like and distressing. There may be a background ache. Excessive stretching of the anal canal may cause a sharp, splitting pain, sometimes described as if something is tearing. This is true if the patient has a fissure!

Uncomplicated haemorrhoids and rectal cancer (see below) are not usually painful, while fissures, abscesses and perianal haematomas generally are.

PRURITUS

Perianal itching is a common symptom and may be accompanied by a burning discomfort, which can be severe if the enzyme-rich small bowel contents make prolonged contact with the perianal skin. Itching occurs in those perianal conditions that produce leakage of mucus, liquid faeces or purulent discharge onto the perianal skin, but may also be caused by a primary skin disease.

NOTE: In children, the most common cause is a worm infestation.

The symptom is frequently worse at night, perhaps because there are no other sensory distractions.

INCONTINENCE AND SOILING

Incontinence may be caused by:

- Sphincter failure.
- Impaction with overflow.
- Extreme urgency.
- Neurological impairment.

A fistula connecting the small bowel or colon with the vagina will cause leakage of either small bowel content or stool. The symptom may be concealed by an embarrassed patient. The nature of the leakage should be recorded as *gas, liquid* or *solid.*

The amount of leakage and the frequency of its occurrence must be ascertained. Questions on 'staining on the underclothes', the need for pads and the passage of a full bowel motion will reveal the extent of the problem. It is important to establish whether the patient has an awareness of the need to 'open the bowels'.

A defective external anal sphincter (voluntary muscle) is associated with a feeling of urgency with inability to retain the stool, while internal anal sphincter dysfunction (of smooth muscle, which is autonomically innervated) is associated with the unconscious passage of small amounts of stool between bowel actions.

DIFFICULTY IN DEFECATION

This should be differentiated from the infrequent passage of hard stool. Here, the patient strains to pass stool and may utilize a variety of body positions or local finger pressure around or in the anal canal to aid defaecation.

PROLAPSE

The patient may notice *something 'coming down'* from either the vagina or the rectum. This may occur sporadically with a bowel action or during walking or standing. Faecal and urinary incontinence commonly coexist.

TENESMUS

This is defined as *a constant intense desire to defaecate*. When the patient tries to evacuate the rectum, either nothing or just a small amount of mucus and loose faeces appears. Tenesmus should always be taken seriously as it may indicate a space-occupying lesion mimicking the presence of faeces, often a carcinoma of the rectum. It can, however, be caused by benign conditions including inflammatory bowel disease and even irritable bowel syndrome.

CHANGE IN BOWEL HABIT

NOTE: Beware of the terms 'diarrhoea' and 'constipation'. When patients use the word constipation, some mean that their bowels are opening less frequently than usual, while others feel that their motions are harder. Diarrhoea has a similar double meaning, either frequent defaecation or loose motions.

Make sure that you find out what the patient means. It is better to record the frequency of bowel action and the consistency of the stool than to use these lay terms.

Many patients, particularly the elderly, complain of a change in bowel habit – some of these patients feel that daily defaecation is a basic human right! All individuals with this symptom must be taken seriously as *bowel cancer frequently presents in this way*. A change to a looser stool is generally more worrying than the development of constipation.

Technique for digital ano-rectal examination

This is commonly called a rectal examination but is actually an examination of the anus and lower rectum. The patient should give clear verbal consent.

PREPARATION (FIGURE 16.1)

Position of the patient

Ensure adequate privacy, *have a chaperone*, and uncover the patient from the waist to the middle of the thighs.

The patient should lie in the left lateral position with the neck and shoulders rounded so that the chin rests on the chest, with the hips flexed to 90° or more, and the knees flexed to slightly less than 90°. The patient's ankles will get in your way if the knees are flexed to more than 90°. If the bed is soft, ask the patient to bring their buttocks to its edge. This makes inspection easier and tips its abdominal contents forwards, which helps bimanual examination.

Equipment

You need a *plastic glove*, some inert *lubricating jelly* and a *good light*. Tissues must be available for cleansing afterwards.

Tell the patient what you are going to do. Explain that you are going to feel inside their 'back passage', which will be uncomfortable but not painful. Ask the patient to relax by breathing deeply and letting their knees go loose.

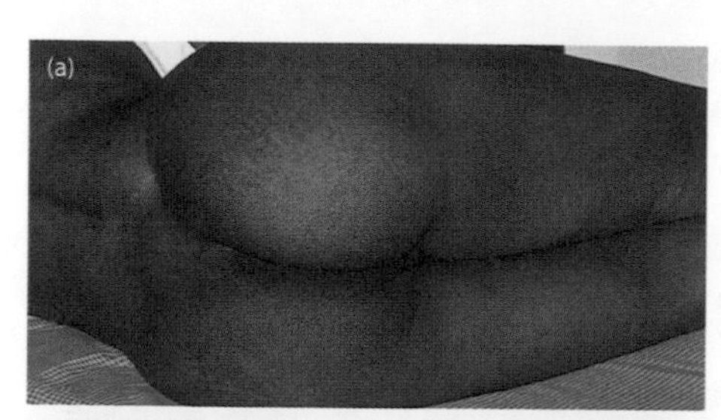

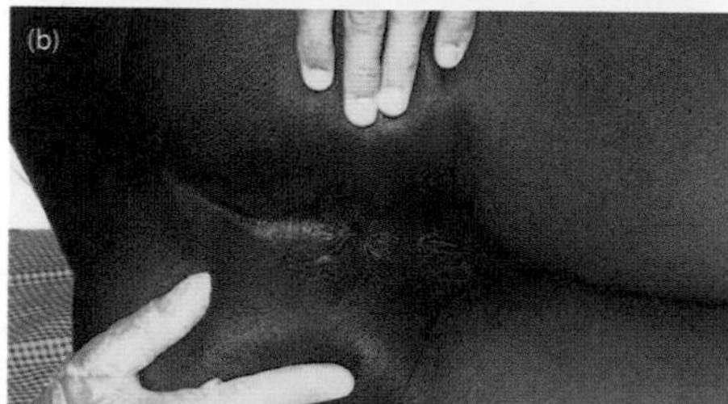

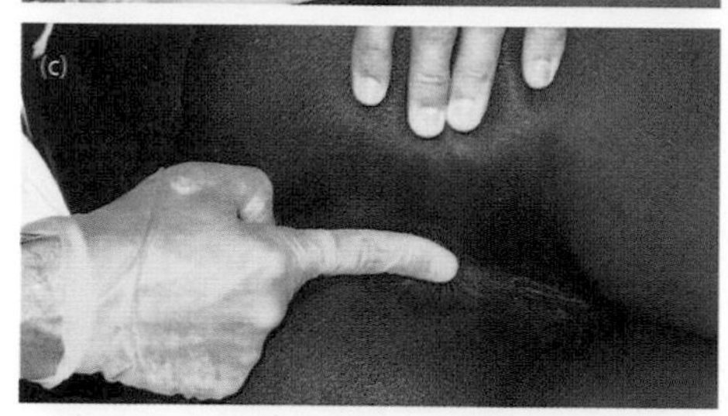

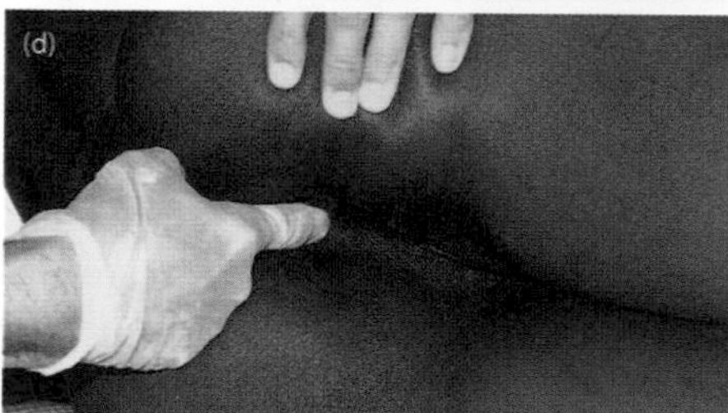

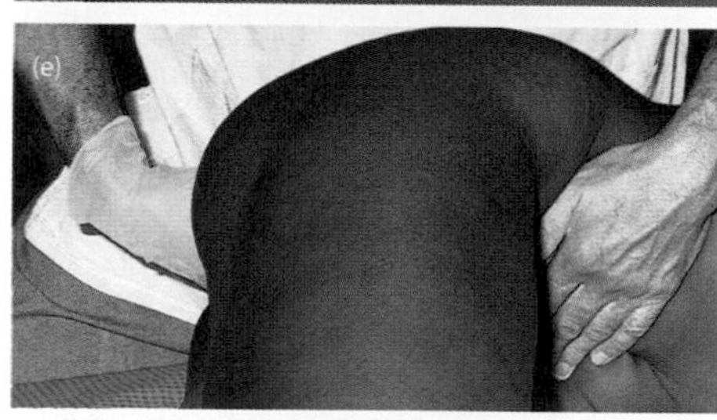

Figure 16.1 THE TECHNIQUE OF ANORECTAL EXAMINATION. (a) Place the patient in the left lateral position, with the hips flexed to 90° and the knees less flexed to 100°. (b) Part the buttocks and inspect the anus and perineum. (c) Place the pulp of your finger on the anus. (d) As you insert your finger, pull backwards to counteract the tone in the puborectalis muscle. (e) After examining the anal canal and rectum, place your hand on the abdomen and examine the contents of the pelvis bimanually.

INSPECTION

Lift the uppermost buttock with your left hand so that you can see clearly the anus, perianal skin and perineum. Look for:

- Skin rashes and excoriation.
- Faecal soiling, blood or mucus.
- Scarring, or the opening of a fistula.
- Lumps and bumps (e.g. polyps, papillomas, condylomas, perianal haematoma, prolapsed piles, rectal prolapse or even a visible carcinoma).
- Ulcers.
- Distortion of the anal canal by an underlying muscular defect.
- Whether the anus appears to gape.
- Whether a fissure is visible on parting the buttocks.

The patient should be asked to cough, which causes the normal anal sphincter to contract. They should then be asked to 'bear down' as if to open their bowels. This tests for prolapse of the bowel wall and for prolapsing piles.

PALPATION

Before carrying out a digital examination, the anus should be inspected, particularly if there is a history of pain on defaecation. This demonstrates whether there is any spasm associated with a fissure, which may be visible.

> **NOTE:** Under no circumstances carry out instrumentation if there is any spasm or a fissure, as this could cause severe pain.

Place the pulp of your gloved right index finger on the centre of the anus, with the finger parallel to the skin of the perineum and in the midline. Press gently into the anal canal but, at the same time, press backwards against the skin of the posterior wall of the anal canal and the underlying sling of the puborectalis muscle. This overcomes most of the tone in the anal sphincter and allows the finger to straighten and slip into the rectum. Never thrust the tip of your finger straight in.

The anal canal

As the finger passes through the anal canal, *note the tone of the sphincter*, any pain or tenderness and any thickening or masses.

> **NOTE:** Patients with fissures or abscesses may have so much spasm that rectal examination is extremely painful. Do not continue in these circumstances. General anaesthetic may be needed for adequate assessment.

The rectum

Feel all around the rectum as high as possible. The mucosa of the anus and rectum should feel smooth, and it is important to elicit the presence of any masses or ulcers. The site of any abnormality should be noted for its level above the anal verge and its position.

If you feel a mass, try to decide if it is:

- Ulcerated or polypoid.
- Within or outside the wall – test the mobility of the mucosa over the mass, which provides a vital distinction.
- Mobile or fixed to other structures, for example the sacrum.

Do not forget to feel the lower rectum, just above the anal canal. Posteriorly, the rectum turns away at a right angle, and it is easy to miss a small abnormality in this area (as it also is at sigmoidoscopy).

Note the contents of the rectum. The rectum may be:

- Full of faeces (hard or soft).
- Empty and collapsed.
- Empty but 'ballooned out'.

Faeces may feel like a tumour but are *indentable*, the only rectal mass that is.

When you can just detect a possible abnormality at your fingertip, ask *the patient to strain* or 'bear down'. This will often move the mass down 1–2 cm or so and bring it within your reach.

The rectovesico/rectouterine pouch

Turn your finger to feel forwards to detect any masses outside the rectum in the peritoneal pouch between the rectum and the bladder or uterus. This is *the pouch of Douglas* (between the rectum and vaginal vault) in the female, and the rectovesical pouch in the male.

Pelvic abscesses are tender and boggy, while malignant pelvic deposits are hard and craggy.

Bimanual examination

Examination of the contents of the pelvis is helped if you feel 'bimanually' between the left hand on the abdomen and the right index finger in the rectum. This gives a much better idea of the size, shape and nature of any pelvic mass. This examination is much more difficult in an obese patient.

The cervix and uterus

These structures are easy to feel per rectum, and on bimanual palpation you should be able to define the shape and size of the uterus and any adnexal masses.

> **NOTE:** A tampon, palpable as a firm mass, can be mistaken for the cervix.

The prostate and seminal vesicles (Figure 16.2)

> **NOTE:** It takes practice to be able to tell the normal prostate and cervix from an abnormal mass, so do not be downhearted if you get it wrong at first.

The normal prostate gland is firm, rubbery, bilobed and 2–3 cm across. Its surface should be smooth, with a shallow central sulcus (median groove), and the rectal mucosa should move freely over it. The *seminal vesicles may occasionally be palpable* just above the upper lateral edges of the gland.

Benign hypertrophy of the prostate produces enlargement of the whole gland, which bulges backwards into the rectum. The central sulcus is palpable

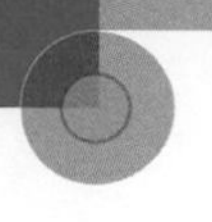

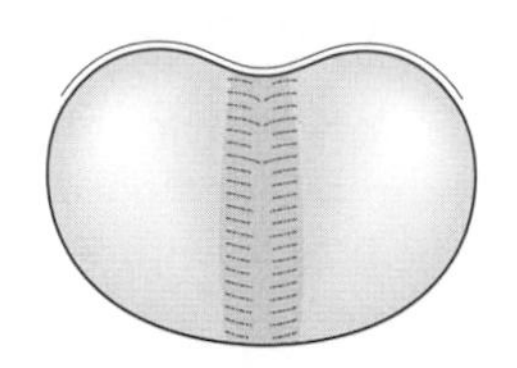

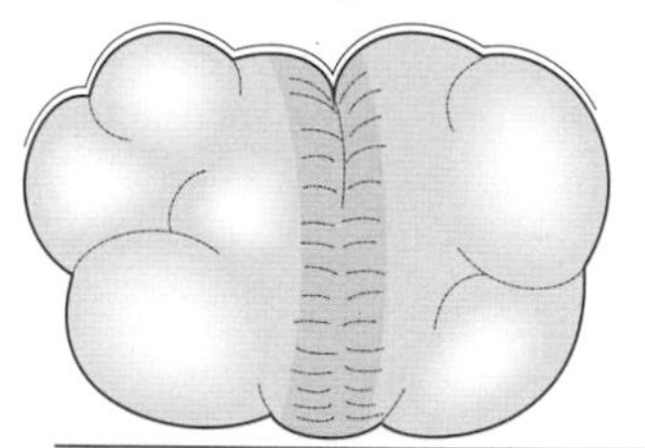

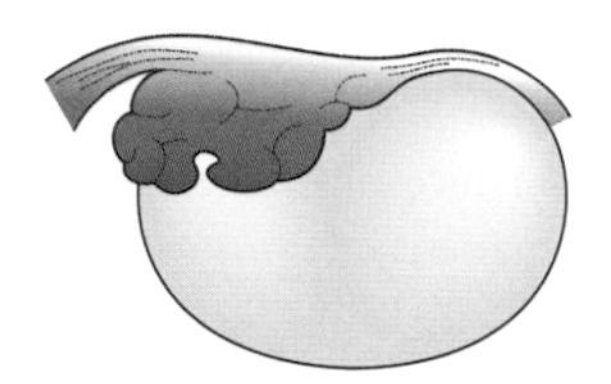

Figure 16.2 The prostate gland.

unless the gland is very large. It may feel lobulated, and the overlying rectal mucosa remains mobile.

Carcinoma of the prostate causes an *irregular, hard enlargement of the gland,* which is often unilateral or *asymmetrical*. The edge of the enlarged area is usually indistinct. Thickening can often be felt either side of the gland and, in advanced cases, can encircle the rectum. The *central sulcus is distorted or obliterated* at an early stage of the disease, and the *rectal mucosa becomes fixed to the underlying gland*.

NOTE: When assessing the prostate, beware of the incompletely emptied bladder, which pushes the prostate downwards and makes it feel bigger than it actually is.

The anal sphincter

The anal sphincter may be assessed for strength at rest and by *asking the patient to squeeze* the examining finger. In females, the vaginal septum is easily felt anteriorly.

The rectal contents

Hard, packed stool is indicative of 'faecal impaction', which often presents with anal discomfort and leakage. An empty ballooned rectum is found in large bowel obstruction.

NOTE: On completion of the examination always inspect the glove for the presence of blood or mucus and note the colour of the faeces.

Sigmoidoscopy and proctoscopy

Sigmoidoscopy and proctoscopy using simple rigid instruments are part of the routine clinical examination of every patient with bowel symptoms.

SIGMOIDOSCOPY

The sigmoidoscope should really be called a rectoscope. It is an illuminated tube, 30 cm in length, that is passed through the anus to inspect the rectum and its lining. It has an obturator with a rounded end to allow introduction, and a sealed lens with a bellows attachment that fits into the end of the tube when the obturator has been removed. Insufflation of air allows the rectal lining to be inspected. *It can usually be passed as far as the rectosigmoid junction* or just beyond. Many patients experience significant discomfort when the sigmoid colon is entered.

Technique of rigid sigmoidoscopy (Figure 16.3)

- No bowel preparation is necessary.
- Position the patient as for a rectal examination, making sure that they are lying as transversely as possible on the couch, with their buttocks at the edge or slightly overhanging. Elderly patients may feel they are going to fall off and need reassurance.
- Explain to the patient what you are going to do. Tell them that they will experience discomfort and a feeling of fullness as air is 'pumped in',

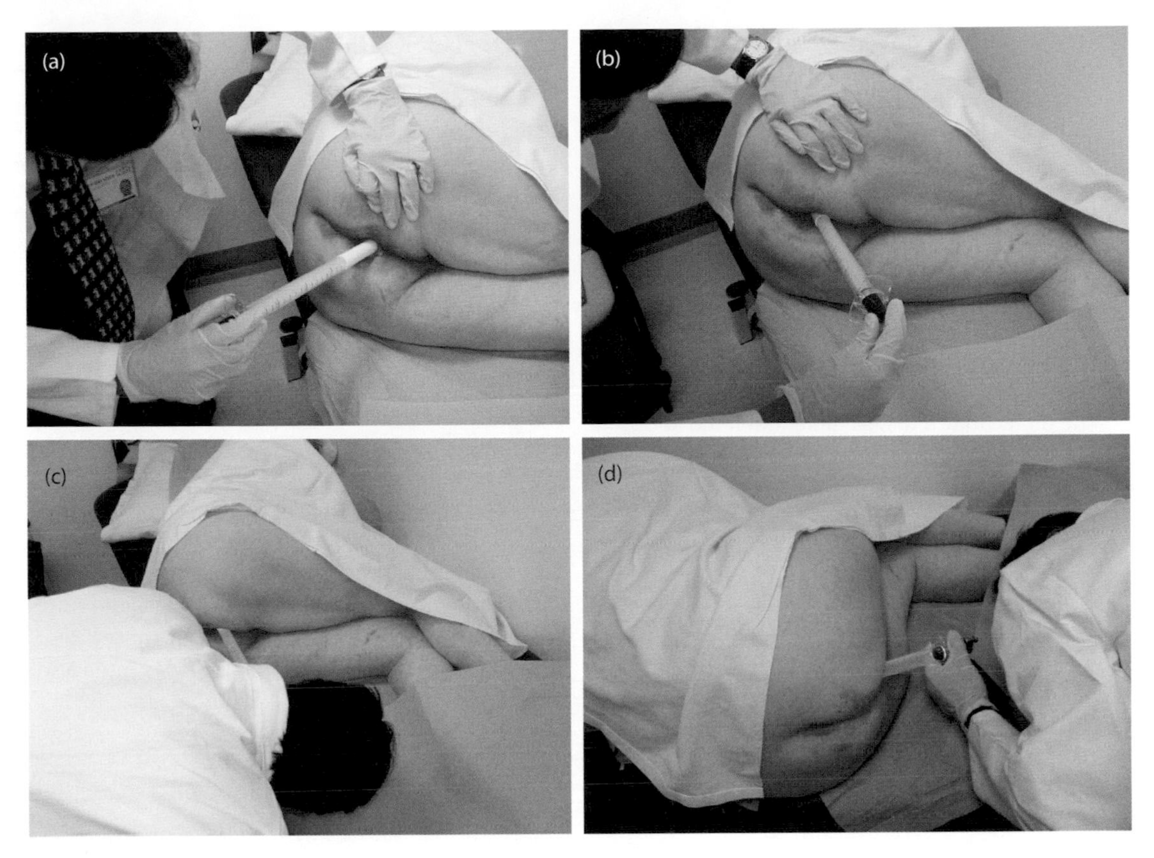

Figure 16.3 SIGMOIDOSCOPY. (a) Position the patient with the body as near transverse as possible, with the legs drawn up and the buttocks at the edge of the couch. Insert the well-lubricated instrument along the axis of the anal canal by aiming it in the direction of the umbilicus. (b) Point the sigmoidoscope backwards to follow the course of the rectum into the sacral hollow. (c) Under direct vision, insufflating air as you go, pass the instrument up the rectosigmoid junction. (d) Carefully inspect the lining of the rectum as you withdraw the instrument.

that you will release this pressure at the end to the examination, and that you will stop at once if there is any pain.

- Check the anus again to make sure there is no fissure or other painful condition.
- *Apply adequate amounts of lubricating jelly to the instrument.*
- Insert the instrument in the direction of the anal canal. This is achieved by pointing it towards the umbilicus.
- Once you have entered the rectum, remove the obturator and attach the light source and bellows. At this point, *change the angle of insertion backwards, to follow the course of the rectum into the sacral hollow.*
- Under direct vision, insufflating enough air to separate the rectal walls, negotiate the instrument to the *rectosigmoid junction*. You will see and work around the three semicircular folds known as *Houston's valves.*
- At the rectosigmoid junction, you will see the rectum narrowing down to the diameter of the colon, which is similar in calibre to the instrument you are using. You will occasionally find a wide-open rectosigmoid junction, which allows you to pass the instrument to its full length without any problem.
- Any gross pathology will be evident as soon as the rectum is entered, but *it is best first to advance the sigmoidoscope to the rectosigmoid*

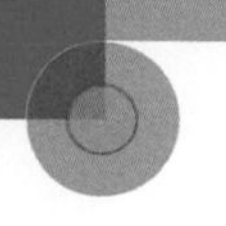

junction and inspect the contents and lining during withdrawal.

- A variable amount of faeces will be present but, in most cases, a reasonable assessment of the rectum and its contents can be made. Are the faeces solid or liquid? Is there any obvious blood or mucus?
- Look at the whole lining of the rectum, searching for *tumours or polyps*. Is the *mucosa shiny, smooth and of normal colour, or is it velvety, granular and reddened, as in proctitis?*
- Carefully inspect the posterior area just above the anal canal. This is a potential blind spot on sigmoidoscopy where it is easy to miss a small polyp. (The same applies to rectal examination.)
- On completion of the examination, make sure all the air is released, and wipe away any lubricating jelly from around the anus.
- Remember that sigmoidoscopy only demonstrates pathology in the lumen or wall of the rectum and does not show lesions outside the wall or in the pelvis.

Flexible sigmoidoscopy (Figure 16.4)

Most conditions of the rectum and some of the lower sigmoid colon can be diagnosed by the rigid sigmoidoscope. The flexible sigmoidoscope has increased the detection rate, as it can be passed further into the sigmoid colon. Bowel preparation *with an enema* is required.

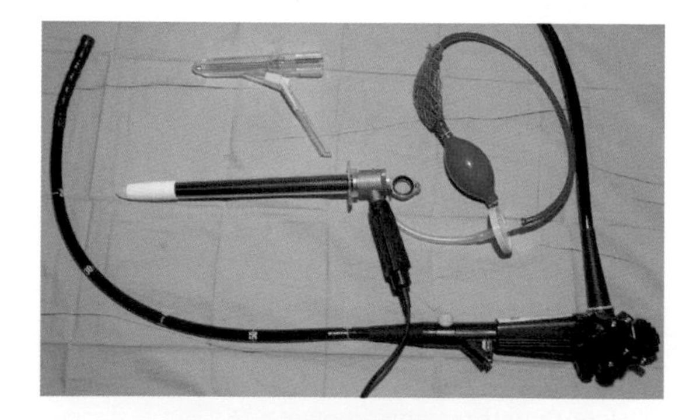

Figure 16.4 SIGMOIDOSCOPES. (a) A flexible sigmoidoscope, rigid proctoscope and rigid sigmoidoscope.

PROCTOSCOPY (FIGURE 16.5)

The proctoscope (or anoscope) is a short-illuminated tube, employed to inspect the anal canal. Its principal use is for the diagnosis and treatment of haemorrhoids. Proctoscopy usually follows immediately after sigmoidoscopy.

Technique of proctoscopy

- Position the patient as for sigmoidoscopy.
- No bowel preparation is necessary.
- Confirm that there is no painful external pathology.
- Insert the instrument in the direction of the anal canal, pointing at the patient's umbilicus.
- Remove the obturator and inspect the anal canal as you withdraw the instrument.
- Before removing the instrument, ask the patient to push down, which may cause haemorrhoids to swell and prolapse into view.

NOTE: Every patient with any rectal complaint must have a proper examination, with either sigmoidoscopy or simple digital examination. You will be considered negligent if you fail to perform a rectal examination on a patient complaining of rectal bleeding.

Revision panel 16.1

POSSIBLE DIAGNOSES OF CONDITIONS THAT PRESENT WITH RECTAL BLEEDING

Bleeding but no anal pain

Blood and looser stool – colorectal carcinoma
Blood after defaecation – haemorrhoids
Blood and mucus – colitis

Bleeding and pain – fissure (or carcinoma of the anal canal)
Blood alone – diverticular disease or angiodysplasia
Melaena – peptic ulceration

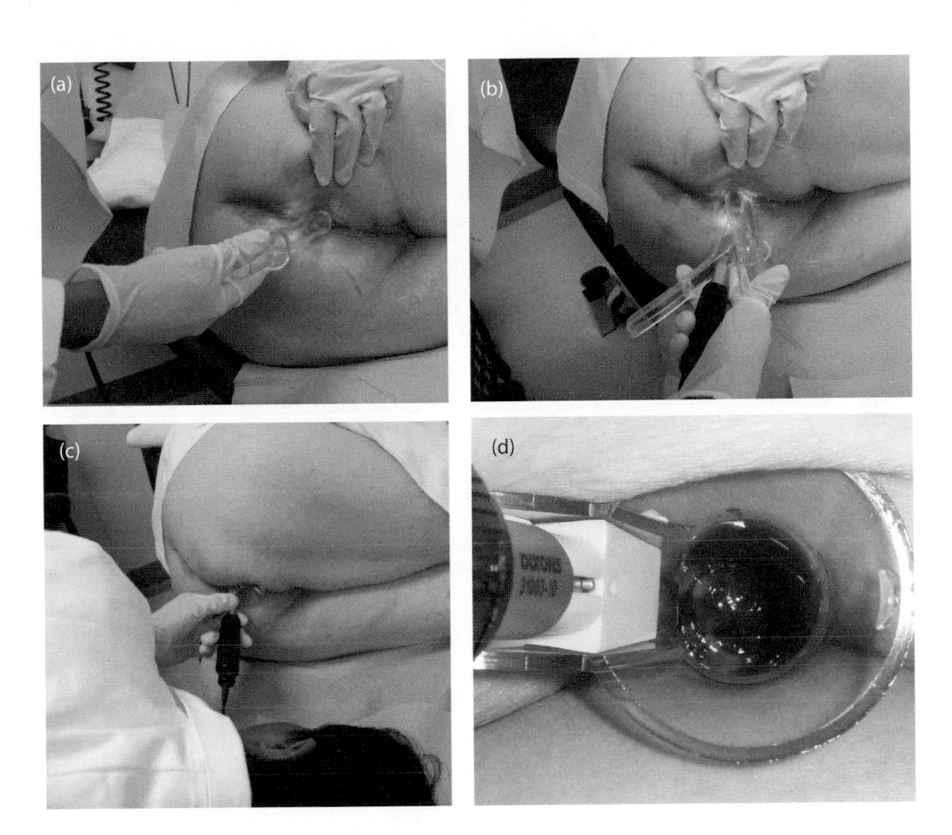

Figure 16.5 PROCTOSCOPY. (a) Insert the proctoscope as you would the finger for a rectal examination, obliquely and from behind, pulling backwards against the puborectalis muscle. (b) Pass the instrument along the axis of the anal canal. (c) Inspect the anal canal as you slowly withdraw the proctoscope. (d) A large haemorrhoid will fall into the lumen of the proctoscope; smaller ones just bulge over its end, an appearance that can be enhanced by advancing the scope 5 mm.

Conditions presenting with rectal bleeding

HAEMORRHOIDS

The mucosa and submucosa of the anal canal fall into *three anal cushions* that help to provide an efficient gas- and fluid-proof seal. The submucosa of the anal canal has a rich blood supply with a cavernous and capillary network of blood vessels covered by a thin epithelium, These *highly vascular cushions can become congested, enlarge, bleed and prolapse*. Abnormal enlargements of the anal cushions are called haemorrhoids (Figure 16.6).

NOTE: They are *not* varicose veins of the anus.

The process of prolapse eventually stretches the overlying perianal skin, often producing an external skin tag. The two together are sometimes termed a *pile mass*. Skin tags may occur in isolation. The general public uses the term 'piles' for any swelling near the anus, and sometimes for anal pain – remember this when taking a history.

History

Age Piles occur at all ages but are uncommon before the age of 20 years. They are extremely rare in children.

Symptoms *Uncomplicated piles do not cause pain.* The two common symptoms are *bleeding* and *a palpable lump* or a sensation of 'something coming out' of the anus (prolapse) after defaecation. They may also cause perianal discomfort and a mucous discharge that leads to pruritus.

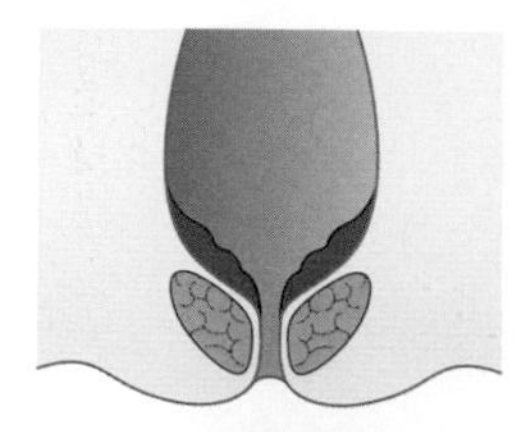

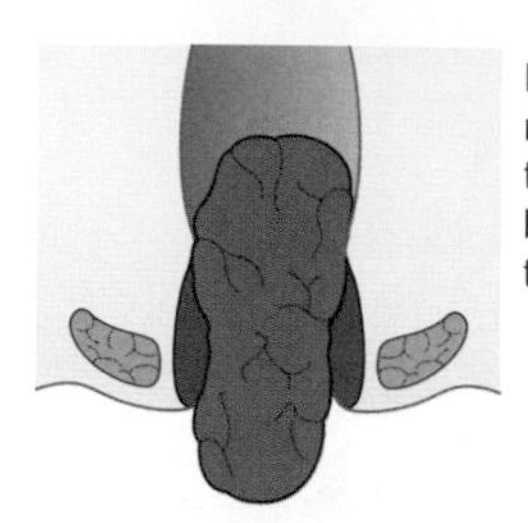

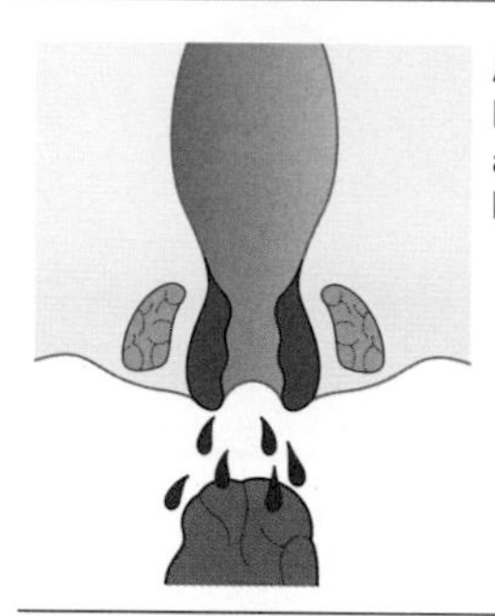

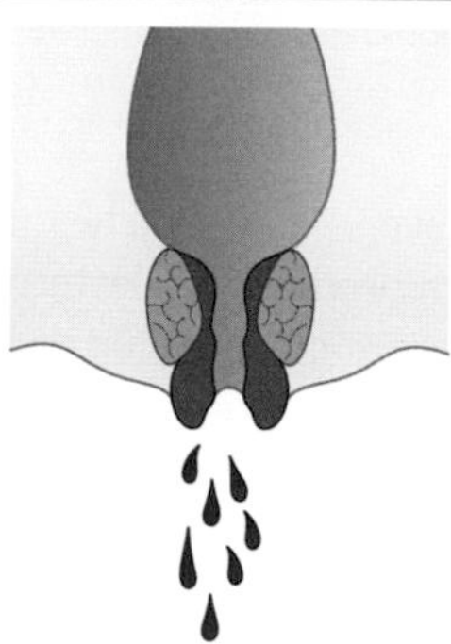

Figure 16.6 The way in which haemorrhoids are caused to bleed.

The *bleeding, which is bright red,* usually occurs after defaecation. It may just streak the faeces or be noticed on the toilet paper. When it is copious, it may splash into the lavatory pan and even result in iron-deficiency anaemia.

If the piles prolapse out of the anus after defaecation, a *swelling is noticed on wiping,* which may return to the rectum spontaneously or may need to be pushed back. If the prolapse becomes permanent, the skin tags often hypertrophy as well, forming a major component of the pile mass.

Pruritus is commonly associated with piles; this is caused by the leakage of mucus from the exposed mucosa onto the perianal skin.

Classification

Piles are categorized into three degrees by the history:

- First-degree piles bleed but do not prolapse.
- Second-degree piles prolapse but reduce spontaneously.
- Third-degree piles prolapse and need reduction or may not go back at all.

Although this distinction is artificial, it does help to guide treatment.

Cause

The geographical incidence of haemorrhoids is inversely proportional to the stool volume, which depends on the amount of fibre in the diet. Piles are rare in Africa, and common in more industrialized nations. The lower volume of stool may lead to more straining on defaecation, which leads to congestion and enlargement of the cushions, although some patients with piles never have any difficulty defaecating and do not complain of straining.

Examination

First- and second-degree piles

After a full examination of the abdomen, you should then carry out an *external inspection of the anus* and perianal skin and perform a digital rectal examination to exclude other rectal conditions.

External skin tags will be immediately visible.

After the *digital rectal examination,* all patients with rectal bleeding must be *sigmoidoscoped* to make sure there is no other serious coexisting pathology.

A *proctoscope is then inserted.* On withdrawal through the anal canal, pale pink mucosa can be seen collapsing over its end (see Figure 16.5d). *Piles are darker bluish–red, and bulge into the end of the instrument.* The multiple longitudinal corrugations are lost, and three deep clefts appear between the bulging piles.

The three 'primary' positions for haemorrhoids are at *3, 7 and 11 o'clock* (with the patient in the lithotomy position), corresponding to the most common sites of the three anal cushions (which are associated with the arterial supply). 'Secondary' piles seen at other positions in the anal canal are usually smaller and *appear between the primary piles.*

> **NOTE:** You cannot palpate haemorrhoids with your finger.

Third-degree piles (Figure 16.7)

These are *bluish–purple, permanently prolapsed swellings*, in the 3, 7 and 11 o'clock positions. Their distinguishing feature is their mucosal covering, recognized by its soft, smooth, mucus-exuding surface. They are usually associated with skin tags, which lie over the true haemorrhoid. If piles remain prolapsed, they ulcerate and bleed.

Thrombosed prolapsed piles

Piles are painful only when complications develop. A pile becomes tense, hard and oedematous if the submucosal vessels thrombose. Defaecation is then painful.

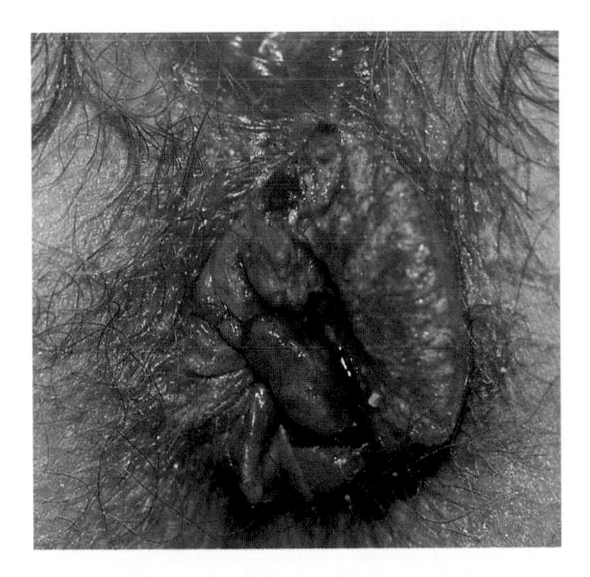

Figure 16.7 Third-degree (prolapsed) haemorrhoids. The epithelium covering the 3 o'clock pile is becoming thick and white. The 7 o'clock pile is bleeding.

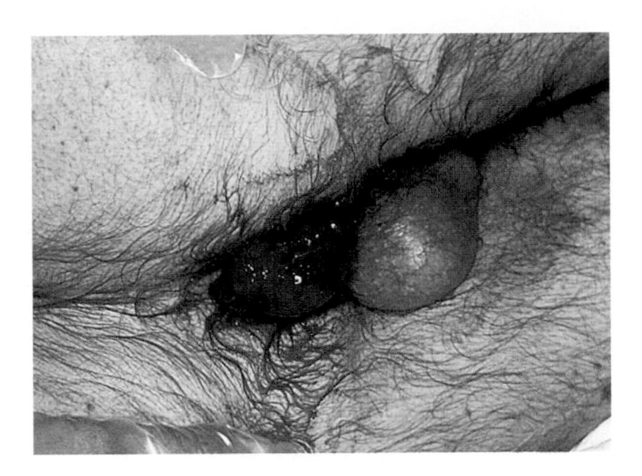

Figure 16.8 Prolapsed, strangulated, thrombosed haemorrhoids. Note the bloody serous discharge.

Inspection reveals *one to three red–purple dark swellings protruding from the anus with oedematous skin tags* (Figure 16.8). The pile mass can eventually become ulcerated.

> **NOTE:** The other common cause of a localized painful anal swelling is a perianal haematoma (see below). This can be distinguished from a mucosa-covered prolapsed haemorrhoid because it is covered by skin.

CARCINOMA OF THE RECTUM

The vast majority of rectal cancers are adenocarcinomas and can be:

- Polypoid.
- Ulcerating.
- Annular stenosing.

History

Age Rectal carcinoma usually develops in middle and old age but can occur in young adults.

Sex It is equally common in both sexes.

Symptoms *Many patients present with rectal bleeding*, usually a small amount of dark red blood streaked onto the surface of the stool. Very occasionally, enough blood accumulates in the rectum to be passed without faeces.

There is usually an associated change in bowel habit. The surface of the tumour produces excessive amounts of mucus, causing liquid motions, often described as 'diarrhoea'.

> **NOTE:** Patients who complain of 'passing water through the back passage' either have a rectal cancer or a villous adenoma (see below) until proved otherwise.

High cancers of the annular variety at the rectosigmoid junction may cause partial obstruction, presenting as *alternating episodes of diarrhoea and constipation.* This is because initial obstruction causes true constipation, followed by irritation of the colon above the tumour by impacted faeces, which liquefy before passing through the carcinomatous stenosis as loose stool.

Tenesmus occurs when a tumour in the lower part of the rectum becomes large enough to be mistaken for faeces. The persistent desire to empty the rectum is often accompanied by the passage of mucus, called 'slime' by the patient.

Small primary cancers may not cause symptoms but can metastasize to the liver. The patient then presents with upper abdominal pain and/or malaise and may have a palpably enlarged liver.

Pain is an uncommon symptom of carcinoma of the rectum, but three types can occur:

- Colic, with distension, caused by high annular tumours obstructing the lumen of the bowel.
- Local pain in the rectum, perineum or lower abdomen, caused by direct spread of the tumour to the surrounding structures, especially the sacral nerves.
- Pain on defaecation, which occurs if the tumour has spread downwards below the mucocutaneous junction into the sensitive anal canal.

Previous history Always ask about any previous large bowel symptoms, particularly recurrent episodes of diarrhoea associated with the passage of mucus and blood. Long-standing *inflammatory bowel disease* increases the risk of malignant change in the colon and rectum after 10 or more years of the disease. The fact that the colitis has been quiescent for many years does not reduce the risk of malignancy. The symptoms of a cancer may be passed off as a recurrence of the colitis and lead to a late presentation.

Family history A small number of bowel cancers can be linked to genetic conditions which increase risk. These include *familial adenomatous polyposis* and *Lynch syndrome*.

Examination

Rectal examination More commonly only the lower edge of a malignant tumour is palpable, unless very low.

The cancer feels hard, has raised, rolled and everted edges and bulges into the lumen of the rectum. The base is irregular and friable. Record the site of the tumour (anterior, posterior or lateral) and estimate its distance from the anal verge. Try to decide if the tumour is fixed or mobile.

Blood and mucus are commonly seen on the glove after the finger has been withdrawn.

When the cancer is in the upper part of the rectum, only its lower edge may be palpable.

Sigmoidoscopy should be carried out in all cases.

General examination *The liver is by far the most common site of distant metastases* from rectal cancer and must always be palpated. Every patient should also have staging investigations.

Rare rectal tumours

These include carcinoid tumours, lymphomas and rectal squamous cell cancers. The symptoms are similar to those of carcinoma.

Malignant pelvic tumours

Bladder carcinomas, carcinomas of gynaecological or prostatic origin and any intraperitoneal malignancy with spread to the pelvis may present with rectal symptoms. The extra-rectal deposits can cause a stricture presenting as constipation, or the tumour mass can cause tenesmus.

Digital examination reveals a hard, craggy mass in the pelvis.

ADENOMAS OF THE RECTUM

Benign adenomas of the rectum may be *solitary or multiple* throughout the colon and rectum and are sometimes of the familial variety. They are *villous* or *polypoid* in shape. In narrow parts of the bowel such as the sigmoid colon, peristalsis draws the adenomas down on a stalk. In the wider rectum, they are usually sessile.

Adenomas have a variable degree of dysplasia, which can undergo malignant change to invasive cancer. This is unusual if the adenoma is less than 3 cm in diameter, but eventually most true adenomas will turn into carcinomas.

The *villous adenoma* is a distinct clinical variety of rectal adenoma, more common in the elderly. There is a *broad base with a frondular (lots of villi) surface that exudes large quantities of mucus*. Growth is slow, and the onset of symptoms is often so gradual that presentation is late. Frail patients with large villous adenomas lose vast amounts of potassium with the mucus and can present with hypokalaemia.

NOTE: Malignant change in the base of the papilloma is common.

History

A *large adenoma* produces *mucous discharge* and diarrhoea with a *variable degree of bleeding*. A small adenoma may bleed or prolapse.

Examination

Adenomas are soft and sometimes difficult to feel on rectal examination, but are always visible on sigmoidoscopy as dark pink, frond-covered tumours.

Not all polyps in the rectum are true adenomas. *Hyperplastic polyps* are most common in the rectosigmoid colon, and are usually less than 5 mm in diameter. On histology, these have long crypts with excess proliferation in the base. Biopsy confirms the diagnosis.

Pseudopolyps are islands of normal mucosa in patients with severe ulcerative colitis. The rolled-up edge of the mucosa appears 'polypoid'.

Rare *hamartomatous polyps* are found in children and can cause intussusception or rectal bleeding. They also occur in Peutz–Jeghers syndrome (see Chapter 15).

SOLITARY RECTAL ULCER

This is a rare condition, with a peak age of between 30 and 40 years, although all ages can be affected. *It is linked to rectal prolapse in nearly two-thirds* of those affected and is thought to be caused by repeated episodes of intussusception, difficulty in defaecation and straining at stool. *The majority of ulcers lie anteriorly about 10 cm from the anal verge.*

Symptoms include *rectal bleeding, the passage of mucus, anal discomfort* and occasionally incontinence. There is almost always some difficulty in evacuation.

The mucosa is usually reddened and oedematous with ulceration in more than half the cases. In half the ulcers, the edge is raised and polypoid, and *it can be easily mistaken for a carcinoma.*

DIVERTICULAR DISEASE

Diverticular disease is often an incidental finding in patients with other colorectal disease (see Chapter 15). It can, however, present with rectal bleeding, which can be acute, massive and fresh. The usually elderly patient feels a little faint, gets lower abdominal pain and then has a desire to defaecate with the passage of a large volume of fresh blood and clots.

This is a fairly common reason for emergency admission. The bleeding usually stops spontaneously, but occasionally the patient may be shocked, and the bleeding can be life-threatening. The bleeding usually comes from an eroded artery in the mouth of a diverticulum, but *angiodysplasia should be considered*. This can be diagnosed by colonoscopy or angiography.

Conditions presenting with anal pain

PERIANAL HAEMATOMA

The name of this condition is well established, even although *it is not a true haematoma but a thrombosis of a vein (thrombosed perianal varix)* in the subcutaneous plexus, probably caused by an injury to

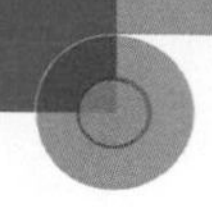

Revision panel 16.2

POSSIBLE DIAGNOSES OF ANAL CONDITIONS THAT PRESENT WITH PAIN

Pain alone

Fissure (pain after defaecation)
Proctalgia fugax (spontaneous pain at night)
Anorectal abscess

Pain and bleeding

Fissure
Crohn's disease

Pain and a lump

Perianal haematoma
Anorectal abscess

Pain, a lump and bleeding

Thrombosed prolapsed haemorrhoids
Carcinoma of the anal canal
Prolapsed rectal polyp or carcinoma
Prolapsed rectum

the vein wall during defaecation. It also occurs after childbirth, from stretching of the perineum.

The thrombus/haematoma causes an inflammatory reaction with pain and oedema.

History

Age and sex Perianal haematomas occur at all ages and are equally common in both sexes.

Symptoms The main symptoms are of *pain and a swelling at the anal margin*. The pain is of sudden onset and subsides gradually over a few days. It is a continuous discomfort, made worse by sitting, moving and defaecation, and is clearly localized to the lump.

The swelling is small and spherical but may gradually enlarge and become more painful.

Bleeding occurs if the skin over the lump ulcerates.

Perianal haematomas may recur.

Examination

Position The lump (occasionally multiple) may be anywhere around the anal margin.

Colour The lump is *deep blue–purple*.

Tenderness The lump is tender.

Shape and size It is initially spherical, and up to 1 cm in diameter.

Surface It is a smooth lump covered by skin, which may be normal or oedematous.

Composition The lump feels rubbery or firm.

Relations It is directly under the perianal skin, and superficial to the external sphincter.

FISSURE-IN-ANO

An anal fissure is a longitudinal split (ulcer) in the skin of the anal canal.

An acute tear is quite a common event in patients with constipation and usually heals quickly. Reopening of the tear when the patient next defaecates causes further pain, leading to an increase in anal sphincter tone that progresses to spasm. This makes the tear more likely to reopen on subsequent defaecation and leads to a vicious circle of tearing–pain–spasm. The base then becomes fibrous and does not heal. It effectively becomes a chronic ulcer of the anal verge.

History

Age and sex Most fissures develop in young males, and in females after childbirth. They are quite common in children, who often pass bulky stools very quickly.

Symptoms Both acute and chronic fissures are *very painful*. The pain begins during defaecation and is often described as a tearing sensation. With a chronic fissure, the spasm pain persists for hours and can be so severe that the patient becomes afraid to defaecate.

Fissures streak the stool with blood and stain the toilet paper. When parents notice rectal bleeding in children, it always causes great alarm. The child rarely complains of the pain, unless questioned directly.

Persistence There may be periods of remission, and eventually the condition either heals or becomes chronic.

Examination

Position The majority of fissures, especially in males, are in the *midline posteriorly*, but some, particularly in females, are anterior. A few are lateral, and both anterior and posterior fissures can coexist.

The diagnosis is made by gently parting the skin of the anus and looking for a split in the anal skin. This may be all that is possible, because further examination is prevented by pain. A small skin tag, often called incorrectly a *sentinel pile*, may be visible at the lower end of the fissure.

Tenderness The anal sphincter is usually in spasm and exquisitely tender. A careful rectal examination is possible in a few patients but is mainly of value in excluding alternative pathology.

Sigmoidoscopy and proctoscopy Never attempt either of these examinations in a conscious patient with a fissure – they would be much too painful. Proctoscopy under general anaesthesia displays the raw base of the fissure.

ANORECTAL ABSCESS

There are two distinct varieties of anorectal abscess:

- In a *perianal abscess*, the swelling is clearly at the anal margin, which it distorts.
- An *ischiorectal abscess* lies lateral to the anus, occupies a much larger space and can track round behind the anus to the opposite side.

The infection that causes both types of abscess probably begins in an anal gland. From here, the pus either tracks down to the perineum between the sphincters to form a perianal abscess or penetrates the external sphincter to reach the ischiorectal fossa. The anal gland is usually destroyed if the abscess is drained externally or bursts quickly, but if it continues to secrete, a fistula will develop. This can then be associated with further episodes of infection.

Abscesses can also form in the intersphincteric space and in the submucosa of the anus. Abscesses in these positions can lead to severe pain with very few external signs.

History

Age Anorectal abscess is most common in patients between 20 and 50 years old, but occurs at all ages, rarely in childhood.

Sex It is more common in males.

Symptoms There is a gradual (often over several days) onset of *severe, throbbing pain*, which makes sitting, moving and defaecation painful.

A tender swelling close to the anus will become apparent to the patient, who may have had previous episodes of infection. If left untreated, the abscess will eventually point and burst.

Systemic effects A patient with an ischiorectal abscess is more likely to be systemically unwell with the general symptoms of an abscess – *malaise, loss of appetite, sweating and even rigors. Pain and tenderness* tend to be greater with a perianal abscess, as the space in which it can expand is confined.

Examination

General examination The patient tries not to move, and lies on their side. There is likely to be tachycardia, pyrexia, sweating, a dry, furred tongue and fetor oris.

Position *A tender red mass* is usually obvious lateral to the anus in the soft tissues between the anus and the ischial tuberosity, although this is less obvious with an ischiorectal abscess.

A perianal abscess may develop anywhere around the anal margin. The distinction between the physical signs of the two types is often blurred.

Tenderness The whole area is usually exquisitely tender.

Colour and temperature The overlying skin eventually becomes hot and red.

Shape, size and composition The surface of the abscess is often indistinct, and its size may be difficult to assess. *Tenderness makes testing for fluctuation impossible.*

Rectal examination This is best deferred until the patient is anaesthetized prior to drainage. The abscess can then be felt to bulge into the side of the lower part of the rectum. Fluctuation and the size of the abscess can then be determined.

Lymph glands The inguinal lymph glands are sometimes enlarged and tender.

Local tissues There may be scarring from previous abscesses and fistulas. Cellulitis and, very occasionally, necrotizing fasciitis may occur.

PELVIC SEPSIS

Infection in the abdominal cavity (see Chapter 15) can result in pus collecting in the pelvis, its most dependent part, particularly after acute appendicitis,

salpingitis (*pelvic inflammatory disease*) and *diverticulitis*. It can also occur after operations, especially after anastomotic dehiscence.

Patients complain of *pelvic discomfort, diarrhoea and tenesmus*. There are general signs of sepsis such as *fever, malaise, lassitude, sweats, rigors and pyrexia*.

Digital rectal examination may demonstrate a tender, hot boggy swelling high in the pelvis.

FISTULA-IN-ANO

A fistula is a pathological track, lined with epithelium or granulation tissue, that connects two epithelial surfaces (see Chapter 4). A fistula-in-ano connects the lumen of the rectum or anal canal with the external perianal skin. It is caused by *an abscess developing in an anal crypt gland in the intersphincteric space that bursts in two directions – internally into the anal canal, and externally through the skin*. Mucus is forced through the fistulous tract as stool is expelled, and this is the mechanism that stops a fistula from ever healing.

Fistulae-in-ano may also be associated with *Crohn's disease* or *ulcerative colitis*. Rarely, a fistula can be caused by direct infiltration and necrosis of a low rectal carcinoma.

Classification

A fistula-in-ano can run through a variety of anatomical planes (Figure 16.9). The important distinction is between low and high fistulas, as the subsequent surgical management is completely different.

A *low* fistula-in-ano *has its internal opening below the anorectal ring*. This is the point where the puborectalis muscle sling fuses with the external sphincter, and is the major muscle involved in maintaining continence. It is more likely that a fistula at this level can be laid open without significant impairment of continence, although there will virtually always be some change in control if enquiry afterwards is careful enough. Particular caution should be employed in females with anterior fistulas as the sphincter is smaller anteriorly.

A *high* fistula-in-ano *joins the rectum above the anorectal ring*. Laying this open would divide the ring and render the patient incontinent.

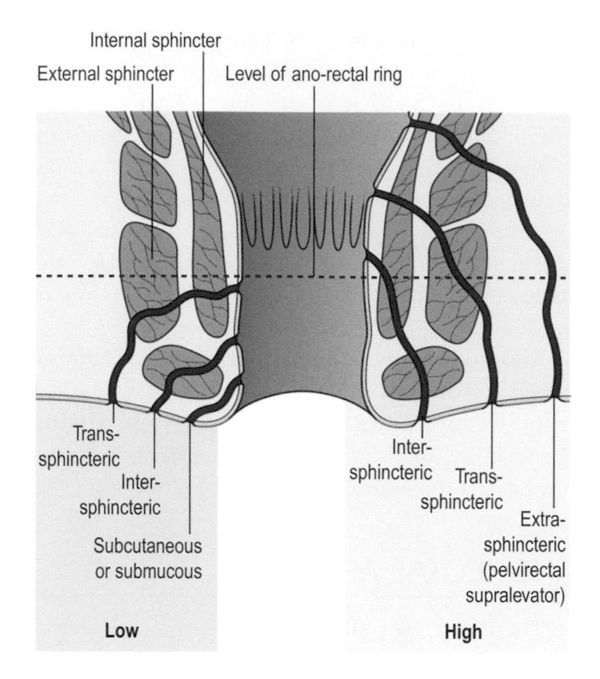

Figure 16.9 The varieties of fistula-in-ano.

History

Age A fistula-in-ano can occur at any time during adult life, and rarely in children.

Symptoms There may be a history of a perianal abscess that has spontaneously burst or has been drained surgically. Some patients with a fistula have never had an abscess but notice a small tender lump in the perineum that discharges pus.

The most common symptom is a watery or purulent discharge from the external opening of the fistula. There may be recurrent episodes of pain if pus collects in the fistulous track. The fistula may appear to heal, but then becomes painful and discharges again, with relief of the discomfort.

The discharge, which can on occasion be blood-stained, may cause pruritus ani.

Other symptoms (direct questions) Up to 70% of patients with rectal *Crohn's disease* develop a fistula, and it is important to enquire about any bowel or abdominal symptoms or systemic upset.

Examination

Position The external opening(s) of the fistula is usually visible as a *puckered scar or a small tuft of granulation tissue* anywhere around the anus (Figure 16.10),

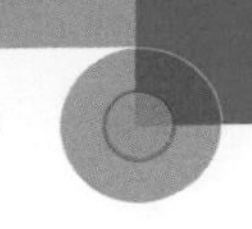

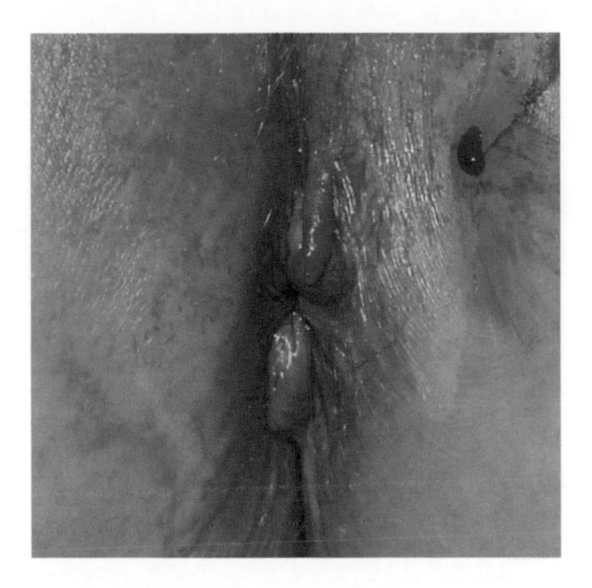

Figure 16.10 An anterior low-level fistula, obeying Goodsall's rule.

usually close to the anal verge, although it is sometimes several centimetres away.

> **NOTE:** *Goodsall's rule* states that the internal opening of an anterior fistula lies along a radial line drawn from the external opening to the anus, but the internal opening of a posterior fistula always lies in the midline posteriorly. Although things are rarely certain in medicine, this rule is reliable

There may be more than one opening, particularly if the patient has Crohn's disease.

Tenderness The external opening of the fistula is not usually painful, but the tissues around it may be thickened and tender.

Discharge The discharge, usually purulent, may be visible on the skin or the underclothes.

Rectal examination The internal opening of the fistula can sometimes be felt as an area of induration or a small nodule beneath the mucosa. If you can feel it, try to decide if the internal opening of the fistula is below or above the anorectal junction, i.e. at the low level or high level.

The *indurated track of the fistula between the internal and external openings is sometimes palpable* beneath the perianal skin but is easier to define under anaesthesia. The track may be palpable between a gloved index finger in the rectum and the thumb of the same hand. Look for coexistent pathology, such as a carcinoma.

Sigmoidoscopy and proctoscopy These are essential to exclude Crohn's disease, ulcerative colitis, a carcinoma of the anus and even tuberculosis. Disappointingly, the internal opening of the fistula is rarely visible.

Lymph glands The inguinal lymph glands are not enlarged.

Local tissues These are indurated and 'violaceous' if the patient has Crohn's disease.

General examination Many of the diseases mentioned above have associated abdominal and general clinical signs, so never confine your examination to the patient's perineum. Examine the abdomen carefully.

PERIANAL CROHN'S DISEASE

Perianal disease can occur in isolation, but many patients are already known to have Crohn's disease elsewhere in the intestine, especially the colon. Bleeding, discharge, pain and faecal leakage can all occur, and fistulas and fissures are also common.

The appearances are protean, with abscesses, complex fistulas and indolent fissures predominating in an indurated perianal region that looks inflamed and 'sore'.

PILONIDAL SINUS

The word *pilonidal* means a nest of hairs. A pilonidal sinus usually, but not always, contains hair. They *are found commonly in the midline skin of the natal cleft, between the coccyx and the anus.* They sometimes develop between the fingers of hairdressers, and occasionally at the umbilicus.

A pilonidal sinus is lined by granulation tissue, not skin, and hair does not grow within it. The hairs in the sinus have often come from the scalp. The midline skin in the natal cleft is tethered, and during walking the motion of the buttocks rubbing together causes shed hairs that are covered in small barbs to be driven into a pre-existing dimple, or to pierce normal skin. When an infection develops, the hairs act as foreign bodies, preventing clearance of infection. *The end result is a chronic abscess that periodically flares up into an acute abscess.*

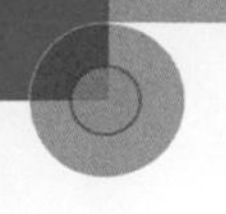

History

Age Pilonidal sinus is rare before puberty and over the age of 40 years.

Sex This condition is far more common in males than in females, and most often develops in dark-haired, hirsute males.

Symptoms The common symptoms are *pain and a swelling in the natal cleft*, often associated with a purulent discharge if the sinus becomes infected. Local discomfort sometimes leads the patient to discover the openings. The pain varies between a dull ache and an acute throbbing pain. An abscess may be the first event. A patient with a pilonidal abscess finds some relief from the throbbing pain by lying prone, in contrast to patients with anorectal abscesses who usually prefer to lie on their side.

Chronic discharge indicates chronic low-grade infection, but between acute exacerbations patients often think the sinus has disappeared.

Examination (Figure 16.11)

Position Pilonidal sinuses arise in the midline of the natal cleft between the coccyx and the anus. They are usually closer to the tip of the coccyx than the anus.

Temperature and tenderness The skin over a pilonidal abscess is red and tender.

The sinus The sinus openings are usually easy to see as *small midline pits* with epithelialized edges. Protruding hairs are rarely seen, but *pouting granulation tissue and purulent discharge are common*. Pressure may produce a small quantity of serous discharge. When the sinus becomes infected, it is indistinguishable from any other type of subcutaneous abscess.

There is palpable subcutaneous induration, corresponding to the extent of the granulation tissue beneath the skin. There may be scars well away from the midline, where previous abscesses have discharged or been incised.

Lymph glands The inguinal lymph glands are not enlarged.

Local tissues The local tissues are normal.

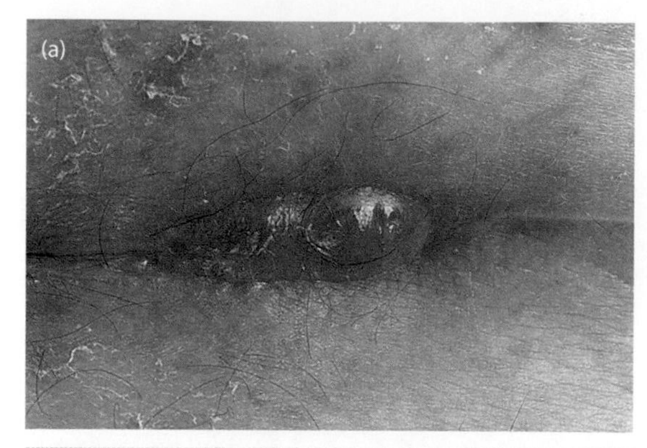

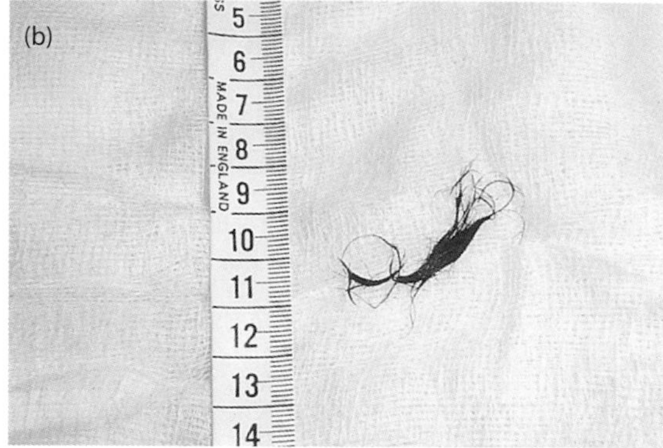

Figure 16.11 PILONIDAL SINUS. (a) The patient is lying on his right side with his buttocks held apart to expose the bottom of the natal cleft. The sinus, which is difficult to see, is the small, pale, central pit. The stiff black hair that commonly covers the buttocks of these patients has been shaved off. (b) The hairs that were removed from the sinus shown in (a).

PROCTALGIA FUGAX

This condition is thought to be caused by a spontaneous spasm (cramp) in the muscles of the pelvic floor, or possibly by a spasm at the rectosigmoid junction. It is often associated with IBS.

It presents with *sudden, severe, cramp-like rectal pain* experienced within the rectum or pelvis rather than the anal canal, which comes on suddenly, often at night. It is of *short duration*, sometimes lasting just a few seconds and rarely longer than 5 minutes. Nothing relieves the pain, but it passes off spontaneously. There may be associated symptoms of a functional bowel disorder (see Chapter 15).

General and rectal examinations are normal. The patient may experience the same pain on sigmoidoscopy as air is insufflated at the rectosigmoid junction.

Conditions presenting as an anal lump with or without pain

The following conditions are not necessarily 'painless', but the lump is the dominant symptom (Revision panel 16.3).

PROLAPSED THROMBOSED STRANGULATED HAEMORRHOIDS

These are very painful and tender (see above).

Revision panel 16.3

POSSIBLE DIAGNOSES OF ANAL CONDITIONS THAT PRESENT WITH A LUMP

A lump and no other symptoms

- Anal warts
- Skin tags

A lump and pain

- Perianal haematoma

A lump, pain and bleeding

- Prolapsed haemorrhoids
- Carcinoma of anal canal
- Prolapsed rectal polyp or carcinoma
- Prolapsed rectum

One or more tense, tender, red–purple mucosa-covered swellings protrude from the anal canal often associated with oedematous skin tags (see Figure 16.8). They may eventually become necrotic and ulcerated.

ANAL SKIN TAGS

Tags of skin, of varying size and shape, are commonly found in the perianal area. They represent an exaggeration of the normal wrinkling of the lax anal skin, which stretches during defaecation (Figure 16.12). They are usually symptomless, but may rub, catch or itch. Patients may complain that skin tags prevent proper cleaning of the perianal area.

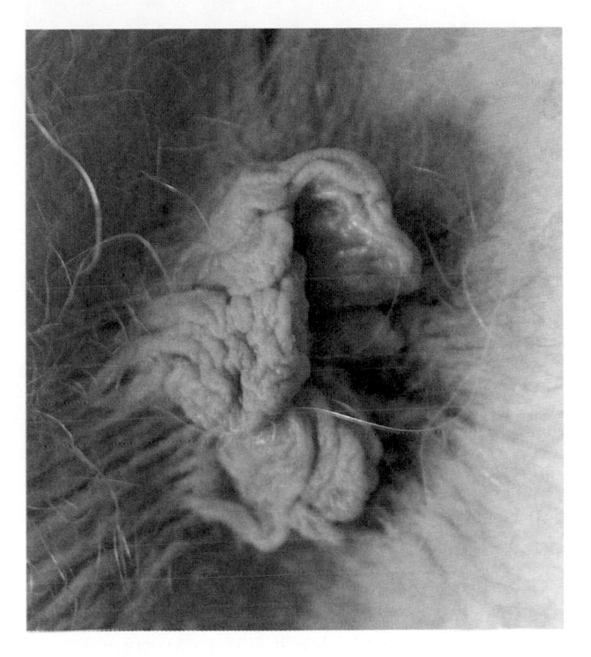

Figure 16.12 Anal skin tags. Many patients call these tags 'piles', but they are not haemorrhoids.

Skin tags in the 3, 7, and 11 o'clock positions are normally part of a pile mass, but *quite large skin tags can occur without piles* and, of course, quite large piles can be present without skin tags.

A tag may develop at the lower end of an anal fissure, called a *sentinel tag* (see above).

Anal skin tags may become polypoid in shape and are called fibroepithelial anal polyps. They must not be confused with adenomatous polyps (see Figure 16.13).

ANAL WARTS

These are multiple, pedunculated, papilliferous skin excrescences that resemble warts elsewhere in the body (Condylomata acuminata) (see Figure 16.14). They may spread over the whole perineum and are caused by the human papilloma virus (HPV) (subtypes 6 and 11), which is carried by 20% of the population and is transmitted by sexual

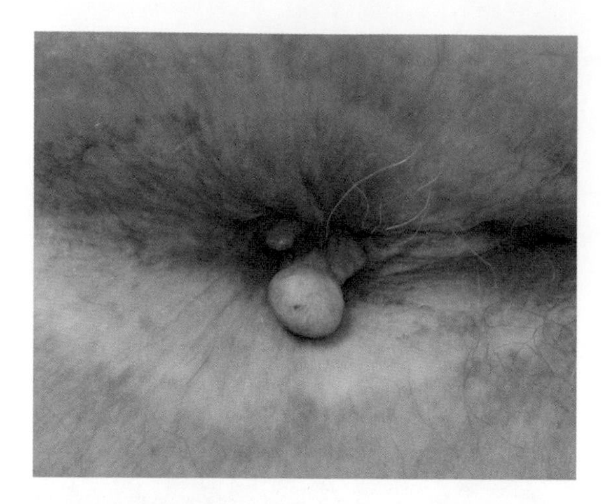

Figure 16.13 An anal polyp. This is clearly fibrous and quite different from an adenomatous polyp, in both level and appearance.

contact. Therefore, they are often associated with other sexually transmitted infections. They also develop in patients whose immune response has been depressed with steroids or organ transplantation, and in HIV.

Condylomata lata are rarely seen nowadays and are a manifestation of secondary syphilis. They are broad-based, flat-topped papules that are highly contagious.

All condylomas cause *irritation, discomfort and pain from rubbing,* and may ulcerate, and bleed. Proctoscopy assesses for intra-anal warts.

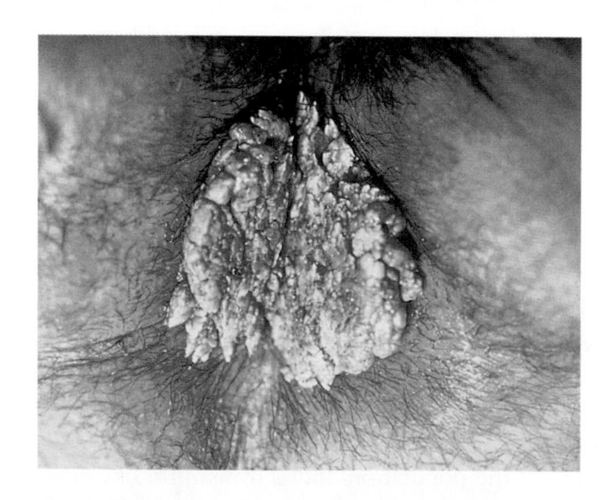

Figure 16.14 Examples of multiple perianal warts.

SQUAMOUS CELL CARCINOMA OF THE ANUS

This is a carcinoma of the anal or perianal skin and is identical to the squamous cell carcinoma found elsewhere in the body (see Chapter 4). It may follow precancerous changes in the local skin known as anal intraepithelial neoplasia. HPV (subtypes 16 and 18) can cause dysplasia of the anal skin and eventually lead to anal cancer. This occurs more frequently in men who have sex with men, and suspicious lesions should be biopsied.

The presenting symptoms depend on how close the cancer is to the anal verge. If it is in the anal canal, it presents with *pain on defaecation and bleeding, or the patient notices a lump* (Figure 16.15). A squamous cell carcinoma does not exude mucus.

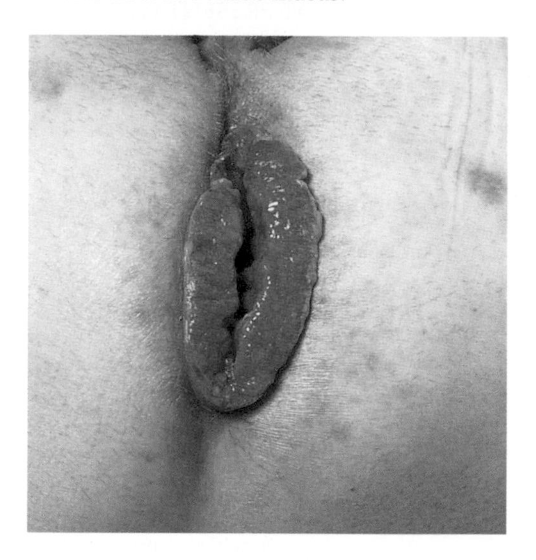

Figure 16.15 A carcinoma of the anal canal that has spread into the skin of the perineum. The patient was still able to defaecate. The patient is in the lithotomy position.

On examination, the tumour often has the appearance of a skin cancer. It can be an ulcer with a raised everted edge, or a plaque, and occasionally it can be circumferential and stenosing. The inguinal lymph nodes should be examined.

Prolapse of the rectum

This is an eversion of the lower part of the rectum through the anal canal. There are two varieties.

FULL-THICKNESS PROLAPSE

With a full-thickness prolapse, the *entire rectal wall, muscle and mucosa become displaced through the anus*. This occurs when the structures in the floor of the pelvis that normally hold the rectum in the curve of the sacrum become weak and lax. Chronic constipation and prolonged straining at stool are other aetiological factors. It is always associated with impaired continence because of weakness and stretching of the anal sphincter. Continence problems precede the prolapse, often for many years.

History

Age Prolapse of the rectum is primarily a disease of the elderly, although it does occur in infants and children.

Sex It is 20 times more common in females than males. Normal anal sphincters are thin anteriorly behind the vagina, and the anal canal may be stretched and damaged during childbirth.

Symptoms The patient complains of a *large lump that appears at the anus after defaecation*, or sometimes spontaneously when standing, walking or coughing. *The lump can usually be pushed back into the rectum* or may reduce spontaneously when the patient lies down.

A prolapsed rectum is *uncomfortable and causes a persistent desire to defaecate*. The prolapsed rectal mucosa *secretes mucus* and, if it remains prolapsed, *ulcerates and bleeds*.

Examination

Colour and shape The prolapsed rectum, which may be up to 20 cm in length, forms *a long tubular mass protruding symmetrically through the anus*. The bowel is not tender and can be handled without causing the patient discomfort. The exposed mucosa is red and thrown into circumferential concentric folds around a central orifice, which is the lumen of the rectum (Figure 16.16).

> **NOTE:** Sometimes you need to ask the patient to strain down to produce the prolapse, and the diagnosis may be missed if this manoeuvre is omitted.

Reducibility It is usually possible to reduce a prolapse with gentle compression and cephalad pressure.

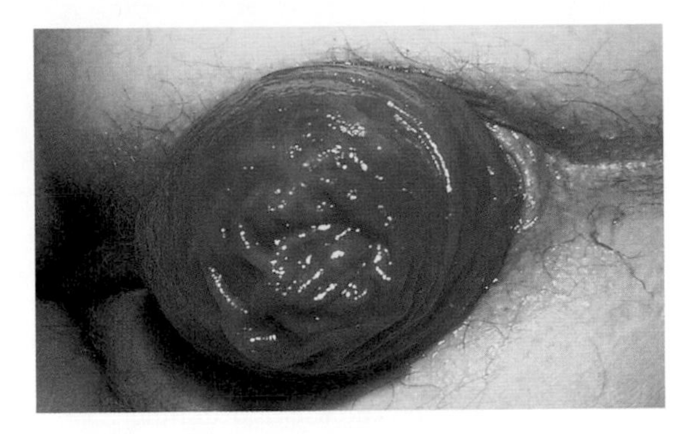

Figure 16.16 A rectal prolapse.

Local tissues The anal sphincter is very lax when it is contracted on the examining finger.

PARTIAL-THICKNESS OR MUCOSAL PROLAPSE

The history is very similar to that of prolapsing piles, and the two conditions do overlap. However, instead of there being purplish anal cushions, pink folds of anal mucosa are seen, with a less circular appearance than a full-thickness prolapse. A mucosal prolapse may not reach the anal verge.

On examination, a *soft painless mass is visible* and palpable at the anal margin; this consists of *two thin mucosal layers*. A *mucous discharge is often the main symptom*, and the redundant mucosa is visible on proctoscopy.

MUCOSAL RECTAL PROLAPSE IN CHILDREN

In children, the mucosa of the bowel is more loosely attached to the muscle layer than in adults. In addition, there is often hypertrophy of the submucosal lymphoid aggregates known as *Peyer's patches*. This may result in prolapse of the anal mucosa.

History

Age The condition usually presents at toilet training but occurs up to puberty.

Symptoms The parents notice a smooth, *soft swelling coming out of the anal margin* after defaecation.

The child may complain of discomfort, and older children may become frightened. *Mucous discharge is common, but bleeding is rare.* The frightened child may try to avoid defaecation, and the rectum then becomes impacted with hard faeces.

Examination The swelling is rarely reproducible in the clinic, and the diagnosis must be made on the history. The only differential diagnosis is the very rare juvenile polyp, which usually presents with bleeding.

The condition often cures itself over time.

Conditions presenting with pruritus ani

This is a symptom rather than a condition. Many people experience an *idiopathic perianal itch,* worse overnight. It is, however, important to seek a cause (Revision panel 16.4).

Associated prolapse or bleeding suggest the presence of haemorrhoids, one of the most common causes of pruritis. Other intra-anal conditions that cause the leakage of small amounts of liquid faeces or mucus cause itching. Contact with the perianal skin produces maceration and excoriation, which leads to 'scratching'. *A vaginal discharge may also be responsible.*

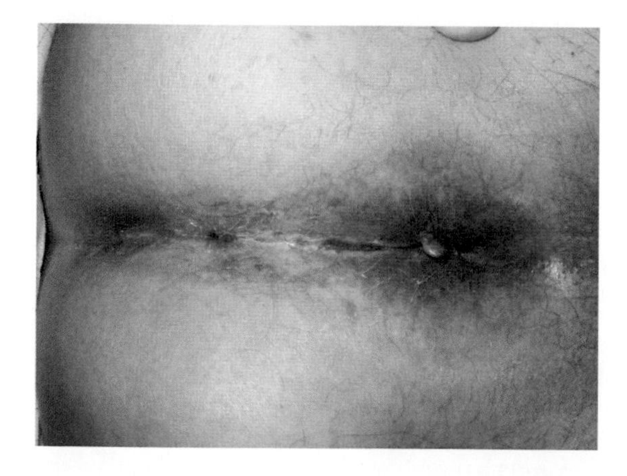

Figure 16.17 Severe pruritis caused by the leakage of mucus from large second-degree haemorrhoids. There is a small skin tag.

Revision panel 16.4

CAUSES OF PRURITIS ANI

Mucous discharge from the anus caused by:

- Haemorrhoids
- Polyps
- Skin tags
- Condylomas
- Fissure
- Fistula
- Carcinoma of the anus

Vaginal discharge caused by:

- *Trichomonas vaginitis*
- *Monilia vaginitis*
- Cervicitis
- Gonorrhoea

Skin diseases

- Tinea cruris
- Fungal infections, especially monilial infections in diabetes

Parasites

- Threadworms

Faecal soiling

- Poor hygiene
- Incontinence
- Diarrhoea

Psychoneuroses

A few patients have a sensitivity to washing powder or other allergens, and some have a high intake of coffee or fizzy drinks.

On examination, there may be *evidence of perianal redness and excoriation* (Figure 16.17), as well as the presence of piles or the opening of a fistula. A *primary skin disorder may be responsible,* and plaques of psoriasis may be visible. *Fungal infection* usually has a very distinctive edge, and microscopy of skin scrapings can be diagnostic.

In children, *threadworms* are a common cause of itching, and may be visible or detected on a stool swab. Generalized causes of itching such as obstructive jaundice should not be forgotten.

Conditions presenting with faecal incontinence

This is defined as an involuntary loss of control of flatus, fluid motions or solid faeces.

Normal continence depends on maintenance of the anorectal angle at rest by the puborectalis muscle, and closure of the anal canal by the internal and external sphincters. The presence of functioning sensory receptors in the anal canal is also important.

The problem is particularly common in older females who have had children, as is prolapse.

Causes of faecal incontinence are:

- Diarrhoea: infective or inflammatory.
- Reduced rectal compliance caused by inflammation, tumour or surgery, for example, low anterior resection or severe IBS.
- Neurological: MS, dementia, spinal trauma, pudendal neuropathy.
- Damage to the anal sphincter from childbirth, anal surgery or other trauma.
- Fistula to the vagina from small bowel (enterovaginal), colon (colovaginal) or rectum (rectovaginal).
- Connective tissue disease, which causes fibrosis and thinning of the internal anal sphincter.
- Autonomic neuropathy, for example, associated with diabetes, which causes weakness of the internal sphincter.

Many patients have more than one of the above factors impacting on their continence.

Some patients have uncontrollable passage of an entire bowel action, often associated with severe urgency of defaecation. This is usually the result of an inability to contract the external sphincter. Others report a more constant leakage of smaller quantities of liquid or solid stool of which they are unaware. This is the result of a defective action of the autonomically innervated internal sphincter. Some patients have a combination of both problems.

Patients with loose stools may be incontinent despite a normal sphincter mechanism. Incontinence can occur in patients with inflamed or irritable bowels, when excessive peristalsis overcomes the anal sphincter in a very 'sensitive' rectum.

When taking the patient's past medical history, ask specifically about surgery on the anus, *pelvic radiotherapy and local or spinal trauma. A detailed obstetric history should also be documented.*

Inspection may demonstrate an excoriated perineum because of the leakage of loose stool.

When there is a large defect in the anal sphincter from an obstetric injury, the pelvic floor usually appears very attenuated. The perineum may appear flat, with the anal verge at the same level as the buttocks. This becomes even more pronounced if the patient is asked to 'bear down', which may reveal a prolapse. The anal canal often gapes. The sphincter pressure may be found to be reduced if the patient is asked to 'squeeze' the examining finger. This requires experience to assess.

HIRSCHSPRUNG'S DISEASE

This inherited condition affects one in 5000 infants. There is an absence of ganglia in Auerbach's plexus in the colonic wall. This produces an abnormal segment of variable length in the large bowel, and results in a functional obstruction.

It is four times more common in males than females, and usually presents in childhood. There is an adult form of the disease, presenting with chronic constipation.

In this condition, neonates fail to pass meconium in the first 24–48 hours of life, and the abdomen becomes distended. The infants develop feeding difficulties, and eventually vomit if left untreated. Older children develop chronic constipation and fail to thrive.

The *abdomen is usually markedly distended*, and a mucus plug is often present on rectal examination. The dislodgement of this plug is often followed by a dramatic decompression of the abdomen. Older children usually have a chronically distended abdomen with an empty rectum.

ANORECTAL ANOMALIES

These occur in approximately 1 in 5000 live births, and the cause is unknown. They can be classified as either *low* or *high* defects, *with or without an associated fistula* to the genitourinary tract. They vary from simple to complex, with the simplest being an anterior anal displacement or the presence of an anal membrane. The most complex include a *persistent cloaca in a female,* or in either sex a very high rectal agenesis with defective anal innervation.

Neonates present with a *failure to pass meconium;* this may leak from the vagina or be present in the urine if a fistula is present.

An absent or 'covered' anus (imperforate anus) should be obvious on careful inspection of the perineum at the routine postnatal examination. The fistula may be visible. Other malformations commonly coexist.

Acknowledgements

The contribution of Ruth McKee to this chapter in the 5th edition is gratefully acknowledged.

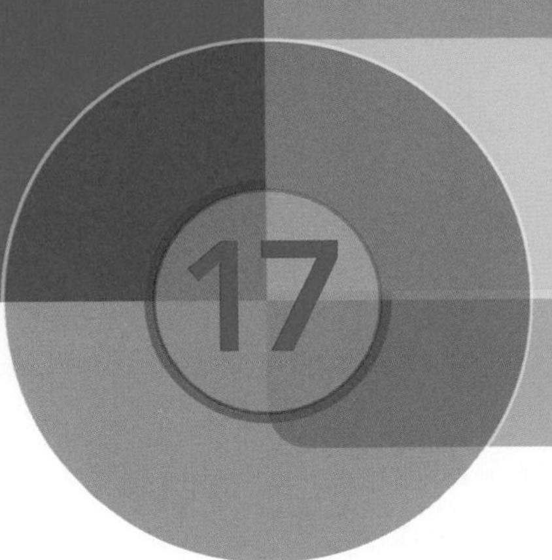

The kidneys, urinary tract and prostate

BEN CHALLACOMBE AND MATTHEW F BULTITUDE

Symptoms of renal and urinary tract disease

It is very important to obtain an exact history of the symptoms of renal and urinary tract disease because the kidney, ureter and bladder are not readily accessible for physical examination.

RENAL PAIN

Site Pain from the kidney is typically felt in the:

- *Loin*: the space below the 12th rib and the iliac crest.
- *Renal angle*: the angle between the 12th rib and the edge of the erector spinae muscle (Figure 17.1).

> **NOTE:** When asked to show you the site of renal pain, *the patient usually spreads a hand around his waist with fingers covering the renal angle and thumb above the anterior superior iliac spine.*

Nature Renal pain can be a *continuous dull ache* or be *sharp and very severe*. Do not use the term 'renal colic'. True colic is autonomically modulated and can only come from distension of the smooth muscle wall of a conducting tube such as the ureter. Because

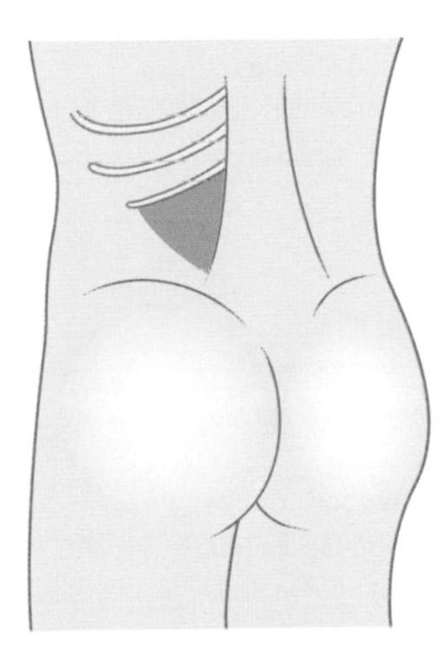

Figure 17.1 The renal angle is the area in the loin between the 12th rib and the edge of the erector spinae muscle.

the intensity of renal pain often fluctuates rapidly, it gets called renal colic, but patients rarely describe it as spasmodic, and *it does not usually disappear completely between exacerbations.*

URETERIC COLIC

Site Pain from the ureter is felt along the line of the ureter (Figure 17.2). *The point where it begins is a reliable indicator of the level of the obstruction.*

In most cases, the pain starts in the loin and then radiates downwards, around the waist, obliquely

Revision panel 17.1

CAUSES OF HAEMATURIA

Kidney

Congenital
Polycystic kidney
Traumatic
Blunt or penetrating injury
Stone
Inflammatory:
- Pyelonephritis
- Tuberculosis

Neoplastic:
- Renal cell carcinoma of the kidney
- Transitional cell carcinoma of the pelvi-calyceal system

Angiomyolipoma
Blood disorders:
- Anticoagulant drugs
- Purpura
- Sickle-cell disease
- Haemophilia
- Scurvy
- Malaria

Congestion:
- Right heart failure
- Renal vein thrombosis

Infarction:
- Arterial emboli from:
  - Myocardial infarct
  - Subacute bacterial endocarditis

Ureter

Stone
Neoplasm: transitional cell carcinoma
Trauma (often iatrogenic)

Bladder

Stone
Blunt or penetrating trauma
Iatrogenic (after endoscopic surgery)
Inflammatory:
- Bacterial cystitis
- Non-specific cystitis or ulceration
- Tuberculosis
- Schistosomiasis (bilharzia)

Neoplastic:
- Carcinoma (transitional cell/adenocarcinoma/squamous cell carcinoma)
- After radiotherapy to pelvis or bladder

Prostate

Benign and malignant enlargement
Acute prostatitis
Post-transurethral resection

Urethra

Traumatic:
- Rupture
- Stone
- Foreign body

Inflammatory:
- Acute urethritis

Neoplastic:
- Squamous cell carcinoma

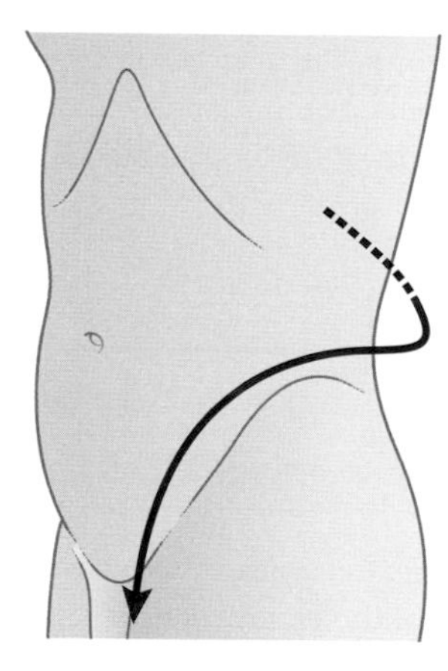

Figure 17.2 Ureteric colic radiates down from the renal angle, along a line parallel to the inguinal ligament, and into the base of the penis, the scrotum or the labium majus.

across the abdomen just above the inguinal ligament, and to the base of the penis, the testes or the labia.

Severity *Ureteric colic is severe.* The patient tries to relieve the pain by *rolling around the bed or walking about* (unlike patients with peritonitis). Patients often say it is the worst pain they have ever experienced, and females may say it is as bad as labour pains. It is accompanied by *sweating*, and often by *nausea* and *vomiting*.

Nature It is a true colic, griping in nature and coming in waves, with pain-free periods between attacks.

HAEMATURIA (REVISION PANEL 17.1)

Blood may be noticed during or after micturition. Minor bleeding may not affect the colour of the urine, or may make it look darker than usual. With heavy bleeding, the urine may be bright red. Old blood or clot in the bladder is usually very dark.

When the blood is coming from the prostate, bladder neck or the lower part of the urinary tract, it may appear only at the end of micturition.

Make sure that female patients have not mistaken menstrual bleeding for haematuria, and remember that there are other rare causes of a red/brown discolouration of the urine, such as:

- Eating large amounts of beetroot.
- Paroxysmal haemoglobinuria.
- Porphyria.
- Medications (e.g. rifampicin).

VESICAL PAIN

This is usually a *dull, suprapubic ache, made worse by micturition.*

Strangury (literally, squeezing urine) is a term used by some to describe a painful desire to micturate, which starts in the bladder and radiates into the urethra. Others use it to describe pain felt at the end of micturition as the patient squeezes out the last few drops of urine. To avoid confusion, do not use the term at all.

FREQUENCY OF MICTURITION

This may be caused by a reduction in functioning bladder capacity following incomplete emptying, or by irritation of the bladder mucosa. It is of greater significance if it wakes the patient from sleep, so *remember to ask about frequency by day and night.*

Dysuria should be used to describe *pain (often burning or stinging) that originates from the urethra during urination.* Do not confuse it with, for example, the abdominal pain experienced on micturition by a patient with appendicitis, which has a totally different cause.

PROSTATIC PAIN

Pain from the prostate gland is *felt deep inside the pelvis, between the legs, in the perineum and sometimes in the lower back.* It is poorly localized, and patients may think it is coming from the rectum, inner thigh or the penile tip.

Diseases of the urinary tract

CONGENITAL ANOMALIES OF THE RENAL TRACT

There are a large number of congenital anomalies of the urinary tract, many of which are symptomless and insignificant. Only some of the more common ones are considered here.

Horseshoe kidney

The incidence of horseshoe kidney is 1 in 400, males being affected twice as often as females.

The kidneys are joined at their lower poles by an isthmus, which is under the inferior mesenteric artery. This prevents them rising to the normal position, and pulls the pelves and ureters to face anteriorly, with the *ureters passing in front of the isthmus.*

The condition is associated with Turner's syndrome, trisomy 18 and other genitourinary abnormalities.

Although impalpable, horseshoe kidneys are at *increased risk of injury from abdominal trauma because of their reduced mobility.* They are usually symptomless, but there is an *increased risk of renal calculi, pelviureteric junction obstruction and infection* because of impaired drainage of the collecting systems.

Pelvic kidney

The incidence of pelvic kidney is 1 in 2000.

One kidney (usually the left) *fails to ascend normally and remains in the pelvis.* There may be contralateral renal agenesis or other anomalies. The condition is very rarely bilateral. The ectopic kidney is usually malrotated, with an anteriorly facing renal pelvis and a short ureter, although the ureteric orifice in the bladder is normal. Most cases are symptomless, but,

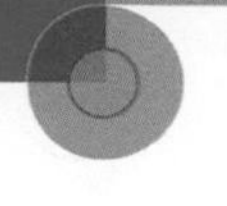

as with horseshoe kidneys, the impaired drainage can cause problems.

Malrotation may occur in normally placed kidneys, when the renal shape may also be abnormal. Again, the complications of impaired drainage may occur.

Duplex kidney/ureter

The incidence of duplex kidney is 1 in 125, with females being affected twice as often as males. The condition is usually unilateral.

There are two separate renal collecting systems draining into two ureters, which may join at the level of the kidney (a *bifid collecting system*) or at some point in their descent (*partial duplication*), or may remain separate all the way to the bladder, giving two ureteric orifices (*full duplication*).

The presentation can be with flank pain, loin mass and (recurrent) urinary infection, but *most are symptomless.*

In a complete duplex, the upper pole ureter enters the bladder below and medial to the lower pole ureter, giving it a longer intramural course. The lower-pole ureter is shorter and enters the bladder more directly. *The upper pole of the kidney is thus prone to obstruction, and the lower to reflux.*

Cross-fused renal ectopia

The incidence is 1 in 1000 births, males being affected twice as often as females. The kidneys are fused and located on the same side. Complications include infection and obstruction causing hydronephrosis and calculi.

HYDRONEPHROSIS

This is *distension of the calyces and pelvis of the kidney* (Revision panel 17.2).

It is often symptomless, but it may produce *renal pain*, may present as *renal failure* or may be detected when investigating the symptoms of the disease causing it.

History

Age Hydronephrosis occurs at all ages.

Symptoms The most common symptom is *pain in the loin*. This is a dull, persistent ache that can be so mild that it is accepted by the patient as backache and ignored, but which gets worse as the hydronephrosis enlarges. If a sudden enlargement occurs, the pain can be severe.

As it is autonomic pain, it is poorly localized and occasionally felt in unexpected sites such as the epigastrium. A patient with this sort of pain will never be able to localize the exact site with a finger, but will place their hand over quite a wide area.

The pain associated with hydronephrosis may be initiated or exacerbated by an increased urine flow. Alcohol and caffeinated drinks are diuretics and may exacerbate the pain, so check this when taking a history.

Revision panel 17.2

CAUSES OF HYDRONEPHROSIS

Unilateral

- Pelviureteric obstruction:
  - Congenital stenosis
  - Pressure from aberrant vessels
  - Stones and tumours in the renal pelvis, occluding the opening into the ureter
- Ureteric obstruction:
  - Stones
  - Tumour compressing or infiltrating the ureter from the cervix, rectum, colon or prostate
  - Tumours of the ureter
  - Ureterocele
  - Schistosomiasis
  - Bladder tumour
- Reflux

Bilateral

- Bladder outflow obstruction:
  - Benign prostatic enlargement
  - Urethral strictures and valves
  - Phimosis (causing chronic retention)
- Malignant invasion of the bladder trigone:
  - Carcinoma of the bladder
  - Carcinoma of the prostate
- External compression from malignant pelvic lymphadenopathy
- Retroperitoneal fibrosis
- Schistosomiasis

Pain is less frequent in bilateral hydronephrosis as the cause usually lies in the lower urinary tract, and distension of the renal pelvis tends to develop slowly.

Congenital pelviureteric junction obstruction is often intermittent and associated with more severe pain.

Only a very large hydronephrosis will cause abdominal distension.

There are usually no general symptoms unless the back pressure damages both kidneys so severely that renal failure and uraemia result.

Examination

The kidney is well hidden in the back wall of the abdomen (retroperitoneum), and *only a large hydronephrosis is palpable. The kidney may be tender, especially if there is coexisting infection*. The features of a palpable kidney are described in detail in Chapter 15.

An enlarged palpable hydronephrosis should:

- Arise from the loin.
- Be reducible into the loin.
- Be palpable bimanually.
- Be ballotable.

ACUTE PYELONEPHRITIS

Pyelitis is an infection in the upper part of the urinary tract caused by bacteria that have come from the bloodstream or up the ureter from the urethra or bladder. It is more common in females because the shorter length of their urethra makes the entry of bacteria into the lower urinary tract more likely.

History

Sex Pyelonephritis is much more common in females than in males.

Age It occurs in children, in females soon after the initiation of sexual activity ('honeymoon cystitis') and during pregnancy.

Symptoms The patient usually complains of a *sudden onset of severe pain in one or both loins*. It may occasionally be felt anteriorly, and on the right-hand side can be mistaken for biliary pain.

Either simultaneously with or before the onset of the loin pain, *micturition becomes frequent and painful*. Although there may be a vague suprapubic ache, the main pain during micturition is felt as a burning sensation along the length of the urethra. The patient may also complain of a painful desire to micturate, with only small volumes of urine produced.

Headache, malaise, nausea and vomiting often begin a few hours before the loin pain.

The urine may become cloudy and even bloodstained.

> **NOTE:** The patient feels ill, hot and sweaty and may, in severe cases, suffer rigors and be clinically septic.

Cause The patient may have had similar attacks and be aware of their relationship to sexual intercourse or pregnancy.

Examination

General features The patient looks ill and may be *flushed and sweating with fever and tachycardia*. The tongue is dry and furred.

Abdomen One or both kidneys are moderately tender when palpated through the abdomen, and the *renal angle is very tender*. Guarding and peritonism will not be found. There may be mild suprapubic tenderness.

The kidneys are not clinically enlarged unless the infection has arisen in a previously hydronephrotic kidney.

Urine The urine may look cloudy and bloodstained. *Red blood cells and pus cells will be seen on microscopy.*

GENITOURINARY TUBERCULOSIS

This is now a rare condition in countries with good access to healthcare, although it has been more common in recent years. It produces fibrosis, scarring, calcification and strictures. Presentation is often late, when chronic damage has already been done.

History

Age It can occur at any age, but is most common in the fourth decade.

Sex It is twice as common in males.

Travel The patient may have travelled to areas where tuberculosis is endemic, but infection can occur from exposure to infected individuals anywhere.

General Patients may complain of *weight loss, night sweats* or *chronic chest symptoms*.

Urological symptoms Tuberculosis can affect anywhere in the urogenital tract, so the range of symptoms is wide. There may be *loin pain* (from ureteric obstruction), *haematuria* or *lower urinary tract symptoms* (from bladder inflammation, fibrosis and scarring).

A history of chronic recurrent urinary tract infection, usually with negative bacterial cultures but pyuria, should raise a suspicion of tuberculosis.

> **NOTE:** The symptoms of genitourinary tuberculosis are non-specific. Therefore, the condition should be borne in mind in any patient with recurrent unexplained urological symptoms or failure to respond to treatment.

Examination

General There will rarely be any physical signs, but there may be evidence of weight loss. The prostate should be examined as prostatic tuberculosis may mimic malignancy, with a firm or hard prostate on palpation.

External genitalia Tuberculous epididymitis is described in Chapter 18.

CARCINOMA OF THE KIDNEY

Correctly called a renal cell carcinoma, and usually of *clear cell, papillary* or *chromophobe* subtypes, this tumour was previously called a hypernephroma because of its macroscopic appearance and site of occurrence. It can present in a huge variety of ways due to local, metastatic, general and paraneoplastic effects.

History

Age Carcinoma of the kidney is uncommon below the age of 50 years.

Sex It is twice as common in males as it is in females. Symptoms are often a late presentation and often these are incidental findings as a result of the increase in the number of imaging studies being performed.

Symptoms

- **Haematuria** This is the most common symptom. The bleeding is usually intermittent, macroscopic and sufficient to stain the urine a pale red colour.

  Occasionally, the bleeding is heavy, and causes ureteric colic as blood clots obstruct the ureter (clot colic).
- **General debility** Many patients with renal carcinoma have no symptoms until metastases or the burden of the primary tumour cause *general malaise, loss of energy and loss of weight.*
- **Bone pain/fractures** Carcinoma of the kidney is one of the cancers that metastasizes to bone, and some patients present with bone pain and pathological fractures.
- **Pain in the loin** When this occurs, it usually signifies advanced disease.
- **A mass** A mass may be felt by chance at a routine examination or by the patient, or it may cause abdominal distension.

Less common symptoms include:

- **Pyrexia of unknown origin** Carcinoma of the kidney should be excluded in every patient who presents with this.
- **Polycythaemia** The tumour cells produce erythropoietin, resulting in polycythaemia. This causes redness of the face and hands, and spontaneous venous and arterial thromboses. To emphasize the multiplicity of symptoms of renal cancer, other patients present with *anaemia* from their haematuria.
- **Varicocele** Occlusion of the renal and testicular veins by direct spread of the tumour along the renal vein can cause an acute onset varicocele (see Chapter 18). There may even be inferior vena caval obstruction, producing oedema of both legs and the abdominal wall.
- **Pain** Sudden severe abdominal pain may indicate acute haemorrhage into the tumour or even spontaneous rupture, with collapse caused by massive intraperitoneal bleeding.
- **Hypertension** of renal origin is a rare complication of renal carcinoma.

Examination

General features The patient may show signs of recent weight loss.

Abdomen *Large tumours* are palpable, and demonstrate the physical signs of an enlarged kidney. There is no tenderness.

Skeleton There may be areas of swelling and tenderness in the bones, at the sites of secondary deposits. Very rarely, such deposits of renal carcinoma are vascular and feel soft with an audible bruit.

Chest There may be a pleural effusion on the side of the tumour if it has spread through the diaphragm.

The usual type of lung metastasis, sometimes solitary, from carcinoma of the kidney has a *'cannon ball' appearance* on thoracic CT or chest X-ray.

NOTE: Although rare, renal tumours are among the most common causes of an abdominal mass in children, accounting for 7% of malignancies.

CHILDHOOD RENAL TUMOURS

Symptoms There may be *abdominal pain* and bloating, as well as *macroscopic haematuria*, usually painless but sometimes producing clot colic. Pressure effects include *anorexia, malaise, lethargy, nausea* and *vomiting*.

Signs An abdominal mass is seen, perhaps with evidence of disseminated malignancy.

Wilms tumour/nephroblastoma

Incidence *The most common childhood renal tumour* occurring in one in 125,000 individuals. A total of 5% of cases are bilateral (either synchronous or metachronous).

Age Peak age is 3–4 years.

Race There is a preponderance of Afro-Caribbean children.

Associated conditions One-quarter of children affected have another congenital anomaly, including hemihypertrophy, cryptorchidism and hypospadias. In some rare syndromes, there is a role for screening for renal masses.

In addition to the symptoms listed above, there may be fever, and occasionally hypertension. The tumours are encapsulated, vascular and generally do not cross the midline, but they may metastasize widely.

Other childhood renal tumours

There are a number of extremely rare kidney tumours that present in the same way as a Wilms tumour, and the diagnosis is often not made until after resection. These tumours usually have a higher rate of relapse and death than classical Wilms tumours.

Renal cell carcinoma can be seen in children and adolescents, often related to von Hippel–Lindau disease, familial renal cell carcinoma or sickle-cell disease.

CARCINOMA OF THE RENAL PELVIS

This is a transitional cell carcinoma of the urothelium, and is identical to the type commonly found in the bladder. It is often associated with tumours elsewhere in the urinary tract, but may be the only manifestation of uroepithelial malignant change.

The condition presents with *haematuria* and occasionally with *clot colic*, with clots described as 'stringy'. There are no physical signs.

RENAL AND URETERIC CALCULI

Stones in renal calyces may lie silent for years and not present until complications such as infection occur. Stones in the ureter usually cause pain.

History

Age Renal and ureteric calculi are found most often between the ages of 30 and 50 years.

Sex They are more common in males than in females.

Occupation They are more common in professionals and manual workers.

Season Urinary calculi develop more frequently in the summer, perhaps initiated by the lower urine flow in warm, dry weather, and an abundance of soft fruits, which are rich in oxalates, an important constituent of calculi.

Symptoms The principal symptoms are *pain and haematuria*.

The pain depends on the site of the stone. *A dull ache in the loin is typical of a renal stone.* A stone in the ureter produces *ureteric colic* (described above), which moves down along the line of the ureter as the stone makes its way to the bladder. All stones start in the kidney. A large stone will not pass the pelvi-ureteric junction. A stone small enough to enter the ureter will often pass through to the bladder, with much patient discomfort as it intermittently becomes jammed and causes colic.

Ninety percent of patients with ureteric colic have microscopic haematuria. Visible haematuria is unusual.

The first indication of the presence of a stone may be acute pyelonephritis, or if the calculous disease has damaged renal function, symptoms of uraemia.

Examination

Abdomen Abdominal examination is difficult during an attack of ureteric colic because the patient is rolling around with tense muscles. There may be secondary abdominal distension, as with other problems that arise in the posterior abdominal wall.

Investigation with CT or ultrasound is needed to make the diagnosis.

Some metabolic disorders predispose to the formation of urinary calculi. The most common (1 in 300) is *hyperparathyroidism* (see Chapter 12). There may be symptoms of hypercalcaemia (thirst, polydypsia, nausea, vomiting and eventually drowsiness).

> **NOTE:** All patients with stone disease should have their serum calcium and uric acid measured.

BLADDER CALCULI

Stones may form in the bladder in association with stasis (usually due to benign prostatic hypertrophy), infection or tumour, or enter from the ureter. There is always a degree of *bladder outflow obstruction* or *bladder dysfunction*, otherwise the stone would have been rapidly voided.

History

Age Bladder stones are *rare in Western countries,* except in middle-aged and elderly males with prostatic problems.

Symptoms The most common symptom is *increased frequency of micturition*, sometimes related to posture. When the patient stands up, the stone falls onto the trigone, causing a stabbing pain and initiating a desire to micturate. During the night, the stone rolls away and the problem resolves.

There is sometimes a history of a *sudden cessation of urinary flow,* which is relieved by lying down.

There may be suprapubic stabbing pain, exacerbated by standing.

Haematuria, particularly at the end of micturition, also occurs.

Many patients have chronic infection, with the *symptoms of cystitis.*

The symptoms caused by the stone are often preceded by the symptoms of its cause, namely bladder outflow obstruction, recurrent infections and bladder tumours.

Examination

There are rarely any physical signs, although very large stones can sometimes be felt on bimanual examination of the pelvis.

Sounding the bladder Bladder stones were common in past centuries and were diagnosed, before X-rays, by passing a metal instrument into the bladder via the urethra and listening to the sound made as it tapped on the stone. The legacy of this is the instrument named a urethral 'sound'.

CYSTITIS

Cystitis is infection of the urine within the bladder, with a concomitant inflammatory reaction in the bladder wall. The common predisposing factors for cystitis are incomplete emptying of the bladder, abnormalities within the bladder and, in females, bacteria migrating up the urethra. In females, there is often a clear relationship with sexual activity.

History

Age Cystitis occurs often in young and middle-aged females, in young males with urethritis and in elderly males with benign prostatic enlargement and bladder tumours.

Symptoms *The usual symptoms are increased frequency and urgency of micturition,* which begin suddenly and persist through the night as well as the day. The patient often wants to micturate every few minutes.

Passing urine causes a *burning or scalding pain along the length of the urethra.* It is often so bad that the patient tries to avoid passing urine. There may be a mild suprapubic ache.

Haematuria is common, with a few drops of bloody urine at the end of micturition. The urine may be cloudy and malodorous.

Examination

Mild suprapubic tenderness is the only physical sign.

> **NOTE:** Remember to look at and dipstick-test the urine, *and to send it for culture.*

URETHRAL SYNDROME

Many females with the symptoms of recurrent cystitis never have bacteria demonstrated in the urine. This collection of symptoms is termed the urethral syndrome. Its cause is unknown and its management difficult.

CARCINOMA OF THE BLADDER

Bladder cancer is *usually a transitional cell carcinoma,* although there are rarer types (squamous cell and adenocarcinoma) that can be more common in certain parts of the world. It rarely produces any physical signs, so the diagnosis must be suspected from the history.

History

Age Bladder cancer occurs throughout adult life, with a peak incidence between 60 and 70 years.

Sex Males are afflicted more often than females, *and smoking is the main risk factor.*

Occupation Some industrial chemicals are excreted in the urine and can stimulate malignant change in the uroepithelium (Revision panel 17.3). The better known ones are *alpha* and *beta-naphthylamine, benzidine* and *xylenamine,* and artificial sweeteners such as *cyclamates.* The industries that use these chemicals (the rubber and cable industries, printing and dyeing) are well aware of the relationship, and chemically induced bladder cancer is now rare.

Revision panel 17.3

RISK FACTORS FOR BLADDER CANCER

Bladder carcinogens

- Smoking
- Aniline dyes
- Alpha- and beta-naphthylamine
- Xylenamine
- Benzidine

Occupations associated with exposure to bladder carcinogens

- Dry cleaners
- Hairdressers
- Leather workers
- Painters and decorators
- Paper and rubber manufacturers
- Dental technicians

Predisposing conditions *Squamous cell carcinoma* may be induced by the chronic irritation caused by *schistosomiasis, bladder calculi* or recurrent infections.

Symptoms In 95% of cases, carcinoma of the bladder presents with *bright red haematuria,* which may be intermittent or occur every time the bladder is emptied. The passage of blood clots may cause pain and difficulty with micturition.

NOTE: Visible haematuria should always prompt investigation.

If the urine becomes infected, the patient will experience a suprapubic ache and burning micturition.

Pain in the loin may occur, as bladder tumours often begin near the ureteric orifice and obstruct the lower end of the ureter.

Pain in the pelvis and lower abdomen, and nerve root pain down the legs, can occur if the tumour spreads through the wall of the bladder into the pelvis.

A small group of patients with bladder cancer present with *frequent and painful micturition,* without visible haematuria, but there will be microscopic haematuria.

NOTE: Never forget that symptoms of cystitis may indicate a bladder tumour, particularly when they persist after treatment. Large tumours can also result in recurrent urinary infection by harbouring bacteria.

Examination

It is unusual to find any abnormality. If the tumour is large, it may be felt bimanually or on rectal examination alone, and if it has spread beyond the bladder, the floor of the pelvis may be indurated.

Examination under anaesthetic is an important part of staging a bladder tumour.

Retention of urine

There are two classic forms of retention of urine, acute and chronic, which are usually easily distinguished.

Acute retention is painful and sudden. Chronic retention is painless, and there is a chronically distended bladder.

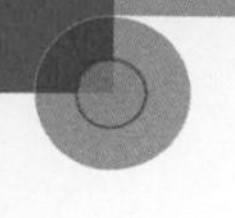

As ever in medicine, things are rarely so discrete. Acute retention may develop in the presence of chronic retention, when the expression *acute-on-chronic retention* is sometimes used.

Acute retention in the absence of bladder outlet obstruction is rare, and occurs only after a surgical operation, anaesthesia or an injury to the urethra. Most patients with acute retention give a history of progressive slowing of the urinary stream caused by narrowing of the bladder outlet or urethra. *This is termed bladder outflow obstruction.*

Patients with *chronic retention* may be symptom free except for the abdominal swelling produced by the large bladder and can present with enuresis (involuntary leakage of urine at night).

> **NOTE:** Acute retention is the sudden, painful inability to micturate.
>
> Chronic retention is an enlarged, painless bladder, whether or not the patient is having difficulty micturating.

The causes of retention are listed in Revision panel 17.4. It is a long list, but *the most common cause by far is prostatic obstruction* (benign or malignant) in middle-aged and elderly males. In hospitals, an operation under general anaesthesia is a common precipitating factor.

Revision panel 17.4

CAUSES OF RETENTION OF URINE

Mechanical

- In the lumen of the urethra, or overlying the internal urethral orifice:
  - Blood clot
  - Stones
  - Tumour
  - Foreign bodies
  - Congenital valves
- In the wall of the bladder or the urethra:
  - Prostatic enlargement (benign and malignant)
  - Trauma (rupture of the urethra)
  - Urethral stricture
  - Urethritis
  - Meatal ulcer
  - Tumour
  - Postprostate biopsy due to prostatic swelling
- Outside the wall:
  - Pregnancy (retroverted gravid uterus)
  - Fibroids
  - Ovarian cyst
  - Faecal impaction
  - Phimosis or paraphimosis

Neurogenic

- Denervation of bladder (e.g. after rectal resection)
- Diabetes
- Postoperative retention
- Spinal cord injuries
- Spinal cord disease
- Multiple sclerosis
- Psychogenic
- Drugs:
  - Alcohol
  - Anticholinergics
  - Antihistamines
  - Smooth muscle relaxants
  - Some tranquillizers

ACUTE RETENTION

History

Symptoms The patient is likely to have symptoms related to one of the causes listed in Revision panel 17.4, as well as suprapubic pain and an inability to pass urine. *The pain is severe and is described as a gross exaggeration of the normal desire to micturate.* The patient is aware that the bladder is overdistended.

Examination

The bladder has usually enlarged sufficiently to become *a palpable, tense, dull, rounded, tender mass arising out of the pelvis* to a point a few centimetres above the pubis (Figure 17.3). Gentle pressure on the swelling exacerbates the patient's desire to micturate. It may however be too tender to palpate, particularly when the abdominal wall is tense or the patient is overweight.

Percussion is useful in deciding whether a patient is in acute retention, as the bladder is always dull.

The bladder may reach up to, or above, the umbilicus if the patient has had chronic retention before the acute episode. A large bladder of this size indicates acute-on-chronic retention.

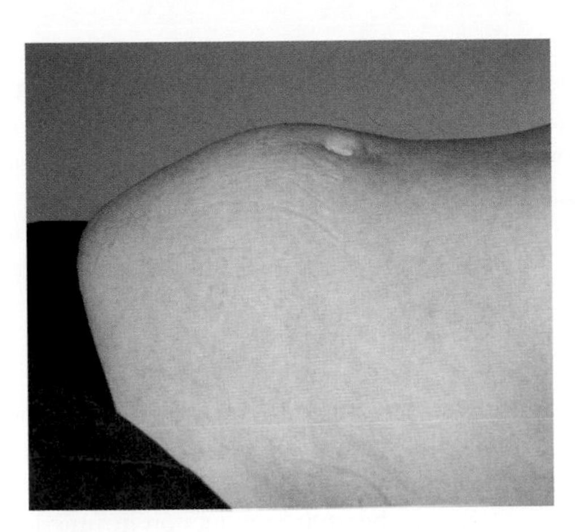

Figure 17.3 Bladder distension.

Rectal examination, if the patient is not too distressed, will reveal that the prostate or uterus is pushed backwards and downwards, with the cystic mass of the bladder filling the front half of the pelvis.

> **NOTE:** You cannot assess the size of the prostate gland, or the pelvis, when the bladder is full. It is better to defer the rectal examination for prostate assessment until after the retention has been relieved with a catheter.

Remember to examine not only the prostate, the urethra and the contents of the pelvis, but also the central and peripheral nervous systems to exclude a neurological cause.

CHRONIC RETENTION

There are two varieties of chronic retention – *high pressure and low pressure.*

In the *high-pressure type,* the cause is obstruction of the bladder outlet. Bladder pressure builds up and, in a proportion of cases, produces dilatation of the ureters and the renal collection systems as well as the bladder. This ultimately results in renal failure, of the postrenal type.

In the *low-pressure type,* the fault seems to lie with the bladder muscle, which is atonic. The vesicoureteric junctions remain competent, and there is no back-pressure effect on the kidneys.

The retention is of the high pressure type if a patient in chronic retention has the symptoms and signs of renal failure.

History

Age and sex Chronic retention is most common in elderly males.

Symptoms The patient may be unaware of his chronic retention, but complains of symptoms related to bladder outflow obstruction, such as *hesitancy, poor and intermittent flow, nocturia and postmicturition dribbling.*

Chronic retention is painless.

Many patients with chronic retention have *dribbling overflow incontinence,* particularly at night. This is not nocturia but leakage while asleep, and is pathognomonic of chronic retention.

Examination

The bladder will be palpable. It is likely to reach at least half way up to the umbilicus. It is not tense or tender, and suprapubic pressure may not always induce a desire to micturate.

The palpable bladder of chronic retention is dull to percussion, will fluctuate and has a fluid thrill.

Look for signs of the cause of the retention in the pelvis, prostate, urethra and nervous system.

BLADDER DIVERTICULA

This is an outpouching of bladder mucosa through a defect in all layers of the muscle in the bladder wall.

Diverticula usually occur just above one or both ureteric orifices. They are caused by outflow obstruction or can be congenital.

Bladder diverticula are rarely palpable because of their position, but they may give rise to a peculiar symptom. When the patient needs to pass urine, the muscle contracts and empties the bladder, but the diverticulum does not empty because its orifice closes as the bladder shrinks. When the patient has finished and the detrusor muscle relaxes, the urine in the diverticulum passes into the bladder, and within minutes the patient feels the need to micturate again (*pis en deux*).

Conditons of the prostate gland

BENIGN ENLARGEMENT (HYPERPLASIA) OF THE PROSTATE GLAND

The inner portion (*transitional zone*) of the prostate gland enlarges during late adult life. As it grows, it

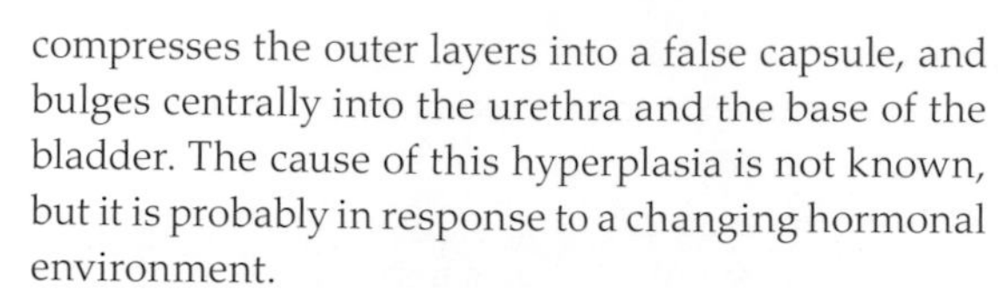

compresses the outer layers into a false capsule, and bulges centrally into the urethra and the base of the bladder. The cause of this hyperplasia is not known, but it is probably in response to a changing hormonal environment.

The voiding symptoms of prostatic obstruction result from either *mechanical obstruction (voiding symptoms)* or *secondary overactivity of the bladder detrusor muscle (storage symptoms)*. They are summarized in Revision panel 17.5.

Revision panel 17.5

SYMPTOMS OF HYPERTROPHY OF THE PROSTATE GLAND

Symptoms of bladder outflow obstruction (voiding symptoms)

Hesitancy
Poor flow
Intermittent flow
Postmicturition dribbling
Sensation of incomplete emptying
Double micturition

Symptoms of bladder and bladder neck irritation (storage symptoms)

Increased frequency of micturition
Urgency
Nocturia
Urge incontinence

History

Age The prostate starts enlarging at the age of 40 years, but symptoms commonly appear between the ages of 50 and 70 years.

Symptoms The cardinal symptom of prostatic obstruction is *a reduced rate of urine flow during micturition, that is, a poor stream.* The condition develops slowly and intermittently, and the bladder compensates by muscular hypertrophy of its wall, which initially overcomes the increased outflow resistance. In consequence, the reduced rate of flow comes on gradually, and you must enquire about this. Ask whether the flow is as good as it was 20 years earlier.

Hesitancy Associated with the reduced urinary flow are two other symptoms, hesitancy and dribbling. *Hesitancy is the inability to start to pass urine.* Straining does not help; it actually prolongs the waiting time before the urine starts to flow.

Dribbling *This is the inability to finish cleanly.* A few drops continue to appear for some time after the main stream has ceased. This goes on until patience is lost, resulting in staining of the underclothing.

Increased frequency What the patient complains of most is increased frequency of micturition, often first noticed when it is necessary to pass urine during the night (*nocturia*). Inadequate emptying of the bladder, and therefore a reduction in functional volume (the additional volume needed to trigger the desire to micturate), is the cause of the frequency.

Urgency In addition to increased frequency of micturition, the patient reports an urgent need to start passing urine as soon as the desire arises. This is called urgency, and is caused by increased bladder pressure.

Haematuria, in the form of a little dark blood at the end of micturition, is a not uncommon symptom, but should be investigated appropriately to rule out bladder or renal malignancy.

A proportion of patients first present with acute or chronic retention, described above.

Examination

Abdomen The bladder will be palpable if there is acute or chronic retention.

Rectal examination Benign hyperplasia causes a diffuse prostatic enlargement. The gland bulges into the rectum, its surface is smooth, but the enlargement is often slightly asymmetrical and the surface bosselated. The consistency of the gland is *firm, rubbery and homogeneous.*

The *median sulcus usually remains palpable,* even when the gland is grossly enlarged, and the rectal mucosa moves freely over the gland. It is not tender.

> **NOTE:** that there may be quite significant prostatic obstruction without gross enlargement of the gland. The key factor in the generation of symptoms is the compression of the prostatic urethra, which may occur with quite modest enlargement.

Remember that a full bladder pushes the prostate downwards and makes it feel bigger.

CARCINOMA OF THE PROSTATE

Adenocarcinoma of the prostate gland usually begins in its outer part (the *peripheral zone*), which permits easy spread into the seminal vesicles and floor of the pelvis. It is commonly quite locally advanced before it causes lower urinary tract symptoms.

History

Age It is predominantly a disease of the elderly. Its incidence increases from the 50s onwards.

> **NOTE:** By the late 80s and 90s it can be found in nearly all males, but in the vast majority it produces no symptoms or signs.

Symptoms The most common presentation is with symptoms similar to those caused by benign prostatic hypertrophy and collectively called voiding symptoms, namely *hesitancy, poor stream, incomplete emptying, coupled with urgency and frequency*. With prostatic cancer, these symptoms tend to progress more rapidly and do not fluctuate in severity, as is so often the case with benign hypertrophy.

A proportion of patients with carcinoma of the prostate present with some form of retention of urine.

It may cause pain in the lower abdomen and perineum if the tumour spreads outside the gland.

Presentation with secondary metastases is common, with local symptoms that are absent or ignored. There may be debility and loss of weight.

Prostatic cancer metastasizes to bone, particularly the *pelvis and lumbar spine*. These bone deposits are nearly always osteosclerotic and osteoblastic, so tend to produce bone pain rather than pathological fractures (see Chapter 6).

> **NOTE:** Do not forget to consider prostatic bone metastases in any elderly male with skeletal pain.

Screening Prostatic cancer may be detected by measuring the serum levels of *prostate-specific antigen*. There is controversy over the value of this investigation as a screening tool, as it has been estimated that, on the basis of this test, there are approximately 1 million males with occult prostatic cancer in the UK, but only 12,000 die from the disease each year. An elevated prostate-specific antigen is now the commonest mode of presentation. A prostate MRI may also be used to clarify prostate cancer risk.

Examination

The bladder will be palpable if there is retention of urine.

Rectal examination The prostate gland may be asymmetrically enlarged or distorted. It is irregular in contour and heterogeneous in texture. Some areas are hard and knobbly; others are soft. The median sulcus may be absent, and the rectal mucosa may be tethered to the gland. However, if the presentation is through a raised PSA level, the prostate often does not feel malignant.

The tissues of the pelvis, lateral to the gland and around the rectum, may be infiltrated by tumour, and it may be possible to feel seminal vesical involvement.

Other physical signs will be those caused by metastases. Carcinoma of the prostate gland sometimes gives rise to metastases in the skin and other unusual sites, as well as in bone. Presentation is occasionally with symptoms of renal impairment, either from retention of urine or direct invasion of the bladder base and obstruction of the ureters.

Conditons of the urethra

URETHRITIS

This produces symptoms of *painful micturition*, with a *purulent discharge from the external meatus*, which is easier to notice in males than in females. It is usually caused by a sexually transmitted disease, commonly *Gonococcus* and *Chlamydia*. If not properly and promptly treated, it heals with a scar, producing a urethral stricture (see Revision panel 17.6).

URETHRAL STRICTURE

These strictures occur as a result of the damage or destruction of the urethral mucosa followed by healing with fibrous scar tissue usually due to infection or trauma (see Revision panel 17.7).

History

Age Urethral strictures occur at all ages. The most common cause *used to be gonorrhoea*, which is a disease of the sexually active, so the strictures that follow it appeared in young and middle-aged males.

Revision panel 17.6

CAUSES OF URETHRAL DISCHARGE

Infection (urethritis)

- *Gonococcus*
- *Chlamydia*
- *Coliforms*
- *Trichomonas*
- *Candida*

Lesions in the urethra

- Warts
- Herpes

Foreign bodies

Revision panel 17.7

THE CAUSES OF URETHRAL STRICTURE

Congenital

- Pinhole meatus
- Urethral valves (not a true stricture)

Traumatic

- Instrumentation (catheterization)
- Foreign bodies
- Prostatectomy (transurethral or radical prostatectomy)
- Amputation of the penis
- Direct perineal injuries

Inflammatory

- Gonorrhoea/non-specific urethritis/chlamydia
- Meatal ulceration/balanitis
- Balanitis xerotica obliterans (lichen scelosus)

Neoplastic

- Primary and secondary neoplasms

Better and quicker treatment of the infection has reduced the incidence of postgonorrhoeal strictures, and the most common cause nowadays is probably *catheterization or surgical instrumentation of the urethra.*

Symptoms The key symptom is *poor urinary flow, with a classical flat and prolonged trace on flow rate measurements. The stream is prolonged, thin and dribbles at its end.* Attacks of cystitis are common, but retention of urine is rare unless there is added pathology such as a bladder calculus.

There may be a *urethral discharge,* which is particularly noticeable in the morning.

Increasing frequency of micturition indicates that the bladder is not emptying completely.

Examination

The bladder is sometimes palpable. Renal failure is occasionally seen.

The penis and urethra usually feel normal because the most common site for stricture is where the urethra passes through the perineal membrane. A stricture caused by scarring of the penile urethra can *sometimes be felt as an area of induration.*

Meatal strictures, common following transurethral operations, are usually visible if the edges of the meatus are gently retracted.

Trauma to the urinary tract

RENAL TRAUMA

The kidneys are protected by the rib cage and are mobile, so injury from blunt trauma is relatively unlikely (see Chapter 5).

There may be flank pain and tenderness, or bruising and haematuria. *The patient may be shocked and haemodynamically unstable.* The diagnosis can be made only with CT imaging, and occasionally at urgent laparotomy. Simultaneous injury to other viscera is common.

BLADDER TRAUMA

Usually only a full bladder will be ruptured in abdominal trauma. The tear is usually intraperitoneal, so urine collects in the abdominal cavity where it does not produce significant peritoneal irritation. The diagnosis is suggested when the (sometimes inebriated) patient does not pass urine and does not feel the need.

URETHRAL TRAUMA

The site of injury may be suspected from the history:

- The penile urethra is occasionally injured during sexual intercourse.

- The bulbar urethra may be injured by falling astride a fairly narrow object.
- The membranous urethra may be damaged and even transected by a pelvic fracture.

Urethral injury is suspected if the patient *is unable to pass urine, or there is blood at the external meatus.*

The findings depend on the site of the injury:

- There will be *tenderness and bruising* at the site of injury to the penile urethra.
- *Bruising and extravasated urine* are seen if the rupture (total or partial) of the bulbar urethra is deep to the membranous layer of the superficial fascia. In this situation, the blood tracks to the perineum, scrotum, lower abdomen and the upper thighs, but only as far as the attachment of the fascia.
- Rupture of the membranous urethra allows the *bladder and prostate to float upwards*. This is theoretically palpable on rectal examination (*high-riding prostate*), but this is likely to be impossible in a patient with a fractured pelvis.

Penetrating trauma of the urinary tract is unusual. The history and site of the entrance wound will suggest the diagnosis, which is usually confirmed on surgical exploration.

18 The external genitalia

ARUN SAHAI AND MATTHEW F BULTITUDE

Examination of the male genitalia

Remember to have warm hands, wear protective gloves and take care to be gentle, especially if the testes are tender.

THE PENIS

Inspection (Figure 18.1)

Note the size and shape of the penis, the colour of the skin, the presence or absence of the foreskin, scarring and the position and patency of the urethral

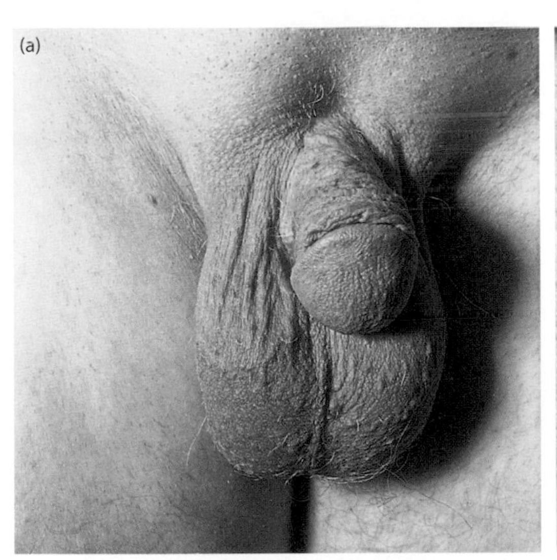

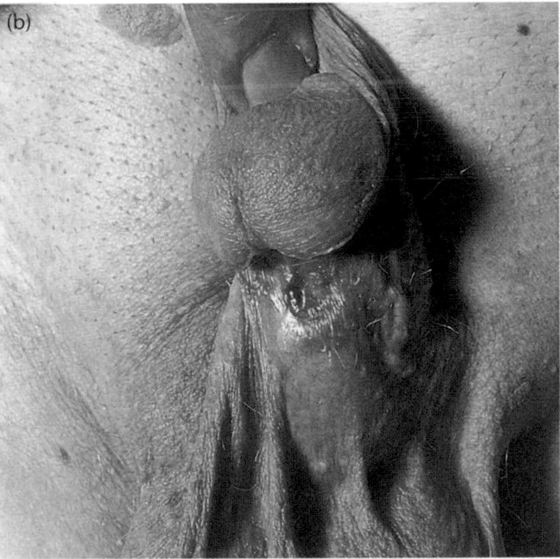

Figure 18.1 EXAMINATION OF THE PENIS. (a) Always look at the ventral surface of the penis. (b) In this patient, this revealed a hypospadias.

meatus. Inspection of the penis in an erect state may also be informative in cases of suspected Peyronie's disease (see later). Some patients may bring a photograph to allow this.

Palpation

Assess the texture of the body of the penis and the whole length of the urethra, right down to the perineal membrane. Palpate the corporal bodies assessing for the possibility of plaque deposition, which feels nodular, or other pathology.

Ask the patient to retract the prepuce to examine the skin on its inner aspect, the glans penis and the external urethral meatus (Figure 18.2).

> **NOTE:** At birth, the foreskin is tethered to the glans penis with only a small opening, so do not try to retract the foreskin of a small child (less than 4 years of age).

THE SCROTAL SKIN

The skin of the scrotum is usually wrinkled and freely mobile over the testes. If it is reddened, tethered or fixed, there is probably a deep abnormality. Do not forget that the conditions that affect hair-bearing skin on any other part of the body – *sebaceous cyst, infected hair follicle and squamous carcinoma – may affect the scrotal skin*.

Remember that the scrotum has a back and front, *and do not forget to examine its posterior aspect* (Figure 18.3).

Should you find a lesion in the scrotal skin, proceed methodically through your examination of any lump or ulcer found elsewhere (see Chapter 1).

THE SCROTAL CONTENTS

The shape of the scrotum and the position of the testes within it can only be observed properly when the patient is standing up, but it is more comfortable for patient and student to perform the major part of the examination with the patient lying supine.

Inspection

Note the size and shape of the scrotum, particularly any *asymmetry, erythema, discharge, scarring* and the *presence and location of both testes*.

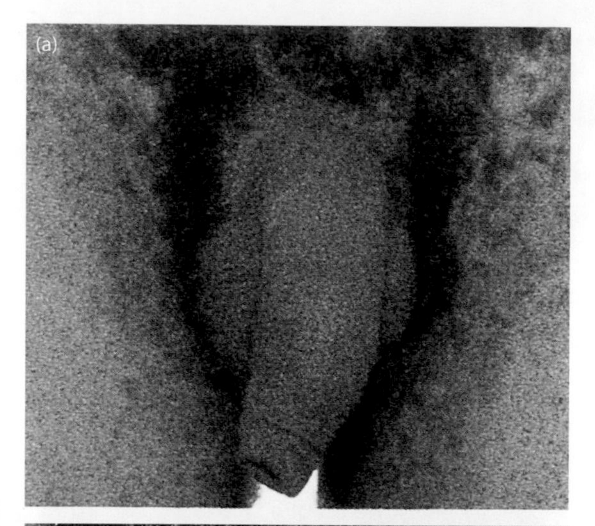

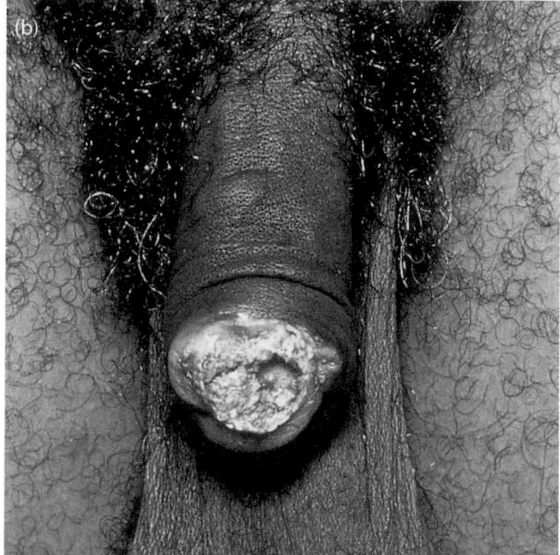

Figure 18.2 EXAMINATION OF THE PENIS. (a) Always retract the prepuce and inspect its inner surface, and the glans penis. (b) In this patient, this revealed a carcinoma.

Palpation

First, is there a testicle on each side?

The scrotal contents are examined by gently supporting the scrotum on the fingers of one or both hands, while feeling the testis and any other lumps between your index finger, which is behind the scrotum, and your thumb, which is in front. Do not squeeze the testis or a lump between your thumb and index finger – let it slip from side to side so that you can feel its shape and surface.

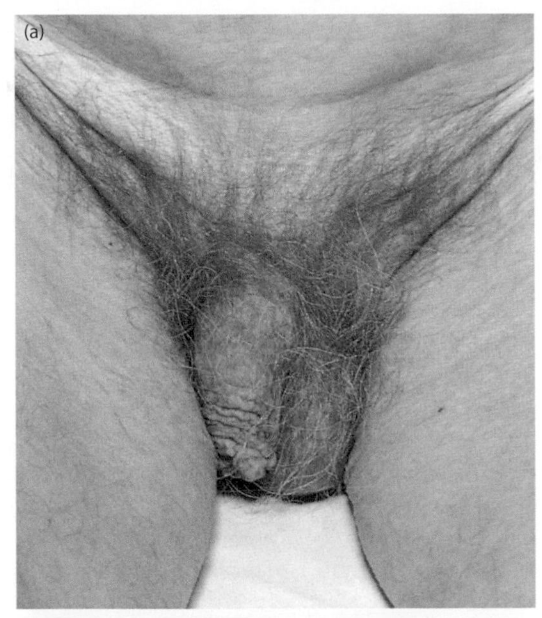

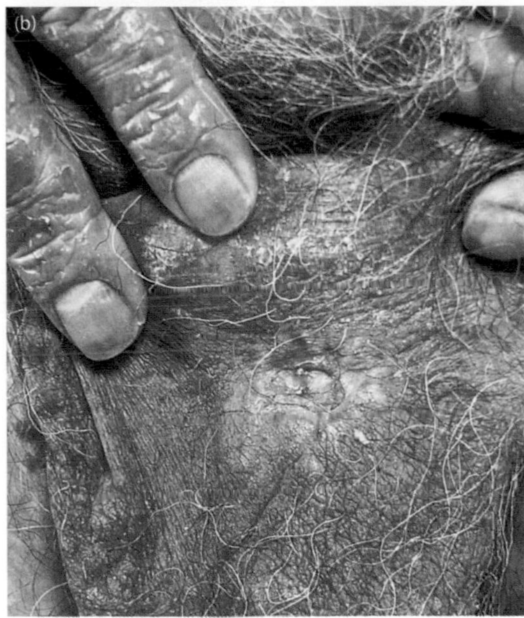

Figure 18.3 EXAMINATION OF THE SCROTUM. (a) Always look at the posterior surface of the scrotum. (b) In this patient, this revealed a squamous carcinoma.

Decide the position and nature of the body of each testis, epididymis (which lies on the posterior border of the tesis) and spermatic cords. If you are unsure if what you are feeling is the testis, ask the patient. The testis has unique sensation.

With knowledge of the anatomy and the pathology of scrotal conditions, it is possible to make an accurate clinical diagnosis in most cases.

There are several characteristics of any scrotal lump that must be determined for all scrotal lumps:

- Can you get above it? (Is the lump confined to the scrotum?)
- Does the lump transilluminate?
- Does the lump have an expansile cough impulse?
- Is the lump separate from the body of the testis?

When you have established the answers to these questions, and have defined the physical characteristics of the lump and its relations to each testis and epididymis, you will be able to make the diagnosis. Record your findings on a diagram similar to that shown in Figure 18.4.

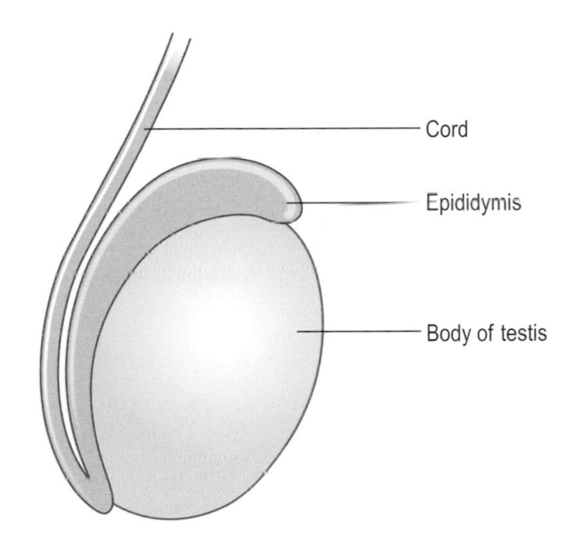

Figure 18.4 If you think of the way in which you will draw the testes, and any abnormality you find, in your notes, it will help you to define the anatomy. Define the cord, the epididymis and the body of the testes.

THE PERINEUM AND RECTUM

Examination of the perineum and rectal examination to feel the prostate is required in many cases (see Chapter 16). If in doubt it is better to do the examination.

LYMPH DRAINAGE

The skin of the external genitalia drains to the inguinal lymph glands (Figure 18.5). The scrotal contents, however, develop in the para-aortic area in the retroperitoneum. During the descent into the scrotum, the arterial blood supply, venous and lymphatic drainage follow the testis. In consequence:

- Lymph from the skin of the penis and scrotum drains to the inguinal glands.
- Lymph from the coverings of the testis and spermatic cord (i.e. the tunica vaginalis and the cremasteric and spermatic fasciae) drains to the iliac glands.
- Lymph from the body of the testis drains to the para-aortic glands.

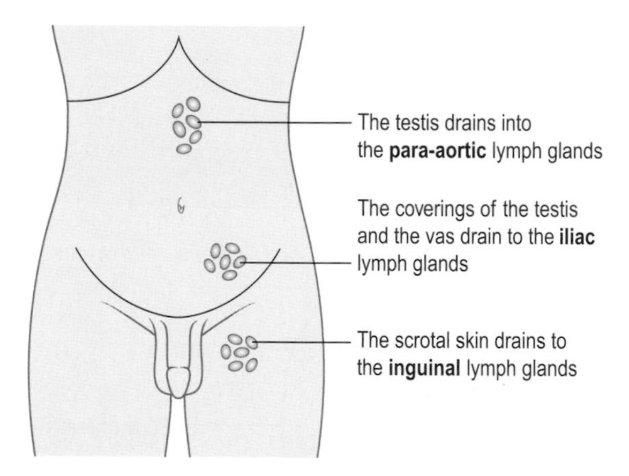

Figure 18.5 The lymph drainage of the testis, its coverings and the scrotum.

Conditions of the penis

PHIMOSIS

Phimosis is a narrowing of the end of the prepuce (foreskin), which prevents its retraction over the glans penis. It may be congenital, or it may develop due to scarring of the skin following infection or trauma.

Natural history of the foreskin

At birth, the foreskin covers and is adherent to the glans penis. The opening may initially be very narrow, like a pinhole. In the first few years of life, the foreskin gradually separates and widens so that, *by the age of 5 years, approximately 90% of males are able to retract it freely and easily.* The mechanism by which this happens is uncertain. Certainly, the normal skin secretions that build up between the foreskin and the glans (smegma) play a part, and there is also stretching from erections and patient self-curiosity.

It is *normal to have a non-retractile foreskin in early childhood.* Even when the foreskin retracts, adhesions between the foreskin and glans may persist into the early teens. There is no 'normal' age beyond which failure to be able to retract the prepuce may be termed abnormal and require treatment, but full retraction should be possible in all adults. So, when does failure to be able to retract become a disease? This is a grey area, and can cause considerable parental concern.

There is one variety of phimosis that is clearly pathological from the beginning, and that is *lichen sclerosis et atrophicus*, formerly known as balanitis xerotica obliterans. In this condition, there is scarring of the tip of the foreskin, presumably from minor tearing and healing with scarring. The appearance is characteristic (Figure 18.6). On gently attempting retraction, *whitish, irregular scarring is seen.* The process usually begins at the tip of the foreskin, but may spread on to the glans and even narrow the urethral meatus.

Symptoms *Ballooning of the prepuce on micturition is usually not abnormal in a young child.* It can only occur when there are no preputial adhesions.

Recurrent balanitis (see below) causing pain and a purulent discharge may occur, but actual urinary tract infection is uncommon, although it is sometimes attributed to phimosis.

Similar symptoms may occur in the adult, but the most common complaint is of *discomfort with erection and during sexual intercourse.*

If a tight foreskin gets retracted, it may not be possible to pull it forwards again; the patient then has a paraphimosis (see below).

Examination

In a child, gently draw back the foreskin and look at the tip. In a normal but narrow foreskin in a small child, the orifice will be small, but the skin

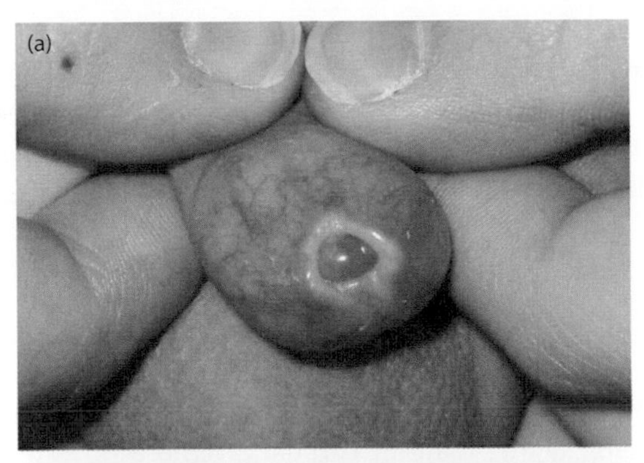

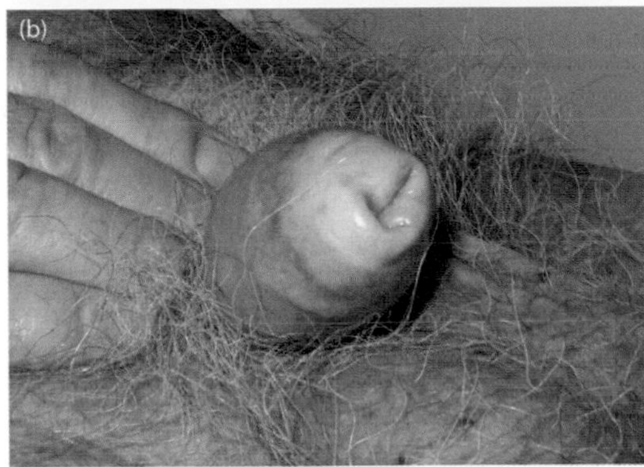

Figure 18.6 TWO EXAMPLES OF LICHEN SCLEROSIS ET ATROPHICUS AND PHIMOSIS. (a) Phimosis in a child with a ring of LSA. Note the white scar tissue that is made prominent as the patient tries to retract his foreskin. (b) Phimosis and LSA in an adult.

will appear normal. As you continue to retract it, the foreskin will not come back completely, but skin on the inside of the prepuce will 'flower' outwards. It is pinker and more delicate than the exposed skin on the outside. If there is any lichen sclerosis et atrophicus, you will see a narrow ring of white scar tissue (Figure 18.6) and will be unable to retract the skin at all.

In children, smegma may build up as yellow masses visible and palpable through the foreskin. This appearance may alarm both parents and referring physicians.

PARAPHIMOSIS

This occurs when the narrowing of the prepuce is just sufficiently tight for it to get stuck behind the glans penis, often during an erection. In this position, it impedes venous blood flow and causes oedema and congestion of the glans, which in turn makes reduction of the prepuce more difficult.

History

Age Paraphimosis usually occurs in young males and sometimes in children. It is a common complication of urethral catheterization at any age. *It is preventable by ensuring that the foreskin is always pulled forward after catheter insertion.*

Symptoms There is swelling and discomfort of the glans penis, with a tender, tight band at the coronal sulcus. It is uncommon for the urethra to be obstructed.

Past history The patient will not usually have been circumcised, but note that in some religious circumcisions the whole of the prepuce is not removed, so recurrent phimosis and hence paraphimosis may occur.

Examination

The diagnosis is usually obvious (Figure 18.7). The *glans penis is swollen and oedematous,* and there is a deep groove just below the corona where the skin looks tight, and may be split and ulcerated.

The condition may be chronic, in which case there may be superficial ulceration and infection of the skin of the glans penis.

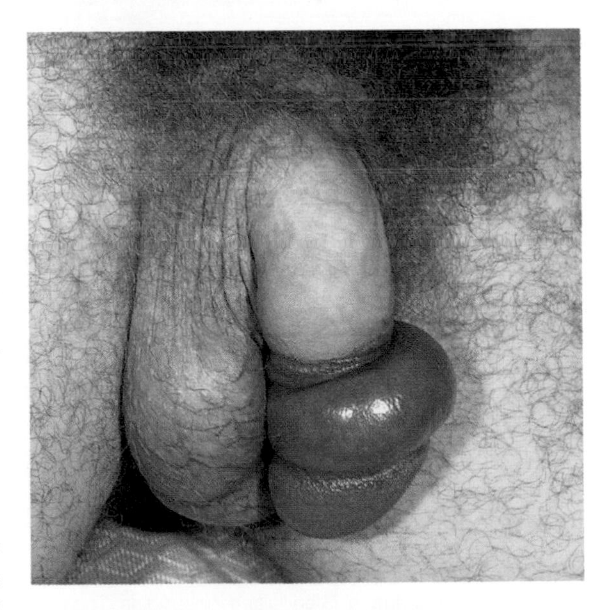

Figure 18.7 Paraphimosis. The retracted, tight, constricting ring of preputial skin is causing oedema of the skin distal to it, and congestion of the glans penis.

HYPOSPADIAS

Hypospadias is a congenital abnormality in which the *urethra opens on the ventral surface of the penis*, proximal to its usual position (Figure 18.8).

The opening may be anywhere along the line of the urethra, from the tip of the penis to the perineum. If the urethral opening is in the perineum, the scrotum is *bifid*. The site of the opening may be classified as *glandular (on the glans), penile (on the shaft)* or *perineal*.

Glandular hypospadias is easy to miss because it causes no symptoms and there is a deceptive vertical slit at the normal site of the urethral opening. The actual meatus may be quite small, and a common site is in the coronal sulcus. Thus, this can be found in the adult who was unaware it was abnormal.

The prepuce has a hooded appearance in proximal hypospadias, because it is deficient ventrally where the urethra emerges. It is vital never to carry out circumcision in a child with any degree of hypospadias, as the preputial skin may be needed for corrective surgery.

Chordee is a descriptive term for a curved penis, commonly associated with hypospadias. The curvature is convex dorsally and is more pronounced the further the urethral meatus is away from the end of the penis. It is caused by the corpus spongiosum being shorter than the corpora cavernosa when the urethral opening fails to reach the end of the penis. It may only be visible on erection.

Chordee in the other direction, convex ventrally, is seen in adults with Peyronie's disease (see below).

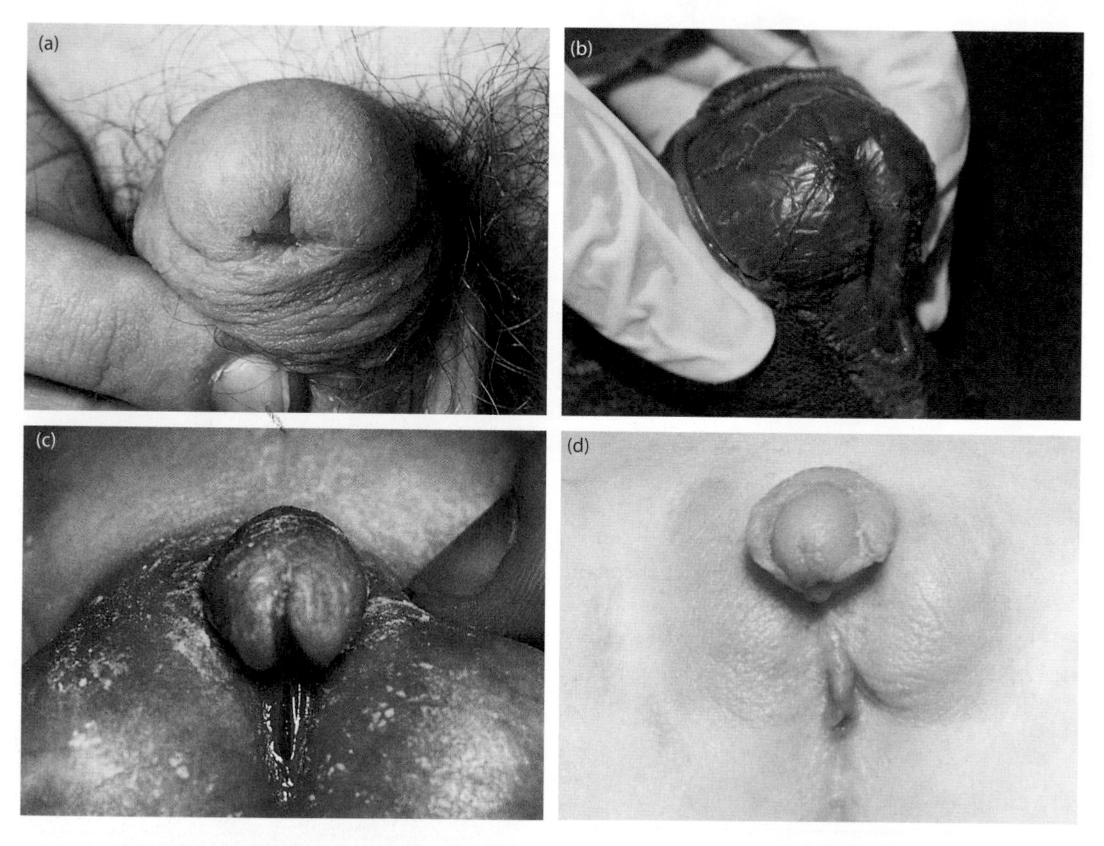

Figure 18.8 HYPOSPADIAS. Note that the external urethral meatus may be on the glans penis, the shaft of the penis or the perineum. (a) Glandular hypospadias. The urethral opening is on the edge of the glans penis. The pit where the opening should be is also visible. (b) Penile hypospadias. The urethral opening is 1 cm below the edge of the glans. (c) Scrotal hypospadias. The urethra opens in the scrotum with the penile urethra deficient ventrally. (d) Perineal hypospadias. The urethral opening is in the perineum. The scrotum is bifid.

EPISPADIAS

Epispadias is the opposite of hypospadias. The urethral opening is on the *dorsal surface of the glans penis* (Figure 18.9). It is extremely rare and is part of a spectrum of deficiencies with abdominal and pelvic fusion in the first months of embryogenesis known as the *exstrophy–epispadias complex*.

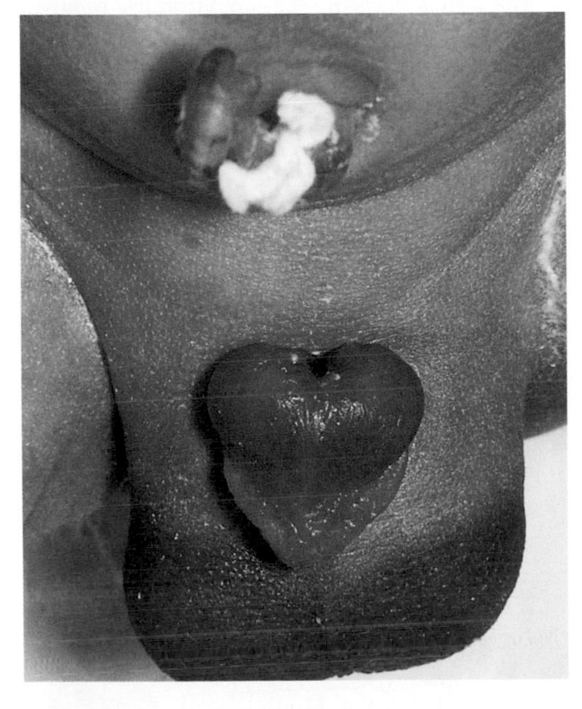

Figure 18.9 Epispadias. The urethra opens on the dorsum of the glans penis, almost on the dorsal aspect of the shaft of the penis.

BALANITIS

Strictly speaking, this is *inflammation of the prepuce,* and the term for inflammation of the glans is posthitis. It is usually caused by bacterial and sexually transmitted infections. Most patients have inflammation of both prepuce and glans, and therefore have balanoposthitis, but in practice the only term used is balanitis. It may be caused by poor personal hygiene and smegma/debris accumulating beneath the prepuce.

Symptoms The patient may complain of *itching, pain or discharge,* almost invariably with difficulty retracting the foreskin.

Examination

The foreskin appears reddened and oedematous, and there may be a purulent discharge. Patients are occasionally febrile and systemically unwell. In children, there will usually be collections of smegma, which may be visible. Look for signs of lichen sclerosis et atrophicus.

In elderly males, remember the possibility that balanitis may be caused by a carcinoma hidden beneath the prepuce, so retract it if possible.

Palpate the glans and the inguinal lymph glands.

Other causes of balanitis

Candidal balanitis is seen particularly in those with *diabetes and immunosuppressed patients.* The glans penis will show itchy red patches. The foreskin has a white appearance with longitudinal fissuring, particularly at the tip (Figure 18.10).

Genital herpes can involve the shaft, glans or foreskin. The vesicles, initially itchy, are soon replaced by shallow, painful erosions. There may be painful inguinal lymphadenopathy.

Drug eruptions are usually painless discolourations, most often seen on the glans penis, and are sometimes the only manifestation of drug hypersensitivity (see Figure 18.11).

Zoon's balanitis, also known as plasma cell balanitis, is a rare, idiopathic, benign, penile dermatosis.

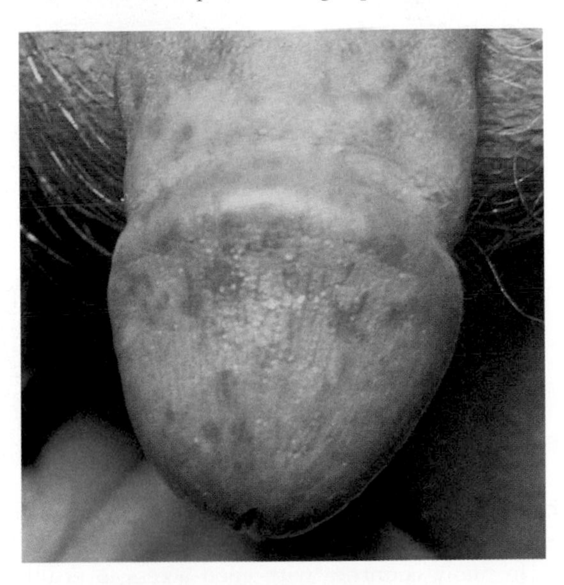

Figure 18.10 Candidal balanoposthitis.

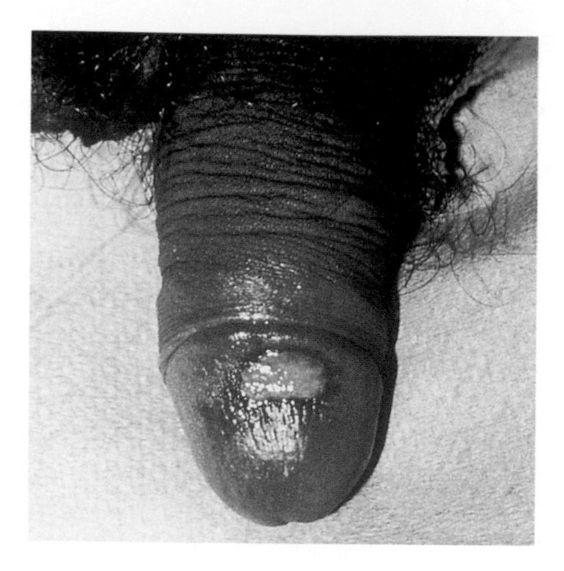

Figure 18.11 A drug eruption. This ulcer was part of a reaction to co-trimoxazole.

There are discrete plaques on both the glans and inner prepuce, which appear moist and erythematous.

Penile warts are caused by the human papilloma virus and are sexually transmitted (Figure 18.12).

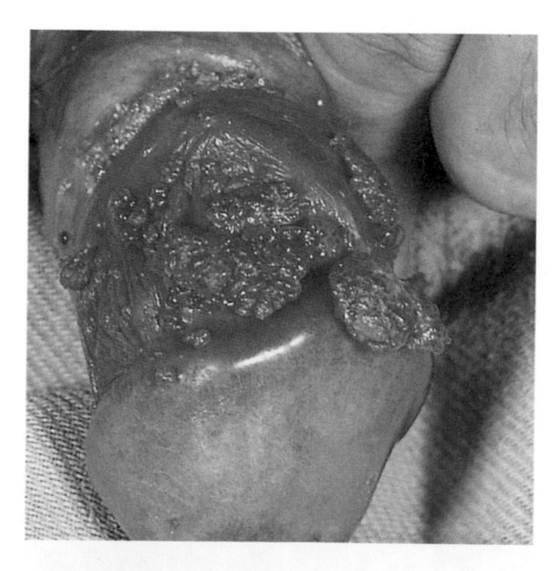

Figure 18.12 Penile warts.

SYPHILITIC CHANCRE

In many countries with good access to healthcare, syphilis is now rare. *The primary sore, known as a chancre, is solitary and always painless.* It usually occurs in the coronal sinus, the prepuce or the frenulum, and produces a serosanguinous discharge.

Beneath an area of superficial ulceration is an indistinct, indurated lump, 5–10 mm in diameter. The ulcer is covered with a slough and has a sloping, indolent edge (see Chapter 1) (Figure 18.13). It is not fixed to deeper structures.

The *inguinal lymph glands are invariably enlarged,* often mainly on one side. They are rubbery and discrete, but not tender.

General examination may reveal no other abnormalities, but a primary sore may still be present should the patient present with the secondary manifestations of the disease 4–6 weeks after the appearance of the chancre.

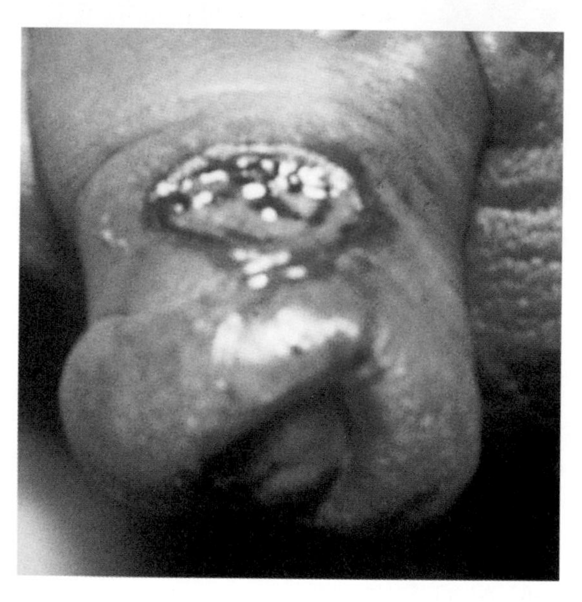

Figure 18.13 A syphilitic chancre on the inner surface of the prepuce.

CARCINOMA OF THE PENIS

Carcinoma of the penis is a squamous cell carcinoma. It is exceedingly rare in males who have been circumcised at birth or in adolescence, as in Jewish and Muslim communities.

It may be preceded by a number of premalignant conditions described below. It invades from the penile skin into the tissues of the shaft of the penis and spreads via the lymphatics.

History

Age Carcinoma of the penis presents in middle or old age, and rarely in young males.

Ethnic group It occurs in cultures that do not practise ritual circumcision.

Symptoms Most patients present with a lump or an ulcer that may be painful, especially if infected.

There is usually a purulent discharge, which may be bloodstained.

The patient may have a phimosis if the primary lesion has become quite advanced before detection.

The inguinal lymph glands may be enlarged by secondary infection or secondary deposits, and may be the first abnormality noticed by the patient. Presentation with distant metastases is rare.

The occasional patient ignores his symptoms until the tumour compresses or invades the urethra and urinary retention occurs.

Examination

Prepuce The patient is usually uncircumcised, and in the UK is commonly elderly and self-neglected. There may be a serous, purulent or sanguineous discharge coming from beneath the prepuce. *If the foreskin cannot be retracted, full examination of its inner surface and the glans penis may require a surgical dorsal slit.*

Deformity The penis may be swollen at its tip owing to the mass beneath the prepuce. In the advanced stages, the tumour may appear through the opening in the prepuce or erode through the preputial skin.

Position The lesion may be anywhere on the skin of the prepuce or the glans penis.

Tenderness The lump or ulcer is not usually tender, except with concomitant infection.

Shape Carcinoma of the penis tends to adopt one of two macroscopic forms: a classic carcinomatous *ulcer with a raised everted edge and necrotic base, or a papilliferous tumour with a wide sessile pedicle and an indurated base* (see Figure 18.14). The microscopic pathology is the same.

Size Patients who can retract their foreskin present earlier.

Composition The *tumour is hard,* especially at its base. Any part of the penis that is infiltrated also feels hard. The surface of the papilliferous variety is soft and friable. It resembles granulation tissue, and bleeds easily.

Relations At first, the tumour is confined to the skin, but it may invade and spread through the whole corpus cavernosum, making it indurated and hard. If it begins on the inner side of the prepuce, it may spread to and through the outer layer of skin.

Lymph glands The inguinal lymph glands of both groins may be enlarged by infection or metastatic deposits.

SKIN CONDITIONS OF THE PENIS

Various skin conditions are associated with an increased incidence of carcinoma of the penis, and the underlying pathological condition is called intraepithelial neoplasia (see Figure 18.15). This is the same as that seen in the female genital tract in the cervix and vulva, and in the perianal skin.

It is now appreciated that various clinical appearances, often classified by their colour (e.g. *leukoplakia*) or eponymously (e.g. *Paget's disease* and *erythroplasia of Querat*), have essentially the same pathology. Any chronic skin eruption on the penis might be penile intraepithelial neoplasia and should be assessed and treated accordingly.

Clinical diagnosis is difficult because any skin disease may occur on the skin of the penis.

Lichen sclerosis et atrophicus particularly mimics intraepithelial neoplasia.

HPV is another risk factor for penile cancer.

PRIAPISM

Priapism is a persistent, usually painful erection. There are two varieties, *low-flow (ischaemic)* and *high-flow.*

Low-flow priapism is seen in previously fit males after sexual activity. It is caused by a failure of the venular spasm that sustains erection to relax, often triggered by intracavernosal injections (e.g. papaverine, alprostadil) or rarely oral agents (e.g. sildenafil). Because of embarrassment, presentation may be late. It may also be caused by haematological disorders such as *leukaemia* or *sickle-cell disease,* which cause thrombosis of the corpora cavernosa, or by obstruction of the venous and lymphatic drainage of the penis by *pelvic malignancy.*

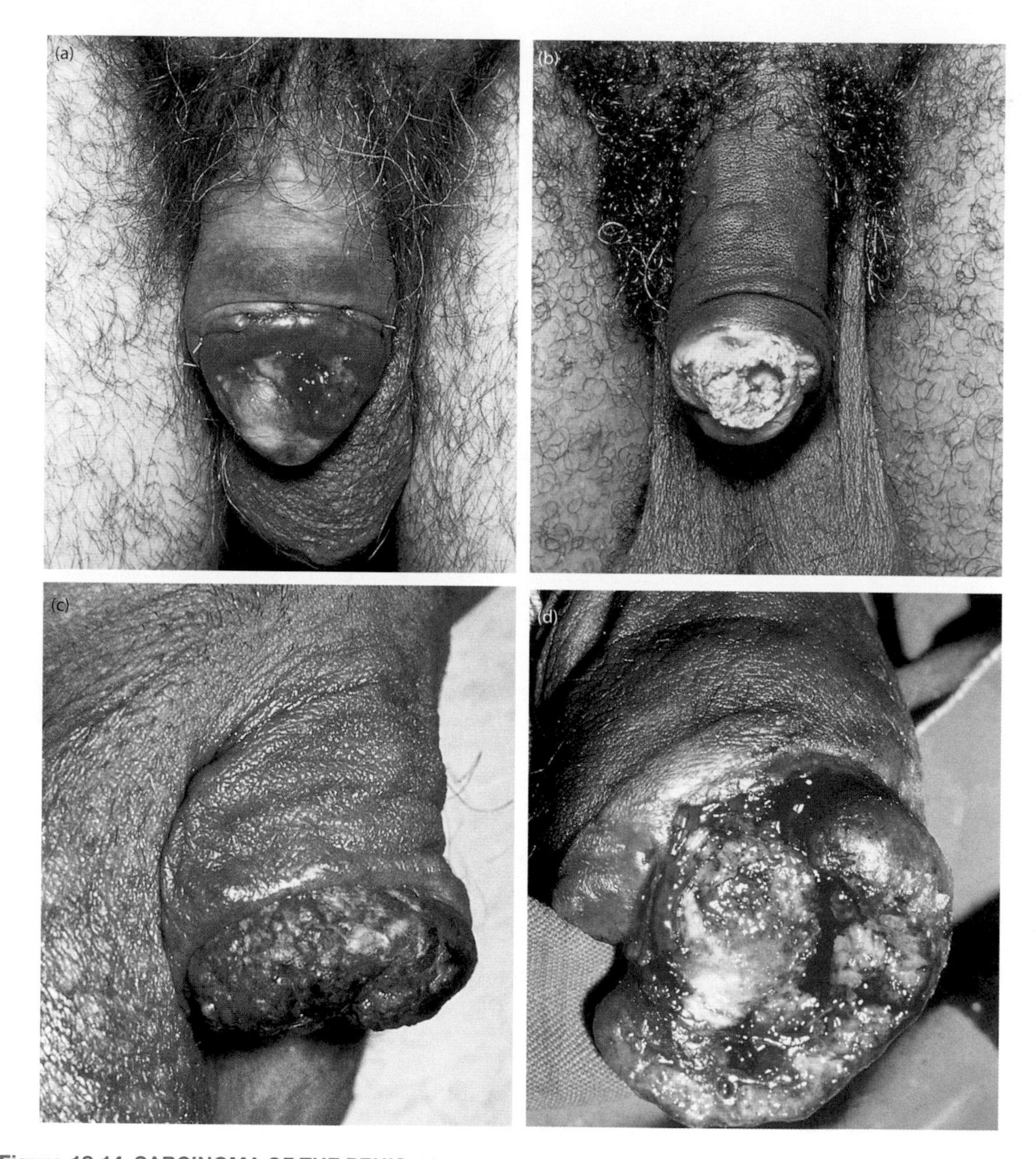

Figure 18.14 CARCINOMA OF THE PENIS. (a) An early carcinomatous ulcer on the glans penis, exposed by a circumcision. (b) A papilliferous carcinoma arising in the coronal sulcus. (c) An advanced infiltrating carcinoma that has invaded the whole thickness of the prepuce. (d) An ulcerating carcinoma that has destroyed half of the glans penis.

The erection seen in priapism is not of the normal pattern and shape. The corpus spongiosum remains soft. *Without immediate surgical treatment, irreversible impotence may result.*

High-flow priapism is not painful or ischaemic and usually results from an *arteriovenous fistula following pelvic trauma.*

PEYRONIE'S DISEASE

This is an idiopathic plaque of fibrosis in one or both of the corpora cavernosa, usually on the dorsal side (Figure 18.16). It occurs in middle-aged males. The symptoms are pain and a curvature of the penis when erect, which can interfere with sexual intercourse.

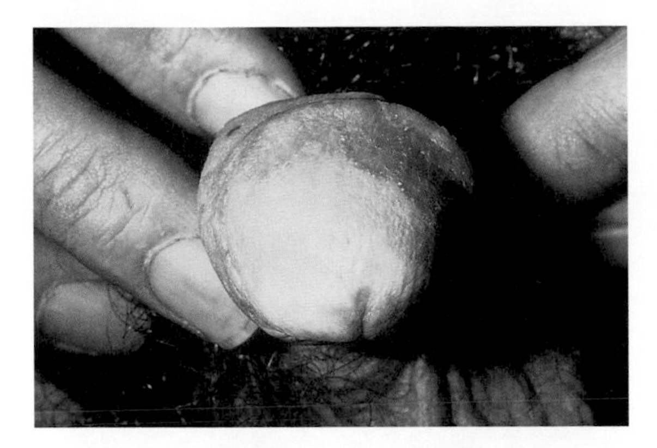

Figure 18.15 An example of penile intraepithelial neoplasia. This variety is commonly called leukoplakia.

The plaque may be palpable when the penis is flaccid, and in the first 6 months the plaques are tender.

The differential diagnosis includes metastatic tumour deposits and sarcomatous soft tissue tumours, but these are rare.

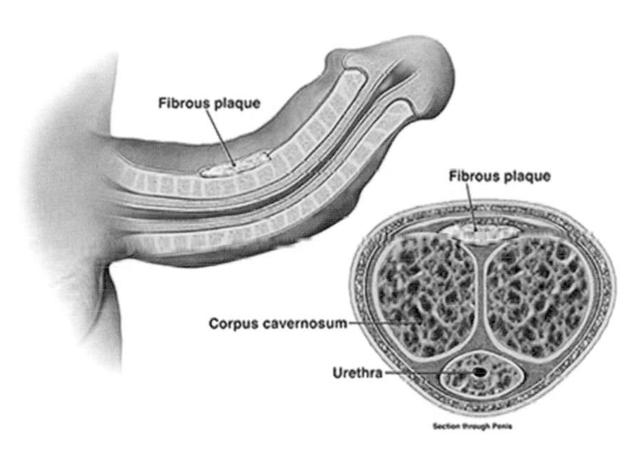

Figure 18.16 Peyronie's disease.

Conditions of the scrotal skin

SEBACEOUS CYSTS

Sebaceous cysts are common in the scrotal skin and are often multiple (Figure 18.17). They have all the features described in Chapter 4. They occasionally become infected, discharge and produce so much granulation tissue that they look like a carcinoma.

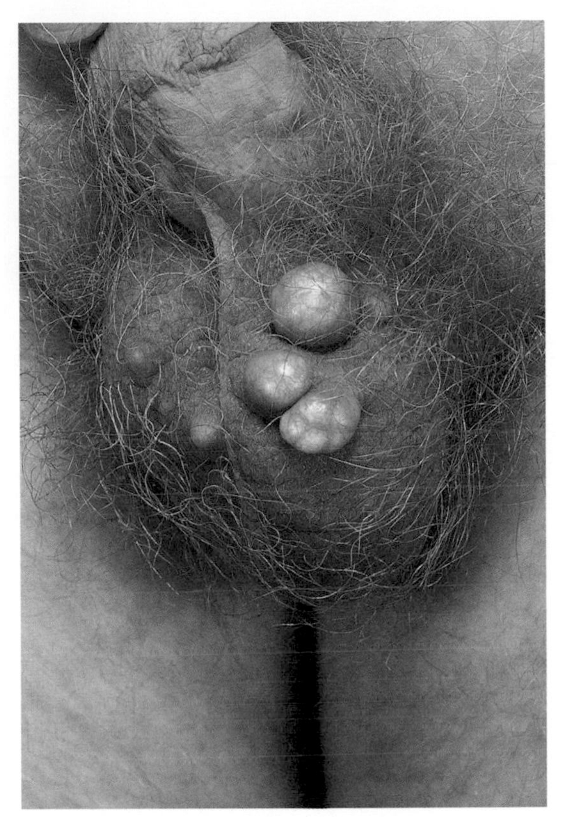

Figure 18.17 Sebaceous cyst.

CARCINOMA OF THE SCROTAL SKIN

This is a squamous carcinoma caused by chronic irritation. Historically, it was caused by frequent contact with *soot (Pott's chimney sweep's cancer)*. The skin must be exposed to these irritants for many years before a cancer develops.

History

Occupation The patient's occupation may be responsible for frequent soiling of the scrotal skin with oil and other carcinogenic hydrocarbons, and should be documented.

Symptoms Presentation is with a *lump or an ulcer*. A purulent discharge may be present. The patient may notice lumps in the groin if the inguinal lymph glands are involved.

Examination

Position A carcinomatous ulcer can occur on any part of the scrotal skin (see Figure 18.18). Industrial

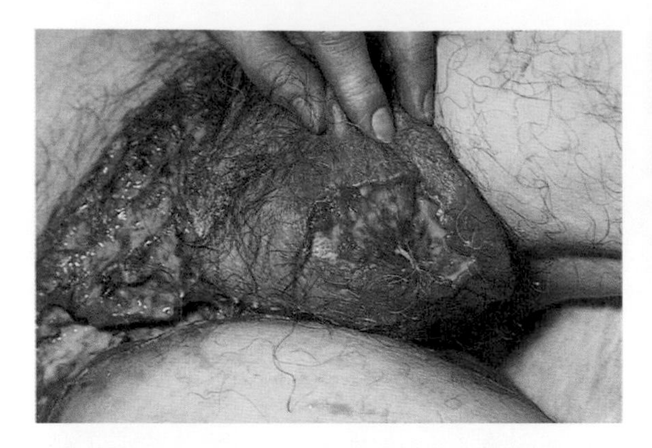

Figure 18.18 A carcinoma of the scrotal skin. Note that it is on the posteromedial surface of the scrotum.

cancers are often located high up in the cleft between the leg and the scrotum, where there is friction and persistent traces of oil. *Always examine the whole scrotum.*

Tenderness The ulcer is usually painless and not tender.

Shape In its early stages, the ulcer is small and circular, but it enlarges in an irregular fashion with an irregular outline.

Edge The ulcer edge is *reddish, friable and typically everted* (see Chapter 9).

Base The base is covered with yellow–grey, infected, necrotic tumour.

Relations In the early stages, the ulcer is freely mobile, but with deep spread to the skin it may become tethered to the underlying testis.

Lymph glands The inguinal lymph glands may be enlarged by tumour metastases or secondary infection.

LYMPHOEDEMA

Swelling of the penis and scrotum caused by excess fluid in the subcutaneous tissue (oedema) is seen in patients confined to bed with heart failure or fluid retention. It also occurs after surgery in the groin or pelvis.

True lymphoedema of the genitalia – oedema caused by the retention of protein-rich lymph in the subcutaneous tissues – is uncommon. It may be associated with lymphoedema of one or both limbs. The cause is obstruction of the inguinal and iliac lymph pathways by secondary or primary malignant disease or, in tropical areas, by worms (*Wuchereria bancrofti*, which causes filariasis) (Figure 18.19).

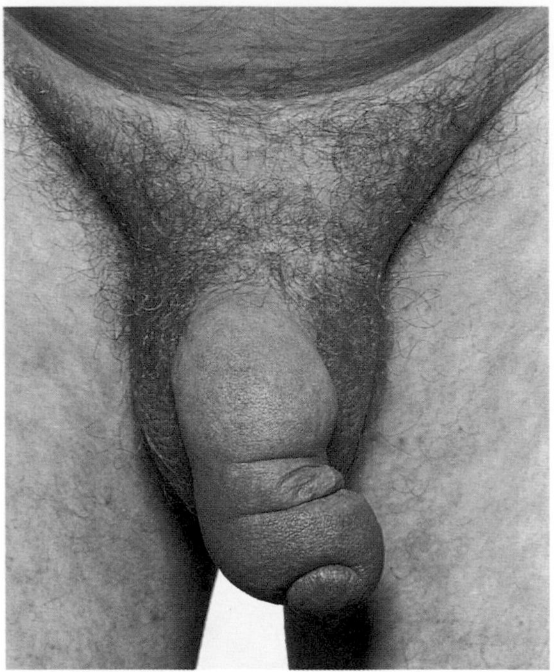

Figure 18.19 Lymphoedema of the penis.

Primary genital lymphoedema is very rare, and is caused by hypoplastic lymphatics.

SINUSES OF THE SCROTUM

Sequelae of scrotal surgery, e.g. wound breakdown or non-healing or advanced disease of the testis or epididymis, can create a sinus between the primary lesion and the skin surface.

Provided the testis is lying in the normal position, disease of the body of the testis tends to spread to the anterolateral surface of the scrotum, whereas disease of the epididymis spreads to the posterior surface.

The most common sinus in the scrotal area is a discharging cutaneous sebaceous cyst.

FOURNIER'S GANGRENE

This highly lethal condition, an example of synergistic gangrene (necrotizing fasciitis), is a disease of the scrotal skin and subcutaneous tissues, and not of the testicles themselves, which are unaffected, protected by the external spermatic fascia. *It primarily affects older patients who are immunocompromised from a wide variety of causes.*

There is infection with a combination of aerobic organisms (e.g. *Escherichia coli*, enterococcus) *and anaerobic organisms* such as *Bacteroides* and *Clostridium*. The combined infection produces toxins that cause tissue necrosis, in which the bacteria can flourish and spread.

The prominent feature is an *acutely unwell patient with septic shock*. The scrotal skin shows *dusky erythema*, which progresses to a *purple blotchy appearance with rapidly spreading black patches of obvious skin gangrene* (Figure 18.20). There is often gas in the subcutaneous tissues, and there is a crackling sensation on gentle palpation (crepitus).

The *mortality is as high as 80%*, because of the comorbidity of the sufferers. Urgent treatment is essential.

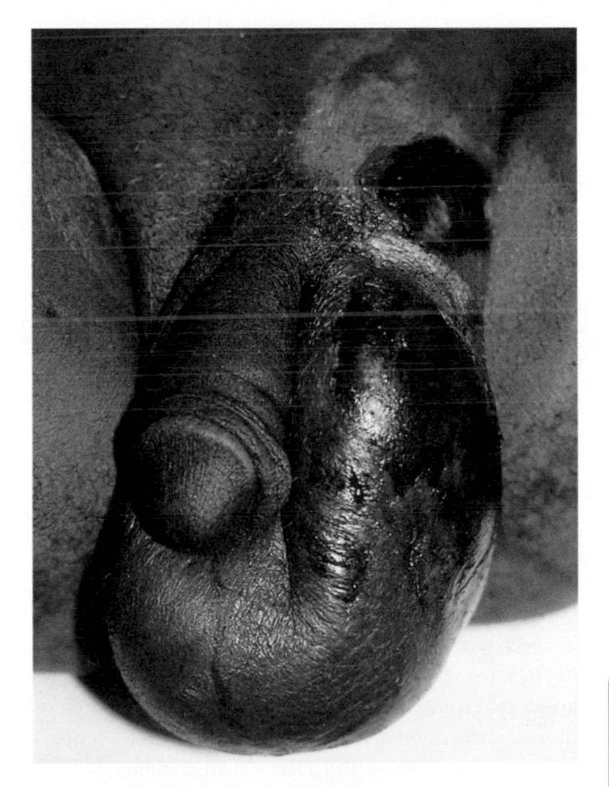

Figure 18.20 Fournier's gangrene.

Conditions of the testes

FAILURE OF NORMAL TESTICULAR DESCENT (CRYPTORCHIDISM)

The testis develops in utero in the posterior abdominal wall. *Its blood supply comes from the aorta, and its veins drain into the inferior vena cava, on the left via the renal vein.*

Lymph drainage is to the para-aortic glands.

Guided by the gubernaculum, the testis descends into the scrotum at between 25- and 30-weeks' gestation. Most testes have reached the scrotum by full term. In premature males, testicular descent may occur during the first 3 months of life.

Examination of the scrotum and groin can be difficult in small babies.

You can only confirm the presence or absence of the testes by careful palpation. A quick glance at the scrotum is not good enough.

By 3 months, only 1–2% of testes cannot be found by an experienced examiner.

When the testis has never been in the scrotum, the scrotal skin on that side will be underdeveloped.

If a testis is not in the scrotum, it may either have found its way to an abnormal site or have stopped somewhere along the route of normal descent:

- *A testis that has descended to an abnormal site is an ectopic testis.* The testis may be in the superficial inguinal pouch, the femoral triangle or the perineum (see Figure 18.21). The mechanism causing descent is normal, but the guidance system has gone wrong. The testis itself is normal.
- *A testis that is in its correct anatomical path but has failed to reach the scrotum is a truly undescended testis* (see Figure 18.22).

The truly undescended testis is small and abnormal, with a separated epididymis and often an associated indirect inguinal hernial sac.

NOTE: The absence of both testes from the scrotum may prompt further genetic investigation to exclude intersex conditions.

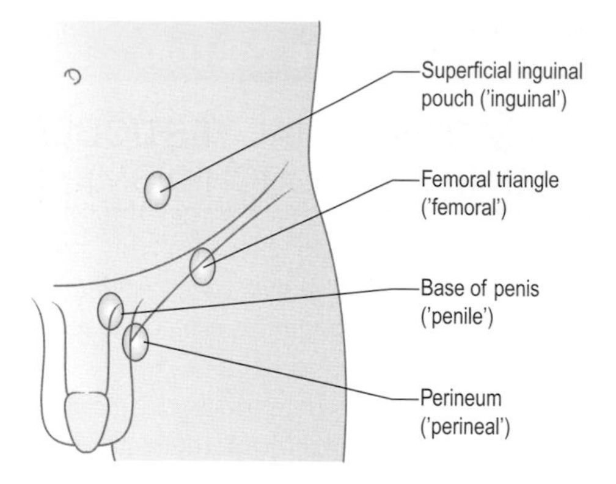

Figure 18.21 The sites where you may find an ectopic testis.

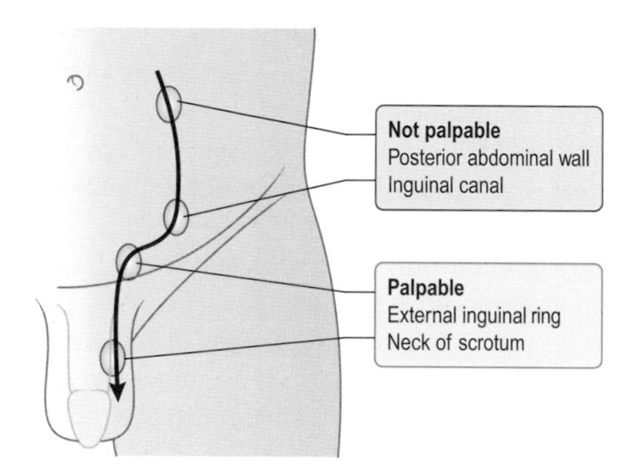

Figure 18.22 The line of normal testicular descent. A truly undescended testis may be found anywhere on this line. If it is above the external inguinal ring, it will be impalpable.

True congenital absence of a testis is rare. The testis is sometimes missing because it has met with a vascular accident, usually torsion (see below) in early or even intrauterine life.

Examination of a child with a missing testis

This can be difficult with a child who does not want to be examined and anxious parents. *Make sure that the room and your hands are both warm.* The child has to be persuaded to lie down.

Inspection The child must be undressed from the waist downwards in a good light. An empty scrotum, with very little development of the scrotal skin because it has never had the testis within it, is usually obvious (Figure 18.23). *A retractile testis is the likely diagnosis* if the testes are visible in the scrotum.

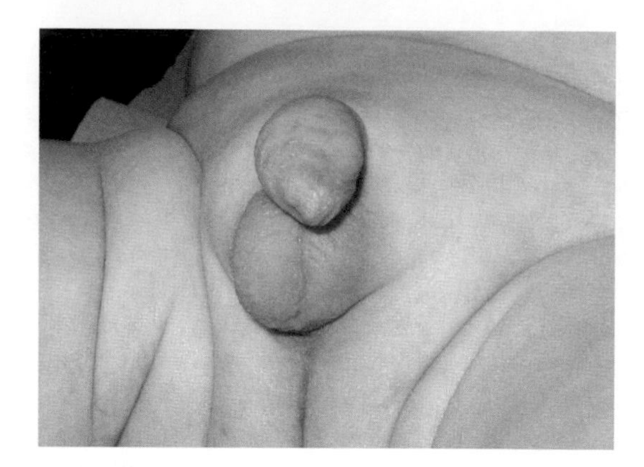

Figure 18.23 This baby has a truly undescended and impalpable left testis. The scrotal skin is very poorly developed compared with the right side, where the testis has fully descended.

If the testis is in the superficial inguinal pouch, it may be visible in a thin patient.

Palpation Try to get the child to relax, as muscular activity makes the dartos muscle contract and draw the testis up towards the groin.

Examine the groin before palpating the scrotum. If you cannot see or feel the testis in the subcutaneous tissues, find out if it is in the inguinal canal by gently sweeping your fingers from the anterior superior iliac spine obliquely across the groin to the pubis, along the line of the inguinal canal and towards the neck of the scrotum; this will *'milk' the testis,* if present, through the external ring. If the testis becomes palpable, catch it gently with the thumb and index finger of your other hand and draw it down to the scrotum. If it is a *retractile testis,* it will move down easily.

> **NOTE:** Should you get the testis down into the scrotum, show it to the parents before you remove your fingers and the testis retracts!

Ectopic testis

History

Age Children in countries with good access to healthcare will usually be *routinely examined at birth* and again in the first year of life. The patient may not discover the abnormality himself until adolescence.

Symptoms *Absence of a testis is the common presenting symptom,* but the child may complain of pain or discomfort if the testis is in a site such as the superficial inguinal pouch, where it is likely to be rubbed or compressed during normal physical activity. *Note that the pain pathway is via the autonomic afferent nerves so, for developmental reasons, pain may be experienced in the groin or even loin.*

Systemic effects If both testes are ectopic, the patient may be subfertile, but he rarely lacks secondary sexual characteristics.

Examination

The side of the scrotum without the testis may be poorly developed, but not as obviously as with a truly undescended testis.

Site *An ectopic testis is nearly always palpable,* although with difficulty in a fat child. A truly undescended testis lying in the inguinal canal or abdomen is not palpable. If the testis is not in the scrotum, you must carefully examine those sites where ectopic testes are known to settle:

- **Superficial inguinal pouch.** *This is by far the most common site in which to find an ectopic testis.* It is also the place to which the retractile testis retreats. An ectopic testis in this site has emerged through the external ring but, having failed to enter the scrotum, turns upwards and laterally to lie in a pouch deep to the superficial fascia. This may be caused by some obstruction at the neck of the scrotum from tight fascia. The testis can be palpated in the subcutaneous tissue just above and lateral to the crest of the pubis and the pubic tubercle.
- **Femoral triangle.** If the testis moves laterally after leaving the external inguinal ring, it can come to rest in the upper medial corner of the femoral triangle. A testis in this site is easy to feel, and is easily misdiagnosed as a lymph gland or even a femoral hernia, although the latter is very rare in children. This variety is sometimes termed *crural,* as it lies in the thigh.
- **Base of the penis.** If the testis moves medially, it will lie at the base of the penis, where it can be easily felt against the underlying pubic bone.
- **Perineum.** Occasionally, the testis passes over the pubis and then backwards, instead of downwards, to lie in the perineum just to one side of the corpus cavernosum of the penis (Figure 18.24).

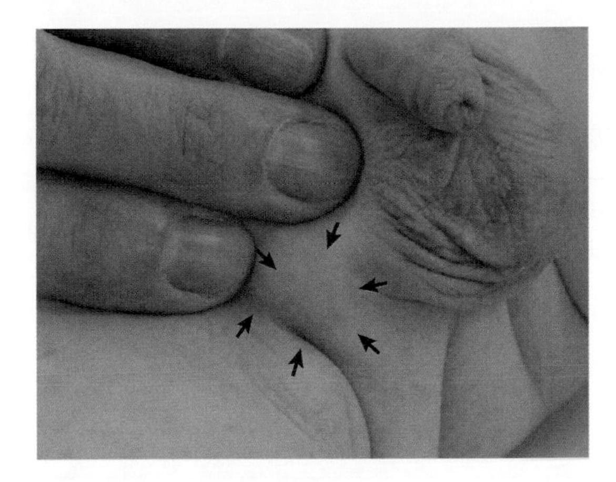

Figure 18.24 Perineal ectopic testicle.

An ectopic testis cannot be manipulated into the scrotum. It is unusual to be able to define the separate features of the body of the testis and the epididymis.

Any enlargement, irregularity or immobility should make you suspect the presence of malignant change in the testis, or make you look for another diagnosis.

Truly undescended testis

History

Age Truly undescended testes are usually noticed in early life at postnatal check ups, but occasionally not until adolescence.

Symptoms *An absence of one or both testes from the scrotum is the presenting symptom.* The parents may notice that the scrotum has not developed – unaware of the absence of the testes. A small proportion of patients present in adult life with *infertility.* Although failure of testicular descent is invariably associated with abnormal spermatogenesis, the hormone-producing cells are usually normal, so the male has a normal puberty and secondary sexual characteristics.

Truly undescended testes are associated with an indirect inguinal hernia, and a groin swelling may be the presenting complaint.

Examination

The scrotum When both testes are undescended, the *scrotum is small and hypoplastic.* If only one testis has descended, it is markedly *asymmetrical* (see Figure 18.23).

Site A truly undescended testis lies somewhere in the line of normal descent but only becomes palpable when it reaches, or is outside, the external inguinal ring.

It cannot be felt within the inguinal canal because the tense overlying external oblique aponeurosis conceals it, and it tends to slip back through the internal ring into the abdomen.

> **NOTE:** Thus, if you can feel a testis lateral to the external inguinal ring, it must be superficial to the external oblique, and is therefore an ectopic testis in the *superficial inguinal pouch* rather than a truly undescended testis.

Some testes that lie in the inguinal canal can be *milked down* to the external ring by gently stroking along the line of the canal, as described above.

The lump *A truly undescended testis is usually smaller than normal.*

In an adult, the appearance of a mass in the line of testicular descent, whether within the abdomen or the inguinal canal, and an empty scrotum should make you suspect malignant change in a truly undescended testis. *The risk of malignant change is many times greater than in a normally descended or ectopic testis***.**

Fixing the testis in the scrotum (*orchidopexy*) does not eliminate this risk, but allows easier self-examination.

The truly *undescended testis* is also more likely to *undergo torsion* than a normally descended testis.

Retractile testes

The cremaster is a strong active muscle during childhood, and the testes of many young children (commonly 2–7 years of age) move freely up and down between the scrotum and the inguinal canal or the superficial inguinal pouch. A cold examining hand may be sufficient stimulus to cause retraction. If the patient is seen when the testis is retracted, it may be *misdiagnosed as a truly undescended testis* and surgical treatment advised. This will be an unnecessary operation because all retractile testes ultimately descend properly, either before or at puberty.

History

The parents notice that the *testis* (frequently both) is *absent from the scrotum.* This situation is often intermittent, and it may be noticed that everything appears normal when the child is warm and relaxed, typically in the bath.

The testis may have been reported in the scrotum at previous routine examinations.

Examination

When the testes are retractile, the scrotum is normally developed.

You should always attempt to manipulate the testis into the scrotum, as described above. If the testis can be persuaded into the scrotum and it rests there when you let go, it is a retractile testis.

> **NOTE:** A testis should only be classified as truly undescended or ectopic if you cannot manipulate it into the scrotum.

The ascending testis

There is also a group of patients in whom the testis has been found and placed in the scrotum to the satisfaction of all, but some while later the parents notice that it is no longer visible and seek further advice. On this occasion, the testis may be palpable in the superficial inguinal pouch and cannot be persuaded into the scrotum. This is termed the *ascending testis* and may require surgery.

HYDROCELE

This is an *abnormal quantity of fluid within the tunica vaginalis* (Revision panel 18.1). There are two varieties:

- *Primary,* of unknown cause (but related to a mismatch in secretion and absorption in the tunica vaginalis).
- *Secondary,* caused by trauma, infection or neoplasm.

Most secondary hydroceles appear rapidly in the presence of other symptoms associated with their cause, *are lax and may contain altered blood.* They are much less common than primary (idiopathic) hydroceles, which develop slowly and progressively and become large and tense.

Revision panel 18.1

CAUSES OF HYDROCELE

Primary

Idiopathic

Secondary

Trauma
Epididymo-orchitis
Tumour
Lymphatic obstruction

History

Age Primary hydroceles are most common over the age of 40 years. *In children, the swelling may be intermittent, and the condition is always associated with a patent processus vaginalis and is a variety of inguinal hernia* (see Chapter 14). It occurs in 2–5% of newborn males, and 90% of cases resolve within 1 year.

Secondary hydroceles occur in an older age group because trauma, infection and testicular neoplasms are more common in this period.

Symptoms *The patient complains of an increase in the size of the testis, or a swelling in the scrotum.* There may be pain and discomfort if there is underlying testicular disease, but idiopathic hydroceles reach a considerable size without causing pain. The patient may complain of the social embarrassment of his large scrotum, which shows through his trousers.

Hydroceles do not affect fertility, although a large one may cause problems during sexual intercourse.

Examination

Position The swelling fills one side of the scrotum but is *within the scrotum,* and the spermatic cord can be felt above the lump. The testis *cannot be palpated separately* because it is within the swelling. This is the cardinal physical sign that distinguishes a hydrocele from an epididymal cyst (Figure 18.25).

Hydroceles may be bilateral.

Colour and temperature The colour and temperature of the overlying scrotal skin are normal.

Tenderness Primary hydroceles are not tender. Secondary hydroceles may be tender if the underlying testis or epididymis is tender.

Shape and size Hydroceles can be enormous and contain as much as 500 mL of fluid. They are ovoid in shape.

Surface The surface is always *smooth and well defined.* Occasionally, a weak spot in the wall gives way to form a small, fluctuant bump – a hernia of the hydrocele fluid through its coverings.

Composition Hydroceles contain a clear, straw-coloured fluid that is rich in protein. *They are fluctuant, have a fluid thrill if they are large enough, are dull to percussion and usually transilluminate* (Figure 18.25b).

They may be tense or lax, depending on the cause.

The wall of a long-standing hydrocele may become calcified, making the mass hard and opaque.

Reducibility Hydroceles cannot be reduced.

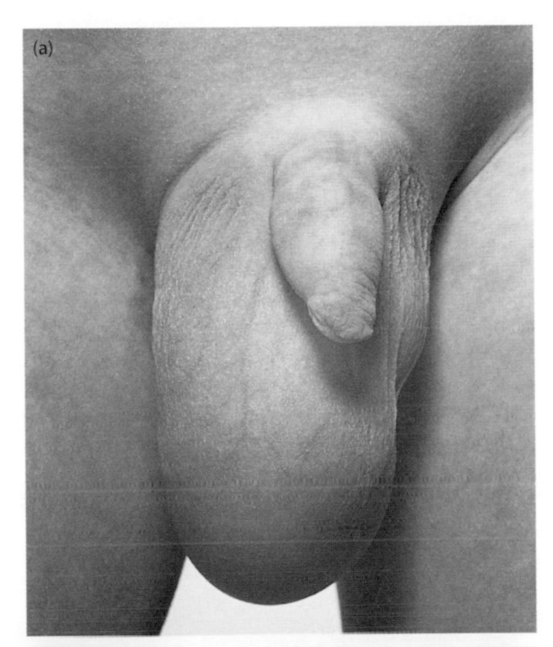

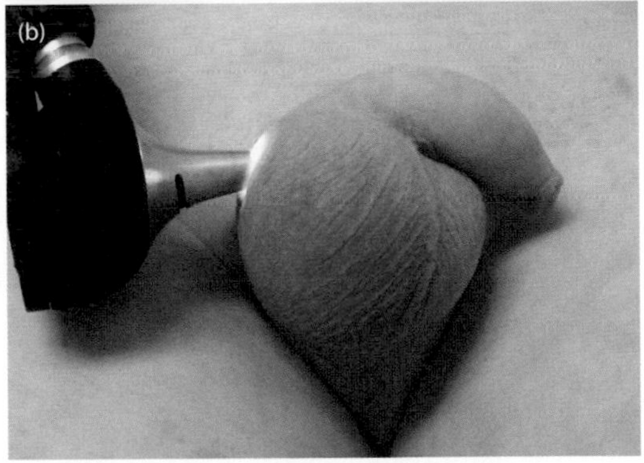

Figure 18.25 HYDROCELES. (a) A large hydrocele. The swelling is confined to the scrotum, is not tender, and is fluctuant and translucent; the testis is not palpable. (b) A transilluminated hydrocele.

Relations The fluid of a hydrocele surrounds the body of the testis, usually making the testis impalpable. The swelling cannot be a hydrocele if you can feel the testis separate from a scrotal swelling.

When a hydrocele is lax, which is seen only in secondary hydroceles, it may be possible to feel the surface of the testis through the fluid.

The spermatic cord can be felt coming down to and running into the swelling. The skin of the scrotum is freely mobile over the swelling.

Lymph glands If you think the swelling is a secondary hydrocele, you should palpate the para-aortic lymph glands in the epigastrium. This is the area of lymphatic drainage of a testicular tumour.

EPIDIDYMAL CYST

Epididymal cysts are *fluid-filled swellings arising from the epididymis*. Their aetiology has not been satisfactorily explained, but they are derived from the collecting tubules.

An *epididymal cyst usually contains clear fluid.* The variety that contains slightly grey, opaque, 'barley water'-like fluid and a few spermatozoa is sometimes termed a *spermatocele*, and may occur following a vasectomy operation (Figure 18.26).

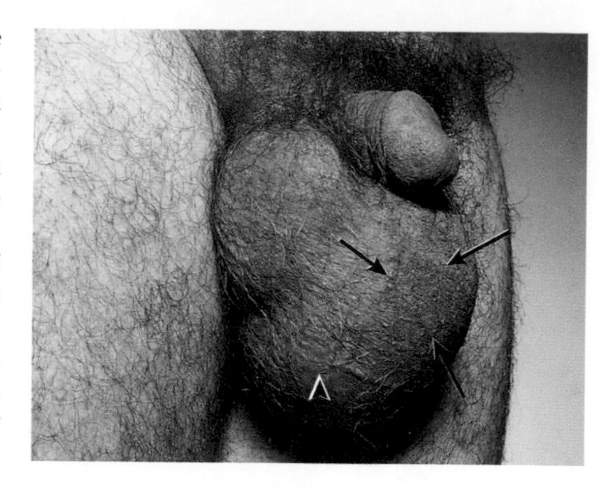

Figure 18.26 Large epididymal cyst (arrow: cyst; arrowhead: testis).

> **NOTE:** As the large majority of cysts connected with the epididymis contain clear fluid, it is usual to call them all epididymal cysts and not use the term 'spermatocele'.

History

Age Most epididymal cysts occur in males over the age of 40 years, but they are occasionally seen in children and adolescents.

Symptoms The main complaint is of *a swelling in the scrotum*, with the occasional patient believing that he has developed a tumour or a third testis.

In older age groups, the swelling is usually *painless*.

Small epididymal cysts in males in their 30s and 40s may be painful and tender.

Development Epididymal cysts enlarge very slowly, but rarely become enormous, unlike primary hydroceles.

Multiplicity They are often multiple or multilocular, and are frequently bilateral.

Fertility Epididymal cysts do not interfere with fertility, but surgery to remove such cysts may do so.

Examination

Position The swelling lies within the scrotum, usually above and slightly behind the testis. *The testis can be felt separately from the swelling.* If the swelling is similar in size to a testis, the patient may identify which of the lumps is which.

The spermatic cord can be felt above it.

Tenderness Cysts are variable with some being very tender and others entirely painless.

Shape Because the cysts are *usually multilocular, the swelling is rarely a perfect sphere.* It is usually elongated and bosselated, and individual loculi may be palpable.

Size Epididymal cysts may vary in size from a few millimetres to 5–10 cm in diameter. They rarely reach the size of the large hydroceles.

Surface The surface is smooth but the contours of individual loculi may be palpable.

Composition These swellings are *fluctuant, have a fluid thrill, are translucent* if large enough to transilluminate and are dull to percussion.

Epididymal cysts cannot be reduced.

Relations *Epididymal cysts are separate from the testis, and therefore the testis remains palpable.*

Most epididymal cysts are connected to the head of the epididymis, so *lie above the testis*, with the spermatic cord descending into or behind them. They occasionally lie at the lower pole.

Lymph glands The regional lymph glands should not be palpable.

Differential diagnosis

The normal epididymis is usually palpable and may be noticed by concerned young males who think they have a testicular tumour. It may on occasion be difficult to say if a swelling is a normal palpable organ or a small cyst.

Tumours of the epididymis itself are so rare as to be virtually non-existent. Any swelling that is clearly in the epididymis is therefore benign.

> **NOTE:** All the signs mentioned in this section on composition are identical to those for hydrocele. The difference between a hydrocele and an epididymal cyst lies in the *relation of the swelling to the testis.*

VARICOCELE

A varicocele is a collection of dilated and tortuous veins in the pampiniform plexus. The condition could be renamed varicose veins of the spermatic cord. *It is much more common on the left.* The right testicular veins drain into the inferior vena cava, but on the left they drain into the renal vein. The left testicular vein (or veins) is a much longer vessel, and it is hardly surprising that its valves can fail and cause a varicocele.

Small symptomless varicoceles occur in 25% of healthy males, on the left side. When the veins become large, they may cause a *vague, dragging sensation and aching pain in the scrotum or groin.* The appearance may embarrass adolescents and young males.

The sudden appearance of a varicocele in middle or old age may be caused by *a renal neoplasm spreading along the renal vein and obstructing the testicular vein.* This is a very rare presentation of carcinoma of the kidney but should not be forgotten, particularly if there are other urinary tract symptoms, especially haematuria.

A *varicocele can be difficult to palpate when the patient is lying down because the veins are empty.* This is one of the reasons why you must always examine the scrotum with the patient standing up (Figure 18.27). The dilated, compressible veins above the testis are then palpable and often visible. *They feel like a 'bag of worms', an accurate description.*

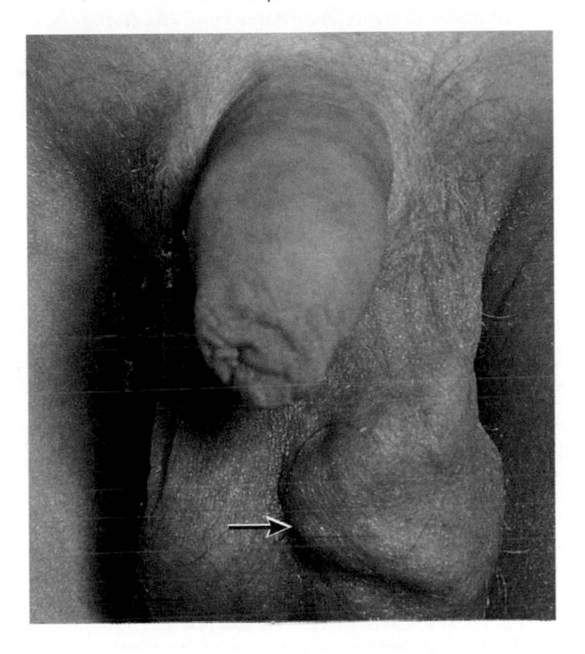

Figure 18.27 A varicocele (arrow). When the patient is standing, the tense, tortuous, distended veins are said to feel like a 'bag of worms'. When the patient is supine, they collapse and are almost impalpable.

The testis below a large varicocele may be smaller and softer than the testis on the normal side.

The effect of a varicocele on spermatogenesis is controversial.

HAEMATOCELE

A haematocele is *a collection of blood within the tunica vaginalis.* The bleeding is usually caused by trauma or underlying malignant disease.

In the acute phase, the mass has the same physical signs as a hydrocele, except that it is *not translucent and may be tender.* When the blood clots, it contracts and forms a small, hard mass, which can cause diagnostic problems.

Acute haematocele

The patient usually but not always gives a clear history of an *injury,* or of vague discomfort in the testis, followed by a painful, rapid swelling of the scrotum. It is a condition particularly associated with *cricket, rugby and cycling.*

The unilateral swelling is tense, tender and fluctuant, but does not transilluminate. The testis cannot be felt separate from the swelling.

Chronic haematocele

When the acute episode is managed conservatively or not recognized, the blood in the tunica vaginalis will clot. As time passes, the clot that surrounds the testis contracts and hardens. This may result in *a hard mass, which is no longer tender* and is not fluctuant. Normal testicular sensation may be lost if the contracting clot causes ischaemic necrosis of the testis.

> **NOTE:** These changes make a chronic haematocele *difficult to distinguish from a testicular tumour,* and investigation or even exploration may be needed.

TORSION OF THE TESTIS

Testicular torsion can occur at any age, and is of two distinct types, *intra-* and *extravaginal.*

- **Intravaginal torsion** The testis twists within the tunica vaginalis itself. *This is the most common type, predisposed to by the 'bell clapper' abnormality in which the testis lies horizontally* (Figure 18.28) and is more mobile because of a longer length of the vessels. This process can be aided by contraction of the spiral fibres of the cremaster muscle.
- **Extravaginal torsion** The entire testis and tunica vaginalis twists on the spermatic cord itself. This is rare and seen in neonates and infants.

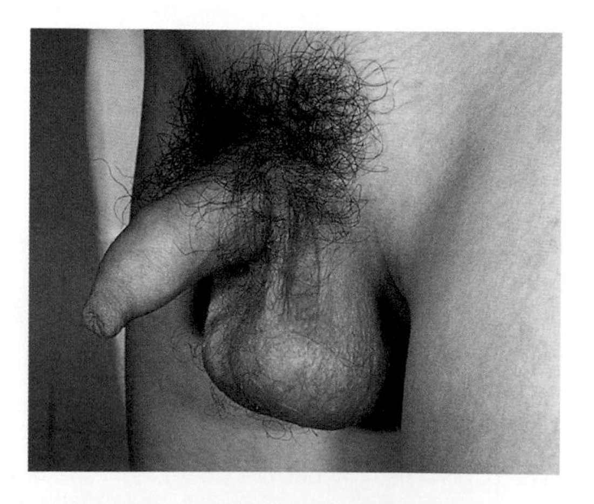

Figure 18.28 A testis hanging horizontally and susceptible to torsion.

The anatomical abnormality that allows torsion is invariably bilateral.

The condition may resolve spontaneously, or may progress to testicular infarction.

History

Age *Torsion presents most commonly in teenagers between 14 and 16 years of age,* but as the cause is a congenital abnormality, it can occur in young children, in neonates and even in utero. It is uncommon in males over 25 years of age but does happen.

Symptoms *The initial symptom is acute severe scrotal pain,* which may be poorly localized, and may radiate to or only be felt in the lower abdomen, loin or groin. This is because it is autonomically modulated, so is referred to the embryological site of origin of the testis. *Nausea and vomiting are common.* In a baby, there may be restlessness and a failure to eat.

Previous attacks The patient may have had similar *mild attacks of pain that subsided spontaneously,* or an episode on the other side that required surgery. Recurrent torsion is possible if the testis has not been appropriately fixed.

Cause Although the majority of torsions seem to occur spontaneously, often in the early hours of the morning, some follow minor trauma.

Examination

Position The swelling is confined to the scrotum. *The affected testis lies higher in the scrotum than the normal testis.* This is a most important physical sign.

Colour The *scrotal skin may be red and oedematous.* Although the latter changes are more commonly associated with epididymo-orchitis, their presence must not dissuade you from making a diagnosis of torsion.

Temperature The skin will feel hot if it is red and hyperaemic.

Tenderness *The testis is exquisitely tender, making palpation very difficult.*

Shape The whole of the testis is swollen, and it is usually impossible to distinguish the contours of the epididymis from those of the body of the testis.

Surface The surface of the testis is smooth, but may be obscured by scrotal oedema.

Composition Because of tenderness, it is usually impossible to elicit the signs that will reveal the composition of the mass in the scrotum. The mass may be the testis, or the testis surrounded by an acute secondary hydrocele.

Local tissues Apart from the scrotal skin, which may be red and oedematous, the other nearby tissues, including the other testis, will be normal. The other testes may be lying horizontally.

Differential diagnosis

Torsion of a testis within the scrotum may be indistinguishable from acute epididymo-orchitis, particularly if there are no urinary symptoms. Epididymo-orchitis usually occurs in an older age group.

Torsion of an undescended testis in the groin may be indistinguishable from *a strangulated inguinal hernia.*

- *Torsion of a testicular appendage* is the most common condition mimicking torsion. There are two appendages (the appendix of the testis and the appendix of the epididymis), and either may tort. The initial symptoms may be identical. The testis is not usually as tender, and sometimes the torted appendage is palpable as a tender nodule, or is visible through the scrotal skin as the 'blue dot sign'. A secondary hydrocele may obscure this.
- *Idiopathic scrotal oedema* is a condition in which the skin and subcutaneous tissues of the scrotum become oedematous, red and inflamed, in most cases as the result of a streptococcal infection. The swelling is confined by the attachments of the scrotal fascia (Figure 18.29). A clinical diagnosis can usually be made, as the testis itself is not tender.

NOTE: When in doubt about a painful scrotal or testicular swelling, make a diagnosis of *torsion*, because failure to explore the scrotum within 6 hours and reduce the torsion will result in the death of the testis. If the diagnosis turns out to be incorrect and the patient has epididymo-orchitis, the surgical exploration will have done no harm, and decompression of the tunica vaginalis may relieve the painful pressure from the secondary hydrocele.

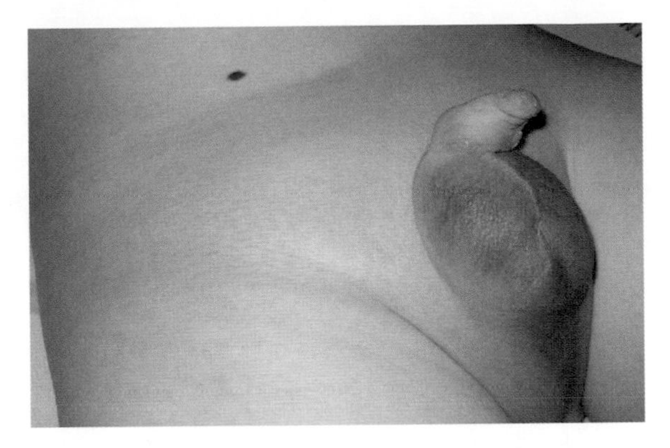

Figure 18.29 A very severe case of idiopathic scrotal oedema. The scrotal skin has lost its wrinkled appearance. Unusually, the oedema has tracked into the groin, the perineum and the other side of the scrotum. The attachment of Scarpa's fascia in the thigh is clearly visible.

There are occasional reports of manual external detorsion. Although possibly successful at times, this does not replace surgical exploration.

ORCHITIS

Acute orchitis, in the absence of epididymitis, is invariably caused by a virus infection, commonly *mumps*. The damage caused by orchitis may leave the patient with a painful testis or render him subfertile, especially if the condition is bilateral. Mumps orchitis may occur without enlargement of the salivary glands, but there is usually a history of contact (see Chapter 12).

Acute epididymo-orchitis

This is primarily an infection of the epididymis, but oedema and inflammatory changes spread into the testis. There is usually an associated urinary tract or sexually transmitted disease.

The common infecting organisms in patients under 40 years old are *Chlamydia trachomatis* and *Neisseria gonorrhoeae*. In older patients, *Escherichia coli* is common.

History

Age This condition can affect all age groups, but is most common in young and middle-aged males. It is rare in children.

Symptoms There is often an *initial flu-like illness, with malaise and fever,* and sometimes deep-seated pelvic pain caused by inflammation of the prostate. The patient then develops severe *pain and swelling in one side of the scrotum,* which usually comes on quite quickly over 30–60 minutes and is sometimes relieved by supporting the scrotum. *Frequency of micturition and painful micturition may indicate the presence of a urinary tract infection.*

Examination

Position The swelling is confined to one side of the scrotum (Revision panel 18.2).

Revision panel 18.2

CAUSES OF A UNILATERAL SCROTAL SWELLING

- Hydrocele
- Epididymal cyst
- Varicocele
- Haematocele
- Orchitis (mumps)
- Epididymo-orchitis
- Testicular tumour

Colour The scrotal skin is red and shiny. After a few days, it turns a bronze colour, and the superficial layers of skin desquamate.

Temperature The scrotal skin feels hot.

Tenderness The testis and epididymis are extremely tender, but the scrotal skin is not. Careful palpation will reveal that the *tenderness is in the swollen epididymis,* and that the body of the testis itself is not so tender.

Shape and size *The whole testicle may be enlarged and tender, and you may be unable to distinguish the epididymis from testis.* This is more likely in the presence of a small secondary hydrocele. If a hydrocele does not form, you should be able to distinguish the testis from the epididymis, which is commonly enlarged to a centimetre or so in width.

In mild cases, the inflammation may be localized to the head or tail of the epididymis.

Surface The surface of the epididymis remains smooth, but will probably be too tender for this to be obvious.

Composition If there is a small hydrocele, the swelling may be fluctuant, with the testis palpable through the fluid.

If there is no hydrocele, you may be able to detect that the body of the testis feels a little more tense than normal. The epididymis is initially soft, but as the inflammation subsides, it becomes hard and craggy.

Relations and local tissues *The skin over the involved testis is oedematous but mobile.* Untreated, the infection may spread beyond the epididymis to the surrounding tissues, and the skin then becomes fixed. If an abscess develops in the epididymis, it may point and discharge through the area of skin fixation. As the epididymis normally lies behind the testis, *epididymal disease involves the skin of the back of the scrotum, so always remember to look at its posterior aspect.*

The *spermatic cord is always thickened and tender* because epididymal infection spreads distally from the urinary tract along the vas deferens.

The other testis should feel normal.

General examination Pay particular attention to the lower urinary tract. Rectal examination may reveal tenderness of the prostate and seminal vesicles, and there may be a palpable bladder. There may also be a fever and a tachycardia.

Tuberculous epididymo-orchitis

History

This condition is now uncommon in the UK, but is still seen in many other parts of the world. The tubercle bacillus reaches the epididymis via the bloodstream or by travelling along the vas from the lower urinary tract. The infection develops slowly, without causing severe or acute pain or tenderness. There may be systemic symptoms of tuberculosis, or only the urinary tract may be clinically involved, with a prior history of tuberculous exposure.

Most patients complain of a lump in the scrotum, and an associated dull, aching pain.

Examination

On examination, the *epididymis is hard, irregular and two or three times its normal size.*

A secondary hydrocele is unusual.

The spermatic cord is thickened as far as you can feel. The vas deferens is often irregular and swollen, and feels like a string of beads. This physical sign is rare, but is diagnostic of tuberculosis.

TUMOURS OF THE TESTIS

There are several varieties of testicular tumour. Around 90% are germ cell in origin, including *seminoma and non-seminomatous germ cell tumours, comprising teratoma, yolk sack tumour and choriocarcinoma.*

The rest are tumours of the sex cord and stromal structures, such as Leydig and Sertoli cell tumours.

Rarely, lymphoma and metastases present in the testes.

History

Age Non-seminomatous germ cell tumours commonly occur between the ages of 20 and 35 years, but seminomas often occur a few years later (age 35–45 years). Both are very rare in childhood and the teenage years. *A scrotal mass lesion in a man 20–45 years of age should be considered a testicular cancer until proven otherwise.*

Symptoms The most common presentation *is a swelling arising from the body of the testis, which is not usually painful.* The occasional patient presents acutely with a *painful, tender testis,* and the diagnosis is not always straightforward, especially if there is a history of minor testicular trauma.

Dull, aching, dragging pains in the scrotum and groin occur in some patients, particularly if the testis is significantly enlarged. Many patients complain that the affected *testicle feels heavy.*

Presentation with distant metastases may occur in many different ways, such as *general malaise, loss of appetite, wasting, abdominal pains and dyspnoea.* Rarely, there may be generalized lymphadenopathy, haemoptysis and headache.

Presentation may be with an abdominal mass.

> **NOTE:** There is a considerably higher incidence of malignant change in the incompletely descended testis. As the testis is not in the scrotum, diagnosis will be difficult and may be delayed.

Examination

Position The swelling is confined to the scrotum.

Temperature and colour The scrotal skin should be normal, except in the extremely rare circumstance in which the tumour has invaded and ulcerated through it.

Tenderness Testicular tumours are *not tender* except in the unusual acute presentation. *Normal testicular sensation may be lost.* Ask the patient about this, as it is an important symptom of a testicular tumour and rarely associated with other conditions.

Shape You may be able to feel *a nodule* that is clearly in the testis and not in the epididymis. A nodule that is in the epididymis is almost never a tumour. Testicular tumours are irregular and variable in shape.

Size Tumours are noticed by the patient when the testis is *clearly larger than its companion.* Large swellings are now uncommon in the UK because of heightened public awareness.

Surface This is usually smooth, but can be irregular or nodular.

Composition Testicular tumours *feel harder* than a normal testis, and are not fluctuant or translucent.

Heaviness is an important physical sign. With the patient lying down, lift the testis with your fingers. Compare with the normal side. A feeling of heaviness is characteristic of a tumour.

Relations The other testis should be normal, but tumours are bilateral in 1–2% of cases. The spermatic cord and the vas deferens should be normal. A very advanced tumour may infiltrate the skin of the scrotum.

Lymph glands Lymph from the testis drains to the para aortic lymph glands. Remember that these glands lie in the abdomen above the level of the umbilicus.

The inguinal glands will only be enlarged if the tumour has spread to the scrotal skin, a rare event.

General examination Pay particular attention to all the lymph glands, especially the *para-aortic and supraclavicular groups.*

Testicular tumours may metastasize anywhere in the body. Unusual swellings may be detected on general examination. Lung metastases are not usually detectable on clinical examination, but are readily visible on a chest X-ray or CT scan.

Differential diagnosis

The testicular swellings likely to be confused with tumours are *acute and chronic epididymoorchitis* and *haematocele.* Worried well patients often present wanting reassurance regarding simple epididymal cysts.

Figure 18.30 outlines a plan for diagnosis of scrotal swellings (see also Figure 18.31).

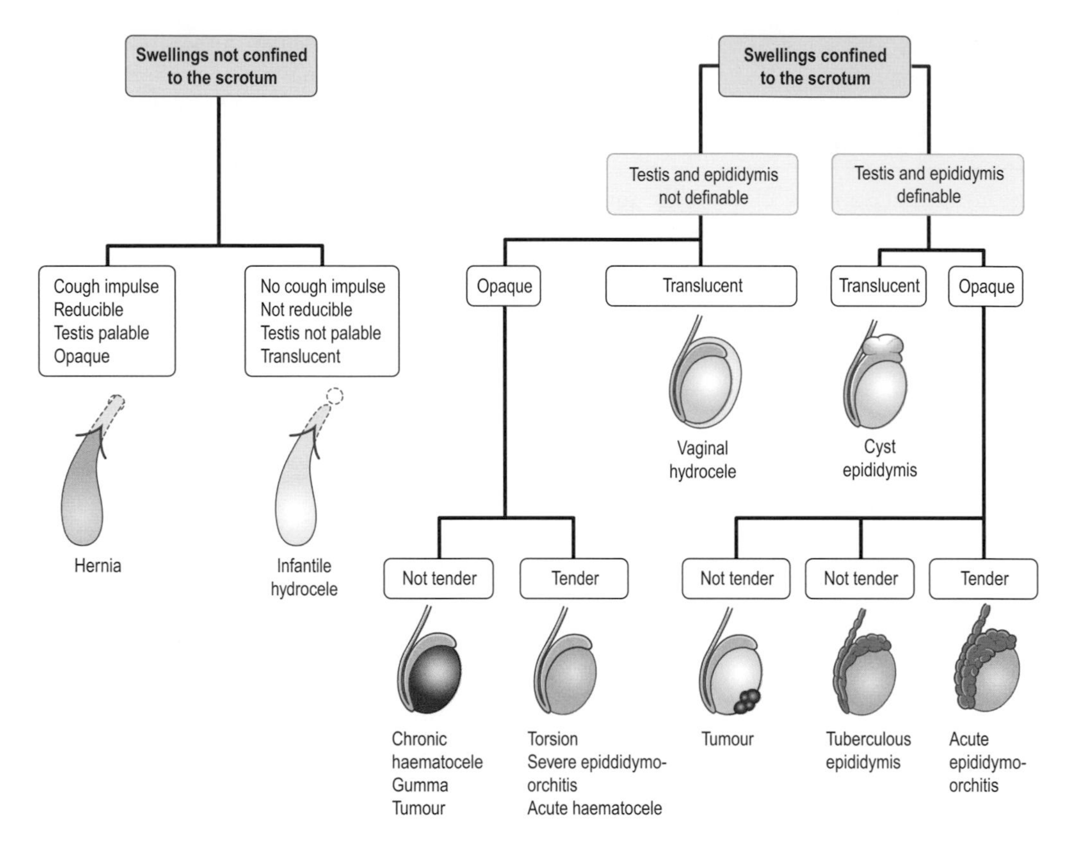

Figure 18.30 A plan for the diagnosis of scrotal swellings.

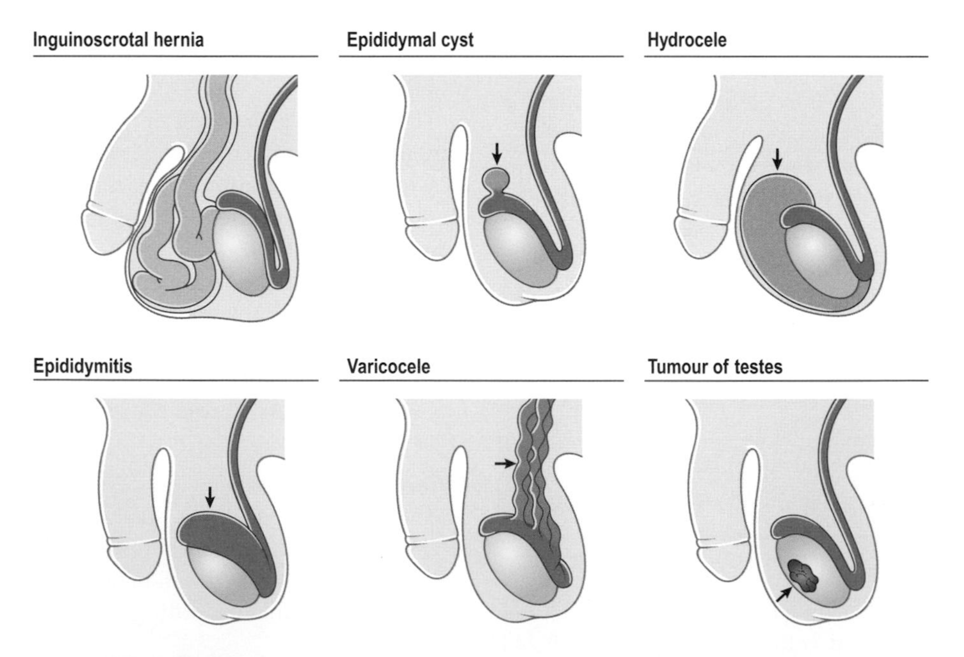

Figure 18.31 Scrotal swellings.

CHRONIC TESTICULAR PAIN

This is a common reason for referral to a surgical clinic. The patient is a young or middle-aged male. The pain may be localized to the testis, or it may radiate to the groin. It may be associated with exercise and movement, or with sitting in certain positions.

Common findings are:

- A mildly tender but otherwise normal epididymis, occasionally associated with a chlamydial urinary tract infection.
- A small epididymal cyst: differentiation from a normal epididymis may be difficult.
- An inguinal hernia: the skin of the scrotum is supplied by the genitofemoral nerve, which may be compressed in the groin by a hernia, causing discomfort referred to the testis.
- Rarely, but significantly, a testicular tumour.
- Nothing abnormal.

The possibilities are many, but, frustratingly for both patient and doctor, there may be no physical signs, and a diagnosis cannot be made. Patients can often be reassured that there is no physical abnormality, and the symptoms usually settle with time.

Erectile dysfunction

The condition is defined as the *persistent inability to achieve or maintain an erection sufficient for intercourse.* This definition is necessarily loose, as what is normal for one may be abnormal for another.

Studies have suggested that as many as one-fifth of males are affected. *Psychogenic factors* (performance anxiety) are common in the young. *Diabetes, cardiovascular disease, obesity and prostatic problems* are factors in older males.

History

Age The incidence increases with age.

Symptoms Enquiry should be made into how long there has been a problem and the suddenness of its onset. Are there early morning erections, and is it better with masturbation? (This helps to differentiate between psychological and pathological causes). Is there any loss of libido, and did the problem occur with previous partners?

General Specific enquiry should be made about *hypertension, diabetes, previous endocrine or neurological problems and pelvic surgery or trauma.*

A full drug history is essential, including alcohol, smoking and prescription, over-the-counter and recreational drug use.

Psychosocial A psychosocial history is vital. Is there occupational stress or financial insecurity? Is the relationship happy, and do both partners want children?

Questionnaire Questionnaires and sexual function scores assess the severity of the condition and monitor the response to treatment. An example is the International Index of Erectile Function.

Examination

General Note factors such as *obesity*, the condition of the *cardiovascular system* and the *abdomen.*

An appropriate *neurological examination* is essential test the genital and perineal sensation, and elicit the bulbocavernosus reflex (see Chapter 3).

Assess secondary sexual characteristics. Is there any *gynaecomastia* or any other signs of hypogonadism? Is there evidence of an *intersex condition* (see page 614)?

Genital The penis should be inspected for signs of deformity, curvature, chordae or phimosis. Are the testes of normal size? Assess the prostate by digital rectal examination.

Male infertility

This is defined as failure to conceive after 1 year of unprotected intercourse.

Approximately 90% of couples will conceive within 1 year. Approximately 20% of infertility is a result of pathology in the male, with 30–40% from combined male and female factors. Infertile females are usually seen and treated by a gynaecologically trained infertility specialist. *It is, however, important to take a history from the female partner.*

History

Age Fertility declines with the age of both partners.

Reproductive history Enquiry should be made into previous fertility, erectile and ejaculatory function, frequency of intercourse and other factors such as contraception and the use of spermicidal lubricants.

Development The age at puberty should be documented. Early (precocious) or delayed puberty may be a sign of an underlying endocrinological disorder such as Kallmann's syndrome or congenital adrenal hyperplasia.

Full medical history Any history of an *undescended testicle or corrective surgery* is important, as is any previous testicular problem such as *torsion, varicocele, tumour, orchitis or sexually transmitted diseases.* Ask about any previous radiotherapy or chemotherapy, and *diabetes.* A recent viral or febrile illness may temporarily impair spermatogenesis. *A full drug history should also be taken.*

Examination

Carry out a full examination as described above for the patient with erectile dysfunction. In addition, examine the patient when he is standing to look for a varicocele. Note the size and consistency of the testes. Feel the vasa, which may be absent or nodular due to previous infection.

Conditions of the female external genitalia

Most complaints about the external genitalia are referred to gynaecologists, but there are two common conditions that quite often appear in a general surgical or urological clinic.

BARTHOLIN'S CYST

The Bartholin's glands are a pair of small glands that lie at the sides of the lower end of the vagina, and whose ducts open on to the inner side of the posterior part of the labium minus. They are normally impalpable. When the duct of a gland is distended by obstruction or infection, it forms a cystic swelling in the posterior part of the labia majora.

URETHRAL CARUNCLE

This is a bright red, polypoid granuloma that arises from the mucosa of the urethral orifice in postmenopausal females. It is very tender and causes painful micturition, dyspareunia and occasional bleeding.

The differential diagnosis is urethral mucosal prolapse, which is purple in colour and not so tender, and rarely urethral carcinoma.

Intersex conditions

An in-depth description of the intersex conditions is beyond the scope of this book. It is a topic that confuses most!

Intersex is divided into:

- Female (46XX) with inappropriate virilization (female pseudohermaphrodite). The most common example is congenital adrenal hyperplasia, which accounts for 85% of all ambiguous genitalia.
- Incomplete virilization of a male (46XY) – a male pseudohermaphrodite.
- Gonadal dysgenesis with abnormal sex chromosomes, e.g. Turner's syndrome (45X0) and Klinefelter's syndrome (47XXY) (see Chapter 1).
- True hermaphrodites, where both ovarian and testicular tissue coexist. This is very rare.

Investigation of a newborn with ambiguous genitalia should take place at a specialist unit. *It is important to recognize life-threatening conditions such as salt-losing aldosterone deficiency in congenital adrenal hyperplasia.*

It is important to recognize the general appearance of older children or adults who may present with related (e.g. infertility) or unrelated problems. Two such disorders are Klinefelter's and Turner's syndromes.

KLINEFELTER'S SYNDROME

Klinefelter's syndrome is a congenital abnormality in which a male has an extra female (X) chromosome. Thus, instead of being a normal XY male, he is XXY, and testosterone production is subnormal.

The patients are tall, with a female distribution of fat around the breast and pelvis, but normal male hair growth on the face and pubis.

The testes are very small and soft, and do not produce spermatozoa, so the patients are sterile.

TURNER'S SYNDROME

Turner's syndrome is a congenital abnormality in which a female has only one female (X) chromosome. Thus, instead of being a normal XX female, she is X0.

There are no skeletal abnormalities, but the patient has a masculine shape – wide shoulders and narrow pelvis – and is invariably shorter than average for a female.

The most distinctive feature, when present, is 'webbing' of the shoulders. This is a thickening of the neck and a prominence of the skin folds that run from the neck to the shoulders.

The breasts and pubic hair are usually underdeveloped.

Acknowledgements

The contribution of Ben Challacombe to this chapter in the 5th edition is gratefully acknowledged.

Index

Page numbers in **bold** refer to figures; those in *italic* refer to tables or boxed text

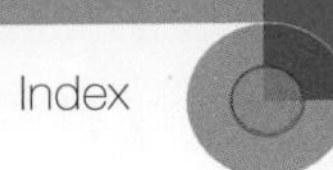

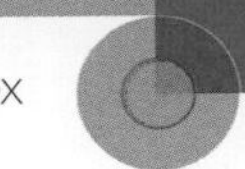

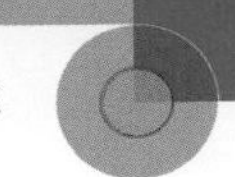

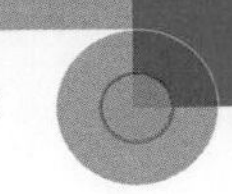

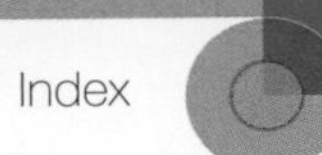

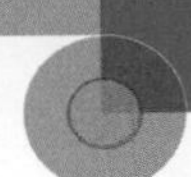

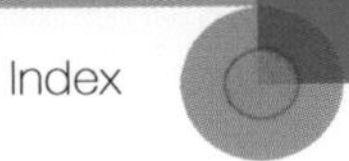

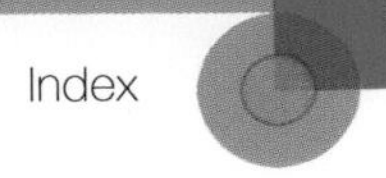